W9-CEV-948

Pulmonary Diseases and Disorders

Volume 1

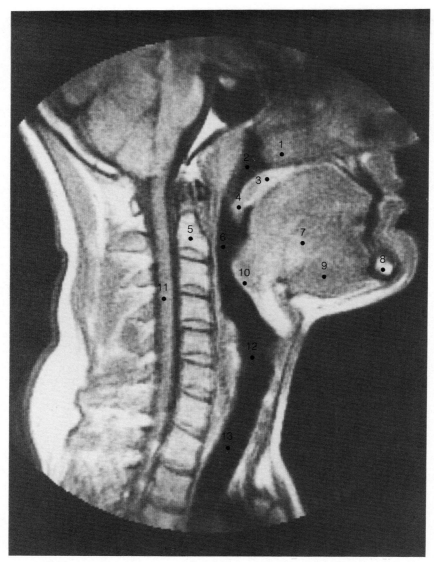

Midsagittal magnetic resonance scan of the neck displays airway from the nasopharynx to the trachea. Adjacent soft tissue anatomy is clearly depicted. 1 = inferior nasal concha; 2 = nasopharynx; 3 = soft palate; 4 = uvula; 5 = C2 vertebral body; 6 = oropharynx; 7 = muscles of tongue; 8 = mandible; 9 = geniohyoid muscle; 10 = epiglottis; 11 = spinal cord; 12 = larynx; 13 = trachea. (Courtesy of Dr. W. B. Gefter.)

Pulmonary Diseases and Disorders

Second Edition

Volume 1

ALFRED P. FISHMAN, M.D.

William Maul Measey Professor of Medicine
Director, Cardiovascular-Pulmonary Division, Department of Medicine
Hospital of the University of Pennsylvania

McGraw-Hill Book Company

New York St Louis San Francisco Colorado Springs Oklahoma City Auckland
Bogotá Caracas Hamburg Lisbon London Madrid Mexico Milan Montreal
New Delhi Panama Paris San Juan São Paulo Singapore Sydney Tokyo Toronto

PULMONARY DISEASES AND DISORDERS

Copyright © 1988, 1980 by McGraw-Hill, Inc. All rights reserved. Printed in the United States of America. Except as permitted under the United States Copyright Act of 1976, no part of this publication may be reproduced or distributed in any form or by any means, or stored in a data base or retrieval system, without the prior written permission of the publisher.

34567890 KGPKGP   92

ISBN 0-07-079982-2 (set)
ISBN 0-07-021132-9 (v. 1)
ISBN 0-07-021133-7 (v. 2)
ISBN 0-07-021122-1 (v. 3)

This book was set in Melior by York Graphic Services, Inc.
The editors were J. Dereck Jeffers and Muza Navrozov;
the production supervisor was Robert R. Laffler;
the cover was designed by Edward R. Schultheis;
the page layout was done by Till & Till, Inc.;
the index was prepared by Irving Tullar.
Arcata Graphics/Kingsport was printer and binder.

Library of Congress Cataloging-in-Publication Data

Pulmonary diseases and disorders.

    Bibliography: p.
    Includes index.
    1. Lungs—Diseases.   I. Fishman, Alfred P.
[DNLM: 1. Lung Diseases. WF 600 P981]
RC756.P826 1988   616.2'4   87-26166
ISBN 0-07-079982-2 (set)

Front cover: Lateral view of resin cast of left human lung, with airways (yellow), pulmonary arteries (red), and pulmonary veins (blue) filled out to fine lobular branches. *(Courtesy of Dr. H. C. Walter Weber, Department of Anatomy, University of Bern, Switzerland.)*

TO LINDA AND HANNAH

NOTICE

Medicine is an ever-changing science. As new research and clinical experience broaden our knowledge, changes in treatment and drug therapy are required. The editors and the publisher of this work have checked with sources believed to be reliable in their efforts to provide information that is complete and generally in accord with the standards accepted at the time of publication. However, in view of the possibility of human error or changes in medical sciences, neither the editors, nor the publisher, nor any other party who has been involved in the preparation or publication of this work warrants that the information contained herein is in every respect accurate or complete. Readers are encouraged to confirm the information contained herein with other sources. For example and in particular, readers are advised to check the product information sheet included in the package of each drug they plan to administer to be certain that the information contained in this book is accurate and that changes have not been made in the recommended dose or in the contraindications for administration. This recommendation is of particular importance in connection with new or infrequently used drugs.

Contents

PART 3   **INTEGRATIONS AND ADAPTATIONS**

PART 4   **APPROACH TO THE PATIENT WITH RESPIRATORY SIGNS
OR SYMPTOMS**

APPENDIXES

VOLUME 2
PAGES 875–1792

PART 8   **NONINFECTIOUS DISORDERS OF THE PULMONARY PARENCHYMA**

PART 9   **PULMONARY CIRCULATORY DISORDERS**

PART 14   MYCOBACTERIAL DISEASES OF THE LUNGS

VOLUME 3
PAGES 1793–2564

PART 15   CANCER OF THE LUNGS

PART 16   **DISEASES OF THE MEDIASTINUM**

Contributors

Masazumi Adachi, M.D., Sc.D.
Professor of Pathology, State University of New York, Health Science Center of Brooklyn; Director of Laboratories, Kingsbrook Jewish Medical Center, Brooklyn, New York

Zalman S. Agus, M.D.
Professor of Medicine, Chief, Renal-Electrolyte Section, Department of Medicine, University of Pennsylvania School of Medicine, Philadelphia, Pennsylvania

Abass Alavi, M.D.
Professor of Radiology, Division of Nuclear Medicine, Department of Radiology Hospital of the University of Pennsylvania, Philadelphia, Pennsylvania

Steven M. Albelda, M.D.
Assistant Professor of Medicine, Cardiovascular-Pulmonary Division, Hospital of the University of Pennsylvania, Philadelphia, Pennsylvania

Murray D. Altose, M.D.
Chief, Pulmonary Medicine, Cleveland Metropolitan General Hospital, Cleveland, Ohio

Nicholas R. Anthonisen, M.D., Ph.D.
Professor and Head, Section of Respiratory Diseases, The University of Manitoba, Winnipeg, Manitoba, Canada

Donald Armstrong, M.D.
Chief, Infectious Disease Service, Memorial Sloan-Kettering Cancer Center, New York, New York

Jeffrey Askanazi, M.D.
Associate Professor of Anesthesiology, Albert Einstein College of Medicine, The Bronx, New York

Marianne Bachofen, M.D.
Department of Anesthesiology, Inselpital, Bern, Switzerland

Joseph H. Bates, M.D.
Chief, Medical Services, John L. McClellan Veterans Administration Memorial Hospital, Little Rock, Arkansas

John Bienenstock, M.D.
Professor of Medicine and Pathology; Chairman, Department of Pathology, Molecular Virology and Immunology Program, McMaster University, Health Sciences Centre, Hamilton, Ontario, Canada

Alan L. Bisno, M.D.
Professor of Medicine, Department of Medicine, University of Miami School of Medicine; Chief, Medical Service, Veterans Administration Medical Center, Miami, Florida

Edward R. Block, M.D.
Professor of Medicine, Division of Pulmonary Medicine, University of Florida College of Medicine; Associate Chief of Staff for Research, Gainesville Veterans Administration Medical Center, Gainesville, Florida

Alvin L. Bowles, Sr., M.D.
Director, Pulmonary Ward, Harper Hospital, Detroit, Michigan

Joseph D. Brain, S.D. in Hyg.
Cecil K. and Philip Drinker Professor of Environmental Physiology and Director, Respiratory Biology Program, Department of Environmental Science and Physiology, Harvard University School of Public Health, Boston, Massachusetts

Kenneth L. Brigham, M.D.
Joe & Morris Werthan Professor of Investigative Medicine; Director, Center for Lung Research, Department of Medicine, Vanderbilt University School of Medicine, Nashville, Tennessee

Peter H. Burri, M.D.
Professor of Anatomy, Institute of Anatomy, University of Bern, Bern, Switzerland

Jerome O. Cantor, M.D.
Assistant Professor of Pathology, Department of Pathology, College of Physicians and Surgeons of Columbia University, New York, New York

Desmond N. Carney, M.D., Ph.D.
Consultant Medical Oncologist, Mater Hospital, Dublin, Ireland

Edwin H. Cassem, S.J., M.D.
Chief, Psychiatric Consultation Service, Massachusetts General Hospital; Associate Professor of Psychiatry Harvard Medical School, Boston, Massachusetts

Randall D. Cebul, M.D.
Associate Professor of Medicine, Henry J. Kaiser Family Foundation Faculty Scholar and Chief, Division of General Medicine, Cleveland Metropolitan General Hospital, Case Western Reserve University, Cleveland, Ohio

Neil S. Cherniack, M.D.
Professor of Medicine and Physiology, Case Western Reserve University; Director, Pulmonary Division, University Hospitals, Cleveland, Ohio

Sanford Chodosh, M.D.
Chief of Medicine and Pulmonary, Veterans Administration Outpatient Clinic; Associate Professor of Medicine, Boston University School of Medicine, Boston, Massachusetts

Jacob Churg, M.D.
Professor Emeritus and Consultant, Department of Pathology, Mount Sinai School of Medicine, New York, New York; Pathologist, Department of Pathology, Barnert Memorial Hospital Center, Patterson, New Jersey; Clinical Professor of Pathology, Department of Pathology, University of Medicine and Dentistry of New Jersey, Newark, New Jersey

James M. Clark, M.D., Ph.D.
Clinical Associate Professor of Pharmacology, Institute for Environmental Medicine, University of Pennsylvania, Philadelphia, Pennsylvania

William D. Claypool, M.D.
Assistant Professor of Medicine, Section of Respiratory and Critical Care Medicine, Department of Medicine, The University of Illinois College of Medicine at Chicago, Chicago, Illinois

Jordan J. Cohen, M.D.
Associate Chairman and Professor of Medicine, University of Chicago Pritzker School of Medicine; Chairman, Department of Medicine, Michael Reese Hospital and Medical Center, Chicago, Illinois

Martin H. Cohen, M.D.
Chief, Oncology Section, Veterans Administration Medical Center; Professor of Medicine, George Washington University Medical Center, Washington, D.C.

Robert W. Colman, M.D.
Professor of Medicine and Director, Thrombosis Research Center; Chief, Hematology-Oncology Section, Temple University School of Medicine, Philadelphia, Pennsylvania

George W. Counts, M.D.
Professor of Medicine, Department of Medicine, University of Washington School of Medicine, Fred Hutchinson Cancer Research Center, Harborview Medical Center, Seattle, Washington

James D. Cox, M.D.
Professor and Chairman, Department of Radiation Oncology, The Presbyterian Hospital in the City of New York, Columbia-Presbyterian Medical Center, New York, New York

Ronald G. Crystal, M.D.
Chief, Pulmonary Branch, National Heart, Lung and Blood Institute, National Institutes of Health, Bethesda, Maryland

Ronald P. Daniele, M.D.
Professor of Medicine and Pathology, Cardiovascular-Pulmonary Division, Department of Medicine, Hospital of the University of Pennsylvania, Philadelphia, Pennsylvania

Arthur M. Dannenberg, Jr., M.D., Ph.D.
Professor (Experimental Pathology), Department of Environmental Health Sciences, Immunology, and Infectious Diseases and Department of Epidemiology, School of Hygiene and Public Health, joint appointment in Department of Pathology, School of Medicine, The Johns Hopkins University, Baltimore, Maryland

Paul T. Davidson, M.D.
Director, Tuberculosis Control, Los Angeles County Department of Health Services, Public Health Programs, Rancho Los Amigos Medical Center, Downey, California

Scott F. Davies, M.D.
Director, Division of Pulmonary Medicine, Hennepin County Medicine Center; Associate Professor of Medicine, University of Minnesota School of Medicine, Minneapolis, Minnesota

Roger M. Des Prez, M.D.
Professor of Medicine, Vanderbilt University Medical School; Chief, Medical Service, Veterans Administration Medical Center, Nashville, Tennessee

Burton F. Dickey, M.D.
Assistant Professor of Medicine, Pulmonary Division, Boston University School of Medicine, Boston, Massachusetts

R. Gordon Douglas, Jr., M.D.
Chairman, Department of Medicine, Cornell University Medical College; Physician-in-Chief, The New York Hospital, New York, New York

Norman H. Edelman, M.D.
Professor of Medicine and Physiology; Chief, Division of Pulmonary and Critical Care Medicine, Department of Medicine, UMDNJ-Robert Wood Johnson Medical School, Academic Health Science Center, New Brunswick, New Jersey

Paul J. Edelson, M.D.
Associate Professor of Pediatrics and Microbiology, Cornell University Medical College; Director, Division of Pediatric Infectious Diseases and Immunology, The New York Hospital, New York, New York

Paul H. Edelstein, M.D.
Associate Professor of Pathology and Laboratory Medicine and Director of Clinical Microbiology, Hospital of the University of Pennsylvania, Philadelphia, Pennsylvania

Gary R. Epler, M.D.
Chairman, Department of Medicine, New England Baptist Hospital; Associate Clinical Professor of Medicine, Boston University School of Medicine, Boston, Massachusetts

David M. Epstein, M.D.
Associate Professor of Radiology, Department of Radiology, University of Pennsylvania, Philadelphia, Pennsylvania

Paul E. Epstein, M.D.
Chief, Pulmonary Division, The Graduate Hospital; Clinical Associate Professor of Medicine, University of Pennsylvania, Philadelphia, Pennsylvania

Robert J. Fallat, M.D.
Director, Division of Pulmonary Medicine, Pacific Presbyterian Medical Center; Associate Clinical Professor of Medicine, University of California, San Francisco, San Francisco, California

George M. Feldman, M.D.
Assistant Professor of Medicine, Renal-Electrolyte Section, Department of Medicine, Hospital of the University of Pennsylvania, Philadelphia, Pennsylvania

Victor J. Ferrans, M.D., Ph.D.
Chief, Section on Ultrastructure, Pathology Branch, National Heart, Lung, and Blood Institute, National Institutes of Health, Bethesda, Maryland

Isaiah J. Fidler, D.V.M., Ph.D
Professor and Chairman, Department of Cell Biology, The University of Texas System Cancer Center; M. D. Anderson Hospital and Tumor Institute, Texas Medical Center, Houston, Texas

Gregory A. Filice, M.D.
Staff Physician, Infectious Disease Section, Veterans Administration Medical Center; Assistant Professor of Medicine, University of Minnesota, Minneapolis, Minnesota

Robert B. Filuk, M.D.
Assistant Professor of Medicine, Stanford University, Palo Alto, California

Sydney M. Finegold, M.D.
Associate Chief of Staff for Research and Development, Veterans Administration Wadsworth Medical Center; Professor of Medicine, UCLA School of Medicine, Los Angeles, California

Aron B. Fisher, M.D.
Professor of Physiology and Medicine and Director, Institute for Environmental Medicine, University of Pennsylvania School of Medicine, Philadelphia, Pennsylvania

Alfred P. Fishman, M.D.
William Maul Measey Professor of Medicine and Director, Cardiovascular-Pulmonary Division, Department of Medicine, Hospital of the University of Pennsylvania, Philadelphia, Pennsylvania

Jay A. Fishman, M.D.
Assistant in Medicine, Massachusetts General Hospital; Instructor in Medicine, Harvard Medical School, Boston, Massachusetts; Visiting Scientist, Yale University School of Medicine, New Haven, Connecticut

William J. Fulkerson, Jr., M.D.
Assistant Professor of Medicine, Duke University Medical Center, Durham, North Carolina

Jack D. Fulmer, M.D.
Director of Pulmonary Research and Professor of Medicine, Division of Pulmonary and Critical Care Medicine, Department of Medicine, The University of Alabama at Birmingham; Staff Physician, Veterans Administration Medical Center, Birmingham, Alabama

John N. Galgiani, M.D.
Associate Professor of Medicine, University of Arizona College of Medicine; Chief, Section of Infectious Diseases, Veterans Administration Medical Center, Tucson, Arizona

Stuart M. Garay, M.D.
Assistant Clinical Professor of Medicine, Department of Medicine, New York University School of Medicine, New York, New York

Jack Gauldie, Ph.D.
Professor of Pathology, Department of Pathology, McMaster University Health Sciences Centre, Hamilton, Ontario, Canada

Ralph T. Geer, M.D.
Associate Professor of Anesthesia and Internal Medicine, Department of Anesthesia, Hospital of the University of Pennsylvania, Philadelphia, Pennsylvania

Warren B. Gefter, M.D.
Associate Professor of Radiology, Department of Radiology, University of Pennsylvania, Philadelphia, Pennsylvania

Jon P. Gockerman, M.D.
Associate Professor of Medicine, Hematology-Oncology Division, Duke University Medical Center, Durham, North Carolina

Roberta M. Goldring, M.D.
Professor of Medicine, Department of Medicine, New York University School of Medicine, New York, New York

Michael A. Grippi, M.D.
Assistant Professor of Medicine and Director, Respiratory Services, Cardiovascular Pulmonary Division, Department of Medicine, Hospital of the University of Pennsylvania, Philadelphia, Pennsylvania

Frederick L. Grover, M.D.
Professor of Surgery, Division of Cardiothoracic Surgery, The University of Texas Health Science Center, San Antonio, Texas

Kenneth R. Hande, M.D.
Associate Professor of Medicine and Pharmacology, Vanderbilt University Medical School; Chief, Medical Oncology, Veterans Administration Medical Center, Nashville, Tennessee

John Hansen-Flaschen, M.D.
Assistant Professor of Medicine, Department of Medicine; Cardiovascular-Pulmonary Division, Hospital of the University of Pennsylvania, Philadelphia, Pennsylvania

Edward F. Haponik, M.D.
Associate Professor of Medicine, Division of Pulmonary and Critical Care Medicine School of Medicine in New Orleans, Louisiana State University Medical Center, New Orleans, Louisiana

P. Kent Harman, M.D.
Chief, Cardiac Surgery, St. Charles Medical Center, Bend, Oregon

Jean E. Hawkins, Ph.D.
Director, Reference Laboratory for Tuberculosis and Other Mycobacterial Diseases, Veterans Administration Medical Center, West Haven, Connecticut

Donald Heath, D.Sc., M.D., Ph.D.
George Holt Professor of Pathology, University of Liverpool, Liverpool, United Kingdom

Joan C. Hendricks, V.M.D., Ph.D.
Assistant Professor of Medicine, Department of Clinical Studies, University of Pennsylvania, School of Veterinary Medicine, Philadelphia, Pennsylvania

Ian T. T. Higgins, M.D.
Professor Emeritus of Epidemiology and of Environmental and Industrial Health, School of Public Health, University of Michigan, Ann Arbor, Michigan

Michael P. Hlastala, M.D.
Professor of Medicine and Physiology and Biophysics, Division of Respiratory Diseases, University of Washington School of Medicine, Seattle, Washington

Peter W. Hochachka, Ph.D.
Professor of The Faculties of Science and Medicine, Department of Zoology and Sports Medicine Division, The University of British Columbia, Vancouver, British Columbia, Canada

Fred D. Holford, M.D.
Associate Professor of Medicine, Cardiology Division, University of Colorado Health Sciences Center, Denver, Colorado

Cyrus C. Hopkins, M.D.
Assistant Professor of Medicine, Harvard Medical School; Hospital Epidemiologist and Physician, Infection Control Unit, Massachusetts General Hospital, Boston, Massachusetts

Leonard D. Hudson, M.D.
Professor of Medicine and Head, Division of Pulmonary and Critical Care Medicine, Department of Medicine, University of Washington, Seattle, Washington

Renato V. Iozzo, M.D.
Assistant Professor of Pathology, Department of Pathology, University of Pennsylvania School of Medicine, Philadelphia, Pennsylvania

Larry K. Jackson, M.D.
Associate Professor of Medicine, Division of Pulmonary and Critical Care Medicine, The University of Alabama at Birmingham School of Medicine; Chief, Pulmonary Section, Veterans Administration Medical Center, Birmingham, Alabama

Brian V. Jegasothy, M.D.
Professor and Chairman, Department of Dermatology, University of Pittsburgh, Pittsburgh, Pennsylvania

Alan H. Jobe, M.D., Ph.D.
Professor of Pediatrics, Harbor-UCLA Medical Center, UCLA School of Medicine, Torrance, California

Waldemar G. Johanson, Jr., M.D.
Professor and Chairman, Department of Internal Medicine, The University of Texas Medical Branch at Galveston, Galveston, Texas

Carol Johnson Johns, M.D.
Associate Professor of Medicine and Assistant Dean and Director of Continuing Education, The Johns Hopkins University School of Medicine; Active Staff Physician, The Johns Hopkins Hospital, Baltimore, Maryland

Bruce E. Johnson, M.D.
Investigator, NCI-Navy Medical Oncology Branch, National Cancer Institute and Naval Hospital, Bethesda, Maryland

Norman L. Jones, M.D.
Professor of Medicine, Ambrose Cardiorespiratory Unit, McMaster University, Hamilton, Ontario, Canada

Robert N. Jones, M.D.
Professor of Medicine, Tulane University School of Medicine, New Orleans, Louisiana

Anna-Luise A. Katzenstein, M.D.
Professor of Pathology, Division of Surgical Pathology, Department of Pathology, The University of Alabama at Birmingham, Birmingham, Alabama

A. B. Kay, M.D., Ph.D.
Professor and Director, Department of Allergy and Clinical Immunology, The Cardiothoracic Institute, Brompton Hospital, London, England

Homayoun Kazemi, M.D.
Chief, Pulmonary Unit, Massachusetts General Hospital; Professor of Medicine, Harvard Medical School, Boston, Massachusetts

Mark A. Kelley, M.D.
Associate Professor of Medicine, Cardiovascular-Pulmonary Division; Vice Chairman, Department of Medicine, Hospital of the University of Pennsylvania, Philadelphia, Pennsylvania

Jeffrey A. Kern, M.D.
Assistant Professor of Medicine, Cardiovascular-Pulmonary Division, Department of Medicine, Hospital of the University of Pennsylvania, Philadelphia, Pennsylvania

Gary T. Kinasewitz, M.D.
Associate Professor of Medicine, Physiology, and Biophysics and Director, Cardiopulmonary Research Center, Department of Medicine, Louisiana State University Medical Center, Shreveport, Louisiana

Jerome I. Kleinerman, M.D.
Professor and Vice Chairman, Department of Pathology, Case Western Reserve University School of Medicine, and Director, Department of Pathology, Cleveland Metropolitan General Hospital, Cleveland, Ohio

Lewis R. Kline, M.D.
Assistant Professor of Medicine, Cardiovascular-Pulmonary Division, Department of Medicine, Hospital of the University of Pennsylvania, Philadelphia, Pennsylvania

Robert A. Klocke, M.D.
Professor of Medicine and Physiology; Chief, Pulmonary Division, Department of Medicine, State University of New York at Buffalo, Buffalo, New York

Michael I. Kotlikoff, V.M.D., Ph.D.
Assistant Professor, Department of Animal Biology, University of Pennsylvania School of Veterinary Medicine, Philadelphia, Pennsylvania

Ann V. Krupinski, B.S., R.CPT
Chief Technician, Pulmonary Diagnostic Services, Cardiovascular-Pulmonary Division, Department of Medicine, Hospital of the University of Pennsylvania, Philadelphia, Pennsylvania

Charles Kuhn III, M.D.
Professor of Pathology, Brown University, Division of Biology and Medicine; Pathologist-in-Chief, Memorial Hospital of Rhode Island, Pawtucket, Rhode Island

Paul Kvale, M.D.
Head, Division of Pulmonary and Critical Care Medicine, and Director, Laser Center, Henry Ford Hospital, Detroit, Michigan

Paul N. Lanken, M.D.
Associate Professor of Medicine, Cardiovascular-Pulmonary Division, Department of Medicine, University of Pennsylvania School of Medicine, and Director, Medical Intensive Care Unit, Hospital of the University of Pennsylvania, Philadelphia, Pennsylvania

Kenneth V. Lieberman, M.D.
Assistant Professor of Pediatrics and Chief, Division of Pediatric Nephrology, Mount Sinai School of Medicine, New York, New York

Glen A. Lillington, M.D.
Division of Pulmonary and Critical Care Medicine, Department of Internal Medicine, University of California, Davis, School of Medicine, Davis, California

H. Kim Lyerly, M.D.
Assistant in Surgery, Department of Surgery, Duke University Medical Center, Durham, North Carolina

Rob Roy MacGregor, M.D.
Chief, Infectious Diseases Section, and Professor of Medicine, University of Pennsylvania School of Medicine, Philadelphia, Pennsylvania

Peter T. Macklem, M.D.
Professor and Chairman, Department of Medicine, McGill University; Physician-in-Chief, Royal Victoria Hospital, Montreal, Canada

Nicolaos E. Madias, M.D.
Associate Professor of Medicine, Tufts University School of Medicine; Chief, Division of Nephrology, New England Medical Center Hospitals, Boston, Massachusetts

Adel A. F. Mahmoud, M.D., Ph.D.
The John H. Hord Professor of Medicine and Chairman, Department of Medicine, Case Western Reserve University; Physician-in-Chief, University Hospitals of Cleveland, Cleveland, Ohio

Lars Malm, M.D.
Assistant Professor, Department of Oto-Rhino-Laryngology, University of Lund, Malmö General Hospital, Malmö, Sweden

Robert L. Mayock, M.D.
Professor of Medicine, Cardiovascular-Pulmonary Division, Department of Medicine, University of Pennsylvania School of Medicine, Philadelphia, Pennsylvania

E. R. McFadden, Jr., M.D.
Argyl J. Beams Professor of Medicine, Case Western Reserve University; Director, Asthma and Allergic Disease Center, University Hospitals of Cleveland, Cleveland, Ohio

David S. McKinsey, M.D.
Clinical Assistant Professor of Medicine, Department of Medicine, University of Missouri-Kansas City; Assistant Director, Department of Infectious Diseases, Research Medical Center, Kansas City, Missouri

Myron R. Melamed, M.D.
Chairman, Department of Pathology, Memorial Hospital for Cancer and Allied Diseases, New York, New York

Robert B. Mellins, M.D.
Professor of Pediatrics, Department of Pediatrics, and Director, Pediatric Pulmonary Division, College of Physicians & Surgeons of Columbia University, New York, New York

Louis F. Metzger, A.B., R.CPT
Associate Director/Technical Affairs, Pulmonary Diagnostic Services, Cardiovascular-Pulmonary Division, Department of Medicine, Hospital of the University of Pennsylvania, Philadelphia, Pennsylvania

Richard D. Meyer, M.D.
Professor of Medicine and Director, Division of Infectious Diseases, Department of Medicine, Cedars-Sinai Medical Center, UCLA School of Medicine, Los Angeles, California

R. Drew Miller, M.D.
Professor of Medicine, Mayo Medical School; Consultant, Division of Thoracic Diseases and Internal Medicine, Mayo Clinic and Foundation, Rochester, Minnesota

Wallace T. Miller, M.D.
Professor and Vice Chairman, Department of Radiology, Hospital of the University of Pennsylvania, Philadelphia, Pennsylvania

Richard P. Millman, M.D.
Assistant Professor of Medicine, Brown University School of Medicine; Director, Pulmonary Function and Sleep Apnea Laboratories, Providence, Rhode Island

John D. Minna, M.D.
Professor of Medicine, Uniformed Services University of the Health Sciences; Branch Chief, NCI-Navy Medical Oncology Branch, National Cancer Institute and Naval Hospital, Bethesda, Maryland

Wm. Keith C. Morgan, M.D.
Professor of Medicine, Chest Disease Unit, University Hospital, University of Western Ontario, London, Ontario, Canada

Adrian R. Morrison, D.V.M., Ph.D.
Professor of Anatomy, Laboratories of Anatomy, Department of Animal Biology, University of Pennsylvania School of Veterinary Medicine, Philadelphia, Pennsylvania

Clifton F. Mountain, M.D.
Professor of Surgery, Department of Thoracic Surgery, The University of Texas System Cancer Center; M. D. Anderson Hospital and Tumor Institute, Texas Medical Center, Houston, Texas

James L. Mullen, M.D.
Director, Nutrition Support Service, and Associate Professor of Surgery, Department of Surgery, Hospital of the University of Pennsylvania, Philadelphia, Pennsylvania

Albert G. Mulley, Jr., M.D., M.P.P.
Chief, General Internal Medicine Unit, Massachusetts General Hospital; Assistant Professor of Medicine, Harvard Medical School, Boston, Massachusetts

David M. F. Murphy, M.D.
Chairman, Department of Pulmonary Medicine, Deborah Heart and Lung Center, Browns Mills, New Jersey

Henry W. Murray, M.D.
Chief, Division of Infectious Diseases, The New York Hospital—Cornell Medical Center; Associate Professor of Medicine, Department of Medicine, Cornell University Medical College, New York, New York

Allen R. Myers, M.D.
Professor of Medicine, Department of Medicine, Temple University School of Medicine, Philadelphia, Pennsylvania

Chuzo Nagaishi, M.D.
Emeritus Professor of Kyoto University, Honorary President, Japanese Association for Thoracic Surgery, Takatsuki City, Osaka Prefecture, Japan

Thomas W. Nash, M.D.
Assistant Professor of Medicine, Divisions of Pulmonary and General Medicine, Department of Medicine, Cornell University Medical College, The New York Hospital—Cornell Medical Center, New York, New York

Harold C. Neu, M.D.
Professor of Medicine and Pharmacology, Department of Medicine, and Chief, Division of Infectious Diseases, Department of Medicine, College of Physicians and Surgeons of Columbia University, New York, New York

Richard H. Ochs, M.D.
Associate Director of Laboratories, Department of Pathology, Bryn Mawr Hospital, Bryn Mawr, Pennsylvania

Yoshio Okada, M.D.
Professor and Head, Second Department of Surgery, Shiga University of Medical Science, Otsu, Shiga Ken, Japan

Gerald N. Olsen, M.D.
Professor of Medicine and Director, Pulmonary and Critical Care Medicine, University of South Carolina School of Medicine, Columbia, South Carolina

Allan I. Pack, M.D., Ph.D.
Associate Professor of Medicine, Cardiovascular-Pulmonary Division, Department of Medicine, Hospital of the University of Pennsylvania, Philadelphia, Pennsylvania

Harold I. Palevsky, M.D.
Assistant Professor of Medicine, Cardiovascular-Pulmonary Division, Department of Medicine, Hospital of the University of Pennsylvania, Philadelphia, Pennsylvania

Michael G. Pearson, M.R.C.P.
Consultant Physician, Mersey Regional Thoracic Unit, Fazakerley Hospital, Liverpool, England

Theodore L. Phillips, M.D.
Professor and Chairman, Department of Radiation Oncology, and Research Associate, Laboratory of Radiobiology, University of California, San Francisco, San Francisco, California

Alan K. Pierce, M.D.
Professor of Medicine, Pulmonary Disease Division, Department of Internal Medicine, The University of Texas Health Science Center at Dallas, Dallas, Texas

Janet E. Price, Ph.D.
Assistant Biologist, Department of Cell Biology, The University of Texas System Cancer Center; M. D. Anderson Hospital and Tumor Institute, Texas Medical Center, Houston, Texas

Donald F. Proctor, M.D.
Professor Emeritus, Environmental Health Sciences, Otolaryngology, and Anesthesiology, The Johns Hopkins Medical Institutions, Baltimore, Maryland

Lynne M. Reid, M.D.
S. Burt Wolbach Professor of Pathology, Harvard Medical School; Pathologist-in-Chief, The Children's Hospital, Boston, Massachusetts

Bruce A. Reitz, M.D.
Professor of Surgery and Cardiac Surgeon-in-Charge, Department of Surgery, The Johns Hopkins Hospital, Baltimore, Maryland

Daniel G. Remick, M.D.
Instructor in Pathology, Department of Pathology, The University of Michigan Medical School, Ann Arbor, Michigan

Herbert Y. Reynolds, M.D.
Professor of Internal Medicine and Head, Pulmonary Section, Yale University School of Medicine, New Haven, Connecticut

Hal B. Richerson, M.D.
Professor of Medicine, Department of Internal Medicine, and Director, Division of Allergy/Immunology, The University of Iowa Hospitals and Clinics, Iowa City, Iowa

Andrew L. Ries, M.D.
Associate Professor of Medicine, Pulmonary and Critical Care Division, University of California, San Diego, San Diego, California

Henrique Rigatto, M.D.
Professor of Pediatrics, Department of Pediatrics, and Director, Neonatal Research, University of Manitoba Health Sciences Centre, Winnipeg, Manitoba, Canada

J. C. Rosenberg, M.D., Ph.D.
Chief, Department of Surgery, Hutzel Hospital, Detroit Medical Center; Professor of Surgery, Wayne State University School of Medicine, Detroit, Michigan

Edward C. Rosenow III, M.D.
Professor of Medicine, Thoracic Diseases and Internal Medicine, Mayo Clinic, Rochester, Minnesota

E. J. Ross, M.D., Ph.D.
Emeritus Professor of Endocrinology, Department of Clinical Pharmacology, University College London and The Middlesex Hospital Medical School, The Rayne Institute, London, England

Milton D. Rossman, M.D.
Assistant Professor of Medicine, Cardiovascular-Pulmonary Division, Department of Medicine, Hospital of the University of Pennsylvania, Philadelphia, Pennsylvania

Charis Roussos, M.D., M.Sc., Ph.D.
Professor of Medicine, Director, Critical Care Division, Royal Victoria Hospital, McGill University, Montreal, Canada

Robert H. Rubin, M.D.
Chief of Infectious Disease for Transplantation, Massachusetts General Hospital; Associate Professor of Medicine, Harvard Medical School, Boston, Massachusetts

Ronald N. Rubin, M.D.
Associate Professor of Medicine and Thrombosis Research, Thrombosis Research Center; Deputy Chairman, Department of Internal Medicine, Temple University School of Medicine, Philadelphia, Pennsylvania

David C. Sabiston, Jr., M.D.
James B. Duke Professor of Surgery and Chairman, Department of Surgery, Duke University Medical Center, Durham, North Carolina

Steven A. Sahn, M.D.
Professor of Medicine and Director, Division of Pulmonary and Critical Care Medicine, Medical University of South Carolina, Charleston, South Carolina

George A. Sarosi, M.D.
Professor and Vice Chairman, Department of Internal Medicine, and Director, Division of General Medicine, University of Texas Health Science Center at Houston, Houston, Texas

Thomas F. Scanlin, M.D.
Director, Cystic Fibrosis Center, The Children's Hospital of Philadelphia; Professor of Pediatrics, University of Pennsylvania School of Medicine, Philadelphia, Pennsylvania

Ralph Scicchitano, M.D., Ph.D.
Instructor in Medicine, Department of Medicine, McMaster University Health Sciences Centre, Hamilton, Ontario, Canada

Robert M. Senior, M.D.
Professor of Medicine, Washington University School of Medicine; Director, Respiratory and Critical Care Division, The Jewish Hospital of St. Louis, St. Louis, Missouri

Elizabeth F. Sherertz, M.D.
Associate Professor of Medicine, Division of Dermatology, University of Florida; Chief, Dermatology Section, Veterans Administration Medical Center, Gainesville, Florida

Dennis A. Silage, Ph.D.
Associate Professor, Department of Electrical Engineering, Temple University; Lecturer, Cardiovascular-Pulmonary Division, Department of Medicine, Hospital of the University of Pennsylvania, Philadelphia, Pennsylvania

James R. Snapper, M.D.
Associate Professor of Medicine, Center for Lung Research, Department of Medicine, and Senior Investigator, the Center for Lung Research, Vanderbilt University School of Medicine, Nashville, Tennessee

Walter E. Stamm, M.D.
Professor of Medicine, University of Washington School of Medicine; Head, Infectious Diseases Division, Harborview Medical Center, Seattle, Washington

William W. Stead, M.D.
Professor of Medicine, University of Arkansas for Medical Sciences; Director, Tuberculosis Program, Division of Health Maintenance, Arkansas Department of Health, Little Rock, Arkansas

James A. Strauchen, M.D.
Associate Professor of Pathology and Associate Professor of Neoplastic Diseases, Mount Sinai School of Medicine, City University of New York, New York, New York

Lotte Strauss, M.D.†
Professor of Pathology, Department of Pathology, Mount Sinai School of Medicine, New York, New York

Morton N. Swartz, M.D.
Chief, Infectious Disease Unit, Department of Medicine, Massachusetts General Hospital, Boston, Massachusetts

J. Peter Szidon, M.D.
Professor of Medicine, Pulmonary Medicine Section, Rush Presbyterian-St. Lukes Medical Center, Chicago, Illinois

Ira B. Tager, M.D., M.P.H.
Associate Professor of Medicine, University of California, San Francisco, Veterans Administration Medical Center, San Francisco, California

†Deceased.

George H. Talbot, M.D.
Assistant Professor of Medicine, Infectious Diseases Section, Department of Medicine, Hospital of the University of Pennsylvania, Philadelphia, Pennsylvania

C. Richard Taylor, Ph.D.
Alexander Agassiz Professor of Zoology, Museum of Comparative Zoology, Harvard University, Cambridge, Massachusetts

Joseph F. Tomashefski, Jr., M.D.
Assistant Professor of Pathology, Department of Pathology, Cleveland Metropolitan General Hospital School of Medicine, Case Western Reserve University, Cleveland, Ohio

Nils Gunnar Toremalm, M.D.
Professor, Department of Oto-Rhino-Laryngology, University of Lund, Malmö General Hospital, Malmö, Sweden

J. Kent Trinkle, M.D.
Professor of Surgery and Head, Division of Cardiothoracic Surgery, The University of Texas Health Science Center, San Antonio, Texas

Gerard M. Turino, M.D.
John H. Keating, Sr., Professor of Medicine, College of Physicians and Surgeons of Columbia University; Director, Department of Medicine, St. Luke's-Roosevelt Hospital Center, New York, New York

Margaret Turner-Warwick, D.M., Ph.D.
Dean, The Cardiothoracic Institute; Professor of Medicine, Department of Thoracic Medicine, Brompton Hospital, London, England

Michael G. Velchik, M.D.
Assistant Professor of Radiology, Division of Nuclear Medicine, Hospital of the University of Pennsylvania, Philadelphia, Pennsylvania

Bruno W. Volk, M.D.
Professor in Residence, Department of Pathology, University of California at Irvine, Irvine, California

Elizabeth E. Wack, M.D.
Clinical Instructor in Medicine, Department of Internal Medicine, University of Arizona College of Medicine, Tucson, Arizona

Peter D. Wagner, M.D.
Professor of Medicine, Section of Physiology, Department of Medicine, University of California, San Diego, School of Medicine, La Jolla, California

Ko-Pen Wang, M.D.
Associate Professor of Medicine and Otolaryngology and Director, Bronchoscopy Research and Training Program, The Johns Hopkins University School of Medicine, Baltimore, Maryland

Peter A. Ward, M.D.
Professor and Chairman, Department of Pathology, The University of Michigan Medical School, Ann Arbor, Michigan

Lawrence G. Wayne, Ph.D.
Chief, Tuberculosis Research Laboratory, Veterans Administration Medical Center, Long Beach, California

John G. Weg, M.D.
Professor of Internal Medicine, Division of Pulmonary and Critical Care Medicine, University of Michigan Medical Center, Ann Arbor, Michigan

Ewald R. Weibel, M.D.
Professor of Anatomy, Department of Anatomy, University of Bern, Bern, Switzerland

Hans Weill, M.D.
Schlieder Foundation Professor of Pulmonary Medicine, Pulmonary Diseases Section, Department of Medicine, Tulane University School of Medicine, New Orleans, Louisiana

Arnold N. Weinberg, M.D.
Professor of Medicine, Harvard Medical School; Physician, Infectious Disease Unit, Massachusetts General Hospital; Director, Medical Department, Massachusetts Institute of Technology, Boston and Cambridge, Massachusetts

Emmanuel Weitzenblum, M.D.
Professor of Pulmonology, Pulmonary Function Laboratory, Department of Pulmonology, Pavillon Laennec, University Hospital, Strasbourg, France

Michael J. Welsh, M.D.
Professor of Medicine, Pulmonary Division and Laboratory of Epithelial Transport, Department of Internal Medicine, The University of Iowa College of Medicine, Iowa City, Iowa

M. Henry Williams, Jr., M.D.
Professor of Medicine, Pulmonary Division, Albert Einstein College of Medicine of Yeshiva University, The Bronx, New York

Curtis B. Wilson, M.D.
Member, Department of Immunology, Research Institute of Scripps Clinic, La Jolla, California

Richard H. Winterbauer, M.D.
Head, Chest and Infectious Diseases Section, Department of Medicine, Virginia Mason Clinic, Seattle, Washington

Theodore E. Woodward, M.D.
Professor of Medicine Emeritus, Department of Medicine, University of Maryland School of Medicine and Hospital, Veterans Administration Medical Center, Baltimore, Maryland

Raymond Yesner, M.D.
Professor of Pathology Emeritus and Director, Autopsy Division, Department of Pathology, Yale University School of Medicine, New Haven, Connecticut

Peter M. Yurchak, M.D.
Associate Clinical Professor of Medicine, Harvard Medical School, Massachusetts General Hospital, Cardiac Unit, Boston, Massachusetts

Muhammad B. Zaman, M.D.
Associate Attending Pathologist, Department of Pathology, Memorial Sloan-Kettering Cancer Center, New York, New York

Warren M. Zapol, M.D.
Anesthetist, Department of Anesthesia, Massachusetts General Hospital; Professor of Anesthesia, Harvard Medical School, Boston, Massachusetts

Preface

The original edition seems to have done what it set out to do. Clinicians were afforded a panoramic view of diseases and disorders of the lungs with an eye toward how the lungs interrelate with other parts of the body, all within the framework of medicine in general. Each entity was considered in terms of the mechanisms responsible for the disturbances, always grasping for therapeutic handles by which the pathologic process might be reversed but often forced to acknowledge that empiricism remained the order of the day. Finally, to ensure balanced perspective, each disease or disorder was depicted critically through the eyes of a seasoned expert.

Why a second edition? In a word, to update and to improve.

THE NEED TO UPDATE

In the eight years since the original edition, new clinical entities have surfaced, concepts and practice of chest medicine have undergone considerable revision, and the scientific underpinnings have shifted ground. In the parlance of Kuhn, many of these changes represent "normal" science and medicine in evolution, entirely in keeping with existing paradigms. Among these are improved preventive measures, such as vaccination against the pneumococcal and influenza virus; fuller exploitation of invasive diagnostic methods, notably bronchoscopy and cardiac catheterization; increasing substitution of noninvasive techniques, such as oximetry, for more traumatic

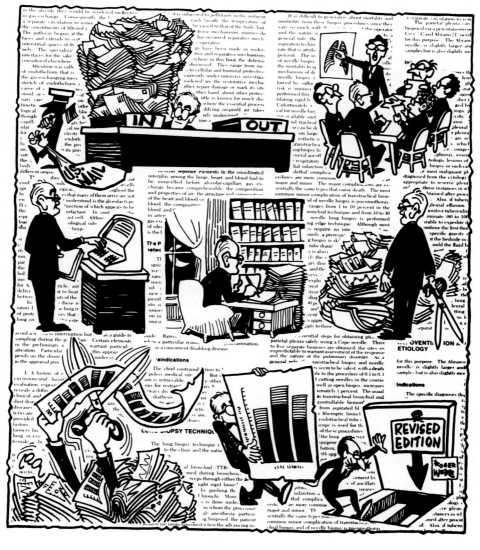

procedures; and new therapeutic modalities, ranging as widely as from antibiotics and replacement of surfactant to chemo- and radiation therapy. A strong case could also be made for "critical care medicine" as a natural outgrowth of normal progress in pulmonary medicine.

In addition to normal progress, the last seven years have been punctuated by the advent of new clinical entities, concepts, and techniques that can no longer be accommodated within traditional patterns of thinking. For example, the immunosuppressive disorders, exemplified in the extreme by AIDS, constitute a revolution in science and medicine that calls for new paradigms about mechanisms of injury and defense and for fresh approaches in management. On a much lesser scale, computed tomography and nuclear magnetic resonance have sent quivers of diagnostic anticipation among pulmonary specialists. And in the wings are impending breakthroughs in the basic sciences that hold promise of bright, new therapeutic modalities: no longer is it fantasy to imagine the identification of the genetic defect responsible for cystic fibrosis or reversing the biochemical defect in α_1-antitrypsin deficiency.

Part of the updating is to signal a broadening of the scientific underpinnings of chest medicine. A decade ago, the weight of chest medicine rested squarely on pathology, physiology, anatomy and, to a lesser extent, biochemistry. As a result, structure-function relationships have become the bedrock of pulmonary medicine. But since then the weight has shifted to include cell biology, molecular biology and molecular genetics, on the one hand, and integrative and developmental biology, on the other. These extensions are evident throughout the book, from chapters devoted to immune mechanisms and mediators to those concerned with sleep disorders.

IMPROVING THE BOOK

In addition to ensuring that its contents are current and comprehensive, and in mobilizing a stellar cast of authors, a considerable effort has been made to enhance the retrieval of the information that it contains. In addition to a precise index, an outline now precedes each chapter and an enlarged, selected, and annotated bibliography points the way to additional references. Regrouping of the chapters helps to identify categories of pulmonary disease, to define essentials and to avoid needless duplication. Fresh illustrations depict lesions and relationships that would be tedious and difficult to define in words. Since many readers had found them useful in teaching, a large effort was made to mobilize proper pictures and to reproduce them well.

THE BOOK AS PART OF A CONTINUING TRADITION

The editor was introduced to chest medicine in the 1950s at the Bellevue Hospital in New York City. At that time, J. Burns Amberson headed the Chest Service; Dickinson W. Richards was Chief of Medicine; André Cournand directed the Cardiopulmonary Laboratory. The setting was replete with seasoned chest physicians and imaginative but disciplined clinical investigators. The patients were seriously ill and needed help. The place was like a beehive: all doors were open; every crowded laboratory was busy. Looking back, Amberson, Cournand, and Richards had created a medical and scientific oasis that centered around pulmonary diseases. It is the animating spirit of these three individuals that sparks the present book.

INDEBTEDNESS TO MANY

As in the original edition, the editor owes much to many. The first acknowledgment has to be to the physicians, scientists, and educators who wrote the individual chapters that make up this book. They also deserve credit for putting up with the editor. Suzanne Markloff was my right hand, gently but firmly steering authors, manuscripts, and all around her in the proper direction. Betsy Ann Bozzarello helped create an environment in which the book could be produced, acting as a buffer, on the one hand, and as an implementor, on the other. Whenever we got into trouble, which was often, Daniel Barrett pitched in to help us meet deadlines. Throughout, Roger Webb sustained all of us with a gentle sense of humor (see the figure, page xxix) and provided drawings that helped in the formidable task of linking the disparate sections of the book into a cohesive text.

The publisher enjoyed the first edition and did all imaginable to help in preparing the second. Robert McGraw was unstinting in the effort to surpass the original work in form and format. Dereck Jeffers and Muza Navrozov helped in the never-ending pursuit of the "final inch," sometimes surging out front, occasionally falling back to push, but always at hand.

Encouragement and indulgence from my family sustained the effort: to Linda, who understood and helped all the way; to Hannah, who took it all in her wobbly stride; to Mark and Jay, who were always there when needed; to Gayle and Martha for a new dimension.

Alfred P. Fishman

Part 1

An Architecture for Physiological Function

Chapter *1*

Structure and Function

Alfred P. Fishman

Examining relationships between structure and function is a natural pursuit of philosophers as well as scientists. The practice can be easily traced back to the ancients, who were better equipped for observation than for testing and who relied heavily in their correlations on keen perceptions and profound reasoning. For more than 1500 years, structural-functional correlations were more a matter of persuasion than of documentation.

Then, in 1628, came William Harvey's "De Motu Cordis." His experiments on the pulmonary circulation not only became the watershed for all of physiology but also were the forerunner of a flood of discoveries that identified the nature of air, respiration, metabolism, the respiratory functions of the blood, and cardiopulmonary interplay.

Clinical medicine has always driven physiology and pathology. As normal structures were unraveled and assigned their proper places and roles in the architecture of form and functions, deviations from the normal were also subjected to scrutiny. Mechanisms of disease and clinicopathologic correlations became the scientific underpinnings, as well as the diagnostic proving grounds, for clinical medicine. Laennec's treatise on "Diseases of the Chest," that related clinical signs to findings at autopsy, quickly took its place as the bible and vade mecum of chest medicine.

BIOLOGIC HIERARCHIES

Until a few decades ago, structure and function could be correlated only at the higher levels in the hierarchy of biologic functions, in organs, tissues, and cells. The predominant instruments were the hand and the eye; how vital parts communicated was considered and tested in terms of the autonomic nervous system and neurohumoral mediators.

We are now in the midst of a scientific revolution. New techniques have made it possible to conceptualize and depict molecules and their arrangements that are too small to visualize. Preoccupation with linkages between organs and tissues has given way to information transfer between cells, between their interiors and surface membranes, and between intracellular molecules and organelles. The microscope and test tube have been succeeded as analytic tools by x-ray diffraction, nuclear magnetic resonance, and computers. Using the concepts of cellular and molecular biology and molecular genetics, protein structure and biologic function are being scrutinized with an eye toward enzymes, growth factors, and components of the plasma membrane. Also in focus are implications of the new understanding for medicine. For example, appreciation of the varying surface proteins of the influenza virus has raised bright prospects for developing drugs to cope with this organism.

Reductionism is the order of this new day. But, as the subsequent sections are intended to show, the same patterns of scientific thought and exploration seem to be operating at the submicroscopic levels as those that came into play 350 years ago with William Harvey's depiction of the circulation of the blood.

THE PULMONARY CIRCULATION

Bridge between the Two Ventricles

Galen's enduring concept of the lungs as a cooling device for the heat-generating heart had to be demolished before the respiratory function of the lungs could surface as a meaningful question. Before Galen (129–200 A.D.) interest in the lungs had been spotty. The Hippocratic Corpus (fifth century B.C.) distinguished between the airways and the vessels that leave the heart (Fig. 1-1). Herophilus and Erasistratos (fourth century B.C.), members of the Museum at Alexandria where human dissection and animal experimentation were practiced, knew of the pulmonary vessels. They, and subsequently Galen, incorporated them into schemes which accounted for generation of humors within the body. But not until the publication in 1628 of William Harvey's *Exercitatio Anatomica de Motu Cordis et Sanguinis* (Fig. 1-2) did the pulmonary circulation begin to gain widespread acceptance as the bridge between the two ventricles. Harvey reasoned convincingly that blood flows in a circle. He based his arguments for the circulation of the blood on anatomic observations coupled with experimentation, quantitative measurements, and calculation. It is true that long before Harvey, visionaries, particularly Ibn Nafis (thirteenth century) and Michael

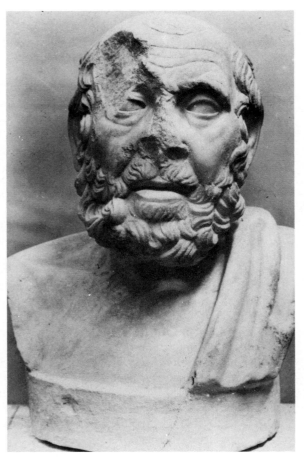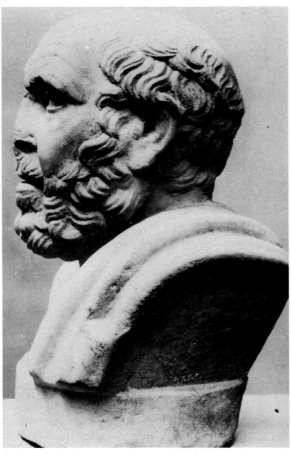

FIGURE 1-1 The Hippocrates of Ostia. The bust of this elderly man was found in a family tomb in excavations near Ostia. This damaged bust is now believed to represent Hippocrates as perceived in antiquity. The bust in the British Museum that was formerly considered to be a representation of Hippocrates is now known to be that of the philosopher Crisippus of Soloi. *(From Cournand, 1964, with permission.)*

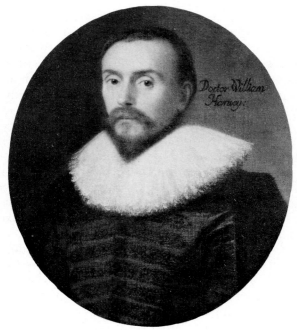

FIGURE 1-2 William Harvey (1578–1657). This portrait was painted in 1626. His discovery of the circulation of the blood marks the beginning of the modern science of physiology. *(From Hamilton and Richards, 1964, with permission.)*

Servetus (1511–1553), had appreciated existence of the pulmonary circulation, but their inspired insights made no impression on the science of their day. It was left to Harvey (Fig. 1-2), 1500 years after Galen, to establish beyond cavil that the pulmonary artery led to fine connections between the right and left sides of the heart. Not until 1660, 3 years after Harvey's death, did Marcello Malpighi show the passage of blood through fine vessels in the lungs: making use of a new technology, i.e., a double convex lens at first and probably a pair of lenses later on, he was able to see blood passing from the arteries to the veins of the lungs, thereby providing final proof of Harvey's concept of the circulation of the blood.

From Air to Tissues

Harvey dealt with the mechanical aspects of the circulation of the blood. Two years after his death, Richard Lower, using a respiration pump devised by Hooke, showed that venous blood became arterialized in transit from the right to the left side of the heart. But the nature of this change was unclear. By the end of the sixteenth century, the traditional concepts of the ancients about four elements had been succeeded by the concept of *phlogiston,* a universal agent that participated in all chemical reactions and was released into the air in the course of combustion. Another century was to elapse before the nature

of the gases involved in external respiration was clarified as a result of advances in chemistry and physics: Black discovered CO_2 (1757); Priestley prepared O_2 (1774), and Lavoisier (1743–1794) discovered its nature; Rutherford discovered N_2 (1772). Lavoisier and his coworkers (Fig. 1-3) not only systematically destroyed the phlogiston theory and proved that O_2, rather than air, was essential for life, but they also showed that combustion and respiration were similar processes. In the course of their investigations, they also introduced quantitative chemistry as the basis for the study of metabolism in animals and human beings. Another one-half century was to elapse before it was accepted that the site of combustion was in the tissues rather than in the lungs, and that hemoglobin was involved in the transport of O_2 from the lungs to the tissues.

Control of the Pulmonary Circulation

By the middle of the eighteenth century, sporadic attempts had been made to examine the mechanical influence of breathing on the pulmonary circulation. However, the behavior of the pulmonary circulation could not be explored systematically until new concepts and technology provided ways to determine cardiac output and to relate pulmonary vascular pressures to pulmonary blood flow. The first major inroad along this line was made in

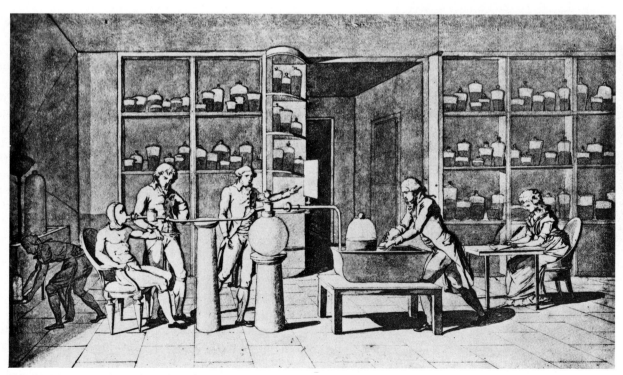

FIGURE 1-3 Scene from the laboratory of Antoine Laurent Lavoisier (1743–1794). He was the first to disclose the true nature of combustion and to show that respiration and combustion were similar processes. His wife is shown acting as his laboratory assistant. *(From Cournand, 1964, with permission.)*

the laboratory of Carl Ludwig (1816–1895). From Ludwig's laboratory flowed a long stream of anatomic and physiological discoveries, techniques, and concepts. His laboratory was also a seat of learning for distinguished forerunners of respiratory physiology: Bohr, Fick, Heger, and Rubner. In the 1850s, pulmonary arterial pressures were determined there using a recording mercury manometer in open-chest dogs. In 1870, Adolph Fick (Fig. 1-4) described, although he did not have the manometric apparatus to measure, the cardiac output. For the Fick principle, mixed venous blood was necessary. For the next three-quarters of a century, refinements in manometric techniques and a variety of indirect methods increased knowledge of pulmonary hemodynamics, but it was not until the 1930s, after the introduction of cardiac catheterization and the standardization by Cournand and Richards of techniques for applying the Fick principle, that the behavior of the normal and abnormal pulmonary circulation could undergo orderly and detailed exploration in unanesthetized, intact human subjects, and ventilation and blood flow could be related in health and disease.

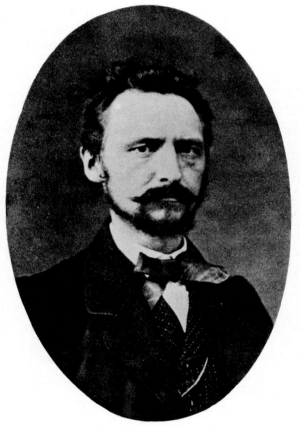

FIGURE 1-4   Adolph Fick (1829–1901). Mathematician, physicist, and physiologist who published in 1870 a brief note that described how to determine cardiac output; he lacked the manometers to put his principle to the test.

ALVEOLAR-CAPILLARY GAS EXCHANGE

After Lavoisier and his contemporaries had succeeded in clarifying the nature of the respiratory gases, the time was ripe for examining how O_2 and CO_2 were transported in blood. In 1851, Funke found hemoglobin in the blood of the spleen. Other investigators began to explore the details of O_2 and CO_2 transport by hemoglobin. But it was only in the twentieth century that Christian Bohr, himself a product of Ludwig's laboratory, began the systematic study of alveolar-capillary gas exchange. At first, O_2 was held to cross the alveolar-capillary membrane by secretion, but it was Bohr's student, August Krogh, aided by his wife and collaborator, Marie Krogh (Fig. 1-5), who provided that alveolar-capillary gas exchange in the lungs took place by diffusion rather than by secretion, thereby laying the groundwork for modern concepts of alveolar-capillary gas exchange. Since then, a succession of brilliant investigators have provided a remarkable synthesis of the processes that are involved in gas exchange in the lungs. Their names are legendary among respiratory physiologists: John Scott Haldane (1860–1936), Sir Joseph Barcroft (1872–1947), and Lawrence J. Henderson (1878–1942) (Fig. 1-6). Their contributions are too voluminous and profound to detail here. A few landmarks warrant mention. Haldane and Barcroft, by ingenious experiments, sorted out the respiratory functions of the blood; Henderson provided the synthesis of blood as a physicochemical system and depicted how this system operated in respiratory exchange and transport both at rest and during exercise.

The regulation of alveolar-capillary gas exchange began to be related to the behavior of the pulmonary circulation in 1946 when Euler and Liljestrand proposed that the local concentration of the respiratory gases within the lungs shaped the distribution of the pulmonary blood flow. According to this idea, local hypoxia, a consequence of local disease, would divert blood to better ventilated parts of the lung for arterialization. This hypothesis was subsequently proved in a variety of ways. Meanwhile the behavior of the pulmonary circulation was explored in one pulmonary and cardiac disease after another. And once the cardiac catheter had provided easy access to the pulmonary circulation, a rash of diagnostic and therapeutic interventions inevitably followed.

FROM HEALTH TO DISEASE

Just as physiology and anatomy have been the traditional basic sciences for the understanding of normal body function, pathology is the science of disease. In concept, the realm of pathology is universal since it is committed to uncovering the causes of disease using any strategy that it can command, but, in principle, its horizons are more cir-

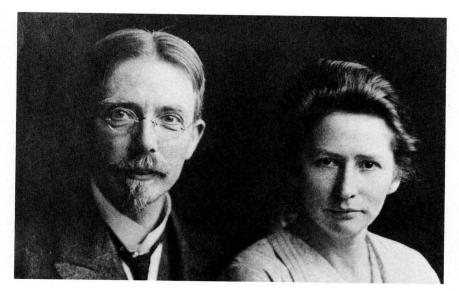

FIGURE 1-5 August and Marie Krogh in 1922 at the time of their first visit to the United States so that August Krogh could deliver the Silliman Lecture at Yale. They demonstrated that diffusion, without secretion, could account for the transfer of O_2 and CO_2 across the alveolar-capillary membranes of the lungs. *(Courtesy of their daughter, Dr. Bodil Schmidt-Nielsen.)*

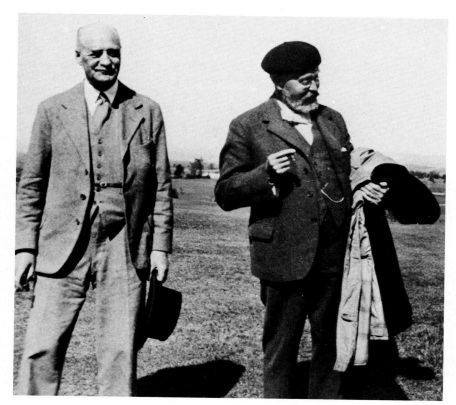

FIGURE 1-6 Two founders of contemporary respiratory physiology. Sir Joseph Barcroft (1872–1947) *(left)* settled, in experiments on himself, that diffusion was the mechanism for gas exchange in the lungs and pioneered current understanding of the respiratory functions of the blood. Lawrence J. Henderson (1878–1942) provided a mathematical analysis of blood as a physicochemical system and stimulated research on the complex interplay involved in respiratory gas exchange during exercise. *(From Cournand, 1964, with permission.)*

cumscribed, largely because pathology has become identified over the years with only one of its components, morbid anatomy.

The association of pathology with morbid anatomy dates back to ancient times. Galen, based on anatomy that he gleaned from animal vivisection and a wide clinical experience, promulgated the doctrine that each alteration in function must correspond to a lesion in an organ; conversely, every lesion in an organ must cause a change in function. For many years after Galen, sporadic attempts were made to explore relationships between structural changes and abnormalities in function, but sustained efforts along this line were periodically interrupted by strictures that religious intolerance imposed upon human dissection. However, in 1761, morbid anatomy assumed the ascendancy role as a scientific basis for medicine.

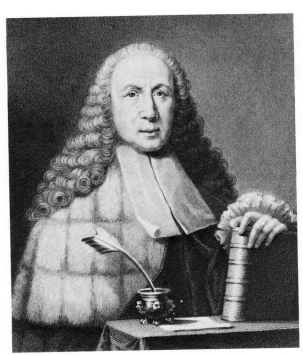

FIGURE 1-7 Giovanni Battista Morgagni. His classic *De Sedibus* contains the clinical and pathologic descriptions of approximately 700 cases. (*Courtesy of the Library of the College of Physicians of Philadelphia.*)

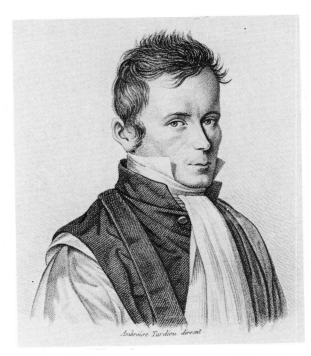

Ambroise Tardieu direxit

FIGURE 1-8 Rene T. H. Laennec (1781–1826). His invention of auscultation and his famous treatise on clinical disorders of the chest laid the foundation for contemporary chest medicine. (*Courtesy of the Library of the College of Physicians of Philadelphia.*)

In that year, Morgagni (Fig. 1-7) published *De Sedibus et Causis Morborum*, a treatise in which clinical syndromes were systematically related to observations that he had made at autopsy. The empiric correlations in this work became the cornerstone of clinical medicine, but the pathologic observations in *De Sedibus* were much more substantial than the clinical, which could be provided only by the physician's senses. In the same year that Morgagni's treatise was published, Auenbrugger's *Inventum Novum* appeared in print, depicting the relationship between anatomic changes in the organs of the chest and abnormal sounds elicited by percussion. However, in contrast to the immediate universal acclaim that greeted *De Sedibus*, Auenbrugger's discovery was not appreciated by the medical world until almost 50 years later when his book was translated into French and popularized by Corvisart, the great clinician of the nineteenth century and physician to Napoleon.

Laennec's (Fig. 1-8) description of a method of auscultation immediately gained widespread attention and acceptance. He was a follower of Morgagni. His book *Diseases of the Chest* was based on the principle of clinicopathologic correlations. The range of diseases of the chest that he covers is extensive: tuberculosis, pneumonia, lung abscess, hemoptysis, bronchitis, bronchiectasis, emphysema, pulmonary edema, cysts, cancer, calcifications, and diseases of the pleura.

However, neither Morgagni nor Laennec distinguished between the *cause of symptoms* and the *cause of disease*. For the former, clinical manifestations are related to static pictures of morbid anatomy; to uncover etiology and pathogenesis, observations have to be made during life, generally by experimentation. This aspect of pathology is identified with Rudolph Virchow (1821–1902), the founder of cellular pathology. Virchow combined physiological thinking, anatomic observation, and animal experimentation in the search for the causes of disease. Virchow discounted metaphysical explanations. His descriptions of thrombosis and embolism began in the autopsy room and were completed in the animal laboratory. After Virchow, animal experimentation has remained an essential component in contemporary pathology.

This is the setting of contemporary chest medicine: structure-function in the sense of Virchow reinforced by clinicopathologic correlations in the sense of Morgagni. It is true that units of structure have grown smaller and smaller; organelles and molecules have succeeded cells as the fundamental sites of abnormal structure; and the idea of function has broadened to include areas of biology far removed from conventional physiology and biochemistry. Nonetheless, progress in medicine is powered by the same mechanisms: science, technology, observations, and experimentation.

BIBLIOGRAPHY

Barcroft J: *Features in the Architecture of Physiological Function.* New York, Hafner, 1934, pp 172–229.
  A classic presentation of integrative biologic interplay at the level of organs and tissues.

Bylebyl J: The growth of Harvey's "De Motu Cordis." Bull Hist Med 47:427–470, 1973.
  An outline of the development of Harvey's work on the heart and blood vessels in relation to the views of his predecessors followed by the author's interpretation of the growth of Harvey's ideas.

Castiglioni A: *A History of Medicine.* Translated from the Italian by EB Krumbhaar. New York, Knopf, 1947, pp 148–178.
  A standard point of departure for reference material on the history of medicine.

Cournand A: Air and Blood, in Fishman AP, Richards DW (eds), *Circulation of the Blood. Men and Ideas.* New York, Oxford, 1964, pp 3–70.
  The growth of ideas about the pulmonary circulature. The role of Michael Servetus is engagingly portrayed.

Fishman AP: Heart, lungs and blood as an integrated system. Circulation (Suppl III), 70:83–87, 1984.
  The organism is viewed as a biologic hierarchy in which each level of organization not only serves a particular, circumscribed function but also contributes importantly to the integrated and coordinated performance of the organism as a whole. The cardiorespiratory apparatus is used to illustrate the concept.

Frank RG Jr: *Harvey and the Oxford Physiologists.* Berkeley, University of California Press, 1980.
  Beginning with William Harvey's pivotal announcement in 1628 of the circulation of the blood, an architecture of physiological functions is built from successive discoveries about the nature of air, respiration, metabolism, combustion, blood, heart and circulation, and the fetus in utero.

Haldane JS, Priestley JG: *Respiration,* 2d ed. New York, Oxford, 1935.
  A classic in the history of respiration by two distinguished pioneers. This book is rich in the tradition of involvement of the investigators as subjects.

Hamilton WF, Richards DW: The output of the heart, in Fishman AP, Richards DW (eds), *Circulation of the Blood. Men and Ideas.* New York, Oxford, 1964, p 72.
  A scholarly essay about the evolution of physiological approaches to cardiac performance.

Harvey W: *Movement of the Heart and Blood in Animals. An Anatomical Essay.* Translated by KJ Franklin. Oxford, Blackwell, 1957.
  A small book that marks the birth of contemporary physiology.

Heinemann HO, Fishman AP: Non-respiratory function of the lungs. Physiol Rev 49:1–47, 1969.
  Based on personal experience and review of the literature, the conclusion is reached that the lung has major nonrespiratory functions, including the processing of biologically active materials that traverse the enormous expanse of pulmonary capillaries.

Henderson LJ: *Blood. A Study in General Physiology.* New Haven, Yale University Press, 1928.
  A monumental study of the physicochemical properties of the blood with particular reference to its respiratory functions.

Klemperer P: The pathology of Morgagni and Virchow. Bull Hist Med 32:24–38, 1958.
  A perspective by a distinguished pathologist-scholar of the evolution of pathology with particular reference to the progression from descriptive pathology to experimental pathology.

Krogh A: *The Anatomy and Physiology of Capillaries.* New York, Hafner, 1959, pp x, xi.
  No one interested in the pulmonary microcirculation can afford to overlook this remarkable presentation of ingenious approaches to understanding the workings of the capillary circulation.

Laennec RTH: *A Treatise on Diseases of the Chest.* New York, Hafner, 1962.
  The seminal volume in the history of chest medicine that based clinical findings on pathology.

Morgagni JB: *Recherches Anatomiques sur le Siege et les Causes des Maladies.* Paris, Caille et Ravier, 1820.
  The beginnings of systematic clinicopathologic correlations. This beginning made its mark on Laennec and subsequent generations of chest physicians.

New Pathways in Science and Technology. Collected Research Briefings 1982–84. New York, Vintage Books, 1985.
  A collection of 21 research briefings prepared under a joint committee of the National Academy of Sciences and Engineering, and the Institute of Medicine. The compendium is intended to identify new directions and new pathways for future scientific and technological advance.

Perkins JF Jr: Historical development of respiratory physiology, in Fenn WO, Rahn H (eds), *Hand-book of Physiology, sec III, Respiration.* Washington DC, American Physiological Society, 1964, pp 1–62.

    A broad perspective by a scholarly respiratory physiologist of the growth of ideas about the respiratory system.

Ryan US: *Pulmonary Endothelium in Health and Disease.* New York, Dekker, 1987.

    An update for the last decade of research on pulmonary endothelium. Structure and function at a cellular level, with a major focus on endothelial cells in culture.

Taylor CR, Karas RH, Weibel ER, Hoppeler H: Adaptive variation in the mammalian respiratory system in relation to energetic demand. Respiration Physiol 69:1–127, 1987.

    A collection of papers by these authors focusing on the hypothesis that structural design is commensurate with functional needs.

Weibel ER: *The Pathway for Oxygen. Structure and Function in Mammalian Respiratory System.* Cambridge, MA, Harvard University Press, 1984.

    A synthesis between the traditional fields of anatomy and physiology using stereological meth-ods to quantify structures and their spatial relationships. A quantitative approach is used to examine the match between structure and function in the transfer from the environment in mitochondria. Questions of design are considered along with those of regulation.

Will JA, Dawson CA, Weir EK, Buckner CK: *The Pulmonary Circulation in Health and Disease.* New York, Academic Press, 1987.

    An up-to-date review, based on a conference, of structure-function relationships of the normal and abnormal pulmonary circulation.

Chapter 2

Design and Structure of the Human Lung

Ewald R. Weibel / C. Richard Taylor

At the end of a deep breath, about 80 percent of the lung volume is air, 10 percent is blood, and only the remaining 10 percent is tissue. Because this small mass of tissue is spread over an enormous area—nearly the size of a tennis court—the tissue framework of the lung must be extraordinarily delicate. It is indeed remarkable that the substance of the lung manages to maintain its integrity in the face of the multitude of insults that inevitably accompany a lifetime of exposure to ambient air and the complex ne-cessity of keeping air and blood in intimate contact, but separate, for the sake of gas exchange.

Part of this success is undoubtedly attributable to the unique design of the lung, which ensures mechanical stability as well as nearly optimal conditions for the performance of the lung's primary function: to supply the blood with an adequate amount of O_2 even when the body's demands for O_2 are particularly high, as during heavy work. There are, however, some problems that limit this performance, such as inhomogeneities in the relations between perfusion and ventilation of the gas-exchange units, basic functions that are, again, related to design properties of the lung, at least in part.

THE LUNG AS AN ORGAN

At total lung capacity, the lungs fill the entire chest cavity and can reach a volume, in the adult human, of some 5 to 6 L, largely depending on body size. Upon expiration, the lungs retract, most conspicuously from the lower parts of the pleural cavity, the posterior bottom edges of the lungs moving upward by some 4 to 6 cm. This preferential lifting of the bottom edges is caused by retraction of the tissue throughout the lungs, the surfaces of which are freely movable within the thoracic cavity.

The structural background for this mobility of a healthy lung is the formation, during morphogenesis, of a

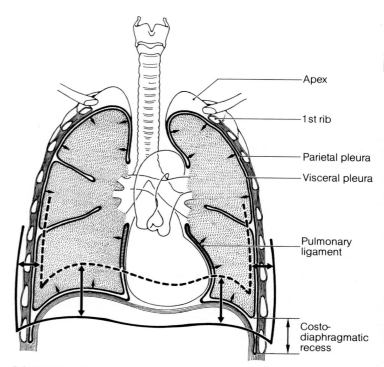

FIGURE 2-1 Frontal section of chest and lungs showing pleural space. Single arrows indicate retractive force, double arrows show the excursion of the lung bases and periphery between deep inspiration and expiration.

serosal space that is lined on the interior of the chest wall and on the lung surface by a serosa, the parietal and visceral pleurae, respectively (Fig. 2-1). However, this serosal space is minimal since the visceral pleura is closely apposed to the parietal pleura with only a thin film of serous fluid intercalated as a lubricant between the two surfaces. Both pleural surfaces are lined by a squamous epithelial layer, often called *mesothelium,* whose surface is richly endowed with long microvilli. It is unknown how the pleural fluid is secreted or how it is maintained as a minimal film. Whether lymphatics in the parietal pleura play an important role in rapidly draining excess fluid is unsettled.

The connective tissue of the visceral pleura consists of three layers. A superficial layer of predominantly elastic fibers follows the mesothelium, thereby forming an elastic "bag" that enwraps each lobe. A deep sheet of fine fibers follows the outline of alveoli and extends into the depth of the lung. Between these sheets lies a bed of loose connective tissue containing free cells (histiocytes, plasma cells, and mast cells) that is often close to lymphatics and to systemic arterial branches from the bronchial arteries.

Each lung is maintained in a stable position within the chest by the hilus, where airways and blood vessels enter from the mediastinum, and by the pulmonary ligament, a long, narrow band of attachment between visceral and mediastinal pleura which extends downward from the hilus. Because of these attachments, a pneumothorax causes the lung to retract and to form a lump of tissue that is attached to the mediastinal wall of the thoracic cavity.

The shape of each lung is congruent with that of the fully expanded pleural cavity. This shape is preformed in lung tissue and is hence also evident if an excised lung is inflated, revealing its three faces: the convex thoracic face apposed to the rib cage, the concave diaphragmatic face modeled by the diaphragmatic dome, and the mediastinal face on which the contours of the heart are impressed beneath the hilus.

As the lungs retract during deflation, the acute edges between the thoracic face and the diaphragmatic and (anterior) mediastinal faces of the lungs withdraw; the thoracic and diaphragmatic leaflets of the parietal pleura become apposed, thereby forming a costodiaphragmatic recess on each side (Fig. 2-1); similarly, as the ventral edges of the lungs retract, the costal and mediastinal pleurae form a recess on each side, corresponding topographically to the borders of the sternum.

The port through which airways and blood vessels enter each lung is the hilus, i.e., the attachment of lung tissue to the mediastinum (Fig. 2-1). The airways reach the two hili by the main-stem, or principal, bronchi (Figs. 2-1 and 2-2); the left main-stem bronchus is longer than the right because it must pass under the aortic arch before it reaches the lung. The two principal bronchi course

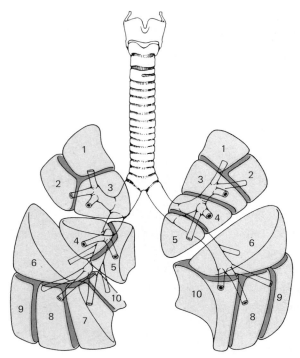

FIGURE 2-2 Bronchopulmonary segments of human lungs. *Left and right upper lobes:* (1) apical, (2) posterior, (3) anterior, (4) superior lingular, and (5) inferior lingular segments. *Right middle lobe:* (4) lateral and (5) medial segments. *Lower lobes:* (6) superior (apical), (7) medial-basal, (8) anterior-basal, (9) lateral-basal, and (10) posterior-basal segments. The medial-basal segment (7) is absent in the left lung. [NOTE: The lungs are represented as slightly turned inward in order to display part of the lateral face (see front cover).]

downward and begin to divide sequentially shortly after entering the lung, first releasing the lobar bronchus to the upper lobe (Fig. 2-2). Since a middle lobe is formed only on the right side, there is no middle lobe bronchus on the left; instead, the corresponding parts form the lingula which receives its airways from the superior bronchus of the upper lobe (Fig. 2-2). The last branch of the stem bronchus goes to the lower lobe.

The pulmonary artery (Fig. 2-3) joins the bronchi while still in the mediastinum; its trunk lies to the left of the ascending aorta, and the right pulmonary artery turns dorsally to course between ascending aorta and right principal bronchus. In the hilus, the right pulmonary artery lies anterior to the right principal bronchus; the left pulmonary artery, however, "rides" on the principal bronchus and crosses over the superior lobar bronchus to the posterior side (Fig. 2-3). From there on, the pulmonary artery branches in parallel with the bronchi; characteristically, each bronchus is associated with one closely apposed pulmonary artery branch, and this relationship is strictly maintained to the periphery, i.e., to the respiratory bronchioles (see front cover).

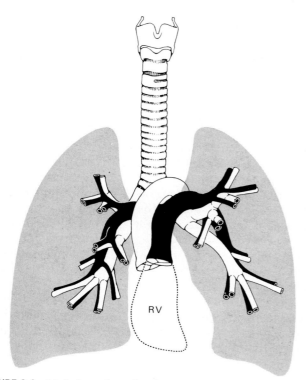

FIGURE 2-3 Main branches of pulmonary artery in relation to bronchi. RV = right ventricle.

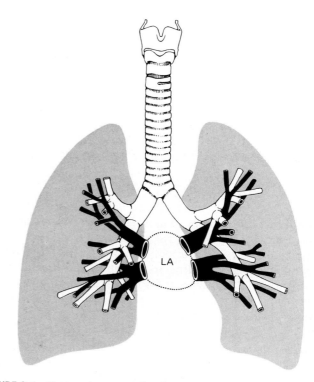

FIGURE 2-4 Two main stems of pulmonary vein penetrate into each lung. LA = left atrium.

In contrast, the pulmonary veins (Fig. 2-4) follow a course independent of the bronchial tree; rather, they lie about midway between two pairs of bronchi and arteries; this position is maintained to the periphery of the airway system. In the hilus these veins are collected on either side into at least two main veins which lead into the left atrium located at the back of the heart.

The airways systematically branch over an average of 23 generations of dichotomous branching, ending eventually in a blind sac (Fig. 2-5). The last six to seven generations of these airways are connected to tightly packed *alveoli*, airway chambers in which gas exchange takes place, whereas the central airways serve the function of conducting the air to the gas-exchange parenchyma. In such a system of sequential branching, the unit of pulmonary parenchyma could be defined according to the portion of parenchyma that is supplied by a particular branch of the bronchial tree, and it is possible to conceive of as many types of units as there are generations, unless clear definitions for such units are proposed. However, two units appear to be natural:

1. The *lobes*, which are demarcated by a more or less complete lining of pleura. There are three lobes on the right (superior, middle, and inferior) and two on the left (superior and inferior).

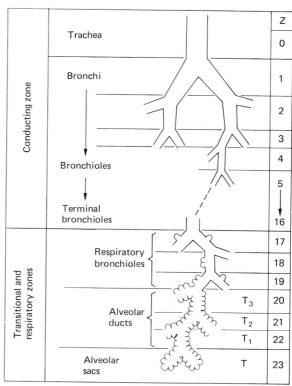

FIGURE 2-5 Airway branching in human lungs by regularized dichotomy from trachea (generation z = 0) to alveolar ducts and sacs (generations 20 to 23). The first 16 generations are purely conducting; transitional airways lead into the respiratory zone made of alveoli. (*After Weibel, 1963.*)

13

2. The *acinus*, which is defined as that portion of pulmonary parenchyma that is supplied by a first-order respiratory bronchiole, i.e., a parenchymal unit in which all airways participate in gas exchange.

Since all other units are somewhat arbitrarily defined, it is not surprising that some ambiguity exists in the literature about their meanings. Nonetheless, a certain convention has been adopted with respect to the following:

1. *The lung segments,* which are considered as the first subdivisions of lobes. Figure 2-2 shows the location and distribution of the segments to the various lobes. The symmetry is imperfect because on the left the two segments corresponding to the right middle lobe are incorporated into the superior lobe as the lingula, and because the medial-basal segment of the lower lobe is generally missing on the left.
2. *The secondary lobule,* an old anatomic unit. It was introduced in the nineteenth century because "lobules" of about 1 cm³ are visible on the surface of the lung. These lobules are delineated by connective tissue septa

that are connected to the pleura. The secondary lobule is difficult to define in terms of the bronchial tree, but it does seem to comprise about a dozen acini, and most often it is said to include the parenchyma that is supplied by about five terminal bronchioles. With reference to bronchograms, secondary lobules are supplied by airway branches that are about 1 mm in diameter.

The pulmonary blood vessels show a characteristic relationship to these units (Figs. 2-3, 2-4, and the front cover). The pulmonary arteries, following the airways, course through the center of the units and finally fan out into the capillaries located in the delicate alveolar septa of pulmonary parenchyma. In contrast, the veins lie in the boundary between units and collect the blood from at least two or three adjacent units. This arrangement applies to acini and secondary lobules (back cover) as well as to lung segments.

Therefore, it is evident that the units of pulmonary parenchyma are bronchoarterial units which share their venous drainage with neighboring units. This architecture has important functional and practical consequences. Except for the lobes, none of the units are separated from each other by complete connective tissue septa.

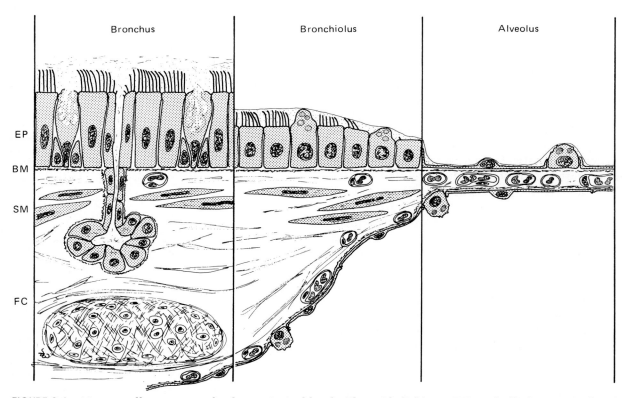

FIGURE 2-6   Airway wall structure at the three principal levels. The epithelial layer (EP) gradually becomes reduced from pseudostratified to cuboidal and then to squamous, but retains its organization as a mosaic of lining and secretory cells. The smooth-muscle layer (SM) disappears in the alveoli. The fibrous coat (FC) contains cartilage only in bronchi and gradually becomes thinner as the alveolus is approached. BM = basement membrane.

ORGANIZATION OF PULMONARY TISSUE

Basic Structural Elements

In looking at the tissue organization of the lung we must first consider that each airway and blood vessel has its own lining by an uninterrupted cell layer. These layers extend all the way out to the gas-exchange region, but they show different properties in conducting as compared to respiratory structures. Likewise, the connective tissue forms a continuum throughout the lung all the way out to the pleura, but it, too, will be differently organized in the different functional zones: whereas it is reduced to a minimum in the alveolar walls, it contributes a number of different ancillary structures to the wall of conducting air-

ways and blood vessels, such as smooth-muscle sheaths or cartilage. This connective tissue space also houses the nutritive vessels and nerves, as well as the elaborate defense system related to lymphatic vessels. However, in the gas-exchange region, very few of these accessory structures are found.

Wall Structure of Conducting Airways

The wall of conducting airways consists of three major components (Figs. 2-6 and 2-7): (1) a mucosa that is composed of an epithelial and a connective tissue lamina, (2) a smooth-muscle sleeve, and (3) an enveloping connective tissue tube, partly provided with cartilage.

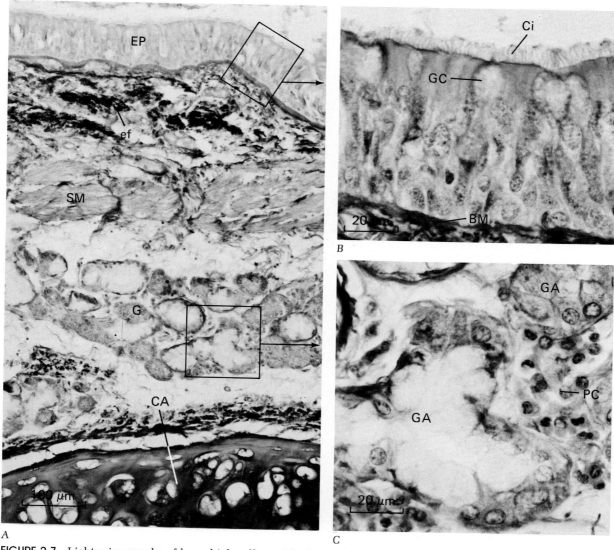

FIGURE 2-7 Light micrographs of bronchial wall. *A.* The layers from epithelium (EP) to cartilage (CA) with elastic fibers (ef), smooth-muscle bundles (SM), and glands (G). *B.* Higher power of pseudostratified epithelium and cilia (Ci). *C.* Details of gland with acini (GA) associated with groups of plasma cells (PC). GC = goblet cell; BM = basement membrane.

Though derived from one and the same anlage, the airway epithelium modifies its differentiation characteristics as we proceed from large bronchi over bronchioles to the alveolar region (Fig. 2-6). A simple epithelium exists as a lining of smaller bronchioles: as we move upward toward larger bronchi, the epithelium becomes higher and some basal cells appear, making the epithelium pseudo-stratified; at the point of transition into the gas-exchange region, that is, at the entrance into the complex of alveoli, the epithelium abruptly becomes extremely thin.

Figure 2-6 also shows that the epithelium is not made of a uniform cell population but that it is, at each level, rather a mosaic of at least two cell types in that secretory cells are interspersed into the complex of lining cells. There are also some additional rarer cells, such as neuro-endocrine cells, that are capable of secreting some media-tors into the blood, or so-called brush cells whose precise function is not yet understood.

If we now take a closer look at the epithelium of larger conducting airways, we see that the lining cells are provided with a tuft of kinocilia at their apical cell face, whereas the secretory cells are goblet cells that produce and discharge a sticky mucus to the surface (Figs. 2-8 and 2-9). This mucus spreads out as a thin blanket on top of the cilia and is capable of trapping dust particles that are entrained in the air entering the lung. Kinocilia (Fig. 2-10) are organelles of movement that are known to beat rhythmically in a given direction and at a frequency of about 20 Hz. In the airway epithelium the cilia are oriented in such a fashion that their beat is directed outward. It is interesting that the cilia of airway epithelia develop fine claws at their tips; with these claws they grasp the mucous blanket in the phase of their forward beat, whereas on their return to the upright position, they glide past the mucous blanket. The result of this is that the mucous blanket, together with trapped foreign material, moves outward or "up the

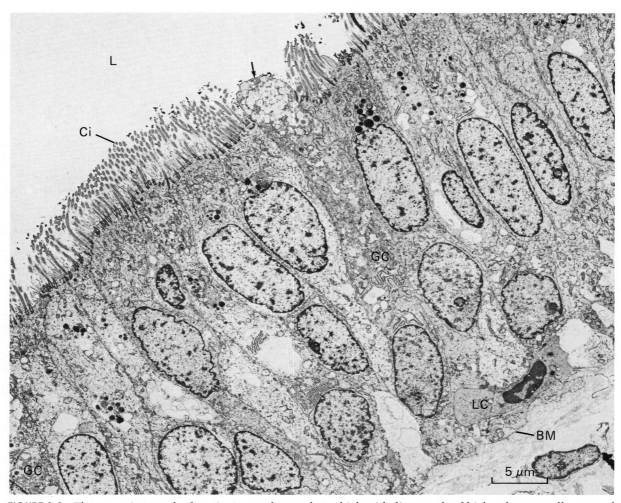

FIGURE 2-8   Electron micrograph of section across human bronchial epithelium made of high-columnar cells, most of which are ciliated (Ci). A goblet cell (GC) is cut lengthwise; note mucous droplets in the process of accumulating at cell apex (arrow) and leukocyte (LC) caught in epithelium in process of diapedesis. L = lumen; BM = basement membrane.

airways" in a steady stream, a feature appropriately called the *ciliary escalator*. Since the lining by ciliated cells is uninterrupted from the bronchioles, up the bronchi to the trachea, this mucociliary escalator ends at the larynx, so that the normal fate of bronchial mucus is to be steadily discharged into the pharynx whence it is swallowed, usually unnoticed. Only when an excessive amount of mucus accumulates in the trachea or in larger bronchi do we have to assist the system by coughing.

The secretory cell population shows a number of specialized features. In the bronchi of all sizes and in larger bronchioles one finds goblet cells interspersed among the ciliated cells; they form the mucus in their endoplasmic reticulum and Golgi complex, store it as droplets in their apical part, and discharge it in bulk (Fig. 2-8 and 2-9). In larger bronchi, one finds, in addition, small mucous glands located in the connective tissue; they are connected to the bronchial surface by long and narrow ducts (Figs. 2-6 and 2-7). In the normal bronchus the glandular acini are relatively small and composed of serous and mucous cells; enlargement of the acini and a relative increase in mucous cells are characteristics of chronic bronchitis. Finally, a special secretory cell appears in the smaller bronchioles, the Clara cell (Fig. 2-11) whose secre-

tory product is still unknown; this cell is rich in smooth endoplasmic reticulum and contains mixed function oxidases that are involved in detoxification of foreign compounds.

The layer of connective tissue in the bronchial mucosa consists predominantly of elastic fibers that are oriented longitudinally; these fibers serve to maintain a smooth outline of the longitudinal profile of the bronchial lumen no matter how much the bronchi are stretched as the lungs are inflated. In this connective tissue lamina there are foci of lymphoid cells; often they form small lymphoid follicles.

Smooth-muscle bundles form a continuous sleeve in the connective tissue underlying the epithelial tube that extends from the major bronchi to the respiratory bronchioles; beyond the respiratory bronchioles, the bundles extend into the wall of alveolar ducts where the muscle fibers lie in the alveolar entrance rings. The bundles have an oblique course and encircle the mucosal tube in a crisscross pattern; hence, their contraction results primarily in narrowing of the lumen.

In the small bronchioles there is little else to the airway wall; the smooth-muscle layer is ensheathed by a layer of delicate connective tissue that is in direct contact

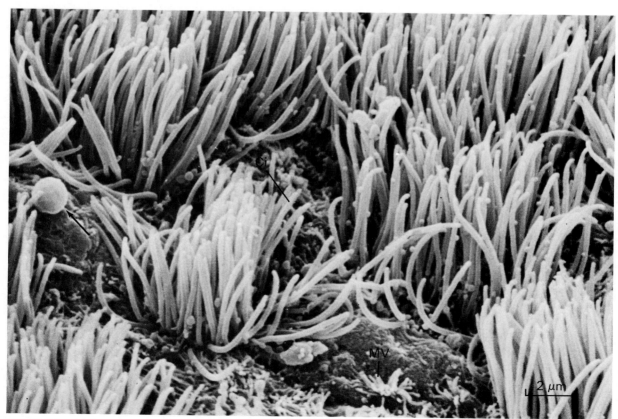

FIGURE 2-9 Surface view of bronchiolar epithelium shows tufts of cilia (Ci) forming on individual ciliated cells and microvilli (MV) on other cells. Note secretion droplet in process of release from goblet cell (arrow).

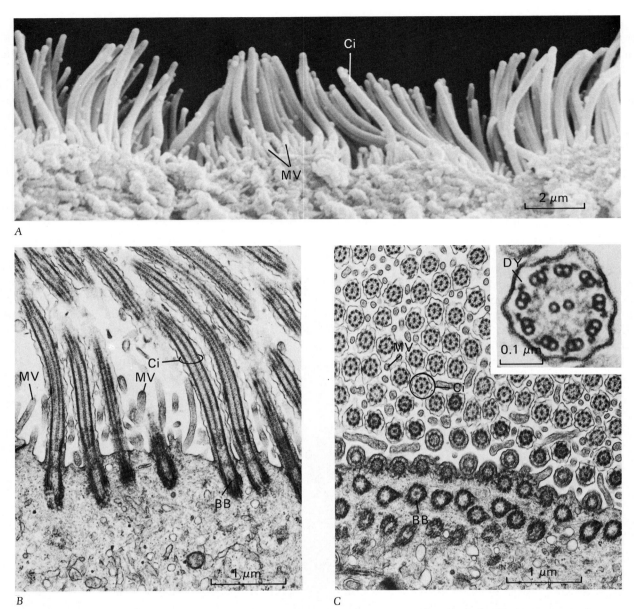

FIGURE 2-10 Cilia (Ci) from human bronchial epithelium seen on sections of epithelial cells in scanning electron micrograph *(A),* and on thin sections in longitudinal *(B)* and oblique cross section *(C).* They are implanted in the epithelial cell by a basal body (BB). Cross-sectioned cilium at high power *(inset, C)* reveals its membrane, which is enveloping a typical set of two axial tubules and nine peripheral duplex tubules with dynein arms (DY) attached. Note abundant short microvilli (MV) interspersed between cilia.

with adjacent alveoli (Fig. 2-6). In the larger bronchioles, and even more in the bronchi, the outer connective tissue sheath forms a strong layer of fibers; in the bronchi, rings or plates of cartilage are incorporated into this layer.

In the respiratory bronchioles, the wall structure is identical to that of terminal bronchioles, except that in some regions the cuboidal epithelium is replaced by an alveolar epithelium of squamous cells (type I cells) closely apposed to capillaries. Very often, these single al-

veoli constitute outpouchings in these regions; sometimes simple "respiratory patches" form in the bronchiolar wall.

Wall Structure of Conducting Blood Vessels

The endothelial lining of pulmonary arteries and veins is basically similar to that of capillaries. It is, however, thicker, and parts of its cytoplasm are richly endowed

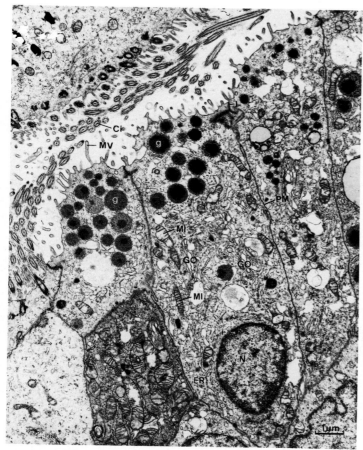

FIGURE 2-11 Clara cells from human bronchiolar epithelium contain dense secretion granules (g) at apex. Note abundant cytoplasmic organelles such as mitochondria (MI), Golgi complex (GO), or endoplasmic reticulum (ER), as well as microvilli (MV) at surface. Cell membranes are closely apposed and form tight junctions (J) at apical edge. Ci = cilia; N = nucleus; PM = plasma membrane.

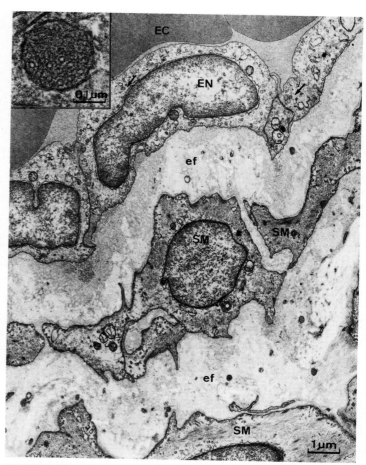

FIGURE 2-12 Part of wall of pulmonary artery from human lung. Endothelial cells (EN) form thick layer; their cytoplasm is rich in organelles. Specific granules of endothelium (arrows), a cross section of one of which is shown at high power in the *inset*, are enveloped by a membrane and contain tubules. The arterial wall is of the elastic type, formed of alternating layers of smooth muscle (SM) and elastic fibers (ef). EC = erythrocyte.

with organelles of various kinds (Fig. 2-12). Clearly, these cells are metabolically more active than those of the capillary endothelium. They are particularly rich in a rod-shaped granule which is specific for endothelial cells, the function of which is to store some factors regulating clotting.

It is said that many of the nonrespiratory metabolic functions of the lung—particularly the transformation of certain bioactive substances, such as angiotensin and prostaglandins—are performed in endothelial cells; the exact site of execution of these functions is not yet known, but caveolae, i.e., invaginations of the surface plasma membrane, have been implicated.

Accessory structures develop in the wall in accord with the functional properties of the vessels. Thus, the wall of the major pulmonary arteries that are close to the heart, and therefore exposed to the pressure oscillations of large amplitude prevailing in the outflow tract of the right ventricle, is of the elastic type, i.e., layers of elastic lamellae are interconnected with smooth-muscle fibers as in the aorta; the tone of the smooth muscle regulates the elastic modulus of the vessel wall, thereby controlling the shape of the pulse wave. In the pulmonary arterial tree, this pattern prevails out to branches of about 1 mm in diameter.

In contrast, branches less than 1 mm in diameter are of the muscular type, i.e., the smooth-muscle fibers encircle the vessel lumen; they can modify the vessel's cross section and can thus regulate blood flow through this vessel. Compared to systemic arteries, the thickness of the pulmonary arterial wall is reduced about in proportion to systolic pressure, i.e., by about a factor of 1:5; in pulmonary hypertension the wall becomes thicker. Although arterioles are a well-defined entity in the systemic vascular bed, where they constitute the major site of arterial resistance, pulmonary arterioles are more difficult to locate and to define. A single muscle layer—the histologic definition of an arteriole—does occur in branches about 100 μm in diameter, but the arterial bed continues out to the precapillaries, which consist of vessels 20 to 40 μm in diameter that lack a complete smooth-muscle sheath. This poverty of smooth muscle contributes importantly to the low resistance to blood flow that is normally afforded by the pulmonary arterial tree.

The pulmonary veins are similar to systemic veins of the upper half of the organism. Their walls are rich in connective tissue and contain irregular bundles of smooth muscle. Larger veins contain a large amount of elastic tissue. In some mammals, e.g., rodents, but not in humans, the larger branches of pulmonary veins have a sleeve of heart muscle fibers that is formed by extensions of left atrial muscle.

Nutritive Vessels and Nerves

The tissue of pulmonary parenchyma is very well supplied with blood; the fact that it is venous is of no disadvantage because O_2 is easily obtained from the air. Thus, nutrient supply from pulmonary arteries, combined with O_2 supply from air, appears to suffice not only for the parenchyma but also for bronchioles and for the smaller pulmonary vessels whose outer surface is almost directly exposed to air. The thicker-walled bronchi, with their glands and cartilage, require a nutrient blood supply from bronchial arteries. These derive, in part, directly from anterior branches of the aorta and partly from the upper intercostal arteries. They course alongside the esophagus and penetrate on both sides into the hilus. The bronchial arteries extend to the most peripheral bronchi but not into the walls of bronchioles. On the other hand, some branches supply large pulmonary vessels, whereas others course along larger septa to reach the pleura. Some bronchial arteries form anastomoses with peripheral branches of the pulmonary arteries. There have been long discussions about the role that such anastomoses may play. It seems that in the normal lung their importance has been overrated. However, in certain pathologic conditions, such as bronchiectasis and tumors, the bronchial arteries, and perhaps the bronchopulmonary anastomoses, appear to play an important role. They also enlarge to form a collateral circulation when branches of the pulmonary artery are obliterated.

Except for a few bronchial veins in the hilar region, the bronchial system does not have its own venous drainage into the systemic veins. Instead, the bronchial veins, which begin as a peribronchial venous plexus, drain into pulmonary veins; this drainage seems to constitute one source of normal venous admixture to arterial blood.

The lung is innervated by the autonomic nervous system. The parasympathetic fibers are derived from the vagal nerves, the sympathetic fibers from the upper thoracic and cervical ganglia; together they form the pulmonary nervous plexus in the region of the hilus before entering the lung. The fiber bundles follow the major bronchi and blood vessels, finally penetrating into the acini; some nerves also supply the pleura. In addition, motor nerves influence the smooth-muscle tone of airways and blood vessels, and sensory nerves are involved in reflex functions (e.g., cough reflex, Hering-Breuer reflex). Moreover, the secretory function of glands, as well as of type II alveolar epithelial cells, is at least partly under control of this nervous system. Nerve fibers are easily found in the wall of bronchioles and bronchi, where they often follow the course of bronchial arteries. However, fibers in alveolar septa are small and scarce.

The Cells of the Alveolar Region

BASIC DESIGN OF A GAS-EXCHANGE BARRIER

Efficient gas exchange in the lung depends on a very thin barrier of very large surface between air and blood. Nevertheless, this barrier must be built of the three minimal tissue layers: an endothelium lining the capillaries, an epithelium lining the airspaces, and an interstitial layer to house the connective tissue fibers. The guiding principle in designing these cells must evidently be to minimize thickness and maximize extent. However, there is definitely a limit to this, set by the need to make the barrier and its constituent cells strong enough to resist the various forces that act on it—capillary blood pressure, tissue tension, and surface tension, in particular. Furthermore, the barrier must remain intact for a lifetime, and this requires continuous repair and turnover of the cells and their components.

In spite of this delicacy of tissue structure we find that three-fourths of all the lung cells by volume or weight are contained in the pulmonary parenchyma (Table 2-1).

TABLE 2-1
Estimated Cell Volumes in the Human Lung

Cell or Tissue	Volume, ml	Percent Septal Tissue
Tissue (excl. blood)	284	—
Nonparenchyma	99	—
Alveolar septa	185	—
Cells	213	—
Nonparenchyma	50	—
Alveolar septa	163	—
Parenchymal cells	163	—
Alveolar epithelium type I	23	12.6
Alveolar epithelium type II	18	9.7
Capillary endothelium	49	26.4
Interstitial cells	66	35.8
Alveolar macrophages	7	3.9

SOURCE: Weibel, 1984a.

We also note that epithelium and endothelium make up about one-fourth each of the tissue barrier in the alveolar walls, whereas interstitial cells amount to 35 percent; the interstitial space with the connective tissue fibers make up no more than 15 percent of the barrier.

THE CELLS LINING THE BARRIER

If we now first look at the cell layers bounding the barrier, we note that by far the major part of the barrier surface is lined, both on the air and on the blood side, by simple layers of squamous cells. This histologic description is sufficient for the endothelium whose cell population is uniform. The epithelium, however, is a mosaic of different cell types, and one therefore finds a small fraction of the total surface—only a few percent (Table 2-2)—to be occupied by secretory cells; one usually calls the squamous lining cells type I and the secretory cells type II

alveolar cells or pneumocytes. A rare third cell, the brush cell, is also found in some specific regions near the terminal bronchiole; its function is as yet unknown.

The squamous lining cells (the capillary endothelium and the type I epithelial cells) show very similar design features (Fig. 2-13). In terms of cell biology they are rather simple cells. Their small compact nucleus is surrounded by a slim rim of cytoplasm that contains a modest basic set of organelles, a few small mitochondria, and some cisternae of endoplasmic reticulum, the picture of a quiescent cell with no great metabolic activity.

At the edge of the perinuclear region a very attenuated cytoplasmic leaflet emerges (Fig. 2-13) and spreads out broadly over the basal lamina. This leaflet is made essentially of the two plasma membranes of the apical and basal cell face, respectively, with a very small amount of cytoplasmic ground substance interposed (Fig. 2-14). Rarely does the leaflet include any organelles, except for

TABLE 2-2

Morphometric Characteristics of Cell Population in Human Pulmonary Parenchyma

Cell Population	Percent of Total Cell Number*	Average Cell Volume, μm^3	Average Apical Cell Surface, μm^2
Alveolar epithelium			
Type I	8	1764	5098
Type II	16	889	183
Endothelium	30	632	1353
Interstitial cells	36	637	—
Alveolar macrophages	10	2492	—

* Total cell number in human lung 230×10^9.

SOURCE: Data from Crapo, Barry, Gehr, Bachofen, Weibel, 1982.

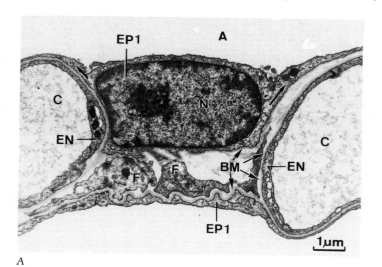

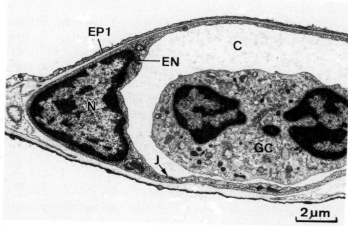

A   *B*

FIGURE 2-13   *A.* A type I alveolar epithelial cell (EP1) from human lung. The nucleus (N) is surrounded by very little cytoplasm which extends as thin leaflets (arrows) to cover the capillaries (C). Note the basement membranes (BM) of the epithelium and endothelium (EN) which become fused in a minimal barrier. Interstitial space contains fibroblast processes (F). *B.* An endothelial cell (EN) of capillary (C) is similar in basic structure to a type I epithelial cell (EP1). The nucleus is enwrapped by little cytoplasm, but thin leaflets extend as capillary lining (arrow). Note the intercellular junction (J) and a white blood cell/granulocyte (GC) in the capillary. *(From Weibel, 1984a.)*

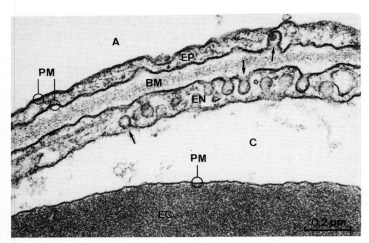

FIGURE 2-14 Thin, minimal tissue barrier between alveolar air (A) and capillary blood (C) is made of cytoplasmic leaflets of epithelium (EP) and endothelium (EN), joined by fused basement membranes (BM). Note that the epithelial and endothelial leaflets are bounded by plasma membranes (PM), as is the erythrocyte (EC). Arrows point to pinocytotic vesicles. *(From Weibel, 1984a.)*

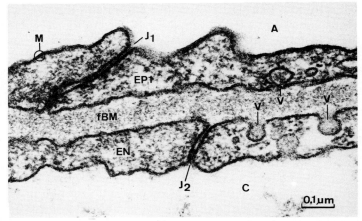

FIGURE 2-15 Minimal barrier part showing intercellular junctions. Between type I epithelial cells (J_1) a "tight" junction is formed by close apposition of the cell membranes over a comparatively wide band; the junction between endothelial cells (J_2) is "leaky" because membranes become apposed over a narrow strip only. Note trilaminar structure of cell membranes (M), the occurrence of pinocytotic vesicles (V) in both epithelium and endothelium (EN), and the fused basement membranes (fBM). C = capillary; A = alveolus; EP1 = type I epithelial cell; M = membrane.

numerous microvesicles that are implied in the transcellular transport of macromolecules.

Terminal bars are formed where the cytoplasmic leaflets of epithelial cells, or of endothelial cells, meet (Fig. 2-15). Here there is a notable difference between these two linings in that the tight junction between epithelial cells constitutes a powerful seal of the intercellular cleft, whereas that in the endothelium is rather leaky, allowing an almost uninhibited exchange of water, solutes, and even some smaller macromolecules between the blood plasma and the interstitial space.

There is another notable and important difference between these two basically similar lining cells: their size. Although the capillary surface is some 10 to 20 percent smaller than the alveolar surface, the capillary endothelial cells are about four times more numerous than type I cells; this means that the surface covered by one type I epithelial cell must be about four times larger, namely, 4000 to 5000 μm^2 as compared to about 1000 μm^2 in endothelial cells (Table 2-2). In some texts, the type I cell is called the *small alveolar cell* because of its small nucleus; clearly this is a misnomer, since the type I cell is a rather large cell indeed, with respect to both surface and cell volume (Table 2-2).

Inspection of the surface of the alveolar epithelium in scanning electron micrographs (Fig. 2-16) reveals that the patches covered by single type I cells are variable in size and that even the largest are much smaller than the 4000 to 5000 μm^2 given above, a number derived by dividing the total alveolar surface by the total number of type I cell nuclei; the one large type I cell seen in Fig. 2-16 has an area of only about 1400 μm^2, and there are not many that are larger. Why is this? There seems to be three to four

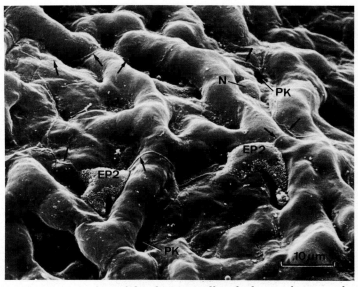

FIGURE 2-16 Surface of the alveolar wall in the human lung seen by scanning electron microscopy reveals a mosaic of alveolar epithelium made of type I and type II (EP2) cells. Arrows indicate boundary of the cytoplasmic leaflet of the type I cell which extends over many capillaries. Note the two interalveolar pores of Kohn (PK) and nucleus (N) of type I cell.

times as many type I cell domains encircled by terminal bars as there are nuclei. Indeed, this observation was made already some hundred years ago by the German pioneer of histology, Albert Kölliker; his interpretation was that part of the alveolar surface was lined by "nonnuclear" cytoplasmic plates rather than by complete cells.

For a modern cell biologist this interpretation cannot be accepted at face value; and it turns out that an alternative explanation is possible: instead of being simple squamous cells, the type I cells are branched cells with multiple apical faces, as shown diagrammatically in Fig. 2-17. Thus, what appears as nonnucleated plates are cytoplasmic domains connected to the perinuclear region by a stalk, spreading out on one side of the alveolar wall or the other; it is evident that several such domains may share a single nucleus.

THE ALVEOLAR SECRETORY CELL: SYNTHESIS OF SURFACTANT

The type II alveolar cell is a conspicuous, but in fact relatively small, cell. Although it is often called the *large al-*

veolar cell, its mean volume is less than half of that of the type I cell (Table 2-2). Its shape is cuboidal, and it has no cytoplasmic extensions (Figs. 2-18 and 2-19). The apical cell surface bulges toward the lumen and is provided, mostly around its periphery, with a tuft of microvilli.

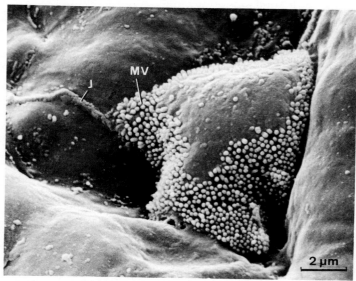

FIGURE 2-18 Higher magnification of a type II cell reveals a "crown" of short microvilli (MV) and a central "bald patch." Note junction lines of type I cells (J) meeting with the type II cell.

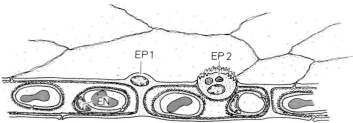

FIGURE 2-17 Diagram of the alveolar wall showing the complexity of a type I epithelial cell (EP1) and its relation to a type II cell (EP2) and endothelial cell (EN). *(From Weibel, 1984a.)*

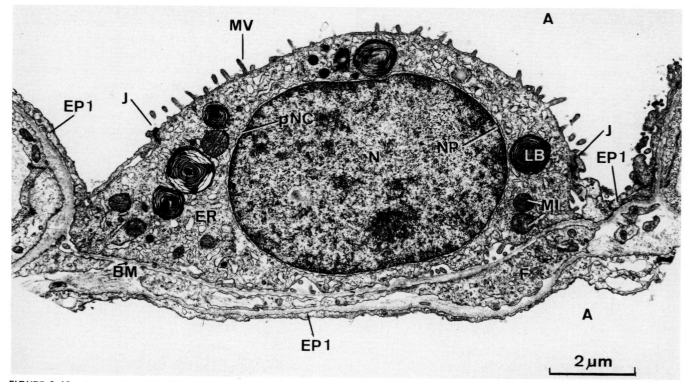

FIGURE 2-19 A type II epithelial cell from the human lung forms junctions (J) with type I epithelial cells (EP1). Its cytoplasm contains osmiophilic lamellar bodies (LB) and a rich complement of organelles: mitochondria (MI), endoplasmic reticulum (ER), and so on. The nucleus (N) is surrounded by a perinuclear cisterna (pNC), which is perforated by nuclear pores (NP). BM = basement membrane; F = fibroblast; MV = microvilli; A = alveolus.

The most conspicuous feature of the type II cell is its wealth of cytoplasmic organelles of all kinds (Fig. 2-19): mitochondria, a lot of endoplasmic reticulum with ribosomes, and a well-developed Golgi complex, surrounded by a set of small lysosomal granules among which the so-called multivesicular bodies—membrane-bounded organelles containing a group of small vesicles—stand out (Fig. 2-20). In addition, there are characteristic lamellar bodies, i.e., larger membrane-bounded organelles that contain a dense stack of phospholipid lamellae which stain black with osmium.

These structural properties are directly related to the type II cell's principal function: the synthesis, storage, and secretion of surfactant, a complex of phospholipids and proteins that spreads in a thin film on the alveolar surface and drastically lowers the surface tension at the air-tissue interface.

The main surfactant phospholipid of the lung, dipalmitoylphosphatidylcholine (DPPC), is a lecithin whose two fatty acid chains are saturated palmitic acid; it lowers the surface tension at an air-water interface by spreading on the surface as a monomolecular film with the hydrophilic polar group immersed in the water and the two hydrophobic palmitic acid residues sticking out. It is well established that the type II cells synthesize DPPC, store it in the lamellar bodies, and secrete it into the thin fluid layer that covers the alveolar epithelium.

In spite of a large number of biochemical studies, it is less certain how the type II cells synthesize DPPC. The problem is that the most common biochemical pathway for the synthesis of lecithins or phosphatidylcholines, the so-called Kennedy pathway, results in phosphatidylcholine where at least one of the two fatty acids is unsaturated. Therefore, DPPC, in which both fatty acid chains are fully saturated palmitic acids, appears like an "unnatural" product which must be made by a two-step procedure, involving remodeling by reacylation.

The site of DPPC synthesis within the type II cells is not yet precisely localized; possible candidates are the endoplasmic reticulum, parts of the Golgi membranes, the multivesicular bodies, or the lamellar bodies themselves (Fig. 2-20); these organelles are arranged in a kind of complex (Fig. 2-21) and could thus establish a spatial sequence for the intracellular processing of phospholipids. It is possible that all sites are involved at one step or another of the complex pathway leading to DPPC. However, one point is beyond doubt: the lamellar bodies are the storage sites for "mature," fully saturated DPPC which becomes "crystallized" into a regular layered stack.

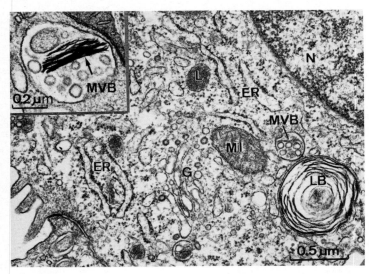

FIGURE 2-20 Cytoplasmic organelles of the type II cell implicated in the synthesis of surfactant are the endoplasmic reticulum (ER), Golgi complex (G), lysosomes (L), multivesicular bodies (MVB), and lamellar bodies (LB). The inset shows a large multivesicular body with a stack of phospholipid lamellae (arrow). *(From Weibel, 1984a.)*

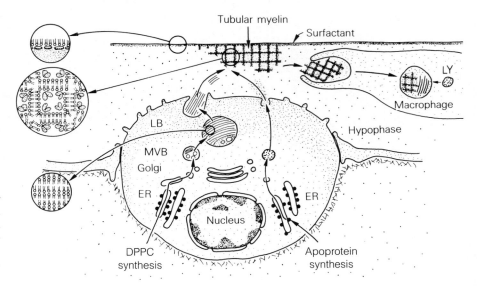

FIGURE 2-21 Schematic diagram of pathways for synthesis and secretion of surfactant DPPC and apoproteins by a type II cell, and for their removal by macrophages. Note the arrangement of phospholipids and apoproteins in the lamellar bodies, in tubular myelin, and in the surface film. *(From Weibel, 1984a.)*

The content of lamellar bodies is eventually secreted into the alveolar surface by exocytosis: the granule membrane fuses with the apical plasma membrane, and the content is discharged (Fig. 2-22). In the alveolar lining layer the once densely packed phospholipid lamellae unravel and become associated with an apoprotein which is probably also synthesized by the type II cells by the usual pathway of protein synthesis in the endoplasmic reticulum (Fig. 2-21). Within the lining layer this lipoprotein complex now forms a new pattern of regular array (Figs. 2-21 and 2-22), so-called tubular myelin, and it can spread on its free surface as a monomolecular film.

Pulmonary surfactant is turned over rather rapidly. Continuous synthesis must therefore be coupled with regulated removal, for which two pathways are known; some of the surfactant leaves the alveolar region over the surface of terminal bronchioles, from where it is removed by the mucociliary escalator; some is engulfed by alveolar macrophages (Fig. 2-21) and broken up in their lysosomes which are known to contain, besides their usual complement of acid hydrolases, phospholipase A_2, the enzyme that cleaves fatty acids from phosphatidylcholine. It is not known whether there are other mechanisms for removing surfactant that has become inactivated, but some recent

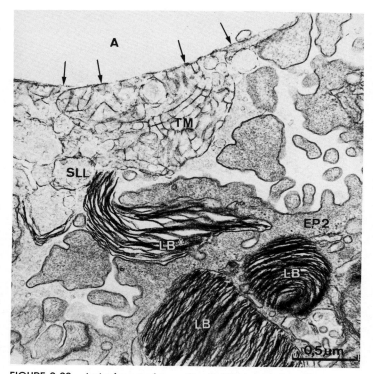

FIGURE 2-22 Apical part of type II cell (EP2) with lamellar bodies (LB); one of these (LB*) is seen in the process of being secreted into the surface lining layer (SLL). The free surface of the lining layer is covered by a thin black film of DPPC (arrows) which is connected with tubular myelin (TM) in the hypophase. *(From Weibel and Gil, 1977.)*

evidence suggests that part of it may be recycled through the type II cells.

A difficult topic is the regulation of surfactant synthesis and turnover. Although "neurohumoral" pathways have been postulated, nothing precise is yet known. Local regulatory effects seem inevitable since surfactant production is stimulated by an increase in ventilation. However, it remains possible that this increased surfactant production is the result of neural effects, since it can also be brought about by stimulation of the vagus nerve and by some neurotransmitters, mainly β-adrenergic agonists. The problem with respect to neural control is that the pulmonary parenchyma contains very few nerve fibers and they have not been shown to be related to type II cells.

There is reasonably good evidence that the potential for surfactant synthesis develops under the effect of some hormones, particularly corticosteroids. In humans, when surfactant begins to be secreted into the lung fluid between the 18th and 25th gestational week, this timely generation of surfactant is critical since, with the first breath, the newborn baby must be able to open instantaneously all of its alveoli and to keep them open. Sufficient quantities of surfactant for this purpose are usually produced by the 28th gestational week, although birth normally takes place at about the 40th week. For this reason premature babies are capable of surviving in a protected environment after the 26th or 28th week. However, in some premature infants survival is threatened because the onset of surfactant production is delayed. These babies rapidly develop a severe, life-threatening disease called the *respiratory distress syndrome* of the newborn; in this syndrome O_2 uptake is compromised by ever-collapsing lungs. It is noteworthy that the surfactant content of the lung can be monitored because the lung fluid communicates freely with amniotic fluid which can be tapped by amniocentesis; when surfactant production has become adequate, one finds the DPPC concentration in amniotic fluid to have risen to a certain level.

KINETICS OF LUNG CELLS: COPING WITH VULNERABILITY

The alveolar epithelium is easily damaged, particularly because each of the very thin type I cells is exposed to air over a much larger surface than any other cell. It is, in fact, astonishing how little seems to happen to this cell which, for example, has only limited potential for repairing membrane defects. But there is an additional problem: the type I cells are not capable of multiplying by mitosis, neither during lung growth when more cells are needed to coat the expanding alveolar surface, nor upon damage in the adult lung when cells need to be replaced. In both instances new type I cells are made by mitotic division and transformation of type II cells which form squamous extensions and lose their potential for surfactant synthesis, a process which takes about 2 to 5 days (see Chapter 3).

This transformation seems to work under normal circumstances. However, under certain conditions this repair mechanism is too slow to cope with excessive damages, so that a syndrome of severe catastrophic respiratory failure develops which requires intensive care, mechanical ventilation, and supplemental O_2 for the patient to survive (see Chapter 142). This syndrome can occur after the lungs have been extensively damaged by toxic fumes; it also occurs occasionally after circulatory collapse, as after severe blood loss or after multiple bone fractures. In these patients, large segments of the type I cell lining of the alveolar surface are destroyed; as a consequence, the barrier has become leaky and the alveoli fill with proteinaceous fluid, so that they can no longer take part in gas exchange. The same type of lung damage and clinical syndrome also ensues after prolonged O_2 breathing (see Chapter 151).

With proper medical care, alveolar edema often resolves within a few days, and the alveoli again fill with air. Nonetheless, gas exchange fails to improve. What has happened is that the repair of the severely damaged alveolar epithelium requires many new cells to be made by division of type II cells. These type II cells form a rather thick cuboidal lining of the barrier surface, and this thick barrier offers a high resistance to O_2 flow. It takes several weeks until a thin barrier is restored by transformation of the cuboidal cell lining into delicate type I cells.

The Defense System of the Lung

At the alveolar level the lung appears to rely heavily on macrophages as primary defense cells; they physically remove from direct contact with pulmonary tissue all sorts of particulate matter that enters the peripheral airways, particularly bacteria and organic or inorganic dust particles. These macrophages are at the forefront of the defense line, in the alveolar surface lining layer, as will be discussed below.

A second defense line, just beneath the alveolar epithelium, is formed by a second set of phagocytic cells. These reside in the interstitial space of the pulmonary parenchyma. In the normal lung, these interstitial histiocytes are not found in alveolar septa; instead, they occur only in the connective tissue sleeves at the periphery, and in the center, of acini. Thus, they are found in regions where lymphatics begin their course toward the major airways in the hilar region where lymph nodes are found. In these juxta-alveolar regions of connective tissue are usu-

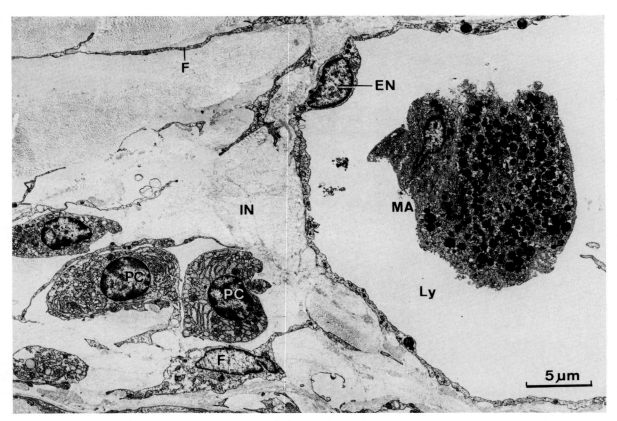

FIGURE 2-23   Perivascular connective tissue with lymphatic (Ly) containing a macrophage (MA) with heterogeneous population of lysosomal granules. Interstitium (IN) contains fibroblasts (F) and plasma cells (PC). EN = endothelium.

ally found the common elements of the defense system (Fig. 2-23):

1. Lymphatic vessels
2. Histiocytes, which may sometimes become permanent residents in the form of storage cells for "indigestible" foreign matter, such as carbon particles and silicates
3. Plasma cells and lymphocytes, indicating that humoral defense factors (specific antibodies) have come into play
4. Leukocytes, which are occasionally seen, but are rare in the healthy lung
5. Mast cells, suggesting that sources of bioactive substances can come into play, particularly in regulating vascular permeability and inflammatory responses

Similar patches of defense cells are also found beneath the ciliated epithelium in bronchi and bronchioles; here *diapedesis* is seen, i.e., lymphocytes and other leukocytes in the process of penetrating the epithelium to reach the mucous blanket. Plasma cells occur in relatively high numbers around the acini of the seromucous glands of bronchi (Fig. 2-7); hence, it is likely that antibodies are being secreted into the mucous blanket by these glands by a process similar to that occurring in the salivary glands or in the glands of the nasal mucosa.

The third defense line is constituted by the lymph nodes which are arranged along the major bronchi and

extend to subsegmental bronchi about 5 mm in diameter (Fig. 2-24). The most peripheral lymph nodes are tiny, a mere 1 to 2 mm in diameter; but closer to the hilus they become larger, and they reach 5 to 10 mm in diameter in the region of the tracheal bifurcation and along the trachea. The lymph nodes from adult human lungs often appear gray or even black because of deposition in the medullary cords of large numbers of macrophages loaded with carbon pigment. This material entered the lungs via the airways, primarily as smoke, soot, or coal dust; depending on the size of the particles, they were either deposited on the surface of conducting airways or reached the alveoli. The further down the deposition, the greater the likelihood that this material cannot be eliminated while in the airways, i.e., within the mucous blanket. The only exit from the pulmonary parenchyma then is via lymphatics, but this exit ultimately leads to the blood, an arrangement that is obviously to be circumvented. Filtering the lymph in lymph nodes and providing a depository for the filtrate in the medullary cords protects the blood, and hence the entire organism, from dissemination of indigestible foreign matter and, as a rule, of infective agents.

Thus, the lymphatic "circulation" of the lungs plays an important defense function. It is unidirectional: it begins as interstitial fluid that seeps from the capillaries and is efficiently drained along the connective tissue fibers toward those connective tissue sleeves in the center and at the periphery of acini where lymph capillaries begin. From there, lymphatic vessels, endowed with valves and an irregular smooth-muscle wall, course in septal structures, in the pleura, and in peribronchial and perivascular sheaths toward the hilar region (Fig. 2-24). Lymph nodes are intercalated in the course of the lymphatics which lead the lymph toward the tracheal bifurcation and then along the trachea into the right and left mediastinal lymph channels. The right channel drains into the right subclavian vein; the left, together with the thoracic duct, into the left subclavian vein. Because of the many anastomoses connecting parallel lymphatics, a particular lymph node receives lymph from various pulmonary regions, but the closest regions tend to predominate.

Macrophages

Alveolar macrophages are the cell population of the surface lining layer. They are free cells, endowed with a high phagocytic capacity, which are transiently attached to the surface of the alveolar epithelium by pseudopodia and can crawl over this surface by ameboid movement (Fig. 2-25). However, they are submerged beneath the surface film of phospholipids (Fig. 2-26) and are, therefore, part of the surface lining layer of alveoli, more specifically of its hypophase.

Alveolar macrophages exert their phagocytic activity within the surface lining layer (Fig. 2-21). Hence, it is not

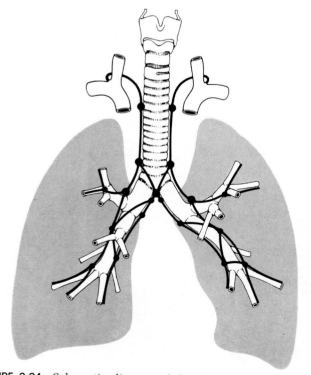

FIGURE 2-24 Schematic diagram of distribution of lymph nodes and main lymphatic channels along bronchial tree.

surprising that their vacuoles contain large amounts of phospholipid material, in part even tubular myelin; a considerable part of these phospholipids is (dipalmitoyl) lecithin. Although it seems likely that this material has been ingested in the process of removing and breaking down the surfactant system, it is possible that macrophages are engaged in surfactant synthesis as well. The presence of tubular myelin in phagosomes tends to support the removal hypothesis because this material has not been observed in type II epithelial cells.

Foreign materials, such as bacteria or dust, that reach the alveoli in aerosols are first intercepted by the lining layer and are then ingested by the alveolar macrophages. Type I alveolar epithelial cells are also capable of phagocytizing small foreign particles, whereas type II cells are not. The acutely diseased lung shows pictures that are reminiscent of phagocytosis by type I cells.

The kinetics of these macrophages is as yet unclear. They seem to be derived from monocytes and therefore, indirectly, from bone marrow cells. They probably reach the alveoli in two steps: first, by settling in the pulmonary interstitial tissue and, second, by migrating from the interstitial tissue into the alveoli where they constitute a partly self-reproducing cell population. Their removal seems to involve two different pathways: (1) some of the macrophages undoubtedly move up the bronchial tree in the mucous blanket and eventually appear in the sputum (heart failure cells, dust cells); (2) others possibly return into the interstitial space; but, in the normal lung, the second path seems to occur exclusively in those alveoli that abut on the connective tissue sleeves around larger vessels and conducting airways, or on interacinar septa, i.e., where the lymphatic capillaries are located. A preferred location appears to be in the respiratory bronchioles at the entrance into the acinus or in the center of the acinus, where dust-laden macrophages tend to congregate; these accumulations may be involved in the pathogenesis of the centroacinar damage that leads to progressive emphysema observed in smokers. In these places, macrophages either settle as carbon pigment-loaded histiocytes or they leave the pulmonary parenchyma via lymphatics (Fig. 2-23) to settle in the lymph nodes. The way in which macrophages and/or their ingested material are transferred from the alveolar surface to the interstitial space is still entirely unknown.

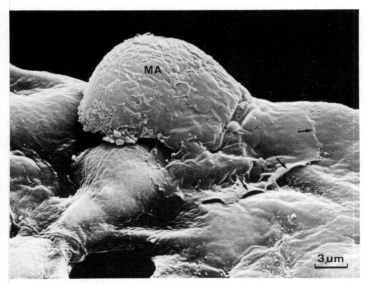

FIGURE 2-25   Alveolar macrophage (MA) seen sitting on epithelial surface of human lung. Note cytoplasmic lamella (arrows) which represents the advancing edge of the cell.

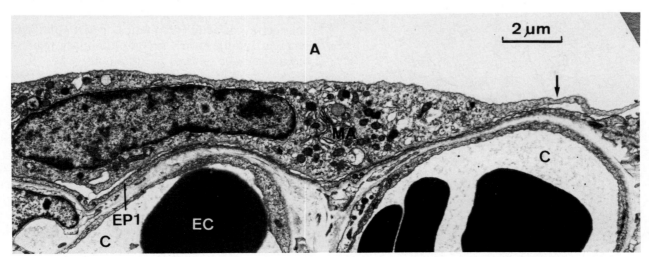

FIGURE 2-26   Alveolar macrophage (MA) fixed in its natural position of flat attachment to the alveolar epithelium (EP1). Arrow points to advancing cytoplasmic leaflet.

DESIGN OF PULMONARY PARENCHYMA

Alveoli and Capillaries

The airspaces and blood vessels of pulmonary parenchyma are designed to facilitate gas exchange between air and blood. To this end a very large area of contact between air and blood needs to be established—for the human lung it is sometimes compared to the surface of a tennis court. Furthermore, the tissue barrier separating air and blood needs to be kept as thin as possible—it is found to be about 50 times thinner than a sheet of airmail stationery. This is important because less than 1 s is available for loading O_2 onto the erythrocytes as they flow through the lung's gas-exchange region.

The first design feature to this end is the formation of alveoli in the wall of all airways within the acinus, i.e., in the gas-exchange units derived from the first-order respiratory bronchiole (Fig. 2-27). In the human lung, there are about 150,000 acini and 300 million alveoli, so that each of the gas-exchange units contains, on the average, some 2000 alveoli connected to about six to eight generations of acinar airways, respiratory bronchioles, and alveolar ducts.

The alveoli are so densely packed that they occupy the entire surface of the alveolar ducts; they are separated from each other by delicate alveolar septa which contain a single capillary network (Fig. 2-28). About half of the space of the septum is taken up by blood which is thus exposed to the air in two adjacent alveoli (Fig. 2-29A). Although the barrier separating air and blood is extremely thin, the capillaries are provided with a complete endothelial lining and the alveolar surface of the septum is lined by an uninterrupted epithelium. As noted above, these two cell linings are very much attenuated over the greatest part of the surface.

To make the barrier very thin the interstitial structures must also be reduced to a minimum (Fig. 2-30). The septal interstitium contains very few cells, mostly slim fibroblasts with long extensions; these contain fine bundles of contractile filaments that serve an unknown mechanical function. The septal interstitium usually does not contain cells of the defense system, nor lymphatics.

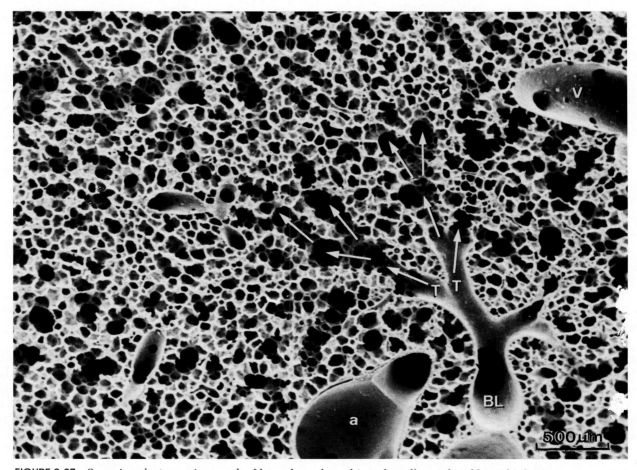

FIGURE 2-27   Scanning electron micrograph of lung shows branching of small peripheral bronchiole (BL) into terminal bronchioles (T) from where the airways continue into respiratory bronchioles and alveolar ducts (arrows). Note the location of the pulmonary artery (a) and vein (V). *(From Weibel, 1984a.)*

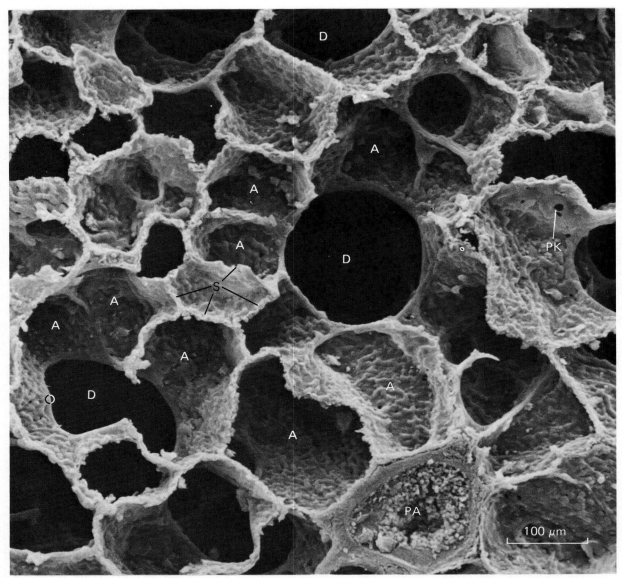

FIGURE 2-28 Scanning electron micrograph of human lung parenchyma. Alveolar ducts (D) are surrounded by alveoli (A), which are separated by thin septa (S). Note small branch of pulmonary artery (PA).

Internal Support of Parenchymal Structures: The Pulmonary Fiber Continuum

This extraordinary reduction of the tissue mass in the alveolar septa inevitably introduces a number of major problems. How is it possible to secure the mechanical integrity of the system if several forces act on the septal tissue with a tendency to disrupt it? Not only must the thin barrier withstand the distending pressure of the capillary blood due both to hemodynamic forces and to gravity, particularly in the lower lung zones; it must also keep the capillary bed expanded over a very large surface, a task that is made difficult because of surface forces that act on

the complex alveolar surface and tend to collapse alveoli and capillaries. These requirements call for a very subtle, economic design of the fibrous support system.

The problem of supporting the capillaries on connective tissue fibers with as little tissue as possible has been solved ingeniously by interlacing the fiber network with the capillary network; when the fibers are taut (Fig. 2-29B), the capillaries weave from one side of the septum to the other. This arrangement has a threefold advantage: (1) it allows the capillaries to be supported unit by unit directly on the fiber strands without the need of additional "binders"; (2) it causes the capillaries to become spread out on the alveolar surface when the fibers are

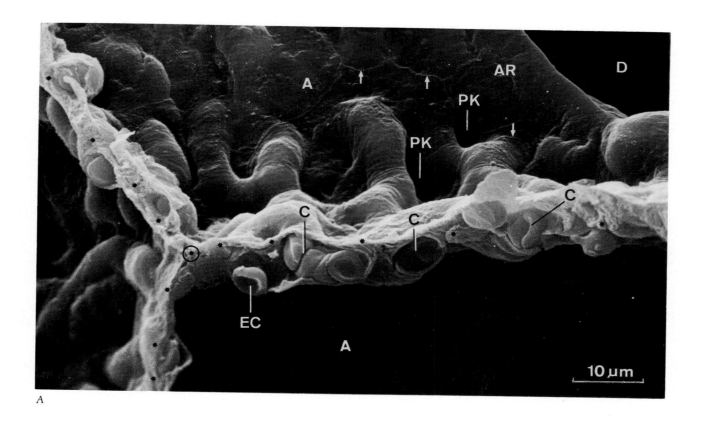

A

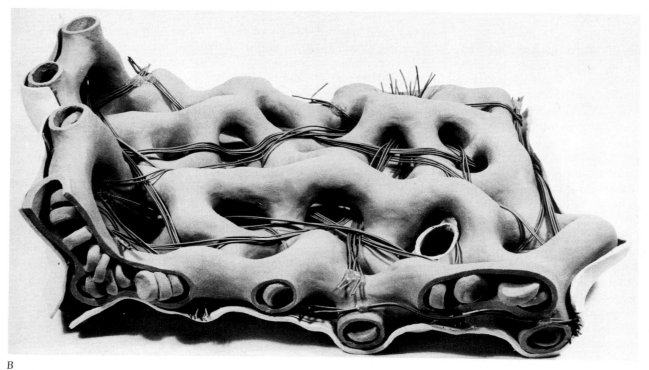

B

FIGURE 2-29 *A*. In the alveolar wall, shown in a scanning electron micrograph from a human lung, the capillary blood (C) is separated from the air (A) by a very thin tissue barrier; asterisks mark thicker barrier parts which contain fiber strands that meet at triple line (circled asterisk). Arrows mark terminal bars in alveolar epithelium. *B*. The model shows the capillary network to be interwoven with the meshwork of septal fibers. PK = pore of Kohn; D = duct; AR = alveolar entrance ring. *(From Weibel, 1984a.)*

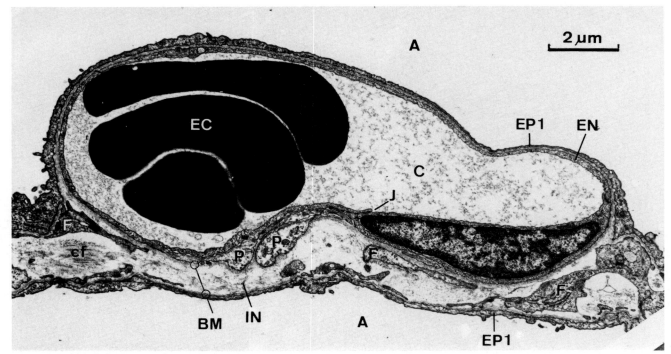

FIGURE 2-30 Alveolar capillary (C) with erythrocytes (EC) from human lung lined by endothelial cell (EN) which is associated with processes of pericytes (P). Substantial interstitial space (IN) with fibers (cf) and fibroblasts (F) occurs on one side only, whereas minimal air-blood barrier is formed on other side by fusion of basement membranes (BM). A = alveolus; EP1 = type I epithelial cell; J = intercellular junction.

stretched; and (3) it optimizes conditions for gas-exchange conditions by limiting the presence of fibers—which must interfere with O_2 flow—to half the capillary surface. The thin section of a capillary (Fig. 2-30) reveals that an interstitial space with fibers and fibroblasts exists only on one side of the capillary, whereas on the other the two lining cells, endothelium and epithelium, become closely joined with only a single, common basement membrane interposed. Therefore, over half of the surface, the capillary blood is separated from the air merely by a minimal tissue barrier made of epithelial and endothelial cytoplasmic sheets with their fused basement membranes (Fig. 2-14).

The principal structural "backbone" of the lung is a continuous system of fibers that are anchored at the hilus and are put under tension by the negative intrapleural pressure that tugs on the visceral pleura. The general construction principle follows from the formation of the mesenchymal sheath of the airway units in the developing lung (see Chapter 3); as the airway tree grows, its branches remain separated by layers of mesenchyme within which blood vessels form. When fiber networks develop within this mesenchyme they will enwrap all airway units and extend from the hilus right to the visceral pleura. Hence, the pulmonary fiber system forms a three-dimensional fibrous continuum that is structured by the airway system and is closely related to the blood vessels. By virtue of the

design of this fibrous continuum the lung becomes, in fact, subdivided into millions of little bellows that are connected to the airway tree (Fig. 2-31); they expand with expansion of the chest because the tension exerted on the visceral pleura by the negative intrapleural pressure becomes transmitted to the bellows' walls through the fiber system.

To try to put some order into this fiber system we can first single out two major components that one can easily identify (Fig. 2-31). First we find that all airways, from the main-stem bronchus that enters the lung at the hilus out to the terminal bronchioles and beyond, are enwrapped by a strong sheath of fibers. These fibers constitute the axial fiber system; they form the "bark" of the tree whose roots are at the hilus and whose branches penetrate deep into pulmonary parenchyma, following the course of the airways. A second major fiber system is related to the visceral pleura which is made of strong fiber bags that enwrap all lobes. The connective tissue septa penetrate from the visceral pleura into pulmonary parenchyma, thereby separating units of the airway tree. Taken together, these fibers have been designated as the peripheral fiber system because they constitute the boundaries between the units of respiratory lung tissue.

The peripheral fiber system subdivides each lung into a number of units that are not simple to define because they form a continuous hierarchy in accordance with the

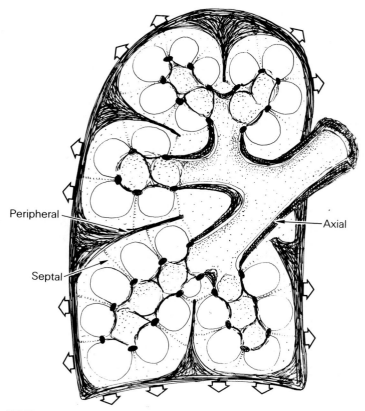

FIGURE 2-31 The major connective fiber tracts of the lung are divided into axial fibers along the airways and peripheral fibers connected to the pleura. They are connected by fibers in the alveolar septa. *(From Weibel and Gil, 1977.)*

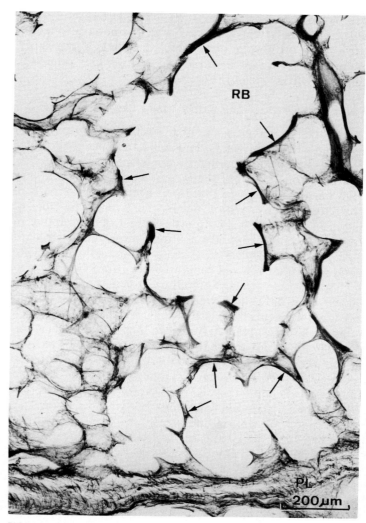

FIGURE 2-32 Connective tissue stain reveals the strong fiber rings that demarcate the alveolar ducts (arrows). *(From Weibel, 1984a.)*

pattern of airway tree branching. At one extreme are the lobes, which are demarcated by a more or less complete lining by visceral pleura with a serosal cleft interposed (Fig. 2-1); at the other are the acini, i.e., the parenchymal units by which the airways participate in gas exchange.

The acinus is the functional unit of the pulmonary parenchyma. The airway that leads into the acinus, the first-order respiratory bronchiole, continues branching within the acinus for about 6 to 10 additional generations (Figs. 2-5 and 2-27). These intra-acinar airways, called *respiratory bronchioles* and *alveolar ducts*, also carry in their wall relatively strong fibers of the axial fiber system that extend to the end of the duct system. But since the wall of intra-acinar air ducts is densely populated with alveoli, these fibers form a kind of network, the meshes of which encircle the alveolar mouths (Figs. 2-28 and 2-32). These fiber rings serve as a scaffold for a network of finer fibers that spread within the alveolar septa (Fig. 2-32). But, since no loose ends are permissible in a fiber system, the septal fiber system must be anchored at both ends, i.e., on the network of axial fibers around the alveolar ducts and on extensions of the peripheral fibers that penetrate into the acinus from interlobular septa. Thus the fiber sys-

tem of the lung is a continuum that spans the entire space of the lung, from the hilus to the visceral pleura (Fig. 2-31). It is put under varying tension as the pleura is expanded by the chest wall and diaphragm.

The continuous nature of a well-ordered fiber system is an essential design feature of the lung. This becomes evident in emphysema: when some fibers are disrupted they cannot be kept under tension; they retract, and larger airspaces form in the process of rearranging the fiber system in the surroundings of the damage. Small foci of emphysema form in most lungs in the course of time.

The fiber system serves mainly as a mechanical support for the blood vessels with which it is intimately associated in an orderly fashion. The pulmonary artery branches in parallel with the airway tree and penetrates into the acinus along the axial fiber system; the pulmonary veins are associated with the peripheral fiber system and are thus located between the airway units. In the alveolar septa the capillary network spreads out as a broad sheet of vessels whose paths are continuous throughout the system of interconnected alveolar walls of the septa. As noted above, these capillaries are intimately related to the septal fiber system (Fig. 2-29).

Parenchymal Mechanics and Tissue Design

As in all connective tissue, the fibers of the lung consist of collagen and elastic fibers. The collagen fibers are bundles of fibrils bound together by proteoglycans; they are practically inextensible (less than 2 percent) and have a very high tensile strength so that they rupture only at loads of 50 to 70 dyn/cm^2, which means that a collagen fiber of 1 mm in diameter can support a weight of over 500 g. In contrast, elastic fibers have a much lower tensile strength but a high extensibility: they can be stretched to about 130 percent of their relaxed length before rupturing.

In the fiber system of pulmonary parenchyma, collagen and elastic fibers occur in a volume ratio of about 2.5:1, whereas this ratio is 10:1 for the visceral pleura. In a relaxed state the collagen fibers are longer than the accompanying elastic fibers so that they appear wavy. Because of the association between rubberlike elastic and twinelike collagen fibers, the connective tissue strands behave like an elastic band: they are easy to stretch up to the point where the collagen fibers are taut, but from there on they resist stretching very strongly.

The elastic properties of the fiber system of the lung can be studied by filling the airways with fluid so as to eliminate the effects of surface tension. This reveals that the lung's fiber system has a high compliance until high levels of inflation are reached and that the retractive, or recoil, force generated by the fiber system amounts to no more than a few millibars at physiological levels of inflation. The actual recoil force in the air-filled lung, reflected by the negative pressure in the pleural space, is appreciably higher, but this is due to surface tension rather than to the retractive force of the fibers.

Surface tension arises at any gas-liquid interface because the forces between the molecules of the liquid are much stronger than those between the liquid and the gas. As a result the liquid surface will tend to become as small as possible. A curved surface, such as that of a bubble, generates a pressure which is proportional to the curvature and to the surface tension coefficient γ. The general formula of Gibbs relates this pressure, Ps, to the mean curvature $\overline{K}$:

$$Ps = 2\gamma\overline{K} \qquad (1)$$

In a sphere the curvature is simply the reciprocal of the radius r:

$$Ps = \frac{2\gamma}{r} \qquad (2)$$

The most critical effect of surface tension is that it endangers stability of the airspaces. In principle, because a set of connected "bubbles," i.e., the alveoli, is inherently unstable, the small ones should shrink and the large ones expand. Therefore, since the 300 million alveoli all connect with each other through the airways, the lung is inherently unstable: why then do the alveoli not all collapse and empty into one large bubble? There are two principal reasons.

The first reason relates to tissue structure. The alveoli are not simply soap bubbles in a froth, but, as noted above, their walls contain an intricate fiber system. Thus, when an alveolus tends to shrink, the fibers in the walls of adjoining alveoli are stretched, thereby preventing the alveolus from collapsing. Alveoli are held to be mechanically interdependent, and this interdependence stabilizes them.

The second reason relates to the fact that the alveolar surface is not simply water exposed to air, but that it is lined by surfactant (Fig. 2-33). This surface coat has peculiar properties in that its surface tension coefficient γ is variable: surface tension decreases as the alveolar surface becomes smaller and increases when the surface expands. Because of this feature, which is due to the phospholipid nature of alveolar surfactant, alveoli do not behave like

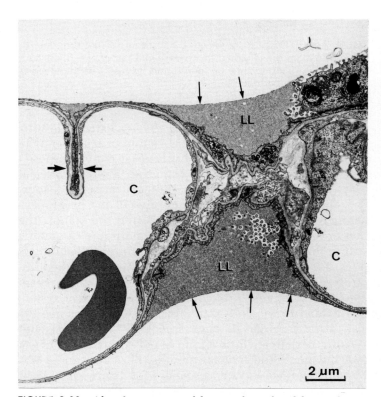

FIGURE 2-33 Alveolar septum of human lung fixed by perfusion through blood vessels shows alveolar lining layer (LL) in crevices between capillaries (C) topped by surfactant film which appears as a fine black line (arrows). Note the type II cell with lamellar bodies and the fold in thin tissue barrier (bold arrows). *(From Weibel: Am J Roentgenology 133:1021–1031, 1979.)*

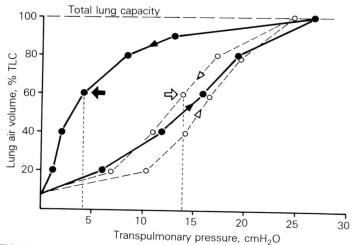

FIGURE 2-34 Comparison of pressure-volume curve of a normal air-filled rabbit lung with that of a surfactant-depleted lung (broken line). The arrows indicate the points at which the lungs shown in Fig. 2-35 have been fixed by vascular perfusion. *(From Weibel, 1984a.)*

soap bubbles whose surface tension remains constant. When an alveolus begins to shrink, the surface tension of its lining layer falls and the retractive force generated at the surface is reduced or even abolished. Combined with interdependence, this property of surfactant allows the complex of alveoli to remain stable.

Which of the two factors for stabilizing pulmonary structure is more important: interdependence or surfactant? It turns out that both are essential. If the lung is depleted of its surfactant lining by washing with a detergent, the pressure-volume curve changes dramatically (Fig. 2-34); on deflation, the lung volume falls rapidly. Samples from lungs fixed at the same volume (60 percent TLC) but derived from either normal or detergent-rinsed lungs reveal that surfactant depletion causes the alveoli to collapse (Fig. 2-35). However, as alveoli shrink in size, the alveolar ducts enlarge, stretching the strong fiber nets at the mouths of the collapsed alveoli. The ducts do not collapse because of interdependence between adjacent units.

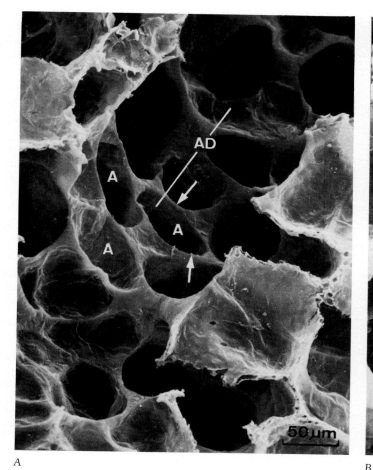

A

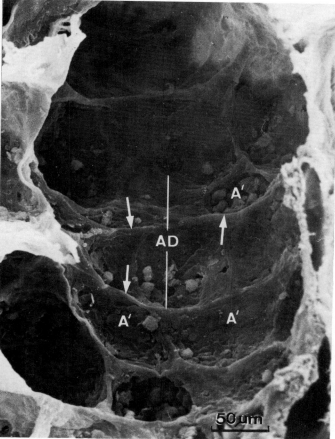

B

FIGURE 2-35 Scanning electron micrographs of normal air-filled (A) and surfactant-depleted (B) rabbit lungs fixed at 60 percent TLC on the deflation curve (Fig. 2-34) show alveoli to be open (A) in *A*, collapsed (A′) in *B*. The alveolar duct (AD) is widened in the surfactant-depleted lung, resulting in a stretching of the fiber strands around the alveolar mouths (arrows). *(From Wilson and Bachofen, 1982.)*

In the normal air-filled lung, both the surfactant properties and interdependence due to fiber tension contribute to stabilizing the complex of alveoli and alveolar ducts. The mechanism is illustrated in Fig. 2-36, which shows a highly simplified diagram of a parenchymal unit. Interdependence is established by the continuum of axial, septal, and peripheral fibers. Surface tension exerts an inward pull in the hollow alveoli where curvature is negative. However, over the free edge of the alveolar septa, along the outline of the duct, the surface tension must pull outward because there the curvature is positive. The latter force must be rather strong because the radius of curvature is very small on the septal edge; but this force is counteracted by the strong fiber strands, usually provided with some smooth-muscle cells, that are found in the free edge of the alveolar septum (Figs. 2-27 and 2-32). Thus interdependence is an important factor in preventing collapse of the complex hollow of the lung where negative and positive curvatures coexist. However, its capacity to do so is limited and requires low surface tensions, particularly upon deflation when the fibers tend to slack. If surface tension becomes too high, the lung's foamlike structure will partly collapse despite fiber interdependence (Fig. 2-35).

Micromechanics of the Alveolar Septum

What are the mechanical factors that shape the alveolar septum in the air-filled lung? As indicated above, the alveolar septum consists of a single capillary network that is interlaced with fibers (Fig. 2-29). When the fibers are stretched, the capillaries bulge alternatingly to one side or the other, thus creating pits and crevices in the meshes of the capillary network.

This irregular surface is evened out to some extent by the presence of an extracellular layer of lining fluid that is rather thin over the capillaries but forms little pools in the intercapillary pits (Fig. 2-33). This lining consists of an aqueous layer of variable thickness, called the *hypophase*, topped by surfactant which forms a film on the surface of the hypophase. The hypophase seems to contain considerable amounts of reserve surfactant material which occurs in a characteristic configuration called *tubular myelin* (Fig. 2-22).

In the alveolar septum the tissue structures are extremely delicate. Therefore alveolar configuration is not determined exclusively by structural features. Instead, it results from the molding effect of various forces that are kept in balance. Figure 2-37 shows how the three principal mechanical forces—tissue tension, surface tension, and capillary distending pressure—interact in the septum. The fibers of the alveolar septum are under tension, the magnitude of which depends on the level of lung inflation. This tension tends to straighten the fibers so that a force (pressure) normal to the fiber axis results; this force shifts the capillaries to one side of the septum or the other (Figs. 2-29*B* and 2-37). The wall of the capillaries is exposed to the luminal pressure, which is determined by the blood pressures in pulmonary arteries and veins; that the luminal pressure of capillaries in a particular region also depends on gravity is indicated by the fact that capillaries at the bottom of the lung are wider than those at the top. If the distending pressure is exerted uniformly over the circumference of the capillary, it will push against the fibers on one side but will cause the thin, opposite side to bulge outward. This effect is to some extent counteracted by surface tension which exerts a force normal to the surface (Fig. 2-37): the direction of the force depends on the orientation of curvature, acting toward the alveolar space in concave regions (negative curvature) and toward the tissue in areas of convexity (positive curvature); its magnitude depends on the degree of curvature and on the value of the surface tension coefficient γ.

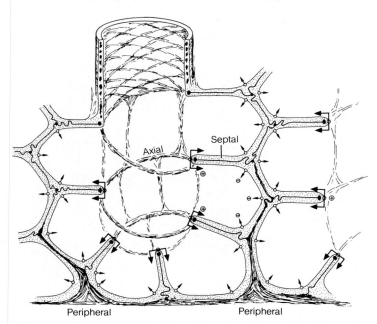

FIGURE 2-36 Model of the disposition of axial, septal, and peripheral fibers in an acinus showing the effect of surface forces (arrows). *(From Weibel, 1984a.)*

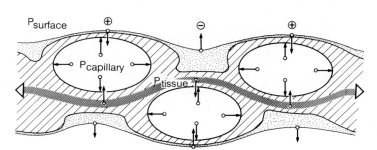

FIGURE 2-37 Model showing the micromechanical forces of surface tension, tissue tension, and capillary distending pressure that shape the alveolar septum. *(From Weibel, 1984a.)*

The alveolar septum achieves a stable configuration when these interacting forces are in balance. Combined forces tend to squash the capillary flat; this happens at high levels of lung inflation when the fibers are under high tension and the surface tension coefficient of surfactant reaches its highest value owing to expansion of the surface. Oppositely, upon deflation the fibers are relaxed and surface tension falls drastically; the capillary distending pressure now exceeds both the tissue and the surface forces. As a result, the slack fibers are bent and weave through the capillary network, whereas the capillaries bulge slightly toward the airspace. Surface tension upon deflation is apparently so low that considerable surface "crumpling" is seen (Fig. 2-38).

The importance of the balance struck among the forces that act on the septum is also shown in Fig. 2-39. The specimen of Fig. 2-39B was fixed under zone 3 perfusion conditions, and all the capillaries are wide, partly bulging toward the airspace (Fig. 2-38). In contrast, the specimen shown in Fig. 2-39A was fixed under zone 2 conditions: in the flat part of the septum the capillaries are squashed flat, because the surface and tissue forces now exceed the vascular distending pressure. However, the capillaries remain wide open in the corners where three septa come together. The distribution of surface forces causes the internal pressure to be lower in the region of these corners, as can be inferred intuitively from Fig. 2-36.

THE LUNG AS A GAS EXCHANGER

Up to this juncture, the principal design features of the lung have been considered with respect to the lung as an organ in its own right. In order to discuss the implications of these design features for the principal function of the lung, i.e., gas exchange between air and blood, our approach must be modified in two ways: (1) the lung must be regarded as a servant of the body, i.e., as one link in the chain of events that provide O_2 for energy production in the cells of the organism, and (2) a quantitative approach is needed to ask essentially, "How much lung is enough to satisfy the needs of the body?"

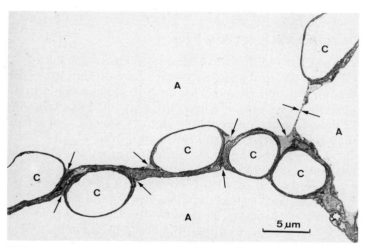

FIGURE 2-38 Alveolar septum of air-filled rabbit lung perfusion-fixed at 60 percent TLC shows empty capillaries (C) which bulge toward the alveolar airspace (A). Note pools of surface lining layer in the crevices between capillaries (arrows) and film spanning across alveolar pore (double arrows). *(From Gil, Bachofen, Gehr, Weibel: J Appl Physiol 47:990–1001, 1979).*

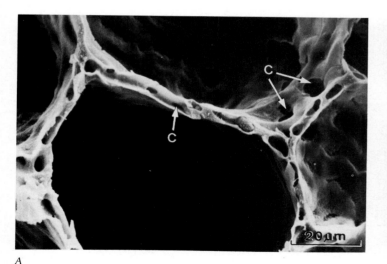

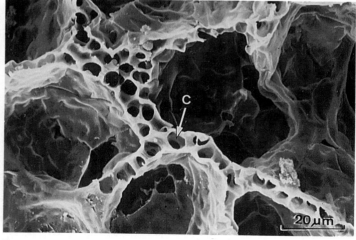

A   *B*

FIGURE 2-39 Scanning electron micrographs of alveolar walls of rabbit lungs fixed under (*A*) zone 2 and (*B*) zone 3 conditions of perfusion. Note that capillaries (C) are wide in zone 3 and slitlike in zone 2, except for corner capillaries, which are wide in either case. *(From Bachofen, Weber, Wangensteen, Weibel: Respir Physiol 52:41–52, 1983.)*

The Lung as Part of the Respiratory System

The O_2 needs of the body are set by the energy requirements of the cells and their mitochondria that produce adenosine-triphosphate (ATP) by oxidative phosphorylation in order for the cell to do work. The process of oxidative phosphorylation requires a flow of O_2 to be maintained from the lung to the cells. It proceeds along the respiratory system through various steps (Fig. 2-40): into the lung by ventilation, to the blood by diffusion, through the circulation by blood flow, and from the blood capillaries by diffusion into the cells and mitochondria, where it disappears in the process of oxidative phosphorylation. A number of basic features characterize this system: (1) under steady-state conditions the O_2 flow rate, $\dot{V}_{O_2}$, is the same at all levels, i.e., O_2 uptake in the lung is equal to O_2 consumption in the tissues; (2) the basic driving force for O_2 flow through the system is a cascade of O_2 partial pressure which falls from inspired P_{O_2} down to near zero in the mitochondria; (3) the O_2 flow rate at each step is the product of a partial pressure difference and a conductance which is related to structural and functional properties of the organs participating in O_2 transfer. It can, for example, be shown that the O_2 flow rate into the O_2 consuming step in the cells is directly related to the volume of mitochondria that engage in oxidative phosphorylation.

With respect to gas exchange in the lung (Fig. 2-41), the O_2 flow rate is determined by the Bohr equation:

$$\dot{V}_{O_2} = (P_{A_{O_2}} - P_{c_{O_2}}) \cdot D_{L_{O_2}} \tag{3}$$

where $P_{A_{O_2}}$ is the P_{O_2} in alveoli, $P_{c_{O_2}}$ is the mean P_{O_2} in pulmonary capillaries, and $D_{L_{O_2}}$ is the pulmonary diffusing capacity or the lung's O_2 conductance. The important point is now that all parameters to the right of this equation may be significantly affected by design features. As indicated previously, O_2 uptake may be affected by the surface available for gas exchange and by the thickness of the barrier between air and blood; an appropriate formulation now has to be made of how these features relate to $D_{L_{O_2}}$. The O_2 partial pressure difference is established by ventilation and blood flow in the gas-exchange units; this relationship may be affected by the design of the airway and vascular trees, particularly by their quantitative properties.

Design of the Branching Tree

The entrance to the lung's airways is the trachea, a single tube; the gas-exchange elements where air and blood are brought into close contact are contained in several million units. Between entrance and periphery lies a meticulously designed system of branching airways which serve to conduct the inspired air into those peripheral channels that carry alveoli in their walls and can thus contribute to the exchange of gases between air and blood (Fig. 2-5).

The pattern of airway branching can be studied on resin casts such as that illustrated on the front cover. Consistently each branch is seen to divide into two smaller branches, i.e., to undergo dichotomous branching. The two daughter branches from the same parent often differ in diameter and/or in length (Fig. 2-42): dichotomy is hence irregular. Nonetheless, morphometric analysis of

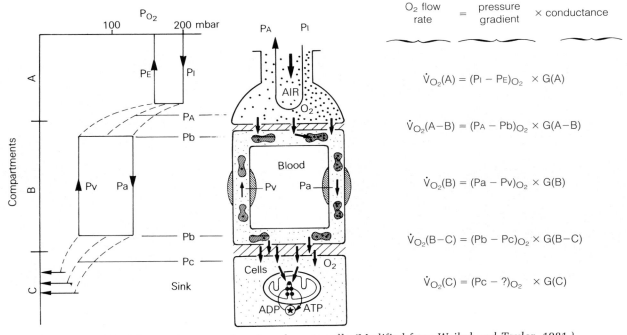

FIGURE 2-40   Model of the respiratory system from lung to cells *(Modified from Weibel and Taylor, 1981.)*

the casts reveals that the progression of airway dimensions from the trachea to the periphery follows strict laws.

There are two ways of approaching such an analysis. In the first place, the pattern of branching is followed from trachea to the periphery: each bifurcation gives rise to a new generation of airways. The number of branches in each new generation is twice that in the parent generation;

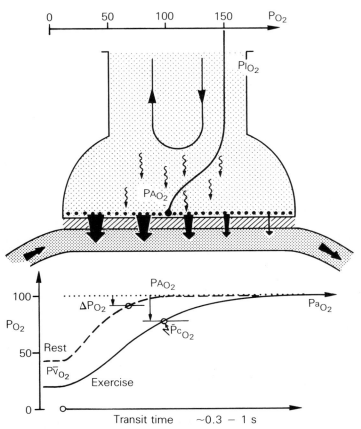

FIGURE 2-41 Model of gas exchange showing gradual rise of capillary P_{O_2} (Pc_{O_2}) as blood flows through capillary until it approaches alveolar P_{O_2} (PA_{O_2}). *(From Weibel, 1984a.)*

the branching ratio of dichotomy is 2. Accordingly, the number (N) of branches in each generation (z) is

$$N(z) = 2z \tag{4}$$

Within each generation, the lengths and diameters of the branches have a characteristic range of sizes; but the mean diameter of the conducting airways (to about the 16th generation) decreases systematically, following a simple law (Fig. 2-43):

$$d(z) = d_0 \cdot 2^{-z/3} \tag{5}$$

where

$d(z)$ = the mean diameter of airways
$\quad$ in generation z
d_0 = the diameter of the trachea

This equation shows that with each generation the airway diameter is reduced by the cube root of the branching ratio 2, a law that is well known in hydrodynamics since it defines an optimal design of a branched system of tubes.

Using this approach, it is possible to construct a model that takes into account irregularities in branching by considering the number of airways of a given diameter, d_μ, that exist in each generation and the number of lengths of bronchial pathway that intervene between the larynx and the particular airways (Fig. 2-44).

The alternative is to regard the airways as a system of tubes converging from the periphery, the acinus, toward the center, the trachea. By adopting an ordering system that has proved useful in analyzing rivers (Strahler system), branches are grouped into orders by size, beginning with the smallest designated as order 1 (Fig. 2-42C). This ordering pattern is particularly well adapted to a system of irregular dichotomy because the size of branches within an order varies less than in the other approach. A branching ratio is determined as the ratio of the number of branches in order μ to that in order $\mu + 1$. Remarkably, the progression of diameters through the various orders is again roughly proportional to the cube root of the branching ratio. Hence, both models yield basically the same result.

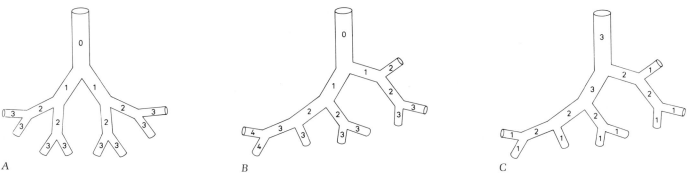

A $\qquad\qquad\qquad$ *B* $\qquad\qquad\qquad$ *C*

FIGURE 2-42 Patterns of airway branching: *A.* Regular dichotomy. *B.* Irregular dichotomy numbered by "generations down." *C.* Irregular dichotomy numbered by "orders up."

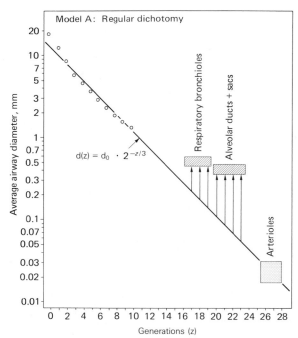

FIGURE 2-43 Average diameter of airways in human lung plotted by generations of regularized dichotomous branching. *(After Weibel, 1963.)*

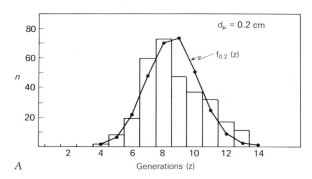

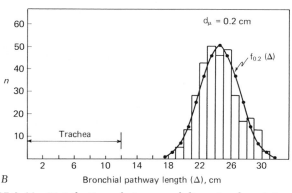

FIGURE 2-44 Distribution of airways of diameter $d_\mu = 0.2$ cm with respect to (*A*) generations of branching and (*B*) bronchial pathway lengths. *(From Weibel, 1963.)*

The general conclusion drawn from this type of analysis is that the diameters of the conducting airways are such as to assure optimal conditions for airflow: from an engineering point of view, the airways of the lung are well designed. The total volume of the conducting airways down to generation 16 (the anatomic dead space) is about 150 ml; it is rapidly flushed by simple gas flow in the course of inhaling 500 ml of fresh air during quiet inspiration. For the larger airways, optimization for flow and its distribution to peripheral units is, therefore, the essential condition for good design.

Figure 2-45 shows the transition of peripheral airways from terminal bronchioles that serve only as conducting tubes to respiratory bronchioles that contain alveoli in their walls. The terminal airways also branch by dichotomy (back cover).

Figure 2-43 shows that the diameters of the most peripheral airways (generations 17 to 23) do not follow the law of reduction by the cube root of 2; the diameters of respiratory bronchioles and alveolar ducts change very little with each generation. Does this arrangement imply less than an optimal design? No, on the contrary, the cube-root-of-2 law relates to optimizing mass flow of a liquid or of air. In the most peripheral airways, mass airflow is only part of the means of transporting O_2 toward the air-blood barrier: since the airways are blind-ending tubes, and since a sizable amount of residual air remains in the lung periphery after expiration, O_2 molecules must move into the residual air by diffusion (Fig. 2-46). But, diffusion of O_2 in the gas phase is best served by establishing as large an interface as possible between residual air and the fresh air that flows in from the trachea. In fact, since the airway diameter remains nearly unchanged, the total airway cross section nearly doubles with each generation beyond generation 16 (Fig. 2-47).

The dimensions of the airway tree influence the ventilatory flow of air in a number of ways. First of all, airflow velocity falls along the airway tree because the total cross-sectional area of the airways increases with every generation (Fig. 2-47); whereas the cross-sectional area of the trachea is about 2.5 cm², that of the 1024 airways in the 10th generation taken together is 13 cm², and as we approach the acinar airways, the total cross section reaches 300 cm². But since the same air volume flows through all generations, the flow velocity falls by more than 100-fold from the trachea to the acini: at rest the mean flow velocity on inspiration is about 1 m/s in the trachea and less than 1 cm/s in the first-order respiratory bronchioles. This shows that in the small airways the transport of O_2 by mass airflow is slower than that by diffusion, since O_2 molecules move through air at a velocity of about 5 cm/s. In exercise the flow velocities are up to 10 times greater, in proportion to the increased ventilation, and, accordingly, mass flow velocity is somewhat greater than molecular velocity at the entrance into the acini (Fig. 2-47).

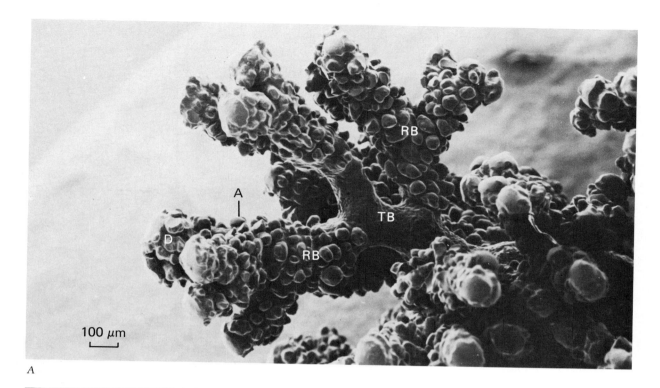

A

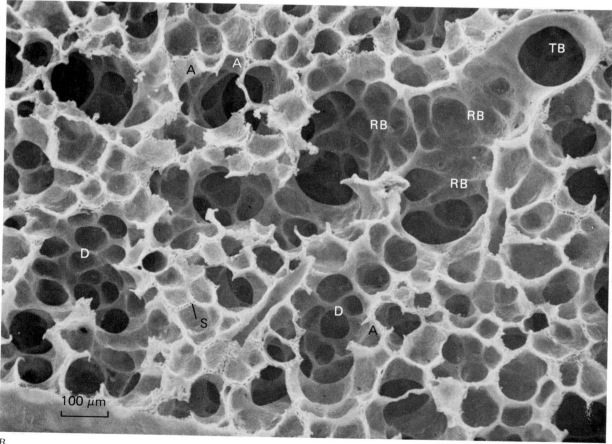

B

FIGURE 2-45 Scanning electron micrographs of airway branches peripheral to terminal bronchiole. *A.* In silicon-rubber cast of cat lung. *B.* In whole tissue preparation of air-filled, perfusion-fixed rabbit lung. Note that branching can be followed from terminal bronchiole to alveolar ducts. A = alveolus; D = alveolar duct; RB = respiratory bronchiole; TB = terminal bronchiole; S = alveolar septum.

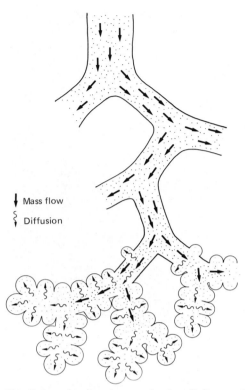

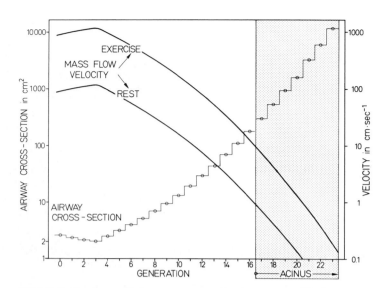

FIGURE 2-47 As total airway cross section increases with the generations of airway branching, the mass flow velocity of inspired air decreases rapidly. (*From Weibel, 1984a.*)

FIGURE 2-46 Oxygen molecules reach alveoli by combined mass airflow and molecular diffusion, the importance of diffusion increasing toward the periphery.

The size of airways also determines the resistance to airflow. The overall resistance is, however, rather small; it is given by the reciprocal of the ratio of ventilatory airflow to the pressure difference between the mouth and alveoli, which is normally no greater than about 1 cmH$_2$O (mbar) or less than 1 mmHg. It is large enough, however, to potentially affect the distribution of ventilation to the many gas-exchange units.

Since the diameter of airways decreases as they branch (Fig. 2-43), one might suspect that their resistance increases toward the periphery. Apparently this is not the case, since the major pressure drop along the airways occurs in medium-sized bronchi; resistance in the small airways is low primarily because the flow velocity falls so rapidly as airways branch (Fig. 2-48). This is further accentuated by the fact that the thin-walled bronchioles become widened as the lung expands on inspiration because they are subject to the tissue tensions in the coarse fiber system of the lung; therefore, airway resistance falls as lung volume increases. When this effect of tissue tension is disturbed, as in emphysema, some small bronchioles may collapse. This causes ventilation of the peripheral lung units to become highly uneven.

Design of the Vascular Trees

In many ways, the course and pattern of dimensional changes in the pulmonary blood vessels resemble those of

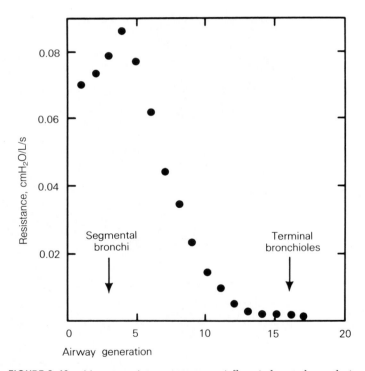

FIGURE 2-48 Airway resistance to mass airflow is located mostly in the conducting airways and falls rapidly toward the periphery. (*Redrawn after Pedley, Schroter, Sudlow, 1970.*)

the airways. The front cover shows that the pulmonary arteries follow the airways closely, out to the smallest branches; together they form the axis of lung parenchymal units of varying order: acinus, lobule, segment, lobe. As indicated previously, the veins are differently disposed, lying in the boundary between two (or three) adjacent units.

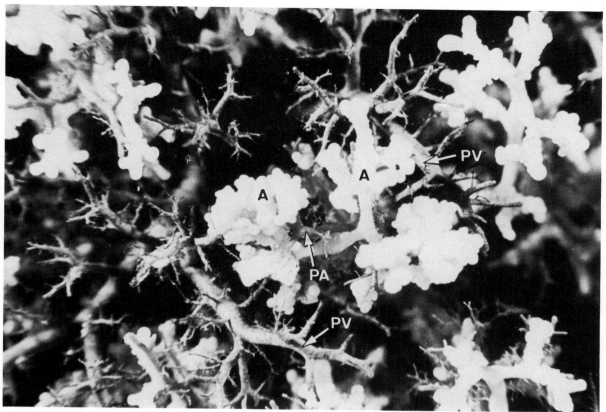

FIGURE 2-49 Detail of cast of airways and blood vessels of human lung shows how pulmonary artery (PA) closely follows the airways (A) to the periphery, whereas the pulmonary vein branches (PV) lie between the units. *(From Weibel, 1984a.)*

The diameter of each pulmonary artery branch also approximates closely that of the accompanying bronchus (Fig. 2-49). Therefore, it is evident that the diameter law presented above for airways must also hold for the first 10 to 16 generations of pulmonary arteries (Fig. 2-43). However, the pulmonary arteries divide more frequently than the airways; very often, small branches leave the artery at right angles and supply blood to the parenchymal units adjacent to the bronchus. From a count of precapillaries, it seems that the pulmonary arteries divide, on the average, over 28 generations, as compared to 23 for the airways. The diameter of these terminal vessels is about 20 to 50 μm; if this range is plotted onto an extension of the graph of Fig. 2-43 to generation 28, it falls on the curve that is obtained by extrapolation from the major branches, $d(z) = d_0 \cdot 2^{-z/3}$. Although no information exists about the entire sequence of dimensional changes throughout the pulmonary arterial tree, this finding suggests that the pulmonary arteries abide by the cube-root-of-2 law from beginning to end. Evidently, the blood is transported to the capillary bed by mass flow only. Therefore, there is no reason to deviate from this fundamental law of design, which minimizes the loss of energy due to blood flow. Parenthetically, this design principle seems to hold also for the systemic arteries.

Not much is known yet about the design of the venous tree. The cast shown on the front cover suggests, however, that it is similar to that of the arterial tree.

The alveolar capillary network of the lung is very different from that of the systemic circulation. Whereas in muscle long capillaries are found to be joined in a loose network, the capillaries of the alveolar walls form dense meshworks made of very short segments (Fig. 2-50). The meshes are so dense that some people believe blood flows through the alveolar walls like a sheet rather than through a system of interconnected tubes. In this *sheet-flow* concept the sheet is bounded by two flat membranes, the air-blood barrier, connected by numerous "posts." When blood flows through this sheet, it is not channeled in a given direction but has freedom to move in a tortuous way between the posts. Although this concept oversimplifies the actual structural conditions, it does provide a useful description of the pattern of blood flow through the alveolar walls and explains why blood flow is not interrupted when some parts of the capillary bed are flattened at high inflation levels, as discussed above (Fig. 2-39); the capillaries which remain open in the corners are simply some channels of this broad sheet. Furthermore, it is important to note that the capillary network or sheet is continuous through many alveolar walls, probably at least throughout

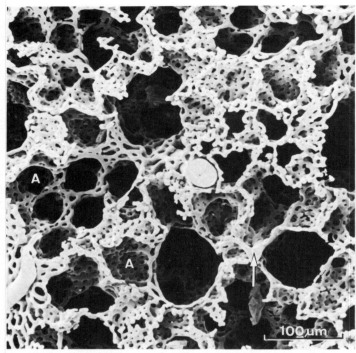

FIGURE 2-50 Alveolar capillary network in walls of alveoli (A) demonstrated by a casting technique. Note larger vessel which leads into network (arrow). *(Scanning electron micrograph courtesy Drs. L. Fischer and P. Burri; from Weibel, 1984a.)*

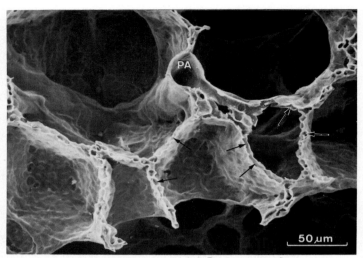

FIGURE 2-51 Scanning electron micrograph of perfusion-fixed rabbit lung shows small pulmonary arteriole (PA) connecting to (empty) capillaries in alveolar walls (arrows). *(From Weibel, 1984a.)*

the entire acinus, if not for greater distances. Hence, it is not possible to isolate microvascular units. Instead, arterial end branches simply feed into this broad sheet at more or less even distances, and veins drain these sheets in a similar pattern (Fig. 2-51). But it must be kept in mind that the arteries reach the acinus along the airways, whereas the veins are in a peripheral location (Fig. 2-49). Therefore, in principle, blood flows through the acinar capillary sheet from the center to the periphery.

The Pulmonary Diffusing Capacity

In discussing the lung as part of the respiratory system, it has been noted that the flow of O_2 from air to blood is determined, according to the Bohr equation, by the product of the P_{O_2} difference between alveolar air and capillary blood and the lung's diffusion conductance or *diffusing capacity* [Eq. (3)]. Whereas alveolar and capillary P_{O_2} are, to some extent, determined by the design of airways and blood vessels, the $D_{L_{O_2}}$ is determined in part by the design properties of the gas exchanger that is constituted by pulmonary parenchyma.

It is well known that the conductance of any conductor, for example, of an electrical wire, can be calculated from its dimensions and its material properties. Accordingly, $D_{L_{O_2}}$ should be proportional to the barrier surface S and inversely proportional to the barrier thickness τ (Fig.

2-41). This ratio multiplied by the permeability coefficient of the lung for oxygen, K_{O_2}, provides a first approximation of $D_{L_{O_2}}$ based on structural parameters, i.e.,

$$D_{L_{O_2}} = K_{O_2} \frac{S}{\tau} \qquad (6)$$

Although it will be shown in the process of developing a morphometric model for $D_{L_{O_2}}$ that this relationship is oversimplified because oxygen passes through a series of barriers before binding to the hemoglobin in the red cell, it does provide a good starting point.

Physiologists also use a functional approach for measuring $D_{L_{O_2}}$. By rearranging Eq. (3), the following formulation emerges:

$$D_{L_{O_2}} = \frac{\dot{V}_{O_2}}{P_{A_{O_2}} - P_{C_{O_2}}} \qquad (7)$$

Thus, if O_2 consumption ($\dot{V}_{O_2}$) and the P_{O_2} in alveolar air and capillary blood ($P_{A_{O_2}}$, $P_{C_{O_2}}$) can be determined, it becomes possible to calculate $D_{L_{O_2}}$ from these functional parameters. In essence, if the measure of $\dot{V}_{O_2}$ and the P_{O_2} gradient can be determined along with S and τ, we have two approaches at hand for estimating $D_{L_{O_2}}$, one based on function, the other on structure. This provides a quantitative way of examining how lung structure affects gas exchange.

MORPHOMETRIC MODEL FOR PULMONARY DIFFUSING CAPACITY

Oxygen crosses a series of barriers as it diffuses from the air in an alveolus to the hemoglobin in a red blood cell. Each barrier presents its own resistance to oxygen flow (Fig. 2-52): (1) resistance of the air-blood tissue barrier (Rt)

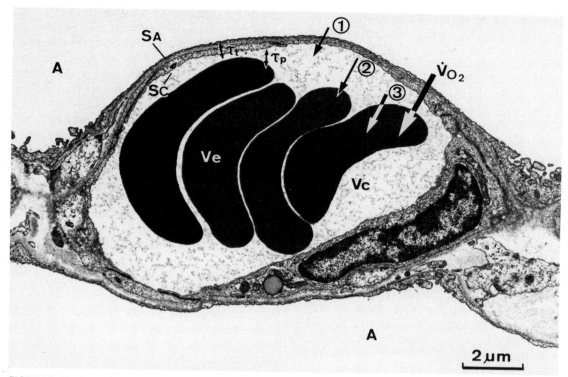

FIGURE 2-52 Morphometric model for calculating diffusion capacity, D. Flow of O_2 ($\dot{V}_{O_2}$) has to traverse in sequence three resistances: (1) tissue barrier, (2) plasma barrier, and (3) erythrocyte interior. *(See text.)*

consisting of alveolar and capillary endothelial cells and interstitial tissue; (2) resistance of the plasma barrier (Rp) consisting of the plasma separating the capillary endothelium from the red blood cell; and (3) resistance of the erythrocyte barrier (Re). The total resistance of the lung (RL) is the sum of all three resistances,

$$RL = Rt + Rp + Re \qquad (8)$$

or, expressed in terms of reciprocals of their conductances,

$$\frac{1}{DL} = \frac{1}{Dt} + \frac{1}{Dp} + \frac{1}{De} \qquad (9)$$

It should be noted that the membrane diffusing capacity DM derives from the sum of the resistances in tissue and plasma:

$$\frac{1}{DM} = \frac{1}{Dt} + \frac{1}{Dp} \qquad (10)$$

Each of these conductances is composed of a physical coefficient and some structural parameters that can be quantified morphometrically, as is shown in Fig. 2-52.

Dt.   The tissue barrier is a sheet of thickness τ which separates two compartments, alveolar air and plasma, over an area S; thus Fick's law determines O_2 flow across this barrier:

$$\dot{V}_{O_2}t = Kt \cdot S \cdot \tau^{-1} \cdot \Delta Pt_{O_2} = Dt \cdot \Delta Pt_{O_2} \qquad (11)$$

where Kt is Krogh's permeation coefficient of the tissue for oxygen (3.3×10^{-8} cm²/min/mmHg) and ΔPt_{O_2} is the pressure head for diffusion across the tissue barrier. Rearranging this equation, we find

$$Dt = Kt\frac{S}{\tau} \qquad (12)$$

As noted earlier in this chapter, the tissue barrier is a complex structure. Its two bounding surfaces are formed by independent cell layers, epithelium and endothelium, and they are related to two independent functional spaces, alveoli and capillaries. The two surfaces are not perfectly matched, and the thickness of the barrier varies considerably. How can we take this into account when calculating S and τ? Oxygen enters the barrier on its alveolar aspect and leaves it on its endothelial aspect; the mean of these two surface areas, (SA + Sc)/2, provides an estimate of the effective area of the tissue barrier. The effect of varying barrier thickness is that the conductance for O_2 will vary from point to point, in fact, about inversely proportional to the local thickness. If the barrier is pictured to be built of a set of units of equal area but varying thickness τ, the overall conductance of the barrier is equal to the mean of the unit conductances, since they are all in parallel. The only variable being the thickness—the reciprocal of which has been shown above to determine the conductance—the relevant estimate of barrier thickness is its harmonic mean, τht, i.e., the mean of the reciprocal local thicknesses. This turns out to be quite important because the value of the harmonic mean thickness of the pulmonary air-blood barrier is consistently about three times smaller than the arithmetic mean thickness τt. For example, in humans τht is about 0.6 μm as compared to 2.2 μm for τt; in the rat it is 0.5 μm versus 1.5 μm. This difference is the result of design features that optimize various functional requirements: although fibers are necessary to support the capillaries, it suffices to locate them in only half of the barrier, so that the other half remains very thin, as noted above (Fig. 2-30). Or, the barrier needs cell bodies with bulky nuclei to keep alive the cell linings; but these can be tucked away into the meshes of the capillary network (Fig. 2-13) where the tissue is already relatively thick because this is where the fiber tracts cross the capillary sheet from one side to the other. Thus the barrier needs to maintain a certain minimal mass to ensure its integrity, and this is reflected in the arithmetic mean barrier thickness; but mass is disposed in such a fashion as to interfere as little as possible with gas exchange. Barrier thickness becomes highly irregular, but this turns out to be an advantage in that it allows the diffusion-effective mean thickness to be three times less than if a barrier of the same total mass were made of even thickness—a remarkable finding!

On the basis of these arguments we find the conductance of the tissue barrier to be

$$Dt = Kt \frac{S_A + S_C}{2\tau ht} \tag{13}$$

where S_A, S_C, and τht are morphometric variables that can be measured on electron micrographs of lung sections using stereologic methods—provided that the micrographs are obtained by proper statistical random sampling.

Dp. The plasma barrier consists of a sheet that is highly variable in thickness. Much of the surface of the red blood cells is "hidden" from the capillary surface by neighboring red cells (Fig. 2-52), so the red cell surface "accessible" for diffusion of oxygen is found to be similar to the capillary surface. Thus, the conductance of the plasma barrier is

$$Dp = Kp \frac{S_C}{\tau hp} \tag{14}$$

The permeation constant for plasma (Kp) and tissue (Kt) are approximately the same.

De. The third conductance, that of erythrocytes, De, is of a different nature in that it involves two coupled events: the diffusion of O_2 within the red blood cell and the reaction of O_2 with hemoglobin. Roughton and Forster developed a simplified expression based on an empirical measure of the rate at which O_2 is bound to whole blood, θ,

$$De = \theta \cdot V_C \tag{15}$$

where V_C is the total capillary blood volume, which can again be estimated on sections by stereologic methods.

The constant θ_{O_2} is problematic for two reasons: the measured values reported in the literature are variable; and it is not really a constant as the O_2 binding rate falls to zero at 100 percent saturation of hemoglobin although it is nearly constant over the range of oxyhemoglobin saturations from 0 to 75 percent. It should also be noted that θ is different for different species because smaller red blood cells bind O_2 more rapidly. Thus, when calculating De, one should use a value for θ that has been determined on that species, and normalize it to the hemoglobin concentration that is observed in that individual. There is as yet no consensus about the true value of θ_{O_2} for human blood, but a value of 1.5 ml O_2/ml/min/mmHg is a currently accepted reasonable estimate for desaturated blood.

MORPHOMETRY AND DIFFUSING CAPACITY OF THE HUMAN LUNG

With this model in hand we can now attempt to estimate the diffusing capacity of the human lung on the basis of morphometric data listed in Table 2-3. These data, obtained by electron microscope morphometry on seven young adults, reveal that the alveolar surface area is 140 m^2, and that the capillary surface is about 10 percent smaller. It should be noted that these values are higher than those most commonly quoted in textbooks derived from light microscope studies which did not adequately resolve the alveolar surface texture. The harmonic mean barrier thickness is 0.6 μm and the capillary volume about 200 ml. Based on these data, DL_{O_2} for the adult human lung is calculated to be about 200 ml O_2/min/mmHg.

These data also allow us to ask the question how the resistance to O_2 diffusion is distributed between the tissue

TABLE 2-3
*Morphometric Information on Normal Human Lung, Obtained by Electron Microscopy**

Body weight	74 ± 4 kg
Body length	177 ± 3 cm
Total lung volume	4341 ± 285 ml
Alveolar surface area	143 ± 12 m^2
Capillary surface area	126 ± 12 m^2
Capillary blood volume	213 ± 31 ml
Air-blood barrier thickness	
Arithmetic mean	2.22 ± 0.19 μm
Harmonic mean	0.62 ± 0.04 μm
Plasma barrier thickness	
Harmonic mean	0.15 ± 0.01 μm
Diffusing capacity	
DL_{O_2}	205 ml O_2/min/mmHg
DM_{O_2}	567 ml O_2/min/mmHg
De_{O_2}	319 ml O_2/min/mmHg

* Mean (±1 SE) of group of eight lungs aged 19 to 40 years, six males and two females.
SOURCE: After Gehr, Bachofen, Weibel, 1978.

barrier and the blood. Table 2-3 shows that the diffusion conductance of the membrane, D_M [see Eq. (10)], is almost twice as large as that of the red cells, D_e, which means that the major resistance to O_2 uptake is in the erythrocytes.

How do these morphometric estimates of $D_{L_{O_2}}$ compare to physiological values? The standard physiological value of $D_{L_{O_2}}$ of a healthy adult at rest is about 30 ml O_2/min/mmHg, thus considerably less than the result obtained by morphometry. However, the comparison is not valid because the O_2 uptake under resting conditions is only one-tenth the amount that the lungs are capable of absorbing during heavy work. A number of physiological estimates of $D_{L_{O_2}}$ in exercising humans have yielded values on the order of 100 ml O_2/min/mmHg. It is evident that these values are closer to the true capacity of the lung to transfer O_2 to the blood by diffusion than is the value obtained at rest. The fact that this is only about half the morphometric estimate is not disturbing, for it is not known whether the true diffusing capacity is completely exploited even during heavy exercise. Inhomogeneities in the distribution of ventilation and perfusion would, for example, limit the degree to which true $D_{L_{O_2}}$ can be exploited.

DESIGN OF THE LUNGS FOR GAS EXCHANGE: IS THERE A MATCH BETWEEN STRUCTURE AND FUNCTION?

Concept and Approach

The principal design features of the lung that we have considered up to this point are: (1) the walls between alveoli are densely populated with blood; (2) the tissue barrier separating air and blood is exceedingly thin—50 times thinner than a sheet of airmail stationery—and is yet tightly organized into three basic layers; (3) the surface of contact between air and blood is very large, approaching in humans the square footage of a tennis court; and (4) the airways and blood vessels are designed in such a way as to allow efficient ventilation and perfusion of the gas-exchange units that number some 300 million in humans.

Intuitively, these structural design features, which determine essentially the pulmonary diffusing capacity, appear related to establishing efficient gas exchange within the lung, and it seems reasonable to expect that they are well matched to functional requirements. Now we must note that the requirements for O_2 flow through the lung are established by the O_2 needs of the cells which perform work, in exercise primarily by the muscle cells where 98 percent of the O_2 taken up is consumed in oxidative ATP production. As a first approximation, it seems reasonable to propose that the lung is designed according to functional needs on the assumption that $D_{L_{O_2}}$ is matched to $\dot{V}_{O_2}$ under conditions of maximal work, i.e., when the limit of O_2 supply to the working muscles is

reached. According to Fig. 2-40, O_2 must flow through several consecutive steps en route from the lung to the mitochrondria. Clearly, each step could limit $\dot{V}_{O_2}$, but in a well-designed system all steps would be expected to reach their functional limit at the same level, i.e., no step should have an excess capacity for O_2 flow.

To test whether this "perfect match" between functional needs and economic design at all levels—which has been called *symmorphosis*—is realized in the organism, is a demanding task. The complexity of the system and the interdependence of the various steps make it impossible to approach it directly. Therefore, we have chosen a comparative approach, exploiting the fact that O_2 needs show large variation in different species of the animal kingdom.

It should be noted that, compared to mammals, the bird lung and the fish gills are very differently designed gas exchangers, particularly with respect to the relation between perfusion and ventilation patterns in the gas-exchange units. The principal advantage of these designs is that the O_2 contained in the ventilating media—air or water, respectively—can be better extracted by blood flow, which is important for birds flying at high altitude, or for fishes swimming in deep waters with a low O_2 content. This is not essential for mammals because O_2 is plentiful in their normal environments. We shall therefore limit the following discussion to mammals which share a basic design of the respiratory system, particularly of the lung and the circulation.

The basic strategy in the approach that follows is to estimate maximal O_2 consumption ($\dot{V}_{O_2max}$) and to set it into relation with the parameters that determine design properties, such as the diffusing capacity of the lung. Although the focus will be on the lungs, it is evident that all steps of the respiratory system must enter our considerations.

Maximal Oxygen Consumption: $\dot{V}_{O_2max}$

The procedure for measuring $\dot{V}_{O_2max}$ of humans under steady-state conditions consists of measuring O_2 consumption of a subject running on a treadmill or bicycling on an ergometer as a function of exercise intensity, i.e., speed or work rate (Fig. 2-53). Oxygen consumption increases linearly with exercise intensity up to a maximal rate ($\dot{V}_{O_2max}$); it does not increase with further increases in exercise intensity but rather stays constant, and the additional energy required to sustain these higher intensities is supplied by anaerobic glycolysis. Lactate, an end product of anaerobic glycolysis, accumulates, limiting the duration of exercise. This procedure for determining $\dot{V}_{O_2max}$ can be applied to animals as well as humans, and it provides very reproducible values.

Large differences in $\dot{V}_{O_2max}$ occur between individuals of the same species (e.g., 1.5- to 2-fold between trained athletes and sedentary individuals), between species of

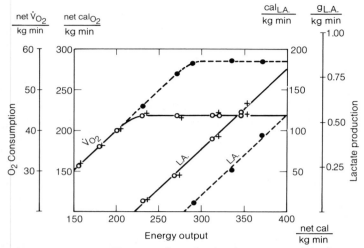

FIGURE 2-53 Rate of lactic acid production (grams per minute) as an effect of exercise (ordinate at right) is plotted as a function of the work intensity and, therefore, of the energy requirement (abscissa). A straight line is obtained that cuts the abscissa at an energy requirement corresponding to 220 cal/kg/min; below this value no production of lactic acid takes place and the energy requirement is met solely by oxygen consumption (shown on the ordinate at left). The broken lines refer to athletes (middle- and long-distance runners) whose maximum oxygen consumption is higher; the line of the lactic acid for these subjects is correspondingly shifted to the right. (*From Margaria, Cerretelli, Di Prampero, Massari, Torelli: J Appl Physiol 18:371–377, 1963.*)

the same size (e.g., 2- to 3-fold between dogs and goats or horses and cows), and between species of different body size (e.g., 10- to 15-fold between mice and cows). These large differences in $\dot{V}_{O_2max}$ provide us with the tools for testing the principle of symmorphosis which predicts a quantitative match in $\dot{V}_{O_2max}$ and structure determining the conductances for oxygen flow at each step in the flow of oxygen through the respiratory system diagrammed in Fig. 2-40.

Differences in $\dot{V}_{O_2max}$ occur particularly as a result of exercise training. This is evidenced in Fig. 2-53: at low energy requirements $\dot{V}_{O_2}$ is the same for untrained and trained persons; in the athletes trained for endurance running $\dot{V}_{O_2}$ reaches the plateau at a markedly higher level, and accordingly lactic acid production takes off at higher energy requirements. This indicates one important feature that has now been demonstrated both for humans and for animals, namely, that the respiratory system is adaptable to functional needs, in that the limit for O_2 supply to the working muscles can be pushed to higher values of $\dot{V}_{O_2max}$ when the energetic demands imposed on the muscles are increased. Moreover, it takes only a few weeks of relatively intense training—running at 70 percent of $\dot{V}_{O_2max}$ for 20 min every day—to reset the level.

Thus the performance of the respiratory system as measured by the limit to O_2 flow, i.e., the $\dot{V}_{O_2max}$, shows considerable variation. It is now pertinent to assess the extent to which the structures which support O_2 flow at the different levels of the system are adapted to the functional needs, i.e., to what extent they can be considered to be limiting factors for O_2 flow.

Structure-Function Relations at the Level of Muscles: Mitochondria and Capillaries

Oxygen is consumed in the mitochondria in the process of oxidative phosphorylation which occurs in a well-controlled manner: the production of 6 mol ATP requires 1 mol O_2. This is clearly at the basis of the straight-line relationship between energy requirement and $\dot{V}_{O_2}$ shown in Fig. 2-53. The fact that $\dot{V}_{O_2}$ reaches a limit ($\dot{V}_{O_2max}$) and that additional ATP required by higher work loads is produced anaerobically (leading to higher lactate output) suggests that the mitochondria themselves may set the limit to aerobic metabolism.

This can be tested in trained and untrained humans by taking small muscle biopsies and determining the mitochondrial content of their muscle cells (Fig. 2-54). An almost direct proportionality has been shown to exist between mitochondrial volume and $\dot{V}_{O_2max}$, as demonstrated in Fig. 2-55. Particularly convincing are the long-term studies where both parameters are followed during the course of training on bicycle ergometers. Similar studies have also been carried out using rats as an animal model for training with similar results, i.e., a direct proportionality between $\dot{V}_{O_2max}$ and mitochondrial volume. Thus, at the level of the muscle's metabolic machinery there appears to be a good match between structure and function during training.

This proportionality can also be demonstrated by comparing different animal species. Taking first an allometric approach, the total volumes of mitochondria in three muscles (two important locomotory muscles and the diaphragm) have been found to scale in direct proportion to $\dot{V}_{O_2max}$ in a group of animals ranging in body mass from 500 g to 250 kg (Fig. 2-56). This same strict proportionality between $\dot{V}_{O_2max}$ and mitochondrial volume is also observed when comparing pairs of mammals of the same body mass but with widely differing energy requirements, such as dog and goat, or horse and cow. The result is therefore consistent: the limit to O_2 consumption is directly related to the quantity of mitochondria that are available to perform oxidative phosphorylation.

The second structural factor which determines O_2 flow in the muscles is the capillary network which must maintain an adequate supply of O_2 to the muscle cells (Fig. 2-54). The capillaries form more or less dense networks between the muscle cells (Fig. 2-57); the O_2 flow rate depends primarily on two features: the distance from the capillary to the mitochondria and the volume of blood available for unloading O_2. These features are directly related to the length of the capillaries in the unit volume of muscle.

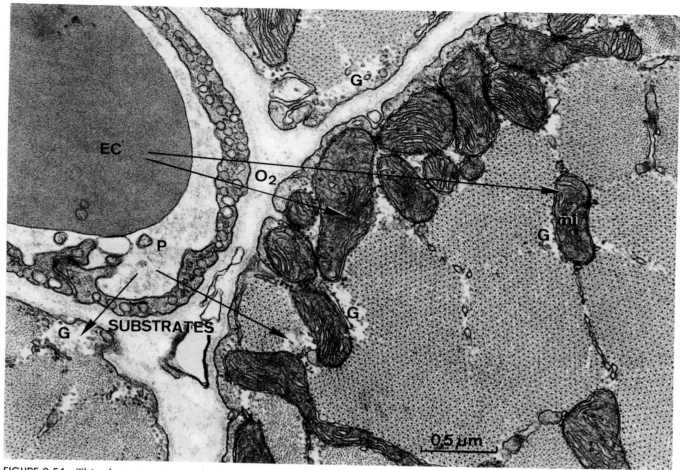

FIGURE 2-54 This electron micrograph of a capillary with its adjacent muscle fibers shows the pathways for O_2 supply from the erythrocyte (EC) to the mitochondria (mi) and for substrates from the plasma (P) to intracellular glycogen deposits (G). *(From Weibel, 1984a.)*

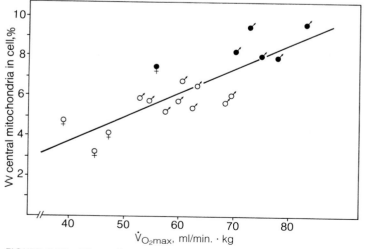

FIGURE 2-55 The volume density of mitochondria in leg muscle cells is proportional to $\dot{V}_{O_2max}$ in a population of untrained (open circles) and trained (full circles) humans. $Vv_{cmi} = (0.118 \cdot \dot{V}_{O_2max}) - 0.928$; $r = 0.82$; $s_{yx} = 1.002$. *(From Hoppeler, Lüthi, Claassen, Weibel, Howald: Pflügers Arch 334:217–232, 1973.)*

The length of capillaries in muscle is directly related to the volume of mitochondria. This has been shown for a wide range of species and different muscles, i.e., from the skeletal muscle of cows to the heart muscle of the shrew in which 45 percent of the volume is occupied by mitochondria (Fig. 2-58); indeed in all muscles studied to date there are about 4 μm^3 of mitochondria for every μm^3 of capillary blood! Thus it appears that, in muscle, the O_2 consumer (the mitochondria) and the O_2 supplier (the capillaries) are directly related to $\dot{V}_{O_2max}$. Therefore, both can be considered to contribute equally to the limitation of O_2 flow.

Structure-Function Relations in the Lung

THE LUNG AND THE O_2 NEEDS OF THE BODY

The first evidence that the lung may also be adapted to the O_2 needs of the body came from comparative and experimental studies in which morphometric $D_{L_{O_2}}$ was used as

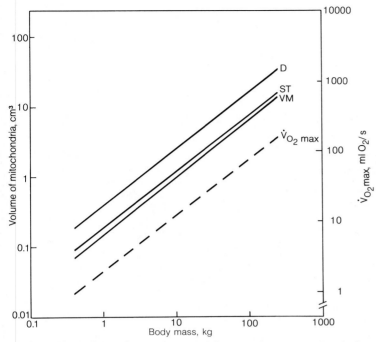

FIGURE 2-56 When the total mass of the muscles is considered, the total volume of mitochondria in the muscles becomes proportional to total $\dot{V}_{O_2 max}$. *(From Mathieu, Krauer, Hoppeler, Gehr, Lindstedt, Alexander, Taylor, Weibel: Respir Physiol 44:113–128, 1981.)*

a compound parameter of lung structures. It was shown that the horse has a higher morphometric $D_{L_{O_2}}$ than the cow in accord with its higher O_2 needs; similarly, the dog's $D_{L_{O_2}}$ is larger than that of humans, when expressed per unit body mass. A particularly striking case is that of the Japanese waltzing mice; their well-known hyperactivity results in higher $\dot{V}_{O_2}$; $D_{L_{O_2}}$ is increased about in proportion to the increase in O_2 needs (Fig. 2-59). The same proportionality between $\dot{V}_{O_2}$ and $D_{L_{O_2}}$ was found in mice in which a waltzing syndrome was induced by drug treatment during early growth (Fig. 2-59). Other studies have also shown that hyperactivity or cold exposure during growth lead to increase in $D_{L_{O_2}}$ as $\dot{V}_{O_2}$ increases. In this context, it is noteworthy that the lung will also adapt to changes in ambient P_{O_2}: animals raised at high altitude develop a larger gas-exchange surface than those raised at sea level; in contrast, chronic hyperoxia leads to a reduction in $D_{L_{O_2}}$.

The important insight gained from these studies is that during growth lung structure is capable of adapting to altered functional needs. This adaptability is further supported by the observation that removal of 25 percent of the lung by bilobectomy in young rats results in compensatory overgrowth of the remaining lobes so that, in the end, the lobectomized animals have the same $D_{L_{O_2}}$ as the controls (Fig. 2-60).

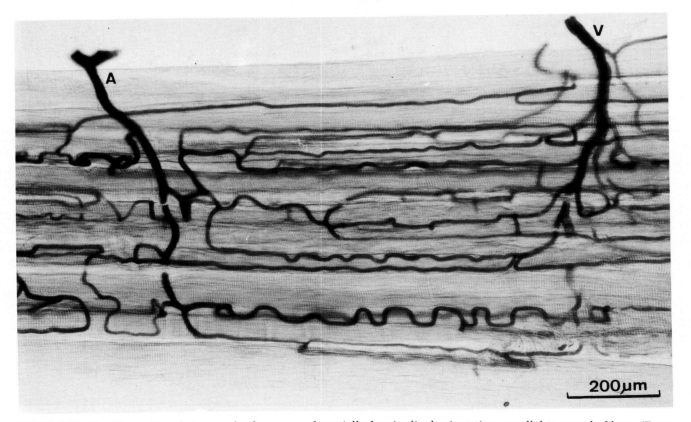

FIGURE 2-57 Capillary network in muscle shows a preferentially longitudinal orientation, parallel to muscle fibers. *(From Weibel, 1984a.)*

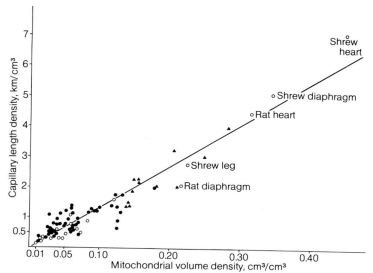

FIGURE 2-58 Capillary length per unit volume of muscle fibers is linearly proportional to mitochondrial volume density in fibers. $N_A(c, f) = -0.11 \cdot 10^4 + 122.9 \cdot 10^4 \cdot V_V(mt, f)$. *(Data from Hoppeler, Lindstedt, Uhlmann, Niesel, Cruz-Orive, Weibel: J Comp Physiol B 155:51–61, 1984.)*

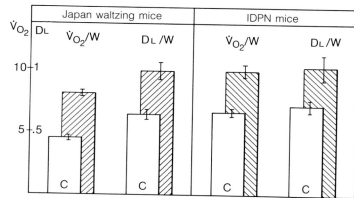

FIGURE 2-59 Increase of O_2 consumption and morphometric D_L in Japanese waltzing mice and in mice rendered waltzers artificially by treatment with β-iminodiproprionitrile (IDPN). *(From Burri, Weibel: in Hudson WA (ed), Development of the Lung. New York, Dekker, 1977, pp 215–268.)*

THE LUNG AND MAXIMAL $\dot{V}_{O_2}$

The problem with older studies along this line is that $\dot{V}_{O_2max}$ was not estimated. They are therefore not conclusive with respect to whether the lung is adapted to limiting levels of $\dot{V}_{O_2}$. More recent studies have revealed several distinctive features. First, training young rats on a treadmill resulted in a 20 to 30 percent increase in $\dot{V}_{O_2max}$; although this increase was paralleled by a proportional increase in muscle mitochondria, $D_{L_{O_2}}$ remained essentially unchanged. Second, in a recent study of goats and dogs of about 28 kg body mass, the $\dot{V}_{O_2max}$ of the dogs was found to be 2.5 times larger than that of the goats, but $D_{L_{O_2}}$ in the dogs was only 1.5 times larger than in the goats (Table 2-4). A similar result was obtained when ponies were compared with calves. However, in both series, the mitochondria in muscles were found to be proportional to $\dot{V}_{O_2max}$. Thus these studies have revealed a possible mismatch between $D_{L_{O_2}}$ and $\dot{V}_{O_2max}$. The relation between the parameters of the structural design of the lungs and their functional needs, as expressed by the limit

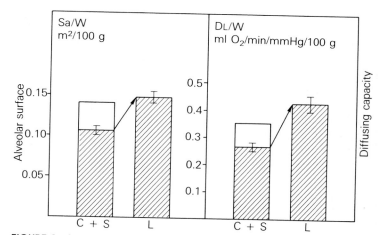

FIGURE 2-60 Following removal of 25 percent of the lung in rats 6 weeks old, the remaining lung makes up for the lost diffusing capacity by compensatory overgrowth. *(Data from Burri, Sehovic: Am Rev Respir Dis 119:769–777, 1979.)*

to O_2 consumption, does not appear to be as simple as it had appeared from earlier studies.

Before looking deeper into this question, it is pertinent to point out that a similarly enigmatic mismatch between $D_{L_{O_2}}$ and $\dot{V}_{O_2max}$ was observed when comparing

TABLE 2-4

The Match between $\dot{V}_{O_2max}$ and $D_{L_{O_2}}$ Compared in Similar-Sized Animals with Different Aerobic Potential

Species	M_B, kg	$\dot{V}_{O_2max}/M_B$, ml O_2/min/kg	$D_{L_{O_2}}/M_B$, ml O_2/min/mmHg/kg	$\dot{V}_{O_2max}/D_{L_{O_2}}$ mmHg
Dog	28	136.2	7.08	19.2
Goat	28	54.0	4.78	11.3
Ratio dog/goat		2.52	1.48	1.7

SOURCE: After Weibel, Marques, Constantinopol, Doffey, Gehr, Taylor, 1987.

animals of different body size, from mice to cows. Although 2- to 3-fold differences in $\dot{V}_{O_2max}$ do occur among animals of the same size, much larger (10- to 15-fold) differences accompany differences in body size. These large differences have been used as another approach to examine the match between structure and function in the lungs.

The basic tool for comparing animals of different size is allometry. In allometry one compares the power function $Y = a \cdot M_B{}^b$, which describes how any functional or structural parameter Y varies with body mass M_B. The exponent b is usually referred to as the *scaling factor* of the parameter Y. In a comparison of 22 species ranging in M_B from 7 g to 260 kg, we found that the scaling factor b for $\dot{V}_{O_2max}$ was 0.8 (Fig. 2-61), not significantly different from the scaling factor of 0.75 found for resting oxygen consumption, $\dot{V}_{O_2std}$, 50 years earlier. On average, $\dot{V}_{O_2max}$ is a nearly constant multiple of 10 times $\dot{V}_{O_2std}$ over the entire range of body size. It is convenient to plot allometric functions on logarithmic coordinates where they become straight lines with the slope being the scaling factor b, and this is done for both $\dot{V}_{O_2max}$ and $\dot{V}_{O_2std}$ in Fig. 2-61.

Before proceeding further, it seems worthwhile to remember that the last step in the respiratory cascade of Fig. 2-40, i.e., the mitochondria of muscles which consume the oxygen, varies with the same scaling factor as does the $\dot{V}_{O_2max}$ (Fig. 2-56). This observation suggests that the size of the mitochondrial O_2 sink in muscles is proportional to the body's capacity for oxygen uptake even in animals whose metabolic rates differ greatly because of differences in body size.

With this relationship in mind, $D_{L_{O_2}}$, the lung's conductance for diffusive gas exchange (step A-B in the cascade, Fig. 2-40), can be examined. When calculated according to the morphometric model, a scaling factor of b is obtained that is clearly different from the 0.8 for $\dot{V}_{O_2max}$ (Fig. 2-62). The consequence of these different slopes is that a 30-g laboratory mouse has the same amount of diffusing capacity per unit body mass as does a 300-kg cow, but O_2 flows through this unit diffusing capacity at 15 times the rate under conditions of maximal oxygen uptake (Fig. 2-63). This enormous difference is in accord with recent findings on the dog and goat; $D_{L_{O_2}}$ of the lung does not appear to change with differences in maximal rates of oxygen flow across the lung. Does one then have to conclude that large animals, such as humans and cows, have pulmonary diffusing capacities that are far in excess of their functional needs, or is there some other explanation of the apparent mismatch between structure and function?

TESTING THE MORPHOMETRIC MODEL FOR $D_{L_{O_2}}$

The question that immediately comes to mind is: Has a basic error been made in the formulation of the morphometric model of $D_{L_{O_2}}$? As indicated above, the principal features in the structural design of the lung seem to be optimized for gas exchange (i.e., large surface areas for exchange, short diffusion distances). It seems reasonable

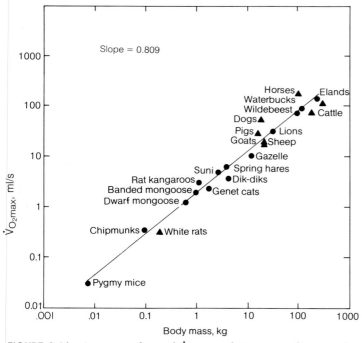

FIGURE 2-61 Average values of $\dot{V}_{O_2max}$ of 21 mammalian species increase with body mass to the power of 0.81. *(From Taylor, Maloiy, Weibel, Langman, Kamau, Seeherman, Heglund: Respir Physiol 44:25–37, 1981.)*

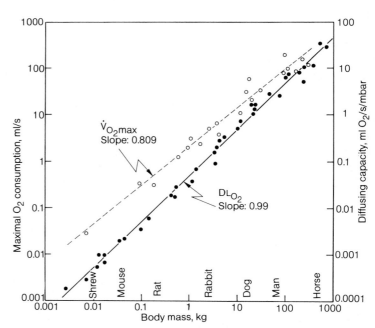

FIGURE 2-62 Allometric plot of pulmonary diffusing capacity and $\dot{V}_{O_2max}$ for mammals. *(From Weibel, 1984a.)*

to expect that these design features are necessary for gas exchange. A direct comparison of diffusing capacity measured from functional parameters according to Eq. (3) with that measured according to the morphometric model could resolve the question.

It is extremely difficult to measure the term (P_{CO_2}) directly. For this reason, most functional measurements of the diffusive conductance of the lung utilize carbon monoxide. The carbon monoxide binds to hemoglobin so

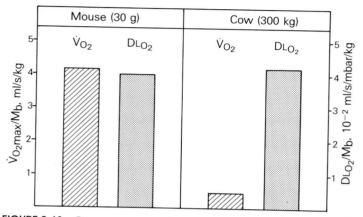

FIGURE 2-63 Oxygen consumption and pulmonary diffusing capacity per unit body mass in mouse and cow compared. *(From Weibel: Am Rev Respir Dis 128:752–760, 1983.)*

avidly that for practical purposes the $P_{C_{CO}}$ is zero. Equation (3) can be rewritten for $D_{L_{CO}}$ as

$$D_{L_{CO}} = \frac{V_{CO}}{P_{A_{CO}} - P_{C_{CO}}} = \frac{V_{CO}}{P_{A_{CO}}} \qquad (16)$$

Since both CO uptake and alveolar P_{CO} are relatively easy to determine, a direct measurement of $D_{L_{CO}}$ can be made independently of any structural measurements. It is also possible to revise the morphometric model of diffusing capacity for CO instead of O_2 on the assumption that the diffusion of CO from alveolar air to erythrocytes is basically governed by the same factors which apply for O_2:

$$\frac{1}{D_{L_{CO}}} = \frac{1}{D_{t_{CO}}} + \frac{1}{D_{P_{CO}}} + \frac{1}{\theta_{CO} V_c} \qquad (17)$$

A direct comparison of $D_{L_{CO}}$ measured morphometrically and physiologically on the same animals has recently been completed on a series of canids spanning a nearly 10-fold range in M_B (4-kg foxes to 30-kg dogs and wolves). It shows that both measurements of $D_{L_{CO}}$ have the same scaling factor (Fig. 2-64A) with the morphometric value being consistently twice that of the physiological. When $D_{L_{CO}}$ and $\dot{V}_{O_2max}$ are compared on the same canids, the same disparity of scaling factors is found as when $D_{L_{O_2}}$ and $\dot{V}_{O_2max}$ were compared, i.e., $D_{L_{CO}}$ increases much more steeply with M_B than does $\dot{V}_{O_2max}$ (Fig. 2-64B). A similar outcome was obtained previously

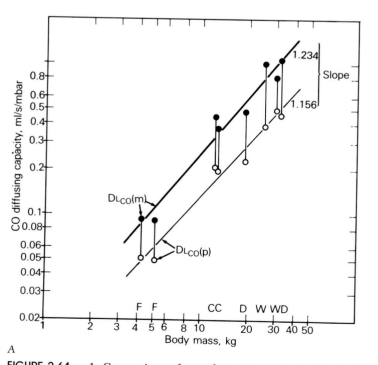

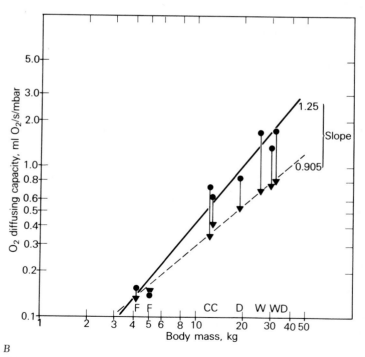

A

B

FIGURE 2-64 *A.* Comparison of morphometric and physiological CO diffusing capacity of the lung in four species of canids: foxes (F), coyotes (C), dogs (D), and wolves (W). *B.* Comparison of morphometric O_2 diffusing capacity with maximal O_2 consumption in the same species. ● = $D_{L_{O_2}}$ (morph. θ std.); ▼ = $\dot{V}_{O_2max}$. *(From Weibel, Taylor, O'Neil, Leith, Hoppeler, Langman, Baudinette: Respir Physiol 54:173–188, 1983.)*

when a large collection of physiological data was analyzed by allometry.

These experiments indicate that (1) the morphometric model for D_L and the functional measurements of D_L agree; and (2) D_{LO_2} and $\dot{V}_{O_2max}$ are discordantly related to body size.

DOES ALVEOLAR P_{O_2} CHANGE WITH BODY SIZE?

Before rejecting the concept of a structural-functional match for gas exchange across the lung, it seems worthwhile to consider other possibilities. For example, the pressure head for diffusion of oxygen might fall as the size of the lung increases in larger animals. If the Bohr equation [Eq. (1)] is rearranged and allometric scaling factors are applied, ($P_{AO_2} - P_{cO_2}$) is found to decrease with increasing size with a scaling factor of -0.2:

$$P_{AO_2} - P_{cO_2} = \frac{\dot{V}_{O_2max}}{D_{LO_2max}} \propto \frac{M_B^{0.8}}{M_B^{1.0}} \propto M_B^{-0.2} \quad (18)$$

How might this decrease in pressure head occur? A number of mechanisms exist whereby P_{AO_2} might decrease with increasing body size. P_{AO_2} is the P_{O_2} at the alveolar surface of the air-blood barrier, which is determined by ventilation and by diffusion of O_2 through the gas phase of residual air. In larger animals, ventilation is slower and the volume of residual air is larger, a combination that might cause P_{AO_2} to be lower.

Another mechanism could cause P_{AO_2} to be lower in larger animals. The conventional model for the gas-exchange unit shown in Fig. 2-41 is too simple; it does not consider that the gas-exchange units are arranged in series

along the pathway of alveolar ducts, whereas all capillary units are perfused in parallel (Fig. 2-65). The possible consequence of this arrangement is that P_{AO_2} may be lower in gas-exchange units at the periphery of the acinus than in its central parts because O_2 is being extracted from the air all along the acinar pathway; this could well contribute to ventilation-perfusion mismatch that is one of the limiting factors of gas exchange. The theoretical analysis of such a model of series ventilation and parallel perfusion of the gas-exchange units of an acinus suggests strongly that the P_{O_2} profile should fall along the pathway and that the slope of this profile should depend on the absolute length of the pathway, as shown in Fig. 2-66, with the result that the mean P_{AO_2} could well be lower in larger lungs.

The only evidence in support of this concept relates to the length of the acinar pathway. Figure 2-67 shows that the length of this pathway depends strongly on body size, being about seven times longer in humans than in the mouse. Preliminary measurements indicate that the acinar pathway length, the distance to be covered mostly by diffusion of O_2 in the air phase, increases with body mass to the power 0.2. It is noteworthy that the difference between the scaling factors for D_{LO_2} and $\dot{V}_{O_2}$ is also about 0.2. Measurements of both P_{AO_2} and P_{cO_2} are therefore necessary before rejecting the notion of a structure-function match in the lung.

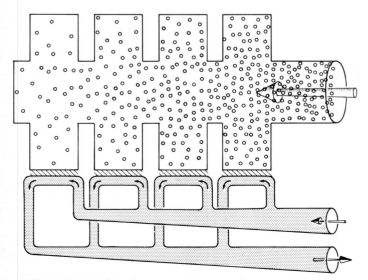

FIGURE 2-65 Model of acinar pathway with gas-exchange units in series ventilation parallel perfusion arrangement.

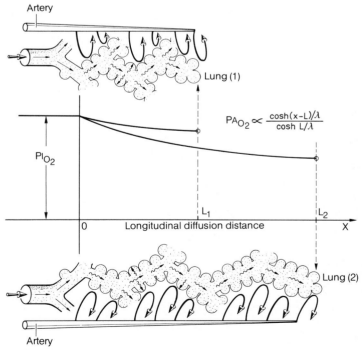

FIGURE 2-66 Model to show how the different acinar pathway length could—hypothetically—cause size-dependent differences in mean alveolar P_{O_2}. (*After Weibel, Taylor, Gehr, Hoppeler, Mathieu, Maloiy: Respir Physiol 44:151–164, 1981*).

THE P$_{O_2}$ OF THE BLOOD AS IT TRAVERSES THE LUNG:
COMBINING STRUCTURAL AND FUNCTIONAL MEASUREMENTS

As the blood flows through the lung capillaries, its P$_{O_2}$ increases from mixed venous to arterial P$_{O_2}$ as a function of O$_2$ uptake. The time course of the P$_{O_2}$ increase is determined by the diffusing capacity D$_{L_{O_2}}$, by the properties of hemoglobin, and by the P$_{O_2}$ of mixed venous and alveolar blood, as well as the rate of O$_2$ uptake. Figure 2-68 shows that the transit time, calculated by dividing capillary volume by cardiac output, becomes shorter as $\dot{V}_{O_2}$ increases;

at $\dot{V}_{O_2max}$ it is about 0.3 s. Accordingly, loading the O$_2$ onto the blood is completed at rest well before the blood leaves the capillary, both in dogs and in goats. However, at $\dot{V}_{O_2max}$, the dog uses all its capillary length for oxygen uptake so that its blood just reaches the P$_{O_2}$ of arterial blood as it exits from the lung (Fig. 2-68). In contrast, goat blood reaches arterial P$_{O_2}$ long before it leaves the lung; only about one-third of the lung appears to be utilized for oxygen uptake even at $\dot{V}_{O_2max}$ (Fig. 2-68). If these calculations for the goat are correct, then it should be possible to

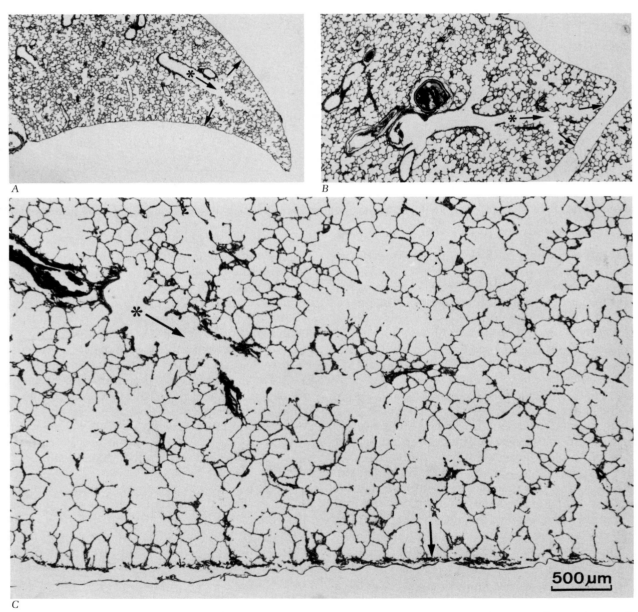

FIGURE 2-67 Acinar pathways in (*A*) mouse, (*B*) rat, and (*C*) human lungs recorded at same magnification. Asterisk marks center of acinus at end of terminal bronchiole, and arrow marks a terminal alveolus beneath the pleura. (*From Weibel, 1984a.*)

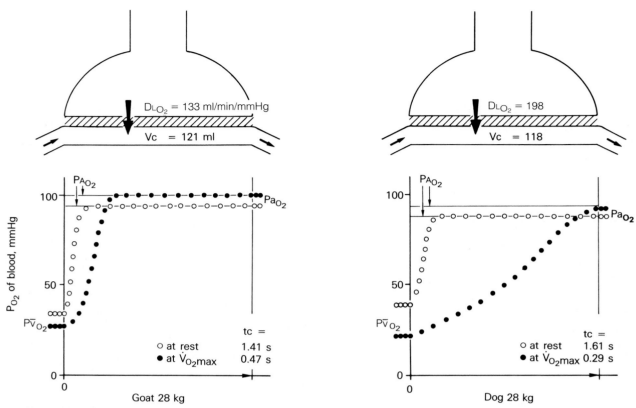

FIGURE 2-68 Bohr integrals of P_{O_2} for blood passing through the pulmonary capillaries in goat and dog, at rest and at exercise, respectively.

decrease the pressure head for diffusion of oxygen drastically without reducing oxygen flow across the lung. In fact, using the morphometric value for $D_{L_{O_2}}$, it seems reasonable to predict that there will be excess diffusing capacity for O_2 across the lung until alveolar P_{O_2} is reduced to approximately 40 mmHg. In recent studies, this prediction was tested by reducing the inspired P_{O_2} of goats exercising at $\dot{V}_{O_2max}$: it was found that $\dot{V}_{O_2max}$ did not decrease until alveolar and arterial P_{O_2} dropped to approximately 40 mmHg; at this P_{O_2} capillary blood equilibrated with alveolar air just prior to leaving the lung.

These hypoxia experiments in the goat help support the validity of the morphometric model for calculating diffusing capacity. Similar calculations can be made for humans exercising at $\dot{V}_{O_2max}$, both at sea level and at altitude: the human lung, like that of the goat, appears to have two to three times as much capacity as it utilizes for maximal oxygen uptake at sea level. However, the entire diffusing capacity of the lungs is needed at altitudes of about 3000 m.

To What "Function" Is Lung Structure Matched, If to Any?

The lung appears to be matched to its main functional task, the uptake of O_2. On this basis, as indicated above, the hypothesis of *symmorphosis* was formulated by

Weibel and Taylor in 1981. This hypothesis proposes that all structures—including the components of the respiratory system—are gauged or adapted to the functional demand imposed on them; moreover this adaptation should be revealed when the system operates at its limit. Although this hypothesis was found to apply to the mitochondria of working muscles and also to the muscle capillaries when related to $\dot{V}_{O_2max}$, the relationship was limited for heart muscle where, instead of being closely related to the $\dot{V}_{O_2max}$ of the whole body, the mitochondrial content appears to be more closely related to the work of the heart at $\dot{V}_{O_2max}$. This is an important new insight because it indicates that functional demand may be a complex function rather than a simple parameter such as $\dot{V}_{O_2max}$.

With respect to the lung, the picture is rather complicated. Only in two instances, in the dog and in the pony, has the diffusing capacity of the lung matched the $\dot{V}_{O_2max}$. In all other instances, the lung appears to have excess diffusing capacity. This was particularly true for the goat (Fig. 2-68). These observations indicate that the lungs can maintain $\dot{V}_{O_2max}$ even at appreciable levels of hypoxia.

Why does this excess diffusing capacity exist in humans, for example? Perhaps it results from the design of the lung being determined during growth when the rate of oxygen uptake is higher. If $D_{L_{O_2}}$ remained the same, while cardiac output doubled with training, then a match is approximated between structure and function: transit time is halved, and almost all of the diffusing capacity of the lungs is utilized. This interpretation is supported by measurements of arterial P_{O_2} which begin to fall at $\dot{V}_{O_2max}$ in the most highly trained athletes. So the human lung is perhaps adapted to levels of aerobic work much higher than what we "normal civilized adults" usually perform.

In this respect it is important to note one fundamental difference between the mitochondria of muscle cells and the gas exchanger of the lung. Muscle mitochondria can be increased by intense training even in adult humans or in mature animals. However, the lung is adaptable only during the early growth phase (cf. Chapter 3); no additional alveolar surface or alveolar capillary volume can be formed at later stages. So the lung may be well designed if it sets up, during early growth, a capacity for O_2 transfer which is matched to "potential O_2 needs" in the adult, a contention that is perhaps supported by the observation made above with respect to diffusion limitation of $\dot{V}_{O_2}$ in highly trained athletes.

Alternatively, the design of the lung may not be simply related to $\dot{V}_{O_2max}$. Instead, it may have to satisfy more complex functions. It has been noted above that the driving force for O_2 diffusion may have to be considered and that this important parameter may depend on lung size. Furthermore, the lung must allow the entire cardiac output to pass its capillary bed; the mean capillary transit time is determined by the ratio of the capillary volume to cardiac output. So an additional functional requirement is that the capillary transit time must be adjusted to the O_2-hemoglobin reaction rate of the blood.

It is evident there is no easy explanation for the disparity of the findings on the structure-function relationships. However, the notion that the design of the lung is adapted to functional requirements remains attractive because observations on pulmonary disease have shown that respiratory function becomes rapidly impaired when an appreciable part of the lung's potential for O_2 uptake is lost. Therefore, it seems worthwhile to gain a deeper understanding of the factors that determine how much lung and how much diffusing capacity is needed to sustain life under various conditions. This is a great challenge, one that has to be met by looking beyond the lung and considering it as an essential and critical part of the respiratory system.

ACKNOWLEDGMENTS

The discussion on structure-function match includes new results obtained notably by Richard Karas, James Jones, Kevin Conley, and Hans Hoppeler, published after completion of this manuscript. We gratefully acknowledge the assistance by Ms. G. Reber.

BIBLIOGRAPHY

Agostini E: Mechanics of the pleural space. Physiol Rev 52:57–128, 1972.
Reviews the forces acting between thoracic and visceral pleura and the distribution of pressures.

Bachofen M, Weibel ER: Alterations of the gas exchange apparatus in adult respiratory insufficiency associated with septicemia. Am Rev Resp Dis 116:589–615, 1977.
Electron microscope study of lung tissue changes in different stages of human ARDS.

Bachofen M, Gehr P, Weibel ER: Alterations of mechanical properties and morphology in excised rabbit lungs rinsed with a detergent. J Appl Physiol 47:1002–1010, 1979.
Demonstrates the importance of low surface tension for stabilizing alveoli.

Bienenstock J, Clancy RL, Perey DYE: Bronchus-associated lymphoid tissue (BALT): Its relation to mucosal immunity, in Kirkpatrick CH, Reynolds HY (eds), *Lung Biology in Health and Disease, vol 1, Immunologic and Infectious Reactions in the Lung.* New York, Dekker, 1976, pp 29–58.
Reviews the origin, distribution, and makeup of lymphoid tissue in the lung, and its contribution to immune defense.

Brain JD, Proctor DF, Reid LM: *Respiratory Defense Mechanisms.* New York, Dekker, 1977.
Monograph with chapters reviewing all aspects of respiratory defense, from phagocytosis to immune defense.

Burri PH: Lung development and histogenesis, in Fishman AP, Fisher AB (eds), *Handbook of Physiology: The Respiratory System I.* Washington, American Physiological Society, 1985, pp 1–46.
Reviews the pre- and postnatal development of the lung with an emphasis on tissue transformation in view of building alveoli and capillaries. References.

Clements JA, Hustead RF, Johnson RP, Bribetz I: Pulmonary surface tension and alveolar stability. J Appl Physiol 16:444–450, 1961.
Classic paper demonstrating variable surface tension and its role in stabilizing alveoli.

Clements JA, King RJ: Composition of the surface active material, in Crystal RG (ed), *Lung Biology in Health and Disease,* vol 2, *The Biochemical Basis of Pulmonary Function.* New York, Dekker, 1976, pp 363–387.
  Reviews composition, function, and biochemistry of pulmonary surfactant.

Crapo JD, Barry BE, Gehr P, Bachofen M, Weibel ER: Cell number and cell characteristics of the normal human lung. Am Rev Respir Dis 125:332–337, 1982.
  Evaluates the human lung cell population morphometrically.

Dejours P: *Principles of Comparative Respiratory Physiology,* 2d ed. Amsterdam, Elsevier North-Holland, 1981.
  Extensive and in-depth review of respiratory physiology, particularly of the insight gained by taking a comparative approach, extending it to nonmammalian systems.

Fox B, Bull TB, Guz A: Innervation of alveolar walls in the human lung: An electron microscopic study. J Anat 131:683–692, 1980.
  Describes the occurrence and morphology of nerve fibers in lung parenchyma.

Fung YB, Sobin S: Pulmonary alveolar blood flow, in West JB (ed), *Bioengineering Aspects of the Lung.* New York, Dekker, 1977, pp. 267–359.
  Discusses mechanics of the pulmonary capillaries and its functional consequences on blood flow, proposing sheet flow concept.

Gehr P, Bachofen M, Weibel ER: The normal human lung: Ultrastructure and morphometric estimation of diffusion capacity. Respir Physiol 32:121–140, 1978.
  Describes the fine structure and morphometry of normal human lungs and estimates their diffusing capacities.

Gluck L, Kulovich MV, Eidelman AI, Cordero L, Khazin AF: Biochemical development of surface activity in mammalian lung. VI. Pulmonary lecithin synthesis in the human fetus and newborn and etiology of the respiratory distress syndrome. Pediatric Res 6:81–99, 1972.
  Describes possibilities to assess fetal lung maturity from biochemical analysis of amniotic fluid.

Gomez DM: A physico-mathematical study of lung function in normal subjects and in patients with obstructive pulmonary diseases. Med Thorac 22:275–294, 1965.
  Discusses on theoretical grounds the relative role of mass airflow and diffusion to get O_2 into the alveoli.

Guntheroth WG, Luchtel DL, Kawabori I: Pulmonary microcirculation: Tubules rather than sheet and post. J Appl Physiol 53:510–515, 1982.
  Demonstrates architecture of pulmonary capillary network by scanning electron microscopy.

Hitchcock KR: Lung development and the pulmonary surfactant system: hormonal influences. Anat Rec 198:13–34, 1980.
  Experimental study on the influence of steroid hormones on fetal lung maturation, particularly with respect to the onset of surfactant synthesis.

Holland RAB, Van Hezewijk W, Zubazanda J: Velocity of oxygen uptake by partly saturated adult and fetal human red cells. Respir Physiol 29:303–314, 1977.
  Estimates O_2 uptake velocity of human blood, leading to calculation of coefficient θ_{O_2}.

Hoppeler H, Lindstedt SL: Malleability of skeletal muscle tissue in overcoming limitations: Structural elements. J Exp Biol 115:355–364, 1985.
  Discusses the adaptation of muscle fibers, their mitochondria, and their capillaries, to different levels of functional demand.

Hoppin FG, Hildebrandt H: Mechanical properties of the lung, in West JB (ed), *Bioengineering Aspects of the Lung.* New York, Dekker, 1977, pp 83–162.
  Reviews lung mechanics from a physiological point of view. References.

Horsfield K, Dart G, Olson DE, Filley GF, Cumming G: Models of the human bronchial tree. J Appl Physiol 31:207–217, 1971.
  Describes models of the bronchial tree based on "orders up" concept.

Kapanci Y, Assimacopoulos A, Irle C, Zwahlen A, Gabbiani G: "Contractile interstitial cells" in pulmonary alveolar septa: A possible regulator of ventilation/perfusion ratio? Ultrastructural immunofluorescence and in vitro studies. J Cell Biol 60:375–392, 1974.
  Describes the occurrence and distribution of contractile fibrils in pulmonary interstitial cells, and proposes one possible interpretation of their role.

Karas RH, Taylor CR, Jones JH, Reeves RB, Weibel ER: Adaptive variation in the respiratory system in relation to energetic demand. VII. Flow of oxygen across the pulmonary gas exchanger. Respir Physiol 69:101–115, 1987.
  Compares gas exchange in dogs and goats by Bohr integration.

King RJ: Utilization of alveolar epithelial type II cells for the study of pulmonary surfactant. Fed Proc 38:2637–2643, 1979.
  Discusses biochemical pathways for surfactant synthesis.

Kleiber M: *The Fire of Life: An Introduction to Animal Energetics.* New York, Wiley, 1961.
  Classic monograph summarizing the author's extensive investigations into the dependency of metabolic rate and related functions on body size.

Lauweryns JM, Baert JH: Alveolar clearance and the role of the pulmonary lymphatics. Am Rev Resp Dis 115:625–683, 1977.
  Detailed description of the pulmonary lymphatics.

Mead J: Mechanical properties of lungs. Physiol Rev 41:281–330, 1961.
  Classic review of the relative importance of tissue and surface forces for lung mechanics.

Pedley TJ, Schroter RC, Sudlow MF: The prediction of pressure drop and variation of resistance within the human bronchial airways. Respir Physiol 9:387–405, 1970.
  Locates major airway resistance in conducting airways.

Piiper J, Scheid P: Comparative physiology of respiration: Functional analysis of gas exchange organs in vertebrates. Int Rev Physiol 14:219–253, 1977.
  Reviews the biophysical basis and the efficiency of fish gills and bird lungs in comparison to the mammalian lung.

Rahn H, Fenn WO: *A Graphical Analysis of Respiratory Gas Exchange.* Washington DC, American Physiological Society 1955, pp 1–38.
  Classic concept of the respiratory system and its integral functioning. O_2-CO_2 diagram.

Ryan US, Ryan JW: Correlations between the fine structure of the alveolar-capillary unit and its metabolic activities, in Bakhle YS, Vane JR (eds), *Metabolic Functions of the Lung.* New York, Dekker, 1977, pp 197–232.
  Describes metabolic the roles of pulmonary endothelial cells, particularly angiotension conversion. References.

Saltin B, Gollnick PD: Skeletal muscle adaptability: Significance for metabolism and performance, in Peachy LD, Adrian RH, Geiger SR (eds), *Handbook of Physiology. Skeletal Muscle.* Baltimore, Williams & Wilkins, 1983, pp 555–631.
  Extensive review of the functional and structural changes induced in muscle by exercise training. References.

Schmidt-Nielsen K: Scaling. *Why Is Animal Size So Important?* Cambridge, University Press, 1984.
  Explores the basic approach of allometry to find dependencies of various functions on body mass.

Schürch S, Goerke J, Clements JA: Direct determination of volume and time dependence of alveolar surface tension in excised lungs. Proc Nat Acad Sci USA 75:3417–3421, 1978.
  Direct measurement of local surface tension in alveoli by microscopic method, showing its variability.

Sleigh MA: The nature and action of respiratory tract cilia, in Brain JD, Proctor DF, Reid LM (eds), *Respiratory Defense Mechanisms,* part I. New York, Dekker, 1977, pp 247–288.
  Molecular structure and function of kinocilia with an emphasis on bronchial mucosa.

Stahl W: Scaling of respiratory variables in mammals. J Appl Physiol 22:453–460, 1967.
  Analyzes the dependency on body mass of a large range of physiological variables related to respiration, computing allometric regressions.

Stossel TP: The mechanism of phagocytosis. J Reticuloendothel Soc 19:237–245, 1976.
  Describes the fundamental process of phagocytosis by cells, particularly by macrophages.

Taylor CR, Karas RH, Weibel ER, Hoppeler H: Adaptive variation in the mammalian respiratory system in relation to energetic demand. Respir Physiol 69:1–127, 1987.
  A series of eight papers assessing the contributions made by structural and functional parameters of the entire respiratory system from lung to mitochondria in increasing the aerobic potential in "athletic" mammalian species, dogs and ponies.

Wagner DD, Olmsted JB, Marder VJ: Immunolocalization of von Willebrand protein in Weibel-Palade bodies of human endothelial cells. J Cell Biol 95:355–360, 1982.
Identifies von Willebrand factor as main content of specific endothelial granules.

Weibel ER: *Morphometry of the Human Lung.* Heidelberg, Springer, 1963.
Besides a general approach to lung morphometry, a model for the bronchial tree is developed (Chapter 11).

Weibel ER: Morphometric estimation of pulmonary diffusion capacity. I. Model and method. Respir Physiol 11:54–75, 1970/71.
Proposes model and method for estimating pulmonary diffusing capacity from morphometric data.

Weibel ER: *Stereological Methods, vol 1, Practical Methods for Biological Morphometry.* London, Academic, 1979.
Review of stereologic methods, with technical details and references.

Weibel ER: *The Pathway for Oxygen.* Cambridge, Harvard University, 1984a.
Puts the lung into the perspective of the respiratory system and the demand of the body set by the energy needs of working cells. Chapters 8 to 12 expand on development, cell biology, airways and blood vessels, lung mechanics, and the lung as gas exchanger. References.

Weibel ER: Lung cell biology, in Fishman AP, Fisher AB (eds), *Handbook of Physiology, sec. 3: The Respiratory System, vol I: Circulation and Nonrespiratory Functions.* Washington, American Physiological Society, 1984b, pp 47–91.
Expands on the morphology and function of the cell population of the lung. Extensive references.

Weibel ER: Functional morphology of lung parenchyma, in Macklem P, Mead J (eds), *Handbook of Physiology, sec. 3: The Respiratory System, vol III: Mechanics of Breathing, part 1.* Washington, American Physiological Society, 1986, pp 89–111.
A comprehensive review of pulmonary morphology as it relates to pulmonary mechanics.

Weibel ER, Palade GE: New cytoplasmic components in arterial endothelia. J Cell Biol 23:101–112, 1964.
Description of specific granules of endothelium.

Weibel ER, Gil J: Structure-function relationships at the alveolar level, in West JB (ed), *Bioengineering Aspects of the Lung.* New York, Dekker, 1977, pp 1–81.
Attempts to establish the interdependence of lung mechanics and tissue design of pulmonary parenchyma.

Weibel ER, Marques LB, Constantinopol M, Doffey F, Gehr P, Taylor CR: Adaptive variation in the mammalian respiratory system in relation to energetic demand. V. The pulmonary gas exchanger. Respir Physiol 69:81–100, 1987.
Shows that "athletic" animals achieve a higher maximal O_2 consumption by increasing the diffusing capacity and the pressure head for diffusion.

Weibel ER, Taylor CR: Design of the mammalian respiratory system. Respir Physiol 44:1–164, 1981.
A series of nine papers investigating the match between maximal O_2 flow rate (III) and the structures for O_2 diffusion from the lung (V) to mitochondria (VII) and capillaries (VIII) in muscle, based on a study of African mammals ranging from 500 g to 250 kg in body mass.

West JB: Stresses, in West JB (ed), *Regional Differences in the Lung.* New York, Academic, 1977, pp 281–322.
Reviews the distribution of forces in the lung as they affect alveoli and capillaries.

West JB, Wagner PD: Pulmonary gas exchange, in West JB (ed), *Bioengineering Aspects of the Lung.* New York, Dekker, 1977, pp. 361–457.
Reviews extensively the physiological basis for gas exchange in the lung, discussing particularly the effects of ventilation-perfusion inequality.

Wilson TA, Bachofen H: A model for mechanical structure of the alveolar duct. J Appl Physiol 52:1064–1070, 1982.
Proposes a new model for the mechanics of pulmonary parenchyma, linking the effects of surface and tissue forces.

Chapter 3

Development and Regeneration of the Lung

Peter H. Burri

DEVELOPMENT AND GROWTH OF THE LUNG

The onset of respiration at birth represents a major caesura in pulmonary development. However, because development of the lung is a continuous process which proceeds from early fetal life into postnatal life (Fig. 3-1), it is a step that is more dramatic functionally than structurally.

The staging of pulmonary development is based on the morphologic changes that the prospective airway system undergoes. Because maturation proceeds metachronically from the proximal to the peripheral portions of the airway tree, there can be considerable overlap between the stages. Figure 3-1 also illustrates that although the beginning of pulmonary development can be relatively clearly defined by the first appearance of the future trachea, there is no clear limit as to when it ends during childhood: the age at which alveolar formation stops is unknown; furthermore, even after alveolization is completed, the gas-exchanging tissues undergo a process of maturation that is open-ended with respect to the age of the lung.

Organogenesis

Following fertilization, the germ cells soon segregate into a cluster of trophoblastic cells to which a few embryoblastic cells adhere. Figuratively, the trophoblastic cells may be viewed as the future placenta, whereas the embryoblastic cells, after differentiating into the three germ layers, will form the human embryo.

Most organs are destined to be laid down between the fourth and eighth week after fertilization by differentiation from the germ layers. This generalization also applies to the lungs, which appear around the 26th day of gestation as a ventral bud of the foregut. In the region of the future esophagus, two lateral grooves, the "laryngotracheal sulci," deepen, join each other, and separate the lung bud from the gut except in its most proximal part, the prospective hypopharynx. The bud rapidly divides di-

FETAL AND POSTNATAL LUNG DEVELOPMENT AND GROWTH

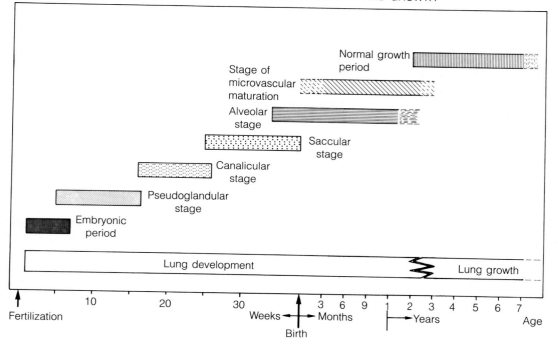

FIGURE 3-1 Stages of human lung development and their timing. Note overlapping between stages, particularly between the alveolar stage and the newly introduced stage of microvascular maturation. Open-ended bars indicate uncertainty as to exact timing. *(From Zeltner and Burri, 1987.)*

chotomously, and both branches grow into the surrounding mesenchyme. The process of dichotomous division is repeated many times, and the future airways, covered by mesenchyme, push into the primitive pleuroperitoneal cavity. It is interesting to note that at this stage the tubular branching pattern already reflects the hierarchy of the future conducting airways. The lobar bronchi are formed by the 37th day; 4 days later all the segmental bronchi are laid down.

As is evident from the above description, the high columnar epithelium of the tubular sprouts is of endodermal origin, whereas the mesenchyme is derived from the third germ layer, the mesoderm. This double origin of lung tissues is critical, since the entire development of the lungs seems to be characterized by a unique interaction between epithelium and mesenchyme. Indeed, removal of mesenchyme from the tip of a bud in these early phases of development and transplanting it to the side of a higher-ordered segment abolishes further branching at the tip and induces a new branch at the site of transplantation. Later on, during maturation of the surfactant system, the interplay between differentiating pneumocytes and mesodermally derived interstitial cells seems again to be decisive. Recently the possibility has been raised that contacts between epithelial and mesenchymal cells continue to regulate type II cell proliferation and differentiation in the postnatal period.

During the fourth week of gestation the heart starts to beat, the first organ to assume its function in the embryo. The development of the pulmonary vessels takes advantage of the earlier development of the systemic circulatory system. The pulmonary arteries develop as buds from the sixth pair of aortic arches and connect to the vascular plexus forming in the pulmonary mesenchyme. The sixth left and right aortic branches are destined to pursue different pathways of development (Fig. 3-2): whereas the proximal (ventral) parts of the arches will be integrated into the pulmonary arterial tree to form permanent parts of the pulmonary vasculature, the distal or dorsal parts will disappear completely on the right side and form the Botallo's ductus arteriosus on the left side. By connecting the pulmonary artery to the aortic arch, the ductus arteriosus enables the right ventricular output to bypass the pulmonary vascular bed during fetal life. Shortly after birth the duct closes, redirecting the entire cardiac output to the lungs.

The pulmonary veins are derived from a single evagination of the left atrium, which divides several times and connects to the pulmonary vascular bed. Subsequently, the original bud and its first- and second-order branches are fully incorporated into the left atrium, so that finally, from each lung, a pair of veins delivers the oxygenated blood to the left heart.

At around 7 weeks the period of organogenesis can be considered as merging imperceptibly with the period of lung development.

Fetal Lung Development

This period lasts till birth and comprises three phases of development, the names of which are derived from the changing morphology of the airway tubes: pseudoglandular, canalicular, and terminal sac (or saccular).

PSEUDOGLANDULAR STAGE

From the fifth week to the end of the 16th week the developing lung looks like a tubular gland; this is the pseudoglandular stage (Fig. 3-3). Until the end of this stage, the tubular tree preforms, through growth and branching, all the conductive airways down to their last generations, i.e., to the future terminal bronchioles.

According to Boyden, transition to the next stage is determined by the first appearance of the pulmonary acinus. Although this transition is well defined, a precise estimation of gestational age cannot be made from it. This is because differentiation usually proceeds centrifugally and the speed of growth varies during a developmental period, accelerating toward the end of a stage. Furthermore, animal studies have shown that upper lobes develop faster than lower lobes; in humans, the difference between the times of development of the lobes of the lungs can be estimated to be of the order of 2 weeks.

Proximally, the airway tubes are lined by a very high columnar epithelium. The height of the cells decreases

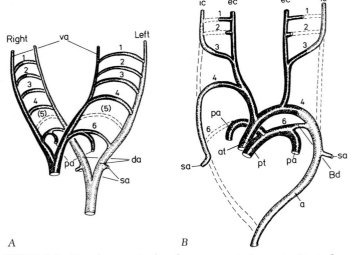

FIGURE 3-2 Development of pulmonary arteries. A. Ventral arteries (va) and dorsal arteries (da) are interconnected by six pairs of aortic arches numbered 1 to 6. Pulmonary arteries (pa) bud off from sixth pair of aortic arches and grow into the nearby pulmonary mesenchyme. Notice that formation of the aortic arches is sequential; they are never present simultaneously. Furthermore, the fifth pair is never formed. sa = subclavian artery. B. Fate of developing arterial vessels. Some segments regress and disappear (white); others develop and grow preferentially. a = aorta; at = aortic trunk; pa = pulmonary artery; pt = pulmonary trunk; Bd = Botallo's ductus arteriosus; ec = external carotid artery; ic = internal carotid artery; sa = subclavian artery.

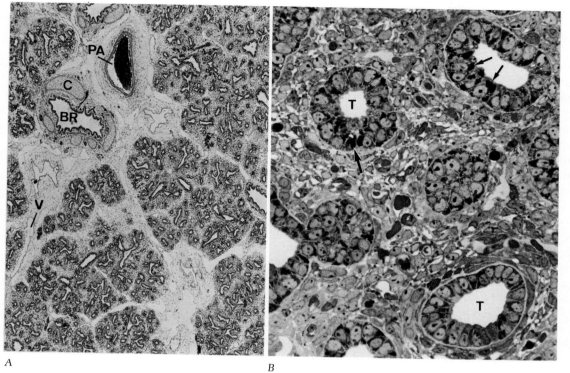

A

B

FIGURE 3-3 Pseudoglandular stage of human lung. *A.* Gestational age 15 weeks. Clear bands of loose mesenchyme containing veins (V) indicate septation of lung into segments and lobules. Denser mesenchyme surrounds the tubular sprouts. PA = pulmonary artery; BR = bronchus with embryonal cartilage (C). Light micrograph, ×25. *B.* Higher magnification of pseudoglandular stage in rat lung. Tubules (T) are lined by high columnar epithelium with large amounts of glycogen (dark spots, arrows). The mesenchyme is highly cellular and contains a loose capillary meshwork. Light micrograph. ×450.

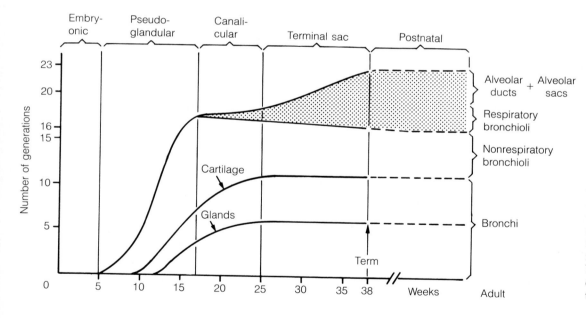

FIGURE 3-4 Timetable of airway development. The diagram from Bucher and Reid (1961) has been modified to fit the dichotomous airway tree model of Weibel (1963). The respiratory portion of the airway system represented by the dotted area develops between week 16 and birth, mostly by centrifugal growth and branching. A few generations of respiratory branches may be formed by centripetal transformation of nonrespiratory into respiratory bronchioles.

continuously toward the periphery, reaching a cuboidal shape in the terminal branches. Mitotic figures are common. The cytoplasmic organellar machinery looks relatively simple: mitochondria, many free ribosomes and a little rough endoplasmic reticulum, some lipid droplets, and large patches of glycogen. Remarkably, the epithelial barrier appears to be tight from the early stages of development: in freeze-fracture preparations, the morphology of the junctional complexes does not differ during development to full term; conversely, gap junctions are present early in gestation and disappear during the canalicular stage as the epithelial cells differentiate. Therefore, it may be that electrical coupling between cells plays a role in cellular differentiation.

The first ciliated goblet and basal cells appear in the central airways. Similarly, cartilage and smooth-muscle cells are found first in the trachea, in condensed areas of the mesenchyme. From the trachea, differentiation spreads toward the periphery so that cartilage is commonly found in the main bronchi around week 10 and in segmental bronchi in week 12 of gestation (Fig. 3-4). However, cartilage formation continues almost up to the end of the canalicular stage.

Mucous glands and goblet cells appear almost simultaneously in the airway epithelium. They develop from solid epithelial sprouts that invade the mesenchyme underneath the epithelium. At around weeks 12 to 13 (Fig. 3-4), mucous glands are found in bronchi, and at week 14, mucus formation can be detected in the trachea.

During the pseudoglandular stage, the vascular system develops along with the bronchial tree, so that by the end of this stage all the preacinar vessels, arteries, and veins have assumed the characteristic pattern of the adult lung. In principle, arteries follow airway branching rather closely, whereas the veins run interaxially, within the mesenchyme, where they demarcate future segments and subsegments. However, the average number of generations in the arterial tree is greater than in the airway system: on the average, more than 28 generations in the arterial tree versus 23 in the airways. In addition to the conventional arteries that follow the bronchi and bronchioles, there are other branches, i.e., "supernumerary" arteries, that split off at right angles. Usually these branches are smaller vessels which irrigate the "recurrent" gas-exchange tissue adjacent to the conducting airways.

CANALICULAR STAGE

The canalicular stage lasts from week 17 to week 26 and comprises the most important steps in the development of the fetal lung. During this stage, lung morphology changes dramatically, due primarily to the differentiation of the pulmonary epithelium, the formation of the typical air-blood barrier, and the beginning of surfactant synthesis and secretion. These alterations have most important functional consequences: at the end of the canalicular stage, the lung has reached a stage of development that, in principle, enables it to exchange gas. Before these developmental steps, a prematurely born infant has no chance to survive. However, as clinical experience unfortunately shows, at the end of the canalicular stage survival is by no means assured.

At the beginning of this stage, the future gas-exchange region of the lung can be distinguished from the conductive tubules of the airway tree. Boyden has characterized this step as "birth of the acinus," i.e., the transition from the pseudoglandular to the canalicular stage. This early acinus is composed of several, very short generations of tubules arranged in clusters and taking origin from the last segment of the conducting airways, a prospective terminal bronchiole. The acinar borders are recognizable because of rarefaction of the mesenchyme (Fig. 3-3A). At this stage in mice, immunofluorescent techniques have also disclosed precursors of the type II cell at the periphery of the airway tree.

In the subsequent weeks, the distal segments of the airways grow in length and widen at the expense of the mesenchymal mass. The cuboidal, glycogen-rich epithelium lining the tubules starts to flatten out: in some cells the junctional complexes localized around the cell apex are shifted to the lower half of the intercellular clefts. Where this happens, the cell develops cytoplasmic attenuations that soon become so thin that they are invisible under the light microscope (Fig. 3-5). No wonder a controversy went on for years about whether the airspaces of mature lungs were lined by a continuous epithelium. This problem was rapidly solved by the first electron-microscope investigations of the lung by Low in the early 1950s.

Important changes in the microvasculature accompany, or even precede, the attenuation of the epithelium. The capillaries, which originally form a three-dimensional network in the mesenchyme, rearrange around the tubules, and it seems that, where capillaries come into close contact with epithelium, the cuboidal cells differentiate into type I cells. In this way, the first, thin portions of the future air-blood barrier are formed. The mechanisms responsible for this process are unknown: whether the capillary contact initiates differentiation of the epithelium, or vice versa, is an open question. Nonetheless, it

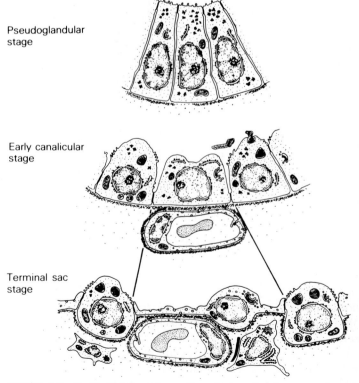

Pseudoglandular stage

Early canalicular stage

Terminal sac stage

FIGURE 3-5 Epithelial transformation during development. In the pseudoglandular phase the columnar epithelium is tall. During the canalicular phase two cell types appear: the prospective secretory and lining cells. *(From Burri and Weibel, 1977.)*

seems very likely that the two events are linked since they coincide so closely in time.

The epithelial cells that remain cuboidal develop into type II cells, the secretory cells of the peripheral airspaces that will produce the pulmonary surfactant. Within their cytoplasm, these cells accumulate groups of lamellated bodies that, in turn, are often associated with multivesicular bodies. Lamellar bodies correspond to the intracellular storage form of the surface-active material present in the alveolar surfactant. Therefore, in all species, the appearance of lamellated bodies in type II cells precedes the presence of surfactant material in the airspaces. In most mammals lamellated bodies appear when pregnancy is about 80 to 85 percent over. In humans, the lamellated bodies are already present at about 60 percent of total gestation time, i.e., during the sixth month of development.

Type II cells are also the progenitor cells of the type I cells in adult lungs. Therefore, it is not surprising that a few, small, lamellated bodies have been found in the cytoplasm of immature epithelial cells *before* they start to differentiate into type I or type II cells, respectively. In cytokinetic experiments using tritiated thymidine, it has been shown that during lung development, early type II cells, i.e., cells resembling type II cells, represent the stem cells of the type I and type II pulmonary epithelium.

At the outer edges of the airspaces, the cuboidal cells of the epithelium remain undifferentiated. Almost until birth, the last airway generations continue to grow and to branch, a process obviously requiring an immature epithelium that can even persist beyond birth (Fig. 3-6). Throughout this stage, the blood vessels grow in length and diameter, and new branches follow the developing peripheral airway tree.

TERMINAL SAC, OR SACCULAR, STAGE

This stage lasts from about week 24 to almost term. At the beginning of this stage, the peripheral airspaces consist of clusters of saccules. These saccules are commonly referred to as "terminal sacs"; they are destined, however, to give rise to the last generations of airspaces, i.e., on average, three generations of prospective alveolar ducts and one generation of alveolar sacs.

Each new generation of this pathway is originally formed as a blind ending saccule. However, as soon as it divides distally it is no longer a saccule, but an open-ended channel. As is discussed in the section on postnatal development, the morphology of all these channels and saccules undergoes change until the postnatal period when the formation of the alveoli is complete. Therefore, these structures are termed *transitory ducts* and *transitory saccules*, respectively, or more generally, *transitory airways or airspaces*.

Also at this stage, within the mesenchyme, one or two populations of fibroblastic cells have differentiated. Not only are these cell types responsible for the deposition of extracellular matrix and fibers, but they presumably also, by way of interactions with the epithelial cover, play a role in epithelial differentiation and in the control of surfactant secretion.

Owing to the expansion of the canaliculi in the previous stage and of the transitory airways in the present stage, the interstitial tissue is somewhat attenuated. Nonetheless, the intersaccular and interductular septa are still relatively thick and contain two or even three layers of capillaries. The interstitium is highly cellular. Because its content of collagen is low, the fetal lung is delicate and fragile; under mechanical stress, it ruptures much more rapidly than the adult organ.

Finally, in anticipation of the next stage during which the alveoli will be formed, the interstitial cells start to produce elastic fibers along the interductular and intersaccular walls. Elastin is found first in extracellular bays of large fibroblastic cells rich in organelles. The deposits

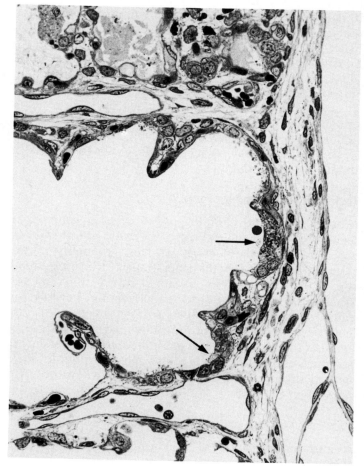

FIGURE 3-6 Periphery of gas-exchange region in human lung aged 26 days. The cuboidal epithelium persists at the uttermost periphery (arrows). Light micrograph, ×425.

later extend throughout the septal walls of the parenchyma, from the peribronchial and perivascular sheaths, to the pleural sac.

Keeping pace with the intense growth of the gas-exchange region during this stage, the vascular tree grows in length and diameter and by adding new generations. Measurements on arteriograms by Hislop have shown that arterial diameter is practically constant at a given distance from the end of the arterial pathway. This is true, irrespective of age, either fetal or postnatal. One practical consequence of this regularity in arterial diameter at a fixed distance from the end is that the vessel of a given size that supplies a larger portion of a lobe in an early fetal lung is apt to supply only an acinus in a child's lung.

In late fetal life, the wall structure of the arteries is similar to that of adult lungs. Proximal arteries are elastic in type with many elastic lamellae strutted to each other by smooth-muscle cells that are arranged obliquely between the elastic sheets. Smaller arterial vessels show a transitional structure, the muscular component becoming increasingly prominent at the expense of the elastic component. Finally, the muscle layer of the media becomes irregular and assumes a spiral configuration. This configuration explains the "partially muscular" arteries seen in histologic sections. Unfortunately, there are no strict relationships between vessel diameter, size of the region supplied, and character of the wall structure; these relationships differ from one pathway to the other.

Intrapulmonary veins are practically devoid of smooth-muscle cells until the end of the canalicular period. In the following weeks, however, a thin muscle layer is formed which, at birth, extends down to vessels of about 100 μm in diameter.

Postnatal Lung Development

Around birth, the complete set of airway generations seems to be present. However, the most peripheral airways are still relatively short. The pulmonary parenchyma consists of several generations of transitory ducts and, as the last generation of each pathway, the transitory saccules. At birth, these structures are on the way to being transformed into alveolar ducts and sacs, respectively, by the process of alveolization. Although recent reports indicate that in humans the formation of alveoli *starts* during late intrauterine life, the alveolar stage of lung development is discussed in this section, because most alveoli (more than 85 percent) are formed after birth.

ALVEOLAR STAGE AND STAGE OF MICROVASCULAR MATURATION

Because of the scarcity of human material properly sampled and fixed for ultrastructural studies, many of the general laws and principles that govern the development of the alveoli have been largely derived from animal studies. Between submission and printing of this chapter, we were able to complete a combined morphologic and morphometric ultrastructural investigation of the lungs of seven children of ages between 1 and 64 months. The study confirmed that, although the timing of events is different in animals and humans, the developmental process involved in alveolar formation and maturation of the lung does not differ in structural essentials. The following description will therefore be based on the rat lung, which has proved to be a particularly useful model in this regard.

At birth the parenchyma of the rat lung consists of smooth walled channels and saccules corresponding to transitory ducts and definitive terminal saccules, respectively. The interductular or intersaccular septa are straight and relatively thick. Three weeks later, the parenchymal structures are much more complex: the septa are slender, and the airspaces are irregularly delineated (Fig. 3-7). This transformation is due to a honeycomblike partitioning of the airspaces into smaller units by a septation process. The newly formed units are the alveoli, and the walls delineating them represent prospective interalveolar septa. The process is nicely visualized by scanning electron microscopy (Fig. 3-8).

Besides alveolization, there is another marked difference between the newborn and the adult rat lung. The relatively thick septa present at birth and after alveolization contain two capillary networks, one on each side of a central layer of connective tissue. In contrast, the septa of the adult lung are not only thinner, but their central axis of connective tissue has disappeared; a single capillary meshwork makes up almost the entire width of the septum. This means that the capillary system has to be completely rearranged after birth.

Morphologic investigations supported by quantitative stereological analyses have led to the following picture of postnatal lung maturation. To begin with, as described above, the newborn rat lung is practically devoid of alveoli. The airspaces correspond to transitory ducts and sacs. The septa between ducts and sacs are called *primary* septa to distinguish them from the *secondary* septa that appear later to form the interalveolar walls. Within the first few days, the lung increases in volume by simple expansion of its airspaces. In the second half of the first postnatal week, the proliferative activity of the cells in the primary septa increases. As a result, a multitude of small ridges and crests appear along the primary septa. These secondary septa subdivide the airspaces into smaller units, the alveoli. As a consequence, the transitory ducts become alveolar ducts, and the terminal saccules become alveolar sacs (Fig. 3-9).

The new partitions increase tremendously the complexity of the airspaces and, hence, the alveolar surface area (Sa). With simple isotropic growth (expansion of airspaces in proportion to the increase in lung volume), Sa would be expected to increase to the two-thirds power of lung volume (VL). As Fig. 3-10 shows, Sa, plotted double

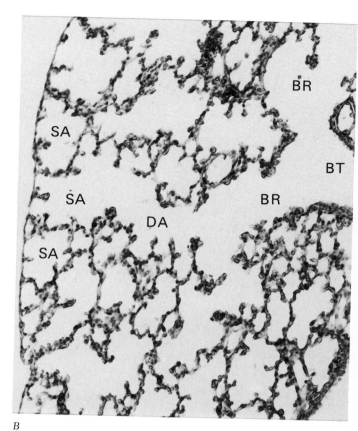

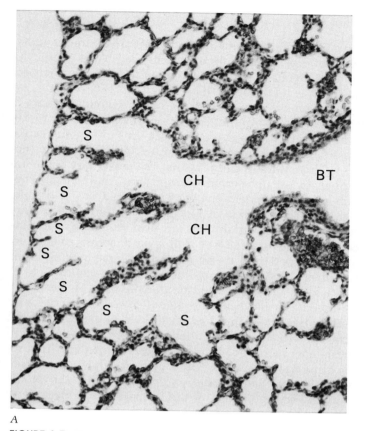

A

B

FIGURE 3-7 Termination portion of the airways of the rat lung. *A.* One day after birth. A terminal bronchiole (BT) divides into smooth-walled channels (CH) which terminate into small airspaces called saccules (S). No true alveoli are present. ×200. This figure can be directly compared with *B,* taken at the same magnification and showing the corresponding structures on postnatal day 17. *B.* Seventeen days. The terminal bronchiole (BT) now opens into respiratory bronchioles (BR). The originally smooth-walled channels have elongated and have transformed into alveolar ducts (DA). The saccules of *A* have been partitioned into alveolar sacs (SA) surrounded by alveoli.

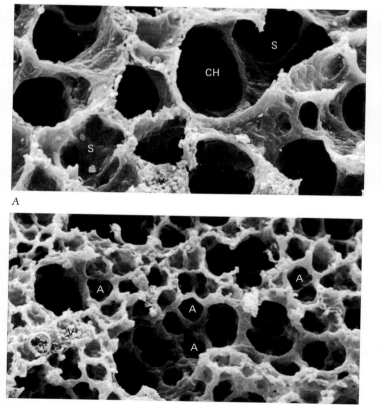

A

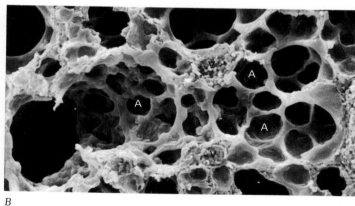

B

C

FIGURE 3-8 Series of scanning electron micrographs taken at the same magnification (×260) showing formation of alveoli. V = blood vessels containing erythrocytes. *A.* Lung parenchyma at day 4. Relatively large holes correspond to smooth-walled channels (CH) or saccules (S). No alveoli are present. *B.* Lung parenchyma at day 8. Within 4 days, numerous small, rounded outpocketings have formed that can now be called alveoli (A). *C.* Lung parenchyma at day 18. Alveoli (A) appear to be deeper and polygonal in shape. More mature aspect of lung parenchyma.

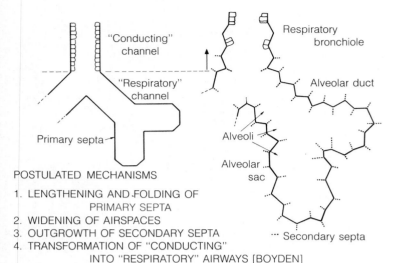

POSTULATED MECHANISMS

1. LENGTHENING AND FOLDING OF PRIMARY SEPTA
2. WIDENING OF AIRSPACES
3. OUTGROWTH OF SECONDARY SEPTA
4. TRANSFORMATION OF "CONDUCTING" INTO "RESPIRATORY" AIRWAYS [BOYDEN]

FIGURE 3-9 The formation of alveoli.

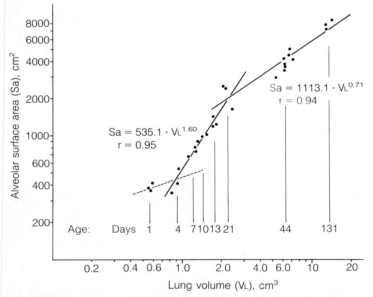

$$Sa = 1113.1 \cdot V_L^{0.71}$$
$$r = 0.94$$

$$Sa = 535.1 \cdot V_L^{1.60}$$
$$r = 0.95$$

FIGURE 3-10 Postnatal increase in "alveolar" surface area. The alveolar surface area (Sa) is plotted double-logarithmically against lung volume (V_L). Steep increase in alveolar surface area between days 4 and 21 corresponds to phase of alveolar formation and septal remodeling. r = correlation coefficient. (*After Burri et al., 1974.*)

logarithmically against lung volume, increases with V_L to the power of 1.6. This high rate of increase in internal surface area is explained by very conspicuous changes in the morphology of the airspaces. In the rat, the septation process is so rapid that the bulk of alveoli are formed within approximately 10 days. However, this does not preclude the formation of additional alveoli later on. Interestingly, the rapid increase in alveolar surface area is paralleled by changes in the subcellular level in type II cells. The total mass of lamellated bodies is augmented in proportion to the increase in the area of the gas-exchang-

ing surface so that lamellar body volume divided by total surface area remains almost unchanged. As a result, the entire respiratory surface is covered with a film of surfactant that is constant in thickness.

It seems that the formation of the secondary septa is closely linked with the deposition of elastic fibers in the primary septa. Indeed, in cross sections of forming septa, elastic tissue can regularly be found in the tip of the septum. This strongly suggests that the secondary septa are formed by an upfolding of tissue from the primary septum, pulling up one of the two capillary layers, as is illustrated by the diagram of Fig. 3-11. Therefore, secondary septa contain invariably, as do primary septa, a double capillary network and a central layer of connective tissue.

The interstitial tissue of postnatal rat lung contains two clearly defined fibroblastic cell types: a cell with lipid inclusions (LIC) that is located at the base of the newly formed crests and has little sign of secretory activity, and a fibroblastic cell that has no lipid vacuoles (NLIC) but does contain a well-developed machinery for protein synthesis and secretion. Whereas the LICs contain lipoprotein lipase and may be the source of this chylomicron-degrading enzyme in the endothelial cells, the NLICs seem to be responsible for the formation of collagen and

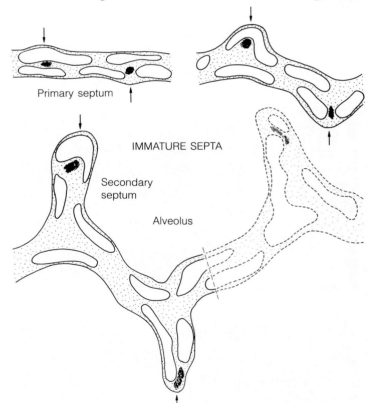

FIGURE 3-11 Formation of secondary septa. Secondary septa are formed by lifting off one of the two capillary layers of the primary septum (arrows). Deposition of elastin (dark spots) is closely linked with alveolar formation. Notice that secondary septa also contain a double capillary network.

elastin. In adult lungs, the LICs apparently have disappeared; their fate is unknown, but it has been speculated that the LICs could represent the progenitors of the contractile interstitial cells of the adult lung.

Shortly prior to, and also during, the onset of septal formation, DNA synthesis increases preferentially in cells located in the region of the forming crests. Autoradiographic studies with H3-thymidine have shown that the rate of DNA synthesis is high first in the mesodermally derived cells, such as the interstitial and endothelial cells; a few days later (at the age of 1 week), type II cells exhibit the highest activity. In the developing—as well as in the adult lung—type I cells proved to be unable to divide. By the age of 2 weeks all labeling indices in the types I and II cells are back to low levels.

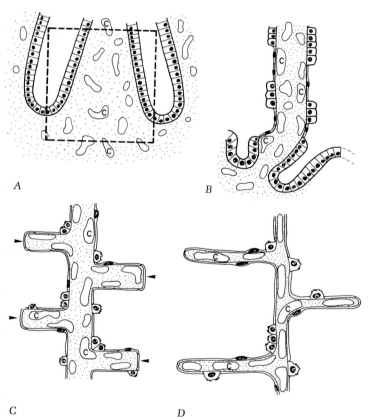

A

B

C

D

FIGURE 3-12 Fetal and postnatal development of the pulmonary capillary bed. *A.* Pseudoglandular stage with capillary network (c). Development of structures within frame is shown in *B* to *D.* *B.* Canalicular stage. Mesenchyme with capillaries is sandwiched between widening canaliculi. Capillaries begin to arrange around canaliculi. At sites of epithelio-capillary contact, thin air-blood barriers develop through differentiation of the epithelium. At the tip of the still-growing canaliculi the cuboidal epithelium is maintained for further branching and growth. *C.* Perinatally, the secondary septa develop from the primary septa (arrowheads). All septa are of the primitive type, i.e., contain a double capillary network (c) and a central layer of connective tissue. *D.* Mature lung with mostly a single capillary network meandering along the interalveolar septa. The interstitial layer is very thin. *(From Burri, 1984.)*

Nonetheless, alveolar surface area continues to increase at a high rate during the third week. It is likely that this further gain in surface area is obtained by restructuring the available tissue mass rather than by further proliferative activity. Such a redistribution of tissue is highly plausible because the morphology of the alveolar septa undergoes marked change during the third week: low and thick septa change to high and slender ones; the double capillary layer disappears in most places; and, despite an increase in the size of the lung, the total mass of interstitium decreases. The reduction in interstitial tissue mass is likely to be functionally linked to capillary restructuring.

A diagram of capillary development during the fetal and postnatal periods may help to clarify the changes in the pulmonary microvasculature. Figure 3-12 illustrates schematically that the loose three-dimensional capillary network formed in early stages of lung development is rearranged around the peripheral airspaces of the canalicular stage. The intervening mesenchyme thins out, bringing the pericanalicular capillary networks of adjacent tubules close together, leading to the formation of the capillary bilayer in the intersaccular septa (Fig. 3-13A). Since the secondary septa that form later also contain a double network, shortly after alveolar formation practically all septa are of the primitive or immature type. It has been assumed that the further thinning of the central interstitial tissue layer could lead to intercapillary contacts and to capillary fusions. This latter process combined with growth would finally end up in the classic adult septal morphology (Fig. 3-13B).

Boyden has postulated an additional mechanism for formation of alveoli: the centripetal transformation of the terminal bronchioles (purely conductive airways) into respiratory bronchioles (gas-exchanging airways). In support of this proposition, Boyden has described a flattening of the cuboidal epithelium in terminal bronchioles followed by local outpocketings of the new air-blood barrier; these first shallow depressions subsequently deepen to form true alveoli. Whether this is a completely different mechanism of alveolization or whether formation of secondary septa also occurs is not yet settled. The consequence of this process is that the average number of purely conducting airway generations would decrease after birth (Fig. 3-4).

Based on animal experiments, the developmental steps of the alveolar stage consists of three phases: (1) a phase of lung expansion, that prepares for (2) a phase of tissue proliferation and formation of interalveolar septa, and (3) a phase of restructuring of the septa. During this last phase, the height of the interalveolar walls increases in conjunction with deepening of the alveolar cups. In addition, the parenchymal microvasculature is reduced from a double to a single intraseptal network.

In humans, alveolization starts during the late fetal period, but the bulk of alveolar formation occurs postna-

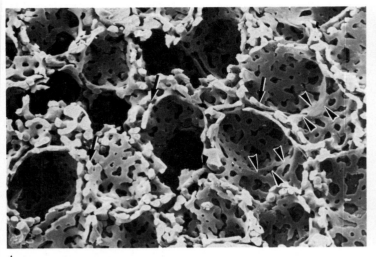
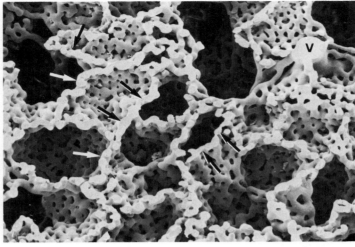

A   B

FIGURE 3-13 Mercox cast of pulmonary capillary bed of rat. *A.* Lung aged 7 days. Tissues are digested away; the vascular structures outline the saccular airspaces. The intersaccular walls contain two well-defined capillary networks (arrows). Secondary septa are low (arrowheads). Scanning electron micrograph, ×250. *B.* Lung aged 139 days. Same technique as above. Interalveolar septa contain a single and dense capillary network (arrows). V = collecting venule. Scanning electron micrograph, ×270.

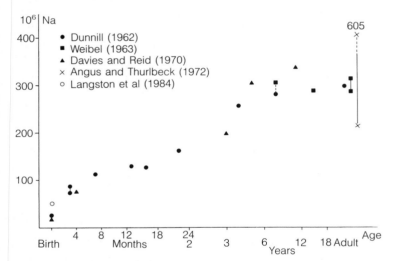

FIGURE 3-14 Number of alveoli in human lungs. Data from various authors as indicated. The most recent publication indicates that 50 million alveoli are present at birth. Note that the adult range is reached at around 4 years of age.

tally (Fig. 3-14). The newborn human lung contains about 50, the adult lung about 300 million alveoli: individual variations are large. In the past, it was generally assumed that alveolization would be completed by the age of 8 years. More recently, the figure of 2 years was advanced, and most recent findings indicate that the figure is likely to be even lower. Although at 1 month the human lung looks very immature (Fig. 3-15A and Fig. 3-16A) (and, except for airspace size, compares well with the lung of a 1-week-old rat), the parenchyma of a 6-month-old lung

already has large regions in which interalveolar septa are slender (Fig. 3-15B). This finding strongly suggests that the stage of massive alveolar formation had passed and that capillary remodeling is already taking place over wide areas by 6 months of age.

In summary, alveolar formation in the human lung starts in late fetal life and is probably completed within the first 12 to 18 postnatal months. As in the rat, the human alveolar stage of development is followed and partially overlapped by a stage of microvascular maturation, which is supposed to end somewhere between 2 and 5 years of age (Fig. 3-1). In this phase, the double capillary network present in the parenchymal septa during the first months of life is reduced to a single-layered system by a complex process combining capillary fusion with capillary network growth (Fig. 3-16B).

Growth of the Lung

As indicated in the previous section, the alveolar stage of human lung development seems to end sooner than previously assumed, but it remains difficult to define clearly when normal growth of the lung starts. For a large part, the difficulty is technical: alveolar counting procedures are problematic because of the uncertainty in identifying more than 70 to 80 percent of alveoli in histologic sections; indirect estimates of alveolar number, such as those based on the alveolar surface complexity, are confounded by the formation of new septa, by deepening of the alveoli, and by an increase in the surface irregularities of existing septa. Turning to the rat lung, the question of when alveolar formation is fully completed cannot be answered either. The rat lung looks mature during the third postnatal

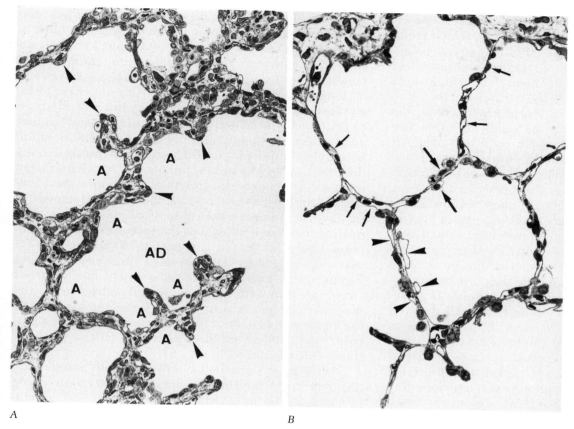

A

B

FIGURE 3-15 Development of pulmonary parenchyma in human lung. *A.* Alveolar formation in human lung aged $3\frac{1}{2}$ weeks. Thick and short secondary septa (arrowheads) bulge from the broad primary septa and subdivide the saccular airspaces into alveolar ducts (AD) with small alveoli (A). Light micrograph, ×250. *B.* Pulmonary parenchyma of a child aged 5.8 months. The interalveolar walls are already slender: they show mostly a single capillary network (short arrows) that appear alternately on either side of the septum (long arrows). In places, a double capillary network seems to be present (arrowheads). Light micrograph, ×360.

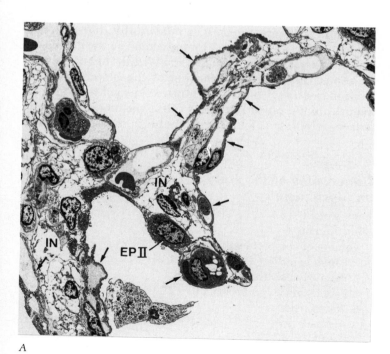

A

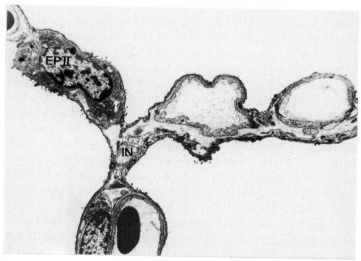

B

FIGURE 3-16 Transmission electron micrographs comparing parenchymal septa in the lung of a child. *A.* Human lung, 32 days. The septa are broad and primitive in type (arrows pointing to double capillary layer). *B.* Human lung, $6\frac{1}{2}$ months. The septa are now slender, the interstitial tissue mass being markedly reduced. IN = interstitium; EP = epithelial cell of type II. Magnification: *A* = ×960, *B* = ×2580.

week. After the third week, the airspace surface area increases with lung volume $V_L^{0.71}$ (Fig. 3-10), which is not significantly different from the $V_L^{0.67}$ that would be expected if the airspaces were to undergo proportional growth thereafter. In rats, as in humans, a slow increase in alveolar number far into adult age is conceivable.

According to quantitative morphometric data, the growth of the human lung can be subdivided into two phases. In the first phase, between birth and about $1\frac{1}{2}$ years of age, the growth rates of the various parenchymal compartments differ widely; they are obviously strongly influenced by the concurrent developmental processes. For example, the airspace and capillary volumes grow faster than lung volume, mainly at the expense of the parenchymal tissue mass. In the second phase, which lasts from $1\frac{1}{2}$ years until body growth stops, the lung grows in a highly proportional fashion. The lung volume increases to the power of one to body weight, and the pulmonary compartments augment linearly with lung volume. Most importantly, the surface area for gas exchange and the morphometrically determined pulmonary diffusion capacity increase both to the power of 1 to body mass.

Unlike the parenchyma for gas exchange, the structure of the conducting airways is mature at birth except for the terminal bronchioles, part of which transform into respiratory bronchioles, as has been described above. Whereas the branching pattern does not change with age, it is not yet clear whether the bronchial tree grows proportionally after birth. In one study, the relationship between diameter and relative distance from the hilus was found to remain almost constant throughout childhood. In a more recent analysis, this was true only after the age of 1 year, whereas during the first year of life, the larger bronchi showed a faster growth rate than the smaller conducting airways. Detailed studies of the airway epithelium of hamsters and rhesus monkeys indicate that the airway lining is largely mature at birth. Though there is some postnatal functional maturation, most developmental changes occur prior to birth.

During fetal life, blood flow through the lung is limited to between 10 and 15 percent of the cardiac output. Clearly the most important vascular event accompanying the onset of air breathing is the closure of the ductus arteriosus and the shunting of the entire cardiac output through the lung. The ductus arteriosus, first obstructed by muscular contraction, is anatomically closed within a few weeks by the fibrotic organization of an intravascular clot. The ligamentum arteriosum represents the tombstone of this important prenatal structure.

After birth, the wall thickness of pulmonary arteries decreases relative to their diameter. In small vessels (up to 200 μm in diameter), this decrease occurs very rapidly. It was assumed that the dilatation was due to a decrease in muscle tone. A recent study performed in pigs, however, relates the vascular dilatation more to a concurrent exten-

sive rearrangement and shape change of the vascular smooth-muscle cells than to a change in muscle tone. In the larger arteries in humans, the thinning of the wall occurs less abruptly; the transformation takes several months. After 1 year of age, the central pulmonary arteries no longer change their relative wall thickness appreciably; instead, they grow more or less proportionally.

Although the central vessels that accompany the conductive airways do not multiply after birth, the situation is completely different for the peripheral vessels. During the first 1 or 2 years of life, intra-acinar arteries undergo intense development and growth as they follow the extensions of the peripheral airspaces; therefore, the number of small vessels increases both absolutely and relatively. The relative increase implies that the increase in number increases per unit area of lung section. From the age of 5 years onward, the relative number decreases again, reflecting the enlargement of the alveoli. The newly formed vessels are thin-walled and are partially muscular or nonmuscular in type, because muscle formation lags behind the increase in diameter. Thereafter, muscularization proceeds gradually toward the periphery, a process that continues into adulthood.

Veins have a smaller amount of smooth muscle than do arteries. But, in principle, the same observations apply to veins as well as to arterial development and growth.

Dimensions of the Adult Lung

Table 3-1 summarizes the dimensions of adult human lung. In a direct comparison of the quantitative data of adult and newborn lungs, it is noteworthy that with age the volume proportion of interalveolar septa decreases and the airspace volume increases. Within the interalveolar septa, the volume proportion of the blood compartment increases with growth at the expense of tissue mass: the arithmetic mean thickness of the air-blood tissue interface, which is calculated by dividing total tissue mass

TABLE 3-1

Dimensions of the Human Lung Based on Morphometry*

Body weight, kg	74 ± 4
Lung volume, L	4.3 ± 0.3
Volume of compartments	
Parenchyma, L	3.9 ± 0.3
Parenchymal tissue, ml	298 ± 36
Parenchymal capillaries, ml	213 ± 31
Surface areas	
Airspace, m²	143 ± 12
Capillary, m²	126 ± 12

*Values represent mean values ± standard errors. Eight human lungs were used.

SOURCE: Based on data from Gehr et al., 1974, and Crapo et al., 1982.

by the alveolar surface area, decreases from around 5 μm at birth to 2.5 μm in the adult; the harmonic mean thickness of the air-blood-tissue barrier, a measure of the effective diffusion distance, remains unaffected by all the structural alterations of development.

Pathology of Lung Development

Little is known about the mechanisms regulating development and/or growth of the lung as it pertains to the various forms of congenital malformations and defects of the respiratory system. Current understanding can be summarized under two headlines: (1) hormonal control and (2) influence of mechanical factors.

Molecular biology has, as yet, had little impact in clarifying pulmonary developmental pathology. Although it is understood that mechanical factors, such as those consequent to a defect in a diaphragm, can evoke untoward consequences in the development and performance of a neighboring system, and that molecular influences as well as mechanical intrusions of abdominal contents into the thorax are probably involved, the connections at a molecular level have not yet been unraveled.

Congenital defects of the lung depend not only on the type of noxious factor, but also on the timing of the insult. As a rule, when injuries are inflicted during the first 4 months of development, the structures mostly affected will be the "nonparenchyma," particularly the airways. Later on, the parenchyma is the target. The primary site of mishap can be outside the lungs (e.g., malformations of diaphragm or heart failure) or within the lungs; with the lungs, the affected site can be in the airway or in the vascular system. Even if the initial derangement can be well targeted, the resulting situation is always very complex. Interdependence of the developing structures is strong because the presence and maturity of one element is required for the development of the other. Therefore, it is the rule that a single mishap generates a whole cascade of anomalies, making it difficult to distinguish a posteriori between cause and effect. Although it is not within the scope of this chapter to review and catalog pulmonary malformations, as a reminder of what can go wrong in pulmonary development, Table 3-2 presents a list of anomalies and attempts a crude classification. Treatment of developmental anomalies, if any is available, will mostly be surgical, directed at correcting a malformation. As it may often entail the removal of lung tissue, the next section, "Regeneration of Lung Tissue," deals more specifically with the consequences of lung tissue resection, as investigated in animal experiments. Here it will suffice to point out that in the very young, the lung has a great capability of compensating for lung tissue removed surgically, as long as the remaining lung tissue is normal. Unfortunately this is often not the case in pulmonary malformations because the remaining tissue is hypoplastic.

REGENERATION OF LUNG TISSUE

Obviously the durability of pulmonary structure throughout life can be achieved only because lung tissues are able (to a certain degree) to repair injuries inflicted by various

TABLE 3-2
Congenital Lesions of the Lungs according to the Sites of the Primary Lesions

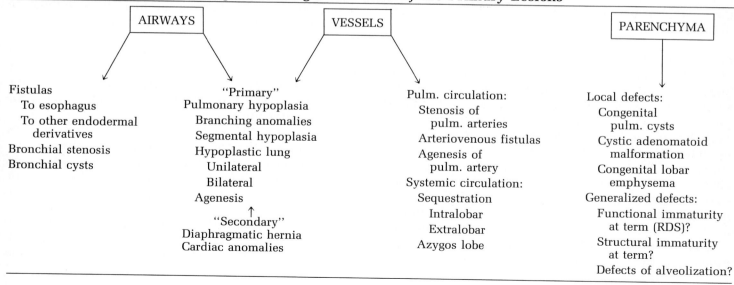

AIRWAYS	VESSELS	PARENCHYMA

Fistulas
  To esophagus
  To other endodermal
    derivatives
Bronchial stenosis
Bronchial cysts
	"Primary"
	Pulmonary hypoplasia
	  Branching anomalies
	  Segmental hypoplasia
	  Hypoplastic lung
	    Unilateral
	    Bilateral
	  Agenesis
	↑
	"Secondary"
	Diaphragmatic hernia
	Cardiac anomalies
		Pulm. circulation:
		  Stenosis of
		    pulm. arteries
		  Arteriovenous fistulas
		  Agenesis of
		    pulm. artery
		Systemic circulation:
		  Sequestration
		    Intralobar
		    Extralobar
		  Azygos lobe
			Local defects:
			  Congenital
			    pulm. cysts
			  Cystic adenomatoid
			    malformation
			  Congenital lobar
			    emphysema
			Generalized defects:
			  Functional immaturity
			    at term (RDS)?
			  Structural immaturity
			    at term?
			  Defects of alveolization?

types of noxious agents. For the lungs, the noxious agents can be airborne or blood-borne microorganisms or chemical compounds. Additionally, structural alterations and impairment of lung function can be caused by physical factors such as mechanical trauma, changes in pulmonary vascular pressures, physical obstruction of the airways, or restriction of intrathoracic volumes. Responses to such types of lung damage and the related repair processes are discussed elsewhere in this book. The following addresses only a very special type of "lung repair," the "regenerative" reaction of the remaining pulmonary tissues to resection of lung tissue. Because quantitative structural data on the lungs of lobectomized patients are scarce, consideration of this problem relies completely on results obtained in animal models.

All experiments performed so far in a large number of laboratories show that the remaining lung is able to undergo some kind of compensatory growth following pneumonectomy. The findings demonstrate the enormous plasticity of lung tissue. Highly debated, however, are the following issues: (1) the extent of the quantitative recovery, (2) the functional capability of the regenerated tissue, (3) the structural features of the response (do existing airspaces enlarge or are new alveoli formed?), and (4) the differences in the responses of the young and of adults.

The operation most frequently performed in experimental animals is the left-sided pneumonectomy; alternatively, the upper and middle lobes of the right lung have been resected. In all species tested, the response has been basically the same. And, in all, it seems that the most important determinant of the magnitude of the regenerative response is the amount of tissue resected.

After surgery, the remaining lung increases in volume within hours and in weight within a few days. The volume increase observed during the first 48 h is due exclusively to overinflation of the peripheral airspaces. Interestingly, it is the alveolar ducts that are first affected by the dilatation; the alveoli become enlarged a couple of days later.

Biochemical changes precede changes in tissue mass during the first four postoperative days. First, the activity of cAMP-related enzymes increases during the first three postoperative days; between days 2 and 6, rates of DNA synthesis increase rapidly, indicating the onset of tissue proliferation. Peaks in mitotic activity occur around the sixth day; in parallel, collagen synthesis increases within the interstitium. According to scanning electron microscopy, and more recently, morphometry, the interalveolar septa are thickened while dilatation of the airspaces has regressed. Three days later (day 9), the morphology of the lung is back to control: within the pulmonary parenchyma, the relative and the absolute amounts of tissue, the capillary blood volume, and the gas-exchanging surface areas are all within normal limits.

The similarity of preoperative and recovery values means that the regenerated tissue was distributed in such a way that the original dimensions of the gas-exchange apparatus were completely restored. Therefore, it is not surprising that the "morphometric pulmonary diffusing capacity" calculated from these data fell within the normal range. These findings suggest that the regenerative response could result in restoration of functional capacity. But whether the functional capacity really matches the structural capacity remains to be determined by physiological measurements.

Although the parenchymal structures were rapidly restored, some nonparenchymal parameters did still differ from control $6\frac{1}{2}$ weeks after bilobectomy. The volume densities of the airways and of the blood vessel compartments were significantly smaller than in control animals. These differences could hint at possible functional imbalances between alveolar ventilation and blood flow. It appears that the parenchymal structures have a greater adaptive potential than do the nonparenchymal structures. An analogous observation has been made in humans with respect to the adaptive response to hypoxia: in Peruvian highlanders, pulmonary function measurements indicated that the larger lungs of this high-altitude population were not matched by increases in airway diameters.

It is highly plausible that young individuals would tolerate pneumonectomy better than would adults. Indeed, a lesser regenerative response in adult animals than in younger animals has been reported many times. After left pneumonectomy, the rate of increase in DNA synthesis was lower, and the gain in lung weight delayed, in older rats. In addition, the weight of the remaining lung did not reach the presurgery levels: in young individuals, the weight of the remaining lung did recover fully. In our own experiments with bilobectomies in rats, however, the extent of the regenerative response was the same in young and adult animals. This indicates that the amount of lung tissue removed (25 percent of total lung volume in bilobectomy versus 37 percent in left pneumonectomy) may represent, besides age and species, an important factor determining recovery. Yet, the possibility remains that the adult rat is a special case, since portions of its thoracic cage never ossify completely, thereby allowing for the continued growth of the thorax, and possibly also of the lungs, far into adulthood.

In humans, the remaining lung increases in volume, but never up to the original dimensions described in animal experiments. In a follow-up study of children and adults who had undergone resection of pulmonary tissue 5 to 25 years previously, a few patients showed exceptional changes in the size of the remaining lung. One patient who was left with only the right upper lobe after resection, showed a three- to fourfold increase in the volume of the remaining right upper lobe, radiologically and by pulmonary function tests; moreover, the diffusing capacity for carbon monoxide reached three-quarters of that calculated for the whole lung. These observations imply that in addition to functional remodeling, considerable structural recovery had also occurred.

Morphometric analysis of the remaining lung after pneumonectomy in humans has, to our knowledge, been performed to date in only one patient; the remaining lung showed no evidence of alveolar multiplication; the airspaces were widened, but there were no signs of tissue destruction.

It is often erroneously assumed that a postpneumonectomy recovery should imply alveolar multiplication in order to be of any functional benefit. Therefore, formation of new alveoli has always been an important issue in most work dealing with lung regeneration. Despite the efforts made to clarify the point, however, the results remain controversial, largely because of the technical difficulties in alveolar counting. For example, as indicated above, it is indeed extremely difficult to properly define an alveolus in a histologic section; three-dimensional reconstructions of pulmonary parenchyma using light microscopy have shown that large errors occur due to misinterpretation of alveolar ducts and alveoli. Furthermore, conventional alveolar counting is unreliable because, as is evident during alveolar formation, alveoli may alter their shape. New counting procedures, based on the disector or selector techniques, afford the prospect of overcoming difficulties related to alveolar shape; however, if it is true that different regions of the pulmonary parenchyma show different patterns of reaction, sampling problems will remain. In one experiment involving a left-sided pneumonectomy, central alveoli were reported to enlarge and subpleural alveoli to multiply. For these reasons, it may continue to be difficult to answer the question of alveolar multiplication merely by counting alveoli or airspaces.

Scanning electron microscopy (SEM) has added another approach to explaining the morphology of the adaptive response to resection of pulmonary tissue. It demonstrated that alveolar formation was not necessary to produce the apparent morphologic recovery of the lung. Instead, expansion of the volumes and surfaces of existing alveoli accounted for the quantitative structural changes observed after bilobectomy.

Finally, with respect to alveolar formation, a very important structural implication or consequence has to be mentioned. Knowing the mode of alveolar formation (secondary septa folding up from primary ones), it is to be expected that additional secondary septa (i.e., new alveolar partitions) can be formed only from immature septa that contain a double capillary network. Unless a new mode of alveolar formation is postulated, lung parenchyma that consists uniquely of mature interalveolar walls has no structural basis for the formation of additional secondary septa; i.e., alveolar formation is closely linked with the degree of septal maturity. A recent SEM investigation of methacrylate casts of the pulmonary vasculature in the adult rat lung has identified the presence of isolated septa that have retained the primitive morphology and, perhaps with it, the ability to form new secondary septa. This structural finding has to be taken into account in the debate on adaptive alveolization.

ACKNOWLEDGMENTS

The author gratefully acknowledges the assistance of Dr. K. Conley, Dr. J. Caduff, Ms. R. M. Fankhauser, Ms. A. Keller, Ms. C. Probst, and Mr. K. Babl in preparing the manuscript.

BIBLIOGRAPHY

Adamson IYR, King GM: Epithelial-mesenchymal interactions in postnatal rat lung growth. Exp Lung Res 8:261–274, 1985.
The authors investigate the number of foot processes of type II epithelial cells contacting interstitial cells and relate it to switching from epithelial proliferation to differentiation.

Bachofen M, Weibel ER: Alterations of the gas exchange apparatus in adult respiratory insufficiency associated with septicemia. Am Rev Respir Dis 116:589–615, 1977.
An investigation of nine patients dying in different stages of respiratory distress syndrome. The study presents the ultrastructure of acute, subacute, and chronic alterations due to septicemia.

Berger LC, Burri PH: Timing of the quantitative recovery in the regenerating rat lung. Am Rev Respir Dis 132:777–783, 1985.
Presents the quantitative data in support of the scanning electron microscopic study of Burri et al., 1982, cited below.

Boyden EA: Development and growth of the airways, in Hodson WA (ed), *Lung Biology in Health and Disease*, vol 6, *Development of the Lung*. New York, Dekker, 1977, pp 3–35.
A review of airway development providing a good insight into Boyden's reconstruction studies of developing acinar structures.

Brody JS, Kaplan NB: Proliferation of alveolar interstitial cells during postnatal lung growth: Evidence for two distinct populations of pulmonary fibroblasts. Am Rev Respir Dis 127:763–770, 1983.
More specific description of the two populations of interstitial cells in the postnatal rat lung.

Brody JS, Vaccaro C: Postnatal formation of alveoli: Interstitial events and physiologic consequences. Fed Proc 38:215–223, 1979.
The first description of two interstitial cell types in the postnatal rat lung.

Bucher U, Reid L: Development of the intrasegmental bronchial tree: The pattern of branching and development of cartilage at various stages of intra-uterine life. Thorax 16:207–218, 1961.
The first of two of the most topical papers on the early development of airways and their structural components in human lung.

Bucher U, Reid L: Development of the mucus-secreting elements in human lung. Thorax 16:219–225, 1961.
The second of two of the most topical papers on the early development of airways and their structural components in human lung.

Burri PH: The postnatal growth of the rat lung. III. Morphology. Anat Rec 180:77–98, 1974.
Detailed morphologic analysis of rat lung growth explaining the morphologic alterations related to alveolar formation.

Burri PH: Development and growth of the human lung, in Fishman AP, Fisher AB (eds), *Handbook of Physiology. The Respiratory System I.* Baltimore, Williams & Wilkins, 1985, pp 1–46.
Comprehensive article on the topic with a complete list of references.

Burri PH, Dbaly J, Weibel ER: The postnatal growth of the rat. I. Morphometry. Anat Rec 178:711–730, 1974.
Provides the quantitative data corroborating the morphologic description of the paper cited above.

Burri PH, Pfrunder B, Berger LC: Reactive changes in pulmonary parenchyma after bilobectomy: A scanning electron microscopic investigation. Exp Lung Res 4:11–28, 1982.
Describes the morphologic alterations following resection of lung tissue and proposes a model explaining why morphologic "recovery" is possible without alveolar formation.

Caduff JH, Fischer LC, Burri PH: Scanning electron microscopic study of the developing microvasculature in the postnatal rat lung. Anat Rec 216:154–164, 1986.
A scanning electron-microscopic study of pulmonary microvasculature casts presenting a new concept for the growth of the pulmonary microvasculature.

Crapo JD, Barry BE, Bachofen M: Cell numbers and cell characteristics of the normal human lung. Am Rev Respir Dis 126:332–337, 1982.
Presents additional data on the same eight human lungs investigated by Gehr et al. cited below. Emphasis lies on the analysis of the various cell populations of the lung.

Cruz-Orive LM: Particle number can be estimated using a disector of unknown thickness: the selector. J Microsc 145:121–142, 1987.
Carries the recent developments in particle counting a step further.

Gehr P, Bachofen M, Weibel ER: The normal human lung ultrastructure and morphometric estimation of diffusion capacity. Respir Physiol 32:121–140, 1978.
So far the only study presenting ultrastructural quantitative data on eight normal adult human lungs. The study is completed by the one of Crapo cited above.

Gil J, Reiss OK: Isolation and characterization of lamellar bodies and tubular myelin from rat lung homogenates. J Cell Biol 58:152–171, 1973.
The authors present data to clarify the link between lamellar bodies of type II cells and the surface-active material of the alveoli.

Hansen JE, Ampaya EP: Lung morphometry: A fallacy in the use of the counting principle. J Physiol 37:951–954, 1974.
By comparing counting results obtained on sections with those obtained after three-dimensional reconstructions, the authors point to the mistakes made in alveolar counting.

Haworth SG, Hall SM, Chew M, Allen K: Thinning of fetal pulmonary arterial wall and postnatal remodelling: Ultrastructural studies on the respiratory unit arteries of the pig. Virchows Arch A 411:161–171, 1987.
Presents interesting data relevant to the drastic pressure changes in the pulmonary arteries after birth.

Hislop A, Muir DCF, Jacobsen M, Simon G, Reid L: Postnatal growth and function of the preacinar airways. Thorax 27:265–274, 1972.
An analysis on the postnatal growth of the airways with an attempt to relate airway dimensions to function.

Hislop A, Reid L: Growth and development of the respiratory system—anatomical development, in Davis JA, Dobbing J, Heinemann W (eds), *Scientific Foundation of Paediatrics*, 2d ed. London, Medical Books, 1981, chap 20, pp 390–432.
Review of pulmonary development with excellent information about the development of the pulmonary vasculature. Bibliography refers to individual reports by same group on pulmonary arteries and veins in the fetus and child.

Horsfield K, Gordon W, Kemp W, Phillips S: Growth of the bronchial tree in man. Thorax 42:383–388, 1987.
Investigates the postnatal changes in diameter, length, and branching ratios of the airway system in nine children between 5 weeks and 17 years.

Kapanci Y, Assimacopoulos A, Irle C, Zwahlen A, Baggiani G: "Contractile interstitial cells" in pulmonary alveolar septa: A possible regulator of ventilation/perfusion ratio? J Cell Biol 60:375–392, 1974.
The original paper showing that interstitial cells have contractile filaments and may have other functions in addition to producing and maintaining the fibrous system of the lung.

Kauffman SL, Burri PH, Weibel ER: The postnatal growth of the rat lung. II. Autoradiography. Anat Rec 180:63–76, 1974.
A study on the cell kinetics during the postnatal growth of the rat lung. It is proposed that type II cells represent the stem cell population of the alveolar epithelium in the growing lung.

Langston C, Kida K, Reed M, Thurlbeck WM: Human lung growth in late gestation and in the neonate. Am Rev Respir Dis 129:607–613, 1984.
The authors present new data on the alveolization process of the human lung and on its timing.

Low FN: The pulmonary alveolar epithelium of laboratory mammals and man. Anat Rec 117:241–246, 1953.
This paper and Anat Rec 113:437–443, 1952, report the first electron-microscope studies of lung tissue. They ended the debate about the existence of the alveolar epithelium.

Mercurio AR, Rhodin JAG: An electron microscopic study on the type I pneumocyte in the cat: Differentiation. Am J Anat 146:255–272, 1976.
An analysis providing the criteria for the early detection of differentiating type I pneumocytes.

Otani EM, Newkirk C, McDowell EM: Development of hamster tracheal epithelium: IV. Cell proliferation and cytodifferentiation in the neonate. Anat Rec 214:183–192, 1986.
Analysis of epithelial cell type frequencies in hamster trachea said to match closely the situation in human bronchi.

Plopper CG, Alley JL, Weir AJ: Differentiation of tracheal epithelium during fetal lung maturation in the rhesus monkey Macaca mulatta. Am J Anat 175:59–71, 1986.
Detailed ultrastructural follow-up of cellular development in the airway epithelium of a higher mammalian species.

Post M, Torday JS, Smith BT: Alveolar type II cells from fetal rat lung organotypic cultures synthetize and secrete surfactant-associated phospholipids and respond to fibroblast-pneumonocyte factor. Exp Lung Res 7:53–65, 1984.
Interesting cell culture model on type II cells capable of responding to fibroblast pneumocyte factor.

Spooner BS, Wessells NK: Mammalian lung development: Interactions in primordium formation and bronchial morphogenesis. J Exp Zool 175:445–454, 1970.
Beautiful experiments making the point that the pulmonary mesenchyme plays a key role in mammalian lung development.

Sterio DC: The unbiased estimation of number and sizes of arbitrary particles using the disector. J Microsc 134:127–136, 1984.
A revolutionary approach for the counting of particles in sections.

Weibel ER: *Morphometry of the Human Lung.* Heidelberg, Springer Verlag, 1963.
The most cited "classic" on lung morphometry.

Weibel ER: Morphometric estimation of pulmonary diffusion capacity. I. Model and method. Respir Physiol 11:54–75, 1970/71.

The original paper describing the model for the calculation of amorphometric diffusion capacity.

Zeltner TB, Burri PH: The postnatal development and growth of the human lung. II. Morphology. Respir Physiol 67:269–282, 1987.

Companion paper to Zeltner et al., 1987, cited below. First paper to describe the ultrastructural changes in the postnatal human lung; proposes a new stage of microvascular maturation following the alveolar development.

Zeltner TB, Caduff JH, Gehr P, Pfenninger J, Burri PH: The postnatal development and growth of the human lung. I. Morphometry. Am Rev Respir Dis 67:247–267, 1987.

The first quantitative ultrastructural study of human postnatal lung development.

Chapter *4*

The Lungs in Later Life

Allan I. Pack / Richard P. Millman

Structural Features
    The Thorax
    The Lungs

Lung Mechanics
    Elastic Properties of the Lungs and Chest Wall
    Airway Function
    Respiratory Muscle Function

Pulmonary Function Tests
    Lung Volumes
    Maximal Expiratory Flow Rates
    Maximal Voluntary Ventilation
    Normal Values

Gas Exchange
    Arterial P_{O_2}
    Arterial P_{CO_2}

Control of Ventilation

Exercise Responses

Sleep

One of the most significant demographic trends of the twentieth century is what has been described as the "graying of the population." The older population is increasing, and will continue to increase, at a rate far faster than the rest of the population. Thus, not only has the number of elderly grown, but so also has the proportion of the total population of those 65 years or over (Table 4-1). Predictions by the U.S. Bureau of Census indicate that this trend will continue into the twenty-first century and, indeed, accelerate as those born during the "baby boom" reach this age group (Table 4-1).

The physiology of the elderly as a group differs from that of younger people. In addition, they differ with respect to the manifestations of disease, the natural history of disease, and the pharmacokinetics of medications. This chapter is concerned with the physiological performance of the pulmonary system in elderly individuals.

However, defining physiological change with age is a difficult problem. Physiological function at a particular age is determined not only by the aging process itself, but also by the life-style that the subject adopts, e.g., whether physical exercise is performed regularly. Intercurrent disease or the effects of other noxious agents can cause function to deteriorate. This is particularly important for the performance of the respiratory system where a lifetime of breathing air contaminated with industrial pollutants and cigarette smoke takes its toll.

One way by which these complicating elements can be taken into account is by appropriate experimental design, e.g., using only lifelong nonsmokers. However, this precaution has not been taken in many of the studies done until now that purport to show effects of aging on the respiratory system. Study design is problematic. Cross-sectional studies of consecutive age groups entail the risk of using biased samples, i.e., survivors, at the elderly end of the spectrum. Longitudinal studies may give totally different estimates of physiological decline as compared to cross-sectional studies. However, they are both expensive and time-consuming. It is against this background of problematic studies that current understanding of the changes in pulmonary performance with advancing age must be viewed.

STRUCTURAL FEATURES

Any consideration of functional changes must first begin with what is known about changes in structure.

The Thorax

The thoracic cage stiffens with advancing age: the ribs decalcify, the costal cartilages calcify, and arthritic changes develop in the joints between the vertebrae and ribs. In addition, the chest often becomes barrel-shaped because of dorsal kyphosis and an increase in the antero-posterior diameter of the thorax; some degree of kyphosis has been reported in 68 percent of individuals who are more than 75 years old. The deformity is thought to result from degenerative changes in the intervertebral disks that lead to an increase in spinal curvature. Since a barrel-

TABLE 4-1
*Actual and Projected Growth of the Older Population**

Year	Total Population All Ages	65 Years and Over	
		Number	Percent of Total Population
1920	105,711	4,933	4.7
1950	150,697	12,270	8.1
1980	226,505	25,544	11.3
2010	283,141	39,269	13.9
2040	307,952	66,643	21.6

* Numbers are in thousands.
SOURCE: U.S. Bureau of Census.

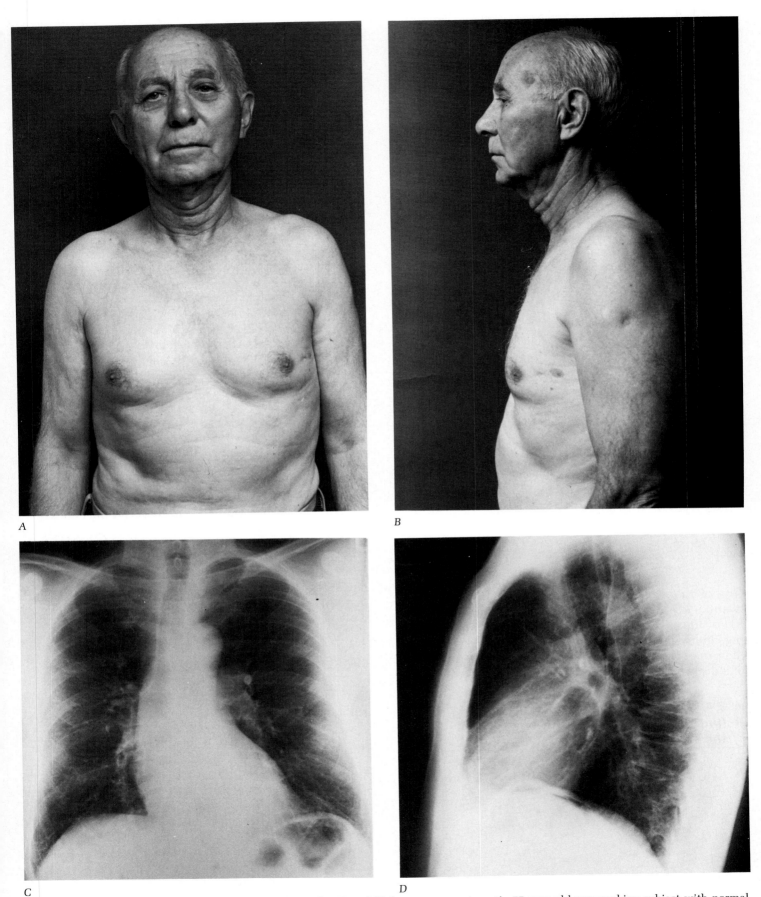

A

B

C

D

FIGURE 4-1 Photographs (*A* and *B*) and chest radiographs (*C* and *D*) from an asymptomatic 75-year-old nonsmoking subject with normal ventilatory function for his age. The normal appearances of the lung fields, diaphragm, and spinal contours are typical of most active, healthy elderly people. *(From Peterson and Fishman, 1982.)*

chest deformity also occurs in pulmonary emphysema, this led to coining of the term *senile emphysema*. However, elderly subjects with this deformity do not have any of the other hallmarks of emphysema and the phrase "senile emphysema" has fallen into disuse. Kyphosis is by no means an inevitable outcome of aging, as is shown by a picture of an elderly subject and his chest radiographs in Fig. 4-1.

The Lungs

The basic architecture of the lungs is preserved, and their dry lung weight changes little, if at all, with age. The large conducting airways are little affected, though their cartilages sometimes calcify and the anatomic dead space probably increases slightly. The mean diameters of bronchioles less than 2 mm in internal diameter decrease progressively after age 40, presumably due to a decrease in elastic recoil that keeps them open. Opposite changes occur in the dimensions of the alveolar ducts: alveolar ducts dilate in the elderly and the term *ductesia* has been introduced to describe this phenomenon. Ductesia is common in the elderly, probably related to the loss of elastic fibers around the alveolar duct region.

The major change in the gas-exchanging surface is a decrease in internal alveolar surface with age. Since the number of alveoli do not change, this overall reduction implies a decrease in the surface area of individual alveoli. Lung geometry is rearranged so that individual alveoli appear flattened. The biomechanical properties of strips of alveolar tissue from aged lungs studied in vitro are also different: the maximal extensibility ratio, i.e., final tissue length/initial length, decreases during tissue stretching even though there is no evidence of fibrosis. The decrease in this ratio presumably reflects an increase in initial resting length rather than in the maximal length that can be attained.

Alterations in the supporting connective tissue of the lung are widely held to be responsible for these changes. However, no consensus exists about the nature of these changes. Part of the problem stems from differences in experimental design, particularly in frames of reference: early studies, which expressed their results as a fraction of the weight of dry lung tissue, indicated that the elastin content of the lungs increased with age while the collagen content remained unchanged. However, when the results are expressed in terms of volume of inflated lung, then an opposite conclusion is reached, i.e., the total elastin content is unaffected while collagen content declines. This latter interpretation is easier to reconcile with physiological determinations of the elastic properties of the lungs.

LUNG MECHANICS

Elastic Properties of the Lungs and Chest Wall

Most, but not all, studies have concluded that the elastic recoil of the lungs decreases with age. In elderly individu-

als, the relationship between transpulmonary pressure and lung volume (expressed as a percentage of total lung capacity) is shifted to the left (Fig. 4-2); the decrease in static recoil is greater at higher lung volumes (Fig. 4-3). However, the slope of the relationship between pressure and volume, i.e., the pulmonary compliance, is, in general, not altered in the elderly (Fig. 4-2).

The changes in the elastic properties of the lung are relatively small and are counterbalanced during breathing by alterations in the elastic properties of the chest wall. The compliance of the chest wall decreases with age. One convenient way in which to view the changes in the elastic properties of the lung and chest wall during aging is the pressure-volume diagram (Fig. 4-4). This diagram compares the PV curve of the chest wall (W) and lungs (L) in a 20 year old and 60 year old. The compliance of the total system (RS) is less in the older adult. Also, the 60-year-old individual does 20 percent more elastic work at a given level of ventilation than does the 20 year old; moreover, in the older individual, 70 percent of the work is done in moving the chest wall as compared to only 40 percent in the younger person.

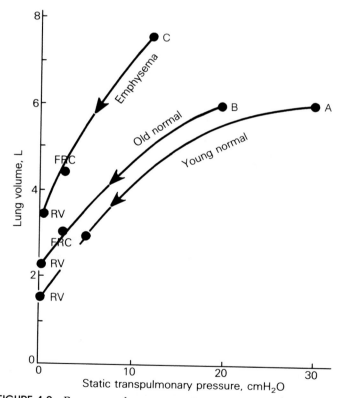

FIGURE 4-2 Pressure-volume curves for the lungs of young (A) and old (B) asymptomatic nonsmoking women, compared with that for patients with emphysema (C). The static pressure-volume curve is shifted to the left in elderly subjects although less so than in emphysematous subjects. There is at a given lung volume a loss of elastic recoil pressure with age, but no change in the slope of the relationship between pressure and volume (pulmonary compliance). FRC = functional residual capacity; RV = residual volume. (*From Peterson and Fishman, 1982.*)

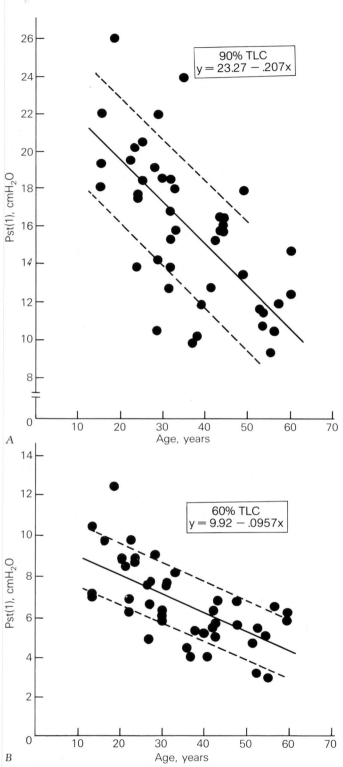

FIGURE 4-3 Reduction in static elastic recoil pressure with increasing age. Data are given for a lung volume of 90 percent of TLC (*A*) and a lung volume of 60 percent TLC (*B*). In both panels, individual data points as well as the regression line ± one standard error are shown. Reduction in pressure is greater at higher lung volumes. Pst(1) = static pulmonary pressure; TLC = total lung capacity. (*From Turner et al., 1968.*)

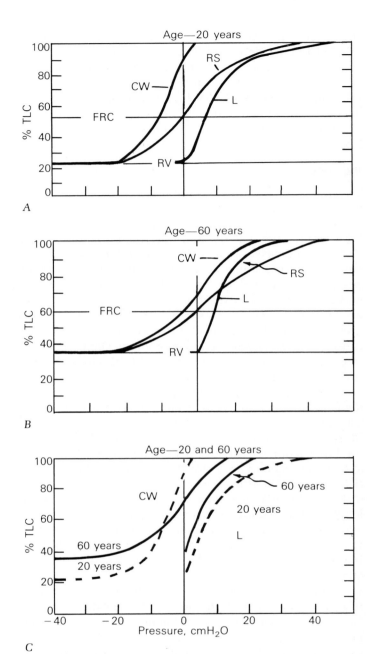

FIGURE 4-4 Pressure-volume relationship of lung (L), chest wall (CW), and total respiratory system (RS) for typical young (*A*) and older (*B*) adults. (Both are compared in *C*.) Data for chest wall are from study of Mittman et al. and for the lung from Turner et al. In *C* panel the solid lines are for the 60-year-old subject, the dashed lines for the 20-year-old. FRC = functional residual capacity; RV = residual volume. (*Modified from Turner et al., 1968.*)

This change in chest wall compliance affects not only the work of breathing, but it is evident in Fig. 4-4 that the altered shape of the pressure-volume curve of the chest wall also contributes importantly to the increase in the residual volume in the elderly. Finally, the abdominal contribution to breathing in the elderly is greater than that of the thorax.

Airway Function

Even though the elastic work of breathing (for a given ventilation) increases in the elderly, the resistive work of breathing remains unchanged. This resistive work is primarily related to the resistance of the major airways. In contrast to the unchanged resistance of the large airways, the aging process does affect the function of the small airways. Because of the decrease in elastic recoil with age, the smaller airways offer less resistance during expiration toward residual volume: closing volume, expressed as a percentage of vital capacity, increases linearly with increasing age (Fig. 4-5). The increase is such that in persons older than 65 years, small airways generally close in the dependent parts of the lung during normal tidal breathing, i.e., at volumes above functional residual capacity. These effects are magnified in the supine position so that small airways typically close during tidal breathing in subjects over 44 years of age. Such closure of small airways during tidal breathing has implications for gas exchange. Furthermore, it offers a plausible explanation for the increase in frequency dependence of compliance that has been described in the normal elderly.

Respiratory Muscle Function

In general, maximal inspiratory pressures and expiratory pressures decrease with age. However, in the extensive study by Black and Hyatt, the regression of maximal inspiratory and expiratory pressures with age proved to be significant only in females older than 55 (Fig. 4-6). Al-

though the mechanism underlying this decrease has not been elucidated for the respiratory muscles, the decrease in function of the limb muscles with age is associated with a decrease in the number of muscle fibers and a reduction in the size of the remainder; the atrophy preferentially affects the fast-twitch anaerobic fibers.

PULMONARY FUNCTION TESTS

Lung Volumes

The changes in the mechanics of the respiratory system lead to alterations in the pulmonary function tests. The stiffening of the chest wall and the decrease in the force of the inspiratory muscles cause a reduction in vital capacity that progresses with increasing age. The stiffening of the chest wall also contributes to the progressive increase in residual volume (Fig. 4-5); an additional, indeed more important, factor in the increase in residual volume is the increasing tendency for the smaller airways to collapse at the lower lung volumes. The increase in residual volume and decrease in vital capacity are almost exactly balanced so that total lung capacity is unaffected by aging (Fig. 4-5). As a consequence, the ratio of residual volume to total lung capacity increases with advancing years.

So, too, may the ratio of functional residual capacity to total lung capacity increase with age. But the increase is less since the functional residual capacity (FRC) increases

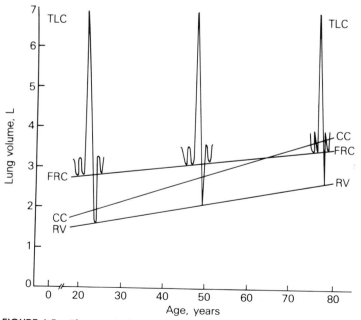

FIGURE 4-5 Changes in lung volumes with age. CC = closing capacity; FRC = functional residual capacity; RV = residual volume; TLC = total lung capacity. *(From Peterson and Fishman, 1982.)*

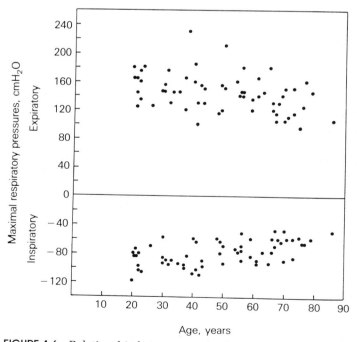

FIGURE 4-6 Relationship between maximal expiratory pressure *(top panel)*, maximal inspiratory pressure *(bottom panel)*, and age established in a study of 60 normal females. Regression with age was significant above 55 years of age. *(From Black and Hyatt, 1969.)*

only slightly, or not at all, with age (Fig. 4-5). The small effect of age on the FRC is a consequence of age-related changes in the PV curves of the lung and chest wall (Fig. 4-4): with advancing age, at lung volumes close to the FRC, the elastic recoil of the chest wall (that tends to move it outward) is virtually unaltered so that any increase in FRC is secondary to a reduction in the elastic recoil of the lung.

Maximal Expiratory Flow Rates

The decrease in elastic recoil of the lungs also contributes to the reduction in flow rates measured during a maximal expiratory flow volume maneuver (MEFV). Although flow rates tend to be depressed at all lung volumes, differences are most marked, and sometimes decrease only significantly, at lower lung volumes (Fig. 4-7), i.e., in the effort-independent region of the curve; in this region, flow is determined by the magnitude of elastic recoil (the driving force) and the resistance of the airways upstream of the equal pressure point. The changes in maximal expiratory flow rates are responsible for the decrease in the commonplace measures of pulmonary function, e.g., FEV_1 and $\dot{V}_{max,50\%}$ (Fig. 4-8).

Maximal Voluntary Ventilation

Maximal voluntary ventilation decreases with age, by approximately 30 percent between 30 and 70 years of age. Particularly important in this decline are the decrease in respiratory muscle force and the decrease in compliance of the respiratory system.

Normal Values

These changes in function, which are a concomitant of the normal aging process, affect the prediction of "normal." Many of the regression equations in common use for normal values do not apply to individuals of advanced years, since the data on which they are based were obtained from younger age groups. One important example of the inadequacy of extrapolating criteria for normalcy is the use of values of FEV/FVC of less than 70 percent as evidence of obstructive airways disease. Although this usage is helpful for middle-aged individuals, it may be useless in elderly individuals who are well and have no evidence of cardiopulmonary disease.

GAS EXCHANGE

The changes in the mechanical performance of the lung affect its gas-exchanging function. Particularly important in this regard is the closure of small airways during tidal breathing in elderly subjects; this results in a maldistribution of ventilation. The maldistribution is, as expected,

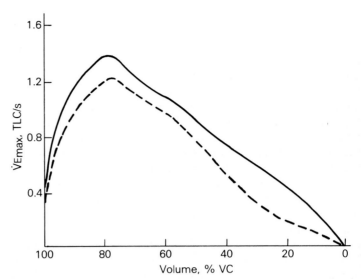

FIGURE 4-7 Maximal flow-volume curves for normal elderly (mean age, 63 years) and young (mean age, 25 years) women (—, young women; ––, elderly women). Differences in flow rates were significant only at lung volumes below 30 percent of the vital capacity. (*From Peterson and Fishman, 1982.*)

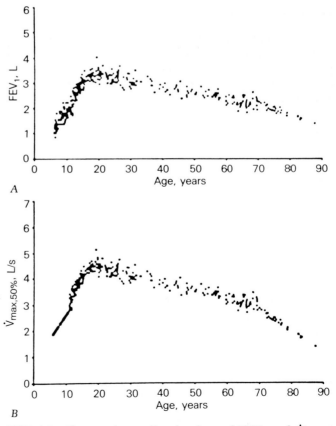

FIGURE 4-8 Changes in predicted values of FEV_1 and $\dot{V}_{max,50\%}$ with age. The initial effects (up to age 20) represent changes due to growth, whereas thereafter there is a decline that accelerates in later life. The data shown are for females. (*Modified from Knudson et al., 1983.*)

less when the elderly subjects use larger tidal volumes in breathing, since at large tidal volumes the effects of airway closure are reduced. Closure of small airways, accompanied by maldistribution of ventilation, is more marked in the basal parts of the lung because of the effects of gravity on the topographic distribution of pleural pressure.

Arterial P_O2

These changes in distribution are thought to underlie the increase in the alveolar-arterial difference in P_{O_2} that occurs with age. Increase in closing volume correlates with increase in venous admixture; closure of small airways produces areas in which ventilation-perfusion ratios are low, thereby increasing the alveolar-arterial difference in P_{O_2} and decreasing arterial P_{O_2}. The effect in the elderly of the low ventilation-perfusion ratios is magnified by the characteristic reduction in cardiac output that occurs in the elderly and the consequent widening of the venous-arterial difference for oxygen; a given amount of venous admixture in this circumstance produces a larger fall in arterial P_{O_2} than when the cardiac output is normal.

The decrease in arterial P_{O_2} with age has been demonstrated in many studies. However, the slopes of the relationship between arterial P_{O_2} and age differ, partly because of differences in the position in which they were performed, i.e., in the supine or sitting position, and their different effect on airway closure (Fig. 4-9). One of the largest of such studies was done by Sorbini et al. using nonsmoking Italian subjects without cardiopulmonary disease from a rural area who were studied in the supine position. The arterial P_{O_2} decreased progressively with age: in those who were more than 60 years of age, the average arterial P_{O_2} was 74.3 mmHg; even a value of 67 mmHg fell within the normal range. The dependence of P_{O_2} on age that Sorbini et al. demonstrated, when corrected to a barometric pressure of 760 mmHg, was expressed by the equation

$$Pa_{O_2} = 109 - 0.43 \text{ (age)} \tag{1}$$

Age-related reductions in arterial P_{O_2} do not appear to be related to alterations to oxygen diffusion in the lungs since diffusion equilibrium is so rapid: the diffusing capacity of the lungs would have to be severely compromised before an end-capillary difference in P_{O_2} could occur. Nevertheless, the diffusing capacity of the lung does decline with age. The reduction is most marked in the supine position, presumably reflecting the effect of posture on airway closure. This reduction in diffusing capacity can be detected at 40 years of age, when the membrane component of diffusion decreases (Dm), presumably because of the decrease in alveolar surface area (see above). In later life, pulmonary capillary blood volume (Vc) also decreases, thereby intensifying the decrease in diffusing capacity.

Arterial P_CO2

Changes in distribution within the lung also influence CO_2 exchange. But unlike oxygen, arterial P_{CO_2} does not change with age. This is a consequence of age producing offsetting effects on the determinants of arterial P_{CO_2}. As discussed in Chapter 13, P_{CO_2} is determined by the balance between metabolic CO_2 production and alveolar ventilation. The latter, in turn, depends on the magnitudes of total ventilation and physiological dead space. With advancing age, the minute ventilation at rest remains unchanged even though the physiological dead space (VD/VT) does increase because of ventilation-perfusion mismatching within the lung. As a result of these changes, alveolar ventilation is less in the elderly. However, total metabolic activity also decreases with age, due largely to a decline in muscle mass.

CONTROL OF VENTILATION

The ventilatory responses to hypoxia and hypercapnia decrease in the elderly (Fig. 4-10). The peripheral chemoreceptor response to acute hypoxia and the central response to acute hypercapnia are depressed by about the same amount, i.e., 51 percent and 41 percent, respectively.

But measurements of ventilatory response do not, per se, prove alterations in the neural control of ventilation. The ventilatory response depends not only on the efferent outflow to the respiratory muscles but also on the performance of the respiratory muscles and the mechanical load presented by the respiratory system. In the elderly, the known reduction in the isometric strength of the respiratory muscles and the decrease in the compliance of the

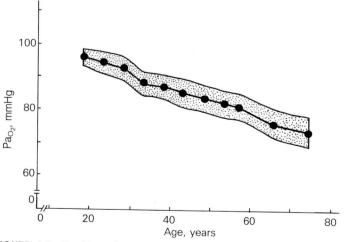

FIGURE 4-9 Decline of arterial P_{O_2} with age in nonsmoking subjects. Filled circles are mean values and shaded areas ± one standard deviation. *(Modified from Sorbini et al., 1968.)*

total respiratory system lead to a reduction in ventilation (for a given neural outflow to the muscles). But the reduction in the ventilatory responses of the elderly cannot be explained solely on this basis: ventilatory responses as reflected in the occlusion pressure (P_{100})—a measurement unaffected by alterations in lung mechanics—are both depressed by approximately 50 percent in elderly individuals exposed to either isocapnic hypoxia (peripheral chemoreceptors) or hyperoxic progressive hypercapnia (central chemoreceptors) (Fig. 4-11). Although these re-

sults indicate that the reduced total respiratory system compliance in the elderly cannot explain the observed reductions in ventilatory response, they do not exclude a role for alterations in muscle strength. But the changes in respiratory muscle strength were too small to be assigned an appreciable role. The reduction in the ventilatory response in the elderly seems to be due primarily to alterations in the central nervous system mechanisms that control efferent outflow to the respiratory muscles.

Alterations in central mechanisms in the elderly are also thought to underlie reduced perception of impediments to ventilation. In the elderly, perceptions of both resistive and elastic loads, as judged by magnitude scaling, are less than those of younger control subjects. That this reduced perception does not simply reflect reduced awareness of the force that the respiratory muscles have to generate to overcome the resistive or elastic loads — a physical stimulus that has been proposed as an important determinant of such respiratory sensations — is indicated by the fact that, in the elderly, the estimation of force, per se, is no different from that of young adults. These reductions in perception of sensory information in the elderly are not unique to respiration since they have been described for other sensory systems, e.g., vision, touch, and weight discrimination.

EXERCISE RESPONSES

Even though the ventilatory responses to acute hypoxia and hypercapnia are reduced in the elderly, somewhat surprisingly the ventilatory response to exercise is in-

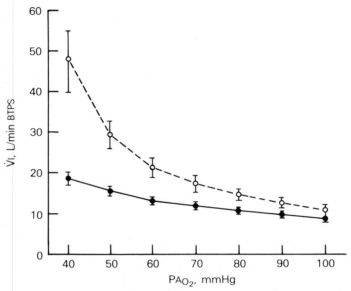

FIGURE 4-10 Ventilatory responses to progressive hypoxia under isocapnic conditions in normal young (open) and elderly (filled) adults. (*From Kronenberg and Drage, 1973.*)

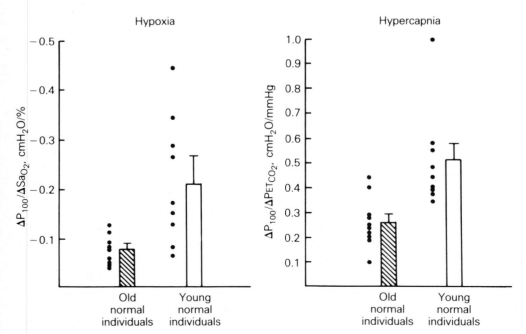

FIGURE 4-11 Occlusion pressure responses to progressive isocapnic hypoxia (*left panel*) and progressive hyperoxic hypercapnia (*right panel*) in young and elderly subjects. Individual data points and mean and standard error of the mean are shown. (*From Peterson et al., 1981.*)

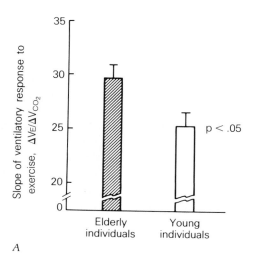

A

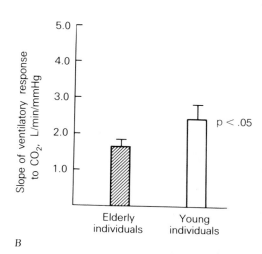

B

FIGURE 4-12 Differences in ventilatory response to exercise ($\Delta\dot{V}_E/\Delta\dot{V}_{CO_2}$) (left panel) and hypercapnia ($\Delta\dot{V}_E/\Delta P_{ET_{CO_2}}$) (right panel) in same groups of elderly and young subjects. Opposite effects of age on the two responses are shown. (From Brischetto et al., 1984.)

creased. This was suggested by early studies on exercise that showed the ventilatory equivalent for oxygen to be higher in the elderly and shown more convincingly in recent studies that compared ventilatory responses to CO_2 and exercise in matched groups of young and elderly subjects: elderly subjects had an increased ventilatory response to exercise (Fig. 4-12A) and a decreased ventilatory response to CO_2 (Fig. 4-12B). Despite the increase in ventilation in the elderly at a given level of exercise or CO_2 production, exercise remained essentially isocapnic. This increased ventilation during exercise presumably compensates for the known increase in physiological dead space with age, thereby maintaining eucapnia. The mechanism which mediates this adjustment is unclear. However, the opposite effects of age on the ventilatory responses to exercise and to chemical stimuli render unlikely a chemoreceptor-linked mechanism.

At any given level of work, the increased ventilation in the elderly during exercise causes them to use a larger fraction of their ventilatory reserve since the maximal voluntary ventilation also decreases. However, more important than the respiratory parameters in limiting exercise performance is the decrease in cardiovascular function with age: both the maximal heart rate that can be achieved during exercise and the maximal cardiac output decrease. These, together with the abnormalities in oxygen exchange between air and blood, are responsible for a decrease in the maximal oxygen uptake and in the anaerobic threshold during exercise. Cross-sectional studies indicate that maximal oxygen uptake declines at a rate of around 0.45 ml/kg per min each year, whereas the estimate from longitudinal studies is about double. A decrease in maximal oxygen uptake takes place even in athletic individuals who continue to exercise. However, not unexpectedly, at all ages, maximal oxygen uptake is greater in individuals who are athletically active.

SLEEP

Respiration during sleep is also different in the elderly; indeed, sleep itself changes with age. Electroencephalographic (EEG) studies have demonstrated that the elderly have different sleeping patterns than do younger adults. In particular, total nocturnal sleep time is shorter in the elderly, although they spend a longer time in bed, i.e., sleep efficiency decreases with age. The shorter duration of sleep is caused by more frequent, and longer, episodes of nocturnal awakenings: although normal cycling from non-rapid eye movement (NREM) to rapid eye movement (REM) sleep is preserved, the amount of time spent in stages 3 to 4 slow wave sleep decreases markedly with advancing age. One hypothesis to account for the increased frequency of nocturnal awakenings in the elderly is that these arousals are related to an increased frequency of apneas.

In younger individuals, the change in alveolar ventilation that occurs when the subject falls asleep correlates with the responsiveness while awake to hypercapnia: those with low responses have greater increase in alveolar P_{CO_2} with sleep. As indicated above, the ventilatory responses to acute hypercapnia and hypoxia are reduced in the elderly. On this ground, one might predict that the elderly would have greater increments in alveolar P_{CO_2} than would younger adults upon falling asleep. However, when ventilation is measured in healthy young and elderly adults awake and asleep, no significant difference is found between the mean ventilations of the two groups, while awake, in stages 1 to 2 sleep, or in stages 3 to 4 sleep (Fig. 4-13).

Several reasons can be offered to explain why mean ventilation during sleep does not fall more in the elderly than the young. First, mean ventilation measured during each sleep stage may be a poor indicator of the changes in

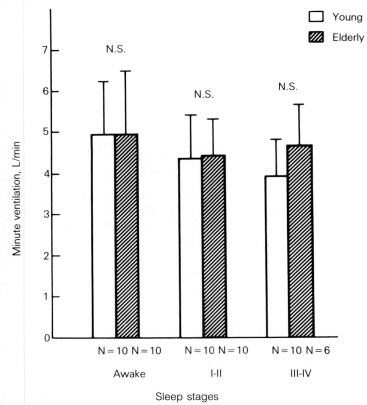

FIGURE 4-13 Mean ventilation in young and elderly nonsmoking adults awake, in stages 1 to 2 sleep, and in stages 3 to 4 sleep. No significant differences between young and old were found. The smaller number of elderly subjects in stages 3 to 4 sleep is because four of the elderly with sleep apnea had no stages 3 to 4 sleep on the night of study. (From Shore et al., 1985.)

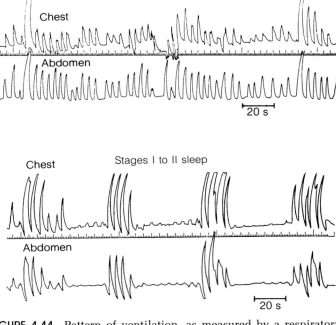

FIGURE 4-14 Pattern of ventilation, as measured by a respiratory inductance plethysmograph, awake and in stages 1 to 2 sleep in an elderly subject with central sleep apnea. Abdominal and chest motions are shown. (Modified from Shore et al., 1985.)

respiratory control that take place with sleep; ventilation becomes much more variable during sleep, particularly in stages 1 to 2 sleep, so that measurements of mean ventilation may obscure changes that take place. Also, the interpretation of a change in ventilation during a particular state of sleep is confounded by the definition of state; in the elderly, arousals are often seen in the EEG, and the sleep state is poorly consolidated; as a result, stages 1 to 2 sleep in the young may not be analogous to the same stage in the elderly. Finally, the possibility exists that ventilatory responses may not decrease in the elderly during sleep as they do in young adults.

During sleep, the pattern of ventilation is irregular in the elderly much more often than in young adults; repetitive periodic apneas occur in 35 to 40 percent of the elderly. The apneas tend to occur predominantly in male subjects, may be either central or obstructive, occur primarily during stages 1 to 2 sleep, and appear to be an extension of the periodic breathing seen in both young and elderly adults during stages 1 to 2 sleep (Fig. 4-14).

Why periodic breathing progresses in certain elderly subjects to periodic apneas during stages 1 to 2 sleep is not clear. One mechanism proposed for the central type is a decrease in arterial P_{CO_2} below the apneic threshold. For the obstructive type, unlinking of diaphragmatic and upper airway muscle activity has been suggested, so that contraction of the diaphragm, and the negative pressure that it produces, causes the upper airways to collapse.

Apneic episodes in the elderly typically terminate in manifestations of arousal on the EEG. However, not all arousals are associated with apnea. No difference in the number of arousals occurs in elderly subjects with or without apnea, even though the elderly, as a group, undergo significantly more transient arousals than do young adults. Thus, while apneas and arousals may be associated, apnea is not the sole mechanism that leads to sleep fragmentation in the elderly. Other processes such as nocturnal myoclonus (leg jerking during sleep) may be as, or more, important. The clinical importance of these apneas in the elderly is dealt with in greater detail in Chapter 83.

BIBLIOGRAPHY

Altose MD, Leitner J, Cherniack NS: Effects of age and respiratory efforts on the perception of resistive ventilatory loads. J Gerontol 40:147–153, 1985.
Confirms observations that perception of resistive loads is reduced in the elderly. This difference is not explained by altered perception of the intensity and duration of the forces generated by the inspiratory muscles. Contains useful discussion with respect to previous work on this topic.

Andreotti L, Bussotti A, Cammelli D, Aiello E, Sampognaro S: Connective tissue in aging lung. Gerontology 29:377–387, 1983.
Collagen content of the pulmonary parenchyma decreases with increasing age, but there is no change in elastin content. Contains good discussion of earlier work in this area.

Black LF, Hyatt RE: Maximal respiratory pressures: Normal values and relationship to age and sex. Am Rev Respir Dis 99:696–702, 1969.
Normal values for isometric strength of respiratory muscles, effects of age, and differences between male and female subjects.

Brischetto MJ, Millman RP, Peterson DD, Silage DA, Pack AI: Effect of aging on ventilatory response to exercise and CO_2. J Appl Physiol 56:1143–1150, 1984.
In same group of elderly subjects there is an increase in ventilatory response to exercise and decrease in response to inhaled CO_2.

Carskadon MA, Dement WC: Respiration during sleep in the aged human. J Gerontol 36:420–423, 1981.
About 38 percent of asymptomatic elderly subjects had more than five episodes of apnea per hour sleep.

Dement WC, Miles LE, Carskadon MA: "White paper" on sleep and aging. J Am Geriat Soc 30:25–50, 1982.
Up-to-date review on changes in sleep with increasing age.

Edge JR, Millard FJC, Reid L, Simon G: The radiographic appearance of the chest in persons of advanced age. Br J Radiol 37:769–774, 1964.
Survey of chest radiographs in asymptomatic subjects at least 75 years of age.

Georges R, Saumon G, Loiseau A: The relationship of age to pulmonary membrane conductance and capillary blood volume. Am Rev Respir Dis 117:1069–1078, 1978.
The diffusing capacity falls with age due initially to changes in membrane diffusing capacity (Dm). Later this fall is exaggerated by reductions in pulmonary capillary blood volume (Vc) as well.

Hodgson JL, Buskirk ER: Physical fitness and age, with emphasis on cardiovascular function in the elderly. J Am Geriatr Soc 25:385–392, 1977.
Useful review of earlier classic work on effects of aging on maximum oxygen uptake and how this is affected by physical conditioning.

Holland J, Milic-Emili J, Macklem PT, Bates DV: Regional distribution of pulmonary ventilation and perfusion in elderly subjects. J Clin Invest 47:81–92, 1968.
In elderly, distribution of ventilation at functional residual capacity is not preferential to lower lobes because of effects of airways closure.

Klocke RA: Influence of aging on the lung, in Finch CE, Hayflick L (eds), *Handbook of the Biology of Aging.* New York, Van Nostrand Reinhold, 1977, pp 432–444.
General review that concentrates particularly on changes in lung structure, lung mechanics and gas-exchange function of the lung with age.

Knight H, Millman RP, Pack AI, Shore ET, Gur RC, Doherty JU: Clinical significance of sleep apnea in the elderly. Am Rev Respir Dis 136:845–850, 1987.
Although apnea during sleep in the elderly may be associated with an increase in daytime sleepiness, it need not result in other physiological or neuropsychologic disturbances.

Knudson RJ, Lebowitz MD, Holberg CJ, Burrows B: Changes in the normal maximal expiratory flow-volume curve with growth and aging. Am Rev Respir Dis 127:725–734, 1983.
Prediction equations developed for effect of age on a number of spirometric variables by cross-sectional study of large sample (697) of nonsmokers.

Kronenberg RE, Drage CW: Attenuation of the ventilatory and heart rate responses to hypoxia and hypercapnia with aging in normal men. J Clin Invest 52:1812–1819, 1973.
Now classic study that first demonstrated reductions of similar magnitude in ventilatory response to hypoxia and hypercapnia in older male subjects.

Leblanc P, Ruff F, Milic-Emili J: Effects of age and body position on "airway closure" in man. J Appl Physiol 28:448–451, 1970.
Increase in closing volume with age. Seated closing volume typically exceeds FRC by age 65; while supine this occurs by age 44.

Mahler DA, Rosiello RA, Loke J: The aging lung. Clin Geriatr Med 2:215–225, 1986.
Lung elasticity decreases, stiffness of the chest wall increases, and respiratory muscle strength declines. These alterations contribute to gradual, but progressive, reductions in forced vital capacity, expiratory flow rates, diffusing capacity, gas exchange, ventilatory drive, and respiratory sensation.

Mauderly JL: Effect of age on pulmonary structure and function of immature and adult animals and man. Fed Proc 38:173–177, 1979.
Concise review of changes in lung structure and function (mechanical and gas exchange) with growth and senescence both in humans and other animals (largely dogs).

Mittman C, Edelman NH, Norris AH, Shock NW: Relationship between chest wall and pulmonary compliance and age. J Appl Physiol 20:1211–1216, 1965.
Classic study that indicates that the major change in lung mechanics in the elderly is decrease in chest wall compliance.

Muiesan G, Sorbini CA, Grassi V: Respiratory function in the aged. Bull Eur Physiopathol Respir 7:973–1009, 1971.
Useful relatively complete review on earlier literature on changes in pulmonary function with advancing age.

Munsat T: Aging of the neuromuscular system, in Albert ML (ed), *Clinical Neurology of Aging,* New York, Oxford University Press, 1984, pp 404–424.
Useful review on changes in morphology, electrophysiology, and bioenergetics of skeletal muscle with age.

Niewoehner DE, Kleinerman J: Morphologic basis of pulmonary resistance in the human lung and effects of aging. J Appl Physiol 36:412–418, 1974.
Shows decrease in average bronchiolar diameter in later life.

Pack AI, Silage DA, Millman RP, Shore ET, Chung DCC: Spectral analysis of ventilation in elderly subjects awake and asleep. J Appl Physiol 64:1257–1267, 1988.
Elderly individuals who develop apnea during sleep have an increased propensity for periodic breathing while awake.

Peterson DD, Fishman AP: The lungs in later life, in Fishman AP (ed), *Update: Pulmonary Diseases and Disorders,* New York, McGraw-Hill, 1982, pp 123–136.
More extensive bibliography than is presented here.

Peterson DD, Pack AI, Silage DA, Fishman AP: Effects of aging on ventilatory and occlusion pressure responses to hypoxia and hypercapnia. Am Rev Respir Dis 124:387–391, 1981.
Study that confirmed and extended that of Kronenberg and Drage. Reduction in the ventilatory response in the elderly is not explained by stiffening of the chest wall and reduction in inspiratory muscle force.

Schmidt CD, Dickman ML, Gardner RM, Brough FK: Spirometric standards for healthy elderly men and women. Am Rev Respir Dis 108:933–939, 1973.
Relatively large study (532 subjects, ages 55 to 94) to establish normal values for spirometry for this age group. FEV/FVC of <70 percent cannot be used to diagnose obstructive lung disease above age 60.

Shore ET, Millman RP, Silage DA, Chung DCC, Pack AI: Ventilatory and arousal patterns during sleep in normal young and elderly subjects. J Appl Physiol 59:1607–1615, 1985.
Central and obstructive apneas during stages 1 to 2 sleep appear to be an extension of normal periodic breathing routinely seen during light sleep.

Sorbini CA, Grassi V, Solinas E, Muiesan G: Arterial oxygen tension in relation to age in healthy subjects. Respiration 25:3–13, 1968.
Age widens the alveolar-arterial O_2 difference and lowers resting arterial P_{O_2}.

Thurlbeck WM, Angus GE: Growth and aging of the normal human lung. Chest 67:3S–6S, 1975.
Brief review of changes in lung structure with age.

Turner JM, Mead J, Wohl ME: Elasticity of human lungs in relation to age. J Appl Physiol 25:664–671, 1968.
Confirms reduction in elastic recoil with age. Useful review of earlier literature and discussion on consequences of changes in elastic properties of lung and chest wall.

Chapter 5

The Upper Respiratory Tract

Lars Malm / Nils Gunnar Toremalm

The upper respiratory tract comprises the nasal cavities and paranasal sinuses, the pharynx and larynx. From a phylogenetic point of view, the eustachian tube and the middle ear should also be considered a part of the respiratory tract. This is especially important from a clinical standpoint because of the intermittent gas exchange between the environmental air and the middle ear. The region as a whole can suitably be divided into seven different parts according to their special features related to the different functions and connections with other organs (Fig. 5-1). The common characteristic of this irregular anatomic system is the epithelial layer with its extraordinary capacities for active and passive exchange of heat and moisture and the mucociliary transportation of secretions.

Most of the modification of the inspired air occurs in the nose, where the inspired air is considerably cleaned, warmed, and humidified by the aerodynamic patterns of flow and by the nasal mucosa.

MORPHOLOGY

The Nose

The interior shape of the nose and the quality of the mucosal lining are of vital importance for the function of the lower airways. The two nasal cavities are nearly equal and are separated by the nasal septum. The lateral wall of the cavities usually has three turbinates, or conchae, an arrangement that considerably increases the mucosal area and contributes to the airflow patterns. Figure 5-2, which includes a schematic drawing of the anterior lateral wall, illustrates five cross sections of the nasal cavity. The smallest cross-sectional area, the internal ostium, is also the narrowest passage of the entire upper respiratory tract. The nostrils can be widened actively by spreading the alar cartilages (Fig. 5-2).

The vestibular region of the nose is lined with a stratified squamous epithelium like the skin, which explains why skin diseases, such as furuncles and contact allergies, can appear. From the internal ostium to the anterior edge of the inferior turbinate, the epithelium is transitional or intermediate in type. Further back, the walls are lined with a typical airway epithelium, which is pseudostratified and columnar. The respiratory epithelium in the nose consists mainly of four types of cells, which are in contact with a basement membrane; the ciliated columnar cells, the nonciliated columnar cells with microvilli, the goblet cells, and the basal cells. Clara cells, and some other epithelial cells that are found in the lower respiratory tract

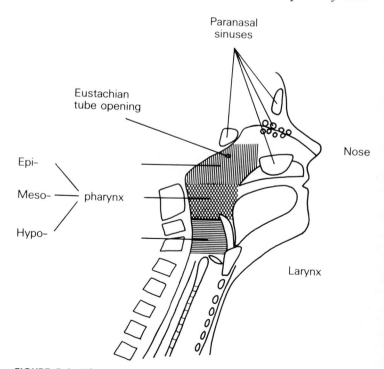

FIGURE 5-1 The seven regions of the upper respiratory tract (see text).

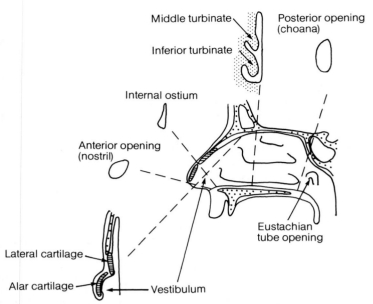

FIGURE 5-2 Lateral aspect of a nasal cavity with five cross sections including the septum.

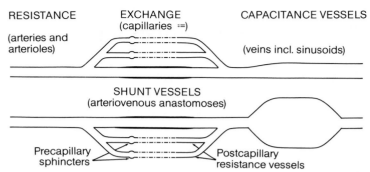

FIGURE 5-3 Schematic drawing of a functional classification of nasal blood vessels.

have not been discovered in the human nose. In the middle part of the inferior turbinate about 20 percent of the epithelial cells are ciliated. Cells with microvilli dominate, and the proportion of goblet cells is only 10 percent. The number of ciliated cells increases posteriorly toward the nasopharynx.

In the upper part of the nasal cavities, the olfactory epithelium consists of three types of cells. The olfactory cells are supplied with peripheral processes that reach the surface and central processes that contain axons and penetrate the cribriform plate of the ethmoid. The olfactory mucosa also includes supporting and basal cells.

The basement membrane of the nasal mucosa separates the epithelial cells from the lamina propria, also called the submucosa. This layer contains blood vessels, lymph vessels, glands, nerves, and connective tissues. Below the submucosa, close to the cartilage or bone, there is a perichondrium or periosteum, respectively.

Two types of blood vessels are richly represented in the nasal mucosa: sinusoids and arteriovenous anastomoses (Fig. 5-3). The sinusoids, which are relatively large venous vessels equipped with smooth muscles throughout their length and richly innervated by adrenergic nerves, allow rapid changes in the thickness of the mucosa. The arteriovenous anastomoses, or shunt vessels, also allow rapid changes in the distribution of the blood. Both of these types of blood vessels are critically important for the exchange of heat and moisture between blood and air breathed through the nose. The occurrence of fenestrated capillaries just below the surface epithelium is probably also of importance for regulating the humidity of the inspired air.

The anatomic variety in the structure of the blood vessel structures is relevant to understanding particular nasal functions. A countercurrent arrangement of nasal arteries and veins found in the camel helps to reduce the loss of heat and water by breathing, while in feline animals it assists in regulating the temperature of the brain. In humans the latter function has no relevance, but the former is probably not without importance, although the ability of the human nose to humidify and warm the inspired air is stressed more often in the literature.

A functional classification of nasal blood vessels is reflected in the terminology—resistance vessels, exchange vessels or capillaries, and capacitance vessels—and is illustrated in Fig. 5-3. The tone of the resistance vessels regulates the blood flow through a tissue, while the tone of the capacitance vessels controls the blood volume or content and consequently also much of the thickness of the mucosa. This classification of nasal blood vessels is justified by the abundance of sinusoids. It is adequate also from a pharmacologic point of view, as some drugs mainly affect the capacitance vessels and others mainly the resistance vessels.

The lymph vessels of the vestibular part of the nose drain into submandibular nodes. The drainage from the rest of the nose collects in lymph nodes mostly situated parapharyngeally.

The glands of the nasal respiratory mucosa are mainly of two types. The serous anterior nasal glands open close to the internal ostium, whereas the numerous small seromucous glands are evenly distributed throughout the entire respiratory mucosa. The secretions reaching the nasopharynx do not originate from these two sources alone: fluids are also added from the paranasal sinuses, nasal goblet cells, and tear ducts.

The nerves of the respiratory mucosa have been studied extensively during the last two decades as a result of the simultaneous development of new histochemical methods capable of revealing extremely minute amounts of peptides. Most of these studies have been performed in the nose because of relatively easy access to nerve fibers

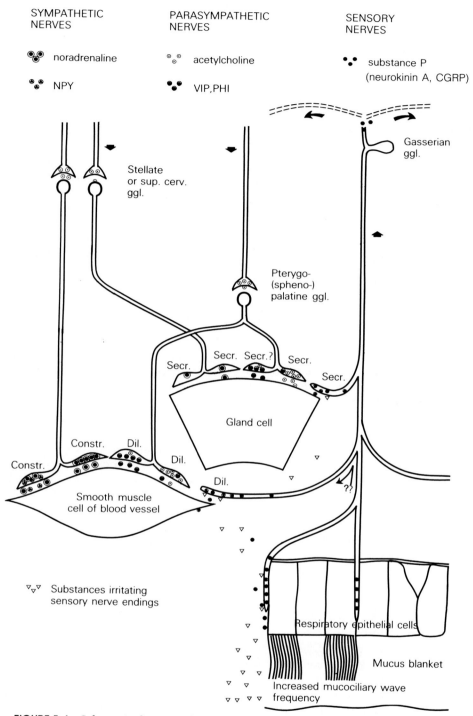

SYMPATHETIC NERVES

noradrenaline

NPY

PARASYMPATHETIC NERVES

acetylcholine

VIP,PHI

SENSORY NERVES

substance P (neurokinin A, CGRP)

Stellate or sup. cerv. ggl.

Pterygo- (spheno-) palatine ggl.

Gasserian ggl.

Secr.   Secr.   Secr.?   Secr.

Secr.

Gland cell

Constr.   Dil.

Constr.

Dil.

Dil.

Dil.

Smooth muscle cell of blood vessel

??

Substances irritating sensory nerve endings

Respiratory epithelial cells

Mucus blanket

Increased mucociliary wave frequency

FIGURE 5-4 Schematic drawing of the innervation and effects of nerve stimulation of the nasal mucosa (see text).

and ganglia. However, the results are also relevant for the lower respiratory tract. A summary of the innervation of the nasal mucosa is illustrated in Fig. 5-4.

Although the cholinergic (parasympathetic) innervation of arteries, arterioles, arteriovenous anastomoses, and glands is quite rich, it is sparse around venous vessels and sinusoids. The postganglionic fibers to the lower and main part of the nose originate in the pterygopalatine ganglion, situated just posteriorly to the maxillary sinus. The corresponding nerve fibers to the upper part or the nasal mucosa originate in the ciliary ganglion.

The classic transmitter of postganglionic parasympathetic neurons is acetylcholine. Two peptides that are also considered to be neurotransmitters, VIP (vasoactive intestinal peptide) and PHI (peptide with N-terminal histidine and C-terminal isoleucine) have been demonstrated in the cell bodies of the pterygopalatine ganglion and in the nerve endings; in at least some neurons, these peptides probably coexist with acetylcholine. VIP and PHI dilate blood vessels. VIP probably augments the fluid secretions released by acetylcholine and perhaps also changes the composition of the secretions as in salivary glands.

Adrenergic (sympathetic) innervation is very rich around the sinusoids, and an abundance of such nerves is also found around small arteries, arterioles, and arteriovenous anastomoses. Sparse but obvious adrenergic innervation exists close to the glands. A clinically important finding is the occurrence of continuous impulse traffic in the sympathetic nerves by which the neurotransmitter noradrenaline is continuously released to the nasal blood vessels; this sympathetic discharge maintains the tone of the vessels, especially of the sinusoids. Some antihypertensive and antipsychotic drugs result in congestion of the nasal mucosa because of their effect on the α adrenoreceptors of the smooth muscles of the vessels.

Adrenergic nerves also seem to have more than one neurotransmitter. Recently a peptide called neuropeptide Y (NPY) was demonstrated in adrenergic nerves. NPY is vasoconstrictive by itself and probably augments the effects of noradrenaline.

A dense plexus of nerve fibers close to and within the epithelium of the nasal mucosa is considered to belong to the sensory innervation. Sensory nerves also contain neurotransmitters. Substance P has been demonstrated in central branches of the trigeminal nerve as well as in peripheral branches in the nasal mucosa. This peptide is strongly vasodilatory and evokes edema. Secretory and mucociliary effects are also known.

Animal experiments have shown that certain gases and substances such as ether, formalin, and cigarette smoke can affect the nasal mucosa via sensory nerves containing substance P. These neurons are also sensitive to capsaicin, a pungent substance found in a large variety of hot red peppers. Capsaicin initiates reflexes like sneezing and simultaneously releases substance P. It seems as if the local release of substance P in the nasal mucosa by vasodilatation and edema, together with increased secretion and increased mucociliary activity, is an attempt to eliminate inhaled irritants. Thus, it cooperates with some of the respiratory reflexes passing the central nervous system. Other reflexes initiated in the nose, such as cardiovascular ones, may use sensory neurons resistant to capsaicin which therefore may not contain substance P.

This new information concerning nasal innervation and blood vessel control relates not only to nasal defense mechanisms but probably also to the defense mechanisms of the lower respiratory tract.

The Eustachian Tube and the Middle Ear

The eustachian tube openings to the epipharynx lie at the same level as the posterior end of the inferior turbinates. The tubes differ from the ostia of the paranasal sinuses in that they are closed most of the time. They open only during swallowing and yawning, when equalization of the air pressure in the middle ear and the atmosphere takes place. A continuously open eustachian tube causes very disturbing hearing sensations, among which hearing one's own voice "as in a barrel" is the most common. The eustachian tubes are lined with respiratory mucosa that contains ciliated cells that propel secretions toward the nasopharynx, a function which does not seem necessary for pressure equalization. In the middle ear the epithelium contains more ciliated cells near the openings of the tubes. The epithelium is mainly cuboidal with scattered ciliated cells in the middle ear; it becomes squamous in the mastoid cells.

The Paranasal Sinuses

The paranasal sinuses are airspaces in the facial bones that open into the nose. They are all lined with a respiratory mucosa that is similar to the nasal respiratory mucosa, except that the sinusoids are smaller and a larger proportion of epithelial cells are ciliated. Most of the paranasal sinuses have their openings below the middle turbinate.

The anatomic proximity of the paranasal sinuses to the oral cavity, the orbit, and the meninges is of special clinical importance with respect to infectious complications, trauma, and surgery. Like the nasal mucosa, the lymphatic drainage of the mucosa of the paranasal sinuses is to the submandibular, retropharyngeal, and upper deep cervical glands.

The Pharynx

The nasopharynx begins at the posterior openings of the nasal cavities, the choanae, and continues to the level of the soft palate. It is mainly lined with pseudostratified columnar ciliated epithelium that changes to squamous epithelium approximately where the uvula and the soft palate touch the posterior and lateral walls during swallowing. The posterior wall contains adenoid tissues, which in small children may grow to a size that impairs nasal breathing and necessitates removal. The adenoid tissues form part of the Waldeyer's tonsillar ring, the remainder consisting of the pharyngeal and lingual tonsils. Both tonsils and adenoids contain numerous germinal centers that are mainly vascular; they are involved in the development of immune defense, especially in children.

The oropharynx is of major interest for the upper digestive tract. The mucosa is richly supplied with small salivary glands and submucosal lymphatic tissues. The muscular system around the oropharynx is involved in swallowing and plays no active role in ventilation. However, the soft palate and the base of the tongue may impede ventilation during snoring. The pharyngeal tonsils contribute to the lymphatic defense mechanism against nosocomial infections.

The hypopharynx continues to the glottic aperture in the midline and to the piriform sinuses laterally. The loosely attached mucosa undergoes large changes in shape and depth following the elevation of the larynx during swallowing.

The Larynx

The larynx is covered with a cuboid columnar epithelium above the level of the vocal cords and consists of cartilages, ligaments, and muscles. The former consists of three unpaired parts (the thyroid, the cricoid, and the epiglottic cartilages) and three paired parts (the arytenoid cartilages and the small corniculate and cuneiform cartilages). The conus elasticus is a circular stabilizing ligament connecting the larynx to the trachea. The cricoid ring constitutes the second smallest rigid part of the upper airways. The laryngeal muscles are divided functionally into an extrinsic and an intrinsic group. Among the extrinsic laryngeal muscles, the sternothyroid depresses the larynx and the thyrohyoid elevates it.

The pharyngotracheal muscles are attached to the posterior part of the larynx and are essential for swallowing. The mechanical properties of the intrinsic muscles are illustrated schematically in Fig. 5-5. The posterior cricoarytenoid muscles are abductors of the vocal folds. Adduction is brought about by the lateral cricoarytenoid muscles together with the interarytenoid and the thyroarytenoid muscles.

The larynx is innervated by two branches of the tenth cranial nerve, i.e., the superior laryngeal and the inferior laryngeal or recurrent nerves. The external branch of the superior laryngeal nerve supplies the cricothyroid mus-

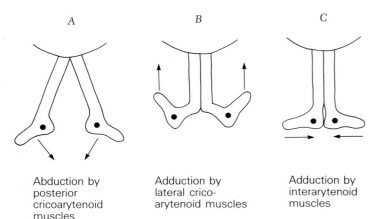

FIGURE 5-5 The mechanical effects of the intrinsic laryngeal muscles on the arytenoid cartilages and vocal folds.

cle. The internal branch, however, is strictly sensory and is responsible for reflexes evoked from the mucosa. This branch can be blocked by subcutaneous injections of a local anesthetic in order to reduce local pain and irritating coughing initiated from mucosal receptors. The recurrent nerves contain motor and sensory fibers. All the other intrinsic muscles are innervated via the recurrent nerves which, because of their extended looping course into the thoracic cavity before reaching the larynx, are easily damaged by surgery and by mediastinal diseases. The blood supply to the larynx is via the superior and inferior thyroid arteries. The vocal folds divide the lymphatic drainage of the larynx into a supraglottic and a subglottic part. The supraglottic drainage goes to the upper deep cervical glands. The subglottic drainage goes to the retrotracheal and lower deep cervical glands.

The subglottic space belongs to the laryngeal region and is of special interest for ventilation and air conditioning. The vocal folds constitute a functional stenosis that increases turbulence during inspiration. Because of poorer conditioning of the inspired air, dryness, irritation, coughing, secondary edema, and formation of crusts in the subglottic region are more apt to occur during mouth breathing than during nasal breathing. This phenomenon is considered subsequently in the section on upper respiratory tract diseases.

FUNCTION

A very important function of *the nose* is to provide for *olfaction.* Patients with nasal polyps are often more disabled by the loss of smell than by the loss of nasal breathing. In most mammals two areas of the nose are involved in olfaction. One is situated in the upper part of the nose and contains sensory cells that are stimulated by airborne molecules. This is the best known sense of smell. Stimulation can change the pattern of breathing. The other sense of smell, which is vestigial in humans, is of great importance for sexual behavior. It is located in the vomeronasal or Jacobson's organ, which is situated in the floor of the nasal cavity and reacts to pheromones dissolved in secretions.

The nose has a *cleansing* function for inspired air. The more inspired air that is in contact with the nasal mucosa the more efficient is the cleansing. Consequently, adequately narrow passages favor turbulent inspiratory airflow in the turbinated portion of the main nasal passage. When water-soluble gases, microorganisms, and other particles in the inspired air meet the secretion of the respiratory mucosa, immunologic and phagocytic activities are initiated and the adhered material is transported to the oropharynx. The nasal defense system, based on humoral antibodies, mucosal and tissue mast cells, phagocytic cells, and other cellular and humoral mechanisms, does not differ from that of the lower respiratory tract.

Mucociliary function resides in most of the upper respiratory tract and constitutes an essential part of the total defense system against inhaled particles and chemical pollutants. Much of our knowledge about this transport mechanism has been gained from studies of the nose and paranasal sinuses. The movements of the cilia are well coordinated into about 1500 to 2000 wiping movements a minute. ATP is the energy source. The ATP stored in the mitochondria of the cells makes it possible for the cilia to continue to beat for several hours without any blood supply if the environmental conditions are suitable. This makes it possible to use the mucociliary function for various experimental purposes, e.g., in vitro toxicity studies.

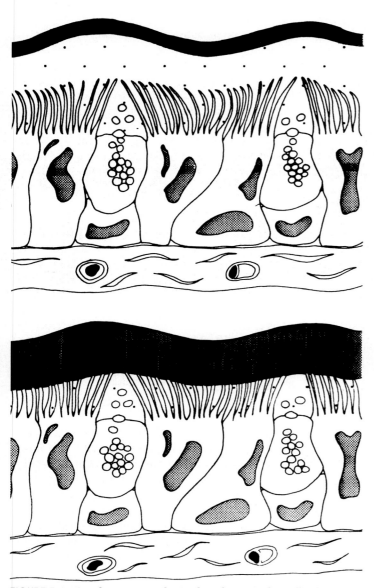

FIGURE 5-6 Freely moving cilia within the periciliary fluid (*above*) and immobilized cilia due to increased amounts of mucus (*below*). The transportation rate is compromised in both cases.

The cilia move within the watery periciliary fluid produced by serous glands and probably also by transudation. The free ends of the cilia are provided with brushlike extensions that grasp the undersurface of the floating, and more or less continuous, layer of mucus next to the lumen. The wave movements are transferred from the cilia to the mucus and can be studied indirectly by observing fluctuating surface light reflections under the microscope. If the amount of periciliary fluid is increased, the cilia move excellently but without improving transportation. If the periciliary fluid is reduced, or if the mucus layer thickens, the ciliary movements are obstructed (Fig. 5-6).

Thanks to the effective air conditioning capacity of the nose this function is normally seldom compromised, not even during inhalation of extremely cold, hot, or dry air. The transportation rate of the mucus varies locally and changes from time to time.

According to Proctor and Andersen, under normal conditions, the transportation rate in the nose may vary between 3 and 25 mm/min. Therefore, it is difficult to evaluate the true mucociliary capacity simply by studying the transportation of radioactively labeled particles or of saccharin and dye indicators. Any transport time through the nose exceeding 30 min is abnormal. Even if the nasal cilia are protected from dryness, they remain extremely sensitive to pollutants, such as tobacco smoke and sulfur dioxide.

The nose also has a *conditioning function* for the inspiratory air. Active warming and moistening of the inspiratory air at rest seems more important than recovering heat and water from the expiratory air, but the latter cannot be ignored. The extent to which water from the expired air is recovered is shown in Fig. 5-7, for a 24-h respiratory volume of 15 m^3 of ordinary room air.

The tracheobronchial mucosa does not have the same air-conditioning capacity as the nose. A practical consequence after tracheotomy is that the inspired air needs to be moistened, for example, by using a heat and moisture exchange (artificial nose).

About four to five times more heat is required for evaporating water than for warming the air. Under comfortable room conditions (20 to 24°C and 50 percent relative humidity), about 400 kcal (1674 kJ) is required to humidify and warm inspiratory air. According to Cole et al., this corresponds to one-sixth of the average adult's daily heat output.

Since at −20°C inspiratory air can be warmed to around 30°C in the pharynx, it is easy to understand that breathing in extreme climates can consume much of the heat of metabolism. In a cold, dry climate the quotient of evaporated and condensed water increases. In desert animals, as much as 90 percent of the water evaporated to the inspiratory air can be recovered from condensation during expiration.

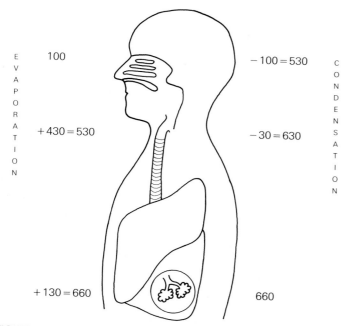

FIGURE 5-7 The daily water vapor content (grams per 15 m³) of inspired air (evaporation) and expired air (condensation) during normal nasal respiration. At 21°C and relative humidity of 35 percent, the 15 m³ of ambient air contains about 100 g of water in the form of vapor. As may be seen *(left)*, during nasal inspiration about 430 g is added by means of evaporation from the mucous membranes in the upper air passages. Only 130 g is supplied from the zone below the larynx. The air in the lungs is almost fully saturated at body temperature so that the 24-h respiratory volume (15 m³) contains altogether 660 g of water at 37°C. The warm and moist expired air *(right)* is primarily cooled during passage through the nose. Part of the moisture condenses on the walls of the nose, where the temperature of the nasal mucous membrane is 3 to 4°C lower than body temperature. Nonetheless, the expired air contains more than 500 g of water when leaving the body by normal nasal respiration. Only 130 g (20 percent) of water from the expired air condenses, chiefly in the nose.

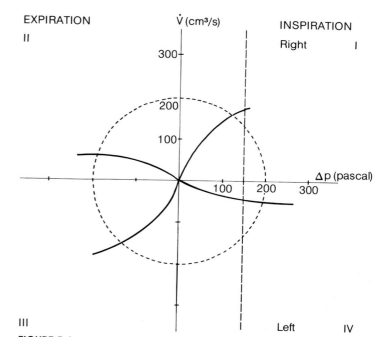

FIGURE 5-8 Pressure flow curves of the right and left nasal cavities. The nasal airway resistance can be given, e.g., at a pressure of 150 Pa or at a circle with radius 200 Pa and 200 cm³/s.

A relative measure of the size of the air passages in the nose is given by the *nasal airway resistance*. The usual method for recording nasal airway resistance is known as *rhinomanometry*, although it ought to be called rhinorheomanometry, since the measure is based on the quotient between transnasal pressure and nasal airflow. Most of the nasal airway resistance (about 70 percent) originates from the internal ostium, which limits its importance as a measure of the size of the air passages as a whole. Unlike that of the lower respiratory tract, the rhinomanometric pressure flow curve is not linear: because of the turbulent airflow, the resistance increases with increasing flow. The methods recommended by the Standardization Committee of the European Rhinologic Society for recording and charting the resistance of the nasal passages are illustrated in Fig. 5-8. Many other methods are described in the literature. One that uses a microprocessor to calculate the work and power for the air

passing through the nose enables simple comparisons with other resistive segments of the airway.

Although the nasal airway resistance of the entire nose remains fairly constant for hours during emotional and physical rest, the resistance of a cavity usually fluctuates. The venous erectile tissues of the nasal mucosa exhibit periodic alternation between congestion and decongestion, thereby causing the main airflow to shift from one nasal cavity to the other. This shift is found in about 80 percent of human subjects and also in animals.

The nasal cycle was described before the end of the last century. It usually recurs every 2 to 4 h. Most people are not aware of their own nasal cycle, unless there are factors, such as a common cold, that increase congestion. The cycle depends on sympathetic nerve activity under the influence of a hypothalamic center. The purpose of the nasal cycle is not known, although proposals have been advanced. A probable explanation is that the mucosa of one cavity rests while that of the other takes over most of the conditioning and cleansing activity.

The increased airway resistance of the entire nose during recumbency is probably caused by increased venous pressure and distension of the vessels. Good advice to people who have difficulty sleeping because of a stuffy nose is to raise the upper end of the bed, thereby reducing the venous pressure in the head region. Lying on a side also affects the nasal mucosa; the mucosa of the lower cavity becomes congested within a few minutes, while the mucosa of the upper cavity is decongested This phenomenon can easily be checked by applying the thumb to each nostril in turn to judge the ease, or difficulty, in breathing. The effect of position is mediated by a reflex initiated from skin receptors, just as pressure applied to an armpit by a crutch causes ipsilateral nasal congestion (a method described in ancient yoga literature).

At birth the nose is practically the only route for respiration. Later, some of the breathing at rest takes the oral path. On increasing physical activity, oral breathing gradually takes over more and more of ventilation, although the nasal airway resistance simultaneously falls markedly. Even with strong activity, 40 percent of the ventilation continues to pass via the nose.

The *larynx* serves several functions such as respiration, phonation, and protection of the lower airways against inhaled particles, secretions, fluids, and food. A closed larynx is also essential for momentary fixation of the chest, e.g., during coughing, vomiting, defecation, lifting, and childbirth, in order to increase pressure in the thoracic and abdominal cavities. The glottic function is also essential for breathing, the aperture of the rima glottidis being regulated automatically via the abductor and adductor muscles. The degree of opening may even influence the acid-base balance of the body by way of determining the arterial P_{CO_2}. When open, the glottis offers little resistance to the airflow; this resistance varies slightly between inspiration and expiration, during panting and deep breathing.

The sphincter function of the larynx takes place at three different levels: at the aryepiglottic folds, the ventricular or false vocal folds, and the true vocal folds.

The *aryepiglottic sphincter* is the most important with regard to protection. During swallowing, the aryepiglottic folds move inward and the epiglottis apparently downward and rearward, thereby facilitating the shunting of a bolus laterally into the piriform sinuses. The elevation of the entire laryngeal skeleton enhances these movements. However, swallowing without aspiration is possible even without an epiglottis because of active or reflex closure of the ventricular and vocal folds. The swallowing reflex is initiated via the ninth cranial nerve as the food touches the hypopharynx, respiration being momentarily arrested. This poses a special problem for some tracheotomized patients, who are able to breath via the stoma during swallowing and, therefore, tend to aspirate.

The *ventricular folds* work as a true sphincter to resist pressure from below. When closed, the intrathoracic pressure can be increased, for example, to facilitate coughing.

The *true vocal folds* can easily be opened by pressure from below, but resist pressure from above. Their vibratory movements are essential for phonation, but in a much more complex fashion than, for example, those of the lips when playing simple wind instruments. The

length, tension, and mass of the vocal folds, together with the resonance of the pharyngeal, oral, nasal, and paranasal cavities, determine the final pitch and timbre of the sound, whereas the respiratory muscles determine the sound pressure.

The laryngeal mucosa is extremely sensitive to external irritants, and it easily triggers coughing and swallowing reflexes. Chevalier Jackson's description of the larynx as "the watchdog of the lungs" is therefore highly significant. Hypersensitive mucosa is often the only cause of nonproductive coughing, a distressing problem that is easily cured by blocking the medial, sensory branches of the upper laryngeal nerves.

The cricoid cartilage is the only supporting structure of the circular airway at this level of the respiratory tract. Its integrity is therefore essential for maintaining an open airway. In contrast, the cartilages of the trachea, often spoken of as tracheal "rings," should be looked upon as open arches from an anatomic and functional point of view. They are narrowed actively by the dominating circularly arranged tracheal muscles, whereas widening of the tracheal lumen is largely the result of the elasticity of the cartilages. The flexible part of trachea—pars membranacea—is of clinical significance because it is easily sucked inward, thereby worsening stridulous ventilation during inspiration.

Reflexes between the Nose and the Lungs

Blowing air through one nasal cavity in laryngectomized patients causes ipsilateral expansion of the thorax, a response that can be inhibited by anesthesia of the nasal mucosa. Other nasopulmonary reflexes have been described above in the section on nasal innervation. Both bronchoconstriction and bronchodilatation occur after nasal stimulation, probably in relation to different types and strengths of stimulation. An increase in intrapulmonary airway resistance occurs in healthy subjects with nasal packings, and it is a common clinical experience that cold air in the nose of patients with bronchial asthma can initiate an asthmatic attack. Although not entirely understood, the existence of nasopulmonary reflexes can certainly not be denied.

DISEASES

As Proctor has pointed out, "symptoms referred to the upper airways may reflect lung disease or conversely, symptoms referred to the chest may originate in the upper airways."

The Nose

Nasal "stuffiness" is a term that can be compared to dyspnea. It is a sensation of difficulty in nasal breathing. The nasal airway resistance is not necessarily increased. On the contrary, it can be very low as in atrophic rhinitis, nowadays an unusual disease in northern countries. In atrophic rhinitis, the cavities are very wide, the mucosa thin and infected. The cause is unknown, other people notice a bad smell (the "stinky" nose), and the patient suffers from "stuffiness."

The word *congestion* is preferred for increased vascular thickness of the mucosa and *obstruction* for any obstacle whatever to breathing (a thick mucosa, polyps, a foreign body, etc.). Congestion seems to be more popular and is used by many as a synonym for obstruction.

Patients with a common cold usually suffer from severe nasal stuffiness. This does not necessarily mean that there is limited air passage through the nose. It is possible that the subjective symptom of stuffiness is more dependent on increased secretion and/or an edema around sensory nerve endings than on congested nasal mucosa. A well-known finding in the common cold is that immediately after sleep there is a sensation of very little secretion and a clear nose. The absence of secretion at that moment indicates that reflexes are involved. It is surprising how little research about these and similar aspects of the common cold is to be found in the literature.

Nasal allergy is also a common disorder. The symptoms are sneezing, watery secretion, and nasal stuffiness. Vasomotor rhinitis (or perennial nonallergic rhinitis) has the same symptoms.

Occupational exposure to irritating fumes and particles may cause nasal stuffiness and nasal discharge. Certain irritants are dangerous. For example, there is an increased incidence of adenocarcinoma of the nose and paranasal sinuses among wood furniture workers. There is also a reported increased risk of nasal carcinoma among nickel workers.

Small children are inclined to put objects in their noses. Unilateral nasal stuffiness with a noxious and sometimes bloody secretion in a small child is always an indication for a thorough inspection of the nose for a foreign body. Similar unilateral symptoms in an elderly person may indicate cancer of the nose or a paranasal sinus. In adults, if there is no blood in the secretions, the first thought is dental empyema via a maxillary sinus.

A deviating nasal septum is a common cause of nasal obstruction, especially in men. If the deviation is due to fracture, the septum (and the external nose) can be corrected within a week by pressure and lifting, without operation. Older fractures necessitate septoplasty or a combined septorhinoplasty, i.e., a surgical correction. However, people without nasal stuffiness seldom have a completely straight septum, so that a deviating septum does not by itself indicate a need for surgery. Rhinomanometry can be recommended to select those patients with nasal stuffiness who have a good chance of improvement by surgical correction. The nasal airway re-

sistance must be determined with the mucosa properly decongested by physical exercise or nose drops, since the firm structures (the cartilage and the bone) are the ones that can be corrected. In acute nasal fractures, it must not be forgotten that the interior of the nose has to be inspected, otherwise, a hematoma of the septum, followed by an infection, can be overlooked. An infected hematoma of the septum that is not treated correctly can easily cause complete breakdown of the septum cartilage, followed by external deformity and severe nasal obstruction.

Pharmacologic agents that have α-adrenergic antagonistic actions are prescribed for hypertension and for certain psychoses and cause nasal congestion. Other drugs used to treat hypertension, such as *Rauwolfia* preparations, also have this disturbing side effect. Diuretics and β-adrenergic antagonists do not cause nasal congestion, and it is sometimes possible to switch to these medications. Patients suffering from nasal stuffiness should always be asked about their intake of drugs.

Rhinitis medicamentosa is a disabling affection of nasal congestion evoked by chronic use of topical vasoconstrictors. It is usually difficult to get the patient to stop the misuse of nose drops, which is the only way to eliminate the problem. However, withdrawal can be facilitated by letting the patient use topical corticosteroids for 2 or 3 weeks. Another threat to the nasal mucosa is the increasing use of aerosols for nasal application of different remedies, such as antihistamines, corticostertoids, pituitary hormones, antidiabetic drugs, and contraceptives. Added preservatives, such as benzalkonium chloride, may be particularly detrimental to the biocellular functions of the nasal mucosa.

Certain hormones influence the nasal mucosa. Hypothyroidism causes nasal congestion by edema and growth of connective tissues. In pregnancy, the nose is congested by edema and dilated blood vessels, especially the sinusoids. Vasoconstrictory nose drops have very little effect during pregnancy because the congestion is due to increased production of progesterone, thereby reducing the sensitivity of α-adrenergic receptors.

The Paranasal Sinuses

Nasal stuffiness, headache, tiredness, and a cough may be the only symptoms of sinusitis, especially in children. Children can seldom localize the pain to pinpoint a particular sinus. In adults, the localization of the headache or pain is often characteristic for each sinus: in the cheek or upper teeth, a maxillary sinus; medially, just below the eyebrow or in the lower forehead, a frontal sinus; in, or behind, the eye, an ethmoid sinus; and, in the parietal region, a sphenoid sinus. It is possible to open all sinuses surgically if pain is excruciating or if abscesses threaten the surroundings. Acute frontal sinusitis is an emergency for the ear, nose, and throat (ENT) surgeon. Surgical intervention in any sinus, except perhaps a maxillary sinus, must be preceded by a radiographic examination. A frontal sinus may be absent in a patient older than 10 to 12 years. Furthermore, except for the maxillary sinuses, the topography of the sinuses varies widely. Only a short distance separates the brain from the frontal sinus; the orbit is close to others and may be involved in sinus affections. The most dangerous condition is acute ethmoiditis in children, causing periorbital edema and, later, a phlegmon. In these children, the eyelids are swollen, particularly in their medial parts. The swollen lids usually cause them to consult an ophthalmologist first.

Polyposis nasi originates from the ethmoidal region. Simple removal of visible polyps reduces nasal obstruction, but the ethmoidal cells are still filled with edematous tissues. Exacerbation of the coexisting chronic ethmoiditis, accompanied by droplet infection to the lower airways, is fairly common. A combination of thorough surgical removal and long-term treatment with topical corticosteroids seems to give the best results. Seldom is the cause of nasal polyposis found. Intolerance to acetylsalicylic acid (aspirin) is the cause in some patients, especially in those who also have bronchial asthma.

The extension of infections, abscesses, mucoceles, cysts, and tumors can necessitate conventional tomography or computed tomography. Experience is also growing with magnetic resonance imaging (MRI) of affections in and around the sinuses.

The experienced physician often can diagnose and treat sinusitis, without radiography, in patients in whom symptoms are less severe. Ultrasound offers the prospect of new, noninvasive, and inexpensive aid in diagnosing affections in the maxillary and frontal sinuses.

In some patients with sinusitis, a decrease in the diameter of the openings to the sinuses probably predates the illness. Therefore, the first treatment before antibiotics is to enlarge the passage. One way is by maintaining an upright position since the blood vessels are then less congested than during recumbency. Another way is to use decongestants. Locally administered decongestants, such as nose drops or spray, are preferable to systemic ones, since the latter have side effects, such as palpitations, hypertension, disturbances in micturition, and even psychoses. The paucity of studies on oral decongestants in sinusitis seems to reflect the consensus that topical decongestants have such easy access to the openings of the sinuses that systemic decongestants are unnecessary. Parenthetically, systemic decongestants have no effect in acute otitis media, in otitis media with effusion, or in the prophylaxis of acute otitis media.

The Ears

There are two reasons why the middle ear has to be mentioned in a chapter dealing with the upper respiratory tract. One is the distribution of the mucous membrane in the whole area, as described above. The other is the complex innervation which includes several connections between the ear and the fifth, ninth, and tenth cranial nerves.

Middle ear infections are a common complication of upper respiratory tract diseases. Inflammatory swelling of the eustachian tube mucosa compromises pressure equalization between the pharynx and the middle ear and facilitates the migration of microorganisms from the nasopharynx. The cause of a middle ear infection is usually the same, i.e., reduced eustachian tube function often in combination with bacterial colonization. Myringitis, retraction of the drum, serous otitis media, acute or purulent otitis media, and glue ear, are usual expressions for different phases of an infection. Aerotitis media is an intermediate form of middle ear dysfunction provoked by pressure changes during airplane descent or scuba diving. People with acute respiratory tract infections should be aware of this phenomenon and avoid such activities when infected.

Otalgia, without involvement of the external or middle ear, may be referred from the nose and molar teeth (trigeminal nerve via the auriculotemporal nerve), the pharynx (glossopharyngeal nerve via the tympanic nerve), or the larynx (vagal nerve via the auricular nerve). These cross innervations must be kept in mind for differential diagnostic purposes regarding symptoms from the upper digestive and respiratory tracts. A cough reflex during irritation of the external auditory meatus is an effect of such a nervous connection.

The Epipharynx

In children the dominating symptom from this region is airway obstruction by adenoid vegetations. The background is repeated nasal infection stimulating the growth of lymphatic tissues. Bacterial colonization of this area, without clinical manifestations, is common. Intermittent nasal infections accompanied by mucopurulent secretions, a nasal voice, and a tendency to oral respiration especially during sleep are typical complaints when airflow is blocked by an adenoid. Adenoidectomy is the most common ENT operation in childhood. Airway obstruction is the only absolute indication for this operation; the possibility that a relationship exists between adenoids and recurrent otitis media is a matter of dispute.

In adults, nasopharyngeal carcinoma is the most difficult diagnostic problem. The tumor starts very silently without pain, obstruction, or bleeding. The disease should be suspected after long-lasting repeated occurrences of otitis media with effusion or a cervical lymph node metastasis without any signs of a primary tumor. In such cases repeated epipharyngeal biopsies are necessary.

The Oropharynx

This is the easiest region to examine by direct inspection. Nevertheless, proper diagnosis is very often overlooked. "Sore throat" and "angina" are two very common descriptions that are hardly accurate. In most instances, it is easy to distinguish acute pharyngitis as a superficial involvement of the mucosa from a true lymphoid infection, i.e., from tonsillitis. This distinction is necessary in order to reduce overconsumption of antibiotics: acute pharyngitis does not require them, whereas tonsillitis does. Tonsillectomy is the second most frequent ENT operation. Not very long ago, the procedure was carried out needlessly or because of doubtful indications. However, surgery is usually reserved for either repeated bouts of tonsillitis for 1 or 2 years or a complicating peritonsillar abscess. Recurrent pain and discomfort in the throat, without other symptoms of infection, may be due to chronic follicular tonsillitis. This diagnosis is sometimes difficult and often overlooked; inspection alone is not sufficient. The tonsils have to be compressed with a spatula in order to expose hidden infected debris and even inspissated epithelial plugs.

A malignant tumor should always be suspected when there is unilateral tonsillar pain, swelling, or ulceration in adults.

The Hypopharynx

Dysphagia is a fairly common symptom that on the one hand may connote disease of the hypopharynx, larynx, or upper part of the esophagus and, on the other, dysfunction of muscles involved in swallowing because of paralysis. Infections accompanied by local edema are common in this region because of the very loosely attached mucosa. Epiglottitis is the most dangerous disease, especially in childhood. However, dysphagia in conjunction with laryngeal obstruction, local pain, and drooling is so obvious that no patient should run the risk of suffocation even if the symptoms develop very quickly.

Malignant hypopharyngeal tumors are usually discovered unduly late because the initial symptoms are not localizing. Proper examination, using a mirror or, preferably, direct inspection is a measure that should be done too often rather than too late.

The Larynx

Functional disorders of voice and speech are not dealt with here. The organic diseases of the larynx have one common symptom: hoarseness. This symptom is so obvious to other people and so tiring for the patient that he or she usually sees a doctor who should be aware of the urgency to refer the patient to a specialist if hoarseness persists for more than 3 weeks.

In children, subglottic laryngitis (pseudocroup) is a common disease following a nasal infection. Steroids are the treatment of choice. Acute laryngitis in adults is a frequent complication of a common cold; it needs no treatment other than temporary rest of the voice.

In childhood, bilateral symmetric benign fibromas are the usual cause of persistent hoarseness; they need no treatment. In adult life, edema of the vocal cords and benign polyps are common causes of chronic laryngitis. However, cancer of the larynx must always be suspected in long-standing cases of hoarseness. Early diagnosis is possible thanks to this persistent, and always obvious, symptom; the physician must not impose any additional delay. Preliminary indirect laryngoscopy must be followed by direct inspection and a biopsy. From having been a typical male disease, laryngeal cancer is now increasing among females, most probably due to their increase in cigarette smoking.

AIRWAY OBSTRUCTION

Recognition

Obstruction of the nasal cavities and epipharynx compromises the normal airflow through the nose, and thereby the air conditioning and cleansing effects, as well as the cellular defense mechanisms, of the nasal mucosa. The drainage of the paranasal sinuses is also impaired, and the quality of the voice is changed. Although snoring, insomnia, and even hypoxemia may occur, there is no danger of total airway obstruction and suffocation. However, medical or surgical treatment to restore physiological patency of the nasal passages is indicated in order to avoid lasting damage to the mucous membranes of the deeper airways. Anterior and posterior rhinoscopy, possibly by flexible fiberoptic instruments, as well as rhinomanometry, allergy provocation tests, and radiographic examinations, may be necessary to obtain a realistic basis for rational therapy in individual patients.

The need for recognition of hypopharyngeal and laryngeal obstructive diseases may be more urgent, especially in childhood. Subglottic laryngitis (pseudocroup), epiglottitis, fulminant laryngotracheitis, and foreign bodies in the larynx or the upper part of the esophagus must be kept in mind when children present manifestations of respiratory distress, including coughing and dysphagia.

In adults, symptoms of laryngeal stenosis following edema, infection, or tumors are less fulminant. However, if a foreign body sticks just above the vocal folds, laryngeal spasms may occur, thereby creating a dangerous situation. Following blunt laryngeal trauma, the patient should always be observed for a few hours because of the latent risk of secondary internal hematoma or edema.

Inspiratory distress, with stridulous respiration is typical of obstructive diseases in the upper respiratory tract. Circumoral pallor, vibrating nares, and retraction of the supraclavicular, intercostal, and epigastric regions are typical signs of impending exhaustion.

Emergency Measures

Immediate orotracheal intubation is the procedure of choice. If this is impossible because of lack of assistance or instruments, a cricothyrotomy (coniotomy) has to be done through the membrane between the lower margin of the thyroid cartilage and the prominent cricoid. In adults, the knife should be inserted about 1 to 1.5 cm through the skin and the membrane. At this level there is no danger of esophageal perforation thanks to the posterior cricoid plate (Fig. 5-9). The incision can be kept open by the shaft of the knife, a pair of scissors, or any other available instrument.

Ordinary tracheotomy is performed about 1 to 2 cm below the laryngeal skeleton. This intervention is more dangerous and has to be planned as an elective operation with free airway and the necessary instruments, lighting, and assistance. In some patients, especially in those suffering from respiratory insufficiency, a permanent tracheotomy may be necessary. Nonetheless, a useful voice can be maintained by using a speech valve fitted to the cannula. In all intubated and tracheotomized patients, prophylactic artificial humidification of inspired air is necessary in order to compensate for the loss of heat and humidifying capacity of the nose. The benefits of tracheotomy are a decrease in dead space, less complicated adaptation to a respirator, and easy cleaning of bronchial secretions. The disadvantages are nasal bypass of inspired air, ineffective coughing, and reduced rigidity of the tracheal wall, which always causes instability and tracheal stenosis that is more or less noticeable, after decannulation.

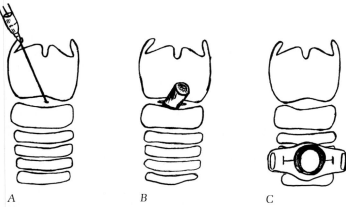

FIGURE 5-9 Puncture of conus elasticus for local anesthesia or aspiration of secretions for bacterial culture *(A)*. Acute laryngostomy (coniotomy) with an accidental piece of rubber tube *(B)* and a routine tracheotomy with an ordinary tracheal cannula *(C)*.

UPPER AIRWAY INVOLVEMENT IN SYSTEMIC DISORDERS

Signs of systemic diseases and abnormalities can be found in the upper airways. This is important in view of the ease of access, especially to the nose, for inspection and biopsy.

Absence of cilia or defective ciliary function can be congenital, as in Kartagener's syndrome, a rare condition consisting of chronic rhinosinusitis, chronic bronchitis with bronchiectasis, and situs inversus. Kartagener's syndrome is part of primary ciliary dyskinesia, also called the "immobile-cilia syndrome," that includes situs inversus. Primary ciliary dyskinesia is a genetic disorder that is autosomal and recessive and can be recognized when the cilia are examined under the electron microscope; the sperm tail is also defective. Cystic fibrosis is another disease with defective mucociliary function and should come to mind if nasal polyps are found in a child. Acquired ciliary defects caused by local infections by rhinoviruses, *Mycoplasma,* and *Bordetella* are well known, but certain systemic infections, e.g., those caused by some influenza viruses, also damage cilia.

Signs of chronic systemic infections can appear in the upper airways. Acquired immunodeficiency disease (AIDS) presents various upper airway and oral symptoms, which have to be detected early. Tuberculosis can be found in the larynx in the form of swelling and erosive ulcerations or in the middle ear as a continuous purulent discharge. Tuberculosis in these regions occurs only in patients with active pulmonary infection and is rarely seen. Other infectious granulomatous diseases that may be manifested in the mucosa of the upper airways are mycoses, such as coccidioidomycosis and histoplasmosis. A very rare finding nowadays is destruction of the nasal cartilages due to congenital syphilis.

Among the granulomatous lesions affecting the mucosa of the upper airways, without signs of infection, are sarcoidosis, berylliosis, and idiopathic midline granuloma. Among the systemic diseases that feature vasculitic lesions in the upper airways are Sjögren's syndrome, polyarteritis nodosa, rheumatoid arthritis, and lupus erythematosus.

Wegener's granulomatosis is characterized by necrotizing granulomatous vasculitis, which occurs in the upper and lower respiratory tracts, and by either focal or proliferative glomerulonephritis. Any other organ can also be affected. It is important to diagnose this disorder as early as possible since untreated patients with granulomatosis die within 12 to 24 months of the onset of clinical symptoms, whereas the majority of patients treated with the cytotoxic drug cyclophosphamide, either alone or with corticosteroids, often undergo complete remission. The diagnosis is often not made until a biopsy has been taken from the nasal mucosa, even though the mucosa appears almost normal to the naked eye. More often, the patients usually have rhinosinusitis in association with mucosal crusting.

BIBLIOGRAPHY

Cauna N, Hinderer KH: Fine structure of blood vessels of the human nasal respiratory mucosa. Ann Otol Rhinol Laryngol 78:865–885, 1969.
   The ultrastructure of the capillaries of the nose is considered with respect to the function of the nose.

Clement PAR: Committee report on standardization of rhinomanometry. Rhinology 22:151–155, 1984.
   Recommendations of the European Rhinologic Society for recording and charting resistance of the nasal passages.

Cole P, Fastag O, Niinimaa V: Computer-aided rhinomanometry. Acta Otolaryngol (Stockh) 90:139–142, 1980.
   The use of a microprocessor to calculate the work and power for air passing through the nose.

Eccles R, Lee RL: The influence of the hypothalamus on the sympathetic innervation of the nasal vasculature of the cat. Acta Otolaryngol (Stockh) 91:127–134, 1981.
   The nasal cycle is controlled by a hypothalamic center operating via the sympathetic nervous system.

Fauci AS, Haynes BF, Katz P, Wolff SM: Wegener's granulomatosis: Prospective clinical and therapeutic experience with 85 patients for 21 years. Ann Intern Med 98:76–85, 1983.
   Review of current therapy of Wegener's granulomatosis including use of cyclophosphamide.

Greenspan D, Greenspan J, Pindborg J, Schödt M: *AIDS and the Dental Team.* Munksgaard, Copenhagen, 1986.

Juliusson S, Bende M: Rhinomanometry at selection for adenoidectomy. Rhinology 25:63–67, 1987.
   Rhinomanometry was found to be a useful method for the selection of children for adenoidectomy.

Lundberg JM, Fahrenkrug J, Hökfelt T, Martling CR, Larsson O, Tatemoto K, Anggård A: Co-existence of peptide HI (PHI) and VIP in nerves regulating blood flow and bronchial smooth muscle tone in various mammals including man. Peptides 5:593–606, 1984.
   In certain neurons, vasoactive intestinal peptide and peptide with N-terminal histidine and C-terminal isoleucine coexist with acetylcholine.

Malm L: Responses of resistance and capacitance vessels in feline nasal mucosa to vasoactive agents. Acta Otolaryngol (Stockh) 78:90–97, 1974.
   A functional classification of the vessels in the nose according to their roles in hemodynamics and gas exchange.

Mygind N, Winther B: Immunologic barriers in the nose and paranasal sinuses. Acta Otolaryngol (Stockh) 103:363–368, 1987.
   This review deals mainly with lymphocyte subsets in the human nasal mucosa and with the common cold.

Proctor DF, Andersen I (eds): *The Nose. Upper Airway Physiology and the Atmospheric Environment.* Amsterdam, Elsevier Biomedical, 1982.
   A comprehensive review of the physiological functions of the nose as part of the respiratory apparatus.

Schmidt-Nielsen K: Counter-current systems in animals. Sci Am 244:118–128, 1981.
   The principle of countercurrent arrangements in the camel serves to illustrate its value as a strategy for conserving heat and water.

Uddman R, Malm L, Sundler F: The origin of vasoactive intestinal polypeptides (VIP) nerves in the feline nasal mucosa. Acta Otolaryngol (Stockh) 89:152–156, 1980.
   Vasoactive intestinal peptide is considered to be a neurotransmitter in the nasal mucosa.

Widdicombe JG: The physiology of the nose. Clin Chest Med 7:159–170, 1986.
   A comprehensive review of the nose in all of its dimensions with special reference to the role of reflexes and mediators in controlling its vasculature.

Chapter 6

Stabilization and Closure of the Upper Airways

Donald F. Proctor

Airway Stabilization and Flow Limitation
   The Nose
   Oronasal Breathing
   The Pharynx
   The Larynx
   The Extrathoracic Trachea

Neurologic Controls

Functions Not Primarily Related to Respiration

Malfunction

Acute Airway Obstruction

The upper (extrathoracic) airways from nostrils to trachea include a series of collapsible passages which can be flow-limiting when pressure within them falls during inspiration. Collapsibility is an essential characteristic of these airways since their closure, as during swallowing, is as necessary to life as the provision of an open path for breathing. In order to understand both the normal function of the upper airways and its failure in disease, it is crucial to bear in mind that, in contrast to the intrathoracic airways, where airflow is the principal function, the extrathoracic airways serve additionally for modification of inspiratory air, olfaction, phonation, the playing of wind musical instruments, deglutition, assisting in the evacuation of abdominal contents, coughing, sneezing, nose blowing, and sucking. Because of the multiplicity of physiological roles to be fulfilled and the elaborate coordination that is required for it to function automatically and properly, it should be no surprise that malfunction or failure should occasionally give rise to clinical disturbances. These range on the one hand from relatively minor symptoms, such as "coffee going down the wrong way" and on the other to serious derangements, such as those seen in sleep apnea and some instances of "asthma."

AIRWAY STABILIZATION AND FLOW LIMITATION

Whereas the bronchi are surrounded by a pressure that is continually changing with the phase and forcefulness of breathing, the pressure surrounding much of the extrathoracic airways approximates atmospheric. To maintain patency during inspiration, the negative pressure within them is counteracted by rhythmic activity in the surrounding muscles. More than a score of muscles in the head and neck play some role in the varied functions involving the upper air and food passages; and, of these, at least 10 serve to open or stabilize the airway (Fig. 6-1). The pharyngeal constrictors keep the entrance to the esophagus closed except during swallowing; palatal muscles are chiefly involved in tightly closing the velopharyngeal valve during swallowing; and all but one of the laryngeal muscles act to close the glottic valve during swallowing. For these muscles to be most effective, their activation must precede the need; i.e., airway closure must occur before, not during, swallowing after aspiration has already begun; and bracing of collapsible airways must come before their collapse during inspiration, not after they are already narrowed.

The Nose

Ordinarily, inspiratory airflow begins at the nostrils. At this locus is the first in the sequence of flow-limiting segments, the nasal valve. The functional need for limiting inspiratory flow at this site is not clear, but it may be related to the entry of inhaled materials which is strongly influenced by the very high linear velocity that is required for air to pass this narrow orifice (and the bend in the airstream just beyond it). The bony and cartilaginous structures of the nasal passages provide some stability, but the richly vascular nasal mucosa which encases them can alter the nasal cross section. In the nasal valve, it is probable that the mucosal vessels of the turbinates swell in response to inspiratory negative pressure. Thus, this entrance to the airway is doubly susceptible to collapse, i.e., through vascular swelling and the mobility of the nostrils; the collapse phenomenon is seen most clearly during a forceful sniff. Although rhythmic activity of the dilator naris muscles does provide some stabilization, nonetheless, when the pressure drop across the nostrils approaches about 10 cmH$_2$O, further inspiratory effort produces no further increment in airflow. If the demand for pulmonary ventilation exceeds that possible during nasal inspiration, the lips are parted and oronasal breathing occurs.

Oronasal Breathing

During oronasal breathing, the high mobile relation between tongue and hard palate is generally set so that the resistance to airflow through the two parallel airways, the naso- and oropharyngeal, is equal. The proportion of oropharyngeal airflow is greater during very heavy exercise; also, during yawning and during the quick, deep inspirations that are interspersed between phrases of singing or

Sella turcica
Sphenoid sinus
Soft palate
Base of tongue
Epiglottis
Hyoid bone
Arytenoid cartilage
Thyroid cartilage
Vocal cord
Cricoid cartilage
Cervical trachea

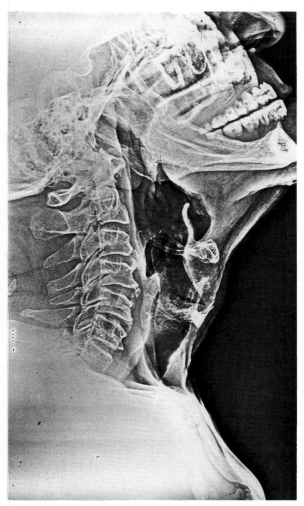

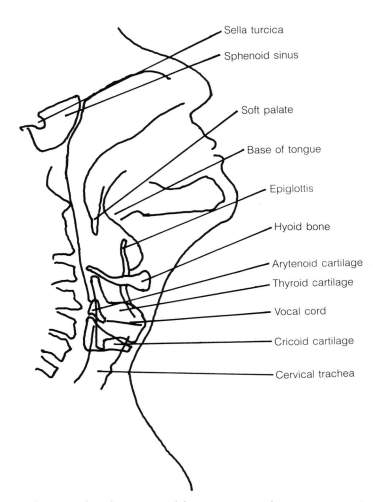

FIGURE 6-1 The upper airways. *Left*, xeroradiograph; *right*, corresponding schematic identifying some of the structures. *(After Proctor, 1977.)*

playing a wind instrument, the oral passage is greatly widened to permit maximal airflow into the mouth. During oronasal breathing the soft palate is delicately controlled to partition airflow between the two parallel airways: its action can totally occlude access of either nose or mouth to pharynx; moreover, tight velopharyngeal closure is essential during swallowing. Positioning of the palate is also important to speech and song; without expiratory closure of the velopharyngeal valve, wind instrument playing (as well as blowing up a balloon) would be impossible.

The Pharynx

The pharyngeal airway is affected by the position of the tongue which under certain circumstances, such as unconsciousness, is strongly affected by gravity. In addition to the muscles of the tongue and those controlling the position of the hyoid bone and mandible, the various pharyngeal constrictors are involved in determining the cross section of the pharynx.

The pharynx appears to be peculiarly susceptible to collapse in response to negative airway pressure. Therefore, its stabilization, especially through rhythmic change in tone in the muscles controlling the position of the tongue and mandible, appears critical for maintaining airway patency. But it must be remembered that the degree of negativity of airway pressure for any given inspiratory flow is related to the resistance to airflow through the nasal passage. Any increase in that resistance will inevitably heighten the tendency toward pharyngeal narrowing. This is equally true of the laryngotracheal airway down to the thoracic inlet. To understand airway stabilization or to discover the cause for airway obstruction, the concept of a sequence of flow-limiting segments from nostrils to thorax is the key.

The Larynx

Although in abnormal circumstances the larynx may be involved in the limitation of inspiratory flow, ordinarily it is the single exception to the sequence of segments that limit flow in the upper airways during inspiration; i.e., the vocal folds normally part slightly during inspiration and come together slightly during expiration. These are both active processes, the cricoarytenoid posticus actively contracting during inspiration and the other (adductor) muscles during expiration. It has been suggested that contraction of the adductor muscles slows expiration. However, the physiological benefit derived therefrom is not clear.

Although control of the laryngeal airway appears to be especially complex (Fig. 6-2), basically there is only one pair of muscles, the cricoarytenoid posticus, that parts the vocal folds and widens the glottic aperture. The others, with one exception, i.e., the cricothyroid muscle, are involved in the vital laryngeal function of airway closure during deglutition. The cricothyroid muscle is ordinarily pictured as being involved in producing glottic closure; indeed, it does serve this purpose when the other laryngeal muscles are inactivated, as in recurrent laryngeal nerve paralysis. But its normal function is probably to stabilize the approximation of the cricoid to the anterior thyroid cartilage during the inspiratory lengthening of the elastic tracheobronchial tree.

The cricothyroid muscles are among those that undergo an increase in tone during inspiration. As noted above, should there be a reduction, or failure, in the action of other muscles controlling the laryngeal airway, the continuing activity of the cricothyroid could account for inspiratory narrowing of the glottis. This type of disparity in the effectiveness of laryngeal muscles seems likely in view of the fact that the cricothyroid alone is innervated by the superior laryngeal nerve whereas the other muscles are innervated by the recurrent laryngeal nerve.

The Extrathoracic Trachea

Although the extrathoracic trachea is vulnerable to inspiratory collapse, normally its lumen is maintained by the tracheal attachment to the strong, complete ring of the cricoid cartilage situated only a few centimeters above the thoracic inlet. If the cricoid cartilage is injured, or if the support of the upper tracheal cartilages is greatly weakened, the extrathoracic trachea may also become flow-limiting during inspiration.

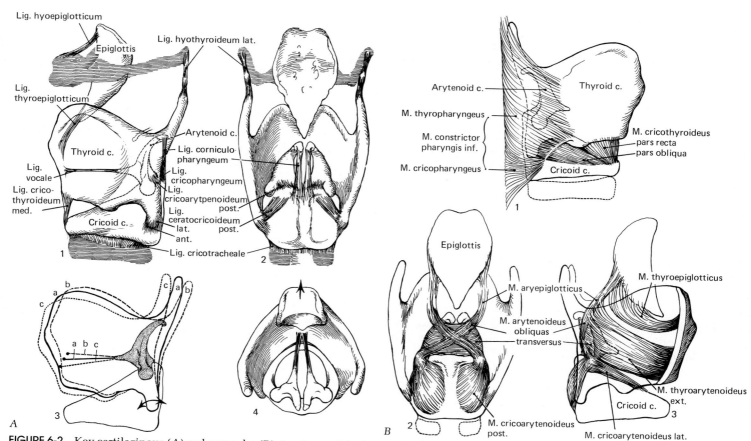

FIGURE 6-2 Key cartilaginous (A) and muscular (B) structures of the larynx. Diagram A shows elongation of the vocal cords when the anterior portions of the thyroid and cricoid cartilages are approximated, as occurs during action of the cricothyroid muscle. (After Proctor, 1964.)

NEUROLOGIC CONTROLS

One particularly interesting aspect of the rhythmic change in tone that occurs in many of the muscles surrounding the upper airways is that tone in them begins to increase before the onset of the inspiratory firing of the phrenic nerves. There is some evidence that the time between the two ("preactivation time") may increase in response to an increase in upper airflow resistance. This appropriate adjustment would require the transmission of sensory information from some locus within the airway to the elements in the central nervous system that control the rhythmic activity in the many accessory respiratory muscles. An abundance of sensory nerve endings exists in the laryngeal region, especially in the subglottic area just below the vocal folds. This region could serve to supply the necessary information about pressure, and perhaps airflow, to modulate the rhythmic changes in tone of the peri-airway muscles.

Speaking teleologically, since these muscles are involved in many functions other than respiratory, it seems desirable for their control to be located separately from the areas that relate breathing to metabolic demand. Such an area in the brain would be a logical site to receive sensory information from the periphery and instructions from the cortex and for overriding the metabolic centers when breathing is directed at activities not primarily respiratory, such as phonation. The effectiveness of the interplay between these two hypothetical, discrete areas of the brain is epitomized by the fact that during singing, despite the gross distortion of breathing pattern that it entails, slight hyperventilation results.

The muscles surrounding the upper airways are innervated by cranial nerves V, VII, IX, X, and XII, and cervical nerves I, II, and III. As noted above, all the laryngeal muscles are innervated by the recurrent laryngeal nerves except the cricothyroid. The superior laryngeal nerves innervate the cricothyroid and carry most of the sensory fibers from the laryngeal region.

FUNCTIONS NOT PRIMARILY RELATED TO RESPIRATION

Phylogenetically the larynx developed as a simple valve to prevent soiling of the airways during swallowing. Its use for phonation was a later development. Over 300 years ago William Harvey wrote:

> So also in deglutition by the elevation of the root of the tongue, and the compression of the mouth, the food or drink is pushed into the fauces, the larynx is closed by its own muscles and the epiglottis, whilst the pharynx, raised and opened by its muscles no otherwise than is a sac that is to be filled, is lifted up, and its mouth dilated; upon which, the mouthful being received, it is forced downwards by the transverse muscles, and then carried farther by the longitudinal ones. Yet are all these motions, though executed by different and distinct organs, performed harmoniously, and in such order, that they seem to constitute but a single motion and act, which we call deglutition.

Harvey compares this to the action of machinery "in which one wheel gives motion to another, yet all the wheels seem to move simultaneously. . . ." In modern terms, the "wheels" represent a complex system of sensory information, elaborate networks in the brain, and multiple efferent pathways to activate selectively and in coordination with the appropriate muscles.

Indeed, the process of swallowing so that the mouth and pharynx are completely cleared of food and fluid while protecting the glottis, subglottic airway, and the nasal passage from being soiled is a complex function. To appreciate the fine control in this region it is instructive to recall that even though tight glottic closure (involving true and false vocal and aryepiglottic folds) is necessary during swallowing or forceful evacuation of abdominal contents, only a loose but finely tuned closure of the true vocal folds is required during phonation. Also, while velopharyngeal and glottic closure must occur in synchrony during swallowing, during phonation the position of the palate must vary.

The crossroads for the periodic interruption of respiratory airflow, for the sake of allowing the passage of food, drink, and respiratory secretions to the esophagus, has until recently been neglected by otolaryngologists, gastroenterologists, and respiratory physiologists. Now all three specialists, with the aid of radiologists, are focusing attention on a variety of clinical problems, such as difficulties in swallowing, dysphagia, reflux, and aspiration.

MALFUNCTION

An important stimulus to the investigation of stabilization and control of the upper airways has been the recognition of sleep apnea and laryngeal asthma as distinct diseases. As is considered in detail elsewhere in this book (Chapter 83), the rhythmic inspiratory activity of several upper airway muscles is disturbed, or deficient, in patients with sleep apnea. Some investigators picture the apnea as occurring during ordinary sleep. But, even though it is well known that airway obstruction sometimes occurs during general anesthesia and in other states of unconsciousness, it seems unlikely that sleep apnea is often attributable entirely to disruption of airway stabilization during ordinary sleep. In some instances, obesity and structural abnormalities of the upper airways have been shown to contribute.

In addition, in some individuals, the intrathoracic airways behave abnormally while awake. Alcohol consumption, and perhaps other sedative drugs, increases the tendency toward obstruction during sleep. Although sleep apnea may prove to be largely a result of less efficient or failed upper airway inspiratory stabilization, the paramount question is whether the fault lies in central nervous control, sensory feedback from the upper airways, efferent pathways that activate the respiratory muscles, or some combination of disorders in the control mechanisms.

The role played by the larynx in some patients with asthmatic manifestations is even more difficult to understand. The larynx may account for added resistance to airflow during either inspiration or expiration or both. In some patients with severe expiratory obstruction, the vocal folds have been seen to actively adduct during that phase of breathing. In this circumstance, perverse activity of the neuromuscular system, rather than inactivity, appears to be involved. Perhaps the normal closure of the glottis during expiration while speaking or singing is related to this type of laryngeal asthma. Also, as noted above, the possibility exists that in inspiratory obstruction of the glottis, persistence of normal inspiratory activity of the cricothyroid muscles coincident with failure of the cricoarytenoid posticus could be responsible.

ACUTE AIRWAY OBSTRUCTION

A special clinical problem is presented by the acute upper airway obstruction seen in croup, epiglottitis, some deep neck infections, and cervical trauma. Significant airway obstruction in the pharyngolaryngotracheal region presents a picture quite different from the chronic obstruction of pulmonary disease. In obstruction involving the pharyngolaryngotracheal region, unless it is complicated by neuromuscular disease, drug sedation, or unconsciousness, the ventilatory effort keeps pace with the degree of obstruction, maintaining normal alveolar ventilation until exhaustion supervenes. For this reason, the physician's attention must focus not on the possibility of cyanosis, but on the prospect of impending exhaustion. Unless an alternative airway is provided through tracheal intubation from above, tracheotomy, or cricothyrotomy, exhaustion may be rapidly followed by respiratory and cardiac arrest (Fig. 6-3).

Severe acute upper airway obstruction is not an occasion either for complicated pulmonary function tests or for the determination of blood-gas composition. Indeed, these may be dangerous delaying tactics. It is better to provide the alternative airway too soon, or even occasionally unnecessarily, than to lose a life through overly cautious delay.

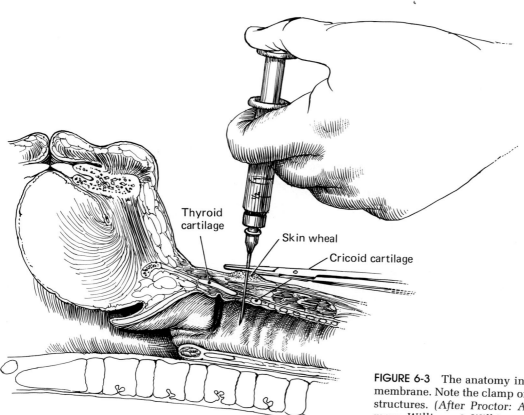

Thyroid cartilage

Skin wheal

Cricoid cartilage

FIGURE 6-3 The anatomy involved in penetrating the cricothyroid membrane. Note the clamp on the needle to avoid injuring posterior structures. *(After Proctor: Anesthesia and Otolaryngology. Baltimore, Williams & Wilkins, 1957.)*

BIBLIOGRAPHY

Anch AM, Remmers JE, Bruce H III: Supraglottic airway resistance in normal subjects and patients with occlusive sleep apnea. J Appl Physiol 52:1158–1163, 1982.
  Evidence for airway stabilization in normal and airway narrowing in abnormal patients.

Brancatisano T, Collett PW, Engel LA: Respiratory movements of the vocal chords. J Appl Physiol 54:1269–1276, 1983.
  Observation of the movements of vocal folds with breathing. Evidence is presented to support the theory that the degree of glottic narrowing during expiration is reflexly modulated by change in lung volume. This modulation may be overcome by voluntary expiratory efforts or during increased chemical drive.

Brouillette RT, Thach BT: Control of genioglossus muscle activity. J Appl Physiol 49:801–808, 1980.
  Inspiratory control of tongue position.

Brown, IG, Bradley TD, Phillipson EA, Zamel N, Hoffstein V: Pharyngeal compliance in snoring subjects with and without obstructive sleep apnea. Am Rev Respir Dis 132:211–215, 1985.
  Patients with obstructive sleep apnea have increased pharyngeal compliance that predisposes to pharyngeal closure during sleep.

Christopher KL, Wood RP, Eckert C, Blager FB, Raney RA: Vocal cord dysfunction presenting as asthma. N Engl J Med 308:1566–1570, 1983.
  Symptoms of asthma related to malfunction of laryngeal muscles.

Collett PW, Brancatisano T, Engel LA: Changes in the glottic aperture during bronchial asthma. Am Rev Respir Dis 128:719–723, 1983.
  Possible malfunction of laryngeal muscles contributing to true asthma.

Euler CV, Lagercrantz H (eds): *Central Nervous Control Mechanism in Breathing.* Oxford, Pergamon, 1979.
  Collection of papers from symposium directed at many of the mechanisms involved in airway stabilization.

Freedman LM: The role of the cricothyroid muscle in tension of the vocal cords. Arch Otolaryngol 62:347–353, 1955.
  One of the few papers describing function of the cricothyroid muscle.

Gleeson K, Zwillich CW, Bendrick TW, White DP: Effect of inspiratory nasal loading in pharyngeal resistance. J Appl Physiol 60:1882–1886, 1986.
  Consideration of factors influencing pharyngeal resistance in humans. Nasal loading causes increased resistance across the segment of the pharynx that collapses in the obstructive sleep apnea syndrome.

Haight JSJ, Cole P: The site and function of the nasal valve. Laryngoscope 93:49–55, 1983.
  Probably the most accurate description of the morphology and function of the nasal valve.

Haponik EF, Smith PL, Bohlman ME, Allen RP, Goldman SM, Bleecker ER: Computerized tomography in obstructive sleep apnea: Correlation of airway size with physiology during sleep and wakefulness. Am Rev Respir Dis 127:221–226, 1983.
  Evidence for malfunction of stabilizing muscles in sleep apnea patients while awake.

Harvey W: An anatomical disquisition on the motion of the heart and blood in animals, in *The Works of William Harvey, M.D.,* Willis R (transl). London, Sydenham Society, 1847, p 32.
  Harvey's early observations on the complexity of deglutition.

Issa FG, Sullivan CE: Reversal of central sleep apnea using nasal CPAP. Chest 90:165–171, 1986.
  Based on the theory that obstructive (OSA) and central (CSA) sleep apneas share common pathophysiological mechanisms, the authors treated eight patients with predominantly central sleep apnea by continuous positive airway pressure (CPAP). They conclude that airway collapse in the supine posture has a key role in the induction of central sleep apnea.

Krol RC, Knuth SL, Bartlett D Jr: Selective reduction in genioglossus muscle activity by alcohol in normal human subjects. Am Rev Respir Dis 129:247–250, 1984.
  Alcohol among influences affecting control of upper airway patency.

Mathew OP, Abu-Osba YK, Thach BJ: Genioglossus muscle responses to upper airway pressure changes: Afferent pathways. J Appl Physiol 52:445–450, 1982.
  Evidence on feedback mechanisms in airway stabilization.

Proctor DF: Physiology of the upper airway, in Fenn W, Rahn H (eds), *Handbook of Physiology, vol 1, Respiration.* Washington, DC, American Physiological Society, 1964, pp 309–345.
A comprehensive overview of the structure-function relationships of the upper airways.

Proctor DF: The Upper Airways II. The larynx and trachea. Am Rev Respir Dis 115:315–342, 1977.
A clear depiction of the structures that make up the upper airways.

Proctor DF: *Breathing Speech and Song.* Vienna; Springer-Verlag, 1980.
Discussion of many aspects of modifications in breathing in connection with phonation.

Proctor DF: All that wheezes . . . (editorial). Am Rev Respir Dis 127:261–262, 1983.
Laryngeal malfunction in relation to asthmatic symptoms.

Proctor DF: The naso-oro-pharyngo-laryngeal airway. Eur J Respir Dis 64 (Suppl 128):89–96, 1983.
Discussion of the sequence of inspiratory flow-limiting segments in upper airway.

Proctor DF, Andersen I (eds): *The Nose, Upper Airway Physiology and the Atmospheric Environment.* Amsterdam, Elsevier Biomedical, 1982.
General survey of nasal physiology in relation to breathing.

Roberts JL, Reed WR, Mathew OP, Thach BT: Control of respiratory activity of the genioglossus muscle in micrognathic infants. J Appl Physiol 61:1523–1533, 1986.
The genioglossus muscle contributes to maintain pharyngeal airway patency in the micrognathic infant.

Robinson RW, Zwillich CW, Bixler EO, Cadieux RJ, Kales A, White DP: Effects of oral narcotics on sleep-disordered breathing in healthy adults. Chest 91:197–203, 1987.
Alcohol and benzodiazepines may increase sleep-disordered breathing by decreasing activity of pharyngeal dilating muscles, favoring the development of obstructive apneas and hypopneas. However, in healthy individuals without suspected sleep apnea, oral hydromorphone in standard dosages does not significantly increase sleep-disordered breathing.

Rodenstein DO, Stanescu DC: Soft palate and oro-nasal breathing in humans. J Appl Physiol 57:651–657, 1984.
Importance of soft palate activity in control of upper airway airflow.

Sant'Ambrogio G, Mathew OP, Fisher JT, Sant'Ambrogio FB: Laryngeal receptors responding to transmural pressure, airflow and local muscle activity. Respir Physiol 54:317–330, 1983.
Study of the sensory feedback system in control of upper airway muscles in relation to breathing.

Santiago-Diez de Bonilla J, McCaffrey TV, Kern EB: The nasal valve: a rhinomanometric evaluation of maximum nasal inspiratory flow and pressure curves. Ann Otol Rhinol Laryngol 95:229–232, 1986.
Premature collapse of the nasal valve is responsible for the symptom of nasal obstruction in many patients with anterior nasal septal deformity.

Sekizawa K, Yanai M, Saski H, Takishima T: Control of larynx during loaded breathing in normal subjects. J Appl Physiol 60:1887–1893, 1986.
Laryngeal movement is tightly coupled with ventilation. However, the size of the laryngeal aperture is strongly influenced by a complex interplay between constricting and dilating mechanisms.

Strohl KP, Hensley MJ, Hallett M, Saunders NA, Ingram RH Jr: Activation of upper airway muscles before onset of inspiration in normal humans. J Appl Physiol 49:638–642, 1980.
Demonstration of preactivation time between stabilizing muscles and phrenic activity.

Suratt PM, McTier RF, Wilhoit SC: Collapsibility of the nasopharyngeal airway in obstructive sleep apnea. Am Rev Respir Dis 132:967–971, 1985.
The pharyngeal airway of awake patients with sleep apnea is more collapsible and has a higher resistance to airflow than normal, and the level of resistance correlates with the degree of sleep-disordered breathing.

Van Lunteren E, Van de Graaff WB, Parker DM, Mitra J, Haxhiu MA, Strohl KP, Cherniack NS: Nasal and laryngeal reflex responses to negative upper airway pressure. J Appl Physiol 56:746–752, 1984.
Other evidence regarding feedback mechanism in airway stabilization.

Wyke B (ed): *Ventilatory and Phonatory Control Systems.* New York, Oxford University Press, 1974.
A record of the proceedings of an international meeting to discuss the current status and possible future directions in the related fields of ventilatory and phonatory controls.

Chapter 7

Production and Control of Airway Secretions

Michael J. Welsh

The normal physiology and pathophysiology of respiratory tract fluid production is a relatively new topic in pulmonary medicine. Only in recent years have investigators focused on the mechanisms and regulation of airway secretion. Consequently, the mechanisms of respiratory tract fluid production and how alterations of secretory function may contribute to the pathogenesis and pathophysiology of disease are just beginning to be understood.

The main function of airway secretions is in mucociliary clearance. Mucociliary clearance is the pulmonary defense mechanism that serves to remove inhaled particulate material from the lung. Effective clearance requires both ciliary activity and respiratory tract fluid. Cilia cover much of the airway surface, and their coordinated beating provides the mechanical force that propels particulate material toward the larynx. As shown in Fig. 7-1, the cilia are immersed in a periciliary fluid layer, or sol phase of the fluid, that is about 6 μm thick. The periciliary fluid is covered by a mucous or gel layer, 5 to 10 μm thick, that exists as a discontinuous blanket, i.e., as islands of mucus. The viscoelastic mucus traps and carries inhaled material, whereas the watery periciliary fluid allows the cilia to move freely, with only the tops of the cilia contacting the overlying mucus and propelling it toward the mouth. The quantity and composition of the periciliary fluid, and perhaps hydration of the mucus, are controlled by the electrolyte transport properties of the surface epithelial cells. The quantity and composition of macromolecules in the mucus are controlled by secretory cells in the surface epi-thelium and submucosal glands. This chapter deals with the production, regulation, and pathophysiology of the airway fluid.

ELECTROLYTE AND FLUID TRANSPORT

Although the morphologic aspects of the airway epithelium are covered in another chapter, it is worth considering two morphologic features that are required for transepithelial transport of salt and water. First, the epithelial cells are joined at their apical surface by tight junctions. The tight junctions and sheet of epithelial cells form a continuous barrier to solute and water movement. However, despite their name, tight junctions do not constitute an impermeable barrier; they have selective permeabilities to ions, other solutes, and water. Thus, solutes and water can move across the epithelium through two pathways: between the cells through the tight junctions, the *paracellular pathway*, or through the epithelial cells, the *cellular pathway*. Second, epithelial cells are polar; the apical membrane, which faces the mucosal or luminal surface, is different from the basolateral membrane, which faces the submucosal or interstitial space. The morphologic differences between the two membranes are paralleled by biochemical and functional differences. Hormone receptors and ion transport processes are located asymmetrically. The segregation of transport processes to one or the other membrane gives the epithelium the capacity for net vectorial transport of electrolytes with water following passively by osmosis.

In vitro studies have demonstrated that canine tracheal epithelium can either secrete or absorb fluid. The active secretion of chloride (Cl^-) underlies the capacity for fluid secretion, whereas active sodium (Na^+) absorption accounts for the ability to absorb fluid. Chloride secretion is an active cellular process; to maintain electro-

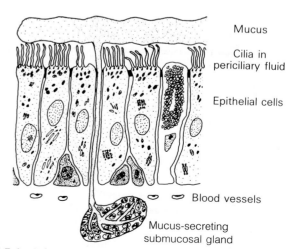

FIGURE 7-1 Schematic representation of the airway epithelium.

neutrality and produce fluid movement, Na^+ presumably follows passively through the paracellular path and water is drawn by osmosis. Conversely, when Na^+ absorption predominates, Na^+ is pumped through the cellular pathway with Cl^- following passively between the cells through the tight junctions. The magnitude of Cl^- secretion and Na^+ absorption, and thus the direction of fluid movement, depends on the neurohumoral environment, the species, and the airway region. In general, more distal airways have a greater rate of Na^+ absorption with minimal, if any, Cl^- secretion. However, the transport properties of small airways, beyond a few divisions, are unknown. In some species, including humans, it appears that the proximal airways primarily absorb Na^+ under baseline in vitro conditions. However, under appropriate conditions they can also secrete Cl^-. The cell type responsible for both Cl^- secretion and Na^+ absorption is most likely the ciliated epithelial cell.

Cellular Mechanism of Electrolyte Transport

The mechanism of ion transport by airway epithelia is graphically depicted in Fig. 7-2. Although the magnitude of secretion or absorption varies, depending on the airway region and experimental conditions, the cellular mechanisms appear similar throughout the airways. Chloride secretion is a two-step process. Chloride enters the cell at the basolateral membrane on an electrically neutral cotransport process against its electrochemical gradient. The energy to drive Cl^- entry comes from the coupling to Na^+ entry, with Na^+ moving down its electrical and chemical gradient. Chloride leaves the cell at the apical membrane, moving passively down a favorable electrochemical gradient through apical membrane Cl^- channels. The energy to support secretion ultimately comes from the basolateral Na^+ pump (Na,K-ATPase), which maintains a low intra-cellular Na^+ concentration and a negative intracellular voltage. The basolateral membrane also contains potassium (K^+) channels, which provide an exit path for the K^+ that enters the cell on the Na^+ pump and on the electrically neutral Cl^- cotransport. The basolateral K^+ channels play an important role in maintaining the negative intracellular voltage that drives Cl^- out of the cell at the apical membrane. Several agents that block specific transport steps have been of value in elucidating the mechanism of Cl^- secretion: loop diuretics block Cl^- entry on the cotransport, carboxylic acid analogs block the apical Cl^- channel, ouabain blocks the Na^+ pump, and barium ion blocks the basolateral K^+ channel.

Sodium absorption is also a two-step process. Sodium enters the cell through apical membrane Na^+ channels, moving down favorable chemical concentration and electrical gradients. Sodium is then pumped out of the cell against its electrochemical gradient by the Na,K-ATPase. Two drugs that have helped investigators understand the mechanism of Na^+ absorption are amiloride, which blocks the apical Na^+ channel, and ouabain, which inhibits the Na,K-ATPase.

Regulation of Electrolyte Transport

Chloride secretion is regulated by a variety of neurohumoral mediators; Table 7-1 lists several agents that stimulate secretion. Most of the agents stimulate secretion from the submucosal surface of the cell. However, the inflammatory mediators, bradykinin, substance P, and leukotrienes LTC_4 and LTD_4 act from either surface, and adenosine acts from the mucosal surface. Thus, secretion can be regulated on a local or regional level by release of mediators from cells in the airway lumen, such as mast cells and macrophages, as well as from cells and nerve terminals in the submucosa.

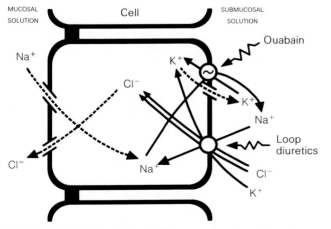

FIGURE 7-2 Model depicting cellular mechanism of ion transport by airway epithelium.

TABLE 7-1

Agents That Stimulate Chloride Secretion in Airway Epithelia

Agent	Surface	cAMP
β-Adrenergic agonists	Submucosal	↑
Prostaglandin E_2	Submucosal	↑
Prostaglandin $F_{2\alpha}$	Submucosal	—
Vasoactive intestinal peptide	Submucosal	↑
Adenosine	Mucosal	↑
Leukotrienes LTC_4 and LTD_4	Mucosal and submucosal	↑ ?
Substance P	Mucosal and submucosal	?
Bradykinin	Mucosal and submucosal	↑ ?

NOTE: Surface = the side of the epithelium on which the agents act; ↑ = an increase; ? = uncertainty; — = no measurable change.

Nearly all the agents shown in Table 7-1 increase cellular levels of cyclic AMP. Moreover, exogenous addition of cyclic AMP or the phosphodiesterase inhibitor, theophylline, stimulates Cl^- secretion. These observations suggest that cyclic AMP may be the second messenger responsible for inducing secretion, perhaps by opening the apical membrane Cl^- channel.

The baseline rate of Cl^- secretion is primarily controlled by prostaglandins produced by the epithelial cells. Indomethacin, a prostaglandin synthesis inhibitor, decreases the baseline rate of Cl^- secretion, decreases intracellular levels of cyclic AMP, and decreases prostaglandin production by the epithelium. Prostaglandins also appear to mediate the secretory response to bradykinin and leukotrienes, because they increase prostaglandin production and the Cl^- secretion induced by these agents is prevented by indomethacin. An increase in intracellular calcium produced by the calcium ionophore A-23187 also stimulates Cl^- secretion. However, in some species the response to an increase in cell calcium may also be mediated by an increase in prostaglandin production because indomethacin prevents the Cl^- secretion produced by the calcium ionophore.

In contrast to the many agents that regulate secretion, little is known about how Na^+ absorption is regulated. Most agents that stimulate Cl^- secretion also decrease the rate of Na^+ absorption. However, the decrease probably results, at least in part, from a decrease in the electrochemical driving force for Na^+ absorption. Given the importance of Na^+ absorption for control of the airway fluid and possible abnormalities of absorption in disease, more work is required to understand how absorption is controlled.

AIRWAY MUCUS

Airway mucus is a complex mixture of macromolecules, including proteins, glycoproteins, electrolytes, and water. The composition of mucus depends on the output of many cell types, including both surface cells and submucosal glands. Surface cells that secrete macromolecules include goblet cells, Clara cells, and probably the ciliated epithelial cells. Secretion from the submucosal glands, which are composed primarily of serous and mucous cells, is carried to the airway surface via the gland ducts. An understanding of the precise physiology and biochemistry of the airway mucus has been hampered by the fact that the end product is the result of several cell types; by the paucity of specific markers or probes for the different macromolecules and cell types; by substantial species differences in cell number, type, and regulation; and by the lack of pure cell culture preparations of the different cells. Perhaps the easiest way to understand the problems is to first consider each of the different cell types involved.

Cellular Production of Airway Mucus

The goblet cell in the surface epithelium contains large electron-lucent secretory granules that stain with Alcian blue and periodic acid Schiff. These stains indicate the presence of acidic and neutral glycoproteins, respectively. Because of the lack of pure preparations, the biochemical composition of goblet cell secretion is only partly defined. One of the most striking features of the morphology of goblet cells is proliferation that occurs in response to irritation or damage of the epithelium. In humans, goblet cell proliferation is characteristically observed in cigarette smokers and patients with chronic bronchitis.

The ciliated cells in the surface epithelium do not contain secretory granules and once were not considered to secrete glycoproteins. However, recent studies have demonstrated that their apical surface is coated with a glycocalyx, the histochemistry of which is unique to the epithelial cell. Moreover, epithelial cells take up radiolabeled glycoprotein precursors, which move to the apical surface and are released from the cell. These observations suggest that ciliated cells also make an important contribution to the final composition of the airway mucus.

Clara cells in the surface epithelium are assumed to be secretory cells because of their characteristic ultrastructural appearance, including the presence of electron-dense granules. However, products of their secretion and the mechanism of regulation are not certain at this time.

The two predominant cell types in the submucosal glands are mucous cells and serous cells. Morphologic, histochemical, and immunocytochemical studies indicate distinct differences between these two cells. Serous cells contain small, discrete, electron-dense secretory granules, whereas mucous cells contain large, often confluent, electron-lucent granules. Although both cell types contain complex carbohydrates, mucous cells are thought to contain more acidic secretions than serous cells and the two cells bind different types of lectins. In addition, serous cells but not mucous cells contain lysozyme, lactoferrin, and antileukoprotease.

Regulation of Mucus Production

The physiological stimuli that regulate macromolecule secretion by goblet cells, ciliated cells, and Clara cells in mammalian airways are largely unknown. Neither stimulation of parasympathetic or sympathetic nerves nor addition of adrenergic or cholinergic agonists has produced unequivocal secretion of the goblet cell contents. Despite the lack of evidence for neurohumoral regulation of secretion, there is good evidence for neurohumoral regulation of goblet cell proliferation during chronic cholinergic or adrenergic stimulation. Irritants appear to be more important than neurohumoral or reflex mechanisms in regulating goblet cell secretion. Cigarette smoke, ammonia, mustard oil, and mechanical factors all induce secretion as well as stimulate goblet cell hyperplasia.

In contrast to secretory cells in the surface epithelium, neurohumoral regulation of macromolecule secretion by the submucosal glands has been convincingly shown. Gland secretion of fluid and mucus is under parasympathetic, adrenergic, and peptidergic (probably vasoactive intestinal peptide) neural control. Several stimuli cause glandular secretion via vagal reflex pathways; mechanical and chemical irritation of the airways, inflammation, hypoxia, and gastric distension all increase mucus output from submucosal glands. In addition to neural control, gland secretion is mediated by local inflammatory mediators that are released from mast cells and neutrophils. Mediators demonstrated to have an effect include histamine and products of arachidonic acid, including cyclooxygenase and lipoxygenase metabolites. Given the variety of agents that are capable of stimulating the submucosal glands and the observation that the gland contains two different cell types, it is reasonable to ask whether the two cell types are regulated differently. Recent studies, summarized in Table 7-2, suggest that this is the case. In addition to different histochemical and immunocytochemical characteristics, there are differences in the number of receptors on the two cell types. Although both cells have muscarinic and β- and α-adrenergic receptors, serous cells have more α receptors and mucous cells have more β receptors. This difference in receptor number is paralleled by differences in the physiological response: α agonists produce a greater degranulation of serous cells and β agonists produce a greater degranulation of mucous cells. In addition, α-adrenergic stimulation produces glandular secretion with a high lysozyme content, low viscosity, and low protein content, whereas β-adrenergic stimulation produces a fluid with a low lysozyme content, high viscosity, and higher protein content. Muscarinic cholinergic stimulation appears to stimulate both cell types because it causes degranulation of both mucous and serous cells and produces secretions that could be explained as the combination of products from both cell types.

TABLE 7-2
Properties of Submucosal Gland Cells

	Serous Cells	Mucous Cells
Granules	Small, electron-dense	Large, electron-lucent
Glycoproteins	Neutral	Acidic
	Lysozyme, lactoferrin	
Hormone receptors	$\alpha > \beta$-Adrenergic	$\beta > \alpha$-Adrenergic
	Muscarinic	Muscarinic
Degranulation	α-Adrenergic	β-Adrenergic
	Cholinergic	Cholinergic
	Substance P	

PATHOPHYSIOLOGY OF RESPIRATORY TRACT FLUID PRODUCTION

The quantity and composition of the respiratory tract fluid is altered in many airway diseases and probably plays an important part in pathogenesis. Abnormalities of airway secretion are briefly considered for a few diseases: manifestations of these diseases are covered in detail in subsequent chapters.

Cystic Fibrosis

Recent work has lead to substantial advances in our understanding of the abnormalities in cystic fibrosis. One of the main clinical manifestations of this disease is thick, tenacious, dehydrated airway secretions. It appears that the abnormal airway secretions result from defective electrolyte transport by the airway epithelium; specifically, airway epithelia are relatively Cl^--impermeable. The sweat gland duct is also Cl^--impermeable, which explains the increased NaCl concentration of the sweat. Although not well characterized, the pancreatic abnormalities in cystic fibrosis could also be explained by a decreased anion secretory capacity. Thus, three of the major organ systems involved in this genetic disease may have a decreased anion permeability. In addition, airway epithelia also exhibit an increased rate of Na^+ absorption, an abnormality that would tend to produce further dehydration of the airway secretions and increase the viscosity of the mucus. The decreased Cl^- permeability of airway epithelia is retained in tissue culture, suggesting that the abnormality is inherent in the epithelial cells themselves, rather than the result of some circulating factor. The Cl^- impermeability of the epithelial cells results from a Cl^--impermeable apical cell membrane, rather than a defect in Cl^- movement through the paracellular pathway or across the basolateral cell membrane. Recent data show that Cl^- channels are present in the apical membrane of cystic fibrosis airway epithelial cells; however, their regulation is abnormal so that they do not open in response to physiological stimuli.

In addition to abnormal electrolyte movement across the surface epithelium, the airways of cystic fibrosis patients show proliferation of goblet cells and hypertrophy of submucosal glands. However, in contrast to the electrolyte transport abnormalities, which are apparent from the time of birth, the hypertrophy of mucus-secreting cells is not present in newborns, but occurs later. This observation suggests that the secretory cell hypertrophy results from irritation, abnormalities in the surface liquid, or perhaps from some signal or reflex initiated in the surface epithelial cells.

Chronic Bronchitis

By definition, patients with chronic bronchitis have increased sputum production. Examination of the airways shows hypertrophy of goblet cells and submucosal glands. The etiologic factors are most likely acute and chronic irritation resulting from inhalation of cigarette smoke or other agents that induce inflammation. Although the mediators and reflex pathways involved are not completely understood, four observations suggest that interactions between the surface epithelium and mucus-secreting and inflammatory cells are important in the pathogenesis of the disease. First, the surface epithelium is the first barrier to make contact with inhaled substances. Second, irritants such as cigarette smoke alter the morphology and function of the surface epithelium. Third, epithelial cells make a variety of mediators, including arachidonic acid metabolites, that may regulate mucus-secreting cells and serve as chemoattractants. Fourth, alterations in the barrier function of surface epithelial cells may allow easier access of inhaled material to the cells in the submucosal space. Understanding the interactions between the surface cells and the submucosal glands (and airway smooth muscle) is likely to provide important new insights into abnormalities in disease.

Asthma

Asthma is another disease in which there is an increase in mucus secretion with subsequent plugging of bronchioles. Although our knowledge of the production of immunologic and inflammatory mediators is steadily increasing, the mechanisms by which mucous secretion increases and cell hypertrophy occurs are not well understood. In animal models there is convincing evidence for allergen and inflammatory modulation of electrolyte and water transport and mucous secretion. However, there is conflicting evidence on whether the barrier function and electrolyte transport properties of the surface epithelium are involved in humans. Better animal models and application of new techniques may also increase our understanding of the pathogenesis of this disease.

BIBLIOGRAPHY

Al-Bazzaz FJ: Regulation of salt and water transport across airway mucosa. Clin Chest Med 7:259–272, 1986.
   A comprehensive overview of the transport of sodium and chloride across the epithelium of the airways. Neurohumoral control mechanisms are invoked to support the idea of switching from active sodium and fluid absorption to chloride and fluid secretion, and vice versa.

Baier H, Moas R, Yerger L, Wanner A: In vivo estimation of tracheal wall water: effects of histamine and carbachol. J Appl Physiol 60:1680–1685, 1986.
   Based on double-indicator dilution principles, a new method is proposed for measuring water content in the tracheal wall by inscribing time-concentration curves with the inert gas, helium, and the water-soluble gas, dimethylether.

Basbaum CB: Regulation of airway secretory cells. Clin Chest Med 7:231–237, 1986.
   Concise summary of current knowledge about factors regulating mucus secretion by surface epithelial and submucosal gland cells. The evidence implicating separate regulation of mucus and serous cells in the submucosal glands is compelling.

Boat TF, Cheng PW: Biochemistry of airway mucus secretions. Fed Proc 39:3067–3074, 1980.
   Provides an excellent review of the biochemistry of mucus.

Boucher RC, Stutts MJ, Knowles MR, Cantley L, Gatzy JT: Na$^+$ transport in cystic fibrosis respiratory epithelia. Abnormal basal rate and response to adenylate cyclase activation. J Clin Invest 78:1245–1252, 1986.
   The airway epithelium of cystic fibrosis patients absorbs Na$^+$ at an accelerated rate.

Breeze RG, Wheeldon EB: The cells of the pulmonary airways. Am Rev Respir Dis 116:705–777, 1977.
   Comprehensive description and review of the literature describing anatomic features of the surface epithelium and submucosal glands.

Cullen JJ, Welsh MJ: Regulation of sodium absorption by canine tracheal epithelium. J Clin Invest 79:73–79, 1987.
   Na$^+$ absorption is both acutely and chronically regulated in the airway epithelium.

Jeffrey PK, Reid L: Ultrastructure of airway epithelium and submucosal gland during development, in Lung Biology in Health and Disease. New York, Dekker, 1977, vol. 6, pp 87–134.
   Anatomic description of airway cells.

Knowles MR, Stutts MJ, Spock A, Fischer N, Gatzy JT, Boucher RC: Abnormal ion permeation through cystic fibrosis respiratory epithelium. Science 221:1067–1070, 1983.
Nasal epithelium excised from cystic fibrosis patients has a higher transepithelial voltage. The increased voltage results from a Cl⁻ impermeability and increased Na⁺ absorption.

Nadel JA, Widdicombe JH, Peatfield AC: Regulation of airways secretions, ion transport and water movement, in Fishman AP, Fisher AB (eds), *Handbook of Physiology,* sect 3: The Respiratory System, vol 1: Circulation and Nonrespiratory Functions. Bethesda, American Physiological Society, 1985, pp 419–445.
Provides a comprehensive review of mucus secretion and ion transport by the airways, with particular emphasis on regulation of mucus secretion by nerves, reflexes, and hormonal and chemical stimuli.

Respiratory Tract Mucus: Ciba Foundation Symposium 54, Amsterdam, Elsevier/North-Holland, 1978.
This book contains articles presented at a Ciba symposium. Chapters cover the structure, function, and biochemistry of mucus. There is also a discussion of abnormalities in disease and animal models.

Van Scott MR, Hester S, Boucher RC: Ion transport by rabbit nonciliated bronchiolar epithelial cells (Clara cells) in culture. Proc Natl Acad Sci USA 84:5496–5500, 1987.
Clara cells in culture form polarized monolayers; Clara cells transport Na⁺ from the apical to the basolateral bathing solution, and the small airways of the rabbit may function in liquid absorption.

Wanner A: Clinical aspects of mucociliary transport. Am Rev Respir Dis 116:73–125, 1977.
Describes measurement of mucociliary clearance and the factors that contribute to effective clearance. Also relates normal physiology to abnormalities found in disease.

Welsh MJ: An apical-membrane chloride channel in human tracheal epithelium. Science 232:1648–1650, 1986.
Airway and sweat gland-duct epithelia are chloride-impermeable in cystic fibrosis. The decreased chloride permeability prevents normal secretion by the airway epithelium. The cells of human tracheal epithelium in culture contain an anion-selective channel that is responsible for the apical chloride conductance in airway epithelia.

Welsh MJ: Electrolyte transport by airway epithelia. Phys Rev 67:1143–1184, 1987.
Review of cellular mechanisms of ion transport by airway epithelia. Focuses on experimental evidence for the individual cell membrane ion transport processes, including in vivo studies, radioisotope flux studies, and cellular electrophysiological studies. Also reviews abnormalities in cystic fibrosis.

Welsh MJ, Liedtke CM: Chloride and potassium channels in cystic fibrosis airway epithelia. Nature 322:467–470, 1986.
Excised, cell-free patches of membrane from cystic fibrosis epithelial cells contain Cl⁻ channels that have the same conductive properties as Cl⁻ channels from normal cells, whereas Cl⁻ channels from cystic fibrosis cells did not open when they were attached to the cell. Regulation of Cl⁻ channels in cystic fibrosis epithelia seems to be defective, and the defect seems to reside at a site distal to cAMP accumulation.

Widdicombe JH, Welsh MJ: Ion transport by dog tracheal epithelium. Fed Proc 39:3062–3066, 1980.
Describes the effect of drugs on Cl⁻ secretion and Na⁺ absorption by tracheal epithelium. Relates these observations to cellular physiology of electrolyte transport.

Widdicombe JH, Welsh MJ, Finkbeiner WE: Cystic fibrosis decreases the apical membrane chloride permeability of monolayers cultured from cells of tracheal epithelium. Proc Natl Acad Sci USA 82:6167–6171, 1985.
Shows that cultured cystic fibrosis cells retain the Cl⁻ transport abnormalities observed in the native epithelium. Localizes the decreased Cl⁻ permeability to the apical cell membrane.

Chapter *8*

Airway Smooth Muscle

Michael I. Kotlikoff

Heightened bronchomotor tone is often a critical element in obstructive airways disease. The rational approach to decreasing bronchomotor tone calls for an understanding of the biology of the smooth muscle of the airways. In recent years advances in the techniques and concepts of cell and molecular biology have provided fresh insights into the cellular and subcellular physiological processes in smooth muscle. Large strides have also been taken in unraveling the biochemistry and regulation of contractile proteins, transduction properties of the sarcolemma, and the pharmacology of neuropeptides, inflammatory agents, and other intercellular messenger substances. From these advances has emerged a clearer picture of the neurohormonal physiological control systems that regulate the activation of airway smooth muscle and the resulting bronchomotor tone. This chapter deals with the factors influencing bronchomotor tone and examines the relative importance of neural and nonneural control systems in airway smooth muscle.

CELL BIOLOGY

The smooth-muscle cells (*myocytes*) of the airways exist in a densely packed, complex, fibrous matrix consisting of collagen, elastin, fibronectin, and basement membrane substance composed of glycoproteins, glycolipids, and glycosaminoglycans. Also present within the smooth-muscle matrix are neural processes, fibroblasts, inflammatory cells, and vascular tissue. When fully relaxed, the myocytes are fusiform, roughly 300 to 600 μm in length

and 3 to 6 μm in central width. While the myocyte is relaxed, the sarcolemma is smooth but, when fully contracted, the membrane bulges out in thousands of saclike vesicles. The sarcolemma exhibits numerous dense bodies, which are attachment sites of actin to the cell membrane, and specialized cell-cell junctions, i.e., nexuses and gap junctions. These junctions are low in electrical resistance and act as direct pathways for intercellular communication. Sarcoplasmic reticulum (SR) and caveolae, or surface vesicles, are numerous in the vicinity of the sarcolemma, whereas mitochondria are more frequently found near the nucleus, which is centrally placed. It is likely that the caveolae and junctional sarcoplasmic reticulum are the major intracellular sources of calcium release that is triggered by excitation. Although the volume of the sarcoplasmic reticulum in vascular smooth muscle constitutes only about 5 percent of the cell total, the calcium content is sufficient to account for the increase in intracellular concentration of Ca^{2+} from approximately 10^{-7} to 10^{-5} M, the level at which contraction is maximal.

REGULATION OF CONTRACTILE PROTEINS

Smooth-muscle cells contain thick (*myosin*) and thin (*actin*) filaments; contraction occurs by a sliding of the parallel filaments. The molecular mechanism of contraction is similar to that of striated muscle in that myosin filaments on which MgATP is bound form cross bridges with actin. However, the regulatory processes that control this interaction appear to be quite different and far more complex in smooth muscle. In skeletal muscle, MgATPase activity is inhibited by troponin and tropomyosin, thin filament regulatory proteins that prevent actin-myosin interaction; in the absence of these regulatory molecules, purified skeletal muscle actin and myosin form crosslinks. In contrast, pure actin and myosin isolated from smooth muscle are inactive; activation occurs by a specific, calcium-dependent phosphorylation of myosin: a light chain component of the myosin molecule is phosphorylated by the regulatory enzyme myosin light chain kinase (MLCK). Although additional regulatory mechanisms, such as direct calcium binding to myosin or troponin, may also be involved, the primary regulator of contractile protein activation in smooth muscle appears to be myosin phosphorylation. The major steps of the regulatory system are outlined below and illustrated in Fig. 8-1.

1. Excitation triggers an increase in cytosolic calcium which, in turn, leads to the binding of calcium to calmodulin, thereby forming an activated complex. This complex binds the cytosolic enzyme myosin light chain kinase.

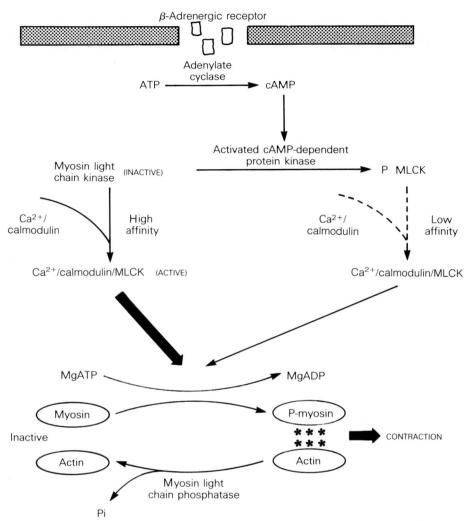

FIGURE 8-1 Biochemical sequence involved in activation of contractile proteins and the mechanism of β-adrenergic regulation.

2. The activated Ca^{2+}/calmodulin/MLCK complex phosphorylates the light chain region of myosin, thereby producing a conformational change in the myosin head.

3. Actin activates myosin ATPase and cross-bridge cycling occurs.

4. Dephosphorylation of myosin light chain by a specific phosphatase terminates the MgATPase activity by altering the conformation of myosin.

Also shown in Fig. 8-1 is the mechanism by which cAMP-dependent protein kinase (A kinase) regulates the affinity of MLCK for calmodulin. One action of A kinase in smooth muscle is the phosphorylation of MLCK, the enzyme which itself phosphorylates myosin; the phosphorylation of MLCK results in a lower affinity of this

enzyme for the Ca^{2+}/calmodulin complex. At any given level of cytosolic calcium, the degree of MLCK activity and the attendant activation of the contractile proteins will be decreased by the coupled stimulation of β-adrenergic receptors and adenylate cyclase.

EXCITATION-CONTRACTION COUPLING

Electrophysiology

A distinguishing feature of airway smooth muscle is its electrical and contractile stability. Unlike gastrointestinal and numerous vascular smooth muscles, airway smooth muscle exhibits neither spontaneous contractions nor slow-wave electric activity when examined in situ or as isolated tissue strips. When stimulated electrically or chemically, airway myocytes do not produce voltage spikes; instead, they exhibit a graded, partial electric depolarization and a contractile response proportional to the stimulus. In response to a supramaximal concentration of acetylcholine, airway myocytes depolarize from a resting transmembrane potential of about -55 to about -35 mV. This electrical stability and graded depolarization result from the strong, outwardly rectifying properties of the cell membrane; i.e., as the cell is depolarized, membrane conductance to outward current increases, thereby limiting further depolarization. Under conditions in which potassium conductance is markedly decreased or eliminated, as during the block of potassium ion channels by tetraethylammonium (TEA), this rectification is abolished and slow-wave activity, spike potentials, and spontaneous contractions are observed.

The recent development of cell disaggregation and patch-clamp recording techniques has greatly enhanced the study of membrane ion channels. Using these techniques, McCann and Welsh have reported single-channel recordings of calcium-activated, potassium channels in canine airway myocytes. A whole-cell experiment from our laboratory, illustrating the response to depolarization of an isolated, patch-clamped myocyte from a ferret's trachea, and the current-voltage relationship of this cell, is shown in Fig. 8-2. It can be seen that an outward (positive) current is evoked by depolarization, and that the amplitude of current increases nonlinearly with depolarization. This current is abolished by TEA applied to the external surface of the cell. Thus, the molecular mechanism for airway smooth-muscle electrical stability appears to be a potassium-channel protein in the membrane; the resulting outward K^+ current counteracts cell depolarization.

A major unanswered question concerns the ionic mechanism that mediates depolarization. For example, the binding of the neurotransmitter acetylcholine to the cell membrane receptor is a fundamental event in the neural activation of airway smooth muscle. The mechanism by which this receptor coupling results in cell depolarization and an increase in cytosolic calcium concentration is not known. We have recently reported patch-clamp measurements of calcium currents in airway smooth-muscle cells. These currents are due to the opening of voltage-dependent calcium channels in the cell membrane. The gating of these or other channels by bronchoactive substances could provide the mechanism for airway smooth-muscle cell depolarization.

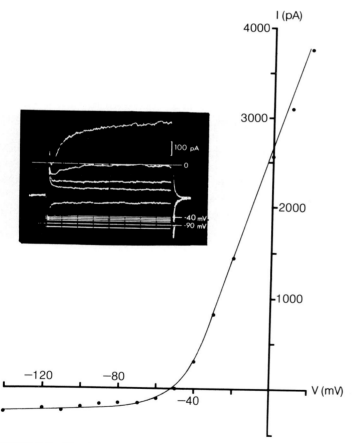

FIGURE 8-2 Steady-state current-voltage (I, V) relationship for an isolated, patch-clamped, ferret tracheal myocyte. The marked change in slope at voltages positive to -60 mV indicates the increased conductance associated with depolarization. Inset shows whole cell currents during voltage clamp. Voltage was stepped for 80 ms from a holding voltage of -90 mV. A slight negative current precedes activation of a positive current in the top trace. *(Unpublished data: MI Kotlikoff, R Mitra, M Morad.)*

Calcium Mobilization

More than one mechanism for increasing cytosolic calcium appears to be available to the airway myocyte. If airway smooth muscle is depolarized by high extracellular concentrations of KCl, the tissue contracts. This depolarization-induced contraction can be blocked by removing extracellular calcium, or by dihydropyridine calcium-channel antagonists, suggesting the importance of extracellular calcium in electromechanical coupling. However, agonist-induced contractions are not completely inhibited either by application of a calcium-free medium or of dihydropyridines, although both partially diminish the contractions.

A functional distinction between depolarization-induced and agonist-induced contractions is also suggested by two findings: (1) at a given transmembrane potential, contraction evoked by acetylcholine (and other agonists) is greater than by KCl, and (2) acetylcholine (and other agonists) can contract airway smooth muscle that has been completely depolarized, and maximally contracted, by KCl. These observations suggest that agonist-induced contraction mobilizes different, or additional, sources of calcium than does pure electrical depolarization. This contraction mechanism, termed *pharmacome-*

chanical coupling (in contrast to *electromechanical coupling*), suggests that increases in cytosolic calcium sufficient to produce contraction can occur by mechanisms other than activation of voltage-sensitive ion channels in the cell membrane. Since dihydropyridine calcium antagonists appear to block voltage-dependent calcium channels, the limited clinical value of these agents in bronchoconstrictive diseases may be due to pharmacomechanical coupling in airway smooth muscle. In addition, since dihydropyridine calcium antagonists exert their effects by binding preferentially to depolarized, open channels, incomplete depolarization of the airway smooth-muscle cell may limit this binding and thereby limit the effectiveness of the antagonists.

Membrane Transduction

The sarcolemma incorporates several mechanisms by which receptor binding of neurotransmitters or other intercellular messengers increases the cytosolic concentration of calcium and the activation of contractile proteins. These membrane transduction systems also process signals that cause relaxation, protein synthesis, cellular secretion, cell division, and other metabolic processes. Three definitive transduction pathways have been established for stimulus-receptor coupling in smooth muscle: (1) calcium-channel proteins in the sarcolemma, (2) a receptor-coupled, membrane phospholipid mechanism (phosphatidylinositol system), and (3) the β-adrenergic/cyclic AMP pathway. A schematic representation of these transduction systems is presented in Fig. 8-3. Information about the specific components of these systems and their physiological functions in airway smooth muscle is currently emerging.

With respect to calcium-channel proteins in the sarcolemma, calcium currents resulting from an inward flow of calcium ions have been recorded in our laboratory from canine tracheal smooth-muscle cells. Voltage-dependent calcium channels are of the transient type, showing low sensitivity to dihydropyridine calcium-channel blockers. In cardiac myocytes, receptor binding of β-adrenergic drugs modifies the kinetics and voltage sensitivity of calcium channels, probably via phosphorylation of the membrane protein. Whether receptor binding of acetylcholine or other agonists can activate, or gate, calcium channels in airway smooth muscle by way of channel phosphorylation, or whether the agonists act by depolarizing the cell through actions on other channels, is still unsettled. The question is important because of the phenomenon of pharmacomechanical coupling: since phosphorylation of the channel alters its voltage characteristics, receptor-triggered kinases could increase the number of channels that are open at any given transmembrane potential. Further, since a receptor-gated calcium current would activate an outward potassium current in airway smooth muscle, external calcium could enter the cell by this mechanism without depolarizing the cell.

The second transduction system involves the production and release of soluble inositol trisphosphate (IP_3) from within the phospholipid membrane. Receptor binding of muscarinic cholinergic or α-adrenergic agonists triggers the breakdown of phosphatidylinositol, a membrane phospholipid, to IP_3 and diacylglycerol. These second messengers appear to initiate diverse cellular functions. IP_3 releases Ca^{2+} from intracellular stores. Diacylglycerol, which remains in the membrane, triggers phosphorylation and activation of a specific protein kinase (C kinase) and results in the generation of arachi-

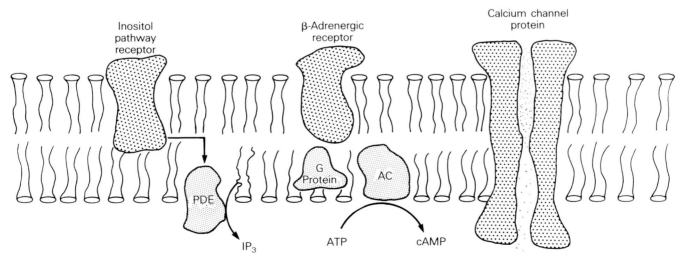

FIGURE 8-3 Schematic representation of membrane transduction systems in airway smooth muscle. Phosphodiesterase (PDE) action on membrane lipids releases inositol trisphosphate (IP_3). Similarly, the membrane bound enzyme adenylate cyclase (AC) catalyzes the release of the second messenger cyclic AMP.

donic acid metabolites in certain cells. This finding of a direct membrane coupling between receptor binding and cellular protein phosphorylation has reordered thinking about phospholipid molecules in the cell membrane, which were previously considered to be passive. Consistent with the idea of a receptor-triggered phosphatidylinositol system is the recent demonstration by Baron et al. that cholinergic stimulation of canine airway smooth muscle causes alterations in phospholipid metabolism. They have proposed that this mechanism may explain, in part, pharmacomechanical coupling in airway smooth muscle.

β-Adrenergic receptor stimulation results in activated adenylate cyclase and increases in cytosolic cAMP; it subsequently activates the regulatory unit of cAMP-dependent protein kinase (A kinase). The established role of this kinase in regulating myosin phosphorylation was described above. Other β-receptor regulatory mechanisms appear to directly influence the concentration of cytosolic calcium by increasing sequestration, decreasing influx, and increasing efflux. Thus, β-receptor stimulation appears to result in stimulation of diverse regulatory pathways that interact to decrease contractility in airway smooth muscle.

NEURAL REGULATION

The neural control of airway smooth muscle is dominated by parasympathetic efferent outflow in the vagus nerve. Preganglionic fibers extend from cell bodies in the ambiguous nucleus and the dorsal motor nucleus of the vagus and synapse in paratracheal and parabronchial ganglia that lie external to the airway smooth-muscle layer. Fibers from postganglionic neuronal cell bodies within the ganglia directly innervate airway smooth muscle and glands. The predominant neurotransmitter at both the preganglionic and postganglionic sites is acetylcholine. Resting neuromuscular tone is maintained by tonic vagal output, as demonstrated by the marked bronchodilation that occurs following bilateral vagotomy, or the bronchoconstriction that occurs following administration of an anticholinesterase. Bilateral vagal stimulation causes marked constriction of the central airways but has little influence on bronchioles and alveolar ducts. Little information, other than reports of various stimuli which result in a vagally mediated bronchoconstriction, is available with respect to the processes that regulate central vagal output. More precise information about the link between complex central integrative processes and vagal output is needed.

Although sympathetic innervation of airway smooth muscle has been demonstrated in several species, it has not been clearly established in human airway smooth muscle, and its physiological role in inhibiting bronchoconstriction is minor. Richardson and Beland have demonstrated that the relaxation of isolated human airway smooth muscle which occurs during field stimulation is not affected by adrenergic blocking agents, demonstrating the existence of a nonadrenergic inhibitory system in human airways similar to that in other species; this system appears to be the principal neural mechanism for bronchodilation in humans. Although the neurotransmitter associated with this system has not been identified, several neuropeptides and purine derivatives have been proposed, including vasoactive intestinal peptide (VIP), adenosine, adenine, and ATP. These are only a few of the numerous neuropeptides that have been demonstrated in the airways by immunocytochemistry (Table 8-1). However, the *physiological* role of these neuropeptides has yet to be ascertained. For example, it is not clear whether peptidergic fibers associated with airway smooth muscle subserve purely sensory functions or if secretion of these bronchoactive peptides contributes to physiological control processes. The coexistence of VIP (a substance which relaxes airway smooth muscle) and acetylcholine in the neurons of the tongue and salivary glands suggests that cholinergic efferent neurons may subserve inhibitory, as well as excitatory, functions in the airways.

In light of the appreciable ganglionic neural processing that operates in other autonomic systems, attention has recently been directed to the role of modulation of ganglionic neurotransmission in peripheral neural control. The presence of catecholamine-containing nerve terminals in human parasympathetic ganglia suggests that the major role of sympathetic innervation may be modulation of parasympathetic neurotransmission. Because of accessibility, the paratracheal ganglia of the ferret have attracted attention as an experimental model. In this species, interganglionic connections are quite extensive and,

TABLE 8-1

Neuropeptides Demonstrated in Human Airways

Peptide	Distribution	Effect
Vasoactive intestinal peptide (VIP)	Fibers in ganglia and fibers to smooth muscle, subepithelium, and blood vessels	Relaxation
Substance P (SP)	Fibers to central airway smooth muscle, blood vessels, and epithelial layer	Constriction, increased vessel permeability
Gastrin-releasing peptide (GRP)	Smooth-muscle layer	Constriction
Neuropeptide Y	Blood vessels, smooth muscle, epithelium	?

SOURCE: Data summarized from Hakanson, Sundler, Moghimzadeh, Leander, 1983, and Laitinen, 1985.

based on electrophysiological behavior, at least two different cell types have been distinguished. An intriguing, but as yet unsubstantiated possibility is that airway ganglia receive afferent input from airway receptors, which modulates neurotransmission, forming a peripheral neural control loop, as has been demonstrated in other autonomic ganglia. Figure 8-4 presents a hypothetical model of neural control of airway smooth muscle, based on available electrophysiological and pharmacologic data.

HUMORAL ACTIVATION

Several features of the electrophysiology, ultrastructure, and neuroanatomy of airway smooth muscles suggest a potential for considerable nonneural excitation. For example, the density of the neural innervation of tracheal and bronchial smooth muscle is much less than that of other smooth muscles that are under direct neural control; moreover, the smooth muscle of the peripheral airways is much less densely innervated than that of the central airways. Also, although nerve endings are located in clefts between myocyte bundles, no close connections (<20 nm), such as those seen in other multi-unit smooth muscles, have been found between nerve endings and

myocytes. Furthermore, individual myocytes are linked by numerous gap junctions or nexuses that constitute low-resistance pathways within the tissue for the spread of depolarization.

These observed facts have led to the suggestion that airway smooth muscle may respond to excitation somewhat like a single-unit syncytium, rather than a multi-unit system under fine neural control. Indeed, neural regulation does appear to occur at a multicellular level, cellular excitation proceeding via the combination of diffusion of neurotransmitter throughout the muscle bundles and the propagation of excitatory junction potentials between cells. These features also suggest the likely participation of extraneural control systems in the physiological activation of smooth muscle. Circulation of humoral substances, many of which may be generated locally, almost certainly modulates neural control in vivo, especially in the lung periphery where neural control is less prominent.

Numerous receptors have been demonstrated in airway smooth muscle. These include specific receptors for norepinephrine, acetylcholine, histamine, prostaglandins, leukotrienes, serotonin, VIP, and other neuropeptides. The presence of specific receptors to these substances, the demonstration of their functional effect when administered intravenously or applied to isolated airway

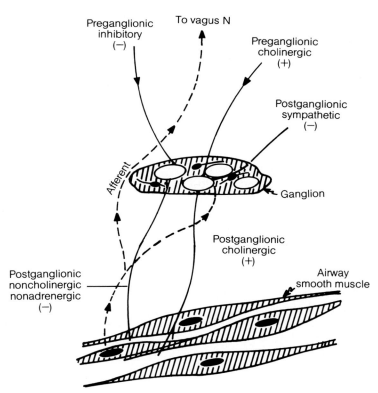

FIGURE 8-4   Hypothetical model of the neural regulation of human airway smooth muscle.

smooth muscle, and the demonstration of the presence or release of these substances following stimuli suggest that they are important as physiological regulatory substances.

In contrast to the lack of evidence for direct sympathetic innervation of human airway smooth muscle, myocytes are well endowed with adrenergic receptors. β_2-Adrenergic receptors are plentiful, and this system is probably the dominant mechanism of nonneural relaxation. Human β-adrenergic receptors are almost entirely of the β_2 subtype, and quantitative autoradiography of canine tissue indicates that their density increases from large to small airways. The possibility exists that the β_2 receptors mediate dilation triggered by circulating adrenal hormones rather than by neurotransmitter released from nerve terminals. Certainly the presence of a high density of β receptors in the smooth muscle of the peripheral airways, which is devoid of demonstrable adrenergic nerve terminals, suggests a high degree of nonneural control.

α Adrenoreceptors, also of two subtypes (α_1 and α_2), are also present in airway smooth muscle; those in the central airways appear to be mostly of the α_2 subtype, whereas the α_1 receptors are more numerous in the lung periphery. Stimulation of α adrenoreceptors causes bronchoconstriction. But, since the density of these receptors is much less than that of the β receptors, their functional effect is difficult to assess.

Humoral control of airway smooth muscle is not limited to the release of adrenal hormones. A rich diversity of cellular communications, including important paracrine and autocrine regulatory systems, is also present. Among these is the well-known immune-mediated release of histamine by mast cells in the course of allergic bronchoconstrictor responses. Histamine receptors are present on smooth muscle: H_1 receptors mediate constriction; H_2 receptors, relaxation. The distribution of these receptors, and hence the net response to histamine, appears to be species—and region—specific. However, the effects of H_2 receptor-mediated bronchodilation are relatively minor, and the functional effect of histamine administration is predominantly one of peripheral bronchoconstriction.

The role of arachidonic acid metabolites on airway smooth muscle has attracted considerable attention during the past decade. Products of the lipoxygenase pathway (leukotrienes) as well as the cyclooxygenase pathway (prostaglandins and thromboxanes) have marked effects on airway smooth muscle; these effects are mediated by specific receptors. The formation and release of these substances are dealt with in Chapter 79. Here suffice it to point out that specific leukotriene receptors for LTC_4 and LTD_4 do appear to exist on the cell membrane. LTC_4, LTD_4, and LTE_4 have potent bronchoconstrictor effects; in humans, aerosolization of these substances causes prolonged, peripheral bronchoconstriction. Some of the bronchoconstrictor effects observed after aerosol challenge may be due to LTC_4 and LTD_4 which appear to increase

the synthesis of prostaglandins and thromboxane. Immunologic challenge also causes the release in vitro of thromboxane A_2 and certain prostaglandins ($PGF_{2\alpha}$, PGD_2, PGG_2, and PGH_2) which are also potent constrictors of airway smooth muscle. Unfortunately, the relative roles of the various products of arachidonic acid metabolism in vivo, under natural conditions, remain to be clarified.

Other prostaglandins (PGE, PGE_2, and PGI_2) appear to participate in the physiological modulation of contraction. Exposure of isolated strips of canine smooth muscle to histamine causes the release of prostacyclin (PGI_2), which decreases the intensity of the bronchoconstriction. PGI_2 also appears to be the principal prostanoid produced by type II alveolar epithelial cells. Similarly, prostaglandins are released in isolated smooth-muscle strips in response to repeated electric stimulation, which may modulate acetylcholine release at cholinergic nerve terminals. Intercellular messenger substances such as interleukins also stimulate smooth-muscle cells to produce PGI_2. Thus, PGI_2 seems to play an important role in the autoregulation of airway smooth muscle during neural- and mediator-induced bronchoconstriction.

Hormonal influences on airway myocytes are not limited to regulation of contraction. The smooth-muscle cell is capable of diverse synthetic activity that is regulated by hormonal substances. In addition to producing contractile proteins, lipids, and matrix components, such as collagen, elastin, and glycosaminoglycans, substances are produced that appear to subserve a wide variety of functions. Myocytes produce fibronectin, somatomedinlike peptides, and prostaglandins E_1 and E_2 that regulate smooth-muscle growth and differentiation; myocytes also produce chemoattractant substances for mononuclear cells. A major regulator of smooth-muscle proliferation and protein synthesis appears to be the cationic polypeptide, platelet-derived growth factor (PDGF), for which specific receptors exist on the cell membrane. PDGF released by platelets promotes entrance into S phase, and subsequent DNA synthesis and cell mitosis. Other regulatory autocoids are currently being identified. They may shed light on the clinically important process of hyperplasia of airway smooth muscle.

SUMMARY

Airway smooth muscle represents the end-effector organ responsible for maintaining normal and abnormal bronchomotor tone. The processes that regulate activation are myriad, existing at a multicellular, cellular, and subcellular level. Furthermore, these processes are not discrete, but interactive. The complexity of the regulatory system is mirrored by the complexity of the associated disease processes. Abnormalities in many of these regulatory processes have been implicated in asthma and other hyperreactive airways diseases. Our present understanding of these regulatory processes has provided a framework for investigation of these disorders. It is likely that future advances will occur through a more complete understanding of the neural and nonneural control systems that regulate airway smooth-muscle function.

BIBLIOGRAPHY

Barnes PJ, Basbaum CB, Nadel JA, Roberts JM: Localization of β-adrenoreceptors in mammalian lung by light microscopic autoradiography. Nature 299:444–447, 1982.
Autoradiographic localization of β receptors in ferret lung.

Baron CB, Cunningham M, Strauss JF III, Coburn RF: Pharmacomechanical coupling in smooth muscle may involve phosphatidyl inositol metabolism. Proc Natl Acad Sci 81:6899–6903, 1984.
Demonstration of agonist-induced phosphatidyl inositol metabolism in canine tracheal smooth muscle.

Bond M, Kitazawa T, Somlyo AP, Somlyo AV: Release and recycling of calcium by the sarcoplasmic reticulum in guinea pig portal vein smooth muscle. J Physiol 355:677–695, 1984.
Measurement of Ca^{2+} in sarcoplasmic reticulum and demonstration of recycling of this store.

Cameron AR, Coburn RF: Electrical and anatomic characteristics of cells of ferret paratracheal ganglion. Am J Physiol 246:C450–C458, 1984.
Electrophysiological properties of neurons of the paratracheal ganglia of the ferret.

Drazen JM, Fanta CH, Lacouture PG: Effect of nifedipine on constriction of human tracheal strips *in vitro*. Br J Pharmacol 78:687–691, 1983.
Dihydropyridine calcium antagonists partially inhibit histamine-induced contraction of human airway smooth muscle.

Farley JM, Miles PR: The sources of calcium for acetylcholine-induced contractions of dog trachealis muscle. J Pharmacol Exp Ther 207:340–346, 1978.
Acetylcholine-induced contractions occur in calcium-free media and in the presence of calcium-channel blocking agents.

Hakanson R, Sundler F, Moghimzadeh E, Leander S: Peptide-containing nerve fibres in the airways: distribution and functional implications. Eur J Respir Dis 131:115–146, 1983.
Review of immunocytochemical localization of neuropeptides in the airways.

Inoue T, Ito Y, Takeda K: Prostaglandin-induced inhibition of acetylcholine release from neuronal elements of dog tracheal tissue. J Physiol 349:553–570, 1984.
Repeated electric stimulation of isolated airway smooth muscle results in prostaglandin release which modulates the contractile response.

Kamm KE, Stull JT: The function of myosin and myosin light chain kinase phosphorylation in smooth muscle. Annu Rev Pharmacol Toxicol 25:593–620, 1985.
Review of contractile regulatory processes in smooth muscle.

Kannan MS, Daniel EE: Structural and functional study of control of canine tracheal smooth muscle. Am J Physiol 238:C27–C33, 1980.
No close connections between nerve ending and smooth muscle cell, sparse innervation, and presence of gap junctions demonstrated by electron microscopy.

Kotlikoff MI: Transient calcium current in isolated canine airway smooth muscle cells. J Physiol (submitted for publication).
Patch-clamp measurement of calcium currents in airway smooth-muscle cells.

Kotlikoff MI, Murray RK, Reynolds EE: Histamine-induced calcium release and phorbol antagonism in cultured airway smooth muscle cells. Am J Physiol (in press).
Internal calcium release induced by histamine and kinetics of cytosolic calcium rise.

Kreulen DL: Integration in autonomic ganglia. Physiologist 27:49–55, 1984.
Review of neural integration mechanisms in peripheral autonomic ganglia.

Kroeger EA, Stephens NL: Effect of tetraethylammonium on tonic airway smooth muscle: Initiation of phasic electrical activity. Am J Physiol 228:633–636, 1975.
Demonstration that tetraethylammonium results in depolarization and spontaneous action potentials.

Laitinen A: Autonomic innervation of the human respiratory tract as revealed by histochemical and ultrastructural methods. Eur J Respir Dis 66:7–42, 1985.
  Histochemical study of cholinergic, adrenergic, and peptidergic fibers in the airways.

Lundberg JM, Hökfelt T: Coexistence of peptides and classical transmitters. Trends Neurosci 6:325–332, 1983.
  Discussion of evidence demonstrating dual neurotransmitter release from a single nerve terminal.

McCann JD, Welsh MJ: Voltage-gated Ca-activated K channels in isolated canine airway smooth muscle cells. Biophys J 47:135a, 1985 (abstract).
  Single-channel recording of potassium-channel activity in isolated canine airway myocytes and demonstration of calcium dependence of channel activity.

Partanen M, Laitinen A, Hervonen A, Toivanen M, Laitinen LA: Catecholamine- and acetylcholinesterase-containing nerves in human lower respiratory tract. Histochemistry 76:175–188, 1982.
  Human airway ganglia contain catecholamine-containing processes.

Richardson J, Beland J: Nonadrenergic inhibitory nervous system in human airways. J Appl Physiol 41:764–771, 1976.
  Relaxation of human airway smooth muscle occurs via a nonadrenergic, noncholinergic neurotransmitter. No functional release of norepinephrine in situ.

Shore SA, Powell WS, Martin JG: Endogenous prostaglandins modulate histamine-induced contraction in canine tracheal smooth muscle. J Appl Physiol 58:859–868, 1985.
  Histamine contraction of isolated airway smooth muscle results in an increase in prostaglandin release.

Somlyo AV, Somlyo AP: Electrical and pharmacomechanical coupling in vascular smooth muscle. J Pharmacol Exp Ther 159:129–145, 1968.
  Formulation of concept of pharmacomechanical coupling.

Stephens NL, Kroeger EA: Ultrastructure, biophysics, and biochemistry of airway smooth muscle, in Nadel JA (ed), *Physiology and Pharmacology of the Airways.* New York, Marcel Dekker, 1980, pp 31–121.
  Review of ultrastructure and mechanics of airway smooth muscle.

Taylor L, Polgar P, McAteer JA, Douglas WHJ: Prostaglandin production by type II alveolar epithelial cells. Biochim Biophys Acta 572:502–509, 1979.
  Prostacyclin is produced by cultured alveolar type II epithelial cells.

Part 2

Physiological Principles

Chapter *9*

Control of Ventilation

Neil S. Cherniack / Allan I. Pack

Major Afferent Systems
  Peripheral Chemoreceptors
  Central Chemoreceptors
  Pulmonary Vagal Afferents

Central Neural Mechanisms

Coordination of the Activity of the Respiratory Muscles
  The Thoracic Muscles
  Upper Airway Muscles

Integrated Responses of the Control System
  Respiratory Adaptation to Altitude
  Hypoxic Depression of Ventilation
  Adaptation to Metabolic Acid-Base Disturbances
  Response to Mechanical Loading
  Response to Bronchoconstriction

Voluntary Control of Breathing and Dyspnea

Breathing is produced by the coordinated action of a relatively large number of muscles. Principal among these is the diaphragm, which generates negative pressure in the thorax, thereby causing inflation of the lung. The diaphragm's action is complemented by that of other inspiratory muscles. Expiration, in turn, involves the coordinated action of muscles of the upper airways, which brakes the rate of airflow from the lung, and of the abdominal and other expiratory muscles, which can act to supplement the expulsive force provided by the recoil of the respiratory system. Since the action of each of these muscles has to be controlled, the control system for breathing has a number of distinct neural outputs (Fig. 9-1).

The action of these muscles is regulated so as to match the level of ventilation to metabolic demand. Since the latter undergoes wide variations during normal behavior, there is a need for feedback systems (Fig. 9-1). Principal among these are the peripheral and central chemoreceptors monitoring the chemical status of the organism. Not only, however, does ventilation have to be set but so, too, does its pattern, e.g., the durations of inspiration and expiration and the magnitude of tidal volume. One might anticipate that ventilatory pattern should be set so as to minimize the work of breathing, and certain evidence suggests that this is so. Control of pattern requires a different

set of afferent information that is provided principally by receptors in the lung monitoring its deformation. Finally, there is a need for more local feedback loops for each of the respiratory muscles to ensure that the central command to the muscle is executed. Such local feedback loops involve segmental reflexes in the spinal cord and are based on information provided by muscle spindles and tendon organs about the mechanical state of the muscle.

Thus, the respiratory control system is a hierarchical one. Neural circuits must match efferent outflow to the need for ventilation (drive component) and generate appropriate oscillatory signals to the inspiratory and expiratory muscles (control of ventilatory pattern). These descending signals can be modulated at the spinal cord by segmental afferent inputs (local control). To accomplish this, the central neuronal circuits produce a variety of efferent outflow signals (multi-output) and receive a large variety of afferent information (multi-input) (for schematic of system, see Fig. 9-1). In this chapter we discuss briefly the functioning of each of the major afferent systems, current knowledge as to the central pattern generator, and the role of the different respiratory muscles. The chapter concludes with consideration of certain of the integrated responses of the total system.

MAJOR AFFERENT SYSTEMS

Peripheral Chemoreceptors

The peripheral chemoreceptors are generally considered to consist of the carotid and aortic bodies. Quantitatively the carotid bodies are considerably more important. Indeed in humans (but not in all species) ventilation does not increase when subjects with denervated carotid bodies are exposed to hypoxia. During normal quiet breathing of ambient air (eupnea), the carotid bodies contribute about 15 percent of the ventilatory drive. They also account for about 30 percent of the ventilatory response to hypercapnia. Finally, the ventilatory response to hypoxia is mostly, if not solely, dependent on the carotid bodies.

The carotid bodies are situated in the neck at the bifurcations of the common carotid arteries (Fig. 9-2). They are supplied by blood from a branch of the external carotid artery, and their venous drainage is to the internal jugular. They have an enormous blood flow when one considers their small mass (of the order of 10 mg in humans): their blood flow is equivalent to 2 L per 100 g/min. Their oxygen uptake is also large, i.e., of the order of 9 ml per 100 g/min. Because of the large blood flow, the arteriovenous difference for oxygen is extremely small (0.2 to 0.5 ml per 100 ml). This large blood flow, coupled with the low extraction of oxygen, makes the carotid body relatively insensitive to variations in oxygen delivery (O_2 con-

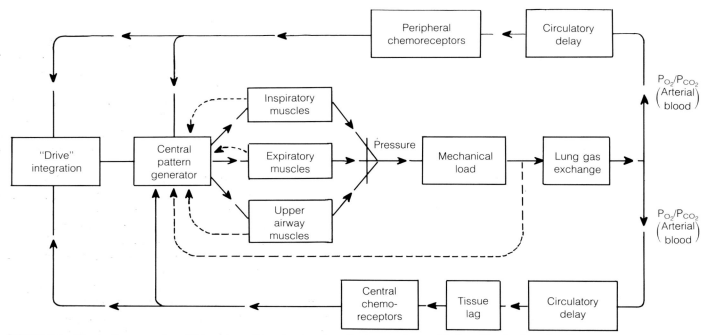

FIGURE 9-1 Block diagram of multi-input, multi-output system that controls ventilation. For further details see text.

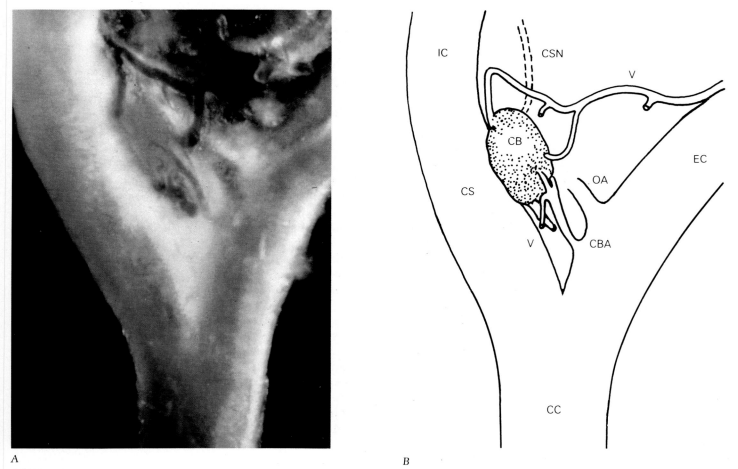

A

B

FIGURE 9-2 A. Photograph (×40) of the carotid body in the rat situated at the bifurcation of the common carotid artery. The organ is highly vascular. B. Schematic representation of the various structures: CB = carotid body; CBA = carotid body artery; CS = carotid sinus; CSN = carotid sinus nerve; CC = common carotid artery; EC = external carotid artery; IC = internal carotid artery; OA = occipital artery; V = vein from carotid body. *(Reprinted with permission from DM McDonald: Peripheral Chemoreceptors in Regulation of Breathing, New York, Dekker, 1981.)*

tent × blood flow). Instead, carotid bodies respond primarily to changes in oxygen tension. Direct evidence for arterial P_{O_2} as the stimulus comes from experiments with carbon monoxide. In contrast to the consistent stimulation by inhaled carbon monoxide of the aortic bodies, which have a lower blood flow per unit mass than do the carotid bodies, relatively few afferent fibers from the carotid body are weakly stimulated.

The carotid bodies respond not only to hypoxia but also to increasing P_{CO_2}. Indeed, there is a complex interaction between these stimuli. At a constant P_{CO_2}, a hyperbolic relationship exists between receptor discharge and P_{O_2} (Fig. 9-3A), whereas at a constant P_{O_2} the relationship between activity and P_{CO_2} is a linear one (Fig. 9-3B). The interaction is such that the receptors become more sensitive to P_{CO_2} with increasing degrees of hypoxia (Fig. 9-3B). In addition to these characteristics, most, but not all, studies indicate that the receptors are sensitive to the rate of change of P_{CO_2}. This rate sensitivity involves carbonic anhydrase in some way since it is abolished by acetazolamide.

The rate sensitivity of the receptors, and their rapid response to changes in P_{CO_2} and P_{O_2}, enable the carotid body to follow respiratory related oscillations in arterial blood-gas tensions. The oscillations in P_{CO_2} in the arterial blood, which can be monitored by using a fast responding pH electrode, seem to be the principal, if not the sole, determinant of oscillations in chemoreceptor discharge. Since the magnitude of oscillations in arterial P_{CO_2} is directly related to metabolic CO_2 production, it has been proposed that this oscillatory signal contains the necessary information to produce the coupling between the metabolic production of CO_2 and the ventilation during exercise. This postulate has been the subject of much

study, but conflicting experimental results lead to a lack of consensus as to its role.

The afferent signals from the carotid body are relayed in fibers in the glossopharyngeal nerve to the medial subnucleus of the nucleus tractus solitarius. The chemoreceptor fibers are both myelinated and unmyelinated. In addition to the afferent fibers, there is both a sympathetic innervation of the carotid body and an efferent pathway in the glossopharyngeal nerve. Stimulation of the sympathetic nervous system leads to an increase in carotid body discharge, an effect that is probably due to local changes in blood flow within the organ. In contrast, increased activity of the efferent glossopharyngeal pathway inhibits chemoreceptor discharge. Thus, the system makes possible direct control of the sensitivity (gain) of the carotid body.

The terminals of the majority of the afferent fibers terminate on glomus cells, i.e., the type I cells. Most of the specific cell types of the carotid body are type I cells (60 to 80 percent in different species). The type I cells appear to be secretory in nature since they contain rough endoplasmic reticulum, aggregates of ribosomes, a well-developed Golgi apparatus, and dense core vesicles. Differences in vesicle size have raised the possibility of subtypes of glomus cells. The glomus cells are arranged in groups (glomerules), and each group is surrounded by the second main cell type of the carotid body, i.e., the sheath, or type II cell. These cells do not appear to be innervated, nor do they contain the dense core vesicles of the type I glomus cell.

The type I cells contain catecholamines, and it seems likely that the catecholamines are contained in their dense core vesicles. The catecholamines that the glomus cells contain are dopamine, norepinephrine, and epi-

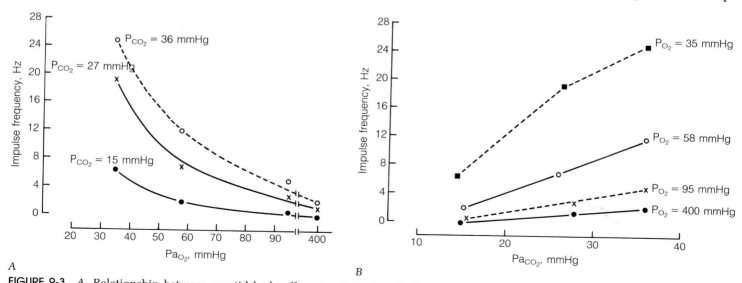

FIGURE 9-3 A. Relationship between carotid body afferent activity (single fiber) and P_{O_2} (at different levels of P_{CO_2}). B. Relationship between single-fiber carotid body afferent activity and P_{CO_2} at different levels of P_{O_2}. (*These data are redrawn from Lahiri, DeLaney: Respir Physiol 24:249–266, 1975.*)

nephrine. Of these, dopamine is the principal one (60 to 90 percent of the total catecholamine present), and its concentration is about the same as that in the adrenal medulla. The carotid bodies can take up circulating catecholamines and their precursors and also synthesize catecholamines from tyrosine. Enzymes responsible for each of the synthetic steps are present in the carotid body, the rate-limiting enzyme being tyrosine hydroxylase, which catalyzes the conversion of tyrosine to dopamine. Hypoxia affects the levels of dopamine in two ways: (1) by causing increased secretion from glomus cells, thereby depleting their content of catecholamine, and (2) over a longer time scale, by causing increased production of tyrosine hydroxylase and, hence, of dopamine. The role of dopamine in the chemoreceptor process remains uncertain: it is not known if it is an essential neurotransmitter or, as seems more likely, if it modulates the chemoreceptor process. What is known is that exogenously administered dopamine depresses chemoreceptor discharge.

Catecholamines are not the only potential neurotransmitter in the carotid body. Also present are 5-hydroxy-tryptamine (serotonin), acetylcholine, and some of the neuropeptides—substance P, VIP, met- and leu-enkephalin. The role of these substances in the transduction process is also unknown. Acetylcholine has been proposed as an essential transmitter since it is present in glomus cells, and exogenously administered acetylcholine stimulates afferent discharge. A plausible scheme can be built around this idea; i.e., hypoxia stimulates glomus cells to release acetylcholine which in turn stimulates sensory endings. However, although plausible, it is unlikely to be correct since pharmacologic blockade of acetylcholine's actions causes no change in the carotid body responses to hypoxia.

Despite many theories, there is currently no agreement as to which component of a carotid body senses the change in oxygen tension. Some propose (see above) that the glomus cell is key. Others favor the sensory nerve terminals as the site of the sensing mechanism and picture secretion from the glomus cell as the modulator of their activity. Even the sheath (type II) cell has been implicated by some; they could serve as chemosensors which respond to hypoxia either by establishing a K^+ gradient that stimulates nearby nerve terminals or by contracting, thereby providing a mechanical stimulus to the nerve endings. Thus, despite considerable investigation, the mechanism of chemoreception by the carotid bodies remains elusive.

Central Chemoreceptors

Knowledge of the functioning of the so-called central chemoreceptors is less complete than for the peripheral chemoreceptors. Indeed, whether the term *central chemoreceptor* should be used is debatable. What is known is that after denervation of the peripheral chemoreceptors,

most of the response to hypercapnia is retained. Also, this central sensitivity to CO_2 is not mediated by the respiratory neurons themselves since, if anything, they are inhibited (hyperpolarized) by the direct effects of increasing CO_2.

That this central chemosensitivity is located in the ventral medulla was originally suggested by experiments involving infusion of acidic cerebrospinal fluid (CSF). More precise localization was achieved by applying pledgets saturated with solutions of low pH directly to different regions of the ventral medulla. Two chemosensitive regions were identified by these experiments. The first (rostral or Mitchell's) area extends caudally from the pontomedullary junction; it is bordered laterally by the roots of the seventh to tenth cranial nerve (Fig. 9-4). The second, smaller (caudal or Loeschcke's) area is situated at the origin of the twelfth nerve (Fig. 9-4). Since ventilation was increased by changes in H^+ ion at the surface and decreased by local application of procaine, it was hypothesized that the chemosensitive elements were close to the surface of the medulla where they were influenced by the pH of the CSF.

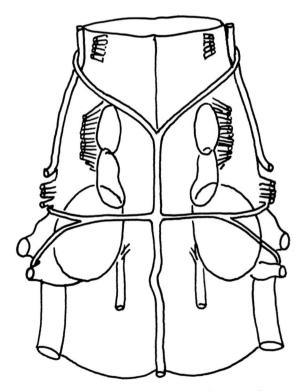

FIGURE 9-4   Outline of various regions on the ventral aspect of the medulla that are associated with the central chemoreceptor mechanism. The largest most rostral area is the chemosensitive area described by Mitchell. The smaller most caudal area is the chemosensitive area of Loeschcke. Between these areas is the region that is known as the intermediate area. (*This schematic is reproduced with permission from Schläfke, Pokorski, See, Prill, Loeschcke: Bull Physiopath Respir 11:277–284, 1975.*)

Certain evidence argues against this hypothesis. First, the changes in pH employed in these experiments were extremely large, whereas the changes in ventilation were small. Second, histologically little is unique about this area. Although some investigators have found cells in this region that increase their firing with increasing H^+ ion, others have failed to find such cells. Thus, the cellular basis of the central chemoreceptors is far from established, and it seems reasonable to regard their precise location as unsettled.

The specific stimulus for the central chemoreceptors also continues to be a subject of debate. The prevailing theory is that the stimulus is uniquely related to hydrogen ion concentration at the receptor site. However, much of the evidence for this view is indirect, based on mathematical predictions of extracellular pH. More recent experiments, using techniques for measuring extracellular pH directly in this region of the brain, have cast doubt on H^+ ion being the unique stimulus since different relationships between stimulation of respiration and H^+ ion concentration are obtained depending on whether the changes in the H^+ ion concentration are produced by respiratory or metabolic perturbations: a given decrease in pH produced by CO_2 inhalation has more marked effects on respiration than does the same decrease produced by metabolic acidosis, suggesting that CO_2 may, per se, have an additional stimulatory action. However, such experiments are somewhat problematic since the precise location of the receptors is unknown so that quantification of the pH "stimulus" can only be approximate.

Between the two chemosensitive areas lies an interesting area, i.e., the *intermediate area* (IA) or "Schläfke's area" (Fig. 9-4). Cooling this small area, or applying procaine to it, markedly depresses ventilation and abolishes the response to inhaled CO_2. These observations have been interpreted to mean that the intermediate area is a site of convergence of fibers from the two adjacent chemosensitive areas as they pass to the respiratory complex in the dorsal medulla. But other evidence suggests that the intermediate area has a more general role in the regulation of ventilation and that its function is not just related to that of the central chemoreceptors. In essence, there is little consensus concerning the roles of these various areas in the ventral medulla and little insight into the cellular bases for the central effects of CO_2 on the ventilation.

Pulmonary Vagal Afferents

Complementing the information from chemoreceptors are afferent systems that provide information about the state of the lungs and of the respiratory muscles; the latter are provided by muscle spindles and tendon organs. The intercostal and abdominal muscles are relatively richly innervated with both muscle spindles and tendon organs, whereas the diaphragm is relatively poor in muscle spindles.

Within the lung there are thought to be four major receptor types: stretch receptors, rapidly adapting ("irritant") receptors, and two receptors that are innervated by nonmyelinated afferents. The last group of receptors is classified according to the receptors' different locations, i.e., either in the pulmonary interstitium (*juxtacapillary*, or *J receptors*) or in the bronchi (*bronchial C receptors*). Although this separation for nonmyelinated afferents may seem somewhat artificial, the responses of the receptors in the two locations to different chemical stimuli are different. Moreover, certain theories center around the role of J receptors in the genesis of the increase in ventilation during exercise and during interstitial edema.

STRETCH RECEPTORS

One of the main receptors in the lung is the pulmonary stretch receptor which shows a slowly adapting response to inflation of the lung that is maintained (Fig. 9-5A). This receptor is situated within the smooth muscle of the airway, and the highest density of receptors is in the more proximal airways. However, receptors in different locations have different reflex effects on ventilation: those in the more distal airways play a major role in modulating the durations of inspiration and expiration, whereas those in the trachea have no such action. Since the transduction

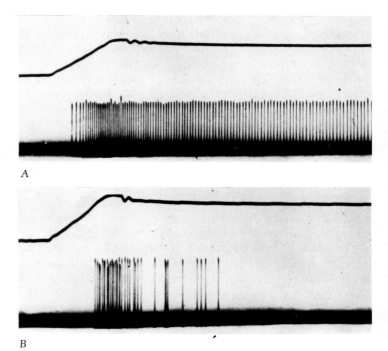

A

B

FIGURE 9-5 Response characteristics of the two major mechanoreceptors in the airways. A. Response of pulmonary stretch receptor. This shows the slowly adapting nature of the response and the continued discharge of the receptor during maintained inflation of the lung. B. Response of rapidly adapting ("irritant") receptor which fires largely during the period while the lung is being inflated and then adapts. *(Reproduced with permission from Knowlton, Larrabee: Am J Physiol 147:100–114, 1946.)*

properties of the receptors in the different locations are similar, this difference in reflex response must be due to their having different central pathways.

The firing of the stretch receptors increases as the lung is inflated, and the receptors continue to fire even when the lung is static (Fig. 9-5A). However, their firing also depends on the *rate* of inflation (dynamic response). At higher lung volumes, the receptor shows more marked sensitivity to changes in flow rate than to changes in lung volume; i.e., those receptors act increasingly as rate receptors at higher lung volumes. Although these overall response characteristics are known, what the receptor actually responds to is not known.

Stretch receptors also exhibit a direct sensitivity to changes in the concentration of carbon dioxide at the receptor site, an effect probably mediated by changes in pH. The implication is that their firing depends on the concentration of carbon dioxide in the airways but not on the concentration in the arterial blood. Low levels of airway carbon dioxide increase firing. The relationship between receptor activity and CO_2 concentration is nonlinear: changes in firing are most marked between 0 and 2% CO_2, whereas virtually no change in firing takes place between 3 and 5% CO_2. Since the concentration of CO_2 in the airways varies throughout the respiratory cycle, i.e., from 0% late in inspiration to 5% late in expiration, this mechanism affords some modulation of the receptors' response during respiration. However, this is not the only mechanism that can produce respiratory related oscillations in receptor activity. For example, efferent modulation of airway smooth-muscle tone during respiration also alters receptor firing. The role of this efferent modulation of stretch receptor firing in reflex control of respiration is unknown.

RAPIDLY ADAPTING RECEPTORS

Efferent modulation of smooth-muscle tone does not affect the firing of the other major mechanoreceptors—the rapidly adapting receptors (also called irritant receptors and deflation or collapse receptors). These receptors are also primarily in the larger airways; indirect evidence indicates that they are situated in the epithelium and submucosa. Although they have been known for four decades, their role remains somewhat enigmatic. Originally identified by their rapidly adapting response to lung inflation (Fig. 9-5B), the receptors quickly became known as *irritant receptors*. This change in nomenclature was based on observations that the receptors respond to a variety of chemical irritants, e.g., ammonia, cigarette smoke, and ether vapor, and to inert dust particles. Their response to inhaled irritants was thought to produce a defense reflex, i.e., coughing, bronchoconstriction, laryngeal constriction, and increased production of respiratory tract mucus. However, recent evidence has challenged this view: (1) a

minority of receptors that respond to lung inflation by a rapidly adapting discharge show any response to inhaled irritants; (2) the firing of the rapidly adapting receptors, although somewhat erratic (compare to carotid chemoreceptors), shows a definite deterministic relationship between the rate and magnitude of inflation on the one hand and receptor activity on the other; it seems strange that the firing of an irritant receptor that "defends the lung" should have such firing characteristics; and (3) other receptors in the airways (bronchial C fibers) that are innervated by nonmyelinated afferents also respond to irritant chemicals; these other receptors are equally likely candidates to mediate defense reflexes.

If the irritant receptor does not defend against noxious challenges, what could be its role? Relevant to this question is the fact that the irritant receptor fires predominantly during the inflation part of the respiratory cycle and that its firing depends strongly on the rate of airflow; also, the firing of the receptor is affected by changes in pulmonary compliance so that decreases in compliance during inflation lead to increased firing of the receptor. Therefore, the rapidly adapting receptor may be responsible for generation of intermittent sighs without which pulmonary compliance decreases progressively.

The possibility also exists that the rapidly adapting receptors may also excite inspiratory neural activity to accelerate lung inflation; this positive feedback would decrease the time lag between neural events in the medulla and mechanical events in the lungs. Although there is no neurophysiological proof that rapidly adapting receptors produce this augmentation, and even though the augmenting effect is apt to be small, the neural circuitry by which the rapidly adapting receptors could mediate such a change does exist.

The rapidly adapting receptors have also been implicated in reflex bronchoconstriction. Chemicals released in asthma, such as histamine, cause bronchoconstriction not only by a direct action on smooth muscle but also by a reflex pathway. That rapidly adapting receptors might be the afferent component of such a reflex is largely based on demonstrations of their marked sensitivity to histamine.

BRONCHIAL C AND J RECEPTORS

A "new" group of nonmyelinated afferent endings appears to be as likely, if not more likely, than the rapidly adapting receptors as mediators of reflex bronchoconstriction in asthma. These endings, identified by Coleridge and Coleridge, innervate receptors in the bronchi. The bronchial C receptors are stimulated by phenyldiguanide and capsaicin, chemicals that are known to increase the firing of nonmyelinated endings. The receptors also respond to a variety of pulmonary autocoids released in asthma and inflammatory disease, i.e., bradykinin, serotonin, prostaglandins [$PGF_{2\alpha}$, PGE_2, PGI_2 (prostacyclin)], as well as to inhaled irritants, such as sulfur dioxide. The sensitivity of the receptors to bradykinin is marked, particularly when bradykinin is infused into the bronchial circulation. Activation of the receptors produces reflex tachypnea, increased tracheobronchial secretion, and bronchoconstriction. The low baseline firing of the receptors may contribute to baseline bronchomotor tone.

In some respects the responses of the receptors identified by the Coleridges are similar to those of the nonmyelinated afferent endings in the pulmonary interstitium described earlier by Paintal, i.e., the juxtacapillary or J receptors. J receptors also respond to chemicals such as phenyldiguanide and capsaicin. However, there are important differences between the bronchial C receptors and the J receptors. In particular, J receptors show only weak stimulation in response to histamine and virtually no response to bradykinin. Whether this represents differences in the receptors themselves, or in the metabolic properties of the different endothelia—since the chemicals are injected into the circulation in these experiments—is unknown.

The particular aspect of the response of the J receptors that has received most attention is their increase in firing during pulmonary congestion. Indeed, Paintal has postulated that congestion is the natural stimulus of the receptors, envisaging that they are sensitive to changes in pressure in the pulmonary interstitium: as left atrial pressure increases, the increments in firing of J receptors are more marked than are those of bronchial C receptors.

The reflex effects of stimulation of J receptors are also somewhat different from those of bronchial C fibers. Stimulation of J receptors produces the *pulmonary chemoreflex*, a triad of apnea, bradycardia, and hypotension. Apnea may not be an integral part of this response but simply a reflection of intense stimulation by bolus injection, since less intense but more sustained stimulation elicits tachypnea rather than apnea. The cardiac depressor effects are marked and are due to both cardiac slowing and a fall in right ventricular stroke volume. Although some cardiac depression also occurs after stimulation of bronchial C receptors, this aspect of the reflex response is modest compared to that for J receptors.

Another feature of the reflex elicited by stimulation of J receptors is inhibition of motoneurons of the spinal cord by a central mechanism; affected by this inhibition are the motoneurons that innervate the respiratory muscles, and those involved in monosynaptic and polysynaptic spinal reflexes. This component of the reflex response, which has been called the J reflex, originally led Paintal to propose that the function of the J receptors is to limit exercise by inhibiting motoneuron discharge whenever alveolar-capillary interstitial pressure increases as the result of interstitial deformation, e.g., by an increase in interstitial water. This hypothesis envisages that the receptors have a protective function to defend against interstitial edema.

However, there are problems with the Paintal proposal. In particular, the J reflex is not unique to J receptors since stimulation of other visceral nonmyelinated afferents, e.g., those in the heart, can also produce these reflex effects. More recently Paintal has proposed that instead of inhibiting exercise, J receptors may facilitate exercise and act as a kind of positive feedback system. At present, the role of the J receptors can only be regarded as unsettled. Indeed, whether these receptors are unique, or just part of a general visceral nonmyelinated system, remains open to debate.

CENTRAL NEURAL MECHANISMS

Since respiration is a rhythmic motor act, the central neural circuits for respiration have to produce a rhythmic efferent outflow. Of the various neural mechanisms that are capable of producing such rhythmic behavior, the prevailing view is that rhythmicity is a property of the synaptic interactions between the various types of respiratory neurons in the network. The rhythm which is generated consists of three phases rather than the conventional two phases (inspiration and expiration). These three phases are inspiration, postinspiration (phase 1, expiration), and late expiration (phase 2, expiration). Identification of these phases is based not only on the different mechanical functions of each (lung inflation, passive expiration with braking of expiratory airflow, and active expiration, respectively) but, perhaps more importantly, on the fact that each is controlled by different components of the neural network. These different components of the cycle are shown on a recording of phrenic nerve activity (Fig. 9-6).

During inspiration, inspiratory neurons in the medulla which are premotor to the phrenic and intercostal motor nuclei display an augmenting discharge. Intracellular recording from such neurons reveals that they receive increasing excitatory postsynaptic activity throughout inspiration. This activity is due, in part, to these neurons reexciting each other, but more to an excitatory input, *central inspiratory activity*, that they receive from an unidentified source. Thus, these premotor neurons are driven by an "upstream" pattern generator.

At the end of inspiration, discharge from these inspiratory neurons is turned off by an off switch. This seemingly simple concept was introduced approximately a decade ago by von Euler and colleagues. It was initially based on examination of relationships between various afferent stimuli, e.g., lung volume, and the duration of inspiration. The concept has since been supported in toto by neurophysiological studies. Inspiratory neurons receive a strong transient inhibition at the end of inspiration (off switch) that terminates the ramp increase of inspiratory neural activity (Fig. 9-6). The source of this inhibition is unknown, although activity has been recorded in cer-

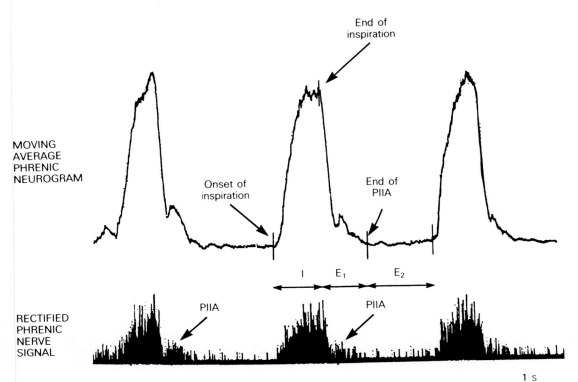

MOVING
AVERAGE
PHRENIC
NEUROGRAM

End of
inspiration

Onset of
inspiration

End of
PIIA

RECTIFIED
PHRENIC
NERVE
SIGNAL

PIIA

PIIA

I   E₁   E₂

1 s

FIGURE 9-6 Different phases of the respiratory cycle shown by a recording of phrenic nerve activity (below) together with its moving average (above). The three phases are inspiration, postinspiratory activity (expiration, phase 1) and late expiration (expiration, phase 2). For further details see text.

tain neurons which fire just at the time of the inspiratory off switch (*late inspiratory neurons*).

However, the off switch is not as totally abrupt as originally conceived. Instead, a period of graded inhibition, when the off switch is reversible, precedes the final off switch. The action of the inspiratory off switch depends on central neural timing mechanisms, akin to a basic clock frequency, whereas certain afferent inputs affect the operation of the switching circuits. One particularly important afferent in this regard is the pulmonary stretch receptor. Increased activity of pulmonary stretch receptors shortens inspiratory duration. As a result, the larger the tidal volume, the shorter the duration of inspiration.

The end of inspiration is followed by a period of postinspiratory activity on the part of certain inspiratory neurons. During this period of declining activity the inspiratory neurons receive both excitatory and inhibitory postsynaptic potentials. This neural activity is associated with active braking of airflow at the beginning of expiration. The duration of this postinspiratory phase of the respiratory cycle seems to be an important determinant of total duration of expiration.

Following the end of the postinspiratory phase of the respiratory cycle, there is a period during which the expiratory muscles may undergo active contraction. In this phase of the cycle, inspiratory bulbospinal neurons receive inhibitory postsynaptic potentials in an augmenting pattern. A particular group of expiratory neurons in the retrofacial nucleus (Botzinger complex) has been shown to be capable of generating this inhibition.

Although the duration of expiration, like inspiration, can be set by intrinsic brain-stem mechanisms, normally it is modulated by afferent inputs. Throughout expiration, there is a decreasing inhibition of the following inspiration. Thus, early in expiration it takes larger stimuli (e.g., pulmonary deflations) to trigger the onset of inspiration than later in expiration. In addition to this intrinsic process, there are various afferent inputs. As in the case of inspiration, afferents from pulmonary stretch receptors are particularly important. Activity of these stretch receptors prolongs expiration, i.e., the Hering-Breuer expiratory promoting reflex. Central processing of this afferent activity is complex and involves a process akin to leaky integration. The time constants of this processing are now known.

COORDINATION OF THE ACTIVITY OF THE RESPIRATORY MUSCLES

The concept that respiratory neurons innervate chest wall muscles which serve to pump air in and out of the lungs, while true, conceals many important relationships.

The chest wall itself is flexible and, although the ribs and the spine act as a framework to preserve its shape, the coordinated activity of the muscles which insert upon the thoracic cage not only brings air to the alveoli, but also prevents the waste of energy that could be caused by chest wall distortion during breathing.

The pharyngeal channels, which air must traverse before arriving at the lungs, also have flexible walls and contain valvelike mobile structures that can be displaced so as to obstruct the airways by the negative and positive swings in pressure that occur during normal breathing. The rigidity and configuration of these channels and their patency again depend on the skeletal muscles of the upper airways. Like the chest wall muscles, the activity of this group of muscles has a respiratory modulation that increases as breathing is stimulated.

The Thoracic Muscles

During quiet breathing the diaphragm is the muscle mainly responsible for the tidal excursions of air. As the diaphragm contracts, it acts on the abdominal contents, which are primarily fluid, to push the abdominal wall outward. At the same time, through its insertions on the lower ribs, it elevates the costal margins and expands the chest cavity.

Even the small transthoracic pressure changes that occur during breathing are sufficient to distort the chest wall. Acting alone, the diaphragm would use energy not only to overcome the resistance of the airways and the stiffness of the chest wall but also to distort the ribs. Contraction of the parasternal intercostal muscles, and perhaps the scalene muscles, prevents this distortion.

Expiration is largely passively determined by the elastic recoil of the chest wall. But it is of interest that usually the inspiratory muscles continue to contract, albeit at a steadily decreasing rate, during early expiration to retard the egress of air from the lungs. The function of this postinspiratory inspiratory activity (discussed above) is unclear. It may help to improve the efficiency of gas exchange and, in infants, in whom the chest wall is extremely pliable, it may help to preserve the constancy of the functional residual capacity by preventing too much air from leaving the lungs during the expiratory period.

It is likely that the diaphragm itself does not behave as if it were a single muscle. The costal portion of the diaphragm seems to be supplied mainly by the upper cervical roots which make up the phrenic nerve, whereas the crural portion of the diaphragm receives its innervation mainly through the lower phrenic roots. Isolated contraction of the crural diaphragm causes primarily expansion of the abdomen, whereas contraction of the costal portion, in addition to causing movement of the abdominal wall, enlarges the rib cage. The crural diaphragm may not only be a respiratory muscle but may also act as part of the sphincter mechanism for the lower esophagus; its contraction compresses the sphincter. In this way, the action of the sphincter is linked with respiration, as is the transdiaphragmatic pressure. For this role the action of the crural diaphragm is coordinated with motor events for the gastrointestinal system. For example, the activity of the crural diaphragm is inhibited during swallowing and vomiting. Such effects on the activity of the costal diaphragm are, however, weak or absent.

The phrenic motor neurons themselves are not strictly homogeneous and have been divided into early firing units, the activity of which begins at the very onset of inspiration, and late firing units, which commence their activity much later in inspiration. It is of interest that the early units are the ones that are responsible for postinspiratory inspiratory activity. The crural diaphragm may contain more of these early units since electrical activity of that part of the diaphragm generally precedes activity in the costal portion.

As respiration increases, the frequency of firing of both the early and late units increases; in addition, more and larger motor units are recruited according to a "size principle." Phrenic neurons supplying larger motor units (which contain more fibers) are recruited later than are phrenic neurons that innervate smaller units (Fig. 9-7). Also, as stimulation of ventilation continues and as ventilation increases, the intercostal muscles are brought into play, the upper intercostals becoming active first and the lower intercostals afterward. The expiratory muscles begin to contract at higher levels of ventilation, and the duration of the postinspiratory inspiratory activity decreases. At high levels of ventilation, the "accessory muscles of respiration," like the sternocleidomastoid, the hyoid muscle, and muscles attaching to the spine, are also brought into play.

The diaphragm, like other skeletal muscles, has less ability to produce force as the velocity of contraction and the degree of shortening increase. The ability of the respiratory system to increase tidal volume is preserved by at least three compensatory mechanisms: (1) motor output to the diaphragm grows greater; (2) as airflow accelerates, reflex mechanisms (possibly from rapidly adapting receptors) further increase motor output; and (3) the recruitment of more muscles helps curtail the load on the diaphragm.

When skeletal muscles are made to contract forcibly over long periods of time, the muscles fatigue; i.e., they are able to generate less pressure. The diaphragm can also become fatigued when it is obliged to develop large pressure changes because of either sustained respiratory stimulation or chronic mechanical impairment of the lungs. Fatigue seems to lead to decreasing tidal volume and, ultimately, to CO_2 retention. Although diaphragmatic fatigue can result from interference with cellular contractile mechanisms, fatigue that is central in origin is also believed to occur. It has been suggested that afferent signals from the diaphragm, originating from unspecified receptors that project to the brain via the phrenic nerves, signal impending fatigue and enable motor output to diminish,

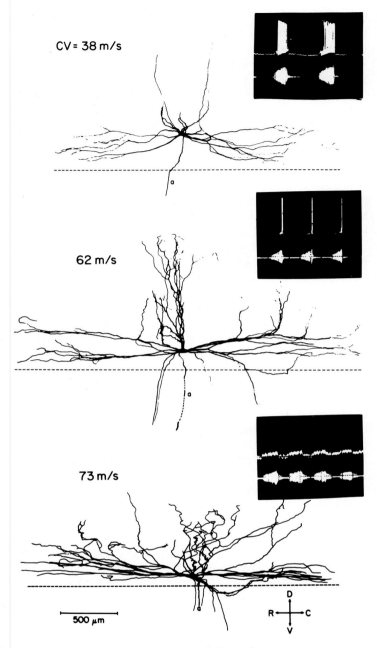

FIGURE 9-7 Examples of structure of these phrenic motor neurons which fire at different times during inspiration. The cellular structures were obtained by reconstruction of structure of neurons labeled by intracellular horseradish peroxidase. The inserts show the intracellular recording from the neuron above and recording of mass phrenic nerve activity *(below)*. CV is the conduction velocity of the axon. The cell in the top panel is the smallest with lowest conduction velocity. It fires throughout inspiration. The cell in the bottom panel is the largest with highest conduction velocity. Its membrane potential is modulated with respiration, but it does not fire during eupnea. The cell in the middle is between these extremes and fires only at the end of the inspiratory burst. These data conform to the size principle. The broken line indicates the ventral margin of the gray matter and a indicates the axon. D = dorsal; V = ventral; R = rostral; C = caudal. *(From Cameron, Averill, Berger: Neurogenesis of Central Respiratory Rhythm, London, MTP Press Ltd., 1985.)*

thereby preventing irreversible damage to the muscle itself.

Upper Airway Muscles

The muscles of the upper airways also serve an important respiratory function. Contraction of the posterior cricoarytenoid muscle during inspiration to open the laryngeal aperture, an important site of airway resistance, increases the efficiency of energy used by the thoracic muscles during breathing. Changes in the laryngeal aperture are thus synchronized with breathing. When respiratory drive is increased, as during exercise or acute hypercapnia, the magnitude of this modulation increases.

In addition to the larynx, activity of the cranial nerves that innervate muscles of the upper airways, such as the alae nasi (the nasal dilator), the genioglossus (the protrussor muscle of the tongue), and the muscles inserting on the hyoid, varies with the breathing cycle. During inspiration these muscles contract, thereby dilating the upper airway passages and overcoming the negative intralumenal pressures produced by shortening of the thoracic muscles. This inspiratory activity may be of particular importance during sleep when the alignment of gravitational forces favors occlusion of the upper airways. Inspiratory activity of the upper airways also begins slightly before the onset of activity of the chest wall muscles. This difference in onset timing within a breath may also help to prevent airway obstruction.

The upper airway muscles seem to be far more susceptible to the inspiratory inhibiting action of pulmonary stretch receptor input than are the muscles of the chest wall. The reduction in stretch receptor stimulation that occurs during airway occlusion increases the inspiratory activity of the upper airway muscles far more than that of either the diaphragm or the intercostal muscles. This heightening of discharge helps to dilate the upper airways and to prevent obstruction during breathing.

INTEGRATED RESPONSES OF THE CONTROL SYSTEM

The afferent and efferent systems described above, coordinated by the central neural circuits, respond to a variety of challenges that face both normal individuals and, more particularly, patients with pulmonary disease.

Respiratory Adaptation to Altitude

Acute exposure to decreased barometric pressure produces an immediate increase in ventilation mediated through the peripheral chemoreceptors which is caused by the reduced partial pressure of oxygen. With continued exposure, ventilation in humans continues to increase for several days resulting in a gradual decrease in arterial P_{CO_2}. This process, called acclimatization, is poorly understood, as is the slow return of ventilation (deacclimatization) when the acclimatized individual returns to sea level pressures. It has been proposed in the past that these ventilatory transients are caused by changes in blood and cerebrospinal fluid bicarbonate concentrations, which return pH from the alkalotic levels produced by acute hypoxic hyperventilation toward more normal levels. But recent studies have failed to find a reasonable correspondence between ventilation and pH. Rather than accounting for the gradual rises and falls in breathing, H^+ concentrations in the blood and cerebrospinal fluid seem to *follow* the ventilatory changes. Recent animal studies show that these slow processes probably depend on the presence of intact peripheral chemoreceptors.

At least three different possibilities may account for ventilatory changes during acclimatization and deacclimatization: (1) slow pH changes may occur at central chemoreceptors that have as yet been undetected by experimental measurements; these changes could take place either in brain interstitial fluid or even within the receptors themselves; (2) over time, hypoxia may produce specific chemical mediators, such as glutamate, which stimulate breathing and appear and disappear slowly; and (3) the gradual breathing changes may not be peculiar to hypoxia; any mechanism that causes active hyperventilation may produce long-lasting stimulation regardless of the initiating mechanism. For example, long-lasting stimulation of ventilation occurs in animals after repeated electrical stimulation of the central ends of carotid sinus nerves.

Hypoxic Depression of Ventilation

If the peripheral chemoreceptors are removed, respiration tends to be depressed by hypoxia. Several different factors seem to contribute to this ventilatory depression: (1) hypoxia, which may be quite severe in some regions of the brain, may interfere with the metabolic function of some neurons in the brain; (2) by dilating cerebral vessels and increasing cerebral blood flow, brain H^+ concentration is decreased, thereby reducing stimulation of the central chemoreceptors; and (3) hypoxia seems to release mediators, such as γ-amino-butyric acid (GABA) and adenosine, that depress breathing. These may overpower the effect of excitatory neurotransmitters that may also be released by hypoxia.

Since the brain is heterogeneous both in its cellular organization and with respect to blood flow rates, the effects of prolonged hypoxia in animals without peripheral chemoreceptors are complex depending on the susceptibility of different brain regions to low oxygen. For example, it has been shown that the cortex generally has an inhibitory action on ventilation, whereas the hypothalamic regions have an overall excitatory effect.

It has been suggested that central depression by hypoxia can occur even when peripheral chemoreceptors are intact. If this proves to be true, it would raise the possibility that depression may contribute to hypoventilation in some patients with hypoxic lung disease.

Adaptation to Metabolic Acid-Base Disturbances

Chronic changes in blood bicarbonate levels which reduce arterial pH increase ventilation and cause hypocapnia. For example, hyperventilation is a feature of diabetic ketoacidosis and renal failure. Conversely, diseases which elevate blood bicarbonate levels and raise arterial pH, such as aldosteronism or hypercalcemia, frequently cause hypoventilation and hypercapnia. As a rule, the arterial P_{CO_2} increases by about 1 mmHg for each milliequivalent per liter change in bicarbonate. The changes in P_{CO_2} help restore pH toward normal.

Although a decrease in P_{CO_2} invariably accompanies metabolic acidosis, P_{CO_2} does not always rise in response to metabolic alkalosis. For example, it is widely held that alkalosis produced by K depletion does not elicit hypoventilation, presumably as a result of the intracellular acidosis that seems to accompany K loss. Also, in hypoxic, hypercapnic patients, complete compensation for metabolic alkalosis is limited by the hypoxia that accompanies hypoventilation.

Like the ventilatory response to altitude, the compensatory responses to chronic metabolic disturbance occur over hours and days rather than immediately. Because of this time course, it seems likely that central, as well as peripheral, chemoreceptors contribute to the ventilatory compensation.

Acidosis either leaves ventilatory responses to inhaled CO_2 unaltered or causes them to increase; ventilatory responses tend to decrease with metabolic alkalosis. In chronic metabolic acidosis, the ventilatory response to exercise remains nearly isocapnic. Because of lower resting levels of arterial P_{CO_2} in the chronically acidotic individual than in the normal individual, ventilation increases more for the same rise in $\dot{V}_{CO_2}$ in the chronically acidotic individual.

Although both peripheral and central chemoreceptors participate in the ventilatory compensations that occur in response to acid-base derangements, the relative role of each is still unclear. In part this uncertainty is caused by the still unresolved question of the location of the central chemoreceptors. It is known that pH changes quite rapidly on the ventral medullary surface when blood is made acid. But the relationship between surface pH and ventilation is quite different in acid-base disturbances than during CO_2 inhalation. As acid is infused into the blood, ventral surface pH falls and ventilation increases (as it does during CO_2 inhalation); but, as the infusion continues, ventilation seems to plateau even though the ventral surface becomes much more acidotic (a similar phenomenon does not occur with CO_2 inhalation). Other complicating factors in acid-base disturbances arise from changes in cerebral blood flow, active and passive movements of bicarbonate between the blood and the brain interstitial fluid, and the buffering capacity of brain. These changes during acid-base disturbances tend to minimize pH changes within the brain as compared to those in blood.

Response to Mechanical Loading

The control system for respiration can also readjust so as to maintain homeostasis in the face of mechanical impediments to breathing. Both resistive loads, mimicking obstructive lung disease, and elastic loads, mimicking interstitial disease, have been used experimentally. But, whether externally applied loads correspond to the mechanical impairments of pulmonary disease is questionable. In particular, the pattern of afferent activity from the lungs and the resulting pattern of ventilation are different in patients with pulmonary disease from those of normal subjects breathing with mechanical loads in place.

Several factors act to maintain ventilation during mechanical loading. First are the factors intrinsic to the respiratory muscles. The force that the muscle develops for a fixed electrical input depends on the length of the muscle (the force-length relationship). As the muscle shortens, less force is developed. The force also depends on the velocity of shortening (force-velocity relationship), with less force being developed as the velocity of shortening increases. During loading, both the magnitude and the velocity of shortening tend to decrease. These intrinsic properties of the respiratory muscles help to compensate for the effects of mechanical loads.

In addition to intrinsic muscular effects, there are reflex neural mechanisms. At the spinal level, reduction in shortening of the inspiratory muscles increases the signal from muscle spindles that, in turn, augments contraction of these muscles. Because the number of spindles in the diaphragm is small, this phenomenon is most marked for the intercostal muscles. During loading, afferent information from pulmonary mechanoreceptors also changes. Since tidal volume is depressed, inspiratory duration tends to be prolonged because of the inspiratory off-switch mechanism (Hering-Breuer inspiratory terminating reflex). This reflex has the characteristics of a negative feedback mechanism since impeding inspiration causes its duration to be prolonged, thereby maintaining tidal volume. However, in humans this mechanism is of little importance in compensating for mechanical loads.

In conscious humans there is another important load mechanism to compensate for an increase in mechanical load. Both resistive and elastic loads elicit an increase in neuromuscular output as reflected in the occlusion pressure. This increase in occlusion pressure occurs in the face of a constant chemical drive; the magnitude of the increase in occlusion pressure is related to the severity of the mechanical load. The intensity of this load-compensating mechanism is variable: in patients with chronic obstructive disease of the airways, no increase in occlusion pressure occurs during flow-resistive loading. When it is present, the mechanism seems to depend on higher, possibly cortical, influences; this aspect of load compensation is abolished by anesthesia.

The final compensation for mechanical loads is provided by the chemoreceptors, peripheral and central. When loads are so severe that hypoventilation ensues, the resulting changes in arterial blood-gas tensions (increase in P_{CO_2}, reduction in P_{O_2}) act to sustain ventilation. The magnitude of this component of the response depends on the gain of the peripheral and central chemoreflexes.

Response to Bronchoconstriction

Major differences exist between the neural responses to bronchoconstriction and the neural responses to loading. In particular, inspiratory muscle activity increases during bronchoconstriction even in anesthetized animals, even though this component of the compensation to external loads is, as noted above, abolished by anesthesia. These differences can be attributed to the different pattern of afferent activity in the two states: during bronchoconstriction, many of the pulmonary receptor systems described above undergo stimulation: both stretch receptors and, more particularly, rapidly adapting receptors can be stimulated by the mechanical changes in the airway walls during bronchoconstriction. In addition, both rapidly adapting receptors and nonmyelinated afferents in the bronchi can be stimulated chemically by a number of autocoids, e.g., histamine and bradykinin, that are released in the lungs in asthma.

During asthma, or induced bronchoconstriction, changes in these afferent systems in the lung cause reflex changes in respiratory timing. The durations of all phases of the respiratory cycle are reduced so that respiratory frequency increases. This shortening of duration is unequally distributed across the different phases of respiration: expiratory duration shortens more than inspiratory duration; within expiration, larger changes take place in the second phase of the expiratory part of the cycle. Indeed, during bronchoconstriction, the duration of the postinspiratory phase of the cycle changes least. Since the work of breathing during airway obstruction is minimized by using slow, deep breaths (lower airflows and, hence, resistive work), these changes in timing during bronchoconstriction are opposite from those produced by afferent stimulation. Thus, part of the reason for the increased work of respiration in asthma is that the respiratory pattern adopted is nonoptimal.

The changes in afferent activity in the lungs described above also change reflexly the magnitude of the inspiratory neural output. For example, vagal blockade abolishes the increase in neuromuscular output. Thus, the increase in inspiratory neural output that occurs during bronchoconstriction is vagally mediated.

Changes in the activity of the inspiratory muscles are not confined to the inspiratory phase of the cycle. During expiration tonic activity of the inspiratory muscles increases. This neural phenomenon leads to an increase in functional residual capacity. Thus, the increase in functional residual capacity in asthma is due not just to mechanical changes within the airways that lead to air trapping, but also to altered neural control of the respiratory muscles. This alteration in the activity of the inspiratory muscles during expiration also seems to be vagally mediated, probably by way of stimulation of the rapidly adapting receptors.

Muscles other than the inspiratory muscles undergo changes in activity. For example, inhalation of histamine narrows the larynx, an effect that is most marked in expiration, thereby contributing reflexly to the increased airway resistance in asthma. This component of the response can be ameliorated by continuous positive airway pressure. It seems unlikely that this reflex narrowing of the larynx serves a useful function in asthma. Instead, as with the changes in respiratory timing, the defense reflexes that are evoked during asthma can superimpose substantial mechanical effects on those produced by the bronchoconstriction, per se.

VOLUNTARY CONTROL OF BREATHING AND DYSPNEA

Normally breathing does not reach the level of awareness except during exposure to severe hypoxia or intense exercise. But patients with lung disease may complain of shortness of breath or dyspnea even at rest. Since dyspnea itself can become an incapacitating symptom, considerable attention has been given to its etiology.

Earlier experiments used breath holding as a model for the investigation of dyspnea. These studies showed that hypercapnia and hypoxia decreased breath-holding times, supporting the idea that increased levels of input promoted dyspnea; conversely, increased lung volume seemed to increase breath-holding time. Since combined blockade of the phrenic nerves and of the vagi seemed to lengthen the time apnea could be voluntarily maintained, these studies led to the idea that contraction of muscles was an important contributor to the sense of dyspnea.

More recent studies have used standard psychophysical tests to evaluate respiratory sensations and then to relate these sensations to dyspnea. These tests have had several goals: (1) to determine the ability of subjects to detect loads applied to the mouth, (2) to scale the respiratory sensations produced either by breathing with a load in place or by changing respiratory pressures and tidal volumes, and (3) to scale the respiratory sensations evoked by increasing ventilation using a variety of maneuvers. Although these approaches have not settled the mechanisms responsible for dyspnea, they have provided fresh worthwhile insights.

With respect to load detection, the ability to sense added loads depends on background mechanical conditions. Resistive loads, for example, are more difficult to detect by patients with increased airway resistance.

The scaling of easily detectable loads depends mainly on the pressure developed while breathing with the load in place, and far less on inspiratory duration and the frequency of breathing. The relationship between respiratory pressure and sensory intensity follows a power law. The sensations produced by pressure changes (produced, for example, by breathing with different efforts against an occluded valve), like the sensations produced by changes in tidal volume, grow disproportionately greater as the magnitude of the stimulus, i.e., change in pressure or tidal volume, increases.

Respiratory effort as well as pressure or tidal volume changes can be scaled, suggesting that subjects can sense intent, i.e., the motor command to the respiratory muscles directly, even if there is little afferent input from the respiratory muscles. Finally, dyspnea seems to be related to the effort (motor command), expressed as a percent of its maximum. Thus, dyspnea increases as the pressures used for tidal breathing increase or the maximal inspiratory pressure decreases, e.g., as by paresis, disease, or respiratory muscle fatigue.

While these observations seem to equate dyspnea with the intensity of the sense of effort and, thus, only indirectly to input, this is probably not the complete story. New observations indicate that dyspnea is less when ventilations are voluntarily increased than when they are produced by chemical stimulation. This suggests that the cognitive factors, and probably affective factors which determine the relative pleasantness of a sensation, as well as sensory intensity, affect the level of dyspnea.

Another important, unresolved issue is whether the sense of dyspnea can induce patients to alter their breathing patterns or to deliberately hypoventilate in order to avoid discomfort. This seems possible since breathing can be controlled voluntarily as well as automatically. Separate pathways to respiratory motoneurons have been described by which the cortex can influence respiratory activity. Moreover, it has been demonstrated that the automatic and behavioral pathways for breathing can be independently altered by disease. Ondine's curse (primary alveolar hypoventilation) is probably mainly caused by an abnormality in the automatic control of breathing. But, on the other hand, patients have been described who have respiratory apraxia; that is, they breathe normally at rest and respond appropriately during exercise but are unable to voluntarily change their breathing. Thus, through voluntary action, patients who are short of breath may be able to alter the way they breathe.

It is also likely that the response of some respiratory sensors (e.g., the carotid body) can be modified by pathways which project from the brain to the receptor.

Some studies suggest that by the judicious use of analgesics the sense of dyspnea can be relieved without causing dangerous hypoventilation. But, much better success in alleviating dyspnea in lung disease patients has been obtained through rehabilitative programs which strengthen or augment the endurance of the respiratory muscles.

BIBLIOGRAPHY

Cherniack NS, Widdicombe JG (eds): *Handbook of Physiology, sect 3: The Respiratory System*, vol III, *Control of Breathing*. Bethesda, MD, American Physiological Society, 1986.
  Definitive recent text on all aspects of control of ventilation.

Cohen MI: Neurogenesis of respiratory rhythm in the mammal. Physiol Rev 59:1105–1173, 1979.
  Extensive review on all aspects of central neurons that are involved in generation of efferent signals to the respiratory muscles. Although somewhat out of date, remains the most complete recent review.

Coleridge JCG, Coleridge HM: Afferent vagal C fibre innervation of the lungs and airways and its functional significance. Rev Physiol Biochem Pharmacol 99:2–110, 1984.
  Extensive authoritative review of properties of nonmyelinated afferents in bronchi and pulmonary interstitium, their reflex effects and role in lung disease.

Euler C von: On the central pattern generator for the basic breathing rhythmicity. J Appl Physiol 55:1647–1659, 1983.
  Brief review on current state of knowledge on central neural mechanisms that generate the respiratory rhythm.

Euler C von, Lagercrantz H: *Neurobiology of the Control of Breathing*. New York, Raven, 1987.
  A collection of papers devoted to new experimental facts and concepts on the neural mechanisms involved in the control of breathing in the fetal, neonatal, and adult stages.

Hornbien TF (ed.): *Regulation of Breathing*. Parts I and II, vol 17, Lung Biology in Health and Disease. New York, Dekker, 1981.
  Contains 22 review chapters by invited experts on various aspects—both basic and applied—on regulation of breathing.

Long S, Duffin J: The neuronal determinants of respiratory rhythm. Prog Neurobiol 27:101–182, 1986.
  Review of known groups of respiratory neurons in the medulla and upper cervical spinal cord. Includes excellent figures. Also touches on upper cervical inspiratory neurons.

Mitchell RA, Berger AJ: Neural regulation of respiration. Am Rev Respir Dis 111:206–229, 1975.
  Good review of the voluntary and involuntary control of respiratory muscles.

Pack AI, Millman RP: Changes in control of ventilation, awake and asleep, in the elderly. J Am Geriatr Soc 34:533–544, 1986.
  A review of the ventilatory control system in the elderly with particular references to the changes that occur during sleep.

Paintal AS: Vagal sensory receptors and their reflex effects. Physiol Rev 53:159–227, 1973.
  Comprehensive review of afferents from the lung emphasizing their effects on breathing.

Richter DW: Generation and maintenance of the respiratory rhythm. J Exp Biol 100:93–107, 1982.
  Clearly written, relatively brief review on neural mechanisms producing respiratory rhythm. Particularly deals with concepts of the respiratory cycle being three phases, as suggested by this author.

Chapter 10

Control of Respiration during Sleep

Allan I. Pack / Lewis R. Kline
Joan C. Hendricks / Adrian R. Morrison

During sleep, in which about one-third of life is spent, relatively major changes occur in the performance of the ventilatory control system. These changes have adverse consequences on two major groups of patients. First, in patients with compromised gas exchange, due to either obstructive or interstitial disease, the hypoventilation that occurs with sleep may lead to arterial hypoxemia. Second, in the sleep apnea syndrome, abnormal respiratory patterns develop during sleep. This chapter reviews the alterations in ventilatory control that occur with sleep and relates them on the one hand to what is known about sleep-related neurophysiological adjustments, and on the other hand to their pathophysiological import. The material in this chapter complements that on control of ventilation (Chapter 9), abnormal breathing patterns (Chapter 25), and sleep apnea syndromes (Chapter 83).

SLEEP STATES AND THEIR CONTROL

Sleep is characterized by recurrent spontaneous episodes of motor quiescence accompanied by increased thresholds to various stimuli. The fact that these episodes are rapidly reversible distinguishes sleep from other states such as coma or torpor. The fact that sleep deprivation is associated with an increased propensity for sleep may be taken as evidence of the "restorative" nature of these episodes—even though the exact functions of sleep are still debatable. An alternative view is that sleeping may be an efficient way to conserve energy.

The classification of mammalian sleep is based on recordings of the electroencephalogram (EEG), the electrooculogram (EOG) for monitoring eye movements, and the electromyographic (EMG) activity of the neck or submental muscles. On the basis of these measurements, combined with behavioral observations, mammalian sleep can be broadly divided into two distinct and very different types—*non-rapid eye movement (NREM) sleep* and *rapid eye movement (REM) sleep*. NREM sleep is also called *synchronized (EEG) sleep, stages 1 to 4 sleep* in human adults, and *quiet sleep* in infants. REM sleep is also called *paradoxical sleep* or *active sleep* in infants. Whereas NREM sleep is characterized by the absence of movement, REM sleep can be recognized by brief phasic motor events, such as eye movements or twitches of the facial muscles and extremities.

The EEG has been used to establish scoring criteria for the stages of sleep based on distinct electrical patterns (Fig. 10-1). Drowsiness exhibits predominately α-wave activity on the EEG. Human NREM sleep is subdivided into the four stages mentioned above: *stage 1:* with the onset of sleep, low-frequency (3 to 7 Hz) theta waves begin to appear; *stage 2:* the presence of sleep spindles and K complexes define stage 2 sleep activity; *stages 3 to 4:* finally, the electrical activity shifts to a characteristic pattern of waves that are very low in frequency ($\frac{1}{2}$ to 2 Hz) and high in amplitude (delta waves). In contrast, during REM sleep, the EEG has a high frequency and low voltage similar to those in wakefulness (Fig. 10-1). In addition, during REM sleep, muscle tone is characteristically absent and rapid eye movements, recorded on the electrooculogram, are present.

The use of standardized scoring conventions has allowed norms to be established for sleep parameters in the various age groups. In general, normal human adults exhibit a 90-min NREM-REM cycle (Fig. 10-2). Most adults, upon falling asleep, will cycle through stages 1 to 3, entering stage 4 about 35 min after the onset of sleep. In the later hours of sleep, episodes of REM can occur more frequently; the later episodes tend to have a longer duration (Fig. 10-2). Total sleep time is less in elderly persons than in younger adults; in particular, the amount of stages 3 to 4 sleep is reduced. The sleep pattern of the human infant,

Awake—low voltage—random, fast

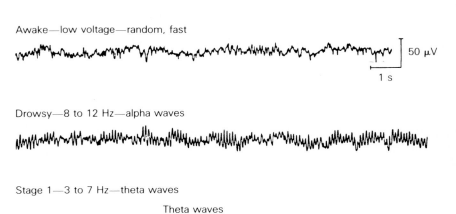

50 μV

1 s

Drowsy—8 to 12 Hz—alpha waves

Stage 1—3 to 7 Hz—theta waves

Theta waves

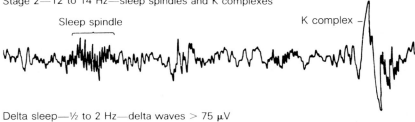

Stage 2—12 to 14 Hz—sleep spindles and K complexes

Sleep spindle

K complex —

Delta sleep—½ to 2 Hz—delta waves > 75 μV

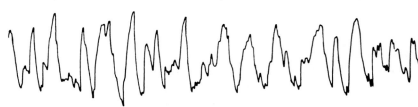

REM sleep—low voltage—random, fast with sawtooth waves

Sawtooth waves   Sawtooth waves

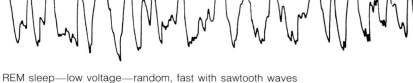

FIGURE 10-1 The electroencephalogram in different states of sleep. *(From Hauri, 1977.)*

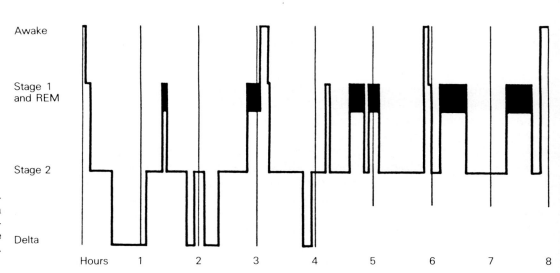

Awake

Stage 1
and REM

Stage 2

Delta

Hours   1   2   3   4   5   6   7   8

FIGURE 10-2 Typical cycling between different stages of sleep in a young adult. As the night progresses, the episodes of rapid eye movement sleep become longer. *(From Hauri, 1977.)*

consisting of 50-min cycles, is also quite different from that of the adult; the REM cyclicity becomes increasingly regular during the first 6 months of life.

Although these ultradian rhythms have been well described, the neurologic basis for these oscillations is not well understood. Animal studies have demonstrated that neural discharge patterns are very different in NREM and REM and that virtually all neuronal groups show clear changes in discharge patterns during transitions in state. Moreover, although there are long periods of motor quiescence during sleep, neuronal discharge is maintained.

Both the lower brain stem and forebrain are capable, independently, of spontaneously organizing alternating periods of NREM sleep and wakefulness. Electrical or chemical stimulation of regions extending from the medulla to neocortex facilitate sleep. However, to date, no neural region has been shown to be essential for NREM sleep, lending credence to the concept that NREM sleep may be regulated by a network of systems involving the forebrain, midbrain, and lower brain stem.

In contrast, studies have shown that REM state control is localized to the midbrain and brain stem, caudal to the inferior colliculi (Fig. 10-3). Decerebrate cats transected through the midbrain are capable of manifesting the elements of REM, including muscle atonia and rapid eye movements. Various neurotransmitters, particularly acetylcholine and serotonin, have been implicated in both the production of atonia and phasic electrical activity that are so characteristic of REM sleep, but a definitive picture has not yet emerged. Thus, both NREM and REM sleep are complex phenomena that require large areas of the brain for full expression. Indeed, there is probably no single neural focus or "pacemaker" that accounts for the cyclic manifestations of either state.

VENTILATORY CONTROL IN NREM SLEEP

Alterations in Set Point and Chemosensitivity

During NREM sleep minute ventilation falls. The fall in ventilation is due both to a slowing of respiratory rate, that was first recognized over a century ago, and to a decrease in tidal volume. The decrease in respiratory rate is related to prolongation of both inspiratory and expiratory durations. Accompanying this fall in minute ventilation is a decrease in alveolar ventilation that causes end-tidal P_{CO_2} to increase by about 2 to 4 mmHg; as expected, the end-tidal P_{O_2} in NREM sleep decreases concomitantly and by the same order of magnitude. These changes in ventilation and in the pattern that occurs during NREM sleep occur even after removal of the major afferent systems for respiration. Therefore, they must be due to changes in the central nervous system. During sleep, the

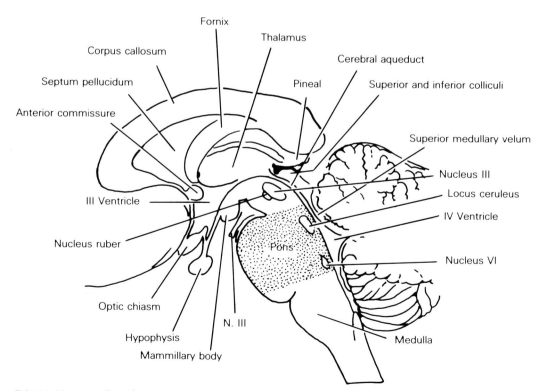

FIGURE 10-3 Outline drawing of a midsagittal section of the brain identifying the regions of the pons (within the stippled area) essential for the manifestations of REM sleep. *[From Carpenter, Sutin (eds): Human Neuroanatomy. Baltimore, Williams & Wilkins, 1983.]*

tonic input to this system, i.e., the "wakefulness stimulus," decreases. The magnitude of the stimulus varies continuously from one state to another. Although the origin of this excitatory input is unknown, it probably originates from the reticular formation. This change in ventilation and P_{CO_2} during NREM sleep has been called an *alteration in set point* and is illustrated schematically in Fig. 10-4.

In NREM sleep, alterations in chemosensitivity also occur. Most observers have found a decrease in the ventilatory response to carbon dioxide during NREM sleep (Fig. 10-4). However, disparity exists between reports in the older and more recent literature about the effect of NREM sleep on the ventilatory response to hypoxia: originally, it was reported that, unlike the CO_2 response, the hypoxic response was preserved in NREM sleep; this would be of considerable pathophysiological significance since increasing the relative gain of the fast-responding peripheral chemoreflex, as compared to that for the more damped central chemoreflex, would tend to make the overall control system more unstable and, therefore, more likely to exhibit periodic breathing. In contrast, recent studies in humans have shown that the hypoxic response is also reduced in NREM sleep. Also, there seems to be a gender difference since the hypoxic response falls more during sleep in men than women.

Alteration in the Apnea Threshold

An even more dramatic change in the chemical system during sleep is the alteration in the apnea threshold. This is defined as the arterial P_{CO_2} at which rhythmic ventilation ceases, i.e., apnea occurs. In the subjects shown in Fig. 10-5, the arterial P_{CO_2} during wakefulness could be lowered to 20 mmHg, without upsetting the rhythmic ventilation. In contrast, during NREM sleep, a reduction in P_{CO_2} of only a few mmHg stopped breathing. Indeed, in some individuals, simply lowering the arterial P_{CO_2} to a level close to that of wakefulness led to apnea. [It is to be recalled that during NREM sleep the arterial P_{CO_2} normally increases by 2 to 4 mmHg above awake levels (see preceding section)]. The duration of the resultant apnea depended on the magnitude of the fall in P_{CO_2} (Fig. 10-5). These data suggest that in NREM sleep the excitatory inputs from the chemoreceptors play a more important role

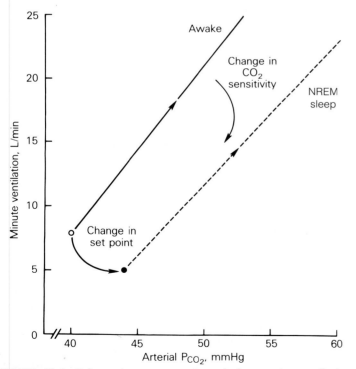

FIGURE 10-4 Schematic representation of changes in ventilation and chemosensitivity during NREM sleep. In NREM sleep, ventilation falls and the arterial P_{CO_2} increases, i.e., the set point of the system is altered. The ventilatory response to carbon dioxide also decreases.

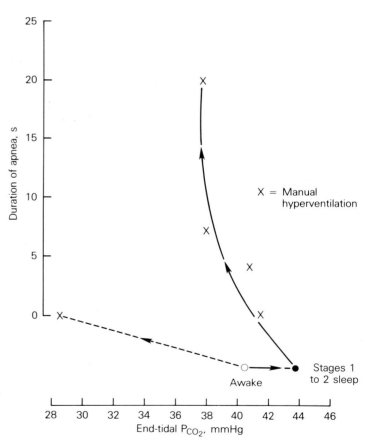

FIGURE 10-5 Change in apnea threshold during sleep. The end-tidal P_{CO_2} while awake and during NREM sleep is shown in the lower right-hand corner. While awake, apnea did not occur even though the end-tidal P_{CO_2} fell below 28 (x) to 20 mmHg (not shown). In contrast, during forced hyperventilation during NREM sleep (manual hyperventilation) an apnea occurred at levels of end-tidal P_{CO_2} that were close to those that obtained while awake. The duration of apnea was correlated with the reduction in end-tidal P_{CO_2}. *(Data modified from Skatrud and Dempsey, 1983.)*

in maintaining rhythmic ventilation than during wakefulness. This presumably is a consequence of the reduction in the wakefulness stimulus. But, whatever the mechanism, the alteration in the apnea threshold has major pathophysiological import: during sleep the operating point of the system is barely above the level of ventilation maintained by the excitatory inputs, i.e., the additional stimulus afforded by the P_{CO_2} is just enough to sustain ventilation during sleep. Consequently, even minor hypocapnia can induce apnea. For example, at high altitude, apneas frequently occur during sleep: because of the ambient hypoxia, the arterial hypoxemia, and the consequent stimulation by the peripheral chemoreceptors, increases in ventilation and, hence, hypocapnia occur; should the apnea threshold be reached, apnea ensues. That hypocapnia is important in producing apnea is evidenced by the fact that, if P_{CO_2} is maintained constant, apneas do not occur during sleep under hypoxic conditions.

Changes in Stability of Ventilation

During NREM sleep, alterations also occur in the apparent stability of the ventilatory control system. In particular, many subjects experience periodic breathing, i.e., there are regular cycles of waxing and waning of ventilation in the lighter stages of NREM sleep (stages 1 to 2). An example of this in an elderly man is shown in Fig. 10-6. During wakefulness (top panel), apart from intermittent sighs, ventilation was regular. In stages 1 to 2 sleep (middle panel), a regular periodicity of ventilation occurred with a cycle time of the order of 60 s. (Cycle time is the interval between successive zeniths or nadirs of ventilation.) In stages 3 to 4 sleep, ventilation once again became regular (bottom panel).

Periodicities such as these are found in many subjects. They are more common in elderly subjects and may be responsible for the high prevalence of sleep apnea in this age group. With increasing age, ventilation may also become more periodic during wakefulness. Indeed, elderly subjects who develop apnea during sleep have more marked periodicities of ventilation while awake than do age-matched controls.

The mechanisms producing these ventilatory oscillations during light sleep are unknown. Their long cycle time (60 s) argues against their being mediated by the peripheral chemoreceptors; e.g., the cycle time of the oscillations in ventilation that occur at high altitude are much shorter (20 s). Whether the oscillations in ventilation are secondary either to an unstable operation of the chemical feedback system (Chapter 25) or to swings in the wakefulness stimulus that accompany oscillations in state is unknown. Nonetheless, such periodicities do have pathophysiological import. At the nadir of the periodicity, ventilation may stop (central apnea). Furthermore, since periodicities affect not only the neural output to the dia-

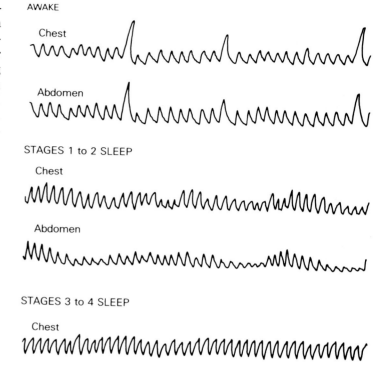

AWAKE

Chest

Abdomen

STAGES 1 to 2 SLEEP

Chest

Abdomen

STAGES 3 to 4 SLEEP

Chest

Abdomen

20 s

FIGURE 10-6 Pattern of breathing in a 77-year-old man while awake and during sleep. During stages 1 to 2 sleep, breathing becomes periodic and reverts to a regular pattern in stages 3 to 4 sleep. Chest and abdominal motions were recorded using a respiratory inductance plethysmograph.

phragm but also to the upper airway muscles, the nadir may be associated with obstructive apnea caused by a greater reduction in the activity of the upper airway muscles than of the diaphragm.

Alterations in Respiratory Mechanics and the Response to Mechanical Loads

Part of the reason for the reduction in ventilation in NREM sleep is the increase in airway resistance that occurs in this state. This increase has been localized to the upper airway. Resistance to airflow between the retroepiglottic space and the mouth increases more than twofold during NREM sleep; in contrast, the flow-resistive properties of the lungs remain unchanged. The increased upper airway resistance has been attributed to narrowing of the pharyngeal airway secondary to hypotonia of the pharyngeal muscles. Reduction in the activity of upper airway muscles, such as the genioglossus, occurs during NREM sleep. Thus, the marked increase in upper airway resistance that occurs in the obstructive sleep apnea syndrome—which even persists during the nonapneic breaths—is likely to be an exaggeration of a phenomenon that occurs during normal sleep. Likewise, in individuals who snore during sleep the increase in airway resistance during sleep (approximately tenfold) exceeds the two- to fourfold increase found in normal individuals.

Therefore, during sleep the respiratory system is subjected to a mechanical load caused by the increase in upper airway resistance. It is, therefore, germane to consider whether normal compensation for such loads is affected by sleep. As discussed in Chapter 9, normal mechanisms for compensating for mechanical loads depend on several factors: (1) the intrinsic characteristics of the respiratory muscles, (2) segmental reflexes involving muscle spindles and intercostal muscles, (3) a neural mechanism that involves higher centers and leads to an increase in inspiratory efferent outflow, and (4) responses to changes in arterial P_{CO_2} and P_{O_2} that are produced by the load. The mechanisms intrinsic to muscles are not affected by sleep, whereas those secondary to changes in blood-gas composition are altered. However, particularly important is whether the increase in the activity of the inspiratory muscles produced by resistive loads, an effect that is abolished by anesthesia, is affected by sleep. Unfortunately, the data concerning this question are conflicting, probably due, in large measure, to methodological differences among studies, e.g., prior sleep deprivation or not, the magnitude of the imposed loads, and the duration of their application. Moreover, all such studies have to contend with the problem that external loads are being added to the natural load that accompanies sleep. The establishment of equivalent conditions for comparing wakefulness and sleep is extremely difficult.

VENTILATORY CONTROL IN REM SLEEP

Alterations in ventilatory control in REM sleep are even more pronounced than during NREM sleep. This is primarily because of the unique physiology of this extraordinary state.

Ventilatory Pattern and Chemosensitivity

The hallmark of REM sleep is irregularities in the breathing pattern. These irregularities are most marked during periods of dense phasic activities, such as eye movements. They are centrally mediated since irregularities persist despite varied manipulations of the different afferents—hypoxia, hyperoxia, metabolic alkalosis, carotid body resection, vagotomy. Although it has been proposed that these irregularities are the consequence of behaviors related to dreams occurring in this state, there is no evidence for this postulate. Indeed, certain evidence suggests that this is not so. Irregularities of respiration are found in

chronically decerebrate animals, implying that mechanisms intrinsic to the brain stem are capable of generating them. Moreover, in REM without atonia, a state that can be produced in experimental animals by lesions in the dorsal pontine tegmentum, no relationship exists between the respiratory changes and the behavioral changes arising from the lack of atonia. Thus, the irregularities of respiration in REM may simply be the result of phasic, relatively unorganized discharges from reticular neurons in the brain stem.

Variability affects not only the respiratory timing intervals but also the amplitude of the ventilatory movements. The effect of the ventilatory movements results from the combined effects of REM on the neural activity of the diaphragm, intercostal and upper airway muscles. These variations are also associated temporally with the occurrence of phasic events: as shown in Fig. 10-7, the reduction in ventilatory movements is more marked for the rib cage than for the abdomen; indeed, during REM, there may be paradoxical movements of the rib cage and abdomen. Such paradoxical movements can result from an intermittent loss of the activity of the rib cage musculature so that the rib cage is sucked inward by the activity of the diaphragm. Alternatively, upper airway obstruction could explain the paradoxical motion, the obstruction being secondary to loss of tone in the muscles of the upper airways.

Since these changes are related to the occurrence of phasic events in REM, the magnitude of ventilation in this state varies with the density of phasic events. Thus, it is not surprising that different investigators have reported increases, no change, or decreases in minute ventilation during REM. Because of the marked heterogeneity of the state, both within an episode and between episodes of REM, it seems impossible to describe average changes that are typical of the state.

This problem also confronts investigation of changes in chemosensitivity during REM. Once again, different studies have reported different results. However, as a rule, a reduction occurs in the ventilatory response to both

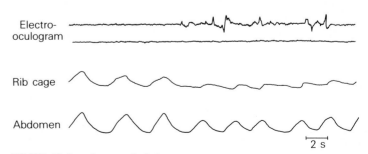

FIGURE 10-7   Chest and abdominal motion as measured by a respiratory inductance plethysmograph in a normal young female subject during REM sleep. Accompanying eye movements (measured by the electrooculogram), the amplitude of excursions of the chest and abdomen decrease. At times, the movements become paradoxical, i.e., the rib cage moves inward (downward on the traces), while the abdomen moves outward.

hypercapnia and hypoxia. But, the responses are not abolished, so that this aspect of homeostasis is still operative during REM, whereas certain other homeostatic functions, e.g., thermoregulation, are lost.

The changes in ventilation during REM may be associated with phasic changes in other autonomic functions, e.g., heart rate, blood pressure. Particularly important with respect to respiration is the increase in cerebral blood flow that occurs in association with phasic activity during REM. This increase reduces P_{CO_2} at the central chemoreceptor. Thus, changes in ventilation in REM may be caused not only by primary neural events but also by changes in the afferent stimuli for respiration.

Motor Control of Skeletal Muscle during REM Sleep

However, alterations in the neural outflow to the respiratory muscles are the important determinants of what happens to ventilation in REM. The mechanisms that produce these alterations are still incompletely understood; more is known about changes during REM in the control of the limb and postural muscles than of the respiratory muscles. This is surprising since study of respiratory muscle control is simpler: respiratory muscles continue to receive a regular descending excitatory potential and to maintain their activity during REM. In contrast, other muscles become atonic, and their motoneurons fire only phasically to produce twitches during bursts of rapid eye movement.

Atonia of nonrespiratory muscles during REM was first discovered in decerebrate cats, then later affirmed in intact cats and humans. The source in the brain stem of the postsynaptic inhibition of cranial and spinal motor neurons has long been ascribed to cells in Magoun's medullary inhibitory area. However, recent work has demonstrated that interactions with the pons must also occur. Even though the pathways involved are not yet well delineated, they are likely to be multiple because, in otherwise intact cats, electrolytic lesions of varying sizes placed within the pontine tegmentum are capable of eliminating the atonia of REM and of releasing a variety of behaviors.

Studies in the 1960s using extracellular recording methods, almost entirely in cats, demonstrated that the excitability of motor neurons is greatly depressed throughout each REM episode; barrages of excitatory influences from the brain stem could overcome the depression, leading to phasic excitations (twitches) of the skeletal muscles. Postsynaptic inhibition was postulated to be the mechanism responsible for the depressed motor neuronal activity. More recently, intracellular studies on minimally restrained cats have confirmed that active postsynaptic inhibition ("hyperpolarization"), rather than mere disfacilitation from the brain stem, is the cause of the motor neuronal inactivation and of consequent muscle atonia.

Although brain-stem discharges are periodically capable of overwhelming the inhibition of skeletal muscle

(best exemplified by the bursts of rapid eye movements), moderate peripheral electrical or natural stimulation is not; both monosynaptic and polysynaptic segmental reflexes are greatly suppressed or absent. The bias toward inhibition is so great that even stimuli that might be considered to be naturally arousing, e.g., electrical stimulation of the reticular formation or sounds, enhance motor neuronal inhibition during the transition from NREM to REM, and then throughout the latter.

This remarkable inhibitory bias of the motor system during REM was first noted by Chase and colleagues studying reflexes in jaw muscles. They demonstrated that stimulation of the reticular formation elicits hyperpolarizing potentials (i.e., tending toward inhibition) in masseteric and lumbar motor neurons during REM, whereas the same stimuli during wakefulness and NREM evoke depolarization; parallel effects on lumbar motor neurons have been obtained by Glenn using auditory stimulation. Chase has suggested that during REM a coupling mechanism between pontomesencephalic reticular activating areas and bulbar inhibiting areas is activated; during wakefulness and NREM sleep, a "gate" is closed to block this mechanism. Thus, a sound during NREM sleep does not trigger inhibition as during REM sleep but, instead, a jerk (startle).

Control of Respiratory Muscles during REM Sleep

These findings, with respect to the control of jaw and limb skeletal muscles, are relevant to changes in the activity of the respiratory muscles during REM. Although it was originally proposed that the diaphragm was spared the atonia of REM sleep, recent evidence suggests that this is not so. Moreover, the dorsal pontine tegmentum seems to be involved not only in the generation of atonia throughout REM but also in the brief flurries of intense inhibition, called fractionations, that can arrest the electrical activity of the diaphragm.

Between the extremes of very brief fractionations and long-lasting inhibition (atonia) is a type of inhibition with a time course of seconds, i.e., intermittent inhibition. In tonic REM, i.e., when there is muscle atonia but no phasic events, the inspiratory firing of the diaphragm EMG is highly reproducible from breath to breath and similar to that in NREM sleep. In contrast, during phasic events, the diaphragm EMG is intermittently inhibited throughout the breath. Occasionally, in contrast with tonic REM, breaths are seen in which the EMG is intermittently excited; the frequency of these altered EMG contours (Fig. 10-8) increases as phasic events increase. During hypoxia or hypercapnia the incidence decreases.

All told, at least three neuronal influences seem to affect the activity of the diaphragm during REM (Fig. 10-9): (1) a descending excitatory input from the respiratory pattern generator, (2) an intermittent inhibitory influence, and (3) an intermittent excitatory influence; these inputs

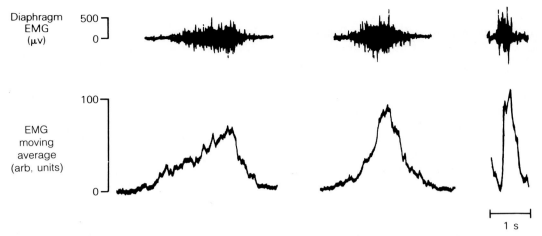

FIGURE 10-8 Different contours of the diaphragm EMG recorded during REM sleep in cats. *Left:* The slope of the EMG is suppressed indicating inhibition. During this inhibition, inspiratory duration is prolonged. *Middle:* The EMG is normal (as shown) throughout most of REM sleep and during all of NREM sleep. *Right:* The upper trace shows a burst of EMG activity in the costal diaphragm. The slope of the moving average EMG is increased, indicating excitation. These alterations in the EMG during REM sleep generally occur in conjunction with other motor events, e.g., eye movements. *(From Kline et al., J Appl Physiol 61:1293–1300, 1986.)*

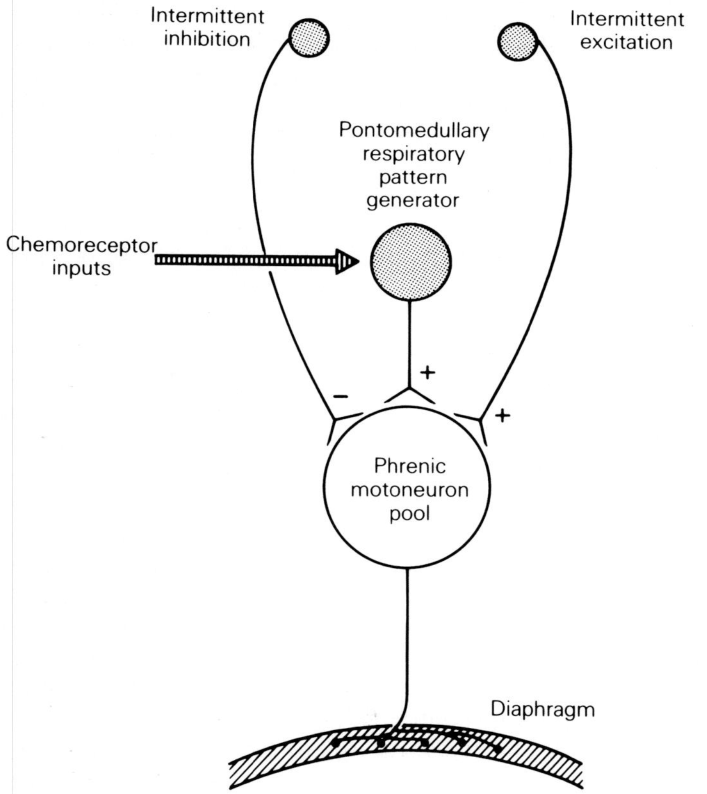

may summate at the phrenic motoneuron pool. Should hypoxia or hypercapnia develop, the relative effects of the inhibitory and excitatory inputs would be lessened since these chemical stimuli enhance the drive produced by the respiratory pattern generator.

This intermittent inhibition also occurs in upper airway muscles and presumably in intercostal muscles. It seems likely, although not yet investigated, that intermittent inhibition in humans may last longer than in the animal species that have been studied. Certainly, periods of hypoventilation in humans that occur in association with eye movements are sometimes relatively long-lasting (Fig. 10-7).

Hypoxemia during REM Sleep in Patients with Pulmonary Disease

The intermittent inhibition of the respiratory muscles during REM can exaggerate alveolar hypoventilation and lead to arterial hypoxemia in patients with pulmonary disease. In such patients, the arterial hypoxemia is usually more profound than in normal subjects. Even when the patients are not hypoxemic while awake, they may be at a point closer to the inflection of the oxygen saturation curve than are normal subjects (Fig. 10-10). As a result, hypoventilation more readily results in desaturation. This effect of hypoventilation is compounded by increased inefficiency of gas exchange during REM. The atonia of the chest wall muscles can lead to a reduction in functional residual capacity. This results in increased ventilation-perfusion mismatching; increases in the alveolar-arterial difference for oxygen occur during REM sleep. Thus, pa-

FIGURE 10-9 Model of possible controlling influences on phrenic motoneurons during REM sleep.

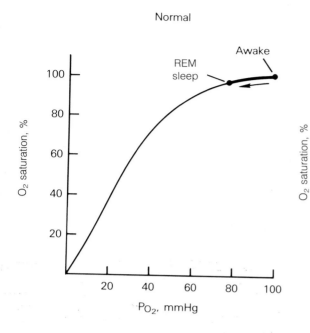

Normal

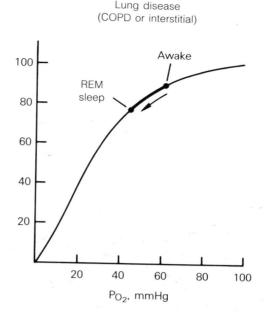

Lung disease
(COPD or interstitial)

FIGURE 10-10 Oxyhemoglobin saturation curves show arterial blood oxygenation both while awake and during sleep. *Left:* Normal individuals. *Right:* Patients with either obstructive or interstitial lung disease. Since the arterial oxygenation in patients is apt to lie close to the "knee" of the curve while they are awake, hypoventilation during sleep is more likely to result in appreciable arterial hypoxemia in the patients than in normal individuals.

tients with either interstitial or obstructive airways disease may develop during REM sleep episodes of arterial hypoxemia that can be corrected by administering oxygen; these may occur despite values for awake arterial P_{O_2} that are within the normal range.

UPPER AIRWAY MUSCLES AND SLEEP

Muscles Involved in Regulating Upper Airway Size

Since intermittent obstruction of the upper airways is an important pathophysiological mechanism in the sleep apnea syndrome, it is pertinent to consider the actions of the muscles that control the size of the upper airways. Airway size is regulated by a number of muscles acting in concert. First, the nasal alae dilate the nose. Like many of the upper airway muscles, the activity of these muscles increases during inspiration so that nasal resistance is kept in phase with the respiratory cycle. The activity of the nasal alae is increased by stimuli, such as hypercapnia, and is decreased during REM sleep.

Second, control of the size of the next level in the upper airway—the pharynx—is more complicated. There are muscles that dilate the pharynx and those that constrict it (Fig. 10-11). The genioglossus increases the size of the pharynx by protruding the tongue. It has both a discharge pattern during inspiration and tonic activity throughout the respiratory cycle. Because its location and bulk make recording of its electromyogram relatively simple, the neural control of the genioglossus muscle has been more extensively studied than has the neural control of any other upper airway muscle. Other muscles, i.e., the

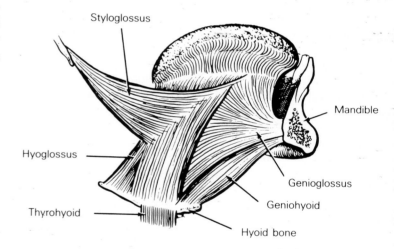

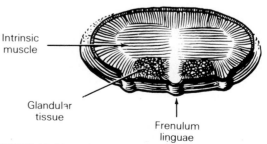

FIGURE 10-11 Schematic representation of the musculature of the tongue and its relationship to the mandible and hyoid bone. *Upper:* Lateral view. *Lower:* Cross section. [From Fletcher (ed), *Abnormalities of Respiration During Sleep,* Orlando, Grune & Stratton, 1986, p 69.]

geniohyoid, tensor palatini, stylopharyngeus, styloglossus, and medial pterygoid, which protrude the mandible, also dilate the pharynx. All these muscles manifest a discharge pattern during inspiration.

The actions of these pharyngeal dilators can be opposed by the actions of pharyngeal constrictors. These (superior, middle, inferior) form a thin muscle covering over the posterior and posterolateral walls of the pharynx. The discharge pattern of these muscles with respect to the respiratory cycle is less certain than for the dilator muscles. However, it does seem likely that these muscles are particularly activated in circumstances that dictate a need to brake markedly the expiratory airflow.

There is no doubt that dimensions at the third part of the upper airways, i.e., the larynx, are modulated in phase with respiration. This has been demonstrated in humans by elegant pictures taken through a fiberoptic bronchoscope. Modulation of the laryngeal aperture is produced by an abductor muscle (posterior cricoarytenoid) and by adductor muscles, such as the thyroarytenoid. The abductor muscle fires during inspiration and continues, with a decrementing pattern, during the early part of expiration. The adductor muscles fire shortly after the end of inspiratory airflow.

These timing patterns for the laryngeal muscles, together with that described above for the other upper airway muscles, cause the upper airways to dilate during the inspiratory phase of the respiratory cycle. As the stimulus to respiration increases, the activity of the dilating muscles increases, and the upper airways enlarge during inspiration. During expiration, the airways narrow; this has been most extensively documented for the larynx. This narrowing, combined with the postinspiratory activity of the diaphragm (Chapter 9), imposes a brake on expiration. The function of this braking of expiratory airflow is not certain, but it may promote gas exchange by prolonging the period during which the interface between resident and airway gas is in the gas-exchanging regions of the lungs.

Controlling Influences on Upper Airway Muscles

The muscles that dilate the upper airways have an inspiratory pattern of discharge. The onset of activity precedes, albeit briefly, the onset of activation of the diaphragm. The time course of their activity also differs from that of the diaphragm: whereas the diaphragm has an augmenting pattern of discharge throughout inspiration, the activity of the upper airway muscles reaches a peak relatively early in inspiration, remaining fairly constant for the remainder of inspiration. This difference in time course is in large part related to the different effects of input from the pulmonary stretch receptors on the activity of the two types of muscle: whereas for the diaphragm these stretch receptors produce an inhibition of firing for only a brief period just before the end of inspiration (graded inhibition), inhibition of the upper airway muscles by this mechanism occurs much earlier in inspiration.

Both the diaphragm and upper airway muscles increase their activity during hypoxia and hypercapnia. However, once again, quantitative differences in response exist between the two types of muscle: for example, in anesthetized dogs, the relationship between increments in hypoglossal activity and P_{CO_2} is curvilinear, whereas that for the diaphragm is linear. Also, a higher threshold obtains for increases in upper airway muscle activity than for the diaphragm; the activity increases with P_{CO_2} and, at high levels of P_{CO_2}, the activity of the upper airway muscles shows larger increases with hypercapnia than does that of the diaphragm. These findings are of considerable pathophysiological significance since small degrees of hypocapnia cause a relative decrease in airway muscle activity, thereby promoting episodes of obstruction.

However, caution must be exercised in extrapolating these observations on anesthetized animals to unanesthetized humans. Anesthesia affects the activity of the upper airway muscles more than that of the diaphragm. Differences in the sensitivity of the two groups of muscles to other chemicals are also known. For example, the same doses of alcohol markedly suppress the activity of the upper airway muscles, while leaving the activity of the diaphragm and the minute ventilation relatively unaffected. This disparity explains the clinical observations of the facilitatory effect of alcohol on snoring and the worsening of obstructive sleep apnea after alcohol ingestion. Certain excitatory chemicals, such as nicotine, protriptyline, and strychnine, also have more marked effects on upper airway muscle activity than on the activity of the diaphragm. Some differences may be consequent to the effects of the agents, such as alcohol and anesthetics, on excitatory inputs from the reticular formation; these inputs differ in importance with respect to the activity of the pre-motor neurons that control the diaphragm and upper airways. In keeping with this concept, arousal produces more marked changes in the activity of upper airway muscles than in the activity of the diaphragm. Again, this disparity is important, this time with respect to the mechanisms that terminate obstructive apnea since the large increase in activity of the muscles that dilate the pharynx upon arousal, e.g., the genioglossus, reopens the airway.

Not surprisingly, in addition to these influences that are centrally mediated, local reflexes are in place to maintain patency of the upper airways. For example, the application of negative pressure to the upper airways increases the activity of the genioglossus EMG and the hypoglossal nerve. More negative pressure elicits greater increments in neural activity. Sectioning of either the superior laryngeal or the trigeminal nerve reduces the magnitude of this response to negative airway pressure, indicating that the afferent pathways for this reflex are complex. In contrast, sectioning of the glossopharyngeal nerve produces the opposite effect; i.e., the increase in hypoglossal nerve activity that occurs during application of negative pressure to the airways is augmented.

These reflex changes in upper airway muscles are often accompanied by changes in other neural outputs. For example, a decrease in the activity of the diaphragm and in respiratory rate has sometimes been found to accompany the increase in activity of the upper airway muscles during application of negative pressures to the upper airways. This reflex reduction in the activity of the respiratory pump also tends to ensure patency of the upper airways. But, to date these reflexes have been studied only in anesthetized animals. Whether these reflexes are blunted during sleep, particularly in subjects with obstructive sleep apnea, is still unknown.

Sleep-Related Changes in Upper Airway Muscle Activity

During sleep there is a reduction in both the tonic and phasic activity of the upper airway muscles. The reductions occur both during NREM sleep and, to a larger degree, during REM sleep, and affect all levels of the upper airways. Activity during sleep decreases in the nasolabial muscles, the genioglossus, and the laryngeal adductor, i.e., the posterior cricoarytenoid. These alterations in muscle activity lead to the increase in airway resistance during sleep that was described earlier. Airway resistance increases during NREM sleep and, even more markedly, during REM sleep. In addition to these changes that persist throughout NREM and REM sleep, the phenomenon described earlier of intermittent inhibition, which occurs in association with phasic events during REM sleep, affects the upper airway muscles. As a result, intermittently throughout REM, there are periods when changes in airway resistance are even more marked.

CARDIOVASCULAR AND PULMONARY INTERACTIONS DURING SLEEP

The alterations described above for sleep affect not only the ventilatory control system but also the cardiovascular system. There are both mechanisms shared by the two systems and interactions between the two systems. Changes in ventilatory control that cause hypoxemia can also cause secondary changes in the function of the cardiovascular system. Likewise, primary cardiovascular events, e.g., changes in blood pressure, may secondarily effect ventilatory control. This section describes the normal changes that occur in the cardiovascular system during sleep and then the alterations that are more marked in patients with the sleep apnea syndrome.

Systemic arterial blood pressure decreases during the early hours of sleep but approaches waking levels later on; during stages 1 to 4 of NREM sleep, the mean blood pressure falls from the awake levels by approximately 20 percent; during REM sleep it sometimes exceeds the awake blood pressure (Fig. 10-12). During REM sleep, wide irregular fluctuations occur in the arterial blood pressure, often associated with phasic events. These circulatory changes are often synchronous with respiratory changes, suggesting a common origin (Fig. 10-13).

The heart rate also shows characteristic alterations during the stages of sleep. In NREM sleep and the tonic component of REM sleep (no phasic events), the heart rate

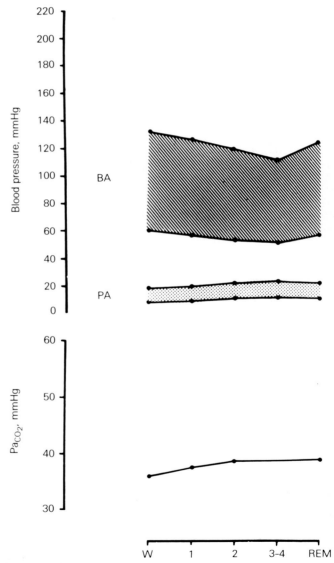

FIGURE 10-12 Normal hemodynamics in the consecutive changes of sleep. BA = systemic arterial pressure; PA = pulmonary artery pressure; W = awake. [*From Lugaresi and Coccagna, in Fishman AP (ed), Pulmonary Diseases and Disorders, New York, McGraw-Hill, 1979.*]

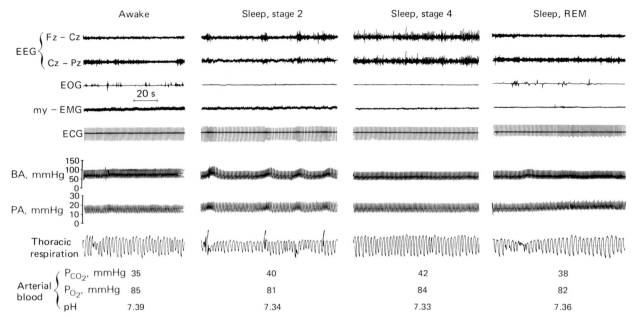

	Awake	Sleep, stage 2	Sleep, stage 4	Sleep, REM

EEG { Fz – Cz / Cz – Pz

EOG

20 s

my – EMG

ECG

BA, mmHg   150 / 100 / 50 / 0

PA, mmHg   30 / 20 / 10 / 0

Thoracic respiration

Arterial blood {
	Awake	Sleep, stage 2	Sleep, stage 4	Sleep, REM
P_{CO_2}, mmHg	35	40	42	38
P_{O_2}, mmHg	85	81	84	82
pH	7.39	7.34	7.33	7.36

FIGURE 10-13 Normal wakefulness and sleep. Polygraphic record in a 40-year-old woman. Respiration becomes periodic in light sleep (stage 2); regular in deep, slow sleep (stage 4); and irregular in REM sleep. Arterial P_{CO_2} increases from 35 mmHg during wakefulness to 42 mmHg during deep, slow sleep. During sleep a slight increase in pulmonary artery pressure (PA) occurs, while systemic arterial pressure (BA) decreases slightly. The first two channels show the EEG. The subsequent channels are electrooculogram (EOG), surface EMG of a chin muscle (my-EMG), electrocardiogram (ECG), systemic (BA) and pulmonary artery (PA) pressures, thoracic respiration, and arterial blood levels. [From Lugaresi and Coccagna, in Fishman AP (ed), Pulmonary Diseases and Disorders, New York, McGraw-Hill, 1979.]

generally decreases. However, during phasic REM sleep wide swings occur, i.e., on the order of 10 to 25 beats per minute. Unfortunately, the effects of sleep in normal individuals on cardiac output, total peripheral resistance, or pulmonary artery pressure remain unknown.

Important adjustments in the autonomic nervous system, involving both sympathetic and parasympathetic outflow, occur during normal sleep. As noted, the heart rate decreases during both NREM and tonic REM sleep, due largely to increased vagal output. The fluctuations in heart rate with the phasic events of REM sleep are due to brief and opposite changes in vagal and sympathetic efferent outflow; in animals, these swings can be eliminated by complete sectioning of the vagi and stellate ganglia.

The impact of sleep on blood pressure, heart rate, and other circulatory parameters can be grave when there is underlying disease. During REM sleep, the outburst of sympathetic activity may predispose patients with coronary arterial disease to angina, accompanied by clinically significant depression of the ST segments on the electrocardiogram. An association exists between dysrhythmias and sleep; among the dysrhythmias that have been observed are sinus arrest, asystole of 3.5 to 17 s, sinoatrial block, premature atrial contractions, atrial fibrillation, recurrent ventricular couplets, multifocal ventricular contractions, ventricular tachycardia, and electrical alternans.

In patients with pulmonary disease, sleep-related changes in cardiovascular parameters are accentuated by the arterial hypoxemia that occurs during sleep. Mild arterial hypoxemia increases sympathetic activity, resulting in a rise in arterial blood pressure, cardiac output, cardiac contractility, and peripheral vascular resistance. Even though the direct effect of hypoxia causes peripheral vasodilatation, the increased sympathetic outflow maintains increased vascular tone and blood pressure. Heart rate responses to hypoxemia are highly variable, but bradycardia is most often seen. Pulmonary artery pressure and pulmonary vascular resistance can also both rise dramatically during episodic hypoxemia with sleep.

Hemodynamic changes during sleep are more profound in patients with the sleep apnea syndrome than in normals. In all stages of sleep, the blood pressure often increases 20 to 30 mmHg during the apneic episodes. Pulmonary artery pressures also increase cyclically during the apneic periods, fluctuating with the level of arterial hypoxemia (Fig. 10-14).

Altered blood gases during apneas cause concomitant increases in sympathetic and parasympathetic tone. An increase in vagal tone, e.g., as manifested by bradycardia, occurs during apnea; atropine completely abolishes the cyclic bradycardia. Occasionally, the increase in vagal tone during apnea "unmasks" a ventricular "irritable" focus. Indeed, in patients with sleep apnea, episodes of

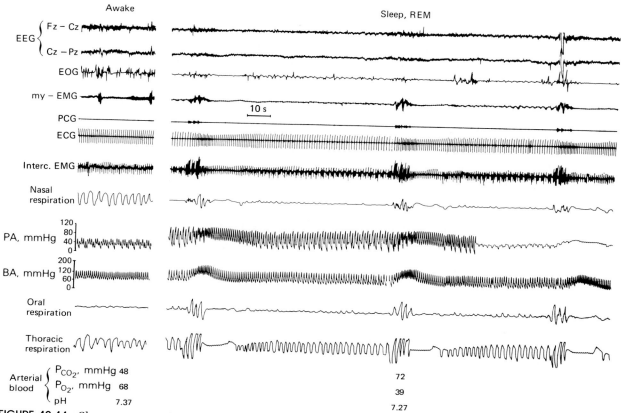

FIGURE 10-14 Sleep apnea syndrome. Polygraphic record in a 46-year-old man. Mixed apneas lasting more than 1 min occur in uninterrupted succession during REM sleep. Arterial P_{CO_2} increases from 48 mmHg during wakefulness to 72 mmHg during sleep. Pulmonary artery pressure increases from a maximum of 40 mmHg while awake to 100 mmHg during REM sleep. Maximum systemic arterial pressure rises from 120 mmHg while awake to almost 200 mmHg during REM sleep. [From Lugaresi and Coccagna, in Fishman AP (ed), *Pulmonary Diseases and Disorders*, New York, McGraw-Hill, 1979.]

sinus arrest or block can mimic the "sick sinus syndrome" and other dysrhythmias.

Mechanical effects of respiration on the circulation during apneas may explain some of the hemodynamic changes. Large negative swings in intrapleural pressure can reduce right atrial pressure and promote venous return to the right ventricle. Concomitantly, outflow from the left ventricle decreases, influencing directly and reflexly both the blood pressure and heart rate.

One important cardiovascular complication of the sleep apnea syndrome is systemic hypertension. As many as 90 percent of patients with the nocturnal sleep apnea syndrome have sustained hypertension during the day. Also, an epidemiologic correlation exists between heavy snoring and hypertension. Many individuals with sleep apnea undergo a return to normal blood pressures after relief of the upper airway obstruction. Additionally, both hypertension and sleep apnea increase in the obese, in the older age groups, and in male subjects.

Up to 50 percent of patients with essential hypertension have been reported to have unsuspected sleep apnea.

These studies have also shown some evidence of amelioration of high blood pressure when apneas are adequately treated. Patients with essential hypertension should have careful histories taken to investigate if sleep apnea is likely.

RESPIRATORY-RELATED AROUSAL MECHANISMS

This chapter emphasizes that ventilation and its control are affected by behavioral state. Thus, an important regulator of ventilation during sleep is a change in the state itself. This is particularly important in disease where termination of an apnea may require arousal to a lighter stage of sleep, or to wakefulness. Appreciation of the importance of arousal in relation to respiration during sleep is relatively recent; Phillipson and Sullivan have called arousal *the forgotten response to respiratory stimuli*.

Although arousal is a change in state, it can be induced by respiratory afferent stimuli. In dogs, for example, hypoxia produces arousal at oxygen saturations of 80 to 90 percent in NREM sleep, whereas in REM sleep lower levels are required. This arousal is mediated by the carotid body since, after carotid body denervation, intense levels of hypoxia are required to produce arousal in NREM sleep (P_{O_2} of the order of 30 mmHg). During REM sleep, arousal rarely occurs even at these levels. However, in humans, hypoxia does not appear to be as important an arousal stimulus: humans have failed to arouse at levels of arterial hypoxemia as low as 70 percent oxygen saturation, i.e., about 40 mmHg. The level at which arousal would occur cannot be tested further for ethical reasons.

In humans, hypercapnia is a more potent arousal stimulus. Even mild degrees of hypercapnia produce arousal; for example, inspired concentrations of 4 to 6 percent CO_2 cause arousal from sleep; in NREM sleep, arousal occurred at an alveolar P_{CO_2} of 55 to 60 mmHg. As with hypoxia in dogs, higher levels, i.e., by 5 to 6 mmHg, are required to produce arousal during REM sleep.

Chemoreceptor inputs are not the only respiratory-related afferents that produce arousal. Stimulation of either the larynx or the tracheobronchial tree can also do so. Again, there is a difference between the arousal thresholds in NREM and REM sleep. For example, 1.0 ml of water instilled into a dog's trachea consistently produces arousal during NREM sleep, whereas up to 10 ml may fail to elicit arousal in the same animal during REM sleep. This response presumably reflects the effects of the afferent input from either "irritant" or nonmyelinated receptors; it is abolished by bilateral vagal blockade.

Arousal thresholds are not constant for a single individual. Repeated application of an arousing stimulus elicits adaptation to its effect and an increase in arousal threshold. As yet, this aspect has received little attention in investigations of respiratory-related arousals. Arousal mechanisms are also affected by sleep deprivation or fragmentation, both of which increase the stimulus threshold for arousal. This is particularly important for individuals with sleep apnea.

Although many of the overall response characteristics of these arousal mechanisms are understood, their neurophysiological basis is not. It is assumed that there are relays between the various respiratory afferent systems and the brain-stem reticular formation that mediate the arousal. Certain areas, such as the amygdala, appear to be involved: both afferent and efferent connections exist between the amygdala and the brain-stem respiratory complex. However, current knowledge of the neural basis for respiratory arousal is rudimentary. This is surprising when considering the importance of arousal. For example, in the sudden infant death syndrome, it is failure of such arousal mechanisms that presumably proves fatal.

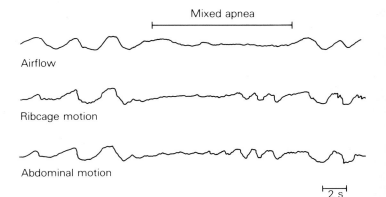

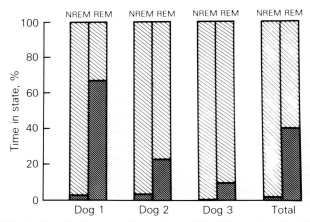

FIGURE 10-16   Results from studies in English bulldogs. *Top:* Simultaneous records from one dog of airflow (thermistor) and of chest and abdominal motions (respiratory inductance plethysmograph). A mixed apnea appears toward the end of the tracings: at the start of the apnea, there are neither ventilatory movements nor airflow. *Bottom:* Results obtained in three dogs. For each animal, the time spent in NREM sleep and in REM sleep during which arterial oxygen saturation was less than 90 percent is shown in black. Most disturbances of breathing during sleep occur in the REM stage.

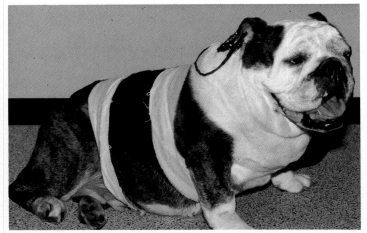

FIGURE 10-15   The English bulldog, a natural model of obstructive sleep apnea.

MECHANISMS PRODUCING APNEA

Apneas during sleep can be caused either by cessation of the action of the respiratory pump muscles (central apnea) or by obstruction of the upper airways. To induce upper airway obstruction, compromise by minimal anatomic changes, e.g., due to obesity, can suffice to occlude the airways during sleep when superimposed on sleep-related reduction in upper airway muscle function. As discussed earlier, this reduction in upper airway muscle function occurs in NREM sleep, particularly at the nadirs of periodic variations in respiratory efferent output. Since such periodicities occur in light sleep, apneas are more prominent in this stage of NREM sleep than in deeper slow-wave sleep. In REM sleep a different mechanism produces reduction in upper airway muscle activity: both reduction in activity throughout this state and "intermittent inhibition," sometimes intense, that occurs in association with rapid eye movements.

These arguments imply that although reduction of upper airway muscle activity is a common mechanism, the central cause of the reduced peripheral neural activity is different in NREM and in REM sleep. This hypothesis is supported by the observation that in individuals with mild obstructive apnea, the obstructive episodes are limited entirely to REM sleep.

Finally, the predominance of obstruction during REM sleep also occurs in an animal model of spontaneous obstructive sleep apnea—the English bulldog (Fig. 10-15). This animal, which snores during sleep, has episodes of apnea that are most common during REM sleep (mixed apnea, Fig. 10-16, *upper panel*). During these episodes oxygen desaturation occurs, and periods of arterial oxygen saturation less than 90 percent are longer during REM sleep than during NREM sleep (Fig. 10-16, *lower panel*). These episodes of desaturation lead to arousal, although the arousal threshold for stimuli in these animals is higher than in other dogs. As in humans with sleep apnea, these animals manifest daytime sleepiness, and the prevalence of hypertension is greater than normal. Animal models of this kind afford the prospect of answering many enigmas of the sleep apnea syndrome.

BIBLIOGRAPHY

Bulow K: Respiration and wakefulness in man. Acta Physiol Scand 59 Suppl 209:1–110, 1963.
Classic, complete study of changes in ventilation, its pattern, and its response to chemical stimuli in humans. In many ways, this study was before its time. Many of the ideas contained within have been rediscovered.

Chase MH: A model of central neural processes controlling motor behavior during active sleep and wakefulness, in Desiraju T (ed), *Mechanisms in Transmission of Signals for Conscious Behavior.* Amsterdam, Elsevier, 1976, pp 99–121.
Discusses activation of coupling mechanism between pontomesencephalic reticular activating areas and bulbar inhibiting areas.

Chase MH, Enomoto S, Hiraba K, Katoh M, Nakamura Y, Sahara Y, Taira M: Role of medullary reticular neurons in the inhibition of trigeminal motoneurons during active sleep. Exp Neurol 84:364–373, 1984.
Authors identified cells involved in generation of atonia of masseter muscles during active sleep. Study suggests that medullary units are the inhibitory neurons responsible for postsynaptic inhibition of trigeminal motoneurons during active sleep.

Cherniack NS: Respiratory dysrhythmias during sleep. N Engl J Med 305:325–330, 1981.
Brief but insightful review on mechanisms that produce abnormal breathing patterns, in particular periodic breathing, during sleep.

Glenn LL, Dement WC: Membrane potential and input resistance in alpha motoneurons of hindlimb extensors during isolated and clustered episodes of phasic events in REM sleep. Brain Res 339:79–86, 1985.
Study of the function of motoneurons during phasic events of REM sleep in cats.

Hauri P: *The Sleep Disorders.* Kalamazoo, MI, Upjohn Company, 1982.
Introductory text on sleep states and disorders of sleep.

Hendricks JC, Kline LR, Kovalski RJ, O'Brien JA, Morrison AR, Pack AI: The English bulldog: A natural model of sleep-disordered breathing. J Appl Physiol 63:1344–1350, 1987.
During sleep, the English bulldog develops disordered respiration and episodes of O_2 desaturation that are worst during rapid-eye-movement sleep. They manifest both central and obstructive apnea.

Kryger MH (ed): Sleep disorders. Clin Chest Med 6:553–718, 1985.
  A few articles on basic physiology of respiration during sleep. Major emphasis is on disordered respiration during sleep.

Lavie P: Rediscovering the importance of nasal breathing in sleep, or shut your mouth and save your sleep. J Laryngol Otol 101:558–563, 1987.
  Nasal breathing plays a major role in the regulation of respiration in sleep.

Lugaresi E, Coccagna G: Sleep, snoring and sleep-apnea syndromes, in Fishman AP (ed), *Pulmonary Diseases and Disorders*. New York, McGraw-Hill, 1980, pp 445–451.
  One of the early accounts of the sleep apnea syndrome that took into account the simultaneous respiratory and circulatory changes that occur during the consecutive stages of sleep in normal individuals and in patients with sleep apnea syndrome.

McGinty DJ, Drucker-Colin R, Morrison A, Parmeggiani PL (eds): *Brain Mechanisms of Sleep*. New York, Raven, 1985.
  Comprehensive recent review of the neurophysiology of mechanisms controlling sleep.

Pack AI, Millman RP: Changes in control of ventilation, awake and asleep, in the elderly. J Am Geriatr Soc 34:533–544, 1986.
  A consideration of periodic breathing in the elderly during sleep in light of physiological mechanisms.

Phillipson EA, Bowes G: Sleep disorders, in Fishman AP (ed), *Update. Pulmonary Diseases and Disorders*. New York, McGraw-Hill, 1982, pp 256–273.
  A review of clinical disorders of breathing during sleep, relating wherever possible the basic knowledge to the clinical problems.

Phillipson EA, Bowes G: Control of breathing during sleep, in Cherniack NS, Widdicombe JG (eds), *Handbook of Physiology, sect 3: The Respiration System, Vol II: Control of Breathing*. Washington DC, American Physiological Society, 1985, pp 649–689.
  Authoritative review on changes in the respiratory control system during sleep.

Phillipson EA, Sullivan CE: Arousal: The forgotten response to respiratory stimuli. Am Rev Respir Dis 118:807–809, 1978.
  Good review of the important, but largely forgotten, arousal response to respiratory stimuli during sleep.

Remmers JE: Control of breathing during sleep, in Hornbien TF (ed), *Regulation of Breathing, Part II*. New York, Dekker, 1981, pp 1197–1249.
  Concise review on neurophysiology of sleep, breathing during sleep, and respiratory disorders during sleep.

Saunders NA, Sullivan CE (eds). *Sleep and Breathing*. New York, Dekker, 1984.
  A monograph that covers almost all topics related to respiration and its abnormalities during sleep.

Skatrud JB, Dempsey JA: Interaction of sleep state and chemical stimuli in sustaining rhythmic ventilation. J Appl Physiol 55:813–822, 1983.
  Provocative study that shows largest change with sleep in ventilatory parameters is in apnea threshold. (See text for further details.)

Smith PL, Bleecker ER: Ventilatory control during sleep in the elderly. Clin Geriatr Med 2:227–240, 1986.
  A review of the normal control of respiration during sleep with aging.

Weil JV, Cherniack NS, Dempsey JA, Edelman NH, Phillipson EA, Remmers JE, Kiley JP: NHLBI workshop summary. Respiratory disorders of sleep. Pathophysiology, clinical implications, and therapeutic approaches. Am Rev Respir Dis 136:755–761, 1987.
  A critical appraisal of the current understanding of the complex interplay between breathing and sleep.

Chapter *11*

Drugs and Mediators in Respiratory Control

Norman H. Edelman

DRUGS

A wide variety of commonly used drugs are capable of modifying respiratory control. Discussed here are the major respiratory depressants and those stimulants which have been thought to be of clinical value.

Although most information about effects of drugs on respiratory control has been developed from studies on animals or relatively healthy humans, e.g., surgical patients undergoing anesthesia, the most important application of this information is to patients with respiratory insufficiency; the differences between the responses of normal individuals and of patients may be substantial. It is well known, for example, that a dose of narcotic analgesic, which has little or no ventilatory effect on normal people, may cause significant further alveolar hypoventilation in the patient with preexisting alveolar hypoventilation. Similarly, respiratory stimulants, which may be effective and well tolerated by volunteer subjects or patients with relatively normal mechanical properties of the lungs and chest wall, may cause considerable dyspnea in the patient whose respiratory mechanics are so severely impaired that increased respiratory drive cannot be translated into increased alveolar ventilation.

Drug Effect on Input to the Respiratory Controller

METABOLIC RATE

Strictly speaking, metabolic rate cannot be considered to be a "source" of afferent input since the precise manner by which metabolism is linked to ventilation is unknown. However, the linkage is quite strong and not ordinarily disrupted. Consequently, any drug or disease state that modifies metabolism is likely to modify ventilation proportionately. An example is therapeutic doses of thyroid hormones. Aspirin in large doses also increases metabolic rate; this component of its effect on ventilation is distinguishable from the ventilatory stimulation caused by direct action on the respiratory neurons. A third example is the effect of modest doses of narcotic analgesics during exercise. Although large doses of these drugs given to the patient at rest have a potent direct depressant effect on brain-stem respiratory neuronal output, modest doses reduce the ventilatory response to exercise by reducing oxygen consumption at a given workload. Interestingly this effect is sufficient to reduce exercise dyspnea in patients with advanced obstructive airways disease.

PERIPHERAL CHEMORECEPTORS

In the nonhypoxic individual, the peripheral chemoreceptors contribute a relatively small fraction to the afferent input involved in sustaining normal ventilation; thus, they are unlikely to be the prime site of action of respiratory depressant drugs. On the other hand, drugs which specifically enhance carotid body output are potentially useful clinically as respiratory stimulants since they may avoid the deleterious effects of general and neural excitation. Thus, doxapram given in clinical doses and the newer drug, almitrine,—both of which act preferentially on the carotid bodies—are more clinically useful as respiratory stimulants than are the older general analeptics.

PULMONARY RECEPTORS

A variety of receptors in the lungs provide potential sites for drug action. In fact, some are defined by the action of chemical substances, e.g., stimulation of parenchymal nociceptors by phenyl diguanide or capsaicin. However, as a rule, these have not been proposed as the main sites of action of the common drugs that have important respiratory actions. A notable exception may be the proposed "sensitization" of lung stretch receptors by diethyl ether, which has been invoked to explain the tachypnea frequently associated with ether anesthesia.

BRAIN-STEM RESPIRATORY NEURONS

These are the sites of several important drug effects. Examples include the depressant effects of opiate drugs and, probably, the depressant effects of certain barbiturates and psychoactive drugs, such as benzodiazepines. The latter is inferred by the depressant action of the application of γ-aminobutyric acid (GABA) to the brain stem, since barbiturates and the benzodiazepines appear to act by binding to GABA receptors.

HIGHER CENTRAL NERVOUS CENTERS

Inferences about the respiratory effects of drugs that act rostrally to the brain stem tend to be rather vague; however, the effects may not be inconsequential. For example, the hyperventilation which is associated with the higher planes of inhalational anesthesia may reflect a selective depressant effect upon the cortex that results in abolition of the ordinarily inhibitory effect of cortical influences upon ventilation.

Drug Effects on Respiratory Output

The output of the respiratory neurons is translated into ventilatory motion by the respiratory muscles; drugs that directly affect muscle function modify respiratory output. Muscle relaxants are obvious examples, but the possibility that similar effects may occur after administering aminoglycoside antibiotics in large doses is apt to be overlooked.

Recently, attention has been drawn to the important role of the dilator muscles of the upper airway in maintaining normal ventilation of the supine patient during sleep. When these muscles fail to activate properly, apnea associated with upper airway occlusion may result. It has become apparent that the dilator muscles of the upper airway may be controlled somewhat differently from the major inspiratory muscles, especially with regard to drug effects. Thus, the major respiratory effect of moderate doses of alcohol is to reduce activation of upper airway muscles and predispose to obstructive apneas during sleep. It has been proposed that selective inhibition of the dilator muscles of the upper airway may be a common effect of many depressant drugs, thereby promoting an increase in the number of episodes of sleep apnea in the susceptible individual.

Multiple and Interacting Effects

Drug actions are frequently not singular, and their multiple actions may be dose-related. Cited above were the multiple actions of aspirin, opioids, and inhalational anesthetics. A useful generalization is that, in large doses, the depressant drugs reduce overall output of respiratory motor neurons, whereas lesser doses produce more selective effects, such as those on the cortex of the brain or on the upper airway. Interaction with the behavioral state of the individual is also an important consideration. Sleep reduces alveolar ventilation by removing the wakefulness stimulus to breathing and, thereby, renders the respiratory

controller more vulnerable to the action of depressant drugs. In addition, the effect of sleep may be selective in that it especially enhances the susceptibility of the dilator muscles of the upper airway to depressant drugs.

Finally, it is important to occasionally consider interacting effects on systems other than respiratory and neural. For example, vasodilator drugs may cause hyperpnea via hypotension that stimulates the baroreceptors and peripheral chemoreceptors. Or, especially in severely ill and hypoxemic patients, marked hypotension may act as a ventilatory depressant as a result of hypoperfusion of the brain and hypoxic depression of neural output.

Assessment of Drug Effects

VENTILATION

In the eupneic patient, minute ventilation is variable and difficult to assess. Thus it is a relatively insensitive measure of drug effects. No method of measurement is ideal. Mouthpieces make possible direct measurements, but they can be used only in alert, cooperative subjects; however, they introduce important artifacts (generally, an increase in tidal volume and a decrease in respiratory frequency) that can modify, or obscure, a drug effect. Indirect measurements of the displacement of the chest wall and abdomen are also possible. These accurately reflect respiratory pattern and may be used in different states of consciousness. They are, however, difficult to calibrate for quantitative measurements of tidal volume, especially when the subject changes positions spontaneously, as during sleep.

ARTERIAL BLOOD-GAS TENSIONS

These may be measured directly by arterial puncture or assessed noninvasively by indirect methods such as ear oximetry (for O_2 saturation) and application of electrodes to the skin surface. Although cumbersome to perform, estimation of arterial blood-gas tensions is an important component of the evaluation of the effect of drugs on ventilation. This is because it is necessary to distinguish between a direct effect on respiratory control and an indirect one through modulation of metabolic rate; blood-gas tensions change when the effect is direct but remain unaltered even though ventilation changes considerably in response to a change in metabolic rate, e.g., steady-state exercise.

MODIFICATION OF RESPONSES TO RESPIRATORY STIMULI

This approach has long been used to assess the effects of drugs on ventilatory control. It has several advantages. Stimuli amplify and stabilize ventilation, thereby rendering the test more sensitive than measurements of eupneic ventilation; comparisons can be made at comparable levels of blood-gas tensions, thereby eliminating the diminution of drug effect brought about by changes in P_{CO_2} as alveolar ventilation changes; and some insight is provided into the mechanism of the drug effect. The disadvantage is that the test is artificial; i.e., drug effects are assessed under conditions that differ from eupneic breathing without external stimuli.

The most frequently used stimulus has been hypercapnia; both steady-state and rebreathing methods have been used effectively. Drug effects are usually described as they modify two attributes of the response to inhalation of CO_2. The "gain" of the response is taken as the slope of the graphic line relating CO_2 tension to ventilation. The "threshold" of the response is that CO_2 tension below which P_{CO_2} ceases to act as a respiratory stimulant. It is rarely measured directly but may be reliably estimated by extrapolation of the ventilation-P_{CO_2} line to zero ventilation in the steady-state test. The rebreathing test provides a less reliable estimate of the CO_2 threshold. Much of the older literature considered effects on gain and threshold to be separate manifestations of drug effects that varied in predominance from drug to drug. However, it now appears that they may be related in a general way. As the dose of depressant drugs is increased, the first effect appears to be a shift of the threshold to higher P_{CO_2} values. As doses are increased, the threshold continues to increase as the gain decreases.

The ventilatory response to hypoxia is more difficult to determine and is more dangerous to test in certain settings. Therefore, it has been used much less often to assess drug effects. However, it is a valuable test since the influence of drugs on the response to hypoxia does not always parallel those on the response to CO_2. For example, the inhalational anesthetic, enflurane, has been shown to have a particularly great propensity for depressing the ventilatory response to hypoxia.

Recently the examination of drug effects on responses to neuromechanical stimuli has provided interesting insights into the mechanisms of their actions. For example, narcotic analgesics readily abolish the augmentation of respiratory muscle effort produced by flow-resistive loads; on the other hand, they enhance the manifestations of the classic Hering-Breuer reflex (lung-volume-dependent shortening of inspiratory time).

Inhalation Anesthetics

SITE OF ACTION

There is general agreement that the major site of action of inhalational anesthetics is within the central nervous system. No more specific site has been clearly identified for their respiratory effects, nor has the action of these agents on a cellular level been elucidated, although some relationship to their lipid solubility has long been noted. Be-

cause of a poor correlation between the anesthetic and respiratory effects, there is some reason to suspect different sites or mechanisms of action. For example, Hickey and Severinghaus have noted that at an anesthetic level of 1.0 MAC (minimum alveolar concentration, a standard measure of depth of anesthesia) cyclopropane reduces the slope of the ventilation-CO_2 response line minimally (to 90 percent of the awake slope), whereas isoflurane reduces the slope profoundly (to 30 percent of the slope while the patient is awake). An important generalization offered by these authors is that anesthetics with the greatest propensity for activation of the sympathetic nervous system manifest the least respiratory depression. Thus, the differential effects may be related to differences in a secondary neural effect, rather than to differences in a primary effect on respiratory neurons.

Several inhalational anesthetics have been studied for their effects on carotid body discharge; no significant modulation has been noted. On the other hand, virtually all inhalational anesthetics increase the manifestation of the Hering-Breuer reflex and most have been shown to increase the discharge of lung stretch receptors at a given lung volume. This effect has been proposed to be responsible for the tachypnea that is characteristic of inhalation anesthesia.

PHYSIOLOGICAL ACTION

All anesthetics decrease alveolar ventilation in a dose-dependent fashion with the exception of diethyl ether which, as the dose is increased, increases alveolar ventilation before depressing it. All anesthetics change ventilatory pattern by decreasing tidal volume and increasing frequency; with a few exceptions, this effect is dose-dependent as well.

All anesthetics reduce the ventilatory response to CO_2. The relative magnitude of this effect as described by Hickey and Severinghaus was, from least to greatest effects: cyclopropane, ether, fluroxene, methoxyflurane, halothane, and isoflurane.

The ventilatory response to hypoxia seems especially sensitive to depression by inhalational anesthetics. Although this characteristic is shared by all agents, a hierarchy of potency, as for the ventilatory response to CO_2, has not been worked out. However, halothane appears to be especially potent in this regard. In one study, clinically useful levels of halothane abolished the ventilatory response to hypoxia. Not only is the ventilatory response to hypoxia, per se, diminished, but also most inhalational anesthetics tend to obliterate the enhancement of the ventilatory response to CO_2; this enhancement is a characteristic of the awake response to hypoxia in humans.

One study has shown that the increased respiratory effort caused by flow-resistive loads is abolished by anesthesia. Although not further tested, this property is probably common to all anesthetic agents since compensation for flow-resistive loads requires intact function at relatively high levels of the neuroaxis.

CLINICAL IMPLICATIONS

With the advent of effective and universally used methods for endotracheal intubation and mechanical ventilation, the choice of inhalational anesthetics is not of major significance when contemplating surgery in a patient with impaired function of the lungs or thoracic cage. Should a choice based on respiratory effects be necessary, diethyl ether remains the least depressant agent. It is important to be aware that when spontaneous breathing is resumed, impairment of respiratory function greatly enhances the potential for anesthetic agents to cause alveolar hypoventilation even during light anesthesia. Thus, preoperative $FEV_{1.0}$ values below 1.5 L/min require considerable attention to the clinical state and to the quantitative criteria for "weaning" prior to discontinuation of mechanical ventilation and extubation.

Opiate Drugs

SITE OF ACTION

The last decade has witnessed remarkable achievements in the determination of the site and mode of action of opiate drugs as a result of the discovery of opiate receptors in neural tissue (three major types are now recognized) and a variety of variably specific endogenous ligands. Opioids or their receptors have now been demonstrated in several structures involved in respiratory control, including the medulla (with increased concentration in the nucleus tractus solitarius and nucleus ambiguus), the carotid bodies, and the vagi (especially the unmyelinated nerve endings which constitute the pulmonary parenchymal "J receptors"). Discrete application of opiates to the brain stem suggests that these agents are active at two sites: the chemosensitive area described by Mitchell, where they primarily reduce tidal volume, and certain pontine areas, where they seem to reduce respiratory frequency.

In some species, action at higher than pontine centers has an excitatory effect (probably through release from inhibitory influences) that is manifest in ventilation as well as in psychomotor activity. Thus, opiates given to unanesthetized felines and ovines cause respiratory stimulation.

PHYSIOLOGICAL ACTION

Despite multiple claims to the contrary, all opiate drugs in current clinical use appear to depress ventilation in general relation to their analgesic potency. In clinically effective doses, they reduce ventilation, primarily through a reduction of tidal volume; larger doses also decrease res-

piratory frequency. The ventilatory response to inhalation of CO_2 is reduced; this is manifested by both an increase in the P_{CO_2} threshold and a reduction in the gain of the ventilation-P_{CO_2} response. Much has been written about the selective effects of certain opiates on these two aspects of the CO_2 response, but differences have proven to be largely related to dose and potency.

Ventilatory responses to hypoxia are readily reduced by opiates, perhaps to a greater extent than the ventilatory response to CO_2. This is also true of the increased respiratory effort response to flow-resistive loads (load compensation). In contrast, the ventilatory response to exercise is largely unaffected by opiates; only a small reduction occurs, consistent with the reduction in metabolic rate.

In recent years, prolonged use of narcotic drugs has become a clinically important issue as a result of their abuse and of their increased use in patients with intractable pain due to incurable disease. Studies of the ventilatory effects of prolonged use of opiate drugs indicate that substantial, but not complete, tolerance develops. In addicts who were being rehabilitated with large daily doses of methadone, alveolar hypoventilation and reduction of ventilatory response to CO_2 were reversed within 5 months. After 8 months of therapy, abnormalities in the compensation for flow-resistive loads could no longer be demonstrated. However, the hypoxia chemoreflex appeared to acquire only partial tolerance since the daily dose of the drug continued to depress responsiveness to hypoxia, even after several years of drug intake.

CLINICAL IMPLICATIONS

The danger of administering opiate drugs to patients with alveolar hypoventilation and/or mechanical impairment of lung and thoracic cage function is well known and cannot be overemphasized. On the other hand, it is now becoming apparent that careful use of opiates in some patients with lung disease may be beneficial. For example, in a group of patients with chronic obstructive airways disease and severe dyspnea but without CO_2 retention, administration of dihydrocodeine reduced ventilation both at rest and during exercise, thereby decreasing dyspnea without producing significant CO_2 retention.

Although opioids are potent respiratory depressants, the availability of an easily given, rapidly acting, and fully effective antagonist agent (naloxone) renders these drugs potentially useful when brief analgesia is required in well-controlled settings. For example, the use of morphine followed by naloxone for electrical cardioversion is recommended for patients with respiratory insufficiency.

Finally, it must not be forgotten that opiates cross the placenta and that infants born of mothers who have been taking this class of drugs are at risk for immediate respiratory depression and, apparently, for development of the sudden infant death syndrome.

Other Respiratory Depressant Psychoactive Drugs

A wide variety of drugs are used for their depressant properties on psychomotor activity and affective state, especially their ability to induce sleep. The major classes considered here are the barbiturates, benzodiazepines, and agents used primarily for recreational purposes, such as alcohol and marijuana.

SITE OF ACTION

The mechanism of action of these agents has been best worked out for the benzodiazepines. They have been shown to interact with the receptors for GABA, an endogenously generated amino acid that has potent depressant effect on neuronal activity. Although respiratory related neurons have been shown to contain GABA receptors, the density of these receptors is far greater in cortical areas. This distribution may explain why cortically mediated effects can usually be obtained in the clinical setting without modification of respiratory activity.

The cellular basis of the actions of the other agents under consideration is less well understood. However, it appears likely that the effects of barbiturates, and possibly some effects of alcohol, are also mediated by the GABA receptor. On the other hand, the depressant effect of massive doses of alcohol may be modified by administration of the opioid antagonist naloxone, implying a role for endogenously generated opioids.

PHYSIOLOGICAL ACTION

In normal individuals, hypnotic doses of barbiturates appear to have little effect on ventilation or on the ventilatory response to CO_2. Larger doses reduce both; toxic doses or those used to provide surgical anesthesia reduce both profoundly. Reduction of ventilatory response to hypoxia appears to parallel the reduction of the ventilatory response to CO_2. Doses sufficient to produce loss of consciousness obliterate flow-resistive load compensation.

The great danger in extrapolating these findings to patients with compromised lung function is perhaps best illustrated by a report of Gold and co-workers. They administered 100 mg of pentobarbital orally to clinically stable patients with obstructive airways disease and hypercapnia. Although no significant effect on ventilation or ventilatory response to CO_2 was observed as much as 135 min later, five of the nine subjects subsequently experienced prolonged drowsiness with further alveolar hypoventilation, requiring hospitalization.

The prototypical benzodiazepine, diazepam, reduces ventilatory responses to CO_2 and hypoxia in clinically relevant doses (about 10 mg, given parenterally). In normal individuals this is without significant effect on ventilation or blood-gas tensions, although an increase in P_{CO_2} may be demonstrated in certain circumstances. Flurazepam has been claimed to be without effect on ventilation and, indeed, most studies show no greater rise in P_{CO_2} with flurazepam-induced sleep compared to that with natural sleep. Reports of unusual sensitivity of patients with obstructive airways disease to the respiratory depressant effects of benzodiazepines have not been prominent in the literature; there are isolated reports of such occurrences and of inordinate respiratory depression in aged individuals. In the latter regard, diazepam has been shown to selectively decrease genioglossal electromyogram (EMG) activity in older individuals. This provides a physiological basis for the observation that benzodiazepines increase frequency and duration of obstructive apnea events during sleep.

Alcohol causes little or no respiratory depression in doses that do not severely alter state of consciousness. However, a depression of responsiveness to CO_2 can be demonstrated. This is reversible by naloxone, implying that part of the effect is mediated by elaboration of endogenous opioids. The same depression of CO_2 sensitivity is induced by marijuana in large doses; tolerance to the depressant effect of marijuana on CO_2 response is manifest after prolonged use. A depression of flow-resistive load detection has been demonstrated for moderate doses of alcohol. Unlike the depression of CO_2 responsiveness, naloxone does not influence this effect of alcohol.

Probably the most important respiratory effect of alcohol is apparently a highly selective depression of respiratory output to the pharyngeal dilator muscles, thereby enhancing in susceptible individuals the tendency toward obstructive apneic episodes during sleep. Perhaps related to this effect is the evidence that moderate alcohol intake may worsen periodic episodes of hypoxemia during sleep in patients with obstructive airways disease who already manifest the phenomenon of obstructive sleep apnea.

CLINICAL IMPLICATIONS

The most prudent approach to the use of drugs with depressant psychomotor properties in patients with either severe mechanical impairment of respiratory function or with CO_2 retention of any cause is the assumption that depression of ventilation is a likely side effect and that these drugs are, therefore, to be avoided. An additional problem is the recently discovered selective depression of motor output to the dilator muscles of the upper airway, thereby enhancing the propensity for obstructive sleep apnea. Thus, as a class, depressant drugs are also best avoided in patients at risk for obstructive sleep apnea.

Nevertheless, the age group in which obstructive airways disease commonly occurs may be expected to complain of true insomnia, i.e., of an inability to sleep that is unrelated to disordered breathing or impairment of gas exchange. In such patients, flurazepam seems to be the drug of choice. It may be prudent to study this type of patient during sleep, before and after administration of the drug, to document both improved sleep patterns and lack of sleep-disordered breathing and gas exchange.

Respiratory Stimulant Drugs

The history of the use of respiratory stimulant drugs has been uneven. A generation or two ago, when the need for such agents was great, only poorly understood, relatively unselective, and therefore frequently ineffective drugs were available. Thus, when effective mechanical ventilation became generally available to treat severe alveolar hypoventilation, use of respiratory stimulants fell into well-deserved disrepute.

Recently, however, there has been a renewed interest in respiratory stimulants. Several factors are responsible for this. We now have a better understanding of the indications for and limitations of respiratory stimulation. On the one hand, it seems possible to identify a subgroup of patients with mechanical impediments to breathing, e.g., obesity and obstructive airways disease, who also have intrinsically low chemical drive and may, therefore, benefit from respiratory stimulation. At the other extreme, it is possible to identify individuals in whom lung dysfunction is so severe that increased alveolar ventilation is not possible or costs as much in CO_2 production as it produces in increased CO_2 elimination; in these individuals respiratory stimulation only results in increased dyspnea. Furthermore, drugs with more selective action have become available, providing the opportunity to employ pharmacologic respiratory stimulation with a wider margin of safety.

The agents discussed below have been used clinically or have the potential for clinical use. Thus, drugs such as aspirin, whose respiratory stimulant properties are only of modest toxicologic interest, are not discussed. Except for the analeptics, the drugs are discussed separately since they do not have readily definable common modes of action.

ANALEPTICS

These agents act by stimulation of multiple areas of the brain, including the respiratory neurons. They also frequently increase the metabolic rate of the entire body. Older agents, such as picrotoxin, that cause convulsions in doses uncomfortably close to those required for stimulation of breathing, are no longer used.

Ethamivan was thought to be a safe and effective ventilatory stimulant; however, much of its effect has been related to an increase in body metabolic rate. It is now rarely used clinically.

Doxapram has a differential effect according to dose: in doses below approximately 1.0 mg/kg, it stimulates ventilation primarily by an action at the carotid bodies; higher doses act centrally and, therefore, increase ventilatory response to CO_2. It has been tested in studies of patients with obstructive airways disease and in patients who became hypoxemic after upper abdominal surgery. The results indicate that increased alveolar ventilation with improved arterial blood-gas tensions can be obtained by administering doxapram to most patients of this kind. The major drawback to the use of the drug is that it must be given parenterally; thus, it is suitable only for short-term use in hospitalized patients. Since this group of patients is probably least suitable for the use of respiratory stimulant drugs, its overall usefulness is limited.

PROGESTERONE

It has long been known that women manifest alveolar hyperventilation during pregnancy and the luteal phase of the menstrual cycle, and that this effect is due to an action of progesterone. Although the mechanism of action is unknown, recent observations suggest that the ventilatory response to progesterone is mediated by estrogen-dependent receptors, as is the case for other effects of the hormone. Physiologically, an increase in ventilatory response to hypoxia and hypercapnia may be demonstrated.

Its major clinical use has been to produce increased ventilation in patients with normal lung function. Thus, it is effective in the obesity-hypoventilation syndrome and in chronic mountain sickness. Some studies report effectiveness in patients with obstructive airways disease. Whether it is useful in the treatment of obstructive sleep apnea is controversial at this time; the weight of evidence seems to be against its effectiveness. Clinically useful doses for respiratory stimulation far exceed those used for treatment of gynecologic disorders; they have ranged from 40 to 80 mg of medroxyprogesterone daily.

ACETAZOLAMIDE

This classic carbonic anhydrase inhibitor has long been known to stimulate ventilation. It probably acts by inhibition of red cell carbonic anhydrase; the impediment to transfer of CO_2 from tissues to blood establishes a new equilibrium, so that tissue P_{CO_2} increases. The resulting acidification is thought to stimulate central chemoreceptors in the brain.

The efficacy of the drug in the obesity hypoventilation syndrome has been demonstrated and it is generally used in this disorder as a second choice to medroxyprogesterone for respiratory stimulation. Usefulness in obstructive airways disease with CO_2 retention has not been established. In addition, some clinicians are reluctant to reduce serum bicarbonate levels in patients who are already at risk of abrupt hypercapnia by an episodic exacerbation of the disease. In our clinic, its use is reserved for correction of inappropriate alkalemia, as may occur when diuretics are used to treat peripheral edema in patients with obstructive airways disease and cor pulmonale.

An interesting use for acetazolamide has been for "preacclimatization" to high altitude. When given about 3 days before ascent to altitude, significant attenuation occurs of the symptoms of acute mountain sickness in susceptible individuals. The symptoms are those of mild brain edema and are presumably due to hypoxia of the brain. Acetazolamide relieves hypoxia of the brain both by ventilatory stimulation and by substantially increasing brain blood flow. The drug has also been reported to be useful in the treatment of the periodic sleep apneas that occur in sojourners at high altitude. In addition, it is reported useful in a (most probably) related condition, central sleep apnea that is unassociated with hypoxia.

THEOPHYLLINE

Although the ventilatory stimulant properties of theophylline are well known, it is not often used primarily for this purpose. An important exception is in the treatment of apnea spells of premature infants.

On the other hand, its usefulness in treating exacerbations of obstructive airways disease may be related, at least in part, to its ability to enhance ventilatory efforts. The improved ventilation may be a consequence of both a direct stimulatory effect on respiratory motor neurons and an indirect effect; the indirect effect is attributed to the fact that clinical doses of theophylline antagonize adenosine, a putative inhibitory neurotransmitter which is present in increased amounts in the hypoxic brain. In addition, theophylline has been shown to ameliorate respiratory muscle fatigue, probably by modulating membrane transport of calcium ion. This could be an important contribution to increased ventilatory effort in patients with severe decompensation of lung function.

ALMITRINE

Almitrine is a new agent that is currently limited to investigational use. This triazine derivative stimulates ventilation by action at the carotid body, thereby increasing responsiveness to hypoxia but not to CO_2. It has been subjected to relatively intense study in patients with obstructive airways disease, and the results are promising. Patients with alveolar hypoventilation that is not "fixed," i.e., amenable to stimulant therapy, are likely to respond to this drug by increasing alveolar ventilation during both the awake and sleeping states. An interesting sidelight is that arterial oxygenation tends to be improved out of proportion to reduction in CO_2 retention; in fact, some patients manifest improved oxygenation without change in arterial P_{CO_2}. This has been attributed to a direct effect on the pulmonary vasculature, presumably to increased hypoxic vasoconstriction that improves ventilation-perfusion matching.

PROTRIPTYLINE

Protriptyline is a nonsedating, tricyclic antidepressant drug that reduces daytime somnolence in the hypersomnolent obstructive sleep apnea syndrome. It is also effective in reducing obstructive apnea episodes during sleep. The action during sleep seems twofold: (1) a reduction of time spent in rapid-eye-movement (REM) sleep so that the number and severity of obstructive episodes decreases (since these are usually more profound during REM sleep), and (2) according to animal studies, a selective stimulation of the dilator muscles of the upper airway during sleep.

GENERAL CLINICAL CONSIDERATIONS

The decision to use pharmacologic respiratory stimulation is rarely simple. All agents have significant side effects and none are uniformly successful. Therefore, alternative therapies, ranging from mechanical ventilation during sleep to phrenic nerve pacing, must be considered.

In our clinic, respiratory stimulants are used in the following settings:

1. Chronic alveolar hypoventilation with normal lungs and chest wall.
2. Chronic alveolar hypoventilation with abnormal lungs or chest wall if suboptimal respiratory drive can be demonstrated. The latter usually requires that two criteria be met: (a) that the patient be able to reduce acutely the arterial P_{CO_2} during voluntary hyperventilation by at least 5 to 7 mmHg, and (b) that the patient demonstrates less than average ventilatory responsiveness to CO_2 and/or hypoxia.
3. Significant disordered breathing during sleep, even in the presence of adequate alveolar ventilation when awake. *Significant* means sufficient disorder to produce considerable arterial hypoxemia or to elicit abnormalities such as cardiac arrhythmias, systemic or pulmonary hypertension, and daytime hypersomnolence.
4. Special conditions, such as sleep apnea at altitude or prophylaxis for acute mountain sickness.

In most circumstances it is necessary to obtain adequate baseline data and to document the efficacy of the drug. This is especially important for treatment of sleep-disordered breathing, since the cardinal symptom, hypersomnolence, is highly subjective and often difficult to evaluate.

NEUROTRANSMITTERS AND NEUROMODULATORS

The study of the chemical basis of transmission of impulses from neuron to neuron has been extraordinarily productive in recent years; dozens of substances have been proposed to perform this function. A *neurotransmitter* is considered to be a substance elaborated by action of a neuronal impulse; the chemical mediator of neuronal transmission binds to a specific receptor on the target dendrite with rapid uptake and inactivation. The term *neuromodulator* is less precise and includes substances elaborated within the central nervous system that may modulate neuronal activity in a more general way, with less organizational specificity and slower onset and decay of action. Single entities such as GABA are thought to subserve both functions, and molecules of the same class may perform either function. For example, among the endogenous opioids the enkephalins probably serve only as neurotransmitters for a variety of pathways of interneurons; the β endorphins may serve a neurotransmitter role but appear to be elaborated as part of the "stress" response and function largely as neuromodulators. Diffuse representation of neurotransmitters is the likely explanation for the frequently conflicting results of experimental studies. Depletion of a neurotransmitter, for example, might have either facilitatory or inhibitory effects on ventilation depending on which aspect of brain function is most modifiable under a specific experimental condition. Further complicating the issue is the recent discovery that single neurons may have receptors for more than one neurotransmitter or elaborate more than one neurotransmitter.

Unlike some systems, no characteristic neurotransmitters have been identified with the neurons of the central nervous system involved in respiratory control. Although much recent work is important and provocative, little has resulted in clinical application. The following are agents which after extensive study appear to have potential pathophysiological significance.

Serotonin

Serotonin is a good example of a putative neurotransmitter that is likely to be involved in modulation of respiration at multiple loci in the brain; however, manipulations of serotonin metabolism have produced complex and conflicting results. Serotonin-containing cells are located in the raphe nuclei of the midbrain, pons, and medulla. They have been implicated in several control systems such as cardiovascular, thermoregulatory, and sleep. Although controversy persists, the weight of current evidence suggests that the net effect of activation of central nervous serotoninergic neurons is to depress ventilation. Stimulation of breathing via the arterial chemoreceptors may result when serotonin agonists are given systematically. The pathophysiological role of serotoninergic nerves in respiratory control remains speculative. Modulation of respiratory responses during REM sleep and of responses to pain and chronic hypoxia have all been proposed.

Dopamine

Currently the most clearly defined and important respiratory effect of dopamine is its inhibition of carotid body activity under euoxic and hypoxic conditions. Haloperidol, a dopamine antagonist, blocks this effect but has little effect of its own, suggesting that elaboration of dopamine may not play a key role in carotid body function. These observations have potential clinical significance since dopamine or its agonists are often given to critically ill hypoxic patients. Like serotonin and the other catecholamines, dopamine has little or no access to the central nervous system when given systemically. Activation of central dopaminergic neurons has generally been reported to have a net depressant effect on ventilation except when large doses of the agonist apomorphine are given. At present there is little evidence that central dopaminergic neurons play a fundamental role in respiratory control.

γ-Aminobutyric Acid (GABA)

Several amino acids have prominent effects on neuronal activity. Glutamic and aspartic acids excite most neurons, whereas GABA, glycine, and taurine are depressant. GABA has been the most well studied.

GABA receptors are distributed widely in the central nervous system. Although the density of these receptors is greater in suprapontine structures than in the brain stem, there are adequate receptors in the brain stem to explain its respiratory effects.

Almost all studies indicate a powerful depressant effect upon respiration when GABAergic neurons are activated. The effect is dose-related and may be observed with levels of the drug which approach those found naturally. Thus, there is good reason to suspect that GABA plays at least a neuromodulatory role in respiration in certain pathophysiological conditions. Two which have been studied are chronic hypercapnia and severe hypoxia. Both states may be associated with respiratory depression, i.e., ventilation which is less than expected for the level of chemical stimuli in the blood, and in both there are elevated levels of GABA in the central nervous system. GABA is important pharmacologically since its receptors are the likely site of action of the benzodiazepines and barbiturates.

Endogenous Opioids

A variety of putative peptide neurotransmitters (the so-called neuropeptides) have been implicated in respiratory control. These include thyrotropin-releasing hormone, substance P, vasoactive intestinal peptide, and the opioids. In addition, angiotensin, bradykinin, cholecystokinin, neurotensin, and oxytocin now all appear to be potential neurotransmitters for control systems which integrate with the respiratory control system. Of these the opioids have been the best studied.

At least three distinct opioid systems have been identified. β-Endorphin neurons have cell bodies in the medial hypothalamus and project rostrally; enkephalins appear in many areas of the brain in local cell groups or short fiber systems; dynorphin neurons arise in the hypothalamus and project to the posterior pituitary. High concentrations of opioid receptors are found in the solitary nuclei and other medullary areas involved in respiratory control. The various opioid systems relate in a relatively but not absolutely specific way to the various receptor types which have been described. Of importance to respiratory control is that the receptors have different susceptibilities to the antagonist action of naloxone, with those thought to be most closely associated with respiratory neurons (i.e., δ receptors) being relatively less sensitive.

With a very few exceptions, activation of the central nervous opioid receptors results in depression of output by respiratory motor neurons. Several studies involving local application of opioid agonists suggest regional specificity of their action; that is, depression of tidal volume can be separated from depression of respiratory frequency. Intracisternal injection of naturally occurring opioid agonists reduces ventilation and ventilatory responses to CO_2 and hypoxia.

In view of the potent depressant potential of opioid agonists and the wide distribution of opioid receptors in the brain stem, the pathophysiological role of the endogenous opioid system in respiratory control seems surprisingly small. Studies involving administration of naloxone to normal adult humans usually fail to reveal any tonic effect of the opioid system on the ventilation or on the ventilatory response to CO_2 and hypoxia. One disease-related role for endogenous opioids has been suggested, i.e., that in certain patients with obstructive airways disease they are responsible for the failure of respiratory effort to increase when flow-resistive loads are added.

Naloxone increases the ventilatory response to hypoxia in obstructive airways disease. However, it remains unclear whether this effect is directly related to the hypoxia chemoreflex or if it results from an increase in load compensation, since the response to hypoxia and flow-resistive loads interact synergistically. In experimental animals, naloxone reverses part of the respiratory depression caused by severe brain hypoxia. On the other hand, the decrease in ventilation that occurs 30 to 60 min after the application of a hypoxic stimulus to unanesthetized humans, and which has been thought to reflect effects of brain hypoxia, is not altered by naloxone.

The evidence for a pathophysiological role of endogenous opioids in setting respiration in the neonatal period is somewhat more convincing. Respiratory depression caused by experimental asphyxiation of newborn rabbit pups is reversible to a considerable degree by naloxone. It is now common clinical practice to use naloxone as part of resuscitative measures in newborn humans with respiratory depression. In the early neonatal period (less than approximately 5 days postpartum), naloxone tends to increase ventilation and ventilatory response to hypoxia. However, the qualitative nature of the characteristic biphasic response to hypoxia in the early neonatal period (stimulation followed by depression to prehypoxic values within 3 to 5 min) is not altered by opioid antagonism. Whether the effects of naloxone in the neonatal period reflect an action of "endogenously" generated opioids, or of opioids received from the mother by placental transfer, is not clear.

A few specific pathophysiological effects are also attributed to endogenous opioids. These include depression of ventilation related to very high opioid levels in the central nervous system of a patient with necrotizing encephalomyelopathy. Single reports have also shown that naloxone reverses the reduction in mean inspiratory flow rate caused by cigarette smoking as well as the reduction in ventilatory responses to chemical stimuli caused by ingestion of moderate doses of alcohol in humans.

BIBLIOGRAPHY

Altose MD, Hudgel DW: The pharmacology of respiratory depressants and stimulants. Clin Chest Med 7:481–494, 1986.
  This article reviews the pharmacology and respiratory actions of depressants and stimulants and the use of these drugs in the management of dyspnea, respiratory failure, and sleep apnea syndrome.

Eldridge FL, Millhorn DE: Central regulation of respiration by endogenous neurotransmitters and neuromodulators. Annu Rev Physiol 43:121–135, 1981.
  A brief review of current thinking on the role of neuromodulators in respiratory control. It is especially valuable because of conciseness and clarity.

Espinoza H, Antic R, Thornton AT, McEvoy RD: The effects of aminophylline on sleep and sleep-disordered breathing in patients with obstructive sleep apnea syndrome. Am Rev Respir Dis 136:80–84, 1987.
Aminophylline reduces central apnea and the central component of mixed apneas but has no effect on obstructive apnea.

Gold MI, Reichenberg S, Freeman E: Respiratory depression in the sedated bronchitis patient: Rapid version of the CO_2 response curve. Anesthesiology 30:492–499, 1969.
A classic paper which describes the delayed deleterious effects of sedation upon alveolar ventilation in chronic obstructive pulmonary disease (COPD).

Hickey RF, Severinghaus JW: Regulation of breathing: Drug effects, in Hornbein TF (ed), *Regulation of Breathing, Part II.* New York, Dekker, 1981, pp 1251–1312.
A good review of the effects of drugs on breathing, with emphasis on anesthetics.

Holaday JW: Cardiovascular effects of endogenous opiate systems. Am Rev Pharmacol Toxicol 23:541–594, 1983.
A good review of the role of opioids in cardiovascular control. It includes several topics of interest to respiratory control as well.

Moser KM, Luchsinger PC, Adamson JS, McMahon SM, Schlueter DP, Spivock M, Weg JG: Respiratory stimulation with intravenous doxapram in respiratory failure. N Engl J Med 288:427–431, 1973.
The best clinical trial of doxapram in patients with respiratory failure.

Mueller RA, Lundberg DBA, Breese GR, Hedner J, Hedner T, Jonason J: The neuropharmacology of respiratory control. Pharmacological Rev 34:255–285, 1982.
The most definitive available review of the neuropharmacology of respiratory control.

Oren J, Newth CJ, Hunt CE, Brouillette RT, Bachand RT, Shannon DC: Ventilatory effects of almitrine bismesylate in congenital central hypoventilation syndrome. Am Rev Respir Dis 134:917–919, 1986.
Almitrine is not a useful ventilatory stimulant in children with the congenital central hypoventilation syndrome.

Pietak S, Weenig CS, Hickey RF, Fairley HB: Anesthetic effects on ventilation in patients with chronic obstructive pulmonary disease. Anesthesiology 42:160–166, 1975.
A good description of the use of anesthetic agents in a high-risk group.

Powles ACP, Tuxen DV, Mahood CB, Pugsley SO, Campbell EJM: The effect of intravenously administered almitrine, a peripheral chemoreceptor agonist, in patients with chronic airflow obstruction. Am Rev Respir Dis 127:284–289, 1983.
A good description of the potential clinical usefulness of almitrine.

Santiago TV, Edelman NH: Opioids and breathing. J Appl Physiol 59:1675–1685, 1985.
A review summarizing recent developments on the effects of opiate drugs and the various endogenous opioid peptides on breathing.

Santiago TV, Pugliese AC, Edelman NH: Control of breathing during methadone addiction. Am J Med 62:347–354, 1977.
A description of the effects of prolonged opiate use on respiratory control.

Scrima L, Broudy M, Nay KN, Cohn MA: Increased severity of obstructive sleep apnea after bedtime alcohol ingestion: Diagnostic potential and proposed mechanism of action. Sleep 5:318–328, 1982.
An important description of the major deleterious respiratory effect of moderate doses of alcohol.

Skatrud JB, Dempsey JA: Relative effectiveness of acetazolamide versus medroxyprogesterone acetate in correction of chronic carbon dioxide retention. Am Rev Respir Dis 127:405–412, 1983.
A good study which demonstrates the relative effectiveness of the two currently major respiratory stimulants.

Sutton FD, Zwillich CW, Creagh CE, Pierson DJ, Weil JV: Progesterone for outpatient treatment of Pickwickian syndrome. Ann Intern Med 83:476–479, 1985.
One of the first definitive demonstrations of the efficacy of a progestational compound in increasing alveolar ventilation in patients with alveolar hypoventilation of nonpulmonary origin.

Woodcock AA, Gross ER, Gilbert A, Shah S, Johnson M, Geddes DM: Effects of dihydrocodeine, alcohol and caffeine on breathlessness and exercise tolerance in patients with chronic obstructive lung disease and normal blood gases. N Engl J Med 305:1611–1616, 1981.
A potentially important paper which shows that pharmacologic depression of respiratory drive in selected nonhypercapnic patients with COPD may reduce dyspnea and increase tolerance without causing CO_2 retention.

Chapter *12*

Pulmonary Mechanics

Murray D. Altose

PULMONARY MECHANICS AND VENTILATION

For venous blood to be properly arterialized, the distribution of air and blood within the lung is automatically matched in order to ensure effective gas exchange across alveolar-capillary membranes. Arterialization involves a series of interrelated processes that begin with the mechanical performance of the ventilatory apparatus, i.e.,

the lungs and chest wall including the rib cage, diaphragm, and abdominal wall. Although the function of each component of the lung and of the chest bellows can be deranged by injury or disease, the design of the ventilatory apparatus provides for considerable reserve. As a result, mechanical derangements are usually quite severe by the time that clinical symptoms appear or arterial blood-gas levels become abnormal.

Depending on the nature of the underlying disorder, assessment of the mechanical properties of the ventilatory apparatus provides several different types of information. In some instances, characterization of the mechanical abnormality provides insight into pathogenesis and affords a quantitative measure of severity. In others, once the nature of the mechanical disorder is understood, the mystery surrounding a life-threatening disorder in gas exchange may be dispelled. Finally, certain breathing patterns make sense only if the mechanical performance of the chest bellows is taken into account.

During breathing, the lungs and chest wall operate in unison. The lungs fill the chest cavity so that the visceral pleura is in contrast with the parietal pleura of the chest wall. The two pleural surfaces are separated by only a thin liquid film that provides the bond holding the lungs and chest wall together.

At the end of a normal exhalation, the respiratory muscles are at rest. The pressure along the entire tracheobronchial tree from the airway opening to the alveoli is equal to atmospheric pressure. The tendency of the lung, however, is to deflate, and lung elastic recoil is directed centripetally. This is counterbalanced by the elastic recoil of the chest wall which is directed centrifugally favoring an increase in volume. These opposing forces generate a subatmospheric pleural pressure of about -5 cmH$_2$O (Fig. 12-1A).

Although it is conventional to consider pleural pressure as a single, mean value that reflects mechanical events within the entire ventilatory apparatus, this is clearly an oversimplification on several accounts: (1) pleural pressure is not directly determinable because normally there is only a potential space between the visceral

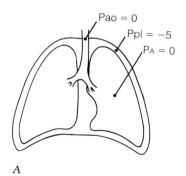
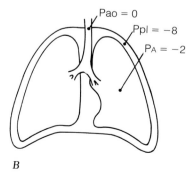
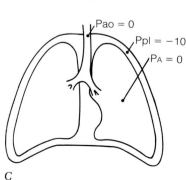

A   *B*   *C*

FIGURE 12-1   Respiratory pressures during a breathing cycle. Ppl is pleural pressure, P$_A$ is pressure in the alveoli, and Pao is pressure at the airway opening.   *A.* End expiration.   *B.* During inspiration.   *C.* End inspiration.

and parietal pleura; (2) on conceptual grounds, distinctions exist between surface and liquid pleural pressures; (3) pleural pressures are not uniform over the surface of the lungs, being strongly affected by gravity; and (4) transmission of pleural pressures at the surface to alveoli located at different depths and loci with the lungs depends on the structural interplay among supporting structures in the alveolar walls (*interdependence*) which resists any inclination of individual alveoli or even a lobule to collapse. Nonetheless, the concept of mean pleural pressure, as generally used in considerations of respiratory system mechanics has proved to be of great practical value.

The contraction of the muscles of inspiration produces the forces that permit the flow of gas along the tracheobronchial tree and the expansion of the lungs and chest. The movement of air into the lungs requires a pressure difference between the airway opening and the alveoli sufficient to overcome the resistance to airflow of the tracheobronchial tree. During spontaneous breathing, the action of the inspiratory muscles causes an increase in the outward recoil of the chest wall. As a result, the pleural pressure becomes more subatmospheric. This pressure change is transmitted to the interior of the lungs so that alveolar pressure also becomes subatmospheric (Fig. 12-1B). In contrast, during artificial ventilation with a positive pressure breathing machine, a supra-atmospheric pressure applied at the inlet to the airways creates the proper pressure gradient between the airway opening and alveoli for airflow.

Expansion of alveoli depends on the achievement of an appropriate distending pressure across alveolar walls. This distending pressure or transpulmonary pressure is the difference between alveolar (P_A) and pleural (Ppl) pressures. As shown in Fig. 12-1A, the transpulmonary pressure at end-expiration ($P_A - Ppl$) is 5 cmH$_2$O. At the end of inspiration (Fig. 12-1C), the transpulmonary distending pressure is higher and the lungs contain more air.

The energy used during inspiration to overcome the elastic resistance of the lungs is stored. Expiration occurs when these forces are released. When the inspiratory muscles relax, the recoil of the lungs causes the alveolar pressure to exceed the pressure at the mouth and air flows out of the lungs. Although expiration during quiet breathing is passive, the expiratory muscles are engaged at high levels of ventilation to assist the movement of air out of the lungs.

LUNG VOLUMES

The lung volumes and capacities (Table 12-1) are considered elsewhere in this book (see Chapter 163). Here it is pertinent to underscore that the end-expiratory position of the lungs is the major reference position for the functional subdivisions of the lungs. When the respiratory

TABLE 12-1
Lung Volumes and Subdivisions

The *functional residual capacity* (FRC) is the volume of air that remains in the lungs at the end of a normal expiration.

The *tidal volume* (TV) is the volume of air that is drawn into the lungs during inspiration from the end-expiratory position (and also leaves the lungs passively during expiration in the course of quiet breathing).

The *expiratory reserve volume* (ERV) is the maximum volume of air that can be forcibly exhaled after a quiet expiration has been completed (i.e., from the end-expiratory position).

The *residual volume* (RV) is the volume of air that remains in the lungs after a maximal expiratory effort.

The *inspiratory capacity* (IC) is the maximum volume of air that can be inhaled from the end-expiratory position. It consists of two subdivisions: tidal volume and the inspiratory reserve volume (IRV).

The *total lung capacity* (TLC) is the total volume of air contained in the lungs at the end of a maximum inspiration.

The *vital capacity* (VC) is the volume of air that is exhaled by a maximum expiration after a maximum inspiration.

muscles are at rest, this position is set by the opposing recoil forces of the lungs and chest wall.

STATIC MECHANICAL PROPERTIES OF THE RESPIRATORY SYSTEM

To assess the elastic properties of the ventilatory apparatus, it is expedient to evaluate the elastic properties of the lungs and chest separately.

Elastic Properties of the Lungs (Pulmonary Compliance)

The change in transpulmonary pressure required to effect a given change in the volume of air in the lungs is a measure of the *distensibility*, or *compliance*, of the lungs. Pulmonary compliance is calculated as the ratio of the *change* in lung volume to the *change* in transpulmonary pressure, i.e.,

$$C = \frac{\Delta V_L}{\Delta (P_A - Ppl)} \qquad (1)$$

where

$$C = \text{lung compliance}$$
$$\Delta (P_A - Ppl) = \text{change in transpulmonary pressure}$$
$$\Delta V_L = \text{change in lung volume}$$

Compliance denotes the ease of stretch or inflation. The inverse of compliance, i.e., *elastance*, refers to the tendency to resist distortion and to return to the original configuration when the distorting force is removed.

In practice, pulmonary compliance is determined by relating the changes in transpulmonary pressures to the changes in lung volume in the course of an expiration after a maximal inspiration, i.e., starting from total lung capacity.

The pressure-volume characteristics of the lung are nonlinear. Thus, the compliance of the lung is least at high lung volumes and greatest as the residual volume is approached (Fig. 12-2). Elastic recoil forces favoring collapse of the lung can be demonstrated throughout the range of the vital capacity, even at low lung volumes approaching the residual volume. If the opposing forces of the chest wall on the lungs are eliminated, as by removing the lungs from the thorax or by opening the chest, the lung collapses to a virtually airless state.

If static measurements of transpulmonary pressure are made during lung inflation rather than deflation, the pressure-volume curve has a different configuration (Fig. 12-3). This indicates that the elastic recoil of the lung depends not only on the lung volume at which the determination is made but also on the "volume history" of the lung.

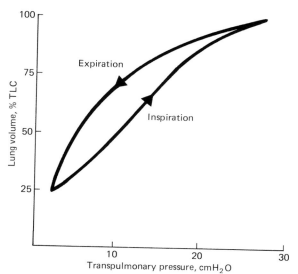

FIGURE 12-3 Pressure-volume curves of the lung during inspiration and expiration.

HYSTERESIS

Difference in the pathways of the pressure-volume curve during inspiration (when force is applied) and expiration (when force is withdrawn) is designated as *hysteresis*. It is a property of all elastic structures. In the lungs, it is due to the elasticity of the tissues and to the properties of the surface material lining the alveolar walls. An additional factor involves the closure of small airways at low lung volumes. Once these airways close, the lung units that they serve will not expand during inspiration until a criti-

cal opening pressure has been exceeded; only then will the closed units inflate. Recruitment of additional lung units as increasing transpulmonary pressure expands the lungs from low lung volume contributes to the hysteresis of the pressure-volume curve.

The elastic behavior of the lung depends on two factors: the physical properties of the lung tissue, per se, and the surface tension of the film lining of the alveolar walls.

SURFACE FORCES

In addition to the elastic properties of the parenchyma, the surface tension at the air-liquid interface of the alveoli contributes importantly to the elastic recoil of the lungs. The intermolecular, cohesive forces between the molecules of the liquid lining of the alveoli are stronger than those between the film and alveolar gas, thereby causing the film to shrink to its smallest surface area. The behavior of this surface film has been examined in experimental animals by comparing pressure-volume relationships of air-filled lungs with those of saline-filled lungs; saline eliminates the liquid-air interface without affecting elastic properties of the tissue. A lung distended with saline requires a lower transpulmonary pressure to maintain a given lung volume than a lung that is inflated with air (Fig. 12-4).

By considering the alveolus to be a sphere, Laplace's law can be applied. Laplace's law states that the pressure inside a spherical structure, e.g., the alveolus, is directly proportional to the tension in the wall and inversely proportional to the radius of curvature, i.e.,

$$\text{Alveolar pressure} = \frac{2T}{r} \qquad (2)$$

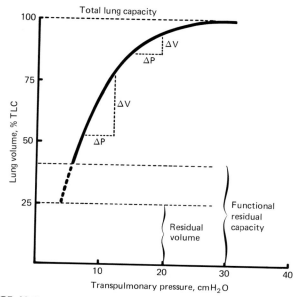

FIGURE 12-2 Pressure-volume curve of the lung. The static elastic recoil pressure of the lung is approximately 5 cmH$_2$O at FRC and 30 cmH$_2$O at TLC. The compliance of the lung ($\Delta V/\Delta P$) is greater at low lung volumes than at high lung volumes.

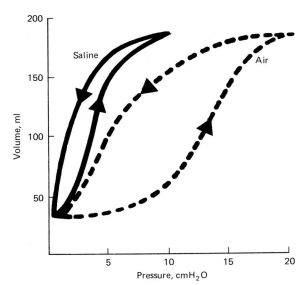

FIGURE 12-4 Comparison of pressure-volume relationships of air-filled and saline-filled excised lungs. Arrows directed upward indicate inflation; those directed downward indicate deflation. Since saline eliminates surface forces at the liquid-air interface without affecting tissue elasticity, the difference in pressure between the two curves, at any lung volume, is that required to overcome surface forces. To maintain a small lung volume, a large proportion of the pressure is used to overcome surface forces. In contrast, at high lung volumes a greater fraction of the pressure is used to overcome tissue elasticity.

where

$$T = \text{tension, dyn/cm}$$
$$r = \text{radius}$$

Abolition of the liquid-air interface by the instillation of saline into the alveolar spaces eliminates surface forces, thereby reducing the transpulmonary pressure required to maintain a given lung volume.

The surface tension of the alveolar walls depends on the lung volume: surface tension is higher at large lung volumes and lower at small lung volumes. These variations in surface tension with lung volume are due to the surface film which contains a special type of surface-active material, *surfactant*. This substance contains differ-

ent phospholipids, notably dipalmitoyl lecithin, and special proteins. It is generated by type II alveolar cells and undergoes a continuous cycle of formation, removal, and replenishment.

Surfactant serves several important functions. The surface tension of surfactant is inherently low and decreases yet further at low lung volumes when the surface area of the film is reduced. The minimization of surface forces, particularly at low lung volumes, increases the compliance of the lung and decreases the work required to inflate the lungs during the next breath. The automatic adjustment of surface tension as lung volume changes also promotes stability of alveoli at low lung volumes: if the surface tension were to remain constant instead of changing with lung volume, the transpulmonary pressure required to keep an alveolus open would increase as the radius of curvature diminished with decreasing lung volume. Therefore, small alveoli would empty into the larger ones with which they communicate, and atelectasis would be a regular occurrence (Fig. 12-5).

PHYSICAL PROPERTIES OF LUNG TISSUE

The elasticity of lung tissue, per se, is due primarily to the elastin fibers in the alveolar walls and surrounding the bronchioles and pulmonary capillaries; they can be stretched to approximately twice their resting length. The collagen fibers contribute much less to the elastic properties: they are poorly extensible and probably act to limit expansion primarily at high lung volumes. Like a stretched nylon stocking, expansion of the lungs appears to involve an unfolding and geometric rearrangement of the fibers and only slight elongation of individual fibers.

As a result of alterations in the elastin and collagen fibers in the lung, the distensibility of the lungs (measured as compliance) increases with age. This is part of the normal aging process. Pulmonary compliance is also increased by the destruction of alveolar walls and the enlargement of alveolar spaces that characterize pulmonary emphysema. In contrast, the distensibility of the lungs is reduced by pulmonary fibrosis, which stiffens its interstitial tissues.

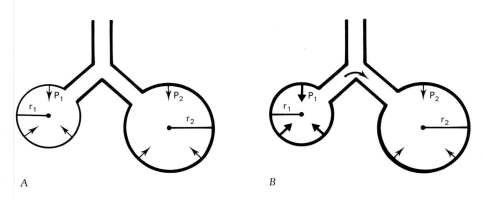

A   *B*

FIGURE 12-5 The effects of surfactant in maintaining alveolar stability. A. Surfactant lowers the tension (T) of the alveolar walls at low lung volumes. Consequently, the transpulmonary pressure (P) of large and small communicating airspaces is the same. $r_1 < r_2$, $T_1 < T_2$, $P_1 = P_2$. B. Without surfactant, the surface tension remains constant as lung volume changes, and the recoil pressure of small airspaces exceeds that of larger ones. As a result, small alveoli tend to empty into larger ones. $r_1 < r_2$, $T_1 = T_2$, $P_1 > P_2$.

Elastic Properties of the Thorax

The elastic recoil of the chest wall is such that if it were unopposed by the lungs, the chest would enlarge to approximately 70 percent of total lung capacity. This position represents its equilibrium or resting position. In this position (when the respiratory muscles are completely relaxed), the pressure difference across the chest wall, i.e., the difference between pleural pressure and the pressure at the surface of the chest, is zero. If the chest were forced to enlarge further, it would, like the lung, recoil inward, resisting expansion and favoring return to its equilibrium position. Conversely, at volumes less than 70 percent of total lung capacity, the recoil of the chest is opposite to that of the lung and is directed outward (Fig. 12-6).

The elastic recoil properties of the chest wall play an important role in determining the subdivisions of lung volume. They may be seriously deranged by disorders such as marked obesity, kyphoscoliosis, and ankylosing spondylitis.

Elastic Properties of the Respiratory System as a Whole

By considering the lung and the chest wall to be in series, the *elastic recoil* pressure of the total respiratory system (Prs) can be calculated as the algebraic sum of the pressures exerted by the elastic recoil of the lung (transpulmonary pressure) and the elastic recoil of the chest wall.

Since the elastic recoil of the lung is determined (under static conditions of arrested airflow) as the difference between alveolar pressure (PA) and pleural pressure (Ppl), i.e., $P_A - Ppl$, and the elastic recoil of the chest wall is determined (while the respiratory muscles are completely at rest) as the difference between pleural pressure and the pressure at the external surface of the chest (Pbs), i.e., $Ppl - Pbs$, the elastic recoil of the entire respiratory system can be expressed as the sum of the two:

$$Prs = (P_A - Ppl) + (Ppl - Pbs) = P_A - Pbs \qquad (3)$$

Thus, a measure of the elastic recoil of the respiratory system is provided by the alveolar pressure provided that the respiratory muscles are completely at rest and the pressure of the body surface is at atmospheric levels.

RELAXATION PRESSURE-VOLUME CURVE

The elastic properties of the entire respiratory system can be determined from the relaxation pressure-volume curve (Fig. 12-7). Functional residual capacity represents the equilibrium position of the lung-chest wall system while the respiratory muscles are relaxed. At this point, the opposing recoils of the lung and chest wall are of equal magnitude, and the recoil pressure of the entire respiratory system is zero. With increases in lung volume above functional residual capacity, the recoil pressure of the entire system becomes positive owing to the combination of an

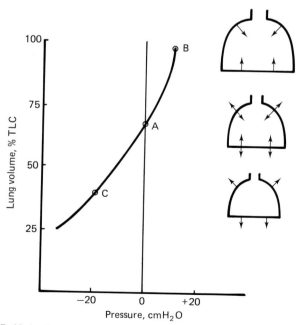

FIGURE 12-6 Pressure-volume relationships of the isolated chest wall. The equilibrium position of the chest wall (A), unopposed by the lungs, is approximately 70 percent of total lung capacity. In this position, the pressure difference across the chest wall is zero. At larger volumes (B), there is inward recoil of the chest wall; at volumes below the equilibrium position (C), the recoil forces of the chest wall are directed outwardly favoring expansion.

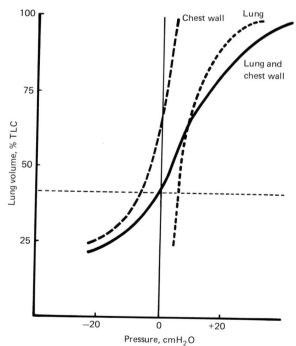

FIGURE 12-7 Relaxation pressure-volume curves. The elastic recoil pressure of the total respiratory system is the algebraic sum of the recoil pressures of the lung and the chest wall. At FRC the recoil pressures of the lung and chest wall are equal but opposite. Since the net recoil pressure is zero, the respiratory system is in a position of equilibrium.

increase in centripetal elastic recoil of the lungs and a decrease in the centrifugal recoil of the chest wall. The net effect favors a decrease in lung volume, and lung volume can be maintained with the airway open to the atmosphere only by the action of the inspiratory muscles. As lung volume exceeds 75 percent of total lung capacity, the recoil of the chest wall also becomes centripetal and the recoil pressure of the chest wall adds to the inward forces acting to diminish lung volume. Total lung capacity represents the lung volume at which the inward passive elastic recoil pressure of the respiratory system reaches the maximum force that can be generated by the inspiratory muscles.

At lung volumes below functional residual capacity, when the centrifugal recoil of the chest wall exceeds the reduced centripetal recoil of the lungs, the relaxation pressure is negative and this net effect favors an increase in lung volume. Lung volumes below functional residual capacity are achieved and maintained by the muscles of expiration.

A switch from the sitting to the supine position decreases functional residual capacity because of the effects of gravity. In the upright position gravity pulls the abdominal contents away from the chest wall. In contrast, in the supine position, the push of the abdominal contents against the diaphragm decreases the centrifugal recoil of the chest wall. The chest wall pressure-volume curve and consequently the pressure-volume curve of the entire respiratory system is displaced to the right.

DYNAMIC MECHANICAL PROPERTIES OF THE RESPIRATORY SYSTEM

The total nonelastic resistance of the lungs consists of the resistance of the airways to airflow (airway resistance), defined in terms of the driving pressure and the resulting rate of airflow, and the frictional resistance of the lung tissues to displacement during breathing (tissue resistance). Normally, tissue resistance makes up only 10 to 20 percent of the total pulmonary nonelastic resistance, but in diseases of the pulmonary parenchyma it may increase considerably.

Airway Resistance

A large fraction of the resistance to airflow is in the upper respiratory tract, including the nose, mouth, pharynx, larynx, and trachea. During nasal breathing the nose constitutes up to 50 percent of total airway resistance. During quiet mouth breathing, the mouth, pharynx, larynx, and trachea constitute 20 to 30 percent of the airway resistance; but they account for up to 50 percent of the total airway resistance when minute ventilation increases, as during vigorous exercise. Most of the remainder of airway

resistance is in medium-sized lobar, segmental, and subsegmental bronchi up to about the seventh generation of airways. Additional branching distally causes a progressive increase both in the number of airways in any generation and in the total cross-sectional area of the tracheobronchial tree. Consequently, in the normal lung, the small peripheral airways, particularly those less than 2 mm in diameter, constitute only about 10 to 20 percent of the total airway resistance.

AIRWAY CALIBER

The airways, like the pulmonary parenchyma, exhibit elasticity and can be compressed or distended. Therefore, the diameter of an airway varies with the transmural pressure applied to that airway, i.e., the difference between the pressure within the airway and the pressure surrounding the airway. The pressure surrounding intrathoracic airways approximates pleural pressure since these airways are tethered to the parenchymal tissue and are exposed to the expansive forces that are involved in overcoming the elastic recoil of the lung.

As the lung volume increases, the elastic recoil forces of the lung increase; the traction applied to the walls of the intrathoracic airways also increases, widening the airways and decreasing their resistance to airflow. Conversely, at low lung volumes, the transmural airway pressure is lower, and airway resistance increases. If the elastic recoil of the lung is reduced, as by destruction of alveolar walls in pulmonary emphysema, the transmural airway pressure at any given lung volume decreases correspondingly; the airways are narrower and airway resistance is greater even though there is no disease of the airways per se.

The effects of a change in transmural pressure on airway caliber depend on the compliance of the airways which, in turn, is determined by their structural support. The trachea, for example, is almost completely surrounded by cartilaginous rings, which tend to prevent complete collapse even when the transmural pressure is negative. The bronchi are less well supported by incomplete cartilaginous rings and plates, whereas the bronchioles lack cartilaginous support. All airways can be stiffened, albeit to different degrees, by contraction of smooth muscle in their walls.

In patients with airway disease, mucosal edema, hypertrophy and hyperplasia of mucous glands, increased elaboration of mucus, and hypertrophy of smooth muscle further compromise airway caliber and increase airway resistance.

PRESSURE-FLOW RELATIONSHIPS: THEORETICAL CONSIDERATIONS

In the lungs pressure-flow relationships are extremely complicated because the airways consist of a system of irregular branching tubes which are neither rigid nor perfectly circular. For purposes of simplification, pressure-flow relationships in rigid tubes are generally regarded as a model for those in the airways.

The driving pressure which produces flow of air into and out of the lung must suffice to overcome friction and to accelerate the air. Acceleration in the lungs is of two types: *local*, i.e., changes in the rate of airflow with time, and *convective*, i.e., acceleration of molecules of air over distance while flow is constant. The driving pressure required for convective acceleration is proportional to the gas density and to the square of the flow rate. It is important during expiration because, as air moves downstream from the alveoli toward the airway opening, the total cross-sectional airway diameter decreases; therefore, molecules of air must accelerate through the converging channels even though the overall flow rate remains unchanged. Also, the driving pressure that produces high expiratory flow rates at large lung volume serves for convective acceleration rather than for overcoming friction.

The driving pressure required to overcome friction depends on the rate and the pattern of airflow. Two major patterns of airflow warrant special consideration: *laminar* and *turbulent*. Laminar flow is characterized by stream-

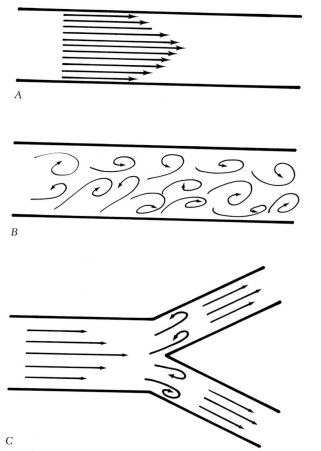

A

B

C

FIGURE 12-8 Patterns of airflow. *A.* Laminar flow. *B.* Turbulent flow. *C.* Transitional flow.

lines that parallel the sides of the tube and are capable of sliding over one another. Also, because the streamlines at the center of the tube move faster than those closest to the walls, the flow profile is parabolic (Fig. 12-8). The pressure-flow characteristics of laminar flow depend on the length (l) and the radius (r) of the tube and the viscosity of the gas (η) according to Poiseuille's equation,

$$\Delta P = \frac{\dot{V}8\eta l}{\pi r^4} \qquad (4)$$

where

ΔP = the driving pressure (pressure drop between the beginning and the end of the tube)
$\dot{V}$ = the flow rate that the driving pressure produces
r = the radius of the tube

The critical importance of tube radius in determining the driving pressure for a given flow is apparent in Eq. (4). If the radius of the tube is halved, the pressure that is required to maintain a given flow rate must be increased 16-fold. Laminar flow patterns occur only in small peripheral airways where, because of the enormous overall cross-sectional area, flow through the individual airways is exceedingly slow.

Turbulent flow occurs at high flow rates and is characterized by a complete disorganization of streamlines, so that the molecules of gas move laterally, collide with each other, and change velocities. Under these circumstances, pressure-flow relationships change. In contrast with laminar flow, the rate of airflow is no longer proportional to the driving pressure. Instead, the driving pressure to produce a given rate of airflow is proportional to the square of flow and is dependent on gas density. Turbulent flow occurs regularly in the trachea.

At lower flow rates during expiration, particularly at branches in the tracheobronchial tree where flow in two separate tubes comes together into a single channel, the parabolic profile of laminar flow becomes blunted, the streamlines separate from the walls of the tube, and minor eddy formation develops. This is referred to as a *mixed*, or *transitional*, flow pattern. In a mixed pattern of airflow, the driving pressure for a given flow depends on both the viscosity and the density of the gas.

Whether airflow is laminar or turbulent is predictable from the Reynolds number (Re), a dimensionless number that depends on the average velocity ($\overline{V}$), the density of the gas (ρ), the viscosity of the gas (η), and the diameter of the tube (D), so that

$$Re = \overline{V}D\frac{\rho}{\eta} \qquad (5)$$

In straight, smooth, rigid tubes, turbulence occurs when the Reynolds number exceeds 2000. Therefore, turbulence is most apt to occur when the average velocity is high, gas density is high, gas viscosity is low, and the tube diameter is large. Since most of the resistance to airflow in the normal lung is in large airways where resistance is density-dependent, breathing a mixture of 80 percent helium and 20 percent oxygen (a mixture that is 64 percent less dense than air) increases airflow at a given driving pressure and substantially decreases airway resistance.

CALCULATION OF AIRFLOW RESISTANCE

The driving pressure along the tracheobronchial tree, i.e., the difference between alveolar pressure and the pressure at the airway opening (mouth) that is required to produce a given rate of airflow into the lungs provides a measure of the flow resistance of the airways, according to the equation

$$\text{Raw} = \frac{P_A - P_{ao}}{\dot{V}} \qquad (6)$$

where

$\dot{V}$ = airflow, L/s
P_A = alveolar pressure, cmH$_2$O
P_{ao} = airway opening pressure, cmH$_2$O
Raw = airway resistance, cmH$_2$O/L/s

FLOW-VOLUME RELATIONSHIPS

Considerable insight into the flow-resistive properties of the airways can be obtained from the relationship between airflow and lung volume during maximal expiratory and inspiratory maneuvers. In practice, an individual inhales maximally to total lung capacity; then exhales as forcefully, rapidly, and completely as possible to residual volume; and then returns to total lung capacity by a rapid, forceful inhalation (Fig. 12-9). During the maximal expiration, the rate of airflow peaks at a lung volume that is close to the total lung capacity; as the lung volume decreases and intrathoracic airways narrow, airway resistance increases, and the rate of airflow decreases progressively.

During the maximal inspiration, the pattern of airflow is different: because of the markedly negative pleural pressure and large transmural airway pressure, the bronchi are wide, and their calibers increase further as lung volume increases. Consequently, inspiratory flow becomes high while the lung volume is still low and remains high over much of the vital capacity even though the force generated by the inspiratory muscles decreases as they shorten.

A family of flow-volume loops is produced by repeating full expiratory and inspiratory maneuvers over the entire range of the vital capacity using different levels of effort (Fig. 12-10). The greater the effort exerted during inspiration, the greater is the rate of airflow over the entire

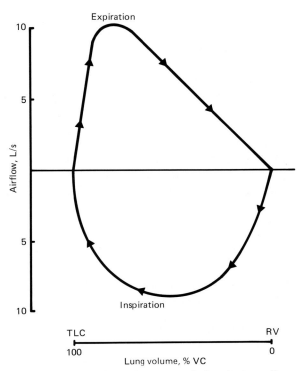

FIGURE 12-9 Maximal expiratory and inspiratory flow-volume loop.

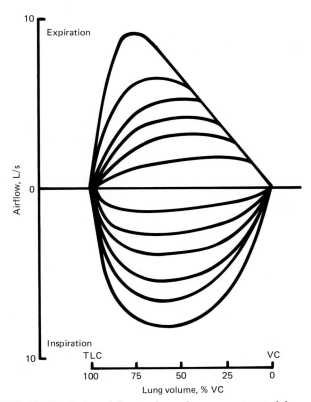

FIGURE 12-10 Series of flow-volume loops constructed from complete inspiratory and expiratory maneuvers repeated at different levels of effort.

range, i.e., from residual volume to total lung capacity. Similarly, during expiration, the rate of airflow increases progressively with increasing effort at large lung volumes close to total lung capacity. At intermediate and low lung volumes, the rate of expiratory airflow reaches a maximum while the effort expended is only moderate; thereafter, airflow does not increase further despite increasing expiratory efforts.

Isovolume Pressure-Flow Curves

Separation of the effects of increasing effort from those of changes in lung volume on the rate of airflow during expiration can be accomplished by using isovolume pressure-flow curves (Fig. 12-11). During repeated expiratory maneuvers performed with various degrees of effort, simultaneous measurements are made of rate of airflow, lung volumes, and pleural pressure. For each lung volume, the rate of airflow is plotted against the pleural pressure, an index of the degree of effort.

As expiratory effort is increased at any given lung volume, the pleural pressure increases toward, and then exceeds, atmospheric pressure; correspondingly, the rate of airflow increases. At lung volumes greater than 75 percent of the vital capacity, airflow increases progressively as pleural pressure increases; it is considered to be *effort-dependent*. In contrast, at lung volumes below 75 percent of the vital capacity, the rate of airflow levels off as the

pleural pressure exceeds atmospheric pressure and becomes fixed at a maximum level. Thereafter, further increases in effort, and in pleural pressure, effect no further increase in the rate of airflow; at these lower lung volumes, airflow is considered to be *effort-independent*. Since the rate of airflow remains constant despite increasing driving pressure, it follows that the resistance to airflow must be increasing in direct proportion to the increase in driving pressure. This increase in resistance is attributed to compression and narrowing of large intrathoracic airways.

Equal Pressure Point Theory: Dynamic Compression of Airways

To illustrate the mechanisms that normally limit airflow during a maximal expiratory maneuver, it is useful to consider a model of the lung where the alveoli are represented by an elastic sac and the intrathoracic airways by a compressible tube, both enclosed within a pleural space (Fig. 12-12).

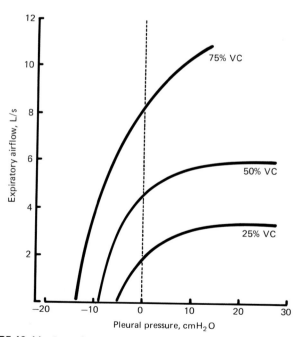

FIGURE 12-11 Isovolumetric pressure-flow curves. At lung volumes greater than 75 percent of the vital capacity, airflow is effort-dependent, i.e., airflow increases progressively with increasing effort. At lower lung volumes, airflow is effort-independent, i.e., airflow becomes fixed at a maximum level and does not increase despite further increases in effort.

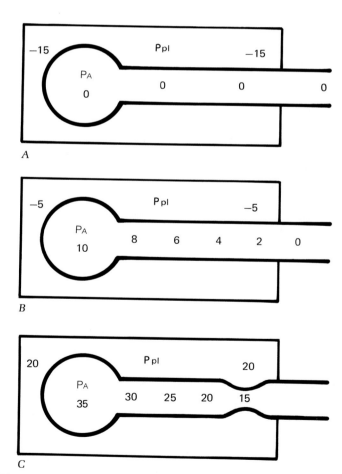

FIGURE 12-12 Schema of the distribution of pleural, alveolar, and airway pressures at rest and during expiration, illustrating the equal pressure point concept. *A.* End-expiration. *B.* Quiet expiration. *C.* Forced expiration.

At a given lung volume, when there is no airflow, pleural pressure is subatmospheric, counterbalancing the elastic recoil pressure of the lung. The alveolar pressure (P_A), which is the sum of the recoil pressure of the lung and pleural pressure (P_{pl}), is zero (Fig. 12-12A). Since airflow has ceased, the pressure along the entire airway is also atmospheric.

At the same lung volume during a *quiet expiration*, pleural pressure is less subatmospheric. Since lung volume and the elastic recoil pressure of the lung are unchanged, alveolar pressure is now positive with respect to atmospheric pressure; airflow occurs. The alveolar pressure is gradually dissipated along the airway in overcoming resistance so that the pressure at the airway opening (P_{ao}) is zero. However, all along the airway, the airway pressure exceeds pleural pressure and the transmural pressure is positive; the airways remain open, and flow continues (Fig. 12-12B).

A *forceful expiration* raises pleural pressure above atmospheric pressure and further increases alveolar pressure (Fig. 12-12C). Airway pressure again falls progressively from the alveolus toward the airway opening. But, at some point along the airway, the *equal pressure point*, the drop in airway pressure is equal to the recoil pressure of the lung; intraluminal pressure and the pressure surrounding the airways are equal and the same as pleural pressure. Downstream, i.e., toward the airway opening, the transmural pressure is negative because the intraluminal airway pressure is less than pleural pressure; the airways are subjected to *dynamic compression*.

The equal pressure point divides the airways into two components arranged in series: an upstream segment, from the alveoli to the equal pressure point, and a downstream segment, from the equal pressure point to the airway opening. Once maximum expiratory flow is achieved, the position of the equal pressure point becomes fixed in the region of the lobar or segmental bronchi. Further increase in pleural pressure by increasing expiratory force simply produces more compression of the downstream segment without affecting airflow through the upstream segment.

The driving pressure of the upstream segment, i.e., the pressure drop along the airways of that segment, is equal to the elastic recoil of the lung. The maximum rate of airflow during forced expiration ($\dot{V}_{max}$) can be expressed in terms of the elastic recoil pressure of the lung (P_L) and the resistance of the upstream segment (R_{us}), as follows:

$$\dot{V}_{max} = \frac{P_L}{R_{us}}$$

Measurements of the rate of airflow during forced expiration form the basis of many tests used to assess the flow-resistive properties of the lung. However, it is evident that the maximum rate of expiratory airflow depends on many factors: the lung volume at which airflow is determined, the force of expiration (particularly at high lung volumes, i.e., above 75 percent of vital capacity), the elastic recoil pressure of the lung, the cross-sectional area of large airways, and the resistance of small peripheral airways.

Wave Speed Limitation Theory

An alternative explanation for airflow limitation during forced expiration is based on principles of wave speed theory. The wave speed theory proposes that flow is limited by the velocity of propagation of pressure waves along the wall of the tube. The velocity of propagation (v) varies proportionally with the cross-sectional area of the tube (A) and the elastance of the tube walls (dP/dA). At a site where the flow rate equals the velocity of propagation of pressure waves, a choke point develops, thereby preventing further increases in flow rate. Where choke points occur in the tracheobronchial tree depends on the lung volume: at large lung volumes, a choke point is situated in the vicinity of the lower trachea; at lower lung volumes, choke points develop more upstream along the bronchial tree. Extension of the neck exerts longitudinal tension and stiffens the trachea, increases wave velocity, and increases maximum expiratory flow rates at large lung volumes.

MECHANICAL DETERMINANTS OF REGIONAL VENTILATION

Pleural pressure in the upright individual is more subatmospheric at the apex than at the base of the lung because of the weight of the lung; the rate of increase in pleural pressure from top to bottom is approximately 0.25 cmH$_2$O per centimeter of vertical distance. Consequently, the transpulmonary pressure, i.e., alveolar pressure minus pleural pressure, is greater at the top than at the bottom of the lung. Therefore, at most lung volumes, the alveoli at the lung apexes are larger (more expanded) than those at the lung bases (Fig. 12-13).

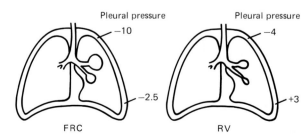

FIGURE 12-13 Pleural pressure gradients in the upright lung at FRC *(left)* and at RV *(right)*. The effect of the gradient on alveolar volumes is shown for each case.

Because of regional variations in lung compliance, ventilation is not uniform, even in the normal lung. By using external scanners after the inhalation of a radioactive gas, such as ^{133}Xe, it has been demonstrated that, within the range of normal tidal volume, lung units are better ventilated, and ventilation per alveolus is greater, at the bottom than at the top of the lung.

At low lung volumes, i.e., near the residual volume, pleural pressure at the bottom of the lung actually exceeds airway pressure and leads to closure of peripheral airways (Fig. 12-13). During a breath taken from residual volume, air that enters the lungs first is preferentially distributed to the lung apexes.

The distribution of ventilation within the lungs and the volume at which airways at the lung bases begin to close can be assessed by the single-breath N_2 washout test (see Chapter 163). This test involves a maximum expiration into an N_2 meter after a maximal inspiration of pure O_2 from residual volume; the changing concentration of nitrogen is plotted against expired lung volume (Fig. 12-14). Because the inspiration starts at the residual volume, the initial portion of the breath containing dead-space gas, rich in nitrogen, is distributed to alveoli in the upper lung zones. The remainder of breath, that contains only O_2, goes preferentially to lower lung zones. Consequently, the concentration of nitrogen is lower in the alveoli at the lung bases than in the alveoli at the apexes of the lungs.

During expiration, the initial portion of the breath consists of O_2 remaining in the large airways; it contains no N_2 (phase I). As alveolar gas containing N_2 begins to be washed out, the concentration of N_2 in the expired air rises to reach a plateau. The portion of the curve where the concentration of nitrogen rises steeply is phase II. The plateau is phase III. Phase III depends on the uniformity of the distribution of ventilation in the lung. If gas enters and leaves alveoli throughout the lung synchronously and equally, phase III is flat. But when the distribution of ventilation is nonuniform, so that gases coming from different alveoli have different N_2 concentration, phase III slopes upward.

At low lung volumes, airways at the lung bases close; only alveoli at the top of the lung continue to empty. Since the concentration of N_2 in the alveoli of upper lung zones is higher than in the alveoli at the lung bases, the slope of the N_2-volume curve increases abruptly, marking the start of phase IV. The volume, above residual volume, at which phase IV begins is the *closing volume*.

Dynamic Compliance of the Lungs

The relationship between changes in volume and changes in pleural pressure during a normal breathing cycle is shown in Fig. 12-15. Airflow momentarily ceases at the end of expiration (A) and at the end of inspiration (C); the change in pleural pressure between these two points reflects the increasing elastic recoil of the lung as the volume of air in the lungs increases. The slope of the line connecting the end-expiratory and end-inspiratory points (AEC in the figure) on a pressure-volume loop provides a measure of the *dynamic compliance* of the lungs.

In normal individuals, dynamic compliance closely approximates inspiratory static lung compliance and remains essentially unchanged even when breathing frequency is increased up to 60 breaths per minute. This indicates that lung units that are parallel with each other

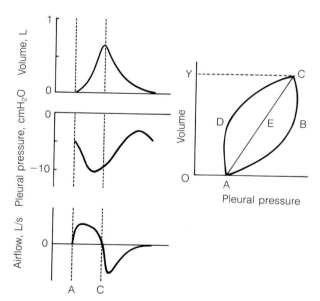

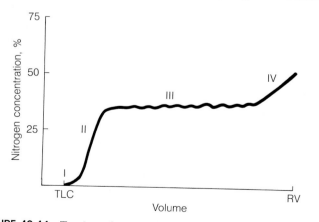

FIGURE 12-14 Tracing of expired nitrogen concentration during a slow expiration from TLC to RV after a full inspiration of pure O_2. The four phases are indicated.

FIGURE 12-15 Individual tracings of tidal volume, pleural pressure, and airflow taken simultaneously during a single complete breath are shown on the left. The relationship between volume and pleural pressure is illustrated by the dynamic pressure-volume loop on the right. Dynamic compliance is determined as the slope of the line AEC. The work of breathing during inspiration to overcome the elastic forces of the lung is represented by the area of the trapezoid OAECY, and the work required to overcome nonelastic forces is represented by the area of the loop ABCEA.

normally fill and empty uniformly and synchronously, even when airflow is high and the change in lung volume is rapid. The rate of filling and emptying of a lung unit depends on its time constant, i.e., the product of its resistance and compliance. In order for the distribution of ventilation in parallel lung units to be independent of the rate of airflow, the resistance and compliance of these units must be matched so that the time constants of individual units throughout the lungs are approximately the same. The time constants of lung units distal to airways 2 mm in diameter are of the order of 0.01 s, and fourfold differences in time constants are necessary to cause dynamic compliance to become frequency-dependent.

Patchy narrowing of small peripheral airways produces regional differences in time constants. At low breathing frequencies, when the rate of airflow is low, ventilation is fairly evenly distributed. However, as the breathing frequency increases, ventilation tends to be distributed to those areas that offer the least resistance to airflow. Therefore, lung units fed by narrowed airways receive proportionally less ventilation than do areas of the lung where the airways remain normal; the change in pleural pressure required to effect the same change in overall lung volume increases. As a result, the dynamic compliance falls.

Measurements of *frequency dependence of dynamic compliance* are time-consuming and technically difficult, but this test has proved useful in the diagnosis of obstruction in small peripheral airways when other conventional tests of lung mechanics are still within normal limits.

WORK AND ENERGY COST OF BREATHING

During breathing, the respiratory muscles do work to overcome the elastic, flow-resistive, and inertial forces of the lungs and chest wall. The elastic work of breathing is done to overcome the elastic recoil of the lungs and chest wall; the resistive work is done in overcoming the resistance of airways and tissues. The mechanical work of breathing can be determined by relating the pressure exerted across the respiratory system to the resulting change in volume, since the product of pressure (P) and volume (V) has the dimension of work, according to the equation

$$\text{Work} = \int P \, dV \qquad (8)$$

Records of pleural pressure and lung volume changes during spontaneous breathing can be used to measure the work of breathing; the work of breathing performed *on* the lungs can be determined from the area of dynamic pressure-volume loop (Fig. 12-15) and fractionated into its elastic and resistive components. During inspiration, the work done to overcome the elastic forces of the lung is determined from the area of the trapezoid OAECY (Fig. 12-15). The area of the loop ABCEA is the work in over-

coming nonelastic forces during inspiration, and the area of the loop OABCY is the total work of breathing during inspiration.

Expiration during quiet breathing is passive since the elastic recoil of the lung suffices to overcome the expiratory airflow resistance. At high levels of ventilation and when airway resistance is increased, additional mechanical work during expiration is required to overcome nonelastic forces. Under these circumstances the pleural pressure exceeds atmospheric pressure, and the loop AECDA extends beyond the confines of the trapezoid OAECY.

Work of Breathing

The work of breathing at any given level of ventilation depends on the pattern of breathing. Large tidal volumes increase the elastic work of breathing, whereas rapid breathing frequencies increase the work against flow-resistive forces. During quiet breathing and during exercise individuals tend to adjust tidal volume and breathing frequency at values that minimize the force and the work of breathing. Similar adjustments are also seen in patients with pulmonary disorders: individuals with pulmonary fibrosis, which is characterized by an increased elastic work of breathing, tend to breathe shallowly and rapidly; those with airway obstruction and increased nonelastic work of breathing usually breathe more deeply and slowly.

The work done on the chest wall during breathing is calculated by subtracting the work performed on the lung from the total mechanical work of breathing. The total mechanical work of breathing cannot be readily measured during spontaneous breathing because the respiratory muscles which perform the work also make up part of the resistance offered by the chest wall. But the total mechanical work can be determined during artificial ventilation by using either intermittent positive airway pressure or negative pressure applied to the chest, provided that the respiratory muscles are completely at rest. For this determination, the change in lung volume is related to the pressure difference across the respiratory system, i.e., differential pressure between the mouth and the body surface. Disturbances of the chest wall such as kyphoscoliosis and obesity usually increase the work of breathing severalfold.

Oxygen Cost of Breathing

In order to perform their work, the respiratory muscles require O_2. The O_2 cost of breathing, which reflects the energy requirements of the respiratory muscles, provides an indirect measure of the work of breathing. The O_2 cost of breathing is assessed by determining the total O_2 consumption of the body at rest and at an increased level of ventilation produced by voluntary hyperventilation or CO_2 breathing. Provided there are no other factors acting to increase O_2 consumption, the added O_2 uptake is attributed to the metabolism of the respiratory muscles.

The O_2 cost of breathing in normal individuals is approximately 1 ml/L of ventilation and constitutes less than 5 percent of the total O_2 consumption. At high levels of ventilation, however, the O_2 cost of breathing becomes progressively greater. There is a dramatic increase in the O_2 cost of breathing at high levels of ventilation in some diseases of the lung, such as pneumonia, pulmonary fibrosis, and emphysema, and in disorders of the chest wall, such as obesity and kyphoscoliosis. The increase in the energy requirement of the respiratory muscles during increased ventilation, concomitant with a decrease in O_2 supply secondary to arterial hypoxemia, probably produces muscle fatigue, thereby limiting the amount of exertion that these patients can sustain.

BIBLIOGRAPHY

Campbell EJM, Agostini E, Davis JN: *The Respiratory Muscles: Mechanics and Neural Control,* 2d ed. Philadelphia, Saunders, 1970.
  Comprehensive review of the contractile properties and mechanical actions of the muscles of respiration.

Clements JA: Surface phenomena in relation to pulmonary function. Physiologist 5:11–28, 1962.
  The surface tension of surfactant stabilizes the lung and prevents atelectasis.

Cournand A, Richards DW, Bader RA, Bader ME, Fishman AP: The oxygen cost of breathing. Trans Assoc Am Phys 67:162–173, 1954.
  The oxygen cost of breathing reflects the oxygen consumption of the muscles of respiration.

Fry DL, Hyatt RE: Pulmonary mechanics: A unified analysis of the relationship between pressure, volume and gas flow in the lungs of normal and diseased human subjects. Am J Med 29:672–689, 1960.
  A description of isovolume pressure-flow curves in health and disease.

Gattinoni L, Pesenti A, Avalli L, Rossi F, Bombino M: Pressure-volume curve of total respiratory system in acute respiratory failure. Computed tomographic scan study. Am Rev Respir Dis 136:730–736, 1987.
  Investigation of the relationship between lung anatomy and pulmonary mechanics in acute respiratory failure suggests that the pressure-volume curve parameters in acute respiratory failure investigate only the residual healthy zones of the lung and do not directly estimate the "amount" of disease (poorly or nonaerated tissue).

Gibson GJ, Pride NB: Lung distensibility: The static pressure-volume curve of the lungs and its use in clinical assessment. Br J Dis Chest 70:143–184, 1976.
  Review of the physiology and clinical evaluation of the elastic properties of the lungs.

Hoppin FG Jr, Hildebrandt J: Mechanical properties of the lung, in West JB (ed), *Lung Biology in Health and Disease,* vol 3, Bioengineering Aspects of the Lung. New York, Dekker, 1978, pp 83–162.
  Detailed review of the mechanical properties of the lung and structural subcomponents, structure-function relationships, and modeling.

Hyatt RE, Black LF: The flow-volume curve: A current perspective. Am Rev Respir Dis 107:191–199, 1973.
  Review of the clinical usefulness of the maximum expiratory flow-volume curve.

Kolobow T, Moretti MP, Fumagalli R, Mascheroni D, Prato P, Chen V, Joris M: Severe impairment in lung function induced by high peak airway pressure during mechanical ventilation. An experimental study. Am Rev Respir Dis 135:312–315, 1987.
  Mechanical ventilation of sheep at peak airway pressure of 50 cm H_2O leads to progressive impairment in pulmonary mechanics.

Macklem PT, Mead J: Resistance of central and peripheral airways measured by a retrograde catheter. J Appl Physiol 22:395–401, 1967.
  Peripheral airways resistance is only a small fraction of the total resistance of the tracheobronchial tree.

Macklem PT, Mead J (eds): *Handbook of Physiology,* sect 3: The Respiratory System, vol 3: Mechanics of Breathing. Bethesda, MD, American Physiological Society, 1986.
  A comprehensive review of current understanding of the mechanics of breathing that explores in considerable depth all of the topics considered in this chapter.

McCarthy DS, Spencer R, Greene R, Milic-Emili J: Measurement of closing volume as a simple and sensitive test for early detection of small airway disease. Am J Med 52:747–753, 1972.
> *Changes on the caliber of small airways can modify the regional distribution of ventilation.*

Mead J: Respiratory flow limitation: A physiologist's point of view. Fed Proc 39:2771–2775, 1980.
> *Review of the tube wave speed theory of airflow limitation.*

Mead J, Takishima T, Leith D: Stress distribution in lungs: A model of pulmonary elasticity. J Appl Physiol 28:596–608, 1970.
> *The peribronchial pressure approximates the pleural pressure.*

Mead J, Turner JM, Macklem PT, Little JB: Significance of the relationship between lung recoil and maximum expiratory flow. J Appl Physiol 22:95–108, 1967.
> *Describes the equal pressure point theory of airflow limitation.*

Milic-Emili J, Henderson JAM, Dolovich MB, Trop D, Kaneko K: Regional distribution of inspired gas in the lung. J Appl Physiol 21:749–759, 1966.
> *The weight of the lung and the effects of gravity contribute to a vertical gradient in pleural pressure.*

Milic-Emili J, Mead J, Turner JM, Glauser EM: Improved technique for estimating pleural pressure from esophageal balloons. J Appl Physiol 19:207–211, 1964.
> *Description of the methods for measuring intrathoracic pressure.*

Mink SN, Wood LDH: How does HeO_2 increase maximum expiratory flow in human lungs. J Clin Invest 66:720–729, 1980.
> *The effects of changing gas density on maximum expiratory flow can be explained by wave speed theory.*

Otis AB: The work of breathing. Physiol Rev 34:449–458, 1954.
> *The mechanical work of breathing can be calculated from dynamic pressure-volume curves of the respiratory system.*

Pride NB: The assessment of airflow obstruction: Role of measurement of airways resistance and tests of forced expiration. Br J Dis Chest 65:135–169, 1971.
> *Review of the physiology of the airways and tests of airway function.*

Rahn H, Otis AB, Chadwick LE, Fenn WO: The pressure-volume diagram of the thorax and lung. Am J Physiol 146:161–178, 1946.
> *A graphic representation of the pressure-volume relationships of the respiratory system.*

Turner JM, Mead J, Wohl ME: Elasticity of human lungs in relation to age. J Appl Physiol 25:664–671, 1968.
> *The elasticity of the lungs progressively falls with advancing age.*

Woolcock AJ, Vincent NJ, Macklem PT: Frequency dependence of compliance as a test for obstruction on the small airways. J Clin Invest 48:1097–1106, 1969.
> *Abnormalities of small airways cause dynamic compliance to fall as breathing frequency increases.*

Chapter *13*

Ventilation, Pulmonary Blood Flow, and Gas Exchange

Robert A. Klocke

The removal of carbon dioxide and provision of oxygen for metabolic needs are dependent on an adequate quantity of ventilation reaching the gas-exchange surface in the lung. Similarly, a sufficient volume of pulmonary blood is required to come into contact with the inspired gas to achieve oxygen and carbon dioxide exchange. Even though the overall quantities of ventilation and pulmonary blood flow are adequate, significant abnormalities in gas exchange may still occur. The distribution of ventilation and blood flow in appropriate quantities to each gas-exchange unit is a crucial requirement for adequate O_2 and CO_2 exchange. Uneven matching of alveolar ventilation $\dot{V}A$ and pulmonary blood flow $\dot{Q}$ at the alveolar level is by far the most common cause of impaired gas exchange.

VENTILATION

Resting ventilatory requirements for gas exchange are approximately 80 ml/min/kg. Under normal circumstances this is accomplished with relatively little energy expenditure, requiring less than 1 ml of oxygen consumption per liter of ventilation. Thus, the oxygen cost of breathing is minimal. Even though the work of breathing per unit ventilation increases modestly, healthy individuals can maintain more than a 10-fold increase in ventilation without difficulty. Hence, a large ventilatory reserve is available, and only extremely severe disease diminishes this capacity to a life-threatening extent. Unfortunately, a large ventilatory reserve provides no guarantee that this inspired volume comes in contact with venous blood in appropriate proportions to permit adequate gas exchange.

Dead Space

Because of the cyclic nature of ventilation, a significant proportion of inspired air never reaches the alveoli but remains in the tracheobronchial tree, only to be exhaled without participating in gas exchange. This portion of the inspired air is termed *anatomic dead space* because it is a consequence of the anatomy of the tracheobronchial tree which mandates to-and-fro ventilation rather than continuous airflow through the lungs. Ventilation of the dead space accounts for a functional loss of approximately one-third of the total ventilation at rest. This fraction decreases to as little as one-tenth of total ventilation with large increases in tidal volume as occurs during exercise. Aside from slight increases associated with increasing tidal volume, anatomic dead space is invariant; it does not change with disease. Hence it plays no causative role in abnormal gas exchange associated with disease.

In contrast, dead-space ventilation of an alveolar nature is an important determinant of deranged blood gases. Normally all ventilation which enters an alveolus exchanges O_2 and CO_2. However, if an alveolus is not perfused with blood, ventilation to this alveolus cannot participate in gas exchange and is wasted; it becomes dead-space ventilation. True alveolar dead space, i.e., ventilation directed to alveoli devoid of all perfusion, probably does exist but is relatively uncommon. A far more likely situation is the hyperventilation of an alveolus relative to its perfusion—excess ventilation beyond that needed to complete respiratory exchange with the blood reaching the alveolus. This circumstance is quite common in disease. For example, in chronic obstructive pulmonary disease the combined total of anatomic and alveolar dead space can rise to one-half to three-fourths of the total inspired ventilation. Excess ventilation to an alveolus is not a complete loss. Although it is of little or no value in terms of oxygen transfer, this ventilation can result in added carbon dioxide excretion. Unfortunately, as the relative excess of ventilation increases, the efficiency of carbon dioxide exchange decreases sharply and a greater proportion of the excess ventilation is wasted.

It is not possible to separate dead-space ventilation into its anatomic and alveolar components without specialized techniques, but this is not important for clinical purposes. Because anatomic dead space is relatively invariant and alveolar dead space is not present to any significant degree under normal circumstances, any increase in dead space by default must result from the presence of alveolar dead space. The two components are usually grouped under the term *physiological dead space*, which is calculated from the CO_2 tensions in arterial blood and mixed expired gas and often expressed as a fraction of the tidal volume:

$$\frac{V_D}{V_T} = \frac{Pa_{CO_2} - Pe_{CO_2}}{Pa_{CO_2}} \qquad (1)$$

Ventilation and Metabolism

The total quantity of ventilation participating in gas exchange is closely linked to metabolism. Normally ventilation rises linearly with corresponding increases in carbon dioxide production. This continues until acidic metabolites from anaerobic pathways of energy production stimulate a further increase in ventilation. This anaerobic threshold normally occurs at a strenuous level of exercise.

The level of metabolic activity and the ventilation effective in removing CO_2 (as opposed to the total expired ventilation) are not easily measured at the bedside. However, their absolute values are less important than their relative relationship which can be easily assessed by measuring arterial P_{CO_2}:

$$\frac{0.863 \, \dot{V}_{CO_2}}{\dot{V}_E (1 - V_D/V_T)} = PA_{CO_2} \approx Pa_{CO_2} \qquad (2)$$

where the term 0.863 is a constant required to express carbon dioxide output $\dot{V}_{CO_2}$, minute ventilation $\dot{V}_E$, and CO_2 tensions in their appropriate units. Equation (2) indicates that the alveolar CO_2 tension PA_{CO_2} reflects the balance between CO_2 production and that portion of the total ventilation which is participating in carbon dioxide exchange. If this effective ventilation increases to match increments of CO_2 production, PA_{CO_2} will remain constant. Unfortunately mean alveolar P_{CO_2} is not easily measured, but for practical purposes it can be assumed to be equal to the arterial P_{CO_2}. This underlies the common usage of the arterial P_{CO_2} as an indicator of the adequacy of ventilation.

Distribution of Ventilation

NORMAL LUNG MECHANICS

Inspired ventilation is not distributed evenly to all gas-exchange units, even in healthy individuals. A number of different factors affect gas distribution, but their effects are relatively small in comparison to abnormalities seen in disease.

Intrapleural Pressure Gradient

With cessation of airflow at end-expiration, alveolar pressure is equal to atmospheric pressure throughout the lungs. Even under normal circumstances there is a vertical gradient of intrapleural pressure within the chest, and pressure surrounding the lung is more negative at the apex of the lung than at the lung base. The distending pressure, the difference between intrapleural pressure and alveolar pressure, is greater at the apex than at the base. Hence, prior to inspiration alveoli at the apex of the lung are relatively more distended and have less potential to be inflated than alveoli at the lung base. As a result, a greater proportion of the inspired breath is distributed to alveoli in the lower portions of the lung.

Airway Closure

During expiration, especially with a maximal effort, small airways in the lung will close and trap gas distal to the point of obstruction. Since the first portion of gas entering alveoli at the start of a breath is inspired from the dead space, alveoli with patent airways initially will receive gas containing CO_2 and possessing an O_2 fraction less than that of inspired air. Alveoli served by airways which open later in inspiration will receive uncontaminated inspired gas. However, since this occurs later in the inspiratory phase, the total volume reaching these airways can be variable. In youth, most airway closure occurs at lung volumes smaller than the functional residual capacity, so that airway closure is not an important factor during normal tidal breathing. However, with advancing age, airway closure occurs at larger lung volumes. In later life, some airways close in the range of normal tidal breathing and affect distribution of ventilation. The lung volume associated with airway closure increases in the supine position. Airway closure occurs in the range of tidal breathing in middle-aged individuals in this posture.

ABNORMAL LUNG MECHANICS

Distortion of the mechanical properties of the lung results in far greater variation in distribution of ventilation. Although the abnormalities in pulmonary mechanics are important in affecting total lung performance, a major factor in determining the distribution of ventilation is the uniformity of changes throughout lung as opposed to the relative degree of the global abnormality. For example, a doubling of total airway resistance will have no appreciable effect on gas distribution throughout the lung if all airways are affected equally. However, if this relatively modest increase in airway resistance is the result of more severe changes in several locations in the tracheobronchial tree, marked nonuniformity of gas distribution will occur.

Altered Resistance or Compliance

Under ideal circumstances when the lung is exposed to an increased intrapleural pressure, all units expand to an equal end-inspiratory volume with the same rate of volume change. As indicated in Fig. 13-1, lung units A and B have normal mechanical properties and both have an equal volume change with time after application of a distending pressure t_0. Even if the inspiratory effort is terminated prior to maximum lung distention t_1, both units have received equal quantities of the inspirate. However, if airway resistance is greater in one unit (C) than another (D), the rate of volume change is substantially less. If the duration of inspiration is sufficiently long t_3, both units will receive the same ventilation. However, shorter inspiratory times (t_1 and t_2) lead to significant reductions in the volume of inspirate directed to unit C. In the case of uniform airway resistance but altered local compliance (unit F in Fig. 13-1), the volume delivered to the abnormal unit (F) is less than that reaching the normal unit (E) at any time during inspiration (t_1, t_2, or t_3). This is the result of the decreased distensibility of the unit with the abnormal compliance.

Altered Time Constants

When both airway resistance and compliance are abnormal, distribution of ventilation becomes more complex. The bottom panel in Fig. 13-1 depicts one lung unit with increased airway resistance (G) and another with decreased compliance (H). With a very prolonged inspiratory effort (t_3), more of the inspired volume will reach the unit with the greater compliance (G), as long as inspiration is long enough to overcome the effect of abnormal airway resistance. With a short inspiratory time (t_1), the effect of the increased airways resistance in unit G predominates and unit H receives more of the inspirate despite its lower compliance. Finally at an intermediate inspiratory time (t_2), the two abnormalities are balanced and both units receive the same quantity of the inspired gas.

The actual rate of alveolar filling in any single lung unit is determined by the interaction of its own airway resistance and compliance. The product of the two factors, termed the time constant since it has the units of time (seconds), determines the rate of alveolar filling (as well as emptying) during respiration. The situation is even more complicated because intrapleural pressure does not change in a stepwise fashion, as assumed in this simple illustration, but rather occurs as a cyclical process. Hence, it is possible that units with markedly different physical properties may be in different respiratory phases simultaneously during rapid changes in intrapleural pressure. This process of alveolar gas leaving one unit to enter another is known as *pendelluft*.

Even diseases which appear to involve the lung in a uniform manner as assessed macroscopically by the radiograph may have substantial variation on a microscopic level. With local alteration of mechanical properties, it is not surprising that inspired ventilation can be distributed to gas-exchange units in a nonuniform manner.

Evidence for Uneven Distribution

Nonuniform distribution of ventilation can be documented by a number of means. Radioactive xenon ventilatory scans have been used to demonstrate macroscopic ventilatory defects to aid in the interpretation of perfusion lung scans. Ventilation lung scans from patients with severe chronic obstructive lung disease provide convincing evidence of nonuniform distribution of ventilation even on a macroscopic level.

In the pulmonary laboratory, assessment of the uniformity of ventilation is usually accomplished with single-breath or multiple-breath nitrogen washouts. In the single-breath test, a maximal inspiration of oxygen is followed by a slow complete expiration with simultaneous measurement of expired volume and nitrogen concentra-

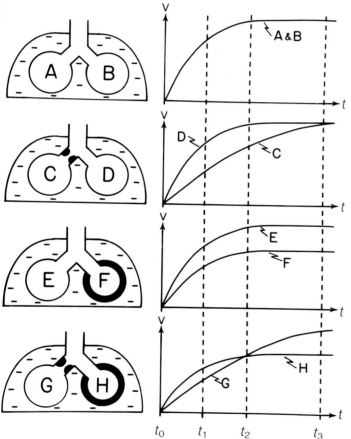

FIGURE 13-1 Effect of mechanical properties on the time course of changes in alveolar volume after the lung is exposed to a negative distending pressure. *Top panel*, alveoli A and B have similar mechanical properties and expand uniformly. *Second panel*, alveolus C has increased local airway resistance which delays alveolar filling compared to the normal alveolus (D). *Third panel*, alveolus F is less compliant. At any point in time it is less distended than the normal alveolus (E). *Bottom panel*, effects of altered resistance (G) and compliance (H) on alveolar expansion. In the graphs, V represents volume and t is time. t_0 is the time of application of the distending pressure and t_1, t_2, and t_3 represent inspiratory times of different duration.

tion at the mouth. The change in nitrogen concentration during expiration of alveolar gas (slope of phase III) and the closing volume (the lung volume at which airway closure takes place) are both utilized to provide an estimation of uniformity. In multiple-breath tests, the rate of dilution of nitrogen (or any other insoluble inert gas) over several minutes also provides an index of the uniformity of gas distribution.

PULMONARY BLOOD FLOW

Similar to the ventilatory reserve, blood flow can increase substantially under normal circumstances to meet body demands. Although blood flow increases with increasing workloads during exercise, it does not exactly parallel changes in ventilation. Ventilation tracks increases in oxygen uptake and carbon dioxide output almost linearly below the anaerobic threshold. On the other hand, oxygen consumption (and carbon dioxide excretion) are maintained at the tissue level by an increase in the arteriovenous content difference as well as an increase in perfusion. In the normal individual this change in mixed venous O_2 and CO_2 are without sequelae, but this is not the case in disease. The effect of any abnormality of pulmonary gas exchange on arterial blood gases is exaggerated by an increased arteriovenous difference.

Compared to the systemic circulation, the pulmonary circulation is a low-pressure conduit. Right ventricular and pulmonary arterial pressures are considerably lower than those seen in their analogues in the systemic circulation. The relative distribution of resistance throughout the various portions of the pulmonary circuit is also quite different from that of its systemic counterpart. Arterial resistance accounts for perhaps one-half or less of the total resistance in the pulmonary circuit. The low resistance in the pulmonary arteries is responsible for transmission of the pulsatile output of the right ventricle all the way to the capillaries. Capillary flow is not only pulsatile, but even ceases momentarily at end diastole in the presence of normal pulmonary pressures and heart rates. The veins as well as capillaries have been demonstrated to offer significant resistance to pulmonary blood flow. This relatively large element of postarteriolar resistance does not normally cause difficulties with transudation of fluid at the capillary level since pressures are low throughout the circuit.

Shunting

In contrast to the cyclic nature of ventilation, pulmonary blood flow is continuous. As a result, there is no large component of perfusion which does not participate in gas exchange in a manner analogous to anatomic dead space.

The closest parallel is shunting of mixed venous blood into the systemic circulation.

EXTRAPULMONARY SHUNTING

The bronchial and thebesian drainage enter the circulation at points distal to the pulmonary gas-exchange vessels, thereby reducing oxygen saturation in systemic blood. Normally this drainage is less than 1 percent of the entire cardiac output, and its effect on arterial blood gases is minimal. The quantity of bronchial drainage can increase in diseases such as bronchiectasis, but it still does not constitute a major problem. Arterial desaturation resulting from abnormalities in pulmonary gas exchange constitutes a far greater problem.

Abnormal connections between the pulmonary and systemic circulations can cause significant hypoxemia. These are most common in congenital cardiac defects such as atrial or ventricular septal defects. These abnormalities are more frequent in pediatric patients and are rare in adults. Although shunting from the hepatic circulation into the bronchial venous drainage has been implicated as a cause of desaturation in cirrhosis of the liver, it is now believed that most hypoxemia seen in these patients results from ventilation-perfusion mismatching.

INTRAPULMONARY SHUNTING

Intrapulmonary shunting is almost nonexistent in healthy individuals. On the other hand, this type of shunting is a major problem in disease. In adult respiratory distress syndrome, for example, as much as 50 percent of the cardiac output can be shunted. For practical purposes, intrapulmonary shunting takes place only at the capillary level. Shunting occurs between arteries and veins in hereditary hemorrhagic telangiectasia, but this seldom causes significant hypoxemia.

Collapse and/or filling of alveoli with fluid in the presence of continued perfusion of alveolar capillaries causes intrapulmonary shunting. A gas-exchange unit which is completely devoid of ventilation will not remain patent because the remaining alveolar gases, including nitrogen, will be absorbed by blood perfusing the alveolus. If an alveolus is perfused but has a sufficient amount of ventilation to prevent collapse, it is more properly grouped as a ventilation-perfusion abnormality rather than as a shunt. Even though both situations produce hypoxemia, the distinction is not merely semantic but has practical importance. In the presence of a true shunt, administration of even large quantities of oxygen has little effect in overcoming the desaturation resulting from the abnormality. In contrast, even a small increase in the inspired oxygen concentration leads to significant improvement when arterial desaturation results from ventilation-perfusion mismatching.

Distribution of Perfusion

EFFECT OF GRAVITY

Gravity results in a nonuniform distribution of perfusion in the vertical direction. In general, perfusion increases from the top to the bottom of the lung, but this increase is not linearly related to the change in vertical distance.

Zone I

Perfusion of lung tissue is dependent on the interrelationships between alveolar, arterial, and venous pressures. As noted previously, the pulmonary circulation is normally a low-pressure circuit. Blood must be pumped as high as the apex of the lung, a distance of 15 to 20 cm above the heart. Since blood has a specific gravity similar to water, a hydrostatic pressure of approximately 15 to 20 cm of water must be overcome for blood to reach the lung apex in the standing position. Thus, in the presence of normal pulmonary arterial pressures (measured at the level of the heart), the pressure in pulmonary arteries in the upper portions of the lung reaches zero (atmospheric pressure). The pulmonary capillaries are exposed not only to pressure from the arterial circuit but also to alveolar pressure. Since these vessels have little structural support, the capillaries will be squeezed shut, and flow ceases when alveolar pressure exceeds arterial pressure. In this portion of the lung, termed zone I, there is no flow because alveolar pressure is greater than arterial pressure (Fig. 13-2). Pulmonary venous pressure plays no role in lung perfusion under zone I conditions. The pulmonary veins enter the left atrium where normally the pressure is approximately atmospheric. Because of the hydrostatic gradient in vascular pressure down the lung, venous pressure at the apex is less than atmospheric and has no effect on control of blood flow.

In reality there can be some flow in zone I for two reasons. First, small pulmonary vessels located at the junction of alveolar walls, so-called corner vessels, are probably not exposed to alveolar pressure alone. It has been postulated that the pressure surrounding these vessels is lower than alveolar pressure owing to the effect of forces which tend to maintain alveolar patency and stability. Indirect evidence supports the concept of flow through corner vessels when alveolar pressure exceeds arterial pressure. Second, pulmonary pressure and flow are pulsatile. The high peak vascular pressure caused by systole is partially transmitted to the capillaries, temporarily causing vascular pressure in the capillaries to exceed alveolar pressure. Current experimental evidence favors the accommodation of pulsatile flow in the pulmonary circulation by two mechanisms—the recruitment of capillaries that previously were not perfused and a transient increase in the rate of flow through the capillaries which are already patent.

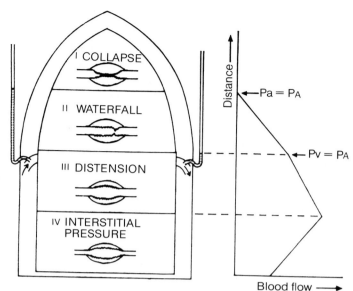

FIGURE 13-2 Four zones of lung perfusion. Zone I has no flow because alveolar pressure exceeds pulmonary arterial pressure, thereby collapsing alveolar vessels. Zone II is present when pulmonary arterial pressure exceeds alveolar pressure and both are greater than pulmonary venous pressure. This is termed the *vascular waterfall* since flow is unaffected by downstream (pulmonary venous) pressure. Zone III is characterized by a constant driving force, the difference between pulmonary arterial and venous pressures. Both are greater than alveolar pressure. Flow increases throughout zone III, even though driving pressure is constant because the absolute pressures lower in the lung distend the vessels to a greater extent, thereby lowering resistance. Zone IV has less flow per unit lung volume for reasons still to be determined. *(From Hughes, Glazier, Maloney, and West, by permission of Respiration Physiology.)*

Zone II

Alveolar pressure is uniform throughout the lung. On the other hand, the local arterial pressure increases from the top to the bottom of the lung because of the hydrostatic gradient produced by the column of blood in the arterial tree extending from apex to base. As the vertical distance above the level of the heart decreases, local arterial pressure increases and finally exceeds alveolar pressure (zone II). Under these circumstances, blood flow is controlled by the difference between arterial and alveolar pressures. Venous pressure still has no effect on flow because it remains subatmospheric at this point in the lung. Perfusion then increases dramatically in a linear fashion with decreasing vertical height because arterial pressure increases linearly with distance but alveolar pressure remains constant. Hence, the driving pressure for flow (Ppa − PA) increases rapidly with decreasing height, and local perfusion follows the same pattern.

Zone III

Eventually, pulmonary venous pressure exceeds atmospheric pressure as vertical height decreases and pressure increases owing to the hydrostatic gradient in the venous side of the circulation. Under these conditions (zone III), both arterial and venous pressure exceed alveolar pressure, and the driving pressure for flow becomes the difference between the two (Ppa − Ppv). Below this point, this driving pressure remains constant. Both Ppa and Ppv increase in direct proportion to the decrease in vertical distance, but their difference remains constant. However, experimental data indicate that pulmonary blood flow increases linearly with decreasing vertical distance under zone III conditions, although the increase may occur at a lower rate than in zone II. Despite the lack of any change in driving pressure in zone III, absolute arterial and venous pressures are greater closer to the lung base. It is thought that these greater absolute pressures cause dilatation of pulmonary vasculature so that greater flow can be achieved with the same difference between Ppa and Ppv.

Zone IV

Investigators have noted a decrease in perfusion at the lung bases and have termed this area zone IV. The size of zone IV increases as lung volume decreases, being greatest at residual volume. The cause for this decreased perfusion is not readily apparent. Speculation attributes its presence to increased interstitial pressure resulting from fluid transudation. Increased interstitial pressure could conceivably cause narrowing of extra-alveolar arteries, thus leading to the decreased flow. The connective tissue framework of the lung may also provide varying support to extra-alveolar vessels as lung volume changes. The exact mechanism underlying the occurrence of zone IV conditions remains unknown.

Effect of Posture

The vertical distance between the top and bottom of the lung is decreased in the supine position. Because the uppermost part of the lung is closer to the heart under these circumstances, arterial pressures usually exceed alveolar pressure in all areas of the lung and zone I no longer exists. Zone II also will be smaller since venous pressure is higher throughout the lung owing to the smaller vertical distance between the uppermost part of the lung and the heart. With increased left atrial (and hence, pulmonary venous) pressure in cardiac failure, zone II may cease to exist also. This is particularly important since accurate assessment of left atrial pressure using the capillary wedge pressure measurement requires that the balloon catheter be placed in a zone II condition. The effect of the supine position on vertical lung height reduces the possible significance of this problem. However, use of positive end-expiratory pressure in ventilated patients or continuous positive airway pressure in patients breathing spontaneously will increase alveolar pressure. If alveolar pressure rises to a value greater than local arterial or venous pressures, zone I and zone II conditions may exist even in supine patients.

HYPOXIC VASOCONSTRICTION

Hypoxia, as occurs with exposure to extreme altitude or severe lack of ventilation, causes vasoconstriction and pulmonary hypertension. This places an increased afterload on the right ventricle and can lead to cor pulmonale and cardiac failure.

In contrast to this global response, local hypoxic vasoconstriction may be beneficial in regulating pulmonary gas exchange. A local decrease in ventilation reduces the ratio of ventilation to perfusion in that area. The resulting decrease in alveolar and end-capillary oxygen tensions contributes to arterial hypoxemia. However, the local reduction in P_{O_2}, even in subdivisions of the lung as small as the primary lobule, leads to local hypoxic vasoconstriction. With an increase in local vascular resistance, blood flow to the area is reduced and diverted to other areas of the lung. The net result of this negative feedback between local oxygen tension and local perfusion is a partial correction of the initial ventilation-perfusion disturbance and improvement in arterial hypoxemia.

Thus, local, as opposed to generalized, hypoxic vasoconstriction is an important compensatory mechanism to correct abnormalities in matching of pulmonary blood flow to alveolar ventilation. If this feedback mechanism worked perfectly, ventilation-perfusion mismatching would not exist. Unfortunately this is not the case. Animal experiments indicate that maximum benefit appears to be achieved in gas-exchange units with moderate reduction of the ventilation-perfusion ratio. Marked reductions in ventilation do not appear to be corrected as well. Information concerning the adequacy of this compensatory process in disease states is totally lacking. The classic extreme of type A ("pink puffer") and type B ("blue bloater") chronic obstructive pulmonary disease are excellent examples of severe disease in which ventilation-perfusion adjustments are adequate to prevent hypoxemia in one case and inadequate in the other. There is no clear-cut explanation for this variability of compensatory mechanisms.

PRIMARY VASCULAR DISEASE

Although mismatching of ventilation and blood flow is often viewed as a problem caused by abnormal distribution of ventilation, disruption of either parameter leads to abnormal gas exchange. In most lung diseases, structural changes in both airways and the vasculature occur, although damage may be greater to one of the two. Pulmonary embolism is the classic example of primary vascular disease affecting the distribution of blood flow. Other predominantly vascular diseases include Wegener's granulomatosis and infarction accompanying sickle cell crisis. However, the vasculature is more commonly affected by diseases that involve the interstitium and are not viewed as "vascular diseases." Interstitial fibrosis of unknown etiology [usual interstitial fibrosis (UIP)] and the collagen vascular diseases can severely disrupt perfusion and lead to altered distribution of pulmonary blood flow. Practically any disease distorting lung structure can lead to uneven perfusion of the pulmonary capillary bed.

$\dot{V}_A/\dot{Q}$ AND GAS EXCHANGE

The major function of the lung is to bring inspired air and mixed venous blood together to achieve exchange of oxygen and carbon dioxide. The characteristics of the ventilatory input into this system can be improved to some extent since the inspired oxygen concentration can be altered. Nothing can be done from the standpoint of carbon dioxide since inspired air is already free of CO_2. The composition of mixed venous blood is beyond ready control. O_2 and CO_2 contents of venous blood are functions of metabolism and cardiac output. Thus, aside from manipulating the inspired oxygen fraction, there is no ability to control the inputs into the system.

The outputs of the respiratory system, expired gas, and arterial blood reflect the efficacy of the lung as an organ of gas exchange. Expired gas is contaminated by dead-space ventilation and does not have a uniform composition throughout expiration. It does not provide much helpful information concerning gas exchange. The oxygen and carbon dioxide tensions of arterial blood are the best indicators of the efficiency of exchange between inspired air and mixed venous blood. Moreover, these tensions indicate the composition of blood delivered to the tissues, a major item of interest.

Overall Ventilation and Perfusion

NORMAL VALUES

Under normal resting conditions alveolar ventilation $\dot{V}_A$ and pulmonary blood flow $\dot{Q}$ are approximately equal, the normal overall $\dot{V}_A/\dot{Q}$ ratio being 0.85 to 0.9. With exercise, ventilation keeps pace with metabolic requirements, but blood flow lags behind. As a result, the overall $\dot{V}_A/\dot{Q}$ ratio may increase to a value as high as 3 to 4 during severe exercise. The linking of alveolar ventilation to metabolic requirements is essential to keep arterial blood O_2 and CO_2 tensions normal. The relatively smaller increment in blood flow during exercise results in higher P_{CO_2} and lower P_{O_2} in mixed venous blood, reflecting altered tissue-gas tensions which are usually tolerated without difficulty. Even though blood flow does not parallel increases in metabolic requirements, arterial blood gases remain normal as long as ventilation keeps pace with alterations in metabolism.

ALTERED VENTILATION AND PERFUSION

A decrease in ventilation (relative to metabolism) causes an increase in alveolar, and hence arterial, P_{CO_2} [see Eq.

(2)]. There is a concomitant fall in the respective oxygen tensions. If ventilation increases, the changes in gas tensions proceed in the opposite directions. These changes occur regardless of any alterations in cardiac output. In the normal lung, for any given metabolic state, alveolar and arterial gas tensions are determined by the magnitude of alveolar ventilation.

Alterations in cardiac output are primarily reflected in mixed venous gas tensions. A reduction in blood flow without a concomitant reduction in metabolism results in lower O_2 and higher CO_2 tissue tensions. The opposite occurs with an increase in blood flow. Alterations in blood flow produce a primary effect on tissue tensions which are reflected in mixed venous blood. Changes in overall perfusion affect arterial blood gases only in an indirect manner, as opposed to the direct effects of ventilatory changes. If alveolar ventilation is appropriate and gas exchange proceeds in a normal fashion, arterial blood gases remain normal regardless of the cardiac output or the mixed venous gas tensions. These latter variables may affect peripheral tissue metabolism and performance, but they have no effect on arterial blood-gas tensions. For this reason arterial blood gases remain essentially normal during strenuous submaximal exercise. In disease states accompanied by abnormal pulmonary gas transfer, cardiac output and metabolism will indirectly affect arterial blood gases through their effects on mixed venous blood composition. The effect of any impairment of gas exchange on arterial blood gases is exacerbated by abnormal mixed venous values.

Extremes of $\dot{V}_A/\dot{Q}$ Mismatching

When ventilation and pulmonary blood flow are distributed in approximately equal quantities to a gas-exchange unit, alveolar and end-capillary P_{O_2} and P_{CO_2} are approximately 100 and 40 mmHg, respectively. If ventilation and perfusion are not matched evenly, gas tensions will become abnormal. The two limiting extremes are represented by alveoli with a complete lack of either ventilation or perfusion.

In the event that an alveolus is ventilated but receives no perfusion, the ratio of ventilation to blood flow is infinite. Because the inspired air does not come in contact with mixed venous blood, there is no uptake of O_2 from the alveolar gas and release of CO_2 into the alveolar space. Thus, with a $\dot{V}_A/\dot{Q}$ of infinity no exchange takes place, and alveolar gas has the same tensions as the inspired gas.

The other extreme is a gas-exchange unit which is perfused but not ventilated ($\dot{V}_A/\dot{Q} = 0$). The lack of inspired air bringing oxygen into the unit precludes any change in O_2 tension in blood perfusing the exchange unit. Similarly, CO_2 tensions in blood and alveolar gas remain unchanged because inspired gas does not reach the alveolus. Under these circumstances blood leaves the unit without alteration, and the alveolar and end-capillary gas tensions are the same as those in mixed venous blood.

Spectrum of $\dot{V}_A/\dot{Q}$ Mismatching

The two extremes of mismatching of ventilation and pulmonary blood flow result in O_2 and CO_2 tensions in an exchange unit which are identical to those of the inputs into the respiratory system—inspired air ($\dot{V}_A/\dot{Q} = \infty$) and mixed venous blood ($\dot{V}_A/\dot{Q} = 0$). These extreme deviations from the normal $\dot{V}_A/\dot{Q}$ relationship are relatively uncommon. However, particularly in disease, mismatching of a lesser degree is extremely common.

When $\dot{V}_A/\dot{Q}$ is increased above unity, the O_2 tension in a gas-exchange unit rises above normal, while the P_{CO_2} falls (Fig. 13-3). As the mismatch worsens and $\dot{V}_A/\dot{Q}$ increases further, the gas tensions bear a closer resemblance to those in the inspired gas. Thus, the possible gas tensions in alveoli with $\dot{V}_A/\dot{Q}$ greater than unity range from normal arterial values to those present in the inspired gas. The degree of mismatching determines the extent of the derangement of the P_{O_2} and P_{CO_2}. As $\dot{V}_A/\dot{Q}$ increases, the P_{O_2} and P_{CO_2} progress toward the inspired values in a monotonic manner (Fig. 13-3).

Similar effects occur when ventilation-perfusion relationships are less than unity, although the changes occur in opposite directions. With decreasing $\dot{V}_A/\dot{Q}$ in an exchange unit, the oxygen tension falls and the carbon dioxide tension rises (Fig. 13-3). As the disparity in matching becomes greater and the $\dot{V}_A/\dot{Q}$ moves from unity toward a value of zero, O_2 and CO_2 pressures no longer are identical to normal tensions but more closely resemble those of mixed venous blood.

Thus the range of P_{O_2} and P_{CO_2} throughout the lung can vary between those of inspired gas to the tensions present in mixed venous blood. The exact P_{O_2} and P_{CO_2} of end-capillary blood in any single gas-exchange unit is determined by the matching of ventilation and blood flow in that unit. Deviations from uniform distribution of ventilation and blood flow result in deviations of P_{O_2} and P_{CO_2} from normal values.

Blood O_2 and CO_2 Contents

Oxygen and carbon dioxide pressures in the gas phase are directly proportional to the O_2 and CO_2 content of the gas. For example, the P_{O_2} in room air (21% oxygen) at sea level is 150 mmHg. Doubling the concentration of oxygen to 42% results in a doubling of the P_{O_2} to 300 mmHg. In contrast, the relationships between O_2 and CO_2 tensions and contents in blood are not linear. The P_{O_2} and P_{CO_2} in the lung determine the contents of the two gases in blood. Thus ventilation-perfusion mismatching will have profound effects on blood O_2 and CO_2 contents by altering the alveolar tensions of these gases.

$\dot{V}_A/\dot{Q}$ ratios less than normal lower the P_{O_2} in blood leaving these alveoli (Fig. 13-3). As illustrated in Fig. 13-4, lower $\dot{V}_A/\dot{Q}$ also decreases blood oxygen content, although the relationship is not proportional to the effect on P_{O_2} because of the sigmoid shape of the oxygen dissociation curve. At elevated $\dot{V}_A/\dot{Q}$ the P_{O_2} increases, but there is minimal effect on O_2 content because hemoglobin is

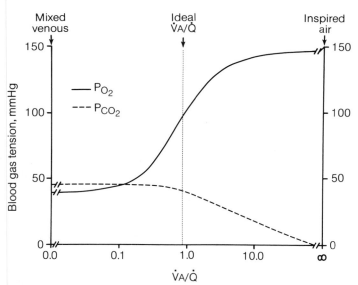

FIGURE 13-3   Effect of the matching of ventilation and blood flow on P_{O_2} and P_{CO_2} in an alveolus and its end-capillary blood. Under ideal circumstances, P_{O_2} and P_{CO_2} are equal to normal arterial values. As $\dot{V}_A/\dot{Q}$ decreases or increases, the gas tensions more closely resemble those in mixed venous blood or inspired air, respectively.

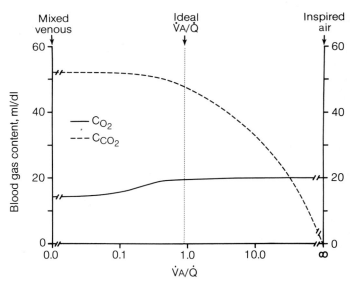

FIGURE 13-4   Effect of the matching of ventilation and blood flow on O_2 and C_{O_2} content of end-capillary blood. Under ideal circumstances the gas contents have normal arterial values. As $\dot{V}_A/\dot{Q}$ decreases or increases, the respective gas contents more closely resemble those seen in mixed venous blood or blood exposed to inspired air.

almost completely saturated above a normal P_{O_2}. Hence, the predominant effect on blood oxygen content of altered matching of ventilation and pulmonary blood flow is seen with low $\dot{V}_A/\dot{Q}$. There is almost no effect at $\dot{V}_A/\dot{Q}$ higher than normal.

In the case of carbon dioxide, the situation is quite different. Elevation of the $\dot{V}_A/\dot{Q}$ above normal decreases both CO_2 tension (Fig. 13-3) and content (Fig. 13-4) in a similar fashion because of the relatively linear nature of the carbon dioxide dissociation curve. Below the normal value, abnormal $\dot{V}_A/\dot{Q}$ relationships lead to an increased P_{CO_2} and CO_2 content in blood, but the effect of the deviation from the ideal value is much less than that seen with elevation of the $\dot{V}_A/\dot{Q}$. As a result, nonuniformity of matching has a proportionately greater effect on CO_2 exchange at higher $\dot{V}_A/\dot{Q}$ as compared to lower values. Although the relative effect of mismatching on blood CO_2 content is smaller at lower $\dot{V}_A/\dot{Q}$, these units still have significant effects on carbon dioxide exchange. Retention of CO_2 above the normal arterial value in blood leaving units with low $\dot{V}_A/\dot{Q}$ leads to hypercapnia unless a corresponding amount of carbon dioxide is excreted elsewhere in the lung.

Normal Dispersion of $\dot{V}_A/\dot{Q}$

Even in the normal lung, ventilation and blood flow are not distributed uniformly. The vertical gradient of intrapleural pressure dictates that the ventilation per unit lung volume increases from the top to the bottom of the lung. The gravity-dependent distribution of perfusion in zones I, II, and III also results in an increase in perfusion from the top to the bottom of the lung. Figure 13-5 illustrates the change in both ventilation and pulmonary blood flow per unit of lung volume. With decreasing vertical distance, there are increases in both ventilation and blood flow, but the relative increase in ventilation is less than the alteration in perfusion. As a result, the ratio of ventilation to pulmonary blood flow decreases from a value greater than normal at the top of the lung to a ratio less than normal at the bottom. Fortunately, the effect of these changes on gas exchange are minimal; arterial oxygen tension is only a few millimeters of mercury less than what would be expected with completely uniform distribution of $\dot{V}_A/\dot{Q}$.

The distribution of the ventilation–blood-flow relationship is illustrated in a topographic fashion in Fig. 13-5. Since nonuniform $\dot{V}_A/\dot{Q}$ distribution in disease may not be dependent strictly on the location of an exchange unit in the lung, it is convenient to express nonuniformity in a statistical manner. Figure 13-6 presents this type of data obtained from a normal individual using the inert gas method of Wagner, West, and their colleagues. A wide range of possible ventilation-perfusion ratios is shown on

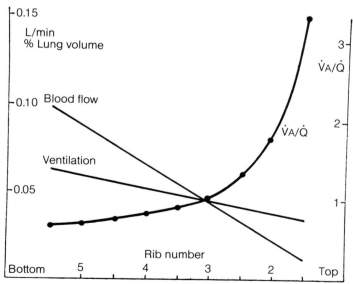

FIGURE 13-5 Effect of vertical height (expressed as the level of the anterior ends of the ribs) on ventilation and pulmonary blood flow (left-hand ordinate) and the ventilation-perfusion ratio (right-hand ordinate). *(From West, by permission of Blackwell Scientific Publications.)*

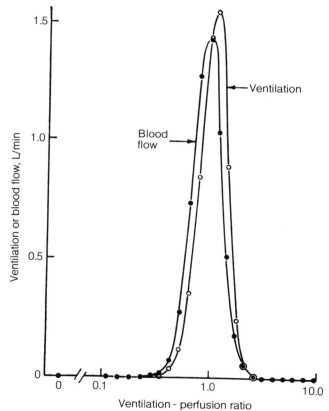

FIGURE 13-6 Distribution of ventilation (open circles) and blood flow (closed circles) to alveoli with different ventilation-perfusion ratios in a normal individual. *(From Wagner, Laravuso, Uhl, West; reproduced from The Journal of Clinical Investigation 54:54–68, 1974, by copyright permission of the American Society for Clinical Investigation.)*

the abscissa. The quantity of ventilation or blood flow directed toward alveoli with these $\dot{V}_A/\dot{Q}$ is plotted on the ordinate. As noted in the figure, all perfusion is directed to units with $\dot{V}_A/\dot{Q}$ grouped around the normal value. No shunt is present. The majority of inspired ventilation is also directed to normal units. This represents alveolar ventilation. The ventilation of the anatomic dead space is not shown in this figure. In addition to the ventilation shown, a portion of the total ventilation entered the tracheobronchial tree but did not reach the alveoli.

$\dot{V}_A/\dot{Q}$ Distribution in Disease

Mismatching of ventilation and pulmonary blood flow is by far the most common cause of hypoxemia. In contrast to the minimal dispersion of $\dot{V}_A/\dot{Q}$ seen in normal individuals as a result of the effect of gravity, nonuniformity of matching in disease is quite severe and can lead to life-threatening hypoxemia. This nonuniformity occurs throughout the lung and is not gravity-dependent. Most frequently these abnormalities are the result of an altered distribution of ventilation caused by abnormal mechanical properties of the lung. Figure 13-7 illustrates the distribution of ventilation and blood flow in six patients with chronic obstructive pulmonary disease. A large segment of perfusion in these patients is directed toward units with relatively normal $\dot{V}_A/\dot{Q}$. However, a significant amount of perfusion also reaches units with abnormally low ventilation-perfusion ratios. Ventilation is also distributed in a nonuniform manner. A large quantity of ventilation reaches alveoli with elevated $\dot{V}_A/\dot{Q}$, as indicated by the large peaks in the right-hand portions of the distributions. As would be expected with alveoli having high $\dot{V}_A/\dot{Q}$, there is relatively little perfusion accompanying these peaks of ventilation. The patients in these examples, like most patients with chronic obstructive lung disease, exhibit a very small shunt. Only two patients had any shunt; one of these was relatively large (12.4 percent of cardiac output). The hypoxemia seen in these patients (mean Pa_{O_2} = 52 mmHg) is predominantly the result of uneven distribution of ventilation with respect to blood flow. Shunting contributes little to the arterial hypoxemia. Figure 13-7 is only one type of $\dot{V}_A/\dot{Q}$ mismatching; a wide variety of patterns are seen in chronic obstructive pulmonary disease.

HYPOXEMIA

Hypoxemia is produced by alveoli with low ventilation–blood-flow relationships. Once such alveoli are present in the lung, hypoxemia is inevitable. The presence of alveoli with elevated ratios cannot compensate for units with low $\dot{V}_A/\dot{Q}$. The reason for this is seen in Fig. 13-8. Both the O_2 and CO_2 dissociation curves are plotted in the figure. The oxygen dissociation curve is sigmoid and essentially flat above a P_{O_2} of 80 to 90 mmHg. Blood leaving alveoli having low $\dot{V}_A/\dot{Q}$ (A in Fig. 13-8) is characterized by a reduced P_{O_2} and O_2 content. Although oxygen tension is elevated in blood leaving units with elevated $\dot{V}_A/\dot{Q}$ (B in Fig. 13-8) oxygen content is not increased substantially (Fig. 13-4) because hemoglobin is already fully saturated. Mixture of blood with normal (B) and reduced (A) O_2 content results in an arterial O_2 content (and pressure) which is lower than normal. Hence, once blood leaves an alveolus with low $\dot{V}_A/\dot{Q}$, the arterial P_{O_2} will be less than normal. The degree of hypoxemia is dependent only on the degree of $\dot{V}_A/\dot{Q}$ inequality and the quantity of blood perfusing the areas with low $\dot{V}_A/\dot{Q}$.

HYPERCAPNIA

In contrast, CO_2 retention is relatively uncommon in ventilation-perfusion mismatching. Blood leaving gas-exchange units with low $\dot{V}_A/\dot{Q}$ (C in Fig. 13-8) has increased P_{CO_2} and CO_2 content. However, perfusion from these units can be balanced by blood that has reduced P_{CO_2} and CO_2 content (Figs. 13-3 and 13-4) leaving alveoli

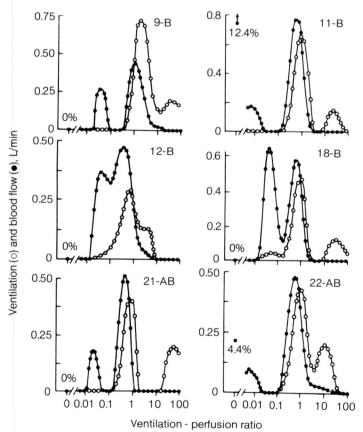

FIGURE 13-7 Ventilation (open circles) and blood flow (closed circles) distribution in six patients with chronic obstructive lung disease. This represents only one of several patterns seen in this condition. *(From Wagner, Dantzker, Dueck, Clausen, West; reproduced from The Journal of Clinical Investigation 59:203–213, 1977, by copyright permission of The American Society for Clinical Investigation.)*

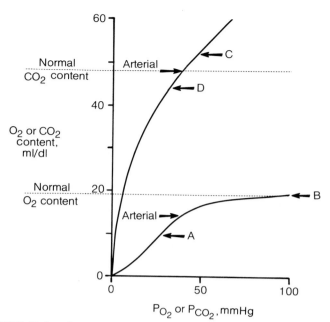

FIGURE 13-8 The carbon dioxide *(upper curve)* and oxygen *(lower curve)* dissociation curves of human blood. Normal CO_2 and O_2 contents are indicated by the dashed horizontal lines. Arterial CO_2 and O_2 contents in the example given in the text are indicated by the arrows.

with high $\dot{V}_A/\dot{Q}$ (D in Fig. 13-8). In contrast to the oxygen dissociation curve, the CO_2 dissociation curve is relatively linear and has no flat portion. Thus, if excess CO_2 is excreted in units with high $\dot{V}_A/\dot{Q}$, compensation can be achieved for CO_2 retention in alveoli with low $\dot{V}_A/\dot{Q}$. The net result of ventilation-perfusion mismatching in most cases is a normal arterial P_{CO_2} but a reduced P_{O_2}.

The ability to excrete an increased amount of CO_2 in alveoli with elevated $\dot{V}_A/\dot{Q}$ is extremely helpful in preventing hypercapnia but, like most compensatory mechanisms, is accompanied by a disadvantage. In this case, an increase in total ventilation over normal is required to maintain eucapnia. Excretion of carbon dioxide from alveoli with excess ventilation in relation to perfusion is not as efficient as normal exchange. This is illustrated in Fig. 13-9. The quantity of ventilation which is necessary to excrete 1 ml of CO_2 is plotted on the ordinate. This index of efficiency is a function of the ventilation-perfusion ratio, which is plotted on the abscissa along with the P_{CO_2} present in alveoli with these $\dot{V}_A/\dot{Q}$ values. The arrow drawn in the figure at a P_{CO_2} of 40 mmHg indicates the efficiency under normal circumstances. It is obvious from Fig. 13-8 that alveoli with $\dot{V}_A/\dot{Q}$ values greater than normal do not excrete CO_2 in a very efficient manner; i.e., at greater than normal $\dot{V}_A/\dot{Q}$ a much larger quantity of ventilation is needed to excrete the same amount of carbon dioxide. As the $\dot{V}_A/\dot{Q}$ increases and approaches infinity, the quantity of ventilation required to excrete CO_2 similarly approaches an infinite value.

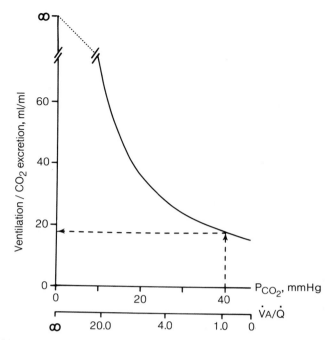

FIGURE 13-9 Ventilation required to excrete 1 ml of carbon dioxide is a function of $\dot{V}_A/\dot{Q}$. The arrows indicate that just under 20 ml of ventilation is required to excrete 1 ml of CO_2 under normal circumstances. As the $\dot{V}_A/\dot{Q}$ of an alveolus increases, the ventilatory requirement to excrete the same amount of CO_2 increases substantially.

If the dispersion of $\dot{V}_A/\dot{Q}$ is not too large and alveoli with $\dot{V}_A/\dot{Q}$ higher than normal do not have extremely elevated values, then the increased ventilation required to excrete CO_2 does not place unreasonable demands on the body and can be achieved by most patients. Accordingly, hypercapnia is not a usual feature of ventilation-perfusion mismatching. However, if an individual has a wide dispersion of $\dot{V}_A/\dot{Q}$, the situation is much more tenuous. If units with extremely high $\dot{V}_A/\dot{Q}$ are present, then an inordinate amount of ventilation may be required to excrete CO_2 to compensate for CO_2 retention in units with low $\dot{V}_A/\dot{Q}$. In this case, the required level of ventilation may exceed the ventilatory reserve of the patient and CO_2 retention will occur. This is usually seen in patients with decreased ventilatory reserve caused by disease of the airways. Under these circumstances, ventilation-perfusion mismatching will cause both hypercapnia and hypoxemia.

Assessment of Uneven $\dot{V}_A/\dot{Q}$ Distribution

It is not possible to completely characterize the distribution of ventilation–blood-flow relationships in an exact manner in a research laboratory. In a clinical setting the difficulty is even greater. Yet there are several possible ways to provide an estimate of the severity of $\dot{V}_A/\dot{Q}$ mismatching. In general, as the detail and precision of the description increases, the complexity of the method similarly increases. Probably the simplest means to assess the severity of ventilation-perfusion maldistribution is to measure the arterial P_{O_2}. The arterial oxygen tension decreases with increasing $\dot{V}_A/\dot{Q}$ dispersion. Most clinicians use this simple approach at the bedside. Obviously, other abnormalities can affect the Pa_{O_2}, so this is not specific for hypoxemia caused by uneven distribution of ventilation and pulmonary blood flow. For reasons mentioned previously, the arterial P_{CO_2} does not reflect $\dot{V}_A/\dot{Q}$ inequality until the abnormality becomes severe.

ALVEOLAR-ARTERIAL O₂ DIFFERENCE

The difference between the alveolar and arterial oxygen tensions provides a slightly better estimate of $\dot{V}_A/\dot{Q}$ dispersion than the Pa_{O_2} because it is unaffected by hypoventilation and the resulting decrease in alveolar oxygen tension. However, $PA_{O_2} - Pa_{O_2}$ is also increased by shunting and diffusion abnormalities so that the index is not specific for $\dot{V}_A/\dot{Q}$ dispersion. Because the alveolar P_{O_2} varies throughout the lung, an actual mean alveolar P_{O_2} cannot be obtained experimentally. Instead it is common to substitute an ideal alveolar P_{O_2}, the P_{O_2} which is present in alveoli with a P_{CO_2} equal to the arterial value. The ideal alveolar P_{O_2} is calculated from arterial P_{CO_2}, the inspired oxygen fraction $F_{I_{O_2}}$, and the respiratory exchange ratio R, the ratio of CO_2 output to O_2 uptake:

$$PA_{O_2} = P_{I_{O_2}} - Pa_{CO_2}\left(F_{I_{O_2}} + \frac{1 - F_{I_{O_2}}}{R}\right) \qquad (3)$$

This calculation of $PA_{O_2} - Pa_{O_2}$ assumes that arterial and alveolar P_{CO_2} are identical. If the respiratory exchange ratio is not measured, a value of R must be assumed. With a normal value of R (0.8) and breathing 21% oxygen at sea level, Eq. (3) simplifies to

$$PA_{O_2} = 150 - 1.2\, Pa_{CO_2} \qquad (4)$$

Interpretation of the $PA_{O_2} - Pa_{O_2}$ is complicated by its dependency on alveolar P_{O_2}. For example, the normal alveolar-arterial O_2 difference is 10 to 15 mmHg when breathing room air but greater than 50 mmHg when inspiring 100% oxygen. Some investigators have used the ratio of alveolar to arterial P_{O_2}, the so-called A/a ratio, to avoid this problem, but this approach has not completely circumvented the problem.

THREE-COMPARTMENT LUNG

Representing the lung as composed of three compartments rather than millions of individual units is an immense simplification, but it provides more insight than viewing the lung as a single, homogeneous organ. One portion of the lung is assumed to have ideal behavior with a ventilation-perfusion ratio equal to the mean $\dot{V}_A/\dot{Q}$ for the whole lung. The alveolar and end-capillary P_{O_2} of such a unit is equal to the ideal alveolar P_{O_2} calculated in Eq. (3).

A second portion of the total blood flow is assumed to be distributed to alveoli which receive no ventilation. This venous admixture is calculated as

$$\frac{\dot{Q}va}{\dot{Q}t} = \frac{Cc_{O_2} - Ca_{O_2}}{Cc_{O_2} - C\bar{v}_{O_2}} \qquad (5)$$

where C refers to oxygen content of blood and the modifiers c, a, and $\bar{v}$ refer to capillary, arterial, and mixed venous samples. Capillary O_2 content cannot be measured but is computed using alveolar oxygen tension. Mixed venous O_2 content is often assumed rather than measured, leading to possible errors of considerable magnitude. Note that the equation for venous admixture is identical with the equation used to calculate shunt ($\dot{Q}s/\dot{Q}t$) when the patient is breathing 100% oxygen. As $\dot{V}_A/\dot{Q}$ dispersion increases, $\dot{Q}va/\dot{Q}t$ becomes larger. The venous admixture, like $PA_{O_2} - Pa_{O_2}$, also is affected by shunting and diffusion abnormalities.

The third compartment in this approach is termed *physiological dead space* and is calculated from Eq. (1), as described previously. Both venous admixture and dead-space concepts treat abnormalities of gas exchange as if they were caused by the extremes of $\dot{V}_A/\dot{Q}$ inequality. This adds to our knowledge but certainly is far from reality since intermediate $\dot{V}_A/\dot{Q}$, rather than the extreme values, are responsible for most abnormal gas exchange.

MULTIPLE INERT GAS ELIMINATION

This technique, alluded to previously, is based on the degree of retention of an inert gas in blood leaving the lung after intravenous administration of the gas dissolved in saline. The retention of an inert gas in blood leaving an alveolus is given by

$$\text{Retention} = \frac{\lambda}{\lambda + \dot{V}_A/\dot{Q}} \qquad (6)$$

where λ is the partition coefficient (relative solubility of a gas in blood) and $\dot{V}_A/\dot{Q}$ is the ventilation-perfusion ratio of the alveolus in question. When the retention in arterial blood of six gases of different solubilities is measured, information such as that shown in Figs. 13-5 and 13-6 can be calculated. This distribution of $\dot{V}_A/\dot{Q}$ throughout the lung is not mathematically exact because only six measurements of retention are used to characterize a lung model composed of 50 compartments, but the technique provides substantial information that permits better understanding of $\dot{V}_A/\dot{Q}$ dispersion. Unfortunately, the methodology and computations used in this technique preclude its routine clinical use.

Clinical Implications

PHARMACOLOGIC INTERVENTIONS

In an acute episode of respiratory or cardiac decompensation, drugs are often used to augment or improve distribution of inspired air and cardiac output. Most drugs utilized in these situations have either a primary cardiac or respiratory effect; they have little or no influence on the other system. Hence, a given pharmacologic intervention will usually affect only one portion of the ventilation-perfusion relationship. Although beneficial from other viewpoints, a given therapy may actually increase $\dot{V}_A/\dot{Q}$ dispersion by its effect on only one factor of the ratio.

In acute respiratory failure, administration of bronchodilators, either by inhalation or a parenteral route, often will decrease airway resistance and lead to better distribution of inspired air. Yet measurements of arterial blood gases in some instances will show a concomitant decrease in arterial oxygenation. This has been attributed to worsening of ventilation-perfusion relationships. It has been postulated that the distribution of ventilation may be improved with respect to the different areas of the lung, but that blood flow which had been distributed in a non-uniform manner does not adjust immediately to the change in ventilation.

Similar effects on arterial oxygenation have been observed following administration of vasoactive agents such as nitroprusside. This drug appears to blunt hypoxic vasoconstriction. The hypoxic vascular response is useful in improving $\dot{V}_A/\dot{Q}$ if perfusion to underventilated areas of the lung is restricted, thereby providing better matching of ventilation and blood flow. Arterial blood gases will remain normal in the face of severe maldistribution of ventilation if blood flow is distributed in a similar, albeit abnormal, pattern. Relief of hypoxic vasoconstriction under these circumstances leads to proliferation of gas-exchange units which are relatively overperfused, i.e., have low $\dot{V}_A/\dot{Q}$ and cause hypoxemia.

Obviously bronchodilators and vasoactive drugs are useful therapeutic modalities, and their use should not be restricted because of potential worsening of ventilation-perfusion matching. However, it is often necessary to supply supplemental oxygen to prevent hypoxemia during the period of adjustment following changes in distribution of ventilation or blood flow.

OXYGEN THERAPY

Mismatching of ventilation and perfusion is extremely common. Fortunately, the hypoxemia accompanying this abnormality usually responds readily to administration of oxygen. The oxygen dissociation curve is expanded in Fig. 13-10 to highlight the portion of the curve involved in O_2 exchange in severe hypoxemia caused by $\dot{V}_A/\dot{Q}$ dispersion. Alveoli with very low $\dot{V}_A/\dot{Q}$ lie on the lower portion

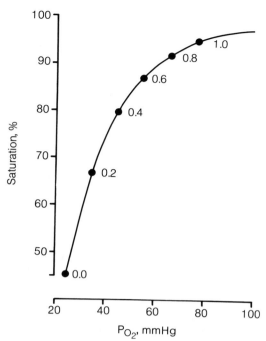

FIGURE 13-10 Expansion of the portion of the oxygen dissociation curve involved in O_2 exchange in severe hypoxemia (Pa_{O_2} = 40 mmHg, $P\bar{v}_{O_2}$ = 26 mmHg). Individual values of $\dot{V}_A/\dot{Q}$ are given at various points along the curve. Note the steep nature of the curve between points associated with low $\dot{V}_A/\dot{Q}$ (0.0 to 0.4).

of the dissociation curve. The low saturation present in blood leaving these alveoli is responsible for arterial hypoxemia. Obviously small increments in alveolar P_{O_2} will cause dramatic increases in oxygen saturation because the dissociation curve is very steep in this area. Administration of oxygen does not change ventilation-perfusion relationships nor increase the ventilation reaching each alveolus, but the higher concentration of oxygen in the inspirate increases the effectiveness of even limited ventilation. Each unit of inspired gas brings additional oxygen to the alveolus, thus raising alveolar and capillary blood P_{O_2}. Despite the lack of change in distribution of ventilation and blood flow, alveoli with low $\dot{V}_A/\dot{Q}$ become much more effective in oxygenating mixed venous blood. This has the effect of moving an alveolus with a given $\dot{V}_A/\dot{Q}$ further up on the O_2 dissociation curve.

It is often argued that intrapulmonary shunting is an extreme $\dot{V}_A/\dot{Q}$ mismatch and should not be considered as a separate pathophysiological mechanism producing hypoxemia. From a practical standpoint, it is helpful to consider the two separately. The hypoxemia of a $\dot{V}_A/\dot{Q}$ mismatch responds to administration of relatively small quantities of oxygen. In contrast, shunting responds poorly, if at all, to large increments in the inspired oxygen. With shunting, alveoli are collapsed and/or filled with fluid. Oxygen in the inspirate cannot reach the alveolar-capillary membrane to allow exchange to take place. Although O$_2$ therapy is utilized, it is important to promote reexpansion of collapsed alveoli to restore O$_2$ exchange with blood perfusing these units.

Diffusion abnormalities cannot be distinguished from mismatching of ventilation and blood flow in clinical circumstances. Practically, this is not a major concern because the hypoxemia associated with abnormal diffusion, like that produced by $\dot{V}_A/\dot{Q}$ dispersion, also responds to small increments in the inspired oxygen concentration.

BIBLIOGRAPHY

Dantzker DR, Brook CJ, Dehart P, Lynch JP, Weg JG: Ventilation-perfusion distributions in the adult respiratory distress syndrome. Am Rev Respir Dis 120:1039–1052, 1979.
  Hypoxemia in the adult respiratory distress syndrome is produced predominantly by shunting, or less often by alveoli with very low $\dot{V}_A/\dot{Q}$. Positive end-expiratory pressure decreases blood flow to these units but also increases ventilation of unperfused alveoli.

Dantzker DR, D'Alonzo GE: The effect of exercise on pulmonary gas exchange in patients with severe chronic obstructive pulmonary disease. Am Rev Respir Dis 134:1135–1139, 1986.
  Worsening of hypoxemia during exercise in patients with severe obstructive airways disease is due to an inadequate ventilatory response (leading to a rise in arterial P_{CO_2}) and the impact of a decreased mixed venous P_{O_2} on the end-capillary P_{O_2} of low V_A/Q lung units and shunt.

Evans JW, Wagner PD: Limits on $\dot{V}_A/\dot{Q}$ distribution from analysis of experimental inert gas elimination. J Appl Physiol 42:889–898, 1977.
  This article describes the limits of accuracy of the multiple inert gas technique for determination of ventilation-perfusion distributions. The main body of the article is descriptive with the underlying mathematical approach contained in an appendix.

Farhi LE: Ventilation-perfusion relationships, in Farhi LE, Tenney SM (eds), Handbook of Physiology, sect 3: The Respiratory System, vol IV: Gas Exchange. Bethesda, American Physiological Society, 1987.
  A chapter in the volume of the Handbook devoted to gas exchange that begins with theoretical considerations indicating that practically every change in ventilation and/or in blood flow affects distribution of ventilation-perfusion relationships, and concludes with practical illustrations.

Grant BJB, Davies EE, Jones HA, Hughes JMB: Local regulation of pulmonary blood flow and ventilation-perfusion ratios in the coatimundi. J Appl Physiol 40:216–228, 1976.
  Local blood flow to subsegmental lung units responded to alterations in ventilation to limit abnormal local $\dot{V}_A/\dot{Q}$. This response is of moderate, not high, efficiency.

Hammond MD, Gale GE, Kapitan KS, Ries A, Wagner PD: Pulmonary gas exchange in humans during exercise at sea level. J Appl Physiol 60:1590–1598, 1986.
  The multiple-inert gas-elimination technique was used to study gas exchange during exercise in healthy subjects at sea level.

Hughes JMB, Glazier JB, Maloney JE, West JB: Effect of lung volume on the distribution of pulmonary blood flow in man. Respir Physiol 4:58–72, 1968.
  Blood flow is not distributed evenly in the lung of normal individuals but is dependent upon vertical height. In addition, lung volume is an important determinant of local blood flow.

Kallay MC, Hyde RW, Smith RJ, Rothbard RL, Schreiner BF: Cardiac output by rebreathing in patients with cardiopulmonary diseases. J Appl Physiol 63:201–210, 1987.
  Noninvasive estimates of cardiac output by rebreathing soluble gases (Qc) can be unreliable in patients with cardiopulmonary diseases because of uneven distribution of ventilation to lung gas volume and pulmonary blood flow.

Munkner T, Bundgaard A: Regional V/Q changes in asthmatics after histamine inhalation. Eur J Respir Dis (Suppl) 143:22–27, 1986.
  One of a series of papers in this issue devoted to changes in ventilation-blood flow relationships in patients with asthma exposed to provocation tests. This paper deals with the immediate changes in regional ventilation and pulmonary blood flow in adults with perennial asthma challenged by histamine inhalation.

Olszowka AJ: Can $\dot{V}_A/\dot{Q}$ distributions in the lung be recovered from inert gas retention data? Respir Physiol 25:191–198, 1975.
  This theoretical study describes the full range of possible $\dot{V}_A/\dot{Q}$ distributions which can be obtained with the multiple inert gas elimination technique.

Riley RL, Cournand A, Donald KW: Analysis of factors affecting partial pressures of oxygen and carbon dioxide in gas and blood of lungs. Methods. J Appl Physiol 4:102–120, 1951.
  The initial, classic three-compartment analysis of ventilation-perfusion abnormalities and their impact on the gas composition of the blood.

Chapter 14

Diffusion, Diffusing Capacity, and Chemical Reactions

Peter D. Wagner

Diffusion across the Blood-Gas Barrier in the Lungs
  The Solubility Ratio (α/β)
  Molecular Weight

Transit Time

The Shape of the Dissociation Curve

Reaction Rates

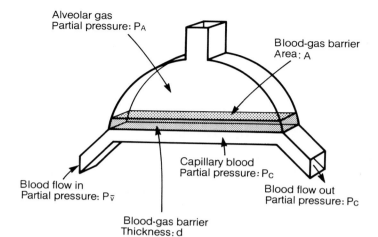

FIGURE 14-1 Idealized scheme of an alveolar unit of gas exchange to illustrate the variables important in diffusion between blood and gas.

Uncertainty was still present as recently as 50 years ago, but it is now accepted that gases cross the pulmonary blood-gas barrier (in either direction) by diffusion along a concentration gradient. This is just as true for gases that undergo chemical reactions in blood (O_2, CO_2, CO) as for all other gases such as N_2 and the inhalational anesthetics. The chemical reaction processes for O_2, CO_2, and CO are, however, not instantaneous and will therefore play a role in the overall rate of equilibration of partial pressure of these gases between alveolar gas and capillary blood.

Both the above components of transfer of gas between alveoli and blood must then be considered. A strong unifying concept can be provided for all gases diffusing across the blood-gas barrier, and this is considered first, but since chemical reactions for O_2, CO_2, and CO are different for each of these species, they must be considered individually.

DIFFUSION ACROSS THE BLOOD-GAS BARRIER IN THE LUNGS

This section illustrates the basic principles that allow one to understand when a gas will become diffusion-limited in its pulmonary exchange. Figure 14-1 shows a simplified gas-exchange unit with diffusion occurring (in the direction of uptake) across an alveolar-capillary barrier of cross section A and thickness d. During normal breathing, alveolar gas has an essentially constant gas partial pressure (P_A), whereas that of the capillary blood (P_c) rises in some fashion from the input (mixed venous) end of the unit to the output (end capillary) end of the unit. The question posed is: What governs the *rate of rise of partial*

pressure of the gas in an element of blood moving through the gas-exchange unit?

Fick's first law of diffusion that describes the quantitative movement of a gas across the barrier allows one to answer this question. This law states that at any instant in time the rate of flow of gas across the blood-gas barrier is the product of a constant D_M (the diffusing capacity of the barrier) and the difference in partial pressures across the barrier ($P_A - P_c$). Thus, as capillary partial pressure P_c rises as an element of blood traverses the capillary, the instantaneous rate of movement of gas into that element is reduced.

It is useful to express this as an equation:

$$\dot{V}(t) = D_M\,[P_A - P_c(t)] \tag{1}$$

where $\dot{V}(t)$ is the instantaneous gas flow across the barrier and $P_c(t)$ the instantaneous partial pressure in an element of blood flowing along the capillary. Both D_M and P_A are (reasonably) assumed to be constant. The diffusing capacity, D_M, is itself made up of several components:

$$D_M = k\frac{A}{d}\frac{\alpha}{\sqrt{MW}} \tag{2}$$

where k is a constant related to the physicochemical nature of the blood-gas barrier, A the cross-sectional area over which diffusion occurs, d the thickness of the barrier, α the solubility of the gas in the barrier, and MW the molecular weight of the gas.

Equation (2) is intuitively evident. For a given barrier structure, the diffusing capacity is doubled if the area A for diffusion is doubled, and so on.

Of special importance is the solubility α. Again intuitively, for a given partial pressure difference across the barrier, the diffusing capacity is directly proportional to the solubility of the gas; the more gas molecules will dissolve in the barrier, the more can cross it per unit time and partial pressure difference.

Now, turning to the left side of Eq (1), which expresses the volume flow of gas into the capillary, $\dot{V}(t)$ can be expressed as a rate of rise of capillary blood concentration $C(t)$:

$$\dot{V}(t) = \frac{dC(t)}{dt} Vc \tag{3}$$

where Vc is capillary blood volume. If we assume that Vc, A, and d, which are all geometric properties of the blood-gas interface, are uniformly distributed along the capillary, we can combine all three equations and use whole lung values for Vc, A, and d:

$$\frac{dC(t)}{dt} Vc = k \frac{A}{d} \frac{\alpha}{\sqrt{MW}} [PA - Pc(t)] \tag{4}$$

Finally, for purposes of discussion, let us consider a gas whose concentration/partial pressure relationship (*dissociation curve*) is linear:

$$C(t) = \beta Pc(t) \tag{5}$$

Here β is the slope of that relationship or the gas solubility in blood. We may then write

$$\frac{dPc(t)}{dt} = \frac{k}{Vc} \frac{A}{d} \frac{\alpha}{\beta} \frac{1}{\sqrt{MW}} [PA - Pc(t)] \tag{6}$$

This equation expresses the rate at which capillary partial pressure changes in time along the pulmonary capillary. Considerable effort has been expended to arrive at Eq. (6) because many critically important conclusions about diffusion limitation can be deduced from it. For example, one can see that for a given lung (i.e., for given values of k, Vc, A, and d), the rate of rise of capillary partial pressure [$dPc(t)/dt$] for a given diffusion gradient [$PA - Pc(t)$] is dependent on two factors only: (1) the *ratio* of solubility of the gas in the blood-gas barrier (α) to that in blood (β) and (2) molecular weight.

The Solubility Ratio (α/β)

From the above considerations of the solubility ratio (α/β), two important conclusions can be drawn. The first is that the dependence of the rate of equilibration is on the ratio α/β and not on absolute values of α and β. Thus all gases having the same ratio of tissue to blood solubilities (and the same molecular weight) will equilibrate at the same rate. Even though DM of Eq. (2) is higher for a more soluble gas because α is greater, its equilibration rate in the capillary is no faster because β is correspondingly higher. In other words, for a soluble gas, more molecules diffuse into the blood per unit time (higher α and DM), but because the blood solubility (β) is correspondingly higher, it takes just as long to raise partial pressure a given amount as for an

insoluble gas with the same α/β ratio and molecular weight. Basically, all inert gases (i.e., all gases except O_2, CO_2, and CO) have very similar α/β ratios that approximate unity.

The second conclusion, ignoring both finite chemical reaction rates (that only further slow down O_2, CO_2, and CO equilibration) and nonlinear dissociation curves particularly of O_2 and CO (see below), is that O_2, CO_2, and CO are much more vulnerable to diffusion limitation than are gases for which the ratio α/β approximates 1.0.

OXYGEN

If β is calculated as the average slope between an arterial P_{O_2} of 100 and mixed venous P_{O_2} of 40, and if the arterio-venous O_2 content difference is assumed to be 5 vol %, $\beta = 5/60$ or 0.083 ml/100 ml/mmHg, whereas, in the same units, α, the tissue solubility, is only 0.003. Thus, for O_2, the ratio of α/β approximates not unity but only 0.036, some 30 times less than for an inert gas, i.e., O_2 equilibrates about 30-fold more slowly than does an inert gas. Under severely hypoxic conditions, where arterial P_{O_2} may be 40 mmHg, mixed venous P_{O_2} 27 mmHg, and the arteriovenous content difference still 5 vol %, β comes to 5/13 or 0.385 ml/100 ml/mmHg and α/β would be 0.008 (or 1/128).

From the principle of tissue/blood solubility ratio indicated above, it is easy to see that O_2 is some 30 times more vulnerable than any inert gas under normal conditions and more than 100 times more so in hypoxia. Classic teaching states that it is the reduction in alveolar P_{O_2} that makes O_2 more susceptible to diffusion limitation in hypoxia. By the above reasoning, it is more correct to state that the increased vulnerability is the consequence of the steeper slope (larger β) of the dissociation curve during hypoxia. Figure 14-2 underscores the significance of this concept; it is neither alveolar nor venous P_{O_2} per se but the dissociation curve slope that determines the rate of equilibration. This figure illustrates hypothetical arterial and venous points that would differently affect diffusive equilibration.

CARBON DIOXIDE

It is usually stated that because CO_2 is some 20 times more soluble than O_2, it is invulnerable to diffusion limitation. While the factor of 20 is approximately true ($\alpha_{CO_2} = 0.067$ ml/100 ml/mmHg in tissue compared to $\alpha_{O_2} = 0.003$), the slope of the CO_2 dissociation curve (β) is also much steeper for CO_2 than for O_2. Thus, under normal conditions, arterial and venous P_{CO_2} are 40 and 45 mmHg, respectively, whereas the venous to arterial CO_2 content difference is about 4.0 ml per 100 ml. Thus, $\beta_{CO_2} = 4/5$, or 0.8, some 10 times greater than that of O_2 under similar normal conditions, as shown above. In other words, the ratio α/β for CO_2 is normally about 0.067/0.8 or 1/12

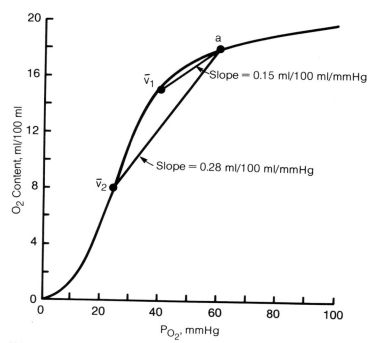

FIGURE 14-2 O_2-Hb dissociation curve showing a single arterial (a) and two mixed venous points ($\bar{v}_1$ and $\bar{v}_2$). Because of the increased slope of the interval a–$\bar{v}_2$ compared to a–$\bar{v}_1$, the rate of approach to equilibrium will be less for the former case. It is neither the arterial nor venous values themselves but the slope of the line joining them that is the most important factor determining speed of diffusive equilibration.

(whereas that for O_2 is 1/28, as shown above). Therefore, CO_2 is *not* 20 times less vulnerable to diffusion limitation as implied in early literature but only 28/12, or 2.3, times less vulnerable (before considering nonlinear dissociation curves and finite chemical reactions).

CARBON MONOXIDE

Similar considerations apply to carbon monoxide. If one accepts that the slope of the CO-Hb dissociation curve is some 250 times steeper than that of O_2 and that one is usually on the steep portion of the CO-Hb curve (or else one could not survive), β_{CO} comes to 250 × 0.385 or about 100 ml/100 ml/mmHg, whereas α_{CO} is only 0.0024 ml/100 ml/mmHg, i.e., even less than α_{O_2}. Consequently, $\alpha_{CO}/\beta_{CO} = 0.0024/100$ or about 1/40,000. Therefore, it is clear that CO is a diffusion-limited gas, with a rate of equilibration 40,000 times less than that for an inert gas, and almost 1500 times less than that for O_2 under normal conditions.

Molecular Weight

The rate of equilibration, other factors being equal, is related to the inverse square root of molecular weight of the gas [Eq. (6)]. For gases like CO (MW 28), O_2 (MW 32), and CO_2 (MW 44), it is apparent that molecular weight is far

less significant than is the solubility ratio α/β. Thus, on the basis of molecular weight alone, CO is faster than O_2 by a factor of $\sqrt{32/28}$, or only 1.07. Compare this to the 1500-fold retardation based on tissue/blood solubility ratio. On the basis of molecular weight, CO_2 is *slower* than O_2 by $\sqrt{44/32}$, or a factor of 1.17, much less than the 2.30 factor *faster* calculated above on the basis of tissue/blood solubility ratios.

TRANSIT TIME

All the above considerations refer to the *rate* at which capillary partial pressure approaches alveolar partial pressure, and the focus has been on a comparison of the inert gases, O_2, CO_2, and CO. However, more important is the final degree of equilibration reached by the end of the capillary: it would not matter how fast or slow equilibration rates were if the residence time of an element of blood were inordinately long.

Transit time can be considered without much further mathematics. Equation (6) is a differential equation describing the rate of movement of a gas at any point along the capillary. To determine the blood partial pressure at the end of the capillary, one need only integrate Eq. (6) over the time spent in the capillary. If we designate zero time at the beginning, the time (T) elapsed after the element of blood has reached the end of the capillary will be $T = V_C/\dot{Q}$, where V_C is the capillary blood volume and $\dot{Q}$ the capillary blood flow. Integrating Eq. (6) between $t = 0$ and $t = V_C/\dot{Q}$ yields a monoexponential function:

$$(P_A - P_{C'}) = (P_A - P_{\bar{V}})\, e^{-[k\,(1/\sqrt{MW})\,(A/d)\,(\alpha/\beta)\,(1/\dot{Q})]} \quad (7)$$

or

$$\frac{P_A - P_{C'}}{P_A - P_{\bar{V}}} = e^{-D_M/\beta\dot{Q}} \quad (8)$$

where D_M is as defined in Eq. (2) and $P_{C'}$ and $P_{\bar{V}}$ are end capillary and mixed venous partial pressures, respectively.

What Eq. (8) says in words is fundamental: the degree to which end capillary pressure approaches alveolar partial pressure in any given capillary is the ratio of D_M, the *diffusing capacity* of the blood-gas barrier, to $\beta\dot{Q}$, the *perfusive conductance* ($\beta\dot{Q}$ is the product of blood solubility β and blood flow $\dot{Q}$ and thus equal to the amount of gas that can be transported per unit time per unit partial pressure of the gas). Therefore, Eqs. (7) and (8) extend the previous arguments concerned with *rate* of equilibration to the *final degree* of equilibration and, accordingly, bring in the additional variables of transit time and blood flow.

In pathophysiological terms, these considerations imply that in a fibrotic area of lung, although D_M is reduced, if its blood flow $\dot{Q}$ were reduced *in proportion*, the ratio $D_M/\beta\dot{Q}$ would be normal: despite the reduced D_M

there would be no failure of diffusional equilibration. Taking this one additional step, it is the *distribution of the ratio of diffusing capacity to blood flow* that will determine the amount of interference to gas exchange attributable to diffusion limitation.

THE SHAPE OF THE DISSOCIATION CURVE

The entire preceding development has used the concept of a linear relationship between content and partial pressure in blood definable by a solubility constant β. A constant value of β makes the equations tractable. However, even though the CO_2 dissociation curve is essentially linear, those for O_2 and CO are clearly not so. The compounding effects of nonlinearity of the dissociation curves are illustrated in Fig. 14-3, showing the O_2-Hb dissociation curve and normal alveolar (A) and mixed venous ($\bar{v}$) points. The preceding theory applies to the average slope assumption corresponding to the straight line between A and $\bar{v}$.

Early in the capillary, the real O_2-Hb curve is steeper than later. As O_2 loading takes place in the capillary, con-

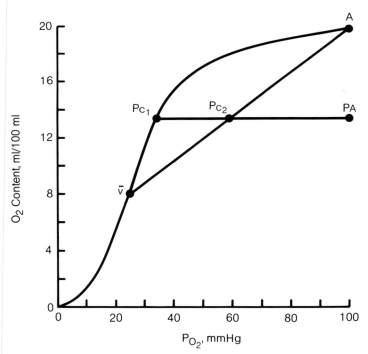

FIGURE 14-3 Illustration of the advantage of the nonlinear shape of the O_2-Hb dissociation curve on O_2 uptake by diffusion in the lung. By the time O_2 concentration has risen from the mixed venous value of 8 to about 14 ml per 100 ml, capillary partial pressure is Pc_1 for the real curve and Pc_2 for the hypothetical linear curve. To complete O_2 loading, the real curve is advantageous because the real driving gradient $PA - Pc_1$, greatly exceeds that for the linear curve, namely, $PA - Pc_2$.

siderable O_2 is added without much loss in the driving difference in partial pressure. Thus, for the real dissociation curve, $PA - Pc_1$ considerably exceeds $PA - Pc_2$, but since the amount of O_2 loaded is the same for Pc_1 and Pc_2, a larger driving gradient is left for completing the remaining loading of O_2. In fact, once on the flat part of the real dissociation curve, a P_{O_2} of about 60, β_{O_2} is effectively quite similar to α_{O_2}, so that equilibration rapidly speeds up. The end result is *more rapid* alveolar-capillary equilibration for the real O_2-Hb curve than would be the case for the example of the linear dissociation curve between the same alveolar and mixed venous points. In other words, the shape of the O_2-Hb dissociation curve is advantageous to loading of O_2 in the pulmonary capillary. Exactly the opposite conclusion holds true for the peripheral capillary where the shape of the O_2-Hb curve retards O_2 unloading by diffusion.

REACTION RATES

To this point, the treatment of diffusion equilibrium has dealt with the basic concept of what determines the rate of equilibration and built on that concept by adding the effects of transit time and the shape of dissociation curve. The remaining major factor is, for the gases O_2, CO_2, and CO, determining their finite rates of chemical reaction in blood.

Oxygen and CO combine with hemoglobin in the red cell and, under most conditions, are negligibly transported in the plasma owing to very low plasma solubilities (equal to tissue solubilities given earlier). For CO_2 the chemical reaction is more complex with different reactions in plasma and the red cell involving both conversion between bicarbonate ion and carbonic acid and combination with terminal amines of proteins (especially hemoglobin) to form carbamino compounds.

Allowing for chemical reactions requires adding equation systems simultaneously to the basic equations developed above. Thus, Eq. (6) applies to transfer between alveolar gas and plasma, and separate but simultaneous equations must be written expressing the rate at which the various chemical reactions for the gas in question take place in plasma and red cells. The simultaneity of the equations ensures internal consistency and mass balance in their evaluation.

For CO, the two components (diffusion across the blood-gas barrier and intraerythrocyte chemical reaction of CO with Hb) can be brought together by the following argument (Fig. 14-4).

If the D_M of Eq. (6) is specifically defined as membrane diffusing capacity, and if θ_{CO} is now defined as the rate of chemical combination between CO and Hb per milliliter of blood per millimeter mercury partial pressure per minute, the following expressions may be written in refer-

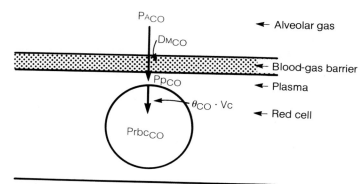

FIGURE 14-4 Diagram to illustrate the series arrangement of the two processes involved in O_2 uptake: (1) diffusion from alveolar gas into the plasma and (2) subsequent chemical reaction with hemoglobin in the red cell. Symbols are defined in the text.

ence to Fig. 14-4 based on the concept of Eq. (1) (Fick's law) and the definition of θ_{CO}:

$$\dot{V}_{CO,alveolus \rightarrow plasma} = D_{MCO} (P_{ACO} - P_{pCO}) \qquad (9)$$

$$\dot{V}_{CO,plasma \rightarrow red\ cell} = \theta_{CO} V_c [P_{pCO} - P_{rbcCO}] \qquad (10)$$

Here, P_{pCO} is plasma CO partial pressure, and P_{rbcCO} is that inside the red cell. Because the relative amount of CO dissolved in plasma is negligible compared to that stored in combination with Hb, it is reasonable to equate both $\dot{V}_{ACO,alveolus \rightarrow plasma}$ of Eq. (9) and $\dot{V}_{CO,plasma \rightarrow red\ cell}$ of Eq. (10) with total CO transfer, $\dot{V}_{CO,alveolus \rightarrow red\ cell}$. Then, rearranging and rewriting these equations gives

$$\frac{\dot{V}_{CO,alveolus \rightarrow plasma}}{D_{MCO}} = P_{ACO} - P_{pCO} \qquad (11)$$

$$\frac{\dot{V}_{CO,plasma \rightarrow red\ cell}}{\theta_{CO} \cdot V_c} = P_{pCO} - P_{rbcCO} \qquad (12)$$

Adding the two equations (11) and (12) yields

$$\dot{V}_{CO,alveolus \rightarrow red\ cell} \left(\frac{1}{D_{MCO}} + \frac{1}{\theta_{CO} \cdot V_c} \right)$$
$$= P_{ACO} - P_{rbcCO} \qquad (13)$$

Finally, if we choose to define a variable D_{LCO} (for total diffusing capacity) by

$$\dot{V}_{CO,alveolus \rightarrow red\ cell} = D_{LCO} (P_{ACO} - P_{rbcCO}) \qquad (14)$$

it becomes apparent that

$$\frac{1}{D_{LCO}} = \frac{1}{D_{MCO}} + \frac{1}{\theta_{CO} \cdot V_c} \qquad (15)$$

Equation (15), originally derived by Roughton and Forster, quantitatively relates the two principal factors determining partial pressure equilibration, namely, D_{MCO} and θ_{CO}, in a manner that allows the combined effects of diffusion and chemical reaction rate to be considered to-

gether. If chemical reaction rates are infinitely rapid, Eq. (15) reduces to the simple statement that diffusing capacity is given by the membrane component [of Eq. (2)].

Equation (15) has the potential of permitting estimates to be made of two variables of considerable interest, D_{MCO} and V_c. This is done by measuring D_{LCO} at two different levels of arterial P_{O_2}, since the relationship between (arterial) P_{O_2} and θ_{CO} is known. Two such measurements provide two simultaneous equations in the two unknowns (D_{MCO} and V_c) that can then readily be solved. One important assumption in this scheme is that altering arterial P_{O_2} does not affect either D_{MCO} or V_c. Because of alterations in pulmonary vascular tone with changing P_{AO_2}, this assumption is highly questionable, and much caution is required before accepting such estimates of D_{MCO} or V_c. Also, as shown in Fig. 14-5 (compiled from several sources), this problem is further compounded by basic uncertainty in the values of θ_{CO}.

A similar concept can be applied to O_2. It turns out that θ_{O_2} varies with red cell P_{O_2}, being high when P_{O_2} is low and vice versa. As a result, there is little deceleration of rate of equilibration of O_2 along the capillary intro-

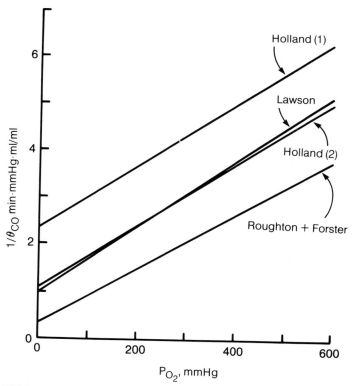

FIGURE 14-5 Relationship between the rate of reaction (θ) between CO and hemoglobin (expressed as the inverse $1/\theta$) and ambient P_{O_2}, from several sources. While the slopes of the relationships are reasonably similar, the intercepts are quite different and reflect incomplete knowledge of all the processes involved in CO movement into the red cell and subsequent combination with hemoglobin. The two curves from Holland reflect different assumptions on cell membrane permeability to CO.

duced by realistic values of θ_{O_2}. However, this is not the case for CO_2 where the bicarbonate-chloride exchange process between plasma and red cells has a half-time of about 0.10 to 0.15 s. This half-time slows CO_2 exchange appreciably so that blood leaving the pulmonary capillary may be not quite in full chemical equilibrium between H^+, HCO_3^-, and carbamino species in plasma and red cells; subsequent readjustment of blood P_{CO_2} after red cells have left the lungs has been estimated at as much as 0.5 mmHg under normal conditions.

All the above statements in reference to chemical re-action rates for O_2, CO_2, and CO must be interpreted with some caution since considerable debate still exists concerning the in vivo rate of chemical reaction for all three gases. At present, it does not seem that reaction rates are primarily responsible for alveolar-end capillary disequilibrium. Probably the most important single factor is the distribution of the ratio of membrane diffusing capacity to blood flow ($D_M/\dot{Q}$), giving rise to areas of the lung with a low $D_M/\dot{Q}$ ratio. This could be due to reduced diffusing capacity D_M, or a rapid transit time (high $\dot{Q}$ in relation to capillary volume), or both.

BIBLIOGRAPHY

Forster RE: Diffusion of gases across the alveolar membrane, in Farhi LE, Tenney SM (eds), *Handbook of Physiology, sect 3: The Respiratory System, vol IV: Gas Exchange.* Bethesda, American Physiological Society, 1987, pp 71–88.
  This chapter is concerned with the diffusion of gases across the alveolar-capillary membrane, focusing primarily on CO and O_2.

Hill, EP, Power GG, Longo LD: Mathematical simulation of pulmonary O_2 and CO_2 exchange. Am J Physiol 224:904–917, 1973.
  A theoretical treatment of rate of equilibration of both oxygen and carbon dioxide along the pulmonary capillary. Separate equations are given for intracellular and extracellular events and for various chemical species.

Hlastala MP: Diffusing-capacity heterogeneity, in Farhi LE, Tenney SM (eds), *Handbook of Physiology, sect 3: The Respiratory System, vol IV: Gas Exchange.* Bethesda, American Physiological Society, 1987, pp 217–232.
  A comprehensive survey of the present understanding of the contribution of heterogeneity in pulmonary diffusing capacity to interpretations of ventilation-perfusion limitations that are based on a homogeneous lung model.

Piiper J: Blood-gas equilibrium of carbon dioxide in lungs: A continuing controversy. J Appl Physiol 60:1–8, 1986.
  A review of recent evidence concerning the occurrence of negative blood-gas partial pressure differences of CO_2 in the lungs. The author concludes that the traditional concept of equal P_{CO_2} in blood and gas still stands.

Roughton FJW, Forster RE: Relative importance of diffusion and chemical reaction rates in determining rate of exchange of gases in the human lung, with special references to true diffusing capacity of pulmonary membrane and volume of blood in the lung capillaries. J Appl Physiol 11:290–302, 1957.
  Benchmark paper introducing the two concepts of physical diffusion and chemical reaction as being linked processes in the uptake dynamics of oxygen along the pulmonary capillary. Includes application of diffusing capacity technique to measurement of membrane diffusing capacity and capillary blood volume.

Wagner PD: Diffusion and chemical reaction in pulmonary gas exchange. Physiol Rev 57:257–312, 1977.
  Comprehensive review of physical and chemical processes involved in dynamics of gas uptake in the lung.

Weibel ER: *The Pathway for Oxygen.* Cambridge, Massachusetts, Harvard University Press, 1984.
  The morphometric estimation of pulmonary diffusing capacity is considered within the total framework of O_2 uptake from ambient air to O_2 delivery to mitochondria.

West JB (ed): *Ventilation, Blood Flow, and Diffusion. Pulmonary Gas Exchange,* vol I. New York, Academic, 1980.
  A review of many factors important to gas exchange in the lung. Particular chapter reference is the historical description of the secretion-diffusion controversy, chapter 1.

Chapter 15

The Nonrespiratory Functions of the Lungs

Alfred P. Fishman

General Effects
  Filter
  Sieving of Emboli
  Sieving of Formed Elements
  Water and Solutes
  Elimination of Volatile Substances

Metabolism
  Endothelium
  Oxygen Consumption and Energy Requirements
  Lipid Metabolism

Blood-Endothelial Interactions
  Angiogenesis
  Biologically Active Substances
  Endogenous Amines
  Chemicals

Hemofluidity and the Lungs
  Proteolysis
  Fibrinolytic Activity
  Disorders of Fibrinolysis
  Thromboplastin
  Heparin

Epilogue

It is remarkable how nonrespiratory functions have been engrafted on the respiratory functions of the lungs. Each element in the architecture of the lungs has been exploited so that respiratory and nonrespiratory functions can be accomplished in parallel. For example, the enormous expanse of endothelial surface is traversed by the cardiac output in such a way that red blood cells slide through capillaries, single file, on a sleeve of plasma; this arrangement enables not only the respiratory gases to exchange between air and blood but also the biologic machinery of the endothelium to interact with plasma constituents.

The nonrespiratory functions of the lungs are exceedingly diverse (Table 15-1). Elsewhere in this volume, considerable attention is paid to the nonrespiratory functions of the airways and airspaces, particularly to their defenses against infection (see Chapters 38, 39, 47, and 86). In this chapter, the focus is primarily on the pulmonary vascular endothelium of the adult lung. Not taken into account is the endothelium of the fetal lung since virtually nothing is known about its form and function during the consecutive stages of gestation. However, the fetal lung differs from that of the adult in many ways: it receives only a small fraction of the cardiac output; it does not participate in gas exchange; and, in contrast to the adult lung, its pulmonary vascular reactivity is exquisitely sensitive to sympathetic and parasympathetic stimuli. Indeed, it seems likely that the nonrespiratory functions of the fetal lung differ markedly from those of the adult lung.

GENERAL EFFECTS

Filter

The lungs act as a filter to rid the blood of particulate matter larger than normal red blood cells. Particles larger in diameter than 75 μm are apt to be caught at the level of the smaller pulmonary arteries (75 to 100 μm). These arteries give off right-angle branches that taper rapidly to diameters of about 50 μm before they lead into the dense capillary network. These rapidly tapering pulmonary arteries have been designated as "catch traps" because they trap microemboli, including carcinoma particles.

The average diameter of human capillaries is of the order of 8 to 9 μm. From these dimensions it is clear that the capillary network provides the smallest pores, as well as the largest area, for sieving. For several reasons, however, these numbers can be used as only a rough guide for predicting the size of particles that can traverse the lung because (1) the calibers of the capillaries are not uniform throughout the lung, so that red blood cells, which seem barely to squeeze through in one part, course through rapidly in another; (2) the rhythmic variation in capillary calibers during breathing may also help to milk arrested particles through the capillary bed, particularly in states

TABLE 15-1

Nonrespiratory Functions of the Lungs

Passive: Structural
  Filter
  Blood reservoir
  Elimination of volatile substances
  Uptake and storage of chemicals
  Water and macromolecular exchange
Active
  Lipid metabolism
  Defense mechanisms
  Hemofluidity
  Biologic interactions with plasma

of exaggerated respiratory effort; (3) the nature of the particle surface, e.g., its surface charge, and its interplay with the endothelial surface will affect its passage along the narrow capillary tubes; and (4) in addition to the large-bore capillaries noted above, there may be larger-bore arteriovenous communications in the pulmonary microcirculation. All in all, these observations do suggest that the bulk of particles ranging between 10 and 75 μm in diameter are apt to be delayed, if not arrested, in the distal pulmonary vascular tree; they also indicate that a widening of the capillary bed—as occurs in states of pulmonary congestion—is apt to decrease the efficiency of the pulmonary capillary bed as a fine filter.

Sieving of Emboli

Emboli from systemic veins are regularly trapped in the lungs. These physiological emboli are of several different kinds, including conglutinated white or red blood cells, fibrin clots, fat, bone marrow and, during pregnancy, placental tissue and amniotic fluid. Tumor cells carried in the circulating blood may also "nestle" in the lung and take root depending on their size, surface characteristics (stickiness), and local conditions. However, the effectiveness of this natural sieve is far from absolute since tumor cells 17 to 19 μm in diameter have been shown to traverse the pulmonary vascular bed.

Emboli that are trapped in the lungs not only cause pulmonary vascular obstruction but also initiate a secondary train of events that may culminate in bronchoconstriction or even pulmonary edema, apparently via humoral and neurogenic pathways. The trapped particulate matter is cleared from the lung by the action of proteolytic enzymes and phagocytosis.

Sieving of Formed Elements

The removal of granulocytes and lymphocytes from blood traversing the lungs has suggested that the lungs play a role in maintaining a stable level of circulating leukocytes. Indeed, the lungs may even operate as a "leukostat" to maintain a preset level of circulating white blood cells. This view is supported by observations on the arteriovenous difference in white blood cells that develops when leukemic blood is given intravenously to normal subjects.

Platelets, like leukocytes, may be removed from or added to blood in the lungs. The added platelets probably originate from megakaryocytes that are retained in the lungs as physiological emboli from bone marrow. Marked intrapulmonary destruction of erythrocytes occurs in disorders such as primary pulmonary hemosiderosis. And, after incompatible transfusions, the lungs trap the remnants of lysed red cells and remove them from the circulation.

Water and Solutes

During the respiratory cycle, inspired air is conditioned by the airways. The effectiveness of this process, which involves adjustment of both the water content and the temperature of the air, depends on patterns of airflow within the respiratory tree. Water loss via the respiratory tract also depends on the temperature and water content of the inspired air, the total volume of air exchanged, and the body temperature. The bronchial circulation, primarily through the submucosal bronchial venous plexus, is part of the water-exchanging apparatus of the airways (Fig. 15-1).

Under usual conditions, about 250 ml of water and 350 kcal of heat are lost from the airways per 24-h period. Water loss is increased during fever and hyperpnea. Hyperpnea is also an effective device for heat dissipation; it is exploited for this purpose by furry animals. The heat used to warm and humidify the inspired air increases caloric requirements in people who live in cold climates.

The temperature and humidity of the air reaching the lung are not only of significance with respect to water balance, but, more importantly, for the proper functioning of the epithelia lining the major airways, since the function of the cilia of the tracheobronchial tree is affected by the humidity within the respiratory tract. Despite wide fluctuations in the temperature of inspired air, the temperature of alveolar air and pulmonary capillary blood seems to be stable. Tracheostomy, which excludes the upper airways, interferes seriously with both the conditioning of inspired air and the recovery of heat and water from the expired air.

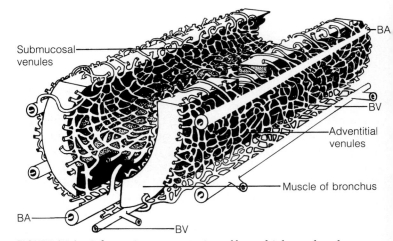

FIGURE 15-1 Schematic representation of bronchial venular plexus. The bronchial arteries (BA) deliver blood to the bronchial venular plexus, part of which lies beneath the mucosa and part beneath the adventitia. The bronchial muscle separates the two layers of the plexus, and connecting vessels link the submucosal and subadvential components of the plexus. Blood leaves the venous plexus via bronchial veins (BV). *(Modified after Fishman, 1972.)*

The lungs also play a part in the excretion of solutes by way of the carbon dioxide that they eliminate. In humans, for example, 15 to 30 osmol of carbon dioxide are produced and eliminated via the lungs every 24 h compared with 0.5 to 1.0 osmol of solute excreted via the kidneys. Carbon anhydrase in pulmonary capillary endothelium promotes the elimination of CO_2. The total solute (CO_2) and water loss via expired air is affected by body temperature, physical activity, and basal metabolic rate.

Carbon dioxide in blood is carried predominantly as bicarbonate ion (more than 60 percent of the whole blood CO_2 and as much as 90 percent of the plasma CO_2 is in the form of bicarbonate). Variations in concentration of this ion alter the total solute concentration, i.e., the osmolality of plasma: a change in the CO_2 content of plasma of 1.0 mM/kg of water alters plasma osmolality by 0.9 mosmol/kg of water. During quiet breathing, arteriovenous differences in plasma solute content caused by the elimination of carbon dioxide are offset by the concomitant increases in the amount of dissolved oxygen, of potassium (released from hemoglobin), and of chloride (from the red cell). However, the arteriovenous difference for CO_2 is affected by abrupt hyper- or hypoventilation, and the osmolality of the plasma changes accordingly.

In essence, the loss of heat and water via the expired air is ordinarily small despite the enormous alveolar surface area, the continuous tidal exposure of the alveolar surface to fresh air, and the huge capillary network through which the entire cardiac output flows. This conservation of heat and water is made possible by effective air conditioning along the upper airways. By exhaling carbon dioxide, the lungs contribute to solute excretion. Indeed, the lungs remove more solute from the body per 24 h than do the kidneys.

Elimination of Volatile Substances

Nonrespiratory metabolites that are volatile at 37°C, pass from blood to air across alveolar capillary membranes in accord with the physical properties of the metabolite and the membrane, and the laws of diffusion.

Several disease entities are associated with a characteristic odor to expired air (diabetic acidosis, liver failure, renal insufficiency, intestinal obstruction). Best known is the presence of acetone in expired air of patients with diabetic acidosis; less familiar is the fact that acetone can also be detected in the expired air of fasting normal individuals, i.e., without diabetes. The acetone content of alveolar air samples can be determined quantitatively, and it has been claimed that its presence in expired air is a more sensitive and reliable index of the state of control of the diabetes than is the determination of ketones in the urine. In hepatic failure, methylmercaptan, a derivative of methionine metabolism, is responsible for the typical odor of expired air, i.e., fetor hepaticus. Ammonia is an-

other metabolite that has been measured quantitatively in expired air; the partial pressures of ammonia in alveolar air and arterial blood are equal, supporting the contention that metabolites volatile at 37°C equilibrate across the alveolar-capillary membrane. Methanol has also been detected in human breath; the origin of this alcohol has not been identified.

The volatility of alcohol has been put to practical use as a basic test for identifying automobile drivers who have had "one too many." The characteristic odor of expired air after a meal spiced with garlic is due to allicin derived from enzymatic degradation of constituents of garlic. A similar odor can be detected in the breath after application of DMSO (dimethyl sulfoxide) to the skin; this is probably due to the fact that one of the intermediates of DMSO is quite similar in structure to allicin. Drugs like paraldehyde, which is volatile at body temperature, also appear in the expired air after oral or parenteral administration.

Volatile compounds have been used for the determination of the circulation time (ether), the cardiac output, the lung volumes (diethyl ether, acetone, alcohol, acetylene, nitrous oxide), and the detection of shunts (krypton). Unfortunately, their usefulness for accurate determination of the cardiac output is limited because of their solubility in tissue fluids. The classic example of this difficulty is acetylene, which, because of its solubility, is distributed in a lung tissue volume that is larger than the volume measured with an inert gas such as helium. As a result, values of the cardiac output measured with acetylene tend to be erroneously low.

METABOLISM

Endothelium

The pulmonary endothelium is part of a continuous vascular lining that extends from one end of the body to another (Fig. 15-2). In different parts of the body, endothelium assumes specialized functions. But overall, the endothelium has three extraordinary attributes that warrant special mention: (1) blood runs continuously over its luminal surface for a lifetime without appreciable clotting or denaturation of its proteins; no synthetic membrane has yet been devised that can duplicate this feat; (2) when appropriately stimulated, endothelium changes character; as part of the reticuloendothelial system, it can switch from indifference to circulating particulates to become intensely phagocytic; and (3) it serves as a metabolic organ that operates uninterruptedly under normal conditions in handling biologically active materials.

For endothelium to conduct its respiratory and nonrespiratory activities, it requires a large surface. Conventional wisdom has gauged the surface area provided by

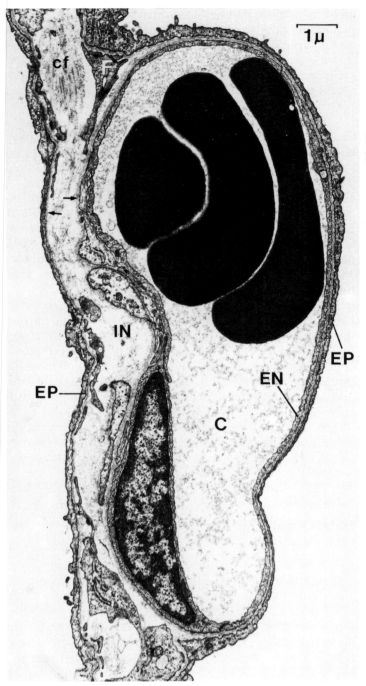

FIGURE 15-2 Transmission electron micrograph of cross section of alveolar capillary (C) from human lung. On the right, the basal laminae of epithelium (EP) and endothelium (EN) are fused; this is the "thin side" of the air-blood barrier. On the left is a distinct interstitial space (IN) containing connective tissue fibers (cf); this is the "thick side" of the air-blood barrier and is characterized by separation of the basal laminae (arrows). F = fibroblast. *(From Weibel and Bachofen, 1979.)*

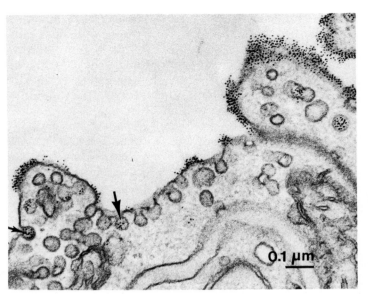

FIGURE 15-3 Pinocytotic vesicles after perfusion of lung with polycationized ferritin. Clusters of the charged ferritin are seen on the endothelial surface. The pinocytotic vesicles are clearly outlined, and some contained the polycationized ferritin (arrows). *(From Pietra et al., 1983.)*

endothelium to be of the order of 70 m². This is clearly an underestimate on two accounts: (1) the luminal surface is punctuated by pinocytotic vesicles (Fig. 15-3), many of which open to the vascular lumen; and (2) the luminal surface is covered by a glycocalyx ("endothelial fuzz") that seems to enlarge greatly the opportunity for contact between endothelium and plasma; the glycocalyx is disposed not only to serve as a molecular gateway to receptors, enzyme domains, and transport molecules on the endothelial surface but also to serve as a matrix for surface reactions.

Oxygen Consumption and Energy Requirements

In the adult, the O_2 consumption of the lungs accounts for as much as 4 percent of the total O_2 consumption of the body. The oxygen consumption of the lungs is of interest for at least two reasons: (1) it affords insight into the metabolic processes that take place in the lungs, and (2) oxygen consumed by the lungs could conceivably introduce an appreciable error in the determination of the cardiac output by Fick principle. The latter possibility is greater in lungs that are the seat of widespread cellular infiltration or neoplasm than in normal lungs.

Oxygen consumed by the lung is probably used not only to satisfy its own basal metabolic needs but also to meet the needs of additional metabolic reactions, i.e., the processing of biologically active substances, e.g., the inactivation of serotonin by deamination.

Although the relative oxygen uptakes by the different cellular elements of the normal lung are unknown, it seems likely that the alveolar macrophages, the type II alveolar epithelial cells, and the mast cells are responsible for most of the uptake since these cells contain the elements commonly associated with high metabolic activity. It has been estimated that there are six to eight type II alveolar epithelial cells per alveolus; assuming that there are 300 million alveoli, the tissue mass of type II cells is about that of the spleen.

Glucose is an important nutrient for the lungs. By providing both acetate and glycerophosphate, glucose supplies precursors for the formation of fatty acids and complex lipids. In addition, the lungs use lactic, pyruvic, acetic, and palmitic acids to form various components of complex lipids. The role of the lungs in handling circulating metabolic intermediates, such as lactic or pyruvic acid, is still unsettled, largely because arteriovenous differences across the lungs are narrow because of the large blood flow; as a result, analytic errors interfere seriously with the determination of arteriovenous differences in metabolic intermediates.

Lipid Metabolism

Lipid metabolism in the lungs has attracted particular attention because of surfactant on the one hand and the prostaglandins on the other (see Chapters 57 and 59). However, the lungs also have other major responsibilities in dealing with lipids: in the de novo synthesis of fatty acids, the esterification of lipids, the hydrolysis of lipid-ester bonds, and the oxidation of fatty acids. The alveolar type II cells are a key site of lipid synthesis, whereas the pulmonary capillary endothelium appears to be importantly involved in the hydrolysis of lipids. Although the sites of oxidation are unknown, except for the kidneys, the lungs have the highest rate in the body of oxidation of palmitate to CO_2.

LIPID SYNTHESIS

In contrast to organs such as the liver where the lipid metabolic pathways are oriented to form both neutral lipids and phospholipids, the lipid metabolic pathways of the lungs are geared primarily to form phospholipids. Phospholipids are typically found in high concentrations in membranous structures. The lungs, because of their enormous surface area, constitute the largest biologic membrane in the body.

HYDROLYSIS OF LIPID-ESTER BONDS

Lipids, especially long-chain fatty acids that have been absorbed in the intestinal tract, enter the bloodstream as chylomicra (glycerides in stable emulsion) via the thoracic duct; therefore, they are obliged to traverse the pulmonary circulation as minute globules that could coalesce to form fat emboli before reaching the systemic vessels. The lungs are important in clearing chylomicra from the bloodstream. One mechanism for doing so are lipoprotein lipases that are situated on the surface of, or within, pulmonary capillary endothelium. Whether other mechanisms exist, such as pinocytosis or effusion through capillary walls or pores, is not known.

PULMONARY SURFACTANT

In addition to the phospholipids in the anatomic membranous structures, the air-tissue interface of the alveolar membrane is coated with a separate phospholipid-rich layer (surfactant). The predominant phospholipid in this lining layer is dipalmityl lecithin, an unusual phosphatide that is highly surface-active. This lining layer lowers and stabilizes the surface tension of the lung as lung volumes undergo change during the respiratory cycle.

The ultramicroscopic and biochemical nature of surfactant is currently a topic of intensive research. Ultrastructurally, the phospholipids related to surfactant are represented by the lamellar bodies of type II cells (in which surfactant is stored) and their extracellular extrusions, the myelin figures (Fig. 15-4) lodged in the surfactant that lines the alveoli or fills alveolar corners. Biochemically, interest has shifted to the apolipoproteins that are associated with surfactant and that are believed to influence the movement of surfactant across the membranes of the type I cells and their organelles.

BLOOD-ENDOTHELIAL INTERACTIONS

Continuous interactions between the constituents of the blood and the endothelium are essential for normal growth and development and for the metabolic activities of daily life. Respiratory gases, water, electrolytes, nutrients, and other molecules move endlessly, in one direction or another, across the alveolar-capillary barrier (Fig. 15-5). Leukocytes migrate across endothelium to the site of injury under the guiding influence of chemotactic substances. Hormones generated in the lungs, e.g., angiotensin II, travel long distances in the blood to engage in biologic processes far removed from their sites of origin. Each metabolic system is governed by elaborate control mecha-

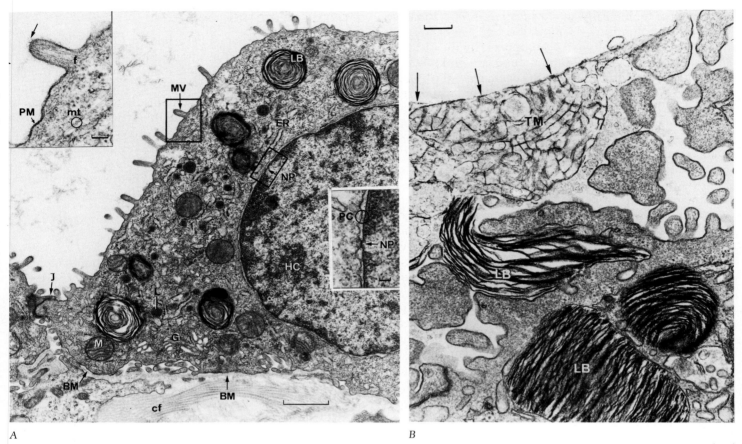

A   *B*

FIGURE 15-4 Type II cell. *A.* Part of a type II cell to show its organization. The nucleus is enwrapped by a perinuclear cisterna (PC) made of two membranes, which is traversed by nuclear pores (NP), shown *(inset, right)* at greater magnification; nuclear content is divided into dense heterochromatin (HC) areas and karyoplasm, which contains euchromatin. Cell surface is made of the plasma membrane (PM) with a subjacent ectoplasmic layer of filaments (f) and a fuzzy coat or glycocalyx (arrow) on the outside *(inset, left).* Cells in epithelia are joined by junctional complexes (J) with terminal bars at the boundary between apical and lateral face; basal face is attached to the basement membrane (BM). Cytoplasm houses a variety of organelles; cf = collagen fibrils; ER = endoplasmic reticulum; G = Golgi complex; L = lysosomes; LB = lamellar body; M = mitochondrion; mt = microtubule; MV = microvilli. Bars: 1 μm; 0.1 μm *(insets).* *B.* Release of lamellar body (LB) from type II cell into surface lining layer, which contains tubular myelin (TM) that is continuous with the phospholipid surface lining film (arrows). Bar: 0.2 μm. *(From Weibel, 1985.)*

FIGURE 15-5 Permeability of the pulmonary vasculature to macromolecules, e.g., plasma proteins. *A.* Potential transendothelial pathways. Water- and lipid-soluble molecules can cross the entire cell (1) or via interendothelial clefts (2) as part of bulk flow. Macromolecules can cross by pinocytotic vesicles (PV) or via the endothelial junctions (EJ) in the interendothelial clefts (2). *B.* "Small pores" in alveolar capillaries. Normal pulmonary capillary pressures. Stroma-free hemoglobin (molecular weight about same as albumin) injected into a perfused isolated lung of dog is arrested at intercellular junctions (arrow). Physiological measurements estimate these small pores to be about 40 Å. Hb = stroma-free hemoglobin injected intravascularly as tracer; EJ = endothelial junction; PV = pinocytotic vesicles; BL = basal lamina; EP = epithelium; ALV = alveolus. *C.* "Small pores" in alveolar capillaries. Same preparation as *A* but mean pulmonary capillary pressure = 50 mmHg. The tracer has now traversed the intercellular junctions because of "stretched pores." Hb = stroma-free hemoglobin injected intravascularly as tracer; EJ = endothelial junction; PV = pinocytotic vesicles; BL = basal lamina; EP = epithelium. *D.* "Large pores" in alveolar capillaries. Most of the plasma proteins traversing the endothelium to enter the pericapillary interstitial spaces do so in pinocytotic vesicles (arrows). These vesicles are believed to be the anatomic equivalent of physiological large pores. BM = basement membrane (basal lamina). *E.* Gaps in bronchial venules. These venules are part of the systemic circulation to the lungs. The gaps appear after injection of histamine (which leaves pulmonary capillaries unaffected). Carbon particles are shown escaping through the gaps. END = endothelium; IS = interstitial space; C = carbon particles. *(From Fishman and Pietra, 1974; Pietra et al., 1983.)*

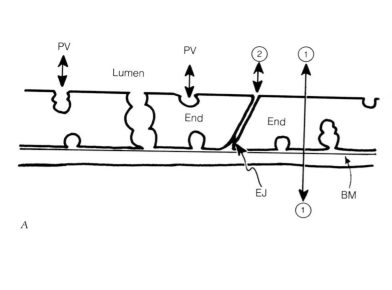

A

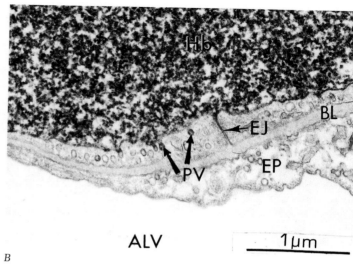

ALV

B

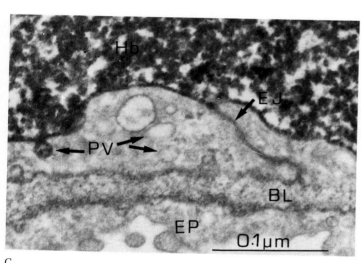

C

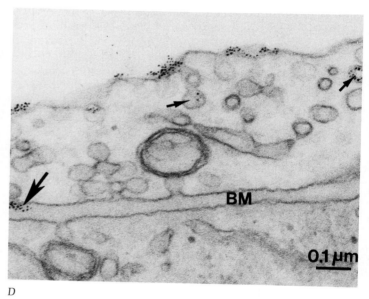

D

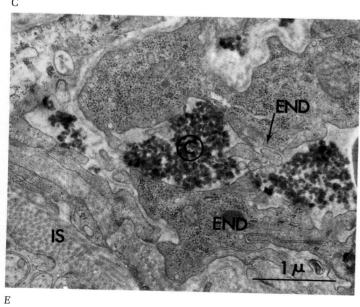

E

nisms that keep the metabolic processes in the lungs within homeostatic bounds. The pulmonary capillary endothelium, interacting with blood constituents, plays a vital role in many of these processes. For example, the pulmonary capillary endothelium is part of an elaborate mechanism for the control of systemic arterial blood pressure: on its luminal surface, the angiotensin converting enzyme degrades bradykinin (a potent vasodilator) to inactive products; the same enzyme also converts angiotensin I to angiotensin II (a powerful vasoconstrictor) (Fig. 15-6). In addition, pulmonary capillary endothelium generates angiotensin III, a hormone that acts on the kidneys to influence blood pressure by way of salt and water balance.

Angiogenesis

The growth of new capillaries is greatly dependent on the activity of endothelial cells. The endothelial cells that line capillaries are usually in a resting state. Their rate of proliferation is so low that turnover times are measured in years. However, these endothelial cells are capable of sudden growth spurts during periods when new capillaries are rapidly forming, e.g., during wound healing. The process of new capillary formation is called *angiogenesis*, and cell turnover times during angiogenesis are measured in days.

Protracted angiogenesis is observed in diverse pathologic states as chronic inflammation arthritis, psoriasis, diabetic retinopathy, and chronic inflammation. In many of these abnormalities, angiogenesis itself contributes to the disease process: in arthritis, new capillaries can invade and destroy joint cartilage; in diabetes, new capillaries in the retina of the eye hemorrhage and cause blindness. Progressive growth of tumors and their ability to form metastases depend on continuous angiogenesis.

Angiogenesis in the lungs is now only a matter of speculation. But, angiogenesis in other tissues undoubtedly has implications for angiogenesis in tumors and chronic inflammatory processes in the lungs. Early in capillary formation, endothelial cells release specific enzymes that punch holes in the vascular basement membrane. Endothelial cells migrate through these holes. The cells align in a linear configuration to form a new sprout. The sprout elongates through interstitial tissue toward an angiogenic stimulus such as a small tumor. Sprout elongation depends on chemotaxis of endothelial cells at the tip of the sprout, division of cells farther back, and production of interstitial collagenases, probably by all the endothelial cells in the sprout.

Endothelial cells and debris-scavenging macrophages play major roles in the inflammatory process and wound healing. Angiogenesis, an automatic feedback system, has

TABLE 15-2

Handling of Biologically Active Materials in the Pulmonary Capillary Bed

Metabolized at endothelial surface without uptake from plasma
Angiotensin I—activated
Bradykinin—inactivated
Adenine nucleotides—inactivated
Metabolized intracellularly after uptake from plasma
Serotonin
Norepinephrine
Prostaglandins E and F
Unaffected by traversing lungs
Epinephrine
Prostaglandin A
Angiotensin II
Dopamine
Vasopressin
Histamine
Vasoactive intestinal polypeptide
Substance P
Prostacyclin
Synthesized within lungs and released into blood
Prostaglandins E and F
Clotting and fibrinolytic factors
Lipoprotein lipase
Discharged from intrapulmonary stores into blood
Histamine
Prostaglandins
Slow-reacting substance of anaphylaxis (leukotrienes C_4 and D_4)
Kallikreins
Eosinophil leukocyte chemotactic factor of anaphylaxis

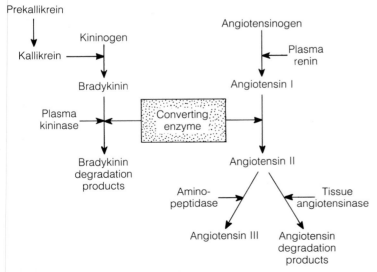

FIGURE 15-6   The metabolic pathways of bradykinin and angiotensin I showing the central role of converting enzyme.

been depicted to control angiogenesis. For example, in the depth of a fresh wound, tissue oxygen levels become extremely low because capillaries have been damaged and blood flow interrupted; macrophages that migrate into the wound secrete angiogenesis factors in a setting that is poor in oxygen. New capillaries are attracted into the wound, oxygen tension rises, and the macrophages then reduce or shut off their stimulation of angiogenesis.

Biologically Active Substances

Blood constituents react with each other as well as with the endothelial lining. In an area of vascular injury, contact of platelets with collagen or macrophages causes them to aggregate; their storage granules then discharge biologically active substances that promote the formation and organization of a clot to plug the breach in the endothelial lining. Enzymes and growth factors released by the aggregated platelets attract other platelets, evoke spasm

and proliferation of adjacent vascular smooth muscle, and draw coagulation proteins to the area for the assembly of the clot. These reactions are controlled by molecular feedback mechanisms. For instance, the activity of thromboxane, released by platelets to promote local vascular constriction and accumulation of other platelets, is modulated in its clot-promoting effects by prostacyclin (an antiaggregating and vasodilator agent) liberated by endothelium.

The lungs seem to distinguish between "local hormones," the actions of which are confined to the vicinity of the site of release, and "circulating hormones" that pass unchanged through the pulmonary circulation. In the category of local hormones are bradykinin, norepinephrine, and serotonin; examples of circulating hormones are epinephrine, isoproterenol, and dopamine (Table 15-2). In abnormal lungs, such as in the adult respiratory distress syndrome, the ability to handle local and circulating hormones is often impaired (Fig. 15-7).

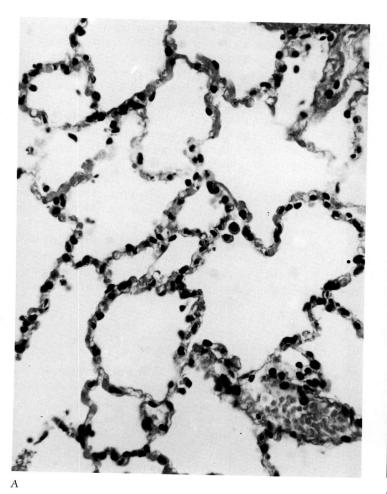

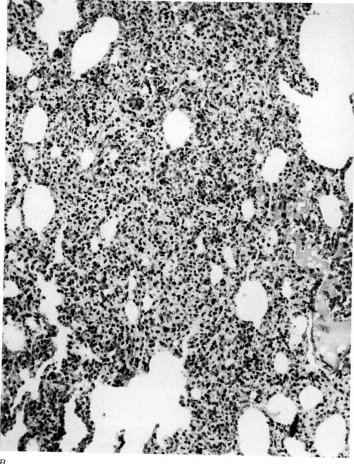

A   *B*

FIGURE 15-7   Abnormal lung in the adult respiratory distress syndrome. In contrast to the normal lung in which a delicate capillary network lies between airspaces (*A*), the microcirculation of the abnormal lung (*B*) is compressed by inflammatory cells and fluid in the airless lung. Should blood percolate through the abnormal lung, it would encounter abnormal endothelium and obliterate airspaces.

Endogenous Amines

Since 1925, when Starling and Verney showed that the lungs had to be included in the circuit of circulation if defibrinated blood through the isolated kidney was to continue, it has been realized that the lungs were involved in detoxification. The substance in question was later shown to be the vasoactive amine, serotonin (5-hydroxytryptamine). In the past decade, the lungs have also been implicated in the processing of other biologically active amines (Table 15-2).

HISTAMINE

The lungs are rich in histamine. In general, their histamine content seems to be related to their mast cell content (Fig. 15-8). Histamine originates from histidine by decarboxylation and is degraded enzymatically by oxidative deamination or methylation. The release of histamine from sites of production within cells probably also involves enzymatic reactions because its release can be modified, or even arrested, either by manipulations that block the reactivity of S—H groups (or S—S bonds) or by oxygen lack.

Much more is known about the pulmonary effects of exogenous than of endogenous histamine. Histamine is commonly released in response to injury and during anaphylactic shock. The outpouring of histamine during anaphylaxis is accompanied by degranulation of mast cells in the lungs and the release of a variety of biologically active mediators: heparin, proteolytic enzymes, lipids ("silico-

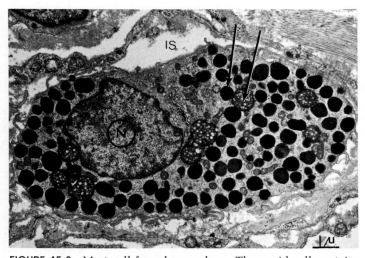

FIGURE 15-8   Mast cell from human lung. The ovoid cell contains many electron-dense granules (arrows). Within the granules may be found heparin, a variety of amines including histamine, and a wide assortment of other biologically active substances: prostaglandins E and F, slow reacting substance of anaphylaxis (leukotrienes), kallikrein, esterases, acid phosphatase, and beta-glucuronidase (lead citrate–uranyl acetate stains). IS = interstitial space; N = nucleus.

reacting substance of anaphylaxis" and prostaglandins), amines (serotonin), proteins (kallikrein), and polypeptides (bradykinin and eosinophil leukocyte chemotactic factor of anaphylaxis).

SEROTONIN (5-HYDROXYTRYPTAMINE)

An efficient removal system for 5-hydroxytryptamine (5-HT) exists in the pulmonary circulation. 5-HT, like norepinephrine, is removed from the flowing blood by a carrier-mediated, sodium-dependent transport system. The 5-HT is rapidly metabolized by oxidative deamination that involves monamine oxidase enzymes. In the lungs, it is difficult to separate the chemical transformation of 5-HT by endothelium from its uptake by platelets.

In patients with metastatic carcinoid, a tumor derived from argentaffin cells, appreciable quantities of serotonin are released into the circulation. These patients are apt to develop lesions of the right side of the heart that may culminate in pulmonic stenosis or tricuspid insufficiency. Histologically, these lesions consist of a peculiar fibrous tissue, characteristically devoid of elastic fibers. The preferential location of these changes in the right heart is consistent with observations indicating that serotonin is retained and inactivated during its passage through the lung. This view is further reinforced by the occasional patient who had both a carcinoid and an atrial septal defect. In these patients all four valves of the heart are apt to be affected, presumably because blood containing serotonin flowed through the atrial communication instead of through the lung to reach the left heart. Serotonin is probably also involved in the "asthmatic" bronchoconstriction that occurs in patients with "malignant carcinoid" and may play a role in the pathogenesis of anaphylactic reactions.

A major difficulty in pinpointing the effects of serotonin is the multiplicity of its effects: pulmonary vasoconstriction, bronchoconstriction, and augmented ventilation; each of these may also be stimulated either directly or reflexly.

VASOACTIVE POLYPEPTIDES

The lungs are involved in the activation, inactivation, and release of circulating peptides. Bradykinin and angiotensin are the two peptides of paramount interest. The pulmonary kinase activity and the angiotensin I converting enzyme activity result from a single enzyme, i.e., converting enzyme (Fig. 15-6). Bradykinin, a vasoactive polypeptide, is formed from bradykininogen by the proteolytic enzyme kallikrein; factor XII is required to activate the bradykininogen.

Parenteral administration of bradykinin elicits profound hemodynamic effects. For example, it stimulates the heart, dilates blood vessels, and produces considerable systemic hypotension; it also increases capillary permeability. Some of these effects may be indirect, e.g., secondary to the release of epinephrine by bradykinin from the adrenal medulla. Polypeptide materials similar to bradykinin are capable of reproducing painful sensations in the skin.

Up to 80 percent of bradykinin infused intravenously disappears during passage through the pulmonary circulation. In the adult lung, bradykinin seems to exert little direct effect on the pulmonary circulation. In contrast, the pulmonary vascular bed of the fetal lamb is exquisitely sensitive to bradykinin, dilating massively in response to minute doses. The greater sensitivity of the fetal lamb than the adolescent lamb to the same doses of bradykinin may be due to the higher initial tone of the pulmonary vessels in the fetus.

Angiotensin I, a decapeptide, is formed by the action of renin, an enzyme present in the juxtaglomerular apparatus of the kidney on angiotensinogen (Fig. 15-6). In turn, converting enzyme splits off the dipeptide His-Leu at the carboxyl terminus to form the octapeptide angiotensin II, one of the most potent vasopressors known. Angiotensin is 10 to 50 times more powerful as a vasoconstrictor than is angiotensin I. Inhibitors of converting enzyme prevent the formation of angiotensin II. Converting enzyme is located on pulmonary capillary endothelial surfaces, making it readily accessible to the flowing blood.

PROSTAGLANDINS

The lungs are a major site of synthesis of the prostaglandins and related substances, notably thromboxanes A_2 and B_2 (Fig. 15-9). Prostaglandins are synthesized by a ubiquitous multienzyme complex, i.e., PG synthetase. Interactions occur between bradykinin and the PG synthetase systems. The lungs are rich in PG synthetase, but the localization of PG synthetase is unclear, except that it can be isolated from microsomal fractions and prostaglandins are readily synthesized and released in response to diverse stimuli: vasoactive peptides, anaphylaxis, histamine, serotonin, mechanical stimulation, and chemical stimulation. Aspirinlike agents inhibit PG synthetase.

The lungs can also inactivate prostaglandins. Prostaglandins of the E and F series are metabolized during passage through the lungs; the extraction of prostaglandins of the A series varies with species. The role played by endothelium in the metabolism of the prostaglandins is unknown. Whether the lungs synthesize and release prostaglandins under physiological conditions is unclear. However, there seems to be little doubt that pathophysiological stimuli, such as extreme hyperventilation, can promote the release of prostaglandins.

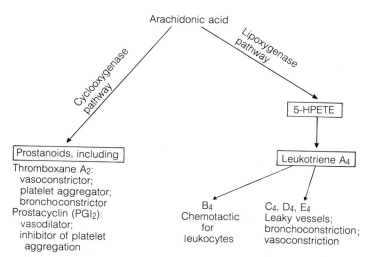

FIGURE 15-9 Some products of arachidonic acid metabolism that affect the lungs. The leukotrienes were formerly known as the "slow reacting substance(s) of anaphylaxis (SRS-A)." 5-HPETE = 5-hydroperoxyeicosatetraenoic acid.

OTHERS

The biologically active agents dealt with above are only a sample of the many substances handled by the endothelium of the lungs. For example, adenosine 5'H-triphosphate (ATP) and adenosine 5'H-monophosphate (AMP) are metabolized by the lungs via phosphate esterase enzymes situated on the luminal surface of pulmonary endothelial cells, and their metabolites appear in the pulmonary venous effluent.

Another example is the uptake of hormones presumably for their own use. Glucocorticoids enhance the production of surfactant by fetal lungs; similar effects can be produced by administering thyroxine.

Chemicals

A wide variety of chemicals that have biologic activity accumulate in the lungs. Among these are narcotics, antidepressants, antihistamines, and herbicides, e.g., paraquat, which is a dipyridyl derivative. Most of these substances (except for paraquat) are "basic amines," some of which contain hydrophobic moieties. The herbicide paraquat accumulates in lung tissue where it inflicts damage primarily by the generation of oxygen radicals. However, its rate of removal, which, like 5-HT, depends on a carrier-mediated transport system, is much slower than that of 5-HT or norepinephrine. Because of its accumulation and persistence in lung tissue, methadone can be administered orally in a single dose per day. Certain amphiphilic drugs, such as imipramine, chloripramine, and chloroquine, accumulate in the lungs and can cause "drug-induced phospholipidosis."

HEMOFLUIDITY AND THE LUNGS

Endothelial cells also participate in maintaining the fluidity of the blood, while ensuring that clot formation occurs locally as needed to limit bleeding; complex sequences of enzymatic reactions ("cascades") either form or dissolve clots. Injured endothelial lining is a mecca for cellular and humoral components of the blood that promote clotting. Prostacyclin generated by the injured endothelium modulates the clotting response; bradykinin, released and destroyed locally, enhances the generation of prostacyclin. And thrombin, the final product in the clotting process, also triggers the anticlotting process. It does so by activating the anticoagulant protein C and by increasing tissue-type plasminogen activator (t-PA) activity. The release of t-PA from endothelium initiates the formation of plasmin, the primary fibrinolytic enzyme of the blood. In turn, platelets release an inhibition of both urokinase and t-PA. Thus, clotting and fibrinolysis are inextricably linked and modulated to form or to lyse thrombi as needed (Fig. 15-10).

Proteolysis

Fibrin is needed for clot formation and the prevention of blood loss (see Chapter 65). Oppositely, the removal of fibrin (fibrinolysis) is a prerequisite for maintaining patent blood vessels. The lung is one of the richest sources of cofactors that either promote (thromboplastin) or inhibit (heparin) blood coagulation; in addition, it contains an activator that converts circulating plasminogen to the proteolytic enzyme, plasmin. The balance between these opposing processes maintains the fluidity of blood.

Without an effective mechanism for ridding itself of aggregated and clotted proteinaceous material, the lungs

would be exceedingly susceptible to occlusive vascular disease. Indeed, removal of clots is accomplished more readily in the lungs than in any part of the peripheral circulation. As a consequence, autologous thrombi, which have been administered intravenously in sufficient quantity to involve most of the pulmonary vascular tree in dogs, cannot be identified histologically in the pulmonary vessels after 2 to 6 weeks.

The proteolytic activity of the lung may not be restricted to fibrinolysis. For example, the disappearance of labeled macroaggregates of human serum albumin from the lungs within a few hours after intravenous injection may be due, at least in part, to proteolytic dissolution. Although it is likely that the mammalian lung contains more than one proteolytic enzyme system, the section that follows is primarily concerned with the fibrinolytic system of the lungs.

Fibrinolytic Activity

In essence the mechanism for fibrinolysis involves a series of reactions in which activators convert the circulating inactive proenzyme, plasminogen (profibrinolysin), to an active proteolytic enzyme, plasmin (fibrinolysin) (Fig. 15-10). The sources of activators include tissues, such as the lung, the formed elements of the blood, and thrombin.

The mammalian lung may participate in the formation and lysis of fibrin clots in one of several ways. First, by preventing clot (fibrin) formation within the pulmonary vessels it may help to maintain hemofluidity within the microcirculation of the lung; second, by fibrinolysis it may free the organ of trapped fibrin emboli; and third, by releasing plasmin activator into the circulation it may contribute to the fibrinolytic activity in circulating blood. The mammalian lung is an unusually rich source of plasmin activator. The activator has been identified in the endothelium of arteries, veins, venules, and capillaries.

Plasmin not only functions as a fibrinolytic enzyme, but also stimulates the formation of highly vasoactive polypeptides (kinins) from circulating precursors. These kinins are generally formed by the action of enzymes, such as kallikrein, that are also present in the lung. By providing plasmin activator and kallikrein, the lung participates indirectly in the formation of the kinins. In addition to a plasmin activator, lung tissue contains an inhibitor of fibrinolysis.

Disorders of Fibrinolysis

Occasionally, fibrinolysis becomes excessive. For example, a bleeding tendency and excessive fibrinolysis occur after manipulation of the lungs during cardiac arrest, pulmonary surgery, and open-heart surgery. In these situations fibrinolysis may be uncontrollable, apparently because of excessive amounts of plasminogen activator in the circulation. That the activator originates in the lungs

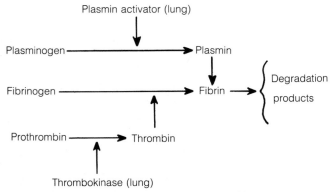

FIGURE 15-10 Fibrinolysis. Plasminogen and fibrinogen are circulating precursors. The lung is rich in tissue activators that convert plasminogen to plasmin (the fibrinolytic enzyme that acts on fibrin). The lung is also rich in thrombokinase, which converts the circulating precursor prothrombin to thrombin, which plays a key role in the conversion of fibrinogen to fibrin. *(From Heinemann and Fishman, 1969.)*

is suggested by the observation that pulmonary venous blood from dogs and humans has higher fibrinolytic activity than does mixed venous blood. It should be noted that at least two other mechanisms may contribute to the bleeding tendency after manipulation of the lungs: one is enhanced fibrinolysis after augmented thromboplastin release; the other is the overconsumption of plasma clotting factors.

Deficient fibrinolytic activity has been found in several diseases and has been implicated in the pathogenesis of two important clinical disorders: hyaline membrane formation in the lung and the pulmonary manifestations of cystic fibrosis.

Thromboplastin

Except for brain tissue, the mammalian lung is the richest source in the body of thromboplastin, a phosphatide-protein complex that promotes the conversion of prothrombin to thrombin. Purification of the microsomal fraction obtained from beef lung produces an enzymelike substance that induces coagulant activity in serum when phospholipid and calcium are added. The thromboplastic activity seems to be an enzyme-dependent reaction with phospholipid acting as a cofactor. The clot-promoting and antifibrinolytic activity of surface-active lipoprotein (surfactant), which has been implicated in the genesis of hyaline membranes, may be due to the fact that surfactant is rich in the phospholipids that have been shown to accelerate clot formation. Accelerated thromboplastin generation is seen in certain diseases, such as carcinoma of the lung, which are associated with a high incidence of thromboembolic complications.

Heparin

This is an acidic, sulfate-containing proteoglycan found in high concentrations in the lungs; in adult humans, the lungs may contain as much as 400 mg of heparin. Indeed, the large content of heparin in beef lungs makes this tissue one of the best sources for its commercial production. Heparin is synthesized in tissues by mast cells; in the lung, as in other tissues, the content of heparin is usually related to the density of the mast cell population.

The chemical homogeneity of heparin is still in doubt. Indeed, heparin from different species—and even different tissues of the same species—may differ in structure. Heparin is removed from the blood by renal excretion, by uptake into the reticuloendothelial system, and by enzymatic inactivation involving heparinase, an enzyme as yet identified only in the liver.

Heparin is a multifaceted molecule. Among its diverse effects can be identified: (1) anticoagulant activity, (2) stimulation of angiogenesis, (3) inhibition of the proliferation of vascular smooth muscle and of mesangial cells, (4) inhibition of the action of complement, (5) modulation

of hypersensitivity reactions, (6) release of lipoprotein lipase, (7) stimulation of pinocytosis and phagocytosis, and (8) control of enzyme binding to endothelial surfaces. This list is only a sampler. But, despite its impressive array of functions, heparin remains a molecule of mystery: What is its dominant biologic function? Is it anticoagulation? How does its role as an anticoagulant relate to its many other activities?

EPILOGUE

It has been shown above that in addition to their role in gas exchange, the lungs play a vital role in the overall economy of the body as well as in self-defense (Fig. 15-11). The apparently simple histologic structure of the alveolar-capillary barriers is deceptive. Situated at the exit from the liver, the lungs are regularly faced with its meta-

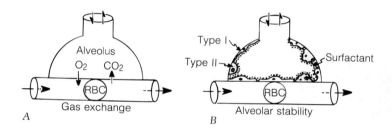

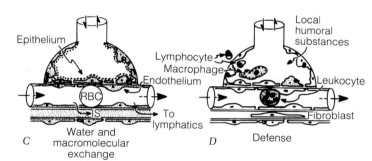

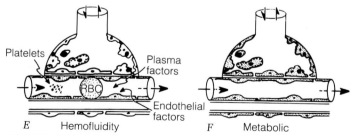

FIGURE 15-11 The nonrespiratory functions of the lungs range from local activities, such as alveolar stability (*B*) and water and macromolecular exchange (*C*), essential for the integrity and functioning of the lungs as an organ, to functions that are essential for the whole body, i.e., defense mechanisms (*D*), maintenance of hemofluidity (*E*), and the processing of biologically active substances (*F*). The respiratory function of the lungs, i.e., gas exchange, is represented in (*A*).

bolic products, often completing the process of handling biologically active materials left unfinished by the liver. On their endothelial aspect, the entire cardiac output is distributed as a thin film for gas exchange and for plasma-endothelium interactions. On their alveolar aspect, each breath exposes the lungs to ambient air; in doing so, the lungs run the risk of drying mucosal linings. Curiously, the lungs, once judged to be relatively inaccessible, have now become the most accessible of all organs: where else is it possible to sample as exhaustively as from the lungs, e.g., mixed venous blood, arterial blood, lymphatic fluid, tracheobronchial secretions, and alveolar washings? Consequently, they are a natural target for research on fundamental biologic problems, e.g., the inflammatory process, as well as their own intrinsic behavior under normal and abnormal conditions.

BIBLIOGRAPHY

Curry FE: Effect of albumin on the structure of the molecular filter at the capillary wall. Fed Proc 44:2610–2613, 1985.
> *A description of the fiber-matrix model of capillary permeability and an investigation of the role played by albumin in the molecular filter.*

Fishman AP: Pulmonary edema: The water-exchanging function of the lung. Circulation 46:390–408, 1972.
> *An early consideration of the turnover of water in the lungs picturing a "third circulation," i.e., of water and macromolecules, as well as the two blood circulations, pulmonary and bronchial.*

Fishman AP (ed): Endothelium. Ann NY Acad Sci 401:1–274, 1982.
> *Endothelium approached as a distributed organ of diverse capabilities. The summing up by Palade (pages 265 to 272) regards endothelium in terms of "a usual, non-differentiated epithelial component and a differentiated (endothelium-specific) component."*

Fishman AP, Pietra GG: Handling of bioactive materials by the lung. N Engl J Med 291:884–890, 953–959, 1974.
> *Structural-functional correlations in the metabolic processing of vasoactive materials by the lungs.*

Gillis CN, Pitt BR: The fate of circulating amines within the pulmonary circulation. Ann Rev Physiol 44:269–281, 1982.
> *The clearance of various biologically active materials by the lungs is altered in pathologic states. This article focuses on the removal of pulmonary amines by injured lungs.*

Heinemann HO, Fishman AP: Nonrespiratory functions of mammalian lung. Physiol Rev 49:1–47, 1969.
> *A comprehensive review of the biology of the lungs leading to the conclusion that they serve important nonrespiratory functions.*

Jaffe EA: *Biology of Endothelial Cells.* Boston, Martinus Nijhoff, 1984.
> *A comprehensive survey of the major facets of endothelial cell physiology based largely on cultured endothelial cells.*

King RJ, Clements JA: Lipid synthesis and surfactant turnover in the lungs, in Fishman AP, Fisher AB (eds), *Handbook of Physiology, sect 3: The Respiratory System, vol I: Circulation and Nonrespiratory Functions.* Bethesda, American Physiological Society, 1985, pp 309–336.
> *This chapter focuses on the role of lipids in maintaining the architecture of the lungs. A subsequent chapter by Y. S. Bakhle and S. H. Ferreira deals with the eicosanoids.*

Philpot RM, Anderson MW, Eling TE: Uptake, accumulation and metabolism of chemicals by the lung, in Bakhle YS, Vane JR (eds), *Metabolic Functions of the Lung.* New York, Dekker, 1977, pp 123–172.
> *A comprehensive overview of the ability of the lungs to concentrate and store chemicals and the toxicologic implications of these accumulations.*

Pietra GG, Sampson P, Lanken PN, Hansen-Flaschen J, Fishman AP: Transcapillary movement of cationized ferritin in the isolated perfused rat lung. Lab Invest 49:54–61, 1983.
> *In accord with the observations of Simionescu, Simionescu, and Palade on microvascular domains elsewhere, anionic sites (domains) are identified on the luminal surface of pulmonary microvascular endothelium. The diaphragms of the pinocytotic vesicles contain highly charged anionic sites that seem to be important in the transport of charged macromolecules.*

Ryan US, Ryan JW, Crutchley DJ: The pulmonary endothelial surface. Fed Proc 44:2603–2609, 1985.
> *A concise review of the complexity of the endothelial surface and of the diverse biologic processes that take place on its aspects.*

Ryan US: *Pulmonary Endothelium in Health and Disease.* New York, Dekker, 1987.
A far-ranging update of the last 10 years of research on the pulmonary endothelium.

Simionescu N, Simionescu M, Palade GE: Differentiated microdomains on the luminal surface of the capillary endothelium. I. Preferential distribution of anionic sites. J Cell Biol 90:605–613, 1981.
An early study of the effect of surface charge on the movement of molecules across the wall of blood capillaries. The results show differentiated microdomains in vascular endothelium that preferentially bind cationized ferritin and presage studies by the same group and others that have reinforced this seminal observation and led to the discovery of active transport of albumin by pinocytotic vesicles across capillary endothelium.

Starling EH, Verney EB: The secretion of urine as studied on the isolated kidney. Proc Roy Soc B 97:321–363, 1925.
The classic paper that implicated a circulating toxic substance (serotonin) in the deterioration of the isolated kidney unless the lungs were included in the circulation.

Vane JR: The release and fate of vasoactive hormones in the circulation. Br J Pharmacol 35:209–242, 1969.
Distinctions are drawn between "local" and "circulating" hormones.

Weibel ER: Lung cell biology, in Fishman AP, Fisher AB (eds), *Handbook of Physiology,* sect 3: The *Respiratory System,* vol 1: *Circulation and Nonrespiratory Functions.* Bethesda, MD, American Physiological Society, 1985, pp 47–91.
The structure of the lungs viewed within the framework of cell biology with remarkable depictions of the variegated cell populations of the lungs.

Weibel ER, Bachofen H: Structural design of the alveolar septum and fluid exchange, in Fishman AP, Renkin EM (eds), *Pulmonary Edema.* Bethesda, MD, American Physiological Society, 1979, pp 1–19.
An analysis of the structure of the alveolar-capillary barrier with respect to its role in water exchange.

Chapter *16*

Blood-Gas Transport

Michael P. Hlastala

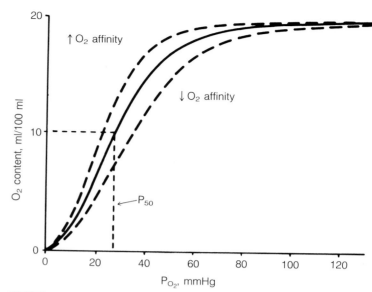

FIGURE 16-1 The oxygen equilibrium curve of human blood. The normal curve (solid line) has a P_{50} (P_{O_2} at 50 percent saturation) of 27 mmHg. Two other curves, one with increased oxygen affinity (decreased P_{50}) and one with decreased oxygen affinity (increased P_{50}), are also shown.

OXYGEN TRANSPORT

The circulatory system provides special mechanisms in order to deliver the large quantities of oxygen required by the peripheral tissues. The major factor is the presence of hemoglobin in blood. Reversible binding of O_2 greatly enhances the effective solubility of O_2 in blood compared to that in other body fluids. In addition to quantitative transport requirements, O_2 must be delivered at a pressure sufficient to allow for its diffusion to the intracellular mitochondria where it is utilized.

Oxygen Equilibrium Curve

The relationship between content and pressure for gases dissolved in blood is linear (Henry's law). Inert gases (such as nitrogen or argon) are carried only in the dissolved form in blood. Oxygen differs from inert gases because of its binding with hemoglobin. Four O_2 molecules can bind with each hemoglobin molecule through a complex interaction that occurs between the four heme components. Binding of an O_2 molecule to one heme site affects the affinity for ligands at other heme sites on the molecule. The resulting S-shaped content-pressure relationship, the O_2 equilibrium curve (also called the O_2 dissociation curve) of blood, is shown in Fig. 16-1. The phys-

iological portion of the curve includes the partial pressures and contents normally seen in arterial blood and in the venous effluent of various organs under both resting and exercising conditions. The flatness of the curve in the arterial range is an advantage because decrements in arterial P_{O_2} (as might be caused by lung disease or excursions to altitude) will still allow for a relatively normal arterial O_2 content. Because of the steepness of the equilibrium curve below 50 mmHg, large quantities of O_2 can be released while the partial pressure of O_2 remains relatively high. Increased O_2 extraction can be achieved with only a relatively small decrease in partial pressure. Although the O_2 content of mixed venous blood is approximately 15 ml per 100 ml of blood (15 vol %) at rest, and may fall to 10 ml per 100 ml during exercise, the O_2 contents of venous blood leaving some organs, such as the heart, are even less. Under pathologic circumstances, venous O_2 content may decrease even further. Adequacy of blood oxygenation can be expressed in a variety of ways. The most common, the arterial P_{O_2}, indicates the partial pressure, but not the content of O_2 in blood.

Oxygen Affinity

The relative affinity of hemoglobin for oxygen, and the position of the O_2 equilibrium curve, can change under a variety of different physiological conditions. However, the sigmoid shape of the curve remains unchanged. A change in O_2 affinity of hemoglobin results in a shift in the position of the equilibrium curve. The magnitude of change in O_2 affinity is indicated by the change in P_{50}, i.e., the oxygen partial pressure needed to achieve 50 percent saturation of hemoglobin. The curve to the left of the normal curve in Fig. 16-1 has a P_{50} of 22 mmHg, indicating that the O_2 affinity is high, since the P_{O_2} required to half-saturate blood is less than normal (27 mmHg). Shifts of the equilibrium curve can be physiologically important—a left shift permits greater O_2 binding, an important factor in O_2 uptake in the fetus in utero or in normal lungs at altitude. However, an increased affinity (lower P_{50}) may impair tissue O_2 delivery since greater binding can limit O_2 release in the periphery. A shift of the curve to the right may enhance O_2 delivery to tissues because oxygen can be delivered while maintaining a higher than normal P_{O_2}, thereby promoting diffusion from the capillary to the cells. Shifts in the curve in either direction are mediated by several factors, all additive in their effect on the position of the O_2 equilibrium curve.

Bohr Effect

An increase in plasma and, therefore, in the intracellular hydrogen ion concentration $[H^+]$ displaces the equilibrium curve to the right. Originally, the shift in the curve was attributed entirely to a change in pH, whether mediated by the addition of fixed acid or a change in P_{CO_2}. However, CO_2 does have a direct effect on O_2 affinity in addition to that associated with a change in pH. This direct effect results from binding of CO_2 to the hemoglobin molecule. But it is small compared to the H^+ effect. A shift of the curve caused by a fixed acid, such as lactic acid, is less than a shift to a comparable pH caused by CO_2.

The Bohr effect assists O_2 exchange to a small extent. In the tissues, addition of CO_2 to blood shifts the O_2 equilibrium curve to the right, releasing O_2 bound to hemoglobin. In the lungs, as the equilibrium curve returns to its normal position with excretion of CO_2, O_2 binding is enhanced. It has been calculated that the Bohr effect accounts for only a few percent of total O_2 uptake, less than assumed previously, because of the small pH changes that occur between arterial and venous blood.

2,3-Diphosphoglycerate

The human erythrocyte contains large quantities of 2,3-diphosphoglycerate (DPG), an organic phosphate that binds to hemoglobin and affects the O_2 affinity. Two different mechanisms are involved: (1) DPG binds more readily to reduced hemoglobin than to oxyhemoglobin, tending to "hold" the molecule in the reduced configuration, and (2) at body pH, the organic phosphate has four negative charges and reduces intraerythrocytic pH by the Donnan effect, since the large DPG molecule does not cross the cell membrane; the reduction in intracellular pH causes a decrease in affinity through the Bohr mechanism.

An increased concentration of DPG is a compensatory mechanism in pathologic states characterized by reduced O_2 transport. The shift of the O_2 dissociation curve to the right facilitates O_2 delivery, maintaining tissue oxygenation despite a reduction in the absolute quantity of O_2 delivered to peripheral tissues.

Blood stored in acid solution is deficient in DPG, leading to questions concerning its efficacy after transfusion in O_2 delivery. Fortunately, normal levels of 2,3-DPG are regenerated in transfused cells within a day after transfusion. In the intervening period, O_2 exchange continues to take place even though efficiency may be somewhat reduced.

Abnormal Hemoglobins

Most hemoglobins have normal equilibrium curves despite differences in amino acid sequence. However, a few hemoglobins are exceptions to the rule and exhibit altered O_2 affinity. Although shifts of the equilibrium curve to the right are common in hemoglobinopathies, this alteration is usually due to other factors, such as increased 2,3-DPG concentration or mean corpuscular hemoglobin concentration.

Carbon Monoxide

Carbon monoxide (CO) has an affinity for hemoglobin nearly 250 times that of oxygen. Although small quantities are produced in the body by the breakdown of heme proteins, CO is important clinically only when it contaminates inspired air (as caused by cigarette smoke or automobile exhaust). Competition between CO and O_2 for ligand-binding sites on hemoglobin reduces the number of sites available for O_2 binding and causes the O_2 equilibrium curve to shift to the left. This combined effect produces a greater deficit in the ability to exchange O_2 than the loss of comparable O_2-carrying capacity in anemia.

The halftime of CO clearance from the body is 4 h. Breathing 100% O_2 reduces the halftime to less than 1 h because of the competition between CO and O_2. Inhalation of 5% CO_2 in O_2 has been used to treat CO poisoning. Although it was once postulated that CO_2 has a specific effect on CO release from hemoglobin, it has now been demonstrated that the faster elimination of CO while breathing CO_2–O_2 mixtures is the result of the hyperventilation produced by CO_2 inhalation. If patients treated with CO_2–O_2 mixtures cannot increase ventilation sufficiently to avoid respiratory acidosis during CO_2 inhalation, this treatment can be dangerous. For this reason, the treatment of choice for CO poisoning is O_2 inhalation, either at ambient pressure or, when available, in a hyperbaric chamber.

CARBON DIOXIDE TRANSPORT

Carbon dioxide is a metabolic by-product which normally is in equilibrium with carbonic acid and must be excreted continuously to avoid acidosis. The body acid-base status depends on ventilatory excretion of CO_2 and the balance of bicarbonate excretion by the kidney.

Carbon Dioxide Equilibrium Curve

The relationship between blood content and partial pressure is much different for CO_2 than for O_2. The total quantity of CO_2 contained in arterial blood is more than twice that of O_2 despite the generally lower CO_2 partial pressures that are involved. Because the slope of the CO_2 equilibrium curve is quite steep, CO_2 partial pressures in venous and arterial blood normally range between 40 and 50 mmHg in contrast to large arterial-venous differences in blood P_{O_2}. The entire CO_2 curve is curvilinear, but over the range encountered under normal conditions the content-pressure relationship is nearly linear (Fig. 16-2). This characteristic helps to maintain efficiency of CO_2 exchange when maldistribution of ventilation of blood flow occurs in the lungs. Even though CO_2 is far more soluble than O_2, there has to be a form of storage of CO_2 in blood other than simple physical solution if CO_2 transport is to be maintained without a very high cardiac output or venous P_{CO_2}. The content of CO_2, i.e., the vertical axis of the CO_2 equilibrium curve, is the sum of these forms: physical solution, bicarbonate, and carbamino.

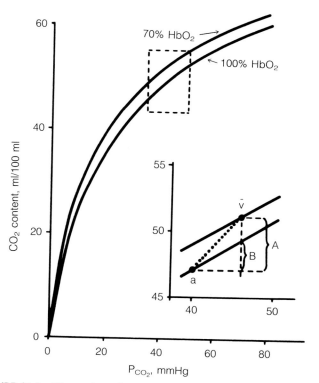

FIGURE 16-2 The carbon dioxide equilibrium curves of completely oxygenated (100% HbO_2) and partially oxygenated (70% HbO_2) human blood. The inset shows the enhancement of pulmonary CO_2 exchange by the Haldane effect.

Dissolved Carbon Dioxide

Approximately 5 percent of total CO_2 content is transported in physical solution in plasma and cell water. This dissolved form is critical for CO_2 transport because molecular CO_2 can rapidly cross cell membranes and be excreted in the lungs. The partial pressure of carbon dioxide, P_{CO_2}, is directly proportional to the quantity of dissolved CO_2. It is indirectly related to CO_2 content through the equilibrium curve.

Bicarbonate

Under the influence of the intraerythrocytic enzyme carbonic anhydrase (CA) which is contained within the erythrocyte, approximately 90 percent of CO_2 entering blood is rapidly converted into bicarbonate ion (HCO_3^-):

$$CO_2 + H_2O \rightleftharpoons H_2CO_3 \rightleftharpoons H^+ + HCO_3^-$$

Catalysis of this otherwise slow reaction permits rapid conversion between the CO_2 and HCO_3^- so that large quantities of CO_2 can be absorbed by blood in the periphery and excreted in the lungs. The H^+ generated by the conversion of CO_2 into HCO_3^- must be buffered to prevent large changes in pH. In blood, this function is performed almost exclusively by binding of protons to hemoglobin.

The plasma bicarbonate level cannot be measured directly since chemical determinations such as the CO_2 content measure CO_2 in all forms. Plasma bicarbonate level is best calculated from the pH and P_{CO_2} of a blood sample. This calculation is more accurate than measurements of CO_2 content, unless the latter are performed anaerobically under precisely controlled conditions.

Carbamino

Another 5 percent of the CO_2 binds directly to amino groups of hemoglobin. Because reduced hemoglobin binds more CO_2 than the oxygenated protein, more CO_2 can be carried in venous blood at any given P_{CO_2}. However, the physiological importance of this process is diminished by binding of 2,3-DPG to hemoglobin (Hb) at a portion of the sites involved in CO_2 binding. Changes in carbamino concentration account for only one-sixth of the difference between arterial and venous CO_2 contents.

Haldane Effect

Oxygenated blood at any P_{CO_2} has a lower CO_2 content than reduced blood at the same partial pressure. This difference, illustrated in Fig. 16-2, is known as the *Haldane effect*. The effect of oxygenation on CO_2 transport is analogous to the Bohr effect but has far greater physiological importance.

Deoxygenation of hemoglobin permits binding of H^+ since reduced hemoglobin is a weaker acid than oxyhemoglobin. In peripheral blood, H^+ formed by the conversion of CO_2 into HCO_3^- is bound to hemoglobin. As a result of this proton binding, at any P_{CO_2} more HCO_3^- is present in blood, and hence its CO_2 content is greater when hemoglobin is reduced. As mentioned previously, direct CO_2 binding to hemoglobin is also facilitated in deoxygenated blood increasing the total CO_2 content in deoxygenated as compared to oxygenated blood. Under normal circumstances, approximately one-third of the Haldane effect is the result of direct binding of CO_2; the remainder is the result of H^+ binding by hemoglobin.

Physiological Importance

The inset in Fig. 16-2 illustrates the importance of the Haldane effect. The change in CO_2 content between nor-mal arterial and mixed venous CO_2 partial pressure in partially oxygenated blood is indicated by bracket B on the right side of the inset. However, under physiological circumstances, the CO_2 equilibrium curve shifts from the position of the partially oxygenated curve to that of fully oxygenated blood. Thus, as is shown by bracket A on the right side of the inset, the shift from one curve to the other produces a greater change in blood CO_2 content between arterial and mixed venous partial pressures. As a result, the changes in venous pH and P_{CO_2} are minimized de-spite transport of large amounts of CO_2. Quantitatively, the Haldane effect has a much larger effect on gas trans-port under physiological circumstances than does the Bohr effect.

BIBLIOGRAPHY

Bauer C: On the respiratory function of hemoglobin. Rev Physiol Biochem Pharmacol 70:1–31, 1974.
   Critical review of the biochemical and physiological aspects of oxygen transport by hemoglobin.

Baumann R, Bartels H, Bauer C: Blood oxygen transport, in Farhi LE, Tenney SM (eds), *Handbook of Physiology*, sect 3: *The Respiratory System*, vol IV. Bethesda, American Physiological Society, pp 147–172, 1987.
   A comprehensive review in typical Handbook style of blood oxygen transport.

Bunn HF, Forget BG, Ranney HM: *Human Hemoglobins*. Philadelphia, Saunders, 1977.
   Description of different human hemoglobins with reference to related clinical abnormalities.

Hill EP, Power GG, Longo LD: Mathematical simulation of pulmonary O_2 and CO_2 exchange. Am J Physiol 224:904–917, 1973.
   Mathematical model of oxygen and carbon dioxide exchange by the lung, which includes the detailed interactions between oxygen and carbon dioxide transport by blood.

Hlastala MP, Woodson RD: Saturation dependency of the Bohr effect interactions among H^+, CO_2, and DPG. J Appl Physiol 38:1126–1131, 1975.
   Description of oxygen saturation dependence of ligand interaction with hemoglobin.

Klocke RA: Carbon dioxide transport, in Farhi LE, Tenney SM (eds), *Handbook of Physiology*, sect 3: *The Respiratory System*, vol IV. Bethesda, American Physiological Society, pp 173–197, 1987.
   A full picture of CO_2 transport by the blood.

Piiper J: Gas exchange and acid-base status, in Heisler N (ed), *Acid Base Regulation in Animals*. New York, Elsevier, pp 49–81, 1986.
   An analysis of factors determining P_{CO_2} and pH in blood and tissues.

Wallis PJ, Skehan JD, Newland AC, Wedzicha JA, Mills PG, Empey DW: Effects of erythropheresis on pulmonary haemodynamics and oxygen transport in patients with secondary polycythemia and cor pulmonale. Clin Sci 70:91–98, 1986.
   The aim of this investigation was to evaluate the effects of reducing packed cell volume on resting pulmonary hemodynamics and tissue oxygenation in 12 patients with polycythemia secondary to hypoxic cor pulmonale.

Part **3**

Integrations and Adaptations

Chapter 17

Homeostasis, Adaptation, and Disease

Alfred P. Fishman

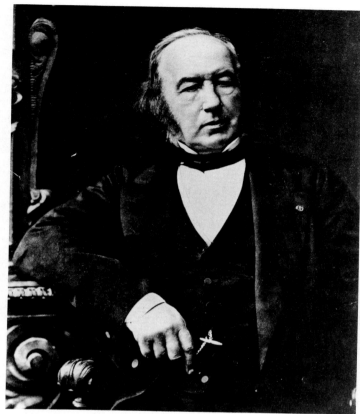

FIGURE 17-1 Claude Bernard (1813–1878) enunciated the principle that stability of the internal environment of the organism in higher vertebrates is prerequisite for the continuation of function at normal levels under conditions that usually prevail in the environment ("free life"). *(From Fishman and Richards, 1964.)*

The physician is obliged to deal with the lungs either as an organ that is the seat of disease or as a failing part of the cardiorespiratory system. Both aspects are covered in this book: as an organ, the lungs are subject to infection, inflammation, and neoplasia; as part of an elaborate mechanism for external gas exchange, disturbances in their function can circumscribe capability for physical activity. It is the integrated performance of the lungs in preserving the internal environment of the body, i.e., the blood and body fluids, that is considered here.

HOMEOSTASIS, THE GROWTH OF AN IDEA

The idea that "all vital mechanisms, however varied they may be, have only one object, that of preserving constant the conditions of life in the internal environment" was advanced by Claude Bernard around 1860 (Fig. 17-1). He envisioned a stable internal environment as a strategy by which the animal organism could maintain a free and independent existence in the face of unremitting challenges arising within from metabolism and from without by a host of deranging influences. This synthesis was reinforced and the concept enlarged by other physiologists, including L. J. Henderson, J. Barcroft, and J. S. Haldane (Fig. 17-2). As summarized succinctly in 1928 by Henderson in his classic monograph, *Blood,*

Protoplasm is a system of exquisite sensitiveness. In order that it may survive it must be protected from too great, or too rapid, or too irregular fluctuations in the physical, physico-chemical, and chemical conditions of the environment. Stability may sometimes be afforded by the natural environment, as in sea water. In other cases an integument may sufficiently temper the external changes. But by far the most interesting protection is afforded, as in man and higher animals, by the circulating liquids of the organism, the blood plasma and lymph, or, as Claude Bernard called them, the *milieu intérieur.* In his opinion, which I see no reason to dispute, the existence and the constancy of the physico-chemical properties of these fluids is a necessary condition for the evolution of free and independent life.

In 1939, Cannon (Fig. 17-3) incorporated the idea of a stable internal environment into the concept of "homeostasis." *The Wisdom of the Body* emphasizes automatic self-

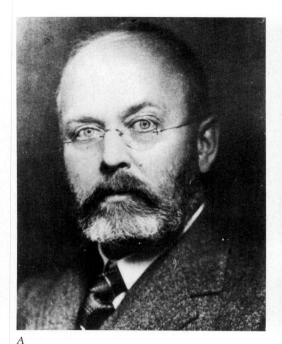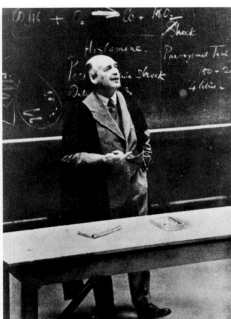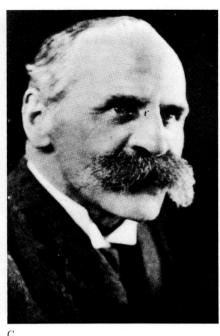

A   *B*   *C*

FIGURE 17-2   *A. Lawrence J. Henderson (1878–1942).   B. Joseph Barcroft (1872–1947).   C. John Scott Haldane (1860–1936). All were pioneers in the conceptualization of the hierarchies of physiological function and their integrations. (A and B from Fishman and Richards, 1964.)*

regulating mechanisms designed to restore the original dynamic equilibrium:

> In an open system, such as our bodies represent, compounded of unstable material and subjected continually to disturbing conditions, constancy is in itself evidence that agencies are acting, or ready to act, to maintain this constancy.

In 1953, D. W. Richards (Fig. 17-4) pointed out that the proponents of the concept of homeostasis were all physiologists concerned with normal body functions. It was true that Bernard had recognized that abnormalities of the same elements which are at play in the healthy individual become operative in disease, and that Henderson and Cannon could see the broader implications of the concept for nonbiologic systems, i.e., social, economic, industrial, and political. However, none of these delved into the idea of disease as a derangement in homeostatic mechanisms.

CHANGING CALLS FOR HOMEOSTASIS IN HEALTH

The normal individual spends little time at complete rest. Even while asleep, the demands on the body economy vary with the depth of sleep. Moreover, the activities of daily life are full of fits and starts. In addition to the diurnal swings, there are larger rhythms in cycles of months or seasons. For the cardiorespiratory system, the complex interplay involved in O_2 uptake at the mouth or O_2 delivery to the tissues is illustrated, in part, by the Morgan-

Murray diagram (see Fig. 63-2), which relates a change in the metabolic need for O_2 to the simultaneous changes in cardiac output, arteriovenous difference in O_2, hemoglobin flow, and diffusing capacity. Similar representations have been used for CO_2 (see Chapter 18).

LIMITS OF HUMAN ADAPTATION

Humans are capable of functioning normally within rather circumscribed limits that are of different kinds. One critical boundary is the architecture of the cardiorespiratory system and the design of the locomotor system. A second is imposed by homeostatic mechanisms. And a third is the body stores of essential ingredients that act as buffers.

Architecture and Design: Optimization

The architecture of the cardiorespiratory system and the intrinsic design of the locomotor muscles impose limits on their capability for adaptation. Disease at any level in the O_2 delivery system—from chest bellows to mitochondrion—may add restrictions of its own. For example, in normal individuals and in patients with different types of cardiac or pulmonary disease, there is an optimal breathing pattern which ensures that the mechanical work done by the chest bellows to accomplish the required minute (and alveolar) ventilation be minimal. Severe spinal deformity, as in kyphoscoliosis associated with dwarfing, increases the elastic work of mobilizing the chest bellows and automatically switches the optimal pattern to one of

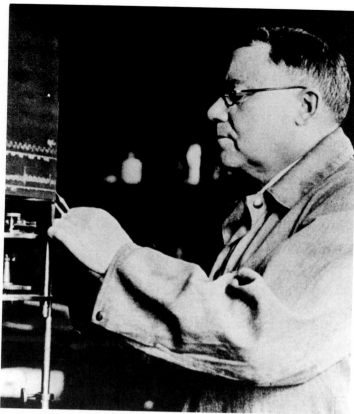

FIGURE 17-3 Walter B. Cannon. Incorporated the idea of stability of the internal environment into the larger concept of "homeostasis" and the self-regulatory processes that it implies. *(From Fishman and Richards, 1964.)*

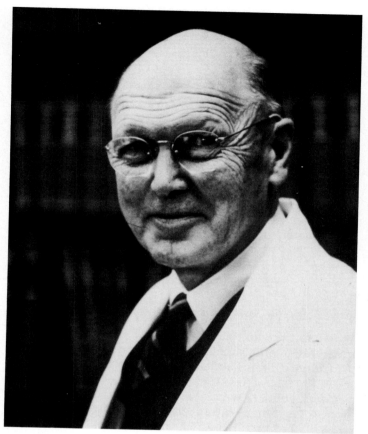

FIGURE 17-4 Dickinson W. Richards (1895–1973). As a physician-scientist, he attempted to relate homeostatic mechanisms and their derangements to clinical disorders.

rapid frequency and small tidal volumes. Although this pattern minimizes the work of breathing, it pays the penalty of alveolar hypoventilation that, in turn, results in respiratory acidosis and arterial hypoxemia and their consequences, i.e., respiratory and cardiac failure. In this way, by adopting a respiratory pattern that minimizes the work, energy cost, and discomfort of breathing, the organism is put at risk of life by severe derangements in the internal environment.

The Bounds of Homeostatic Mechanisms

The call for oxygen can fail to be met at any point in the delivery system, from ambient air to mitochondrion. Ordinarily, the weak link in the O_2 delivery system is the cardiac output, largely because of the restricted potential for increasing stroke volume. But, manipulation of the environment can impose different kinds of limits. The normal range of alveolar gas is schematically represented in the center of the Fenn-Rahn O_2-CO_2 diagram (Fig. 17-5). Outside this central area lies another region in which consciousness is still retained but where performance is increasingly impaired as the border of the region is approached. Beyond the second area, consciousness fades and convulsions follow.

A particular illustration of the limits of human tolerance is provided by the few mountain climbers (all told, about a dozen) who have managed to reach the summit of Mount Everest without resorting to supplementary oxygen. At the peak (altitude 8848 m), the inspired P_{O_2} is about 42 mmHg, arterial P_{O_2} about 28 mmHg, and $\dot{V}_{O_2max}$ about 1 L/min, i.e., about 20 to 25 percent of the sea level value. The feat of reaching the peak is accomplished in the face of a $\dot{V}_{O_2max}$ that barely suffices for the basal metabolism of the climber, limited O_2 diffusion properties of the alveolar-capillary blood interface, and dependence of oxygen exchange in the lungs and tissues on the steep part of the oxygen dissociation curve. However, survival at the brink of endurance is made possible by the striking hyperventilation and the respiratory alkalosis which promotes O_2 delivery to the tissues by shifting the steep part of the O_2 dissociation curve leftward. Somewhat akin to severe exertion at the summit of Mount Everest is the endurance run which is accomplished in the face of severe acidosis and arterial hypoxemia. Here, too, as at the peak of Mount Everest, the limit seems to be set primarily by time spent by blood in the pulmonary capillaries, i.e., by inadequate time for diffusion equilibrium between alveolar air and blood to be reached by the end of the pulmonary capillary.

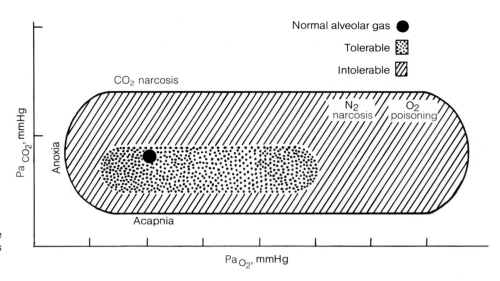

FIGURE 17-5 Schematic representation of the limits of tolerance in terms of alveolar gas composition. (*Modified after Fenn, 1951.*)

Body Stores of Essential Ingredients

As Barcroft pointed out in 1929, "The stability of the internal milieu almost compels the principle of the *storage of materials* [italics added] and of integration in adaptation." Barcroft cites Henderson as saying, "the body seems to contain what may be likened to marshes or swamps into which substances may disappear and be lost to view" and pictures a blackboard behind Sir Michael Forster on which is listed, "Carbohydrates, Fats, Proteins, Salts, Water." Since then, the stores, marshes, and swamps have been extensively explored. With respect to O_2 transfer to the mitochondrion from ambient air, three stores can be identified, i.e., alveolar air, blood, and cells. These are interposed serially between the processes of respiration, circulation, and metabolism (Fig. 17-6).

Modifications in architecture can be part of the adaptive process. For example, $\dot{V}_{O_2max}$ can be increased by modifications in the system at one or more of its consecutive levels. Thus, chronic residence at high altitude is accompanied by an increase in O_2-carrying capacity of the blood, the diffusing capacity of the lungs, and the density of capillaries in muscles. In contrast, neither the ability of the heart to increase its stroke output nor hypertrophy of the respiratory muscles appears to be an important element in this type of adaptation.

HOMEOSTASIS AS A FEEDBACK SYSTEM

The principles that govern man-made control systems apply equally well to the self-regulatory mechanisms of living organisms. The paradigm of a man-made control system is the control of temperature by means of a thermostat which, in turn, is an example of a closed-loop (negative feedback) control system, i.e., one in which any deviation of the controlled output (room temperature) from the desired value automatically signals a change in input (fuel supply that generates heat) to the system in order to minimize the discrepancy between controlled output and desired output. There are two types of feedback: *negative*, which operates to the advantage of the system to minimize the original deviation in the controlled output, and *positive*, which perpetuates the deprivation, promotes instability, and runs the risk of destroying the organism unless turned off by calling another mechanism into play. Clearly, in a biologic system, failure of a negative feedback system or unbridled positive feedback is capable of causing disorder or disease.

Although it is instructive to draw an analogy between man-made and living systems, it should be noted that the living system is infinitely more complex, entailing an

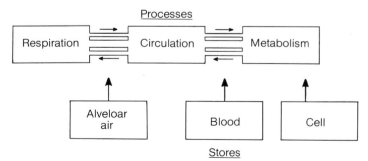

FIGURE 17-6 Processes and stores that maintain stable levels of P_{O_2} within cells. The alveolar air acts as a store for O_2 between ambient air and blood, serving as a tonometer of fairly stable composition. The blood, interposed between alveolar air and metabolizing tissues, has hemoglobin as the store. Within the cells are stores in the form of high-energy phosphates, dissolved O_2, myoglobin, and substrates for metabolic processes. Rearrangements in the distribution of blood by vasomotor activity determine the rate of delivery of O_2 to the different tissues. (*Modified after Weibel, 1984.*)

endless interplay (information transfer) among all levels in the biologic hierarchy, from cell to organ. Also, the sensory part of the regulatory apparatus is almost invariably more intricate than the effectors. Finally, the desired value ("set point") of a biologic parameter often depends on the physiological state, e.g., as dictated by the diurnal rhythm or the level of physical activity: during sleep, arterial P_{CO_2} is kept higher than while awake; while upright, the set point of the arterial P_{CO_2} is lower than while supine. Larger biologic rhythms, such as the monthly cycles in the female, also are associated with different set points for the arterial P_{CO_2}.

PATHOLOGIC DERANGEMENTS AND DISLOCATIONS

The early explorations of homeostatic mechanisms drew heavily on the autonomic nervous system and neurohumoral mediators, such as epinephrine, as integrating and adaptive mechanisms for acute upsets. For more gradual changes, they focused on physicochemical fundamentals, e.g., oxygen, water, osmotic pressure, carbon, and blood sugar. The time was not ripe to incorporate into the architecture of physiological function events at the cellular and molecular levels.

Homeostatic Inadequacy

As indicated above, integrative mechanisms designed to restore the internal environment operate within prescribed limits; disease can restrict the range of control. Also, as long as controls are adequate, the organism benefits; when controls fail, the freedom of the organism is compromised and its life may be endangered. For example, maximal oxygen uptake may have a low ceiling imposed by inadequacies in any of a variety of components of the cardiorespiratory system: cardiac output, ventilation, diffusing capacity, or hemoglobin content (see Chapter 18). More acutely, a high fever, far beyond the bounds of normal temperature control, may prove lethal without artificial cooling of the external environment, i.e., the skin and mucosal membranes.

Homeostatic Excess

In 1953, Richards adopted, from the *Timaeus* of Plato, the Greek word *hyperexis*, "having too much," for the concept of excessive homeostatic responses that, by reason of their excess, lead to bodily injury and death. For example, polycythemia, an adaptive mechanism for ensuring oxygen delivery, can overshoot to cause thrombosis. Similarly, cardiac hypertrophy that is called into play to cope with sustained pressure overload can culminate in heart failure. Finally, the homeostatic vasoconstrictor mechanisms operating to sustain blood pressure in the adult respiratory distress syndrome may deprive vital organs of oxygen and essential nutrients to the extent that failure of organs other than the lungs may determine outcome.

IATROGENIC DERANGEMENTS OF HOMEOSTASIS

Like inexpert manipulations of an automatic thermostat, well-intentioned interventions, especially in the critically ill, have the potential for undermining homeostatic mechanisms. This potential is maximal in the intensive-care setting where urgency dominates therapy. For example, when pulmonary capillaries have been rendered leaky as a result of injury, overzealous administration of fluids intravenously to sustain systemic blood pressure can aggravate pulmonary edema.

BIBLIOGRAPHY

Adair TH, Guyton AC, Montani JP, Lindsay HL, Stanek KA: Whole body structural vascular adaptation to prolonged hypoxia in chick embryos. Am J Physiol 252:H1228–H1234, 1987.
   A study of the role of hypoxia in the development of the blood vascular system in the chick embryo. The results support the hypothesis that prolonged exposure to hypoxia causes the blood vascular system to adapt its structure to allow greater amounts of blood to flow to the tissues at any given perfusion pressure gradient.

Barcroft J: Features in the Architecture of Physiological Function. New York, Hafner, 1972.
   A consideration of the functions that are needed to maintain stability of the internal environment. Barcroft examines integration in adaptation, plus he weighs and illustrates the role of the physicochemical properties of the blood, the storage of materials (oxygen and nutrients), the "all-or-none" phenomenon, and antagonistic and duplicative mechanisms.

Bert P: Barometric Pressure. Translated from the French by Hitchcock MA, Hitchcock FA. Columbus, OH, College Book Company, 1943.
   A fascinating account of Bert's contributions to respiratory physiology. Among these is the proof that the principal symptoms of altitude sickness are due to a low partial pressure of oxygen and not to a reduction in total barometric pressure.

Cannon WB: *The Wisdom of the Body*, 2d ed. New York, Norton, 1932.
   This classic volume on homeostasis presents ideas and summarizes research on the relation of the autonomic nervous system to the self-regulation of physiological processes. Chapter X deals with maintenance of an adequate oxygen supply.

Cherniack NS, Longobardo GS: Oxygen and carbon dioxide gas stores of the body. Physiol Rev 70:196–243, 1970.
   Gas stores help to maintain the level of O_2 and CO_2 tensions in tissues within narrow limits. Stores for O_2 are modest compared with those for CO_2; blood contains most of the O_2 stored in the body. Not only the stored O_2 but also the ability to metabolize anaerobically, to adjust the metabolic rate, and to redirect blood flow from organs to others determine survival when the supply of O_2 from the environment becomes inadequate.

DeFares JG: Principles of feedback control and their application to the respiratory control system, in Fenn WO, Rahn H (eds), *Handbook of Physiology, sect 3: Respiration.* Washington DC, American Physiological Society, 1964, pp 649–680.
   A particularly lucid presentation of biologic feedback that illustrates fundamental principles as they apply to the control of breathing at rest and during exercise.

Dempsey JA: Is the lung built for exercise? Med Sci Sports Exerc 18:143–155, 1986.
   Reviews evidence that the design of the pulmonary system and its pattern of neural integration are intended to satisfy the exercising state. Although the system can adapt physiologically, limits are apparent in homeostatic capabilities in health, in disease, and in alien environments.

Engel BT, Schneiderman N: Operant conditioning and the modulation of cardiovascular function. Annu Rev Physiol 46:199–210, 1984.
   A review that considers the role of operant learning in adaptation. The primary focus is on the role of the central nervous system and conditioning processes in achieving and preserving homeostatic mechanisms.

Fenn WO: Physiology of exposures to abnormal concentrations of the respiratory gases, in Fenn WO, Otis AB, Rahn H (eds), *AF Technical Report 6528, Studies in Respiratory Physiology.* Wright-Patterson Air Force Base, OH, 1951.
   Using the O_2–CO_2 diagram of Fenn and Rahn, the author pictures the normal and abnormal ranges of CO_2 and O_2 in the lungs.

Fishman AP, Richards DW: *Circulation of the Blood. Men and Ideas.* New York, Oxford, 1964.
   The contributors, all distinguished physiologists, trace the growth of ideas in cardiovascular physiology. Each deals with a particular topic to which he has had deep personal involvement as a scientist.

Gordon CJ, Heath JE: Integration and central processing in temperature regulation. Annu Rev Physiol 48:595–612, 1986.
   A review of the neural control of body temperature that illustrates the complexity of the integrative process. A central question remains of how the central nervous system transduces peripheral thermal stimuli to efferent command signals.

Haldane JS, Priestley JG: *Respiration.* Oxford, Clarendon, 1935.
   A classic view of respiratory physiology based on more than 20 years of experimental work, scholarship, and reflection. The underlying assumption is that only through the study of the restorative responses of the body to changes in the environment is it possible to recognize and to interpret disturbance of health and promote the maintenance or restoration of health.

Henderson LJ: *The Fitness of the Environment.* Boston, Beacon, 1913.
   A stable internal environment serves many of the same purposes as a stable external environment and also ensures a proper supply of food for metabolic needs. "Complexity, regulation and food are essential to life as we know it."

Henderson LJ: *Blood, A Study in General Physiology.* New Haven, Yale, 1928.
   After considering blood as a physicochemical system, the author explores organic integration and adaptation among species, at different levels of activity, and in health and disease.

Hochachka PW: *Living Without Oxygen.* Cambridge, Massachusetts, Harvard University Press, 1980.
   A sophisticated but readable account of the adaptations involved in living under oxygen-poor conditions.

Hochachka PW: Balancing conflicting metabolic demands of exercise and diving. Fed Proc 45:2948–2952, 1986.
   During a dive (without exercise) a set of physiological reflexes is evoked as the first line of defense against hypoxia. This reflex is modified when the diving seal also exercises. One modifi-

cation is continued perfusion of the exercising muscles by a regulated release of oxygenated red blood cells from the spleen. A second is a decrease in the metabolism of hypoperfused tissues.

Koshland DE Jr, Goldbeter A, Stock JB: Amplification and adaptation in regulatory and sensory systems. Science 218:220–225, 1982.
   At the level of the cell, biologic systems within the same cell respond to sensory inputs from both the internal and external environments by amplifying signals and by adapting to them. This paper describes the molecular machinery of the cell by which the opposite effects of amplification and adaptation are accomplished.

Lydic R: State-dependent aspects of regulatory physiology. FASEB J 1:6–15, 1987.
   This paper provides a brief and selective review of recent work concerning the alterations in thermoregulation, cardiovascular, and respiratory physiology that occur as a function of different states of sleep and wakefulness.

Richards DW: Homeostasis versus hyperexis: or Saint George and the Dragon. The Scientific Monthly 77:289–294, 1953.
   A challenging essay dealing with the extrapolation of the concept of homeostasis from health and disease.

Salthe SN: *Evolving Hierarchical Systems.* New York, Columbia, 1985.
   In contrast with current trends toward selectionism and reductionism in biology, the author addresses the complexity of biology and nature in terms of hierarchical systems.

Schuitmaker JJ, Berkenbosch A, DeGoede J, Olievier CN: Ventilatory responses to respiratory and metabolic acid-base disturbances in cats. Respir Physiol 67:69–83, 1987.
   It is proposed that in the adaptation of the ventilation to acute metabolic acidosis, the stimulatory effect of the peripheral chemoreceptors is counteracted by a diminished stimulation of the central chemoreceptors.

Sherrington C: *The Integrative Action of the Nervous System,* 2d ed. New Haven, Yale, 1948.
   The central theme is that the nature of the whole organism is determined by the integration of all the parts of which it is composed. A seminal work because of its broad generalization and philosophic insights.

Stern N, Tuck ML: Homeostatic fragility in the elderly. Cardiol Clin 4:201–211, 1986.
   One of many reviews dealing with age-related alterations in homeostatic functions. Set points are readjusted, and limits of performance are decreased by the readjustments.

Weibel ER: *The Pathology for Oxygen.* Cambridge, MA, Harvard, 1984.
   A masterful consideration of structure and function in the mammalian respiratory system. Consecutive levels of organization in the hierarchy of the body are examined with respect to how each is involved in meeting the call for oxygen.

West JB, Lahiri S: *High Altitude and Man.* Washington, DC, American Physiological Society, 1984.
   A monograph based on a symposium that was stimulated by the American Medical Research Expedition to Mount Everest in 1981. The extreme altitude of Mount Everest (altitude 8848 m) places climbers close to the limits of human tolerance. (See also West: Fed Proc 45:2953–2957, 1986, for consideration of lactate levels under this circumstance.)

Chapter 18

Physiological Basis of Exercise Testing

Norman L. Jones

The capacity to exercise depends on a complex functional coordination between many physiological processes. Exercise testing seeks to establish the extent to which these processes respond to the increased energy requirements of exercise. Although in a given subject an abnormality in one process may dominate the capacity to exercise, because of the cooperation between them, adaptation may occur in other processes to minimize the effects. The cooperation or "integration" between processes is a recurring theme in this chapter (see Chapter 17). The interactions are especially important in pulmonary disease where, in addition to functions conventionally classed as *pulmonary*—the mechanics of breathing, ventilation-perfusion matching and the control of breathing—may be added other factors that are less closely related to the lungs, e.g., pulmonary hypertension, impaired cardiac function due to coexisting coronary arterial disease, or poor muscle function secondary to inactivity.

Exercise testing is useful in the objective measurement of impairment and in identifying abnormal physio-logical responses (see Chapter 165). But the power of exercise testing lies in its ability to explore functional interactions between mechanisms in which changes in any one process need to be considered within the context of the total integrated response in terms of the power output capacity ($\dot{W}_{max}$) or the maximum oxygen intake ($\dot{V}_{O_2max}$). Ideally, an exercise test explores all functions to obtain quantitative information regarding their individual contributions to the overall functional impairment. Considered in this light, exercise testing potentially assesses pulmonary function more completely than does any "pulmonary function" test carried out at rest; it also provides information that cannot be obtained readily in any other way.

Although the information obtained during exercise tests is physiological in nature, often there may be diagnostic implications. Where the exercise impairment is qualitatively or quantitatively at variance with the clinical assessment, changes in diagnostic or therapeutic approaches may be suggested. Less commonly, a diagnostic or "pathognomonic" response to exercise may be obtained, as in exercise-induced asthma.

FACTORS CONTRIBUTING TO EXERCISE PERFORMANCE

Muscle Power

During exercise, muscles exert forces to move part or all of the body mass at a velocity for a period of time, often against gravity; in doing so, they accomplish work. The force of 1 newton (N) is exerted on a mass of 1 kg to produce an acceleration of 1 m/s^2. This force, acting through 1-m distance, produces 1 N · m, or 1 joule (J) of work and if maintained for 1 s, generates 1 J/s or 1 watt (W) of power. In some activities, such as stair climbing or pedaling against the braking force of a calibrated cycle ergometer, the power and work performed may be readily calculated. But in other activities, such as running, the forces are less clearly defined; in such situations, measurements of O_2 intake ($\dot{V}_{O_2}$) are used to obtain an equivalent energy output, thereby enabling different activities to be directly compared.

Two main attributes influence the capacity of muscle to perform exercise: *strength*, or the capacity to generate power, and *endurance*, or the capacity to maintain a given power.

The maximum power ($\dot{W}_{max}$) generated during dynamic exercise, as in cycling, is related closely to the size of the muscle and its dominant fiber type. The ability to generate power also depends on the force-velocity characteristics of muscle; thus, in cycling exercise, the maximal power is influenced by the velocity of pedaling. A decline in maximal power occurs with age, related to the diminution in muscle size and in the number of functioning motor units. Strength training has a marked effect in increasing muscle size and the maximum power output.

Although the size of a muscle and the characteristics of its fibers dominate the capacity to generate instantaneous power, the aerobic capacity of the muscle becomes of great importance in maintaining power for more than a few seconds. The relationship between power and the time for which it can be maintained is a parabola (Figs. 18-1 and 18-2); this relationship needs to be kept in mind when considering any aspect of muscular performance, including the energy requirements of everyday activities. The energy required to climb stairs at an ordinary pace is about twice the energy that can be sustained for several minutes. In practice, maximal power ($\dot{W}_{max}$) can be assessed by using an isokinetic ergometer that measures the maximal torque developed during muscle contractions at controlled velocities; aerobic capacity can be assessed by determining maximal O_2 intake ($\dot{V}_{O_2max}$) in an incremental exercise test.

Muscle Metabolism

The chemical energy for muscle contraction is provided by the splitting of ATP to ADP. Because stores of ATP in muscle are small, for exercise to continue ATP has to be resynthesized at an appropriate rate, through energy-yielding phosphorylation reactions (Fig. 18-3). An immediately available source of ATP is creatine phosphate (CP). But this store is also limited and is rapidly depleted during heavy exercise. For continued muscle contraction, energy is obtained from the oxidation of fats and carbohydrates, their use depending on the size of fuel stores and the rate at which the fuels can be made available to muscle (Fig. 18-3). Although the largest fuel store is that of fat in adipose tissue, the rate at which it can be mobilized and carried in blood to muscle is limited. If the supply of free fatty acids to muscle is inadequate, but the maximum rate of muscle utilization has not been exceeded, then fat in muscle is broken down and used as a fuel. Considerations similar to those of fat in adipose tissue apply to glycogen in liver: the rate at which glucose can be liberated and transported to muscle is limited, and the rate at which glucose can be taken up by muscle is also limited. For these reasons the main fuel for heavy exercise, especially if of short duration, is the glycogen store in muscle. The size of the store is influenced by diet and also by activity. However, it can be mobilized almost instantaneously, at the start of exercise.

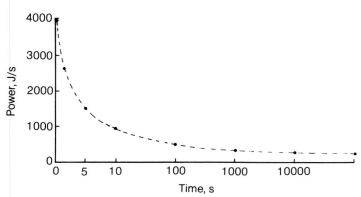

FIGURE 18-1 Power is plotted against the length of time for which it can be maintained by elite athletes.

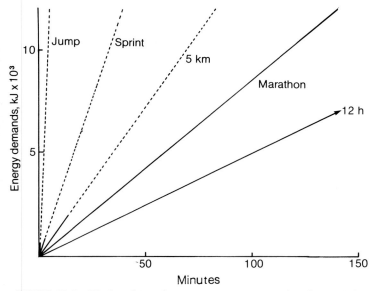

FIGURE 18-2 Work achieved in various activities; the slope of the dotted lines indicates power required for the activity, and solid lines indicate the time taken and total work.

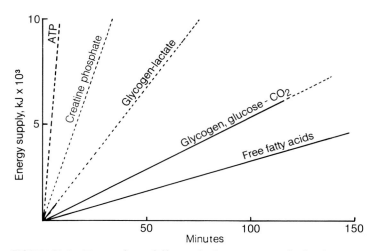

FIGURE 18-3 Energy from different fuel sources, graphed to be comparable to Fig. 18-2. The slope of the lines shows maximal rate of energy flux, and the solid portion shows the total energy available in a given metabolic pathway. Fuels associated with high flux rates (ATP, CP) are present in low concentrations. Large stores (aerobic glycogen and adipose fat utilization) are available only at lower relative rates.

Anaerobic glycolysis generates pyruvate, which may be accepted into the oxidative pathway of the citrate (Krebs) cycle if sufficient oxygen is available and if the activity of the rate-limiting enzyme, pyruvate dehydrogenase (PDH), is sufficient; but if either of these requirements is not met, lactate is formed. The formation of lactate by muscle allows regeneration of nicotine adenine dinucleotide (NAD) from its reduced state, thereby enabling metabolism to continue. However, if lactate ions are not removed from muscle, the process becomes self-limited because enzymes higher in the glycolytic pathway (phosphofructokinase and phosphorylase) are inhibited by decreases in muscle pH. It is important to appreciate that even though lactate production by muscle is an anaerobic process, it is not always secondary to lack of oxygen. Several other factors may influence lactate formation. The most important of these is the net balance between the activity of the rate-limiting glycolytic enzymes, phosphorylase and phosphofructokinase, and the activity of PDH, which controls entry of pyruvate into the citrate cycle; should the glycolytic flux exceed the capacity to metabolize pyruvate, lactate will accumulate. Both the rate at which O_2 can be delivered to muscle and the activation of PDH are increased by exercise training.

Lactate formed by muscle diffuses into the blood; this process is influenced by the acid-base status and by the local circulation. Lactate undergoes extensive aerobic metabolism by cardiac and skeletal muscle and by the liver. Thus, apart from its rate of production, several factors may influence the accumulation of lactate in arterial blood. The point at which arterial lactate concentration increases above resting values has been termed the *anaerobic threshold* (*AT*) or *onset of blood lactate accumulation* (*OBLA*) (Fig. 18-4); although this point in exercise is widely used to identify the power at which oxygen delivery falls short of the demand for oxygen in exercising muscle, as pointed out above, usually this discrepancy is only one of several contributing factors. The point at which plasma lactate concentration increases above resting values is most clearly defined in an exercise protocol in which the intensity of exercise is increased rapidly; if the intensity increases more gradually, the increase in lactate concentration is more curvilinear and a specific point of inflection is more difficult to define. For this reason, some define AT as the $\dot{V}_{O_2}$, or the power output, at which the concentration of lactate in plasma exceeds 2 or 4 mmol/L.

Although anaerobic metabolism plays an important role in heavy, short-term exercise, regeneration of ATP for exercise that is longer than 1 min in duration depends on oxidative phosphorylation.

Oxidative phosphorylation in exercising muscle is linked to the citrate cycle in which the three carbon products of glycolysis and lipolysis are oxidized to regenerate ATP. The following equations express the interrela-

tionships between oxygen consumed, ATP regenerated, and CO_2 produced in the complete oxidation of glucose or glycogen and a representative long-chain fatty acid (palmitic acid).

$$\text{Glycogen}\text{—}C_6H_{12}O_6 + 6O_2 + 36ADP + 36P_i$$
$$\rightarrow 6CO_2 + 36ATP + 42H_2O \quad (1)$$

$$\text{Fat}\text{—}C_{16}H_{32}O_2 + 23O_2 + 129ADP + 129P_i$$
$$\rightarrow 16CO_2 + 129ATP + 145H_2O \quad (2)$$

There are two notable features of these equations: (1) the relationship between oxygen utilized and the number of molecules of ATP resynthesized is slightly different between glycogen ($36ATP/6O_2 = 6$) and fats ($129/23 = 5.6$); in this respect, glycogen is more efficient than fat, and

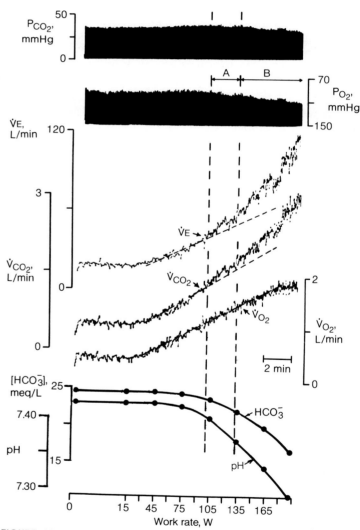

FIGURE 18-4 The *anaerobic threshold* (left-hand dashed line) is defined by an exercise intensity ($\dot{V}_{O_2}$), above which plasma lactate rises to above rest values; there is also an associated fall in bicarbonate concentration, relative rise in CO_2 output and ventilation, with the ventilatory equivalent for O_2 ($\dot{V}_{E_{O_2}}$) increasing. Representative measurements in a healthy subject. (*From Wasserman, 1980, with permission.*)

(2) in a steady state, the production of CO_2 related to oxygen consumption (the RQ) is different between the two fuels; for glycolysis the RQ is 1.0 and for lipolysis 0.7. Therefore, if it is desirable to minimize the CO_2 production for a given rate of ATP resynthesis, fats are preferable. The number of moles of ATP regenerated per mole of CO_2 produced is six for glycogen compared to eight for fat.

Power and O_2 Uptake

In each of the metabolic processes described above, energy is liberated; only part of this energy is recaptured in the high energy bonds of ATP, since heat is also generated. Even when the reactions are carried out in the test tube, they are only 40 percent efficient; in the body as a whole, the *efficiency* of exercise—the relationship between the energy of the oxidations compared to the external energy or work produced—is only about 25 percent.

During exercise, the increase in oxygen uptake ($\dot{V}_{O_2}$) is closely related to the increase in power ($\dot{W}$). In cycle ergometer exercise at any given $\dot{W}$, the $\dot{V}_{O_2}$ is influenced by body size; thus, in obese subjects, the $\dot{V}_{O_2}$ is higher throughout an exercise test than in nonobese subjects; however, the increase in $\dot{V}_{O_2}$ for a given $\dot{W}$ is relatively unaffected by body size (Fig. 18-5). In walking and running, $\dot{V}_{O_2}$ is more strongly influenced by body weight since energy is expended in moving body mass against the force of gravity. The relationship of $\dot{V}_{O_2}$ to the forces exerted in different activities may be expressed in the following equations.

For cycle ergometry in an incremental exercise test,

$$\dot{V}_{O_2} = 3.5Wt + 10.8W \qquad (3)$$

where W is power expressed in watts, $\dot{V}_{O_2}$ in ml STPD/min, and Wt is weight in kg.

For treadmill walking,

$$\dot{V}_{O_2} = 0.9vg \qquad (4)$$

where v is belt velocity in m/min, g is grade in percent incline, and $\dot{V}_{O_2}$ is in ml/kg/min.

For walking on the level, up to a velocity of 120 m/min,

$$\dot{V}_{O_2} = 0.1v + 3.5 \text{ ml/kg/min} \qquad (5)$$

For running on the level,

$$\dot{V}_{O_2} = 0.2v + 3.5 \text{ ml/kg/min} \qquad (6)$$

The peak power ($\dot{W}_{max}$) and maximum O_2 consumption ($\dot{V}_{O_2max}$) are probably the most important measurements obtained in an incremental exercise test. Reductions in the maximum capacity of oxygen transport mechanisms, such as cardiac output and ventilation, are closely paralleled by reductions in $\dot{V}_{O_2max}$; therefore, the determination of $\dot{V}_{O_2max}$ yields an important index of impairment in any mechanism that has reached its adaptive capacity. Classically, $\dot{V}_{O_2max}$ is measured in a test that establishes a maximal value that is not exceeded when a higher power output is attempted; this is a difficult criterion for routine clinical exercise testing. A valid alternative is the peak $\dot{V}_{O_2}$ achieved in an incremental test even though a plateau in $\dot{V}_{O_2}$ may not be reached.

Peak power and $\dot{V}_{O_2max}$ are normally higher in males than females, are influenced by body size and muscle mass, decline with increasing age (Fig. 18-6), and are influenced by the activity of the subject. Thus, the normal expected or predicted values may be obtained from the sex, height, age, and leisure activity of the individual. Impairment may then be defined, as in other function tests, in terms of standard deviations from the predicted value or as a percentage of the predicted value.

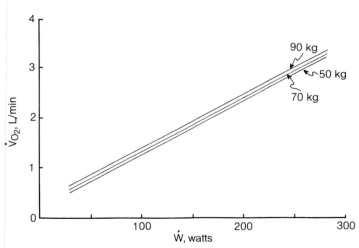

FIGURE 18-5 Oxygen uptake in incremental cycle ergometry in healthy subjects having body weights of 50, 70, and 90 kg.

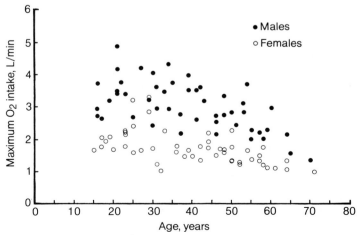

FIGURE 18-6 Maximal $\dot{V}_{O_2}$ in incremental cycle ergometer exercise in healthy females and males aged 15 to 70 years, showing decline with age. The variance in the data is reduced when body size is also allowed for.

CO₂ Production

As can be seen from Eqs. (1) and (2), an equal amount of CO_2 is generated as O_2 is consumed when carbohydrates are oxidized, and about 0.7 of the O_2 consumed when fats are oxidized. To the CO_2 from these aerobic sources is added the CO_2 that is generated from bicarbonate if the H^+ ion concentration increases, as expressed in the conceptual equation

$$H^+ + HCO_3^- = H_2CO_3 = CO_2 + H_2O \qquad (7)$$

This reaction may be considered to occur as a result of lactate acting as a strong ion (La^-): the diffusion of CO_2 from muscle into venous blood is very rapid, whereas the efflux of La^- from muscle occurs at a slower rate (that is influenced by the acid-base status of arterial blood, and may also involve an active carrier system). Since La^- is a strong ion, as it accumulates in the blood, the bicarbonate concentration decreases because of the excretion of CO_2 by the lungs (Fig. 18-4). The metabolic acidosis that develops in heavy exercise may, per se, impair the efflux of lactate from muscle, leading to a rapid fall in muscle pH and promoting muscle fatigue.

The Anaerobic Threshold

As already mentioned, lactate accumulation in plasma is often taken as an indication that the energy needs of exercise exceed the capacity to supply O_2 at a sufficiently high rate. For this reason, the identification of the power output, or the $\dot{V}_{O_2}$, at which this begins to occur may be valuable in the assessment of exercise performance in health and disease. Because accumulation of lactate in the plasma during exercise of increasing intensity is accompanied by excretion of CO_2, there is an increase in ventilation that is out of proportion to the increase in $\dot{V}_{O_2}$. Theoretically this change in the ventilatory response should occur at the same point at which the plasma lactate begins to rise; therefore, it has been termed the *ventilatory anaerobic threshold*. However, in addition to the factors that may influence lactate accumulation, the excess $\dot{V}_{CO_2}$ may be influenced by factors related to the control of breathing and the acid-base status. For this reason, although it is helpful to identify that a ventilatory anaerobic threshold has occurred during an incremental exercise study, the physiological mechanisms underlying the point at which it occurs may vary from subject to subject.

Criteria for the identification of the ventilatory anaerobic threshold include an increase in $\dot{V}_E/\dot{V}_{O_2}$ without change in $\dot{V}_E/\dot{V}_{CO_2}$, and an increase in end-tidal P_{O_2} without a fall in end-tidal P_{CO_2}. Although this point may usually be defined with some precision, often the increase in $\dot{V}_E$ that accompanies an increase in $\dot{V}_{O_2}$ is a smooth curve that allows some latitude in its identification, accounting for the interobserver variability that some have reported. For this reason, identification of the anaerobic threshold

is less important quantitatively in routine exercise assessment than is determination of $\dot{V}_{O_2max}$. The anaerobic threshold is usually expressed in terms of $\dot{V}_{O_2}$ (liters per minute) or as a percentage of $\dot{V}_{O_2max}$; in normal subjects, the threshold occurs at a $\dot{V}_{O_2}$ above 40 percent of the predicted $\dot{V}_{O_2max}$, with an average value in untrained individuals of 58 percent of $\dot{V}_{O_2max}$ (Fig. 18-7).

The concept of the anaerobic threshold has been a useful addition to other exercise measurements, indicating a point at which the adaptation of purely aerobic processes cannot cope alone with the energy demands. Although one may object to the use of *anaerobic* and *threshold* in the strict sense of their meanings, the changing stresses that are imposed on the integrated system as the exercise intensity continues to increase, and particularly on the ventilatory components, makes the observation a valid one in assessing the responses to an incremental exercise test. Also a change in the threshold in a given individual generally accompanies a change in the degree of lactate accumulation, e.g., as a result of training.

O₂ Delivery and CO₂ Removal

For the muscles to continue exercising at a given power output, the required regeneration of ATP has to occur; this regeneration depends on oxygen supply and on the control of muscle pH through the removal of lactate ions and CO_2. Both O_2 delivery and CO_2 removal depend on an adequate alveolar ventilation, the alveolar-capillary transfer of gases, the carriage of the respiratory gases by the blood, the cardiac output, and the distribution of blood flow to the muscles. The interplay among these processes is identified in Fig. 18-8. The same scheme may be used to explore the place of the adaptation that may take place in

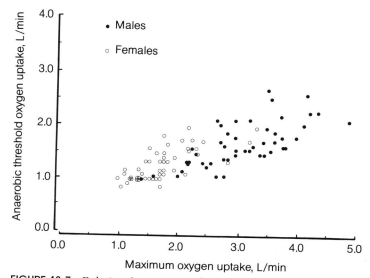

FIGURE 18-7 Relationship between $\dot{V}_{O_2}$ at the ventilatory anaerobic threshold and $\dot{V}_{O_2max}$ in healthy untrained females and males.

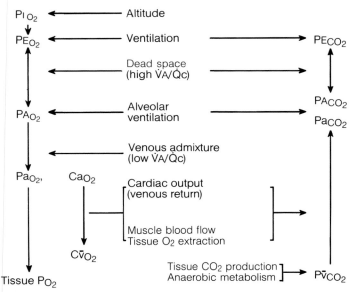

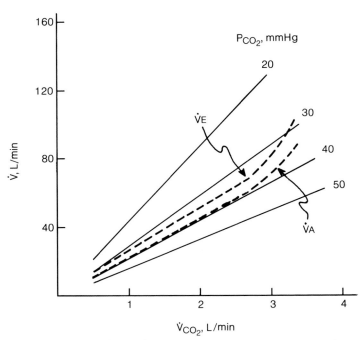

FIGURE 18-8 Processes influencing O_2 and CO_2 transport, to show their influences on pressure gradients of O_2 and CO_2 between inspired air and muscles.

FIGURE 18-9 Ventilation during exercise in a representative subject plotted against $\dot{V}_{CO_2}$, with isopleths of P_{CO_2}. Shown are total ventilation ($\dot{V}_E$), for which isopleths refer to expired CO_2 (P_{ECO_2}), and alveolar ventilation ($\dot{V}_A$), isopleths indicating arterial CO_2 (Pa_{CO_2}). The difference between the two curves ($\dot{V}_E - \dot{V}_A$), when expressed as a proportion of $\dot{V}_E$, represents dead-space ventilation (V_D/V_T ratio).

order to maintain O_2 delivery and CO_2 removal in the face of an impaired process acting as a weak line in the chain (see Chapter 17).

Ventilation and Gas Exchange

In healthy individuals, ventilation ($\dot{V}_E$) during exercise is closely linked to $\dot{V}_{CO_2}$, both during a steady state and in situations where $\dot{V}_{O_2}$ and $\dot{V}_{CO_2}$ are changing rapidly, e.g., at the start of exercise or during experimental variations in power output. At low power outputs, $\dot{V}_E$ increases in parallel with $\dot{V}_{O_2}$ and $\dot{V}_{CO_2}$; however, because of the increase in $\dot{V}_{CO_2}$ that accompanies increases in the concentration of lactate in the plasma, ventilation increases relative to $\dot{V}_{O_2}$ during heavy exercise.

The respiratory control mechanisms during exercise adjust the ventilation so as to maintain Pa_{CO_2} more or less constant at levels of exercise less than about 75 percent of $\dot{V}_{O_2max}$, i.e., the increase in alveolar ventilation ($\dot{V}_A$) parallels the increase in $\dot{V}_{CO_2}$ (Fig. 18-9). However, at very high exercise loads, the Pa_{CO_2} tends to fall indicating that $\dot{V}_A$ has increased relative to $\dot{V}_{CO_2}$. The excess alveolar ventilation has been ascribed to an increasing metabolic acidosis.

Total ventilation ($\dot{V}_E$) is conventionally subdivided into alveolar ventilation ($\dot{V}_A$) and dead-space (V_D) components; dead space is usually expressed as the V_D/V_T ratio. Depending primarily on the increments in tidal volume, the V_D/V_T ratio falls during exercise from resting values of 25 to 35 percent to 5 to 20 percent: at any given level of exercise, the V_D/V_T ratio is increased by a fall in V_T. In addition, ventilation-perfusion ($\dot{V}_A/\dot{Q}_C$) abnormalities tend to increase the V_D/V_T ratio.

The distribution of $\dot{V}_A/\dot{Q}_C$ ratios in the lungs influences the behavior of Pa_{O_2} during exercise; in normal untrained individuals, Pa_{O_2} is usually unchanged or may even increase slightly, at low power outputs; during very heavy exercise, Pa_{O_2} may fall somewhat. Thus, the alveolar-to-arterial ($A - a$) P_{O_2} difference usually does not change during light exercise but does increase gradually, to 30 to 40 mmHg, at $\dot{V}_{O_2max}$. A major reason for the increase in ($A - a$) difference in P_{O_2} during heavy exercise is the decrease in the venous O_2 saturation; in normal individuals, venous admixture ($\dot{Q}_{va}$) during exercise falls from resting values of around 6 percent to less than 3 percent of the cardiac output. In theory, the time spent by blood in the pulmonary capillaries may also determine the degree to which pulmonary arterial blood is oxygenated. At rest, the normal transit time of about 0.75 s allows for full oxygenation; it is conceivable that during heavy exercise, when the transit time may decrease to less than 0.2 s, full equilibration with alveolar O_2 might not be achieved, especially at high altitudes (Fig. 18-10). The decreases in Pa_{O_2} and Sa_{O_2} that occur in athletes exercising at very high power outputs indicate that the diffusing capacity of the lungs has peaked, either because the lung capillary transit time is too short for full oxygenation of the very desaturated venous blood, or because a normal distribution of ventilation-perfusion ratios cannot be maintained. In patients in whom diffusion across the alve-

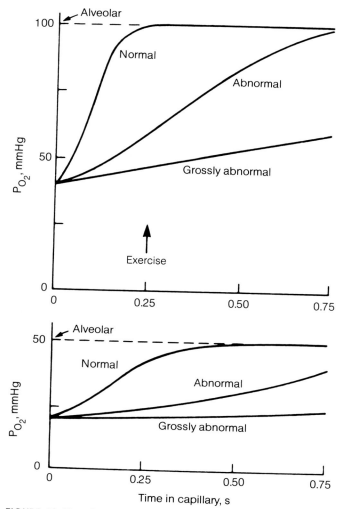

FIGURE 18-10 Theoretical changes in P_{O_2} during passage of blood through the lungs to show effect of shortened transit time in exercise on the difference in P_{O_2} between alveoli and end-capillary blood; the added effects of abnormal pulmonary gas exchange are shown in the upper panel, and the effects of altitude in the lower panel. *(From West: Pulmonary Physiology—The Essentials, Baltimore, Williams & Wilkins, 1974, pp 27–28, with permission.)*

olar-capillary interfaces is impaired, the increase in the metabolic call for O_2 together with the shortened transit time contribute to arterial oxygen desaturation. However, despite the potential for diffusion limitation, abnormal distribution of $\dot{V}_A/\dot{Q}_C$ ratios remains the most important factor contributing to O_2 desaturation in pulmonary disorders.

Pattern of Breathing

The increase in $\dot{V}_E$ during exercise is brought about by an increase in tidal volume (V_T) and in the frequency of breathing (f), and a shortened inspiratory duration (T_I). It seems likely that the pattern of breathing during exercise is adopted as a learned response to minimize the sense of effort arising in the respiratory muscles. The tidal volume increases at low and moderate power outputs to reach a

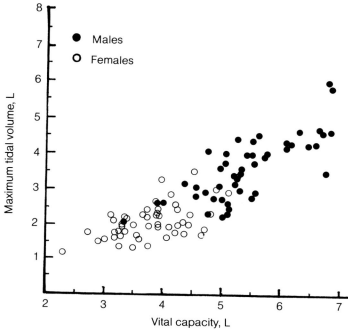

FIGURE 18-11 Maximal tidal volume reached in exercise in healthy adults, related to vital capacity.

relative plateau that is influenced by the size and elastance of the lungs; in normal individuals the maximum V_T is about 60 percent of the individual's vital capacity (Fig. 18-11). Increases in frequency occur primarily during heavy exercise; values of 40 to 50 breaths per minute are often reached. Both T_I and the total duration of breath (T_{tot}) shorten progressively as $\dot{V}_E$ increases; T_I/T_{tot} remains constant at between 30 and 35 percent.

Respiratory Muscles

The changes in breathing pattern during exercise have implications for the demands that are made on respiratory muscles. Progressive increases in V_T mean that the respiratory muscles have to shorten progressively during exercise; increases in inspiratory flow rates imply that the muscles have to increase their velocity of contraction progressively; also, an increase in the frequency of breathing is accompanied by an increase in the frequency of contraction of the respiratory muscles. These changes in the operating characteristics of the respiratory muscles during exercise encroach on their capacity to generate tension and thereby contribute to the sense of respiratory effort during increasing exercise. Although the respiratory muscles may begin to fatigue at very strenous levels of exercise, the accompanying severe sense of effort usually causes the subject to stop exercising before the muscles fail to generate tension. Therefore, even though it is possible, by resorting to inspiratory loading in the experimental situation, to cause normal subjects to exhibit signs of respiratory failure, i.e., an increase in P_{CO_2} and a decrease in Sa_{O_2}, during exercise this seldom occurs under natural conditions, i.e., in the unloaded state.

The tension generated by the respiratory muscles (Pmus) is increased when the impedance to breathing (Z) is increased by an increase in pulmonary elastance (E) or resistance (R). The classic relationships that define Pmus may be expressed as follows:

$$Pmus = E \cdot V + R \cdot \dot{V} + I \cdot \dot{V}^2 \qquad (8)$$

If the small effect of changes in inertia (I) is ignored, Eq. (8) may be rewritten to include variables measured during exercise:

$$Pmus = E \cdot V_T + R \cdot \frac{V_T}{T_I} \qquad (9)$$

This equation indicates that Pmus will increase on the one hand as V_T increases in situations of increased E, and on the other by increases in flow (V_T/T_I) in situations in which R is increased. Adaptive changes in breathing pattern are usually seen in patients with pulmonary fibrosis (increased E), i.e., small V_T and high f, and with chronic airways obstruction (increased R), i.e., relatively well maintained V_T and limited increase in f. An increase in Pmus tends to increase $\dot{V}_{O_2}$ at a given level of exercise, but it seems unlikely that this effect is ever important enough to compromise oxygen supply to exercising skeletal muscle. However, respiratory muscle weakness frequently accompanies pulmonary disorders, thereby contributing to dyspnea and impaired exercise tolerance.

In addition to changes in breathing pattern, pulmonary disorders are usually associated with defects in gas exchange that increase the V_D/V_T ratio, the alveolar-arterial difference in P_{O_2}, and venous admixture; these abnormalities are accompanied by decreases in Pa_{O_2} and Sa_{O_2}. Therefore, during increasing exercise, measurement of $\dot{V}_E$ and determination of blood-gas composition or of the Sa_{O_2} by ear oximetry can yield clinically important information regarding the gas-exchange capacity of the lungs.

Carriage of O₂ and CO₂ by Blood

The characteristics of the oxygen and carbon dioxide dissociation curves for blood are dealt with in Chapter 13. Although changes in the O_2-carrying capacity accompany changes in hemoglobin concentrations, their potential effects are often offset by concomitant changes in blood viscosity: since the total potential delivery of O_2 to muscle is the product of $\dot{Q}_T$ and CaO_2, a decrease in hemoglobin concentration potentially reduces O_2 delivery. However, the associated reduction in viscosity enhances blood flow to muscle; also O_2 extraction by tissues increases, thereby tending to maintain the $CaO_2 - C\overline{v}_{O_2}$ difference. For these reasons, reductions in hemoglobin have to be severe before $\dot{V}_{O_2max}$ falls significantly. Anemia may also influence CO_2 carriage by increasing the arteriovenous P_{CO_2} difference for a given difference in CO_2 content.

Cardiovascular Changes

The increase in $\dot{Q}_T$ during exercise is linearly related to $\dot{V}_{O_2}$ (Fig. 18-12); the O_2 requirements for exercise are met by a combination of an increase in $\dot{Q}_T$ and an increase in O_2 extraction by exercising muscle; concomitantly the arteriovenous O_2 difference ($CaO_2 - C\overline{v}_{O_2}$) widens. Therefore, the normal 10- to 12-fold increase in $\dot{V}_{O_2}$ from rest to $\dot{V}_{O_2max}$ is accompanied by a 4- to 6-fold increase in $\dot{Q}_T$ and a 2- to 3-fold increase in the $CaO_2 - C\overline{v}_{O_2}$ difference. The maximum average $CaO_2 - C\overline{v}_{O_2}$ difference is about 160 ml/L, indicating that exercising muscles can extract O_2 almost completely from arterial blood. There is a postural influence on the response of $\dot{Q}_T$ to exercise, i.e., at any given $\dot{V}_{O_2}$, $\dot{Q}_T$ is about 2 L/min higher in the supine than in the erect position.

The increase in $\dot{Q}_T$ is largely brought about by a three-fold increase in heart rate (f_c), i.e., from 60 to 70 beats per minute at rest to 150 to 200 at $\dot{V}_{O_2max}$, together with 1.5- to 2-fold increases in stroke volume, i.e., from 60 to 100 ml to about 100 to 180 ml. The reduction in heart rate during maximum exercise with age is about 6 to 7 beats per decade, from a value of 200 beats per minute at age 20. As the intrinsic heart rate, i.e., recorded in the autonomically blocked heart, also falls with age to a similar extent, the decrease in maximum heart rate with age is usually ascribed to changes in pacemaker activity. The increase in stroke volume during exercise is largely determined by an increase in the left ventricular end-diastolic volume, together with more complete ventricular emptying; in-

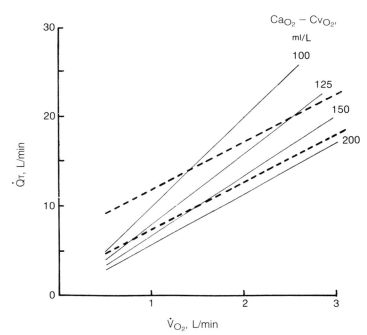

FIGURE 18-12 Cardiac output response to exercise in normal subjects, showing linear relationship to $\dot{V}_{O_2}$, with an intercept that is related to body weight ($0.06 \times$ kg). Isopleths are values of arteriovenous O_2 content difference ($CaO_2 - Cv_{O_2}$).

creases both in cardiac size and in ejection fraction contribute to the larger stroke volume that is found in athletes compared to untrained individuals.

Since the increase in $\dot{Q}_T$ is linearly related to $\dot{V}_{O_2}$, and because the $CaO_2 - C\bar{v}O_2$ difference in maximum exercise is similar in patients with cardiac disorders to that in normal subjects, an indirect assessment of stroke volume in exercise is obtained by the measurement of oxygen pulse ($\dot{V}_{O_2}/f_C$), as shown by a modification of the Fick equation:

$$\dot{V}_{O_2} = \dot{Q}_T(Ca_{O_2} - C\bar{v}_{O_2}) \tag{10}$$

$$\dot{V}_{O_2} = Svf_C(Ca_{O_2} - C\bar{v}_{O_2}) \tag{11}$$

$$\frac{\dot{V}_{O_2}}{f_C} = Sv(Ca_{O_2} - C\bar{v}_{O_2}) \tag{12}$$

Thus, a reduction in $\dot{V}_{O_2}/f_C$ usually indicates a reduction in stroke volume. Normal values for $\dot{V}_{O_2}/f_C$ at maximum exercise may be predicted from the individual's height (Fig. 18-13).

Accompanying the increase in cardiac output during exercise is a fall in systemic vascular resistance, particularly in exercising muscles where autoregulatory vasodilatation appears to occur. Since the increase in $\dot{Q}_T$ is greater than the reduction in resistance, the overall result is an increase in systemic blood pressure during exercise that is linearly related to the increase in $\dot{V}_{O_2}$. The ability to reduce systemic vascular resistance decreases with age; the blood pressure increase during exercise in a 60-year-old is almost twice that found in a 20-year-old (Fig. 18-14). The differences between young and old subjects in blood pressure may be related to the regulation of blood flow to exercising muscle since, in elderly individuals, training leads to a substantial fall in the exercise blood pressure. Pulmonary vascular resistance also increases with age and, in older individuals, pulmonary arterial pressure during exercise increases more than in younger individuals (Fig. 18-15).

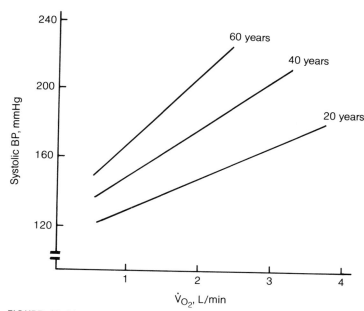

FIGURE 18-14 Arterial systolic blood pressure during exercise to show the effects of increasing $\dot{V}_{O_2}$ and age.

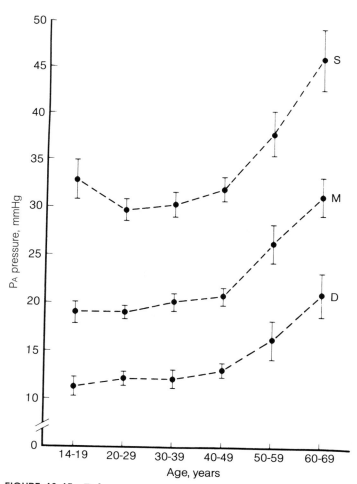

FIGURE 18-15 Pulmonary artery pressures (systolic, diastolic, and mean) at two-thirds of $\dot{V}_{O_2max}$ in subjects of varying age. (*Reproduced from Ehrsam et al., 1983, with permission.*)

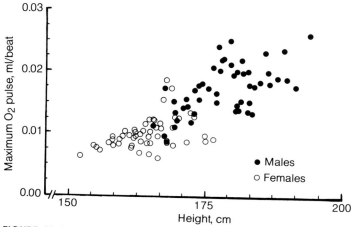

FIGURE 18-13 Oxygen pulse at maximum exercise ($\dot{V}_{O_2max}/f_{cmax}$), related to height in healthy males and females. Part of the variation is accounted for by the effects of age on both $\dot{V}_{O_2max}$ and f_{cmax}.

These circulatory changes manifest some degree of adaptive capacity. For example, if the stroke volume is impaired by a myocardial abnormality, an increase in $\dot{Q}_T$ may still be maintained by increases in f_c. Similarly, a primary defect in the control of heart rate, as in congenital heart block, may lead to an adaptive increase in stroke volume. Although, in principle, a decrease in cardiac output may lead to an adaptive increase in the oxygen extraction by exercising tissues, thereby resulting in a widened arteriovenous O_2 difference, the extent of this adaptation is limited by the O_2-carrying capacity of blood; the maximum arteriovenous difference in O_2 content of about 160 ml/L is seldom exceeded, even in patients with severe cardiac impairment. Therefore, cardiac output at submaximal $\dot{V}_{O_2}$ may often be within the normal range in patients with cardiac disorders, although the *maximum* cardiac output is reduced. In patients with cardiac disease, the reduction in $\dot{V}_{O_2max}$ is a good indication of the extent of reduction in maximal cardiac output.

Acid-Base Control

Heavy exercise imposes a large acid load on the muscles due to increases in lactate production and in P_{CO_2}. If the accompanying fall in muscle pH is not curtailed, enzyme inhibition occurs rapidly and is inevitably followed by fatigue. Control of muscle pH is mainly effected by removal of lactate and CO_2, both being dependent on an increasing muscle blood flow. CO_2 may then be eliminated by the lungs, but the removal of lactate is through oxidation by cardiac and skeletal muscles, liver, and other tissues. Therefore, while elimination of CO_2 is very rapid, the metabolism of lactate is much slower, leading to a metabolic acidosis that is accompanied by a reduction in plasma bicarbonate concentration. In recovery from exercise, the rate of decrease in lactate and of increase in bicarbonate has a halftime of about 20 min—which is shortened by aerobic exercise. Control of muscle pH is also influenced by the movement of strong ions (Na^+, K^+, and Cl^-) between the muscle intra- and extracellular spaces.

INTEGRATION AND LIMITATION

The processes described above each contribute to maximum exercise capacity and, therefore, to the capacity to meet everyday energy demands with minimum effort. The capacity to exercise depends on the integrity of all processes and the linkages that exist between them. The value of exercise testing lies in the opportunity it affords to explore both the function of each process and their linkages, within the framework of the maximum capacity.

Since exercise capacity never depends solely on one process, it is possible for adaptation to occur between processes. The integration between mechanisms may be expressed by a series of Fick equations. The graphic ex-

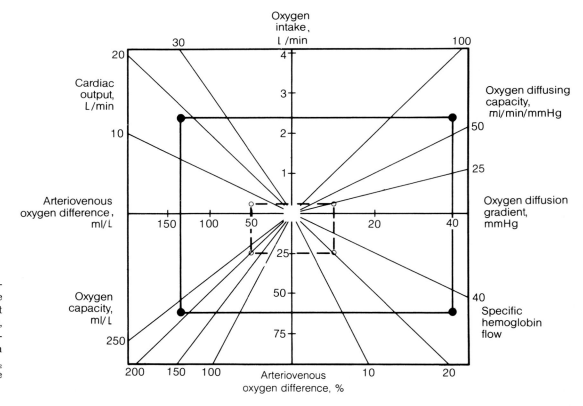

FIGURE 18-16 Barcroft's diagram, modified to show the adaptation of O_2 transport mechanisms (cardiac output, O_2 carriage by blood, and alveolar-capillary O_2 diffusion) in a healthy adult at rest ($\dot{V}_{O_2}$ 240 ml/min) and moderate exercise ($\dot{V}_{O_2}$ 2400 ml/min).

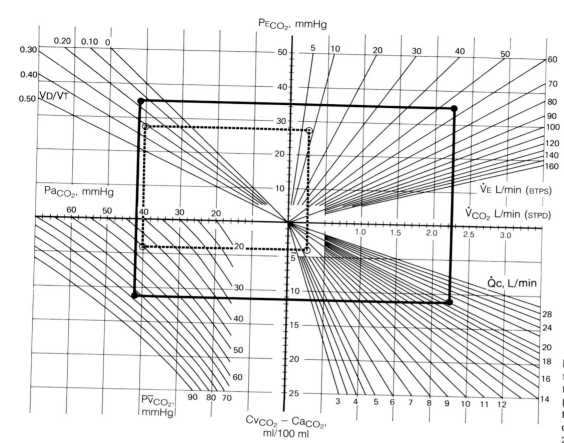

FIGURE 18-17 Graphic presentation of the components of CO_2 transport in a normal subject (ventilation, V_D/V_T ratio, venoarterial CO_2 difference, and cardiac output) at rest and exercise ($\dot{V}_{O_2}$ 200 and 2250 ml/min).

pression of the interrelationships also has a number of attractions. This was first explored by Murray and Morgan in 1925, leading to the classic analysis by Barcroft (1934) in his book *Features in the Architecture of Physiological Function* (see Chapter 17). Both Barcroft's graphic analysis (Fig. 18-16) and the later approach of Margaria et al. (1970) describe the way in which linkage between mechanisms leads to adaptive responses in the total system to maintain oxygen supply. A similar approach was taken to carbon dioxide transport by McHardy et al. (Fig. 18-17).

Clinical Implications of Integration

The linkage between mechanisms has a number of implications for the way in which the total system behaves in different clinical situations, and the ways in which limitation of exercise capacity may occur (Fig. 18-18). Broadly we may identify four types of effect.

1. *Adaptation.* The untoward consequences of one defective process in gas transfer may be lessened by adaptive changes elsewhere in the system. For example, an increase in $\dot{Q}_T$ can sustain O_2 delivery if Sa_{O_2} should fall, e.g., as the result of a disorder in pulmonary gas exchange. Should this adaptation be unavailable, as in a patient in whom ischemic heart disease coexists with

obstructive airways disease and pulmonary hypertension, exercise capacity will be even more seriously impaired. Adaptive interindependence is also evident in the responses to endurance training, in which an increase in muscle aerobic enzymes and a greater utilization of fat as a fuel are accompanied by a decrement in heart rate, an increase in stroke volume, and a reduction in systemic blood pressure. These improvements in oxygen delivery and in muscle aerobic capacity, and the fall in the metabolic respiratory quotient, contribute to a reduction in $\dot{V}_{CO_2}$ for a given $\dot{V}_{O_2}$. The associated fall in $\dot{V}_E$ is the most dramatic physiological effect of training, being accompanied by a reduction in respiratory muscle effort and, therefore, in dyspnea.

2. *Association.* The effect of an impaired process in gas transfer may be accompanied by secondary effects that can become limiting. For example, an impaired response of $\dot{Q}_T$ to exercise is often associated with lactate production that, in turn, causes an increase in $\dot{V}_{CO_2}$ and in $\dot{V}_E$. As a result, the patient with a low cardiac output due to seriously impaired cardiac function may present with breathlessness and apparent ventilatory limitation.

3. *Maladaptation.* When the main defect in exercise capacity lies in the muscles, as in a diffuse myopathy,

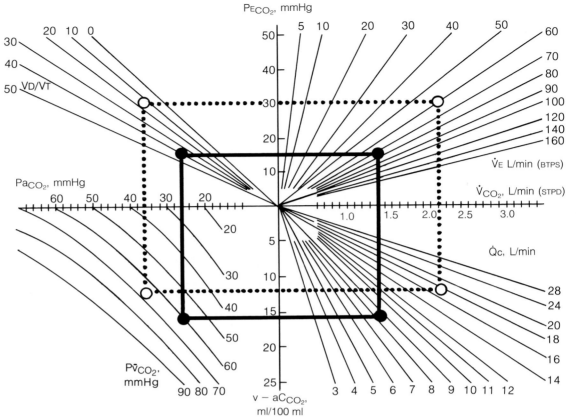

FIGURE 18-18 CO_2 transport in a patient with severe alveolitis (●——●), compared with measurements made in a healthy subject (○· · ·○), both exercising at 60% $\dot{V}_{O_2max}$; $\dot{V}_{O_2}$ in the patient was 1240 compared with 2130 ml/min. In the patient a combination of increased $\dot{V}_{CO_2}$, low cardiac output, alveolar hyperventilation (low Pa_{CO_2}) and high V_D/V_T ratio account for a $\dot{V}_E$ that is *higher* (74 L/min) than in the healthy subject (59 L/min) in spite of the much lower $\dot{V}_{O_2}$.

there is little room for other mechanisms to adapt in order to maintain function. The tachycardia and hyperventilation that occur in this circumstance may be misleading in the identification and assessment of the functional deficit.

4. *Equalization.* The linkage between mechanisms may, in the long term, lead to loss of function in several of the processes that contribute to exercise performance. For example, the enforced inactivity imposed on a patient with a cardiac disorder may result in a secondary fall in the aerobic capacity of the body musculature. If, at this point, the cardiac defect is remedied, as, for example, in coronary bypass surgery, the function of body muscles involved in exercise, rather than cardiac function, may then limit exercise capacity.

Dyspnea

Nowhere is an integrative approach to exercise impairment more important than in assessing dyspnea (see Chapter 165). This is because several factors contribute to the sense of effort in breathing (Fig. 18-19).

1. *The ventilatory demands of exercise.* Ventilation in exercise is the end result of several processes: (a) metabolic production of CO_2, both aerobic and anaerobic; (b) respiratory control mechanisms that influence alve-

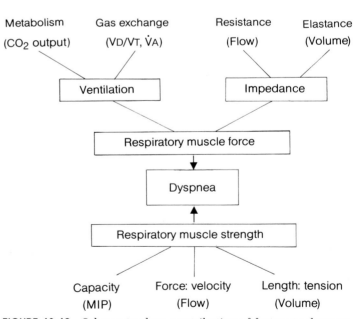

FIGURE 18-19 Scheme to show contribution of factors to dyspnea.

olar ventilation; and (c) pulmonary gas exchange that influences the dead-space-tidal-volume ratio. In many patients with pulmonary disorders, an inordinate pulmonary ventilation at a given exercise level is a major contributing factor to dyspnea.

2. *The impedance to breathing.* Elastic and resistive components that impede the ability to achieve the required ventilation during exercise may be assessed through measurements of the mechanics of breathing. However, in terms of their effect on exercise performance, the vital capacity—representing the capacity to generate a tidal volume—and maximal inspiratory flow—representing the capacity to shorten the inspiratory time—are usually sufficient to identify situations in which the ventilatory capacity is encroached upon by the ventilatory demands of exercise.

3. *The strength of the inspiratory muscles.* Although inspiratory muscle strength may be easily assessed by determining maximum inspiratory pressures, the operating characteristics have to be considered in terms of the length-tension and force-velocity characteristics. As in any skeletal muscle, the maximum tension that can be generated falls as shortening and the velocity of contraction increase, i.e., with larger tidal volumes and increasing inspiratory flow rates.

4. *The pattern of breathing.* The pattern of breathing in terms of tidal volume (VT), frequency (f), inspiratory time (TI), and the duty cycle (TI/Ttot) all contribute to defining the operating characteristics of the respiratory muscles: VT is an index of respiratory shortening, f of frequency of contraction, TI of the duration of contraction, VT/TI of the contraction velocity, and TI/Ttot of the duty cycle of the inspiratory muscles. These measures are easily made during an exercise test.

5. *The sense of effort.* The sense of effort in breathing may be quite precisely assessed by psychophysical measurements that have become an important part of a routine exercise test. Such measures allow the evolution of dyspnea during increasing exercise to be related to the other factors outlined above.

Linkages among these factors are often involved in the pathogenesis of dyspnea (Fig. 18-19): the most severely dyspneic patients are usually found to have an increased $\dot{V}E$ during exercise, increased impedance to breathing, and weak respiratory muscles. In the past, attempts have been made to explain dyspnea in terms of the respiratory muscle work or the oxygen consumption of respiratory muscles. However, both these concepts have proved inadequate because they take no account of the effects of the extent and rate of contraction on the capacity of the respiratory muscles to increase work or oxygen consumption. Instead, dyspnea is related to respiratory muscle effort—the tension generated with respect to the maximum tension-generating capacity of the muscles under the conditions that exist during exercise—as defined in terms of VT, TI, TI/Ttot, and f.

EXERCISE TESTING

As already stated, the power of an exercise test lies in its ability to reveal the function of the total gas-exchanging system as it responds to the metabolic demands for gas exchange between the muscles and inspired air, as well as in describing the function of its component parts. Behind this concept lies another that provides the rationale for the design of a basic, or screening, exercise test: the responses need to be examined starting with the resting state and increasing in several steps to the maximum capacity, which is defined here as the symptom-limited maximum effort. Such a test may be safely carried out on a cycle ergometer or a treadmill, providing that precautions are taken for the test to be stopped if arrhythmia, hypotension, or other serious abnormalities become evident.

The measurements made are generally quite simple but do suffice to give information on the pulmonary, cardiovascular, muscular, and symptomatic responses. For example, to assess the pulmonary responses, ventilation, tidal volume, frequency of breathing, and inspired time are usually determined. To assess pulmonary gas exchange noninvasively, an ear oximeter is often used to measure arterial oxygen saturation. From the cardiovascular point of view, the heart rate and rhythm and the electrocardiograph can be monitored throughout the test and blood pressure measured by sphygmomanometer. The maximal power output and the maximal oxygen uptake assess the aerobic capacity of the muscles to generate power. Symptoms may be quantified using a psychophysical category scale in which patients assign numbers from 0 to 10 to express the sense of effort in the legs and in breathing (see Chapter 165). Measurement of symptom intensity is important, because in most subjects it is symptoms that limit the capacity to exercise.

A completely normal study in which the maximal power output and oxygen intake, ventilation, and the pattern of breathing, heart rate, and blood pressure fall within the normal range (predicted on the basis of sex, age, and height) is a reliable indication that cardiac output, stroke volume, and pulmonary gas exchange are normal; it also excludes a generalized neuromuscular disorder. Abnormal patterns of response allow pulmonary and cardiovascular impairment to be quantified quite precisely. When a low exercise capacity is found without pulmonary or cardiovascular limits having been reached, a primary neuromuscular disorder may be suggested.

Incremental Noninvasive Exercise Testing

Many types of exercise tests have been proposed, some specifically designed for a particular application, such as the diagnosis of coronary artery disease. However, for assessing disability, there is now a consensus that the cornerstone of exercise testing is a procedure in which the exercise level is gradually increased progressively to reach the maximum tolerated intensity in 10 to 20 min; as indicated above, the laboratory must have criteria for stopping the test when untoward signs become evident. Either a calibrated cycle ergometer or a motor-driven treadmill can be used; both allow reproducible and reasonably precise increases in power to be imposed on the subject. For the severely disabled individual, a more appropriate test may be one in which the distance walked in 6 or 12 min is measured.

In a progressive test, it is convenient to increase the power every minute, making measurements at the end of each minute so that the evolution in the exercise responses may be assessed throughout the test, from rest to capacity. Details of measurements are outlined in Chapter 164; the following is a brief list of the information that may be obtained from this type of testing.

1. Increases in oxygen uptake during exercise on a cycle ergometer are related so closely to increases in power output that an abnormality automatically challenges the accuracy of the measurement. In obese individuals, the $\dot{V}_{O_2}$ at any level of work is raised by a constant amount owing to the high resting metabolic rate; also, any condition in which the metabolic rate is high will lead to a high $\dot{V}_{O_2}$ for a given power. The maximal $\dot{V}_{O_2}$ is interpreted with respect to standards that take into account the sex, age, and size of the subject, and if appropriate, the exercise history of the individual.

2. Heart rate at maximal exercise is examined in relation to the subject's age and to $\dot{V}_{O_2max}$; the ratio of these two measurements, i.e., the oxygen pulse ($\dot{V}_{O_2}/f_C$), assesses the maximum stroke volume and is interpreted in relation to sex and height.

3. Increases in systemic arterial blood pressure are interpreted in relation to $\dot{V}_{O_2}$ and the subject's age to obtain information on systemic vascular resistance and myocardial contractility.

4. Increases in $\dot{V}_{CO_2}$ are used to interpret increases in $\dot{V}_E$ and also to identify lactate production.

5. Ventilation is examined to see if increases are appropriate to $\dot{V}_{CO_2}$; if $\dot{V}_{CO_2}/\dot{V}_E$ is low, an increase in $\dot{V}_A$ or the V_D/V_T ratio is suggested; if $\dot{V}_{CO_2}/\dot{V}_E$ is high, alveolar hypoventilation is present. To test if the maximal ventilatory capacity has been reached at maximal exercise, $\dot{V}_{Emax}$ is compared to the $FEV_1 \times 35$; if 80 percent of this value has been exceeded, it is likely that an inability of the inspiratory muscles to increase their power has contributed to the exercise impairment.

6. The pattern of breathing, in terms of V_T, f, and T_I, may be first tested by relating the maximal V_T to the subject's vital capacity, and the inspiratory flow rate (V_T/T_I) to the maximum inspiratory flow rate determined from a maximum flow-volume maneuver at rest.

A low V_T, high f response is accompanied by increases in V_D/V_T ratio.

7. A fall in Sa_{O_2} of more than 2 to 3 percent during exercise is an indication of impaired pulmonary gas exchange and is considered in relation to $\dot{V}_{O_2}$ (percent predicted).

8. Symptoms of leg muscle effort and breathlessness may be reliably quantified by category rating scales that were specifically designed for application to exercise. Usually, as exercise increases, a threshold is reached at 20 to 30 percent of maximum power; the rating then increases linearly. The evolution of the scores, and the comparison between leg effort and breathlessness, give important clues regarding exercise limitation.

Other Techniques in Exercise Testing

Many other measurements may be made during exercise, but the more invasive these become, the more difficult it is to include them in a routine test to be applied to a wide spectrum of patients who have exercise intolerance. For this reason, the more invasive techniques are generally reserved for specific indications or for situations in which a simple noninvasive test has not yielded enough information. Also, some additional measurements are more reliably made in a steady state rather than in the unsteady state that obtains during an incremental test. The following is a short list of the more important of these measurements and their application. The results obtained using all these techniques are considered within the context of the maximum power output, or $\dot{V}_{O_2max}$.

1. Arterial blood gases enable the V_D/V_T ratio and venous admixture to be calculated. Also, when used with the mixed venous CO_2 determined by rebreathing, cardiac output may be derived. The measurements are mainly of help in assessing patients with obscure disability and complex gas-exchange disorders in whom separating pulmonary from cardiac impairment may be difficult.

2. Cardiac output may be determined using a number of techniques to assess a cardiac component to severe disability or where the clinical severity of cardiac impairment is uncertain.

3. Pulmonary artery pressure measurements may be required to establish pulmonary vascular disease and to assess its severity.

4. Radionuclide measurements of right and left ventricular ejection fractions may be helpful in assessing cardiac function in respiratory disorders.

5. In individuals in whom disability is unaccompanied by evidence of cardiac or pulmonary impairment, measurement of maximal isokinetic power will identify a neuromuscular disorder.

6. Measurement of esophageal pressure and lung mechanics is seldom required in the assessment of disability but may be used to quantify the impedance to breathing during exercise.

Although the capacity to exercise may be less important to human survival than it used to be, all activity involves stress on several essential systems that need to function effectively if effort is to be minimized. Impaired function in any of the systems inevitably increases the stress on others and may lead to symptoms that are remote from the initial malfunction. The use of exercise in the laboratory to place the systems under standardized stress affords valuable insights into the function of each system and the remote effects. Because the information cannot be obtained in other ways, and because the results may be directly applied to the assessment of individual disability, exercise testing should be the central technique in any laboratory investigating cardiovascular or pulmonary disorders.

BIBLIOGRAPHY

Altose M, Cherniack N, Fishman AP: Respiratory sensations and dyspnea. J Appl Physiol 58:1051–1054, 1985.

  A summary of a conference held at the National Institutes of Health to deal with the assessment and quantification of respiratory sensations. A major focus was on psychophysical approaches.

Barcroft J. *Features in the Architecture of Physiological Function*. London, Cambridge University, 1934.

  The chapter entitled "Every Adaptation is an Integration" contains a classic description of the linkage between mechanisms in exercise and a graphic approach to the equations involved. (See also Chapter 17 of this volume.)

Bradley CA, Harris EA, Seelye ER, Whitlock RML: Gas exchange during exercise in healthy people. I. Dead space. Clin Sci 51:323–333, 1976.

  This paper and the accompanying paper (Clin Sci 51:335–344) present normal values for gas exchange during exercise.

Cerretelli P, DiPrampero PE: Gas exchange at exercise, in Farhi LE, Tenney SM (eds), *Handbook of Physiology, sect 3: The Respiratory System, vol IV: Gas Exchange*. Bethesda, American Physiological Society, 1987, pp 297–340.

  A comprehensive review of normal gas exchange during exercise with particular reference to the limits of the mechanisms that are involved in the exchange of the respiratory gases in lungs and tissues and in their transport, utilization, and removal.

Dempsey JA, Fregosi RF: Adaptability of the pulmonary system to changing metabolic requirements. Am J Cardiol 55:59D–67D, 1985.

  A review of pulmonary function, chest wall mechanics, and respiratory muscles in exercise.

Dempsey JA, Vidruk EH, Mitchell GS: Pulmonary control systems in exercise: Update. Fed Proc 44:2260–2270, 1985.

  One of a series of papers designed to review recent advances in the understanding of regulatory mechanisms during exercise. The sweep is from molecular biology to integrative neuroscience.

Ehrsam RE, Perruchoud A, Oberholzer M, Burkart F, Herzog H: Influence of age on pulmonary haemodynamics at rest and during supine exercise. Clin Sci 65:653–660, 1983.

  Pulmonary arterial pressures were determined, using right heart catheterization, at rest and exercise in 125 asymptomatic healthy individuals, ranging in age from 14 to 68 years. Increasing age accounted for less than 10 percent of variation in resting values in cardiac output or in pulmonary arterial or wedge pressures. However, pulmonary vascular pressures did increase more in older individuals even though the cardiac output response remained unchanged.

Jones NL: *Clinical Exercise Testing*, 3d ed, Philadelphia, Saunders, 1987.

  A practical approach to exercise as a clinical investigative tool.

Jones NL, Makrides L, Hitchcock C, Chypchar T, McCartney N: Normal standards for an incremental progressive cycle ergometer test. Am Rev Respir Dis 131:700–708, 1975.

  A guide to the prediction of expected responses in the normal population.

Jones NL, McCartney N, McComas AJ: *Human Muscle Power*. Champaign, IL, Human Kinetics, 1986.

  The theme for the book, inspired by the Olympic Games in Los Angeles in 1984, is the mechanisms by which humans achieve and maintain very high power outputs during dynamic exercise. A distinguished group of international exercise scientists are the contributors.

Killian KJ, Jones NL: The use of exercise testing and other methods in the investigation of dyspnea. Clin Chest Med 5:99–108, 1984.

This paper expands on the factors that contribute to dyspnea in pulmonary disorders. The rest of this volume rounds out the picture of limitations to exercise imposed by a variety of cardiopulmonary disorders.

Makrides L, Heigenhauser GJF, McCartney N, Jones NL: Maximal short term exercise capacity in healthy subjects aged 15–70 years. Clin Sci 69:197–205, 1985.

An analysis of indices of maximum aerobic exercise performance in 100 normal subjects (50 men and 50 women) and their relationship to V_{O_2max}. Aging is associated with progressive decrease in V_{O_2max} and an apparently parallel reduction in the "power output capacity" of large muscle groups in leg exercise.

Margaria R, Cerretelli P, Veicsteinas A: Estimation of heart stroke volume from blood hemoglobin and heart rate at submaximal exercise. J Appl Physiol 29:204–207, 1970.

Using a quadrant diagram, the authors are able to determine certain unknown parameters, such as alveolar ventilation, ventilation-perfusion ratio, O_2 pulse, and cardiac output, from other measured or assumed parameters, e.g., $\dot{V}_{O_2max}$, heart rate, alveolar P_{CO_2}, and stroke volume.

McHardy GJR: Diffusing capacity and pulmonary gas exchange. Br J Dis Chest 66:1–20, 1972.

A review of the influence of the diffusing capacity for O_2 on exercise.

Wasserman K, Hansen JE, Sue DY, Whipp BJ: *Principles of Exercise Testing and Interpretation.* Philadelphia, Lea & Febiger, 1987.

Presents an approach to exercise testing based on physiological principles and employs a large number of worked examples to illustrate the interpretation of test results.

Wasserman K: The anaerobic threshold measurement to evaluate exercise performance. Am Rev Respir Dis 129:S35–S40, 1984.

A clear exposition of the concept of anaerobic threshold by its principal protagonist. This paper is part of a symposium on "Exercise Testing in the Dyspneic Patient" that deals with the physiological mechanisms operative during exercise and the pathophysiology of disorders that limit exercise capacity.

Wasserman K: Anaerobiasis, lactate, and gas exchange during exercise: The issues. Fed Proc 45:2904–2909, 1986.

The lead paper in a symposium that identifies the increase in lactate during exercise as a critical biochemical and physiological event that leads to a decrease in intracellular pH, accelerated depletion of glycogen in muscle, and changes in ventilation and gas exchange. The papers that follow provide succinct statements about the current understanding of the metabolic behavior of muscle during exercise as well as about the limits imposed on physical performance by an increase in lactate and a decrease in intracellular pH.

Weber KT, Janicki JS, Fishman AP: Respiratory gas exchange during exercise in the noninvasive evaluation of the severity of chronic cardiac failure, in Braunwald E (ed), *Congestive Heart Failure.* New York, Grune & Stratton, 1982, pp 221–235.

A review of the effects of chronic cardiac disease on respiratory and circulatory performance during exercise. Particular reference is made to the level of ventilation and the anaerobic threshold.

Chapter 19

Lessons from High Altitude

Donald Heath

The Pulmonary Circulation

Response of the Pulmonary Arteries of Animals
to Hypobaric Hypoxia

High Altitude Pulmonary Edema

The Carotid Body

Monge's Disease

Acute Mountain Sickness

Life at high altitude has many lessons for clinicians with a special interest in diseases of the lung and pulmonary circulation. Humans and animals living in these mountainous areas are for the most part healthy, and yet their lungs are exposed for a lifetime to the hypobaric hypoxia consequent upon the diminished barometric pressure. This offers the medical practitioner a remarkable opportunity to assess the physiological and deleterious effects of hypoxia per se without the complicating and confusing effects of the various factors produced by various lung diseases.

It is important to recognize that not all humans and animals living at high altitude are of equal biologic status. The different groups are represented diagrammatically for humans in Fig. 19-1 and for animals in Fig. 19-2. Animals can adjust to the lowered partial pressure of oxygen of ambient air at high altitude by one of two major biologic pathways, acclimatization and adaptation. The term *adaptation* is often used in a loose way in a context where the everyday word *adjustment* would be more appropriate. In this chapter we shall use these terms precisely. *Acclimatization* is a reversible, noninheritable change in the anatomy or physiology of an organism which enables it to survive in an alien environment. Humankind is a species that has to acclimatize to the hypoxia of high altitude (Fig. 19-1). This may be a *natural acclimatization*, as in the Quechua and Aymara Indians of Peru and Bolivia, or it may be the less effective and hard-won *acquired acclimatization*, as in the caucasian lowlander ascending into the mountains. Some animal species living at high altitude also have to acclimatize; the best and most important example is that provided by cattle (*Bos taurus*) (Fig. 19-2). This hard-fought-for acclimatization to hypobaric hypoxia may be lost in both humans and animals (Figs.

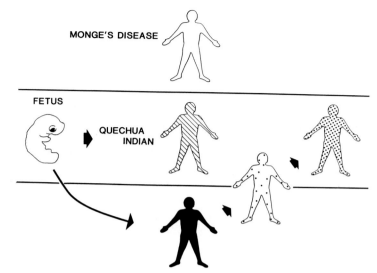

FIGURE 19-1 Diagrammatic representation of acclimatization and loss of acclimatization in humans. Filled figure = life at sea level; cross-hatched = partial adaptation; stippled = acclimatization; open = loss of acclimatization. The upper and middle compartments represent life at high altitude; the lowest compartment, life at sea level. Both the Quechua Indian and the lowlander ascending to high altitude acquire acclimatization, although the process is much longer and more efficient in the natural acclimatization of the native highlander. A minority of Quechuas lose acclimatization and develop Monge's disease. The fetus may be considered to be acclimatized to the hypoxemia of intrauterine life simulating high altitude. The Quechua may show partial adaptation in such phenomena as an increased internal surface of the lung.

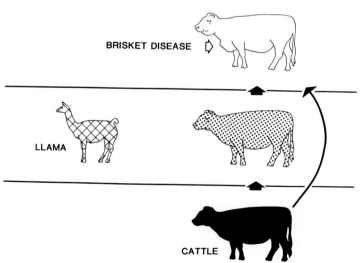

FIGURE 19-2 Diagrammatic representation of adaptation, acclimatization, and loss of acclimatization to high altitude in animals. Filled figure = life at sea level; stippled = acclimatization; open = loss of acclimatization; cross-hatched = full adaptation. The upper and middle compartments represent life at high altitude; the lowest compartment, life at sea level. The llama is fully adapted. High altitude cattle are acclimatized, but some calves in Utah do not sustain acclimatization and develop Brisket disease.

19-1 and 19-2), particularly with aging in humans. Animals exposed to the hypoxic environment of high altitude may, however, respond by the totally different biologic path of *adaptation*. This is a development of biochemical, physiological, and anatomic features which are heritable and of genetic basis, enabling the species to explore the environment of high altitude to its best advantage (Fig. 19-2). If one regards the patient with chronic lung disease and chronic alveolar hypoxia as a subject acclimatizing to hypoxia, it is possible to see how that patient shares certain characteristics with the native highlander. In particular one can see the similarities in the responses of the pulmonary circulation and of the carotid bodies in the two groups.

THE PULMONARY CIRCULATION

At low altitude the human pulmonary vasculature provides a low-resistance type of circulation. Its arteries are thin-walled and its arterioles devoid of any muscular media at all except at the point of immediate origin from the parent muscular pulmonary artery. When babies of Quechua and Aymara Indians in the Andes are born at high altitude, they are exposed from birth to hypobaric hypoxia. As a result, the pulmonary vasculature does not lose the muscularity of the fetal state and persists into adult life. Thus children born and living at high altitude have significant pulmonary hypertension, and a mild elevation of pulmonary arterial pressure persists even into adult life in the native highlanders. We have found that only *some* of the inhabitants of La Paz (3800 m) have muscularized pulmonary arterioles; they are in the main the native Aymara citizens rather than the mestizos and caucasians who have come from outside to live permanently in the city. There is a strong suggestion here of a genetic influence on susceptibility to pulmonary hypertension and muscularization. An individual variation in susceptibility to the effects on the pulmonary circulation is also to be found in the subject at high altitude and in the patient with chronic lung disease.

The site of action of hypoxia on the pulmonary circulation at high altitude and in chronic lung disease is highly characteristic. It affects the terminal portions of the pulmonary arterial tree, bringing about muscularization of the smallest muscular pulmonary arteries of some 200 μm in diameter down to arterioles as diminutive as 30 μm. The sustained alveolar hypoxia of chronic lung disease also exerts its influence in this segment of the pulmonary circulation rather than the larger muscular pulmonary arteries. The involvement of these larger vessels in pulmonary vascular disease, as in plexogenic pulmonary arteri-

opathy, is a feature of quite a different set of diseases such as congenital cardiac septal defects, primary pulmonary hypertension, and cirrhosis of the liver.

The muscularization of the pulmonary arterioles in native highlanders appears to be hardly more than a marker of chronic alveolar hypoxia, for it does not induce significant pulmonary hypertension to diminish their longevity or to interfere with their life-style. The Quechua and Aymara Indians of the High Andes are able to engage in normal daily activities to the extent of playing a vigorous game of football. This is in striking contrast to what occurs in laboratory animals like the rat where exposure for a short period of a simulated altitude of 5500 m may lead to an apparently identical muscularization of pulmonary arterioles which proves to be fatal in inducing congestive cardiac failure. In human chronic obstructive lung disease the same muscularization of the pulmonary vasculature occurs, and the problem is to decide where it lies in this spectrum of functional significance. In deciding this, it has to be kept in mind that even in the healthy highlander the muscularization of the smallest radicles of the pulmonary arterial tree elevates pulmonary vascular resistance enough to prevent the normal regressive changes of the elastic tissue of the media of the pulmonary trunk. Hence there is an abnormal retention of an aortic pattern of elastic tissue in this vessel well on into childhood to the age of 9 years in residents above 4000 m, followed by a transition to a so-called persistent pattern of elastica characterized by alternating fragmented and continuous elastic fibers which may persist into late middle age.

In my experience the degree of development of longitudinal muscle in the intima of pulmonary arteries is limited in the native highlander. The florid development of cellular intimal longitudinal muscle in the pulmonary arteries of patients with emphysema appears to be related more to physical displacement of these vessels around the abnormal airspaces than to chronic alveolar hypoxia.

Another important lesson from high altitude for clinicians interested in pulmonary disease is that the sustained alveolar hypoxia brings about a *hyperplasia of new muscle* in small pulmonary arteries and pulmonary arterioles rather than a constriction of vascular smooth muscle. Hence, if patients with chronic bronchitis and emphysema are treated by long-term oxygen therapy, its possible advantageous effects in reversing muscular changes in the pulmonary vasculature have to be considered in terms of the physical regression of a great deal of vascular smooth muscle rather than in a simple acute reversal of vasoconstriction. When native highlanders with muscularization of their pulmonary arterioles are brought down to sea level, it takes up to 2 years for the regression of vascular smooth muscle in pulmonary arteries to occur completely.

RESPONSE OF THE PULMONARY ARTERIES OF ANIMALS TO HYPOBARIC HYPOXIA

Consideration of the response of the pulmonary arteries of animals to hypobaric hypoxia is valuable in understanding the concepts of adaptation and loss of acclimatization. Their response depends on whether the species in question is acclimatized or adapted to the mountain environment. Some indigenous species like the llama (*Lama glama*), alpaca (*L. pacos*), vicuña (*L. vicugna*) or mountain viscacha (*Lagidium peruanum*) have thin-walled pulmonary arteries (Fig. 19-3) which show an exceedingly weak pressor response to hypoxia (Fig. 19-4). It seems likely that the pulmonary vasoconstrictor response has become reduced by natural selection. It appears that the evolutionary advantage of the mechanism is to constrict the blood supply to underventilated portions of the lung and thus ensure an equal distribution of ventilation-perfusion ratios and the maintenance of the arterial PO_2. In a hypoxic environment, such as occurs at high altitude, the homeostatic necessity for an equality of the distribution of the ratio of ventilation to perfusion becomes less important because of the shape of the dissociation curve for hemoglobin. Thus the advantages of the mechanism for natural selection are minimized. At the same time the disadvantages of global hypoxic pulmonary vasoconstriction become manifest. Pulmonary hypertension increases the afterload on the right ventricle, and sudden increases in the pulmonary arterial trunk can give rise to pulmonary edema which may be fatal, as we shall see below. In this

way, hypoxic pulmonary vasoconstriction becomes an encumbrance to survival at high altitude, and adaptation by natural selection would be expected to be accompanied by a diminution or elimination of the vasoconstrictor response. It would seem that this is, in fact, what has happened to the llama. This viewpoint can be challenged on the grounds that the llama, alpaca, and vicuña are all members of the camel family, which is characterized by a thin-walled pulmonary vasculature, including low altitude species. The same objection, however, cannot be leveled at the example of the yak (*B. grunniens*). This is a member of the cattle family which has, as a group characteristic, a thick-walled pulmonary vasculature. The yak lives at high altitude in the Himalayas and yet has thin-walled pulmonary arteries. This appears to support the concept of reduction of pulmonary vasoconstriction to hypoxia by natural selection.

Members of the cattle family that are not adapted as indigenous mountain species like the yak and which have to acclimatize to high altitude, such as *B. taurus*, may exhibit the opposite problem of a hyperpressor response to the hypobaric hypoxia. Thus in Utah and Colorado calves brought to the mountains for the first time, or some young animals born in the highlands, may develop a condition called *brisket disease*. This picturesque designation refers to the fact that there is edema of the dependent part of the trunk, particularly in the region between the forelegs and the neck, the "brisket" of commerce. Commonly associated with the systemic edema are pleural effusions and ascites, with features of tricuspid incompetence. The clin-

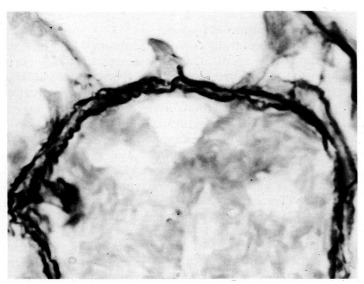

FIGURE 19-3 Part of transverse section of a muscular pulmonary artery from a mountain viscacha (*Lagidium peruanum*) living at an altitude of 4200 m at La Raya in southern Peru. In spite of lifelong exposure to the hypobaric hypoxia of high altitude, there is no medial hypertrophy (elastic Van Gieson, ×1700).

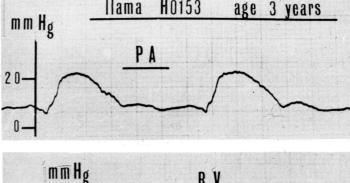
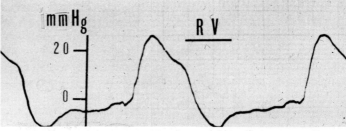

FIGURE 19-4 Pressure tracings from the right ventricle and main pulmonary artery from a 3-year-old llama at Cerro de Pasco (4330 m) in the Peruvian Andes. In spite of lifelong exposure to the hypobaric hypoxia of high altitude, there is no pulmonary hypertension.

ical picture is one of congestive cardiac failure secondary to pulmonary hypertension induced by the environmental hypoxia. It is tempting to explain this all as a loss of acclimatization due to hyperreactivity of thick pulmonary arteries in susceptible individuals. However, there may be additional factors involved for it is a striking fact that brisket disease at high altitude occurs only in this one area of the United States. This district is studded with small water pools and creeks, and in addition large troughs containing salt are spaced at intervals as "salt licks" for the animals. Thus affected cattle are likely to have ingested an excess of salt and it is conceivable that this may play some part in the development of the condition.

HIGH ALTITUDE PULMONARY EDEMA

The pulmonary hypertension and increased muscularity of the pulmonary vasculature in the highlander appear to be unstable when associated with rapid changes in the partial pressure of oxygen in the alveolar spaces, especially when alveolar hypoxia is relieved for a few hours only to be reimposed later. Under such conditions *high altitude pulmonary edema* may suddenly develop. It has been suggested that in this condition there is a leakage of liquid through the small pulmonary arteries which is brought about by a sudden increase in the intraluminal pressure. Such a considerable increase in pressure is rendered possible in native highlanders by the increased amount of muscle in the pulmonary arteriolar walls and by the hypertrophy of the right ventricle. This would explain why high altitude pulmonary edema is most likely to afflict high altitude natives returning to the mountains after a brief sojourn at low level. The influence of exercise in inducing the disease is also consistent with this view since exercise raises the pulmonary arterial pressure even further. Earlier suggestions that the edema was due to left ventricular failure were negated by the finding of normal levels of pulmonary wedge pressure.

In rats hypobaric hypoxia is capable of inducing evaginations of smooth muscle cells in the media of the pulmonary veins which press outward through deficiencies in the internal elastic lamina to press on the undersurface of the venous endothelial cells. These evaginations are devoid of organelles and myofilaments and pass out from the body of the vascular smooth muscle cell between attachment points for actin and myosin filaments. Such evaginations are suggestive of pulmonary venoconstriction in response to hypoxia in experimental animals and in humans at high altitude may play a part in the induction of pulmonary edema. So far as I am aware, muscular evaginations have not been reported in humans. It is, however, at least possible that they occur as the first response of the terminal portions of the pulmonary arterial tree to hypoxia in chronic obstructive disease.

When rats are subjected to simulated high altitude in a hypobaric chamber, they show characteristic ultrastructural changes in the pulmonary capillaries. Small edema vesicles form as a localized swelling of the fused basement membrane of the alveolar wall and project into the lumens of the capillaries. When seen in longitudinal section, these vesicles have an elongated shape similar to that of the capillary into which they project. If such a vesicle is cut in transverse section, without fortuitously including its pedicle, it appears as a round body and gives the spurious appearance of lying free in the pulmonary capillary. The vesicles are covered by a tightly stretched, ultra-thin layer of cytoplasm of the overlying endothelial cell and arise from the edematous zone around the fused basement membrane by means of a pedicle. It is conceivable that large numbers of such endothelial edema vesicles at the venous side of the pulmonary capillary bed could induce hypertension in these small vessels to give rise to edema of the lung.

Direct measurements of the protein in the edema liquid from patients with high altitude pulmonary edema have not been reported. The proposal has been put forward that edema of the lung at high altitude is similar to that induced by multiple pulmonary emboli. In the latter condition there appears to be an extravasation of the liquid from the unobstructed microvessels. The character of the liquid suggests an increased permeability which may be due to injury of the vascular endothelium caused by the high shear stresses induced by an increased velocity of flow. It is possible that such a disseminated obstruction of small arteries may occur in high altitude pulmonary edema due to uneven vasoconstriction or to occlusion with fibrin, which is a well-known histologic feature of high altitude pulmonary edema.

One or more of these mechanisms may lead to a severe pulmonary edema of sudden onset which may overwhelm the newcomer soon after arrival at high altitude especially if he or she engages too quickly after arrival in vigorous exercise. Alternatively, it may affect the native highlander soon after a return to mountains after a brief sojourn to low altitude. Young people are more prone to the disease, but it is rare in infancy. Until about 1950, the acute onset of severe breathlessness far beyond what one would expect to occur in the common form of acute mountain sickness was regarded as due to pneumonia. As early as 1937 it had begun to be suspected that the dyspnea was due to the sudden onset of pulmonary edema. Early reports by Peruvian doctors were followed by the first clear account in the English language in 1960 and by a description of a further 15 patients in the following year.

Factors which exacerbate the condition are the altitude, the rapidity of the ascent, physical exercise, cold, and individual susceptiblity. Symptoms develop usually within a few hours of arrival. Cough, dyspnea, substernal oppression, and cyanosis together with pulmonary crepitations are the prominent clinical features. The chest radiograph shows patchy opacities and some enlargement of the larger pulmonary arterial branches. Treatment with oxygen usually, but not always, leads to a rapid diminution in the pulmonary arterial pressure and amelioration of the condition. The benefit of diuretics or morphine, both popular, is much less certain, and they may even be harmful. Descent to a lower altitude usually has the same beneficial effects as breathing oxygen, but it is not always successful in avoiding a fatal outcome. This is commonly because the condition becomes associated with widespread thrombosis in the pulmonary arteries or cerebral venous sinuses.

THE CAROTID BODY

The carotid body is known to be intimately concerned with chemoreception and probably shares with the adjacent carotid sinus the function of baroreception. In addition to this, the organ probably has as yet undiscovered endocrine functions associated with the secretion of peptides which form the dense osmiophilic cores of the neurosecretory vesicles found in the cytoplasm of its chief cells. It has, for example, been suggested that it is concerned with the secretion of a natriuretic hormone to combat sodium and water retention. With such functions it would be anticipated that the carotid body would be altered both in native highlanders at high altitude and in sufferers from chronic lung disease. The carotid bodies enlarge in native highlanders and in cattle which, like humans, have to *acclimatize* to high altitude (Fig. 19-2). Chronic enlargement of glomic tissue is brought about by hyperplasia of some of its component cells, but the identification of the cell involved in humans at high altitude conflicts with that of the cell implicated in the carotid bodies of patients with chronic lung disease. As far as I am aware, there has been only one report as to the cellular basis of the hyperplasia in native highlanders, and that was in Quechua Indians from the Peruvian Andes. This suggested that the cell involved in the hyperplastic response to the hypobaric hypoxia was the type I (chief) cell. This conflicts with our finding that the cell causing the comparable enlargement of the carotid bodies of patients with chronic obstructive lung disease complicated by hypoxemia is the type II (sustentacular) cell. There is general agreement that the enlargement of the carotid bodies in states of chronic hypoxia is associated with a loss of hypoxic drive. This is true in native highlanders, in patients with chronic lung disease, and in patients with cyanotic congenital heart disease. We interpret the loss of hypoxic drive in subjects with lung disease as being due to compression and even obliteration of clusters of chief cells by hyperplastic sustentacular cells.

In passing it is worthy to note that the carotid bodies of indigenous mountain species, such as the llama and alpaca, do not enlarge in response to chronic hypobaric hypoxia. In such species which are genetically adapted to life at high altitude the histology of the carotid body remains normal.

It is difficult to interpret the functional significance of a hyperplasia of sustentacular cells in response to the sustained hypoxemia of chronic lung disease. These elongated cells are closely related to Schwann cells, and their cytoplasm is packed with intermediate filaments rather than any organelles like neurosecretory vesicles. Their hyperplasia is associated with a proliferation of nerve axons. Some patients with chronic obstructive lung disease and established carotid body hyperplasia show a superadded proliferation of the "dark variant" of the chief cell. We have come to regard the dark variant as a precursor of the chief cell and think it likely that its proliferation is the first response to an acute exacerbation of hypoxemia. We recognize a similarity here to the proliferation of dark cells that we have found in the carotid bodies of cattle living in the vicinity of Cerro de Pasco (4330 m) in the Andes and in patients with a recent reversal of shunt through an intracardiac septal defect. The behavior of the carotid bodies in those living at high altitude is likely to be the same as that in patients with chronic pulmonary disease causing chronic alveolar hypoxia. However, our understanding of the underlying pathology and physiology will remain limited until the role of the peptides in the core of the neurosecretory vesicles in the cytoplasm of chief cells is better understood.

MONGE'S DISEASE

When one walks through the streets of villages and mining towns in the High Andes of Peru, the effects of the sustained environmental hypoxia on erythropoiesis in the healthy Quechua residents are only too obvious. All have deep russety red lips and conjunctivae, and the cheeks show a deep red patch. There are the obvious external manifestations of a hemoglobin level of some 20 g/dl with a hematocrit of 60 percent and a red cell count of about 6.4×10^{12} per liter. Some 4 to 5 g of deoxyhemoglobin need to be present per deciliter of blood for cyanosis to be detected, and hence in the healthy highlander the necessary conditions for its appearance are readily met.

Even the casual visitor, not trained in clinical medicine, is, however, able to pick out a small number of people whose mucosal surfaces appear black rather than deep red, the so-called cardiac negroes (Fig. 19-5). These are the sufferers from *chronic mountain sickness*, or *Monge's disease*, named after the clinician who first described the condition in 1928 as "la enfermedad de los Andes." The

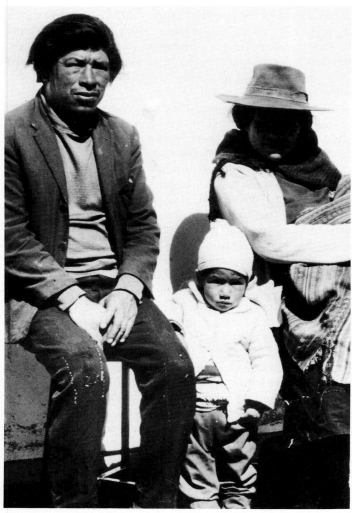

FIGURE 19-5 A sufferer from Monge's disease with his wife and child at Cerro de Pasco (4330 m) in the Peruvian Andes. Note his deeply cyanosed appearance, the hemoglobin level exceeding 23 g/dl. Monge's disease is rare in women and does not occur in children.

no sense be regarded as suffering from cor pulmonale, accentuation of normal hematologic and hemodynamic characteristics can lead to this potentially fatal condition. Monge's disease is rare in women owing to menstrual loss and is not found in children (Fig. 19-5).

Affected subjects suffer headaches, dizziness, parasthesia, and somnolence. The untreated cases described years ago often had striking psychological disturbances such as hallucinations and cerebral crises, but earlier recognition of the disease for what it is and appropriate descent to a lower altitude prevents the development of such extreme manifestations. In addition to the characteristic cyanosed and congested appearance, there is clubbing of the fingernails which commonly show small hemorrhages. The clinical signs of pulmonary hypertension may be demonstrated. There is often a significant elevation of systemic diastolic and mean blood pressure. There may be signs of mild congestive cardiac failure. The fundi show tortuosity and dilatation of venous vessels. Radiology will reveal cardiac enlargement owing to increase in size of the right cardiac chambers which is also detected by ECG. The degree of pulmonary arterial hypertension and the elevation of mean total pulmonary resistance is higher than that found in healthy highlanders. This is associated with muscularization of the pulmonary arterioles and some development of longitudinal muscle in the intima (Fig. 19-6). The cardiac index and pulmonary wedge pressure remain unaltered. The arterial oxygen saturation is even lower than that found in normal highlanders. The total blood volume is elevated. The even further lowering of the partial pressure of oxygen in the alveolar spaces is not due to decreased permeability in the alveolar capillary membrane but to deficient alveolar ventilation. It is this which leads to exaggeration of chronic alveolar hypoxia, more intense pulmonary vasoconstriction, and a greater degree of pulmonary hypertension.

The alveolar hypoventilation has been ascribed to a loss of sensitivity of the respiratory center to carbon dioxide or to an irreversible insensitivity of the peripheral chemoreceptors to hypoxia. This loss of respiratory drive is considered by the Peruvian school to represent a loss of acclimatization to high altitude under the persistent stimulus of chronic hypoxia. It is difficult at the present time to accept or refute this concept because of the lack of data on the pathology of this condition both in the lungs and in the carotid bodies. Three clinicopathologic types of Monge's disease have been recognized. The first, called *chronic soroche*, is said to occur in people who move from sea level to high altitude but never adjust to the change. The second type is the so-called secondary chronic mountain sickness which develops in people who have diseases which are themselves capable, even at sea level, of producing chronic hypoxia and muscularization of the distal portions of the pulmonary arterial tree. Such diseases include gross obesity (the Pickwickian syndrome), kyphoscoliosis, pulmonary emphysema, neuromuscular dis-

basis for the development of this disease is hypoventilation for this exaggerates all the effects of the chronic alveolar hypoxia inherent in a life in the mountains. Monge's disease takes time to develop, and it should be noted that the mean age of the reported cases approaches 40 years. If one is to compare hemodynamic and physiological parameters of cases of chronic mountain sickness with those of healthy native highlanders, the latter should be in the same mature age group. The degree of altitude at which the subject lives is also of importance since the greater the elevation the younger the age at which alveolar hypoventilation may bring about the condition consistent with the development of chronic mountain sickness. The physiological and pathologic features of Monge's disease are but exaggerations of those found in healthy native highlanders of the Andes. However, they are of great clinical importance for, whereas the healthy Quechua Indian can in

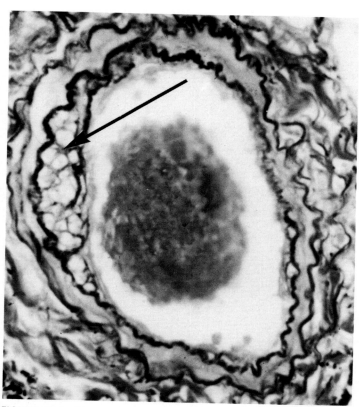

FIGURE 19-6 Transverse section of a pulmonary arteriole from a Quechua Indian who died from Monge's disease. The vessel shows abnormal muscularization so that there is a distinct media of circularly oriented smooth muscle sandwiched between inner and outer elastic laminae. There is a crescentic area of longitudinal muscle which has formed in the intima (arrow) (elastic Van Gieson, ×1000).

sive polycythemia secondary to the fall in ventilatory rate occurring with advancing years. In some ways the hypoventilation of sleep also mimics the physiological basis of Monge's disease.

The simple and effective treatment for the condition is removal to a lower altitude. When a patient with Monge's disease descends to sea level, the symptoms regress rapidly and there are immediate improvements in the hematologic and hemodynamic disturbances. After a further 2 months, the abnormalities have returned virtually to normal. Phlebotomy will lead to some improvement in the systemic arterial pressure. Oxygen has no place in the treatment of the condition for it will achieve little more than a slight temporary and partial alleviation of the pulmonary hypertension.

ACUTE MOUNTAIN SICKNESS

The life-threatening edema which may overwhelm the lung in a minority of lowlanders ascending to high altitude for the first time and in a minority of highlanders returning to their home in the mountains appears to be part of a spectrum of disease. It has a counterpart in the brain where cerebral edema in the same two groups may lead to a variety of symptoms ranging from headache, nausea, and disturbances of vision, to coma. Both of these forms of edema are probably best regarded as extreme examples of a much broader problem which includes acute mountain sickness which afflicts about half of all people ascending to high altitude. This symptom complex has to be carefully distinguished from the bodily sensations of acclimatization which appear to be directly related to hypoxia. In contrast, acute mountain sickness develops in about half of subjects after a time lag of 6 to 96 h and does not seem to be brought about by hypoxia per se but by redistribution of body water. The oliguria of acute mountain sickness is associated with an increased secretion of antidiuretic hormone. Patients with chronic lung disease characterized by sustained alveolar hypoxia do not develop a symptom complex resembling acute mountain sickness. One suspects that in large part this is a function of the time that the body has to adjust to hypoxia, for one can to a large extent avoid acute mountain sickness by a well-planned, gradual ascent to high altitude. The subject of acute mountain sickness is complex, and there is insufficient space here to consider the many physiological and endocrinologic problems that surround the condition.

orders, and pneumoconiosis. Only three reports of the histopathology in fatal cases of Monge's disease have been given since the disease was first described, and each is an example of the secondary form. Hence there is still no confirmation by pathologic examination of the concept that there is a third type, *primary Monge's disease*, occurring in healthy native highlanders who have acclimatized successfully to life at high altitude and then who subsequently develop the features of chronic mountain sickness owing to loss of acclimatization with no organic disease present to explain their increased hypoxemia. It is thus an attractive but unproved concept. An alternative hypothesis to the idea of loss of acclimatization is that chronic mountain sickness is a clinical manifestation of aging at a very high altitude, it being the result of an exces-

BIBLIOGRAPHY

Arias-Stella J, Bustos F: Chronic hypoxia and chemodectomas in bovines at high altitudes. Arch Pathol 100:636–639, 1976.

The paper that first reported that the hypobaric hypoxia of high altitude induces in cattle chemodectomas as well as carotid body hyperplasia.

Anand IS, Harris E, Ferrari R, Pearce P, Harris P: Pulmonary haemodynamics of the yak, cattle, and cross breeds at high altitude. Thorax 41:696–700, 1986.
> *The pulmonary arterial pressure of Ladakhi yaks, at an altitude of about 4500 m, was not significantly different from that found in yaks bred at low altitude. It is concluded that the yak has adapted genetically to high altitude by largely eliminating the hypoxic pulmonary vasoconstrictor response.*

Arias-Stella J, Krüuger H, Recavarren S: Pathology of chronic mountain sickness. Thorax 28:701–708, 1973.
> *Probably the best and most critical account of the pathology of Monge's disease.*

Arias-Stella J, Valcarcel J: The human carotid bodies at high altitudes. Path Microbiol 39:292–297, 1973.
> *The earliest detailed report (excluding abstracts) that the carotid bodies are enlarged in native highlanders.*

Arias-Stella J, Valcarcel J: Chief cell hyperplasia in the human carotid body at high altitude. Physiology and pathologic significance. Hum Pathol 7:361–373, 1976.
> *A sequel giving an account of the histologic features of the enlarged human carotid body at high altitude.*

Dickinson J, Heath D, Gosney J, Williams D: Altitude-related deaths in seven trekkers in the Himalayas. Thorax 38:646–656, 1983.
> *Detailed necropsy findings on seven trekkers in the Himalayas who died from pulmonary or cerebral edema and who also developed thrombosis in pulmonary arteries or cerebral venous sinuses.*

Grover RF, Weil JV, Reeves JT: Cardiovascular adaptation to exercise at high altitude. Exerc Sport Sci Rev 14:269–302, 1986.
> *Exercise training provides an advantage to adaptation to high altitude.*

Harris P, Heath D: *The Human Pulmonary Circulation. Its Form and Function in Health and Disease,* 3d ed. Edinburgh, Churchill-Livingstone, 1986.
> *A comprehensive account of the structure and function of the human pulmonary circulation.*

Harris P, Heath D, Smith P, Williams DR, Ramirez A, Krüger H, Jones DM: Pulmonary circulation of the llama at high and low altitudes. Thorax 37:38–45, 1982.
> *A paper based on field work in the Andes showing that the llama is genetically adapted to high altitude and does not respond to hypobaric hypoxia by pulmonary vasoconstriction.*

Heath D, Moosavi H, Smith P: Ultrastructure of high altitude pulmonary oedema. Thorax 28:694–700, 1973.
> *A description of endothelial edema vesicles protruding into the pulmonary capillaries in rats subject to simulated high altitude.*

Heath D, Smith P: *The Pathology of the Carotid Body and Sinus.* London, Edward Arnold, 1985.
> *An up-to-date account demonstrating the similarities of the changes in the human carotid bodies at high altitude and in chronic lung disease.*

Heath D, Smith P, Fitch R, Harris P: Comparative pathology of the enlarged carotid body. J Comp Pathol 95:259–271, 1985.
> *Paper making the point that the carotid bodies in different species show different structural responses to the same level of partial pressure of oxygen.*

Heath D, Smith P, Jago R: Dark cell proliferation in carotid body hyperplasia. J Pathol 142:39–49, 1984.
> *Paper suggesting that proliferation of dark cells is the first response of the human carotid body to significant hypoxemia.*

Heath D, Smith P, Rios Dalenz J, Williams D, Harris P: Small pulmonary arteries in some natives of La Paz, Bolivia. Thorax 36:599–604, 1981.
> *A study showing that muscularization of the terminal portions of the human pulmonary arterial tree is commoner in the Indian, rather than mestizo or caucasian, section of the population of this city at high altitude.*

Heath D, Williams D, Dickinson J: The pulmonary arteries of the yak. Cardiovasc Res 18:133–139, 1984.
> *This species shows genetic adaptation to hypobaric hypoxia and has thin-walled pulmonary arteries, even though it belongs to a genus characterized by a thick-walled muscular vasculature.*

Heath D, Williams DR: *Man at High Altitude. The pathophysiology of acclimatization and adaptation,* 2d ed. Edinburgh, Churchill-Livingstone, 1981, pp 169–179, 268–281.

A comprehensive account of acclimatization and adaptation to the hypobaric hypoxia of high altitude and their relation to chronic hypoxemia in patients with lung disease.

Hecht HH, Lange RL, Carnes WH, Kuida H, Blake JT: Brisket disease. I. General aspects of pulmonary hypertensive heart disease in cattle. Trans Assoc Am Phys 72:157–172, 1959.

The definitive account of brisket disease in cattle.

Houston CS: Acute pulmonary edema of high altitude. N Engl J Med 263:478–480, 1960.

The first clear account in the English language of high altitude pulmonary oedema.

Houston CS, Sutton JR, Cymerman A, Reeves JT: Operation Everest II: Man at extreme altitude. J Appl Physiol 63:877–882, 1987.

A summary of human experiments at simulated altitude (8840 m) over 40 days in a decompression chamber. This is also the introductory paper to a series of subsequent reports.

Huang SY, Moore LG, McCullough RE, McCullough RG, Micco AJ, Fulco C, Cymerman A, Manco-Johnson M, Weil JV, Reeves JT: Internal carotid and vertebral arterial flow velocity in men at high altitude. J Appl Physiol 63:395–400, 1987.

Cerebral blood flow increases at high altitude after a delay of 18 to 44 h. Subsequently (days 4–12) velocities declined to values similar to those at sea level as hemoglobin concentration and Sa_{O_2} increased to above the initial high-altitude values.

Hultgren HN, Spickard WB, Hellriegel J, Houston CS: High altitude pulmonary edema. Medicine 40:289–313, 1961.

The description in the following year of a further 15 patients.

Monge MC: La enfermedad de los Andes, sindromes eritremicos. An Fac Med Lima 11:314, 1928. (As quoted in Monge MC, Monge CC: *High Altitude Diseases. Mechanism and Management.* Illinois, Charles C Thomas, 1966, p 77.)

The original account of the clinical syndrome of chronic mountain sickness which has since come to bear the author's name.

Moore LG: Altitude-aggravated illness: examples from pregnancy and prenatal life. Ann Emerg Med 16:965–973, 1987.

Emphasis is placed in this article on altitude-aggravated illness or those preexisting conditions that may be adversely affected by reduced O_2 availability at high altitude.

Oelz O, Howald H, Di Prampero PE, Hoppeler H, Claassen H, Jenni R, Bühlmann A, Ferretti G, Brückner JC, Veicsteinas A, Gussoni M, Cerretelli P: Physiological profile of world-class high-altitude climbers. J Appl Physiol 60:1734–1742, 1986.

The functional characteristics of six world-class high-altitude mountaineers were assessed 2–12 months after the last high-altitude climb. It is concluded that elite high-altitude climbers do not have physiological adaptations to high altitude that justify their unique performance.

Singh I, Khanna PL, Srivastava MC, Lal M, Roy SB, Subramanyam CSV: Acute mountain sickness. N Engl J Med 280:175–184, 1969.

An authoritative account of a large series of cases in the Himalayas during the border conflict between India and China.

Staub NC: Mechanism of pulmonary edema following uneven pulmonary artery obstruction and its relationship to high altitude lung injury, in Brendel W, Zink RA (eds), *High Altitude Physiology and Medicine.* Berlin, Springer-Verlag, 1982, p 255.

A hypothesis that the mechanism of pulmonary edema at high altitude may be similar to that induced by multiple pulmonary emboli.

Chapter 20

Diving and Gas Embolism

James M. Clark

Pulmonary Barotrauma
    Possible Sequelae of Alveolar Rupture during Decompression
    Arterial Gas Embolism
    Iatrogenic Arterial Gas Embolism

Pulmonary Decompression Sickness

Continuous Pulmonary Embolism as a Model of Pulmonary Disease

Hyperbaric Oxygen Therapy of Gas Embolism
    Therapeutic Effects of Hyperbaric Oxygenation
    Hyperbaric Oxygen Therapy of Arterial Gas Embolism
      and Decompression Sickness
    Other Medical Applications of Hyperbaric Oxygenation

Limitations Imposed by Oxygen Toxicity

The adverse effects of diving upon the lung and other vital organs originate from two major sources: (1) compression of gas within the lungs and other body spaces as ambient pressure is increased with later expansion of that gas upon return to normal atmospheric pressure; and (2) solution of excess quantities of inert gas in blood and body tissues during exposure to increased ambient pressures followed by evolution of venous and tissue bubbles when decompression occurs too rapidly. The former condition can cause pulmonary barotrauma with arterial gas embolism as its most serious sequela, whereas the latter can cause decompression sickness with manifestations ranging from localized pain caused by joint bubbles to massive neurologic deficits from spinal cord infarction.

PULMONARY BAROTRAUMA

If a diver were to descend while holding his or her breath, the gas within the lungs would be compressed progressively while maintaining a volume that is inversely proportional to the increasing pressure (Fig. 20-1). In order to prevent collapse of the lung to less than residual volume, with tearing of pulmonary parenchyma and blood vessels, the diver is obliged to breath an oxygen-containing gas mixture at a pressure equal to that of the surrounding water. During return to normal atmospheric pressure, compressed gas within the lungs expands exponentially and must be exhaled if alveolar rupture is to be avoided.

The greatest danger of alveolar bursting occurs within the last 33 ft of ascent to the surface, because the relative gas volume doubles during that transition (Fig. 20-1). Theoretically, a critical threshold for alveolar rupture could be reached by ascent from as shallow a depth as 4 ft (1.2 m) after full inspiration at that depth. Fatal arterial gas embolism has occurred following ascent from a depth of 7 ft (2 m).

Possible Sequelae of Alveolar Rupture during Decompression

The sequelae of pulmonary overpressure accidents are determined by the nature and severity of associated tissue trauma, as well as by the volume of expanding extra-alveolar gas. Following rupture of alveolar septa, expanding gas enters the interstitial spaces and dissects along perivascular sheaths, to enter the mediastinum. Gas may also enter the pleural space to cause pneumothorax. Medi-

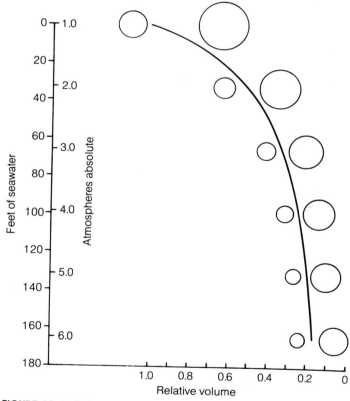

FIGURE 20-1 Relationship of relative gas volume to ambient pressure during compression from 1.0 to 6.0 atm (surface to 165 ft of seawater). Boyle's law states that, at constant temperature, the volume of a gas is inversely proportional to its pressure. Bubbles on the left show the decrease in diameter that would occur during compression without access to a gas source at ambient pressure. Bubbles on the right show expansion that would occur during decompression after restoration of unit volume at a depth of 165 ft. Similar lung volume changes during diving are prevented by inhalation of compressed gas during descent and exhalation of expanding gas during ascent.

astinal gas may further dissect into the pericardial sac, the retroperitoneal space, or the subcutaneous tissues of the neck.

Mediastinal emphysema is often associated with mild substernal discomfort that may be described as a dull ache or a feeling of tightness. Deep inspiration, coughing, or swallowing may exacerbate symptoms, and mild pain may radiate to the shoulders, neck, or back. Unless extensive, mediastinal emphysema is usually not associated with dyspnea, tachypnea, or other signs of respiratory distress. Clinically significant volumes of mediastinal gas have a distinctive appearance on the chest radiograph (see Chapter 136).

Subcutaneous emphysema from pulmonary barotrauma causes swelling and crepitance in the neck and supraclavicular fossae. These signs may be associated with sore throat, dysphagia, or a change in voice tone. Subcutaneous gas can also be demonstrated radiographically. Recompression therapy is not needed for uncomplicated cases of mediastinal or subcutaneous emphysema. If symptoms are bothersome, resolution of gas can be hastened by breathing 100 percent oxygen at normal atmospheric pressure. Gas volumes within the pericardial sac or retroperitoneal space are seldom large enough to be clinically significant.

Pneumothorax is not a frequent complication of pulmonary barotrauma (see Chapter 136). In one series of submarine escape ascents, pneumothorax occurred in about 10 percent of the divers who had lung overinflation syndromes. Recompression of an individual who is known to have a pneumothorax should be avoided if at all possible. Nevertheless, it must be carried out if neurologic symptoms or any other manifestations of arterial gas embolism are present.

Conversion from a simple to a tension pneumothorax will occur if a tear in the visceral pleura remains open during descent, thereby allowing compressed gas to enter the pleural space, and then becomes effectively sealed prior to ascent. Upon decompression, the gas in the pleural space will expand to compress the lung and interfere with venous return. Severe dyspnea, cyanosis, and hypotension may occur, especially when the inferior vena cava is kinked at the diaphragmatic hiatus. This is an emergency that will require immediate recompression to relieve symptoms, and insertion of a chest tube before decompression is resumed. Smaller pneumothoraxes can be managed by inserting a large, 10 to 14 gauge catheter ("angiocath") through the appropriate intercostal space and attaching it to a flutter valve made from a Penrose drain or some other suitable material.

Arterial Gas Embolism

When expanding extra-alveolar gas is forced down a pressure gradient into torn septal vessels, it traverses the pul-

monary veins to the left atrium and left ventricle from which it is ejected into the systemic circulation as foamy particles. Distribution of the gas emboli is determined by their buoyancy relative to blood and orientation of the body with respect to gravity; it may also be influenced by local factors such as turbulence and eddy currents. In the head-up, erect position, most of the embolic air travels to the brain, while the coronary vessels are embolized more frequently with the body in a feet-up, inverted posture.

Cerebral air embolism is a relatively frequent component of lung overinflation syndromes. In a series of 88 divers with pulmonary barotrauma, the incidence of neurologic signs and symptoms was about 75 percent. Electroencephalographic evidence of abnormal neuronal activity after submarine escape training ascents in the absence of associated clinical manifestations indicates that the true incidence of cerebral gas embolism may be even higher than that established on the basis of positive historical and physical findings.

The pathogenesis of cerebral gas embolism involves as a primary event the lodging of embolic gas in arteries and arterioles, causing circulatory arrest with ischemia of the distal tissues. Demonstration of abnormal permeability to protein tracers such as Evans blue dye within 1 to 2 min of air embolism indicates that the bubbles also cause direct endothelial damage at the site of obstruction. Endothelial interaction with active bubble surfaces has been proposed as the basis for this damage.

Clinical manifestations of dysbaric arterial gas embolism have been grouped into two categories based on the initial presentation. The smaller group encompasses critically injured divers who develop apnea, unconsciousness, and cardiac arrest during ascent or immediately after surfacing from a dive. Most of these individuals die even when recompression is initiated within minutes. It is presumed that at least some of these catastrophes are caused by direct embolization of the coronary arteries. Recent experimental evidence also indicates that autonomic influences on the heart and lung can be initiated by brainstem embolization.

The majority of patients with dysbaric arterial gas embolism present with neurologic signs and symptoms, but spontaneous respiration and heart rate are maintained. Just as in the more seriously injured divers, onset of symptoms occurs during ascent or within minutes after surfacing. The clinical spectrum of neurologic disturbances ranges from focal signs, such as monoparesis or discrete sensory deficits, to diffuse brain dysfunction, as manifested by confusion, stupor, or coma. In response to prompt recompression, most patients undergo complete resolution of all neurologic deficits. For reasons that are not well understood, some fail to respond completely or experience initial improvement followed by recurrence of the presenting signs and symptoms. The probability of incomplete response or recurrence is increased as the time between onset of symptoms and initiation of definitive therapy is prolonged.

Iatrogenic Arterial Gas Embolism

Accidental arterial gas embolism is a serious and sometimes lethal complication of many procedures that are widely used in modern medicine. It is often misdiagnosed or recognized only after a delay of several hours. Even when the diagnosis of arterial gas embolism is correctly made, many physicians who are not specifically trained in diving medicine are apparently unaware that hyperbaric oxygenation is *the* definitive and highly efficacious therapy for this condition. No other useful therapy exists. As an example of such unawareness, there are no references to hyperbaric oxygen therapy in at least two surgical texts that contain discussions of cerebral gas embolization as a complication of open heart surgery.

Arterial gas embolism has been reported in association with a variety of procedures including cardiac surgery, intravenous therapy especially with the use of central venous catheters, neurosurgery, pulmonary diagnostic or surgical procedures, surgery of the aorta or cervical arteries, surgical procedures involving the head and neck, hemodialysis, arterial catheterization especially for arteriography, mechanical ventilation, abdominal or retroperitoneal gas insufflation, liver transplantation, and uterine catheterization or insufflation usually during criminal abortion, i.e., if performed under nonmedical, unsterile conditions. Most cases of accidental arterial gas embolism present with focal or diffuse manifestations of brain ischemia. Management is often made more difficult by the existence of concurrent medical or surgical complications. In many patients, hyperbaric oxygen therapy, if administered promptly, completely reverses all neurologic deficits; it is generally remarkably efficacious even when initiated after a delay of several hours.

PULMONARY DECOMPRESSION SICKNESS

The pulmonary form of decompression sickness occurs most frequently after short, deep dives or altitude decompressions. This condition, known to divers as the *chokes*, is manifested by substernal pain, cough, and dyspnea, often associated with extreme malaise. The onset of symptoms is often within minutes after decompression, but it may be delayed for several hours. In some instances, there is only a mild sensation of chest "tightness" that resolves spontaneously. Patients who are more severely affected characteristically manifest a progressive exacerbation of symptoms, entailing rapid, shallow breathing to avoid substernal pain and paroxysmal coughing whenever deep inspiration is attempted. If untreated by hyperbaric oxygenation, pulmonary decompression sickness can terminate in asphyxia, shock, and death.

Although the pathogenesis of pulmonary decompression sickness is not well understood, it apparently involves accumulation in the lung of embolic bubbles along with entrapped aggregates of platelets, fibrin, leukocytes, and erythrocytes.

CONTINUOUS PULMONARY EMBOLISM AS A MODEL OF PULMONARY DISEASE

Development of a unique experimental model of lung disease was stimulated by a series of unexpected observations during deep diving research in human subjects ex-

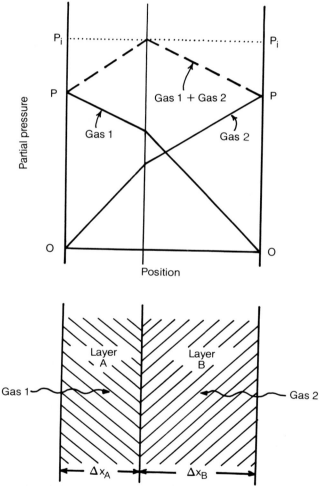

FIGURE 20-2 Supersaturation (and bubble formation) by countercurrent diffusion at the interface of a two-layer system. The two gas reservoirs are large, and their contents are well mixed. In this model, gas 1 (helium) diffuses more rapidly than gas 2 (nitrogen) through layer A (water), and the relative diffusivities of gases 1 and 2 are reversed in layer B (oil). Total gas pressure at any point in the system is the sum of partial pressures of both gases. Bubbles will form at the interface if suitable nuclei are present and if at least one of the two layers is a liquid. *(From Graves, Idicula, Lambertsen, and Quinn, 1973.)*

posed in a hyperbaric chamber to ambient pressures equivalent to depths up to 1200 ft of seawater. When the respired inert gas was nitrogen or neon, with helium as the ambient inert gas at constant ambient pressure, the subjects experienced intense itching in association with maculopapular skin lesions and, on some occasions, developed severe vestibular derangements, with vertigo and nystagmus. The skin lesions were found to be caused by gas bubbles in the skin and subcutaneous tissues; the vestibular derangements were attributed to counterdiffusion of inert gases through the eardrum and middle ear to the inner ear.

Subsequent experiments in pigs and in vitro systems revealed that the development of skin and subcutaneous tissue gas bubble lesions (at constant pressure) was caused by the more rapid inward diffusion of helium from the ambient atmosphere into skin capillaries than outward diffusion of nitrogen or neon from capillaries to atmosphere. The process has been designated *isobaric counterdiffusion gas lesion disease,* and Fig. 20-2 illustrates schematically its probable pathogenetic mechanism. In vivo systems are obviously much more complex than the simple two-layer system shown in Fig. 20-2.

Continuous, steady-state, venous gas embolism can be produced in an anesthetized pig by administration of a normoxic nitrous oxide-oxygen inspired gas mixture with all or part of the pig's body enclosed in a helium-filled bag. This inert gas counterdiffusion model can be used to study adverse effects of gas embolization, interactions of bubble surfaces with blood and vascular constituents, and various methods of therapeutic intervention.

HYPERBARIC OXYGEN THERAPY OF GAS EMBOLISM

In apparently the first medical application of hyperbaric oxygenation in diving, the British Navy began using oxygen inhalation during the early 1930s to hasten inert gas elimination during the final stages of decompression from dives to 300 ft. However, even though it was known by then from animal experiments that oxygen exerts toxic effects on the lungs and central nervous system, the introduction of oxygen decompression as a routine form of treatment was handicapped by the paucity of data concerning oxygen tolerance in humans. This stricture was significantly diminished within the same decade by a series of studies on oxygen toxicity in humans and animals and of oxygen recompression therapy of decompression sickness in anesthetized dogs conducted by A. R. Behnke and colleagues at the Harvard laboratories of Cecil Drinker and Louis Shaw.

Use of oxygen diving for underwater surveillance and demolition during the closing years of World War II greatly stimulated investigation of effects and mechanisms of oxygen toxicity. During the mid-1940s, the times of onset of the signs and symptoms of neurologic oxygen poisoning were observed by K. W. Donald in hundreds of British divers exposed to oxygen pressures ranging up to nearly 4 atm. Working concurrently on different continents, Dickens in London and Stadie, Riggs, and Haugaard in Philadelphia studied biochemical effects of oxygen toxicity in brain slices and other tissue preparations. Many enzymes, especially those with active sulfhydryl groups, were found to be inactivated by increased oxygen pressures.

In a series of investigations during the 1950s, Lambertsen and many collaborators at the University of Pennsylvania obtained extensive data describing in humans the effects of hyperbaric oxygenation on blood-gas transport, pulmonary ventilation, cerebral circulation, and cerebral metabolism. Arterial blood-gas measurements, showing the large increments in oxygen pressure and content that could be achieved in a hyperbaric environment (Fig. 20-3), led to later clinical applications of hyperbaric oxygenation as a means for increasing tumor sensitivity to ionizing radiation, sustaining viability of organs subjected to circulatory arrest for surgical purposes, restoring oxyhemoglobin in carbon monoxide poisoning, and arresting the spread of infection in clostridial myonecrosis.

Therapeutic Effects of Hyperbaric Oxygenation

The oxygen environment of any organ or tissue depends on several interacting factors that influence the balance between oxygen supply and its metabolic utilization. Arterial oxygen content is determined by oxygen partial pressure, hemoglobin concentration, and oxyhemoglobin percent saturation. Oxygen supply to any organ is also highly dependent on the blood flow. Diffusion distance between any individual cell and the nearest capillary is determined by density of the capillary network. Finally, at the mitochondrial end of the oxygen pathway, tissue requirements for oxygen are determined by the level of metabolic activity.

Most of the therapeutic benefits of hyperbaric oxygenation are associated with its capacity for increasing oxygen delivery to hypoxic tissues (Fig. 20-3). Although little additional oxygen can be combined with hemoglobin, which is 97 to 98 percent saturated at normal arterial P_{O_2}, the quantity of physically dissolved oxygen increases linearly with arterial P_{O_2} elevation (about 2.14 ml O_2 per 100 ml blood per atmosphere-inspired P_{O_2}). This important increment in arterial oxygen content is associated with a much larger elevation of the oxygen partial pressure gradient from capillary blood to metabolizing cell. The combined increments in oxygen content and diffusion gradient facilitate oxygen delivery to tissues that, due to ischemia or some other cause, remain hypoxic during air breathing. In many of these states, oxygen breathing at 1.0 atm would also be beneficial. But, the associated in-

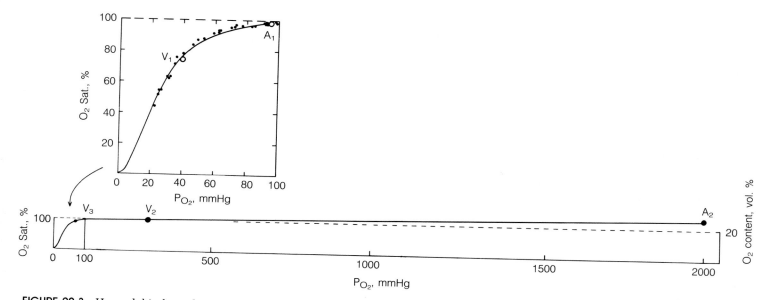

FIGURE 20-3 Hemoglobin-bound oxygen and physically dissolved oxygen in the arterial blood of normal men. *Upper:* A typical range of arterial to mixed venous P_{O_2} (A_1 to V_1) during air breathing and its relationship to oxyhemoglobin percent saturation. The points through which the curve is drawn represent measurements in arterial blood of normal men breathing air or low oxygen gas mixtures. Hemoglobin is an important source of oxygen transport at this level of P_{O_2}. *(From Lambertsen, et al., 1952.) Lower:* The increase in arterial P_{O_2} and the additional oxygen uptake over that bound to hemoglobin when inspired P_{O_2} is increased to 3.5 atm. The additional oxygen is transported as gas physically dissolved in blood water. Fall in P_{O_2} from A_2 to V_2 indicates the decrement across brain capillaries predicted on the basis of same oxygen extraction that occurs during air breathing. Direct measurement shows that brain venous P_{O_2} actually falls to V_3, because brain blood flow is reduced prominently during oxygen breathing at 3.5 atm. *(From Lambertsen, 1978.)*

crements in oxygen content and P_{O_2} are often insufficient to ensure resumption of normal metabolic function in ischemic tissues.

In addition to enhancing oxygen delivery, hyperbaric oxygenation has other therapeutic effects in specific disease states. Resolution of bubbles in decompression sickness and air embolism is greatly hastened by oxygen breathing, because the associated elimination of nitrogen from all body tissues maximizes the outward diffusion gradient for bubble nitrogen. In carbon monoxide poisoning, hyperbaric oxygenation rapidly decreases blood carboxy-hemoglobin concentration and may also oppose CO effects on the cytochrome chain. Hyperoxygenation is also a valuable adjunct in the therapy of clostridial myonecrosis (gas gangrene), because it inhibits multiplication of the anaerobic organisms and, even more importantly, prevents formation of the toxic lecithinase that causes necrotizing myositis. Hyperbaric oxygenation has also been used to increase the radiosensitivity of rapidly growing neoplasms that become hypoxic and, therefore, radioresistant because they outgrow their blood supply.

Hyperbaric Oxygen Therapy of Arterial Gas Embolism and Decompression Sickness

Although arterial gas embolism and decompression sickness have different etiologies and clinical presentations, similar therapeutic principles are applied in both condi-

tions. Primary aims of therapy in both cases are reduction in bubble size, acceleration of bubble resolution, and maintenance of tissue oxygenation. The pressure-oxygenation profile used to accomplish these aims in arterial gas embolism is shown in Fig. 20-4.

The rationale for initial compression to 165 ft is that reduction in bubble size to one-sixth of their original volume will allow at least some bubbles to traverse capillaries and enter the venous circulation to be trapped in the lung. Although the patient cannot safely breathe 100 percent oxygen at 165 ft, administration of 50 percent oxygen throughout this phase will provide hyperoxygenation at a level slightly greater than that afforded by breathing 100 percent oxygen at 60 ft. Oxygen is administered intermittently throughout the remainder of the therapy to accelerate bubble resolution and maintain tissue oxygenation, while avoiding harmful effects of oxygen toxicity by allowing partial recovery during the air intervals. The profile in Fig. 20-4 may be extended in severe cases by adding oxygen intervals at 60 and 30 ft.

Hyperbaric oxygen therapy of decompression sickness, which almost never involves cerebral gas embolism, is often performed by compressing directly to 60 ft without prior pressurization to 165 ft. However, recent experience indicates that the initial exposure to 165 ft may also be beneficial in decompression sickness, especially when severe, or if treatment is delayed for several hours.

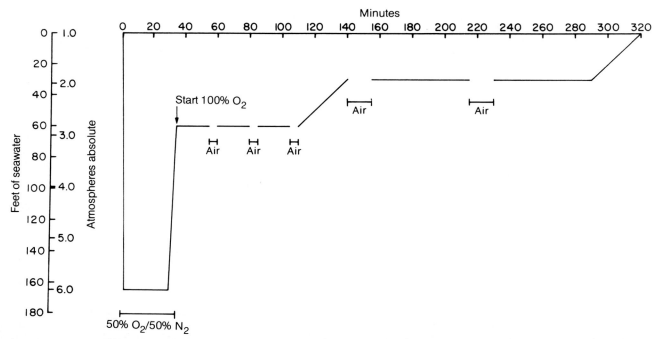

FIGURE 20-4 Pressure-time profile for hyperbaric oxygen therapy of arterial gas embolism and severe decompression sickness. During the initial period of compression to a pressure equivalent to a depth of 165 ft, 50% O_2 in N_2 is administered to the patient for up to 30 min. Upon decompression to 60 ft over a 4-min interval, the patient breathes 100% O_2 and chamber air intermittently for at least 75 min. After a 30-min period of decompression on oxygen to 30 ft, the patient breathes oxygen and air intermittently for at least 150 min, followed by another 30-min decompression on oxygen to normal ambient pressure. *(Modified after U.S. Navy Diving Manual, 1979.)*

In both arterial gas embolism and decompression sickness, increased blood viscosity, hypovolemia, and other systemic effects of bubble interactions with blood components and vessels occur concurrently with the localized tissue ischemia caused by mechanical vascular obstruction. Isotonic fluids are administered intravenously to oppose at least some of these secondary effects. When neurologic symptoms or signs are present, dexamethasone is also given intravenously to reduce swelling of the brain and/or spinal cord. If the patient has other conditions that require medical or surgical intervention, such care is provided concurrently with the administration of hyperbaric oxygenation.

Other Medical Applications of Hyperbaric Oxygenation

Medical uses of hyperbaric oxygenation now extend considerably beyond its initial applications in diving. Several conditions in which there is a physiological and/or experimental basis for its use and in which its clinical efficacy has been demonstrated are listed in Table 20-1. Adjunctive hyperbaric oxygenation has been especially useful in the management of patients with radiation necrosis of bone or soft tissue. Experimental and clinical data indicate that at least part of this therapeutic benefit is related to an oxygen-induced enrichment of the capillary network in tissues that have become hypovascular from radiation

TABLE 20-1

Current Indications for Hyperbaric Oxygen Therapy Approved by Hyperbaric Oxygen Committee of Undersea Medical Society

Gas lesion diseases
 Decompression sickness
 Gas embolism
Vascular insufficiency states
 Radiation necrosis of bone or soft tissue
 Healing enhancement in problem wounds
 Compromised skin grafts or flaps
 Crush injury with acute traumatic ischemia
 Thermal burns
Infections
 Gas gangrene
 Mixed anaerobic-aerobic soft tissue infections
 Chronic refractory osteomyelitis
 Selected refractory mycoses: actinomycosis, mucormycosis
Defects in oxygen transport or utilization
 Carbon monoxide poisoning
 Cyanide poisoning

damage. Improved vascularity and promotion of granulation tissue formation also appear to provide the primary basis for the established usefulness of hyperbaric oxygenation in the preservation of compromised skin grafts and enhancement of healing in problem wounds that do not respond to conventional surgical care. In addition to stimulation of angiogenesis, recent in vitro data indicate that hyperoxia enhances the antibacterial actions of polymorphonuclear leukocytes. Occurrence of a similar effect in vivo would provide an additional mechanism for therapeutic benefits of hyperbaric oxygenation in many of the conditions listed in Table 20-1.

LIMITATIONS IMPOSED BY OXYGEN TOXICITY

During oxygen breathing at increased ambient pressures, rate of intoxication increases progressively in proportion to inspired P_{O_2} elevation. Duration of oxygen exposure at 1.0 to 2.0 atm is limited by pulmonary effects of oxygen toxicity (see Chapter 151). At oxygen pressures of 3.0 atm or higher, visual impairment and convulsions usually occur before development of prominent pulmonary intoxication.

Although the toxic effects of oxygen are numerous and varied (Fig. 20-5), they can be avoided by appropriate administration of hyperbaric oxygen therapy. Early stages of intoxication, even when associated with symptoms and detectable functional alterations, are fully reversible upon exposure termination. The onset of toxic effects is also delayed effectively by periodic interruption of oxygen exposure with scheduled "air breaks" (Fig. 20-4).

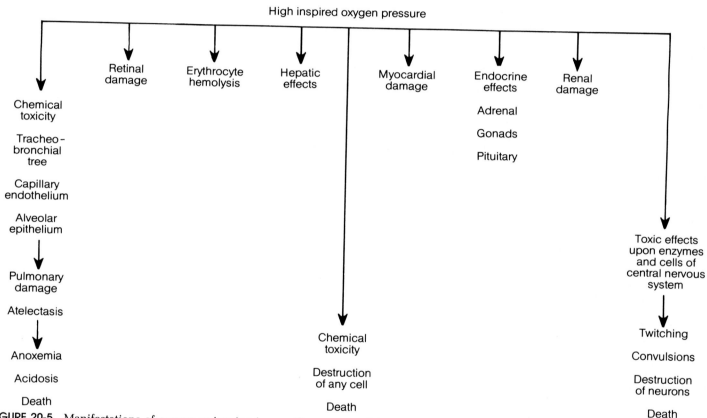

FIGURE 20-5 Manifestations of oxygen poisoning in specific organs and functions. *(Modified after Clark, 1982.)*

BIBLIOGRAPHY

Behnke AR: A brief history of hyperbaric medicine, in Davis JC, Hunt TK (eds), *Hyperbaric Oxygen Therapy.* Bethesda, MD, Undersea Medical Society, 1977, pp 3–10.
  Origins of hyperbaric medicine from perspective of a major contributor.

Brooks GJ, Green RD, Leitch DR: Pulmonary barotrauma in submarine escape trainees and the treatment of cerebral arterial air embolism. Aviat Space Environ Med 57:1201–1207, 1986.
  The reports of all dysbaric incidents occurring during submarine escape training at the Royal Navy's training facility in HMS Dolphin during 1954–84 are reviewed.

Catron PW, Thomas LB, Flynn ET Jr, McDermott JJ, Holt MA: Effects of He–O₂ breathing during experimental decompression sickness following air dives. Undersea Biomed Res 14:101–111, 1987.
  Based on experiments using anesthetized dogs in which decompression sickness was induced, the authors conclude that breathing He–O₂ during decompression sickness resulting from air dive can intensify pulmonary hypertension.

Clark JM: Oxygen toxicity, in Bennett PB, Elliott DH (eds), *The Physiology and Medicine of Diving*, 3d ed. Carson, CA, Best Bookbinder, 1982, pp 200–238.
  Manifestations of pulmonary and central nervous system oxygen poisoning in animals and humans, proposed biochemical mechanisms, and modifying influences.

Dickens F: The toxic effects of oxygen on brain metabolism and on tissue enzymes. Biochem J 40:145–186, 1946.
  Early biochemical studies of oxygen toxicity.

Elliott DH, Kindwall EP: Manifestations of the decompression disorders, in Bennett PB, Elliott DH (eds), *The Physiology and Medicine of Diving*, 3d ed. Carson, CA, Best Bookbinder, 1982, pp 461–472.
  Signs and symptoms of decompression sickness and arterial gas embolism.

Hallenbeck JM, Andersen JC: Pathogenesis of the decompression disorders, in Bennett PB, Elliott DH (eds), *The Physiology and Medicine of Diving*, 3d ed. Carson, CA, Best Bookbinder, 1982, pp 435–460.
  Pathologic effects and proposed mechanisms of decompression sickness.

Kizer KW: Dysbaric cerebral air embolism in Hawaii. Ann Emerg Med 16:535–541, 1987.
  The records of all recompression treatments in Hawaii from 1976 through 1979 are reviewed and both the clinical manifestations and responses to therapy are evaluated.

Lambertsen CJ: Effects of excessive pressures of oxygen, nitrogen, helium, carbon dioxide, and carbon monoxide, in Mountcastle VB (ed), *Medical Physiology*, vol II, 14th ed. St. Louis, Mosby, 1980, pp 1901–1944.
  Summary of physiological and toxic effects of high partial pressures of O₂, N₂, He, CO₂, and CO.

Lambertsen CJ: Effects of hyperoxia on organs and their tissues, in Robin ED (ed), *Extrapulmonary Manifestations of Respiratory Disease.* New York, Dekker, 1978, pp 239–303.
  Physiological and toxic effects of hyperoxia on major organ systems and functions.

Lambertsen CJ, Idicula J: A new gas lesion syndrome in man, induced by "isobaric gas counterdiffusion." J Appl Physiol 39:434–443, 1975.
  Description in humans of isobaric gas counterdiffusion syndrome consisting of dermal lesions and vestibular dysfunction.

Leitch DR, Green RD: Pulmonary barotrauma in divers and the treatment of cerebral arterial gas embolism. Aviat Space Environ Med 57:931–938, 1986.
  A review of case records spanning 20 years reveals 140 cases of decompression pulmonary barotrauma (PBT) in divers. There were 23 cases of uncomplicated PBT and 117 cases of cerebral arterial gas embolism (AGE), of which 58 had respiratory manifestations.

Peirce EC: Cerebral gas embolism (arterial) with special reference to iatrogenic accidents. HBO Review 1:161–184, 1980.
  Clinical manifestations and treatment of cerebral gas embolism caused by accidents associated with a variety of medical, radiologic, and surgical procedures.

Stadie WC, Riggs BC, Haugaard N: Oxygen poisoning. Am J Med Sci 207:84–114, 1944.
  Comprehensive review of early biochemical studies of oxygen toxicity, including many contributions of authors.

Tanoue K, Mano Y, Kuroiwa K, Suzuki H, Shibayama M, Yamazaki H: Consumption of platelets in decompression sickness of rabbits. J Appl Physiol 62:1772–1779, 1987.
  In rabbit decompression sickness, circulating air bubbles were believed to interact with platelets, causing the platelet release reaction; activated platelets presumably participated in the formation of thrombi.

US Navy Diving Manual. Carson, CA, Best Bookbinder, 1979, p 8-25.
  Pressure-time profile for U.S. Navy recompression treatment table 6A.

Ward CA, McCullough D, Fraser WD: Relation between complement activation and susceptibility to decompression sickness. J Appl Physiol 62:1160–1166, 1987.
  The consequences of complement activation and the symptoms of decompression sickness are similar. This report indicates that air bubbles activate the complement system by the alternate pathway.

Chapter 21

Adaptation to Oxygen Limitation

Peter W. Hochachka

Two Divergent Strategies of Adaptation to Hypoxia

Mechanism of Metabolic Arrest

Current Limitations in Applying the Metabolic Arrest Concept

Balancing Metabolic and Membrane Functions

Origin of the Channel Arrest Hypothesis

Coupling Metabolic Arrest with Channel Arrest

Metabolism-Membrane Decoupling in Hypothermia

Diving Response as a First Line of Defense

TWO DIVERGENT STRATEGIES OF ADAPTATION TO HYPOXIA

Recent surveys of animals that are highly tolerant of hypoxia indicate two broad adaptive categories. In one category, typified by species adapted to high altitude and by patients suffering from chronic hypoxia, metabolic mechanisms are directed toward *sustained oxidative function* in the face of potentially chronic limitation in the availability of O_2 and minimal expansion of tissue anaerobic capacities. In these organisms, the fundamental adjustments seem to be designed for high O_2 and substrate fluxes at low O_2 concentration, a strategy that requires "tuning up" of both the O_2 delivery and the cell metabolism parts of the system.

In the second category are many ectotherms (with invertebrate and vertebrate representatives), which direct metabolic strategies toward *sustained anaerobic function* during hypoxia; some of these species have developed such efficient mechanisms of protection against hypoxia that they are often termed *good animal anaerobes* or *facultative anaerobes*. In this adaptive response, two fundamental problems must be resolved, one metabolic, the other membrane-based. In turn, the metabolic problem can be subdivided into two parts: (1) conservation of fermentable substrate and (2) avoidance of self-pollution by production of undesirable end products.

The first part of the problem, i.e., conservation of fermentable substrate, arises from the energetic inefficiency of anaerobic metabolism since the yield of ATP per mole of substrate fermented is always modest compared to oxidative metabolism. For this reason, in most animal tissues, glycogen (glucose) utilization rates vary inversely with O_2 availability (the so-called Pasteur and Crabtree effects*); this means that *if demands for ATP remain unchanged during O_2 lack*, carbohydrate consumption rates necessarily have to increase drastically. In the case of glucose fermentation to lactate, 2 mol of ATP per mole glucose are formed compared to 36 when glucose is oxidized to CO_2 and H_2O; a positive Pasteur effect large enough to make up the energetic shortfall on transition to anoxia would mean about an 18-fold increase in glucose consumption rates; about a 12-fold increase would be required if glycogen were the fermentable substrate.

Facultative animal anaerobes minimize the potentially large depletion of glycogen from tissue stores by (1) storing more glycogen, (2) utilizing more efficient fermentation pathways, and/or (3) depressing ATP turnover rates (i.e., the energy demand) during O_2-limited periods. All three mechanisms are useful in extending anoxic survival time. However, the first two mechanisms in principle cannot extend hypoxia tolerance by more than 3- to 4-fold. In contrast, in some fishes (such as carp, goldfish, and lungfish), processes activated during metabolic arrest can increase tolerance to anoxia by some 5-fold; in hypoxia-tolerant bivalves, by some 20-fold; in diving turtles, by some 60-fold; and in brine shrimp embryos, by orders of magnitude. The limit of the metabolic arrest strategy can be illustrated by estimating the maximum anoxia tolerance of brine shrimp embryos; this limit coincides with entrance into a fully arrested, or ametabolic, state.

Two instructive lessons are learned from the hypoxia adaptation strategies of such animal extremists: (1) *reversing the classic Pasteur effect, so as to allow ATP turnover rates to precipitously drop during anoxia*, appears to constitute the most effective strategy for solving the metabolic problem of substrate conservation, and (2) this mechanism, at least in principle, may be universally applicable, whereas other potentially protective measures, such as energetically improved fermentation pathways, are phylogenetically restricted. Therefore, even in theory, the alternative of energetically improved fermentation pathways does not appear to be a realizable strategy of hypoxia adaptation in those species, such as humans and

*The Pasteur effect is defined as the inhibition of carbohydrate consumption when O_2 concentrations are high and includes the opposite situation: increased anaerobic glycolysis with O_2 is limiting. A reversed Pasteur effect is defined as *decreased or unchanging glycolytic flux when O_2 is limiting*. The Crabtree effect is defined as the inhibition of O_2 consumption by activated carbohydrate fermentation. Current information indicates that several kinds of controlling mechanisms may cause the Pasteur effect and that these may be cell-line or species-specific. However, neither O_2 nor carbohydrate per se play any direct regulatory roles in these effects. Metabolite and enzyme control mechanisms accounting for a reversed Pasteur effect are not well understood.

269

other mammals, that lack the appropriate enzymatic pathways. For this reason, and assuming that factors such as accumulations of end products are controllable, it may be that current estimates of substrate-sparing advantages of metabolic arrest mechanisms for surviving hypoxia may actually be on the conservative side.

The "end products" problem is more difficult to assess because it requires quantifying: (1) the relative effects of organic (usually anionic) end products versus those of H^+ per se, (2) the metabolic sites of H^+ production, (3) the pathways for clearance and subsequent fate of H^+, (4) the H^+ stoichiometry of different fermentation pathways, and (5) the metabolic effects, if any, of net change in strong ion difference, i.e., in concentrations of other strong ions such as Ca^{2+}, Mg^{2+}, K^+, Na^+, or Cl^-. Despite these complexities, it is now evident that the potentially perturbing direct, or indirect, effects of metabolic end products are minimized in "good" animal anaerobes by a few mechanisms that include: (1) the use of fermentation pathways which allow more ATP to be turned over per mole of H^+ generated than in classic glycolysis, (2) tolerance of proton production by improved tissue buffering capacity, (3) minimizing the accumulation of end products by recycling them for further metabolism or excretion, (4) the use of H^+-consuming reaction pathways, and (5) depression of the metabolic rate during anoxia.

Again, it is now clear that all the above mechanisms are advantageous, potentially yielding up to about a several-fold temporal improvement in tolerance to anoxia; yet, it is evident that, by depressing demands for ATP during anoxia (mechanism 5 above), an organism not only reduces the rates of depletion of glycogen (glucose) by relatively fruitless fermentations but it also reduces automatically the rates of formation of anaerobic end products, including H^+. For example, in the case of hypoxic submerged lungfish, the rate of proton production is reduced five-fold because of metabolic depression (primarily in white muscle), whereas in the turtle the process is reduced by nearly two orders of magnitude.

From such analyses of groups of animals that are phylogenetically quite diverse, the conclusion can be drawn that several processes contribute to the hypoxia tolerance of "good" anaerobes. However, of the various biochemical options available to the organism, *metabolic arrest mechanisms yield by far the most effective protection against O_2 lack. Of the known protective strategies, only these resolve both the problem of substrate conservation during anoxia and that of end-product formation.* That is why it was concluded some years ago that for extended survival without oxygen, anaerobic life-support systems (whether considered at the organismal, organ, or cellular level) *must be able to switch down, or even to switch off, metabolically.* To facilitate discussion, we have termed this metabolic switching as *the metabolic arrest concept* by which tissues are protected against hypoxia.

MECHANISM OF METABOLIC ARREST

In principle, metabolic arrest could be achieved by blocking either the ATP-generating, or the ATP-utilizing, arm of the ATP cycle:

ATP synthetases $\begin{matrix} ATP & H_2O \\ ADP & \\ + \\ P_i \end{matrix}$ ATPases
(Energy-yielding   (Cell work functions)
metabolic pathways)

In practice, animal anaerobes seem to rely on blocking the ATP-generating arm, i.e., on blocking the left arm of the above cycle, with a reversed Pasteur effect.

In theory, understanding how the ATP-generating arm is blocked would be enhanced by figuring out how a positive Pasteur effect works. Although the latter problem is still not fully resolved, three approaches are currently being used: (1) conventional allosteric regulation of glycolysis centered primarily at hexokinase (HK), glycogen phosphorylase, and phosphofructokinase (PFK), (2) covalent modification of key regulatory enzymes, and (3) enzyme and pathway compartmentalization.

A fascinating example of the first approach is the aerobic-anaerobic transitions in sperm. This route indicates that a positive Pasteur effect is mediated by a large transfer of control from PFK to HK, with overall flux being accelerated by ATP and glucose 6-phosphate (G6P) deinhibition at the two sites, respectively. The second kind of mechanism for sparking glycolysis at the appropriate time is that of Ca^{2+} influx during hypoxia (see below), with subsequent phosphorylation of phosphorylase b to phosphorylase a. The third approach assumes, in general, that the glycolytic enzymes normally occur in equilibrium between bound and soluble states:

Bound glycolytic   ⇌   Soluble glycolytic
enzymes   enzymes
(More-active forms)   (Less-active forms)

In principle, the only condition needed to cause a Pasteur effect during hypoxia is the shifting of this equilibrium to the left. In the ischemic or hypoxic mammalian heart, a Pasteur effect coincides with a left shift in the equilibrium reaction:

Myofibrillar-bound   ⇌   Solubilizable glycolytic
enzymes   enzymes
(More active)   (Less active)

In contrast, in anoxic bivalves, the equilibrium is right-shifted, which would favor a reversed Pasteur effect, as is observed in these organisms. In effect, these kinds of studies imply that the degree of compartmentalization is controlled and this in turn controls the glycolytic rate. By and large, although some kinetic differences are now recognized, enzyme-binding approaches do not supply any insight into why binding per se should increase the catalytic capacities of glycolytic enzymes.

However, some potential mechanisms do become evident in a special version of the above approach that underscores how specific enzyme-enzyme interactions may influence catalytic rates. The point of departure for these latter studies is the observation that the effective concentrations of active sites of glycolytic enzymes are similar to, or actually higher than, the concentrations of most intermediates and coenzymes in the pathway (starting fuels, end products, phosphagens, and ATP being obvious exceptions). Under such conditions, one way of increasing the flux capacity of a glycolytic pathway is to incorpo-

rate sequences involving enzyme-to-enzyme, direct transfer of substrates or coenzymes. This mechanism is perhaps most conveniently illustrated using glyceraldehyde-3-phosphate dehydrogenase (G3PDH). This enzyme may be involved in a dual coupling for the facilitated transfer of its two products (DPG and NADH) to its two target enzymes, phosphoglycerate kinase (PGK) and lactate dehydrogenase (LDH), respectively. As indicated in Fig. 21-1, coupling of these three enzymes initiates a series of glycolytic cycles in which LDH and PGK enter and leave at specific steps in the process. Pyruvate is reduced to lactate as LDH is cycling through; acyl GPDH phosphorolysis and subsequent ATP synthesis occur while PGK is cycling through; NADH and NAD$^+$ never

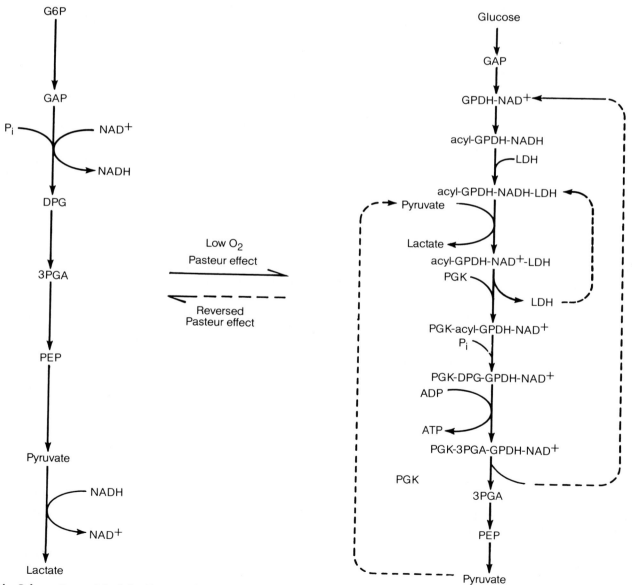

FIGURE 21-1 Schematic model of the Pasteur effect based on the transition from solution-dominated glycolytic function to direct-transfer dominated glycolysis. *(Modified from Srivastava and Bernhard, 1986.)*

need to enter into solution, for GPDH-NAD$^+$, which initiates the entire sequence, is regenerated as 3-phosphoglycerate (3PGA) is released for the next step in the glycolytic path.

In the model shown in Fig. 21-1, the Pasteur effect (activation of glycolytic flux by low O_2 availability) is viewed simply as a transition from solution-dominated, to handoff-dominated, glycolysis, perhaps due to increased availability of pyruvate, NADH, and ADP. In test-tube experiments, such as transition from solution to handoff-dominated GPDH, PGK and LDH function yields an 8- to 10-fold increase in catalytic rates, which could be high enough to account for many, and maybe most, Pasteur effects. For a reversed Pasteur effect, these glycolytic cycles would have to be slowed, presumably by some exogenous signal (increased H$^+$ concentration, for example).

Although Fig. 21-1 provides an intriguing model of how the Pasteur effect might be mediated, it should be clear that the model has not been proven in vivo. As with models based on ratios of bound/soluble glycolytic enzymes, there is no information available on how large a Pasteur effect could be generated by an intact glycolytic path, or on why some cells—even within a single organ such as the kidney—show very large Pasteur effects (e.g., thick ascending limb), some show intermediate ones (e.g., proximal tubules), whereas others (e.g., distal tubules) show very modest ones. It is evident, therefore, that a great deal remains to be done and that a conservative interpretation of the available data would assume no single mechanism for the Pasteur effect. Both its magnitude and its mechanism appear to show a great deal of cell-line specificity that arises from cell specializations and adaptations for specific functions.

In the case of the smooth muscle of arterial walls, the Pasteur effect may even be pathway-specific: one pathway (glucose-lactate) may be fully operational in the presence of O_2, whereas a second (glycogen-lactate) may be normally inhibitive by high O_2 tensions. Cell line and species specificity of the standard Pasteur effect implies a similar degree of specificity for the reversed Pasteur effect and, thus, for metabolic arrest in animal anaerobes in hypoxia. This is a hopeful conclusion, for, in time, this group of organisms may represent a treasury of potentially useful strategies for therapeutic intervention. However, to date, only few attempts have been made clinically to utilize metabolic arrest as a defense against hypoxia.

CURRENT LIMITATIONS IN APPLYING THE METABOLIC ARREST CONCEPT

Although the scientific literature on estivation and hibernation invokes "metabolic arrest" types of concepts to account for protection against hypoxia, these concepts have been more critically tested in clinical studies on cardiac arrest, stroke, acute renal failure (ARF), and liver ischemia. For example, it is commonly assumed that the extent of ischemic myocardial damage varies with the workload or metabolic rate; for this reason, several interventions have been designed to minimize tissue damage by reducing myocardial energy requirements during hypoxia or ischemia. These measures have proved useful to varying degrees, thereby partially living up to the expectations of the metabolic arrest hypothesis. One rather convincing illustration of the usefulness of metabolic arrest is in the use of the ischemic rat kidney as a model for acute renal insufficiency. Ischemic acute renal insufficiency is characterized by reduction in renal blood flow and, thus, by reductions in the delivery of O_2 and substrates to renal tissue. Since the principal ATP-utilizing processes of the kidney are membrane-coupled ion pumps, the metabolic arrest concept requires that any fractional change in demands for ATP by ion pumps should yield a change in hypoxia tolerance of similar magnitude but of opposite direction. In the mammalian kidney, the medullary thick ascending limb (mTAL) of Henle's loop is the most O_2-dependent segment of the nephron; during perfusion of the isolated organ, easily demonstrable hypoxia-induced damage to mTAL cells occurs within about 90 min. However, this sensitivity to hypoxia can be minimized by perfusing with ouabain (a specific inhibitor of Na$^+$,K$^+$-ATPase) or by reducing ion-pumping work by preventing glomerular filtration. Conversely, experimentally increasing membrane permeability by using ionophores increases the energy costs of ion transport and, consequently, increases sensitivity to hypoxia; the hypoxia-induced damage is again avoidable by ouabain inhibition of the Na$^+$ pump. Effective protection can even be achieved against KCN-induced lesions by simultaneous ouabain inhibition of K$^+$ and Na$^+$ pumping.

While such data support the general predictions of the metabolic arrest concept, they also underline a most significant difference: thus far, no metabolically arrested mammalian tissues or organs can sustain severe hypoxia or complete anoxia for more than minutes to perhaps several hours, whereas animal anaerobes are able to sustain comparable or greater degrees of O_2 lack for days, weeks, and, in some cases, even months. Such large differences in hypoxia tolerance between mammalian cells and their homologues in facultatively anaerobic animals means that something is still missing in our understanding of mechanisms for protecting against O_2 lack. Further comparisons of hypoxia-tolerant and hypoxia-sensitive cells and tissues indicate that the missing element is to be found in the coupling between cell membrane functions and cell metabolism.

BALANCING METABOLIC AND MEMBRANE FUNCTIONS

To illustrate the critical role of close coupling between cell metabolism and cell membrane functions in hypoxia-sensitive systems, one of the most convenient models is the mammalian brain, for which the metabolic and membrane functions during various kinds of O_2 limitation are well studied. In the complete cerebral ischemia of cardiac arrest, the electroencephalograph (EEG) becomes isoelectric within 15 to 25 s, producing an electrically silent period that precedes a massive outflux of K^+ from the neurons and a flux of Na^+ into the intracellular fluid (ICF). This breakdown in normal ion gradients is caused by ATP insufficiency (i.e., by the failure of ATP-dependent membrane ion pumping rates to keep up with ion leakage rates); typically it is observable when regional cerebral blood flows are reduced to 10 percent of normal or less. When the $[K^+]$ rises in the ECF to about 12 to 13 mM, the change in membrane potential leads (1) to opening of voltage-dependent Ca^{2+} pores (or channels) and, consequently, (2) to a largely uncontrollable influx of Ca^{2+}, a cation that is toxic when abnormally high concentrations are reached in the cytosol. Although high cytosolic $[Ca^{2+}]$ may disrupt various intracellular functions, its activation of phospholipases appears to be most perturbing to cell structure and to the control of cell metabolism. Three kinds of phospholipases can be activated: A_1, A_2, and C. Increasing concentrations of lysophosphatidylcholine (lysoPC) and free fatty acids soon after ischemia indicate that catalysis by phospholipases of the A class has occurred.

For phospholipase A_2, this catalysis can be written as follows:

H$_2$C—O—palmitoyl $\xrightarrow[\substack{\text{phospho-}\\ \text{lipase A}_2}]{}$ H$_2$C—O—palmitoyl

H C—O—arachidonoyl   H C—OH + arachidonic

        H$_2$O   acid

H$_2$C—O—P—choline   H$_2$C—O—P—choline

    Phosphatidylcholine (PC)   lysoPC

If uncontrolled, this catalysis leads to the gradual hydrolysis of membrane phospholipids and to disruption of cell and mitochondrial membranes and the consequent release of telling free fatty acids, and it further enhances the redistribution of ions in the O_2-limited brain (Fig. 21-2).

Damage initiated by ion flux may also be favored through the action of phospholipase C; its continued catalytic function under O_2-limited conditions is indicated by increasing levels of stearoyl and arachidonoyl diacyl-glycerols coincident with decreasing levels of phosphatidylinositol (PI). The major metabolic pathways responsible for the formation and degradation of PI are illustrated in Fig. 21-3. PI is phosphorylated at the 4 position of its inositol head group by a specific kinase to form phosphatidylinositol 4-phosphate [PI(4)P], which is then further phosphorylated at the 5 position to give PI(4,5)P$_2$, one of the inositol lipids located in the inner leaflet of the plasma membrane. The steady-state concentrations of PI(4,5)P$_2$ are determined by the balance between the activities of these kinases and specific phosphomonoesterases that convert PI(4,5)P$_2$ back to PI (Fig. 21-3); i.e., PI(4,5)P$_2$ levels are determined by the operation of two linked metabolic cycles that entail the continuous addition and removal of phosphates from the 4 and 5 positions of the inositol head group.

In response to various Ca^{2+}-mobilizing hormones, these two metabolic cycles are broken, in a *controlled* way, by the preferential action of phospholipase C upon PI(4,5)P$_2$, thereby releasing diacylglycerol plus water-soluble inositol triphosphate (IP$_3$) as a second messenger to signal the release of Ca^{2+} from the intracellular pools. During hypoxia, the cycles are broken in an apparently uncontrolled way, presumably leading to the same end products.

IP$_3$ released in the process is thought to act as a secondary signal for opening Ca^{2+} channels and for the release of sarcoplasmic Ca^{2+}, thereby increasing the availability of Ca^{2+} in the cytosol, a cascade which may again be self-potentiating (increasing Ca^{2+} levels maintain the catalysis of phospholipase C). Under normal circumstances, diacylglycerol is phosphorylated to phosphatidic acid, which is then converted back to PI. However, in response to appropriate signals, and during hypoxia, diacylglycerol accumulates and is thought to increase Na^+/H^+ exchange, which would effectively slow down the Na^+ exchange-based Ca^{2+} efflux (Fig. 21-3).

Such debilitating cascades initiated by O_2 limitation (Figs. 21-2 and 21-3) are also evident in similar uncontrolled fluxes in other hypoxia-sensitive mammalian tissues and organs. For example, in myocardial ischemia, energy deficiencies and membrane failures are indicated by intracellular fluid (ICF) and extracellular fluid (ECF) changes in $[Na^+]$ and $[K^+]$ as well as by a large influx of Ca^{2+}, a loss of sarcolemmal Ca^{2+}, and a disruption of mitochondrial Ca^{2+} homeostasis. Analogous disruptions of membrane function, with consequent translocation of Ca^{2+} and other ions between intra- and extracellular pools, occur in hypoxic liver, kidney, smooth and skeletal muscle, and presumably generally in mammalian organs and tissues that sustain O_2 shortages, although the process may not be as rapid, or extensive, in relatively hypoxia-tolerant tissues.

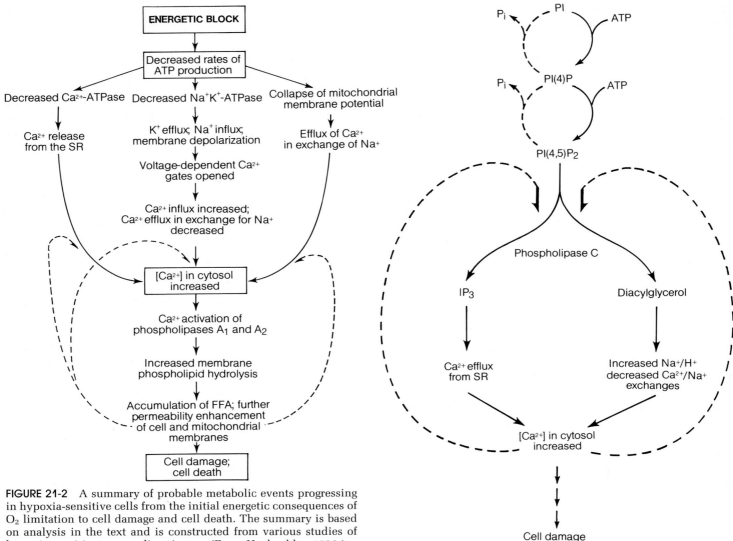

FIGURE 21-2 A summary of probable metabolic events progressing in hypoxia-sensitive cells from the initial energetic consequences of O₂ limitation to cell damage and cell death. The summary is based on analysis in the text and is constructed from various studies of hypoxia-sensitive mammalian tissues. *(From Hochachka, 1986.)*

FIGURE 21-3 Under hypoxic conditions, phosphoinositols decrease in concentration while diacylglycerol levels increase presumably along with inositol triphosphate facilitating increased Ca²⁺ levels in the cytosol. This pathogenic cascade is thought to represent a normally closely tuned signal-transduction system running out of control during O₂ lack. *(From Hochachka, 1986.)*

ORIGIN OF THE CHANNEL ARREST HYPOTHESIS

As in our analysis of metabolic adaptations to hypoxia, the above data on membrane failure in hypoxia-sensitive cells are best appreciated when contrasted with hypoxia-tolerant systems. In such comparative studies of the brain and of other organs of good ectothermic anaerobes during hypoxia, it is observed that, in striking contrast to hypoxia-sensitive cells, failure of membrane function either does not occur at all or develops very much more slowly. These observations are of fundamental importance for they indicate that something about cell membranes in facultatively anaerobic ectotherms is evidently different; when O₂ is lacking, these membranes either: (1) are more impermeable to ions, or (2) their ion-pumping capacity can match the leakage of ions and the drift toward electro-

chemical equilibrium of the ICF and ECF. Stabilized ion gradients almost certainly cannot be due to accelerated ion pumping because ATP turnover rates are lowered in the metabolically arrested states typical of animal anaerobes in the anoxic state. For these reasons, we favor the conclusion that the flux ratio (leakage of ions/pumping of ions) is held at unity during O₂ lack in hypoxia-tolerant cells primarily by adjustments in ion-specific permeability barriers; such adjustments may, in fact, be an expression of a basic difference between cell membranes of hypoxia-tolerant ectotherms and hypoxia-sensitive endotherms. For convenience, and because membrane permeability to ions largely depends on densities of functional, ion-specific pores or channels, we term this basic difference the *channel arrest hypothesis* of defense against hypoxia.

Concepts such as the above are developed because they are heuristic and help to explain previously perplexing data. Accordingly, the channel arrest concept is useful in explaining at least three sets of data that previously were only poorly, or not at all, understood. First, this hypothesis explains well those studies that showed that even if ion gradients do decline in hypoxia-tolerant ectotherms during hypoxia, the process is much slower than in mammals; moreover, in the extreme, ion gradients obviously remain stable even after days of anoxia, even though metabolic arrest keeps ATP turnover rates too low to account for the stability that occurs during ion pumping.

Second, the channel arrest concept provides a better understanding of O_2 conformity. In O_2-conforming cells, tissues, and organisms, in contrast to O_2 regulators whose O_2 uptake is largely independent of O_2 availability down to very low values, the rates of O_2 uptake vary with O_2 availability over broad ranges (despite a very high affinity for O_2 displayed by their isolated mitochondria). The problem arising from O_2 conformity concerns what happens to cell and tissue maintenance metabolism as O_2 availability declines. One possibility is that the required ATP turnover is maintained by anaerobic glycolysis, which would require a positive Pasteur effect. However, O_2 conformity is most commonly displayed by tissues which show a reversed or negative Pasteur effect, e.g., as in ectothermic anaerobes. The only other way for O_2 uptake rates to decrease as O_2 availability decreases is to coordinate a rate reduction in the processes that contribute to maintenance metabolism in the first place. In many cells, major contributions to maintenance metabolism are made by ATP-dependent ion pumping processes. Thus, in O_2 conformers, keeping ion leakage rates and ion pumping rates in balance as O_2 availability decreases means reducing the leakage rates in proportion to reduced rates of ion pumping (i.e., to reduce membrane permeability in proportion to reduced rates of ATP synthesis). Only then can O_2-conforming responses be expressed without a concomitant massive Pasteur effect. In other words, reducing aerobic metabolic rates as O_2 availability decreases is possible if—and only if—the density of functional ion channels decreases concomitantly, for pump and channel fluxes must always remain in balance. Such short-term channel density adjustments are viewed as the underlying mechanism of action of hormones such as aldosterone. The analysis above suggests that similar mechanisms may exist for adjusting maintenance metabolism of hypoxia-tolerant cells to O_2 availability; it also implies that channel arrest is potentially useful not only as a long-term de-

fense mechanism against hypoxia (as in animal anaerobes) but also as a shorter-term defense.

Third, the channel arrest hypothesis sheds new light on recent studies on the origins of endothermy which show (1) that ATP turnover rates and ouabain sensitivities of homologous tissues in mammals are about five times higher than in ectothermic reptiles, but (2) that the permeabilities of mammalian cell membranes, at least in liver, are also some several-fold greater than in the liver of reptiles. We favor the idea that the latter explains the former, i.e., that one cost of endothermy is a higher rate of thermogenesis arising in part from "leaky" membranes and from the consequent necessity for higher ion pumping rates and higher ATP turnover rates. In this view, "leaky" membranes may be adaptive in most endotherms since they form part of a metabolic furnace whereas nonleaky, channel-arrested membranes are adaptive in animal anaerobes because they allow metabolic arrest without risk of dissipated electrochemical gradients. In fact, the implication that leaky membranes are inherent to endothermy and are an important reason for increased hypoxia sensitivity of many mammalian tissues is exactly what is required by the channel arrest concept and appears to supply the link—*stabilized membrane functions*—missing in earlier attempts to extend the hypoxia tolerance of mammalian tissues and cells.

COUPLING METABOLIC ARREST WITH CHANNEL ARREST

We have now arrived at the kind of generalization that this comparative analysis set out to find, namely, that *metabolic arrest + channel arrest = hypoxia tolerance* and that such coupling may be the most basic requirement for establishing in mammalian tissues the hypoxia tolerance of ectothermic anaerobes. The implication for clinical scientists obviously is that intervention strategies should aim at balancing the two functions (leaks and pumps; metabolism and membrane active transporting mechanisms) that are adapted in animal anaerobes for expansion of hypoxia tolerance. It seems a straightforward strategy, pervasively and successfully used by animal anaerobes, but is it transferable to mammalian systems?

Interestingly, interventions with very similar goals have been tried; these maneuvers, in effect, target various Ca^{2+} channels (using channel-specific pharmacologic agents) in order to slow down or prevent uncontrolled Ca^{2+} fluxes and uncontrolled elevation of $[Ca^{2+}]$ in the ICF (Fig. 21-1). Thus, Ca^{2+} channel arrest is conceived as an important defense against hypoxia, and it is often coupled with cold-induced metabolic arrest. Although such interventions applied to all mammalian tissues or organs investigated to date have usually been "protective" against hypoxia for short time periods, they have been of limited success for prolonged protection. It is not yet fully clear where the problem is. One possibility is that hypothermia per se is damaging and its disrupting effects, in combination with those of hypoxia, may well be exaggerated: at the cell level the two stresses are disrupting for a remarkably similar reason, i.e., unregulated metabolic depression becomes uncoupled from membrane function.

METABOLISM-MEMBRANE DECOUPLING IN HYPOTHERMIA

Although it is beyond the scope of this analysis to examine this problem in detail, it should be emphasized that most cold-sensitive cells lose K^+ at low temperature because the temperature coefficient for leakage of K^+ is less than the temperature dependence of ATP-dependent, active accumulation (or of energy metabolism). Therefore, K^+ efflux at low cell temperatures is necessarily blocked less than inward K^+ pumping; as a result, efflux exceeds K^+ influx so that ICF and ECF K^+ ions shift toward their equilibrium concentrations. Na^+ moves in the opposite way, and if this process is not interrupted, it ultimately leads to partial membrane depolarization, the opening of voltage-dependent Ca^{2+} channels, and the influx of Ca^{2+}. Ca^{2+} influx may also be facilitated by Na^+/Ca^{2+} exchange or by damaged (i.e., low-temperature-modified) Ca^{2+} channels behaving as Na^+ channels, a process that would increase $[Na^+]$ in the ICF and set the stage for activated Na^+/Ca^{2+} exchange. Low temperature may also lead to a loss of Ca^{2+} from the sarcoplasmic reticulum (SR), which is again, at least in part, caused by an imbalance between rates of SR Ca^{2+} uptake (by Ca^{2+} ATPase) and rates of Ca^{2+} efflux. In addition, a drop in cell temperature alters the fractional dissociation of imidazole groups on proteins, so that intracellular pH increases and directly activates Ca^{2+} efflux from the SR. The net effect of all these processes would seem to facilitate a gradual increase in $[Ca^{2+}]$ in the cytosol, thus leading to some, and possibly all, the metabolic perturbations shown in Fig. 21-2.

These low-temperature problems are avoided in cold-tolerant cells by maintaining a regulated metabolism and less permeable cell membranes than in cold-sensitive cells, i.e., by utilizing the same strategy as is used by animal anaerobes during anoxia. Although in principle this could be achieved by several means, available evidence indicates that, at least in the long-term, *regulating channel density per unit of membrane surface area may be the commonest way of meeting tissue and cell ion-specific permeability requirements* in different microenvironments or different metabolic states. The common reduction in densities of functional channels may explain the observed permeability differences in cell membranes between cold-tolerant versus cold-sensitive cells and good anaerobes versus hypoxia-sensitive endotherms.

Furthermore, exactly the same considerations hold in principle for membranes of mitochondria and of other intracellular organelles. In the final analysis, it is the inability of cold-sensitive cells to make such channel density adjustments that explains why hypothermia is not very useful for the long term as a metabolic arrest strategy. It also emphasizes the need for metabolic arrest mechanisms *other than hypothermia* for future progress in the application of these protective strategies. Because the coupling of metabolic and channel arrest as a defensive strategy is seemingly wrought with difficulties, one may wonder whether it can ever be successfully utilized with mammalian preparations. It turns out that some tissues in one group of endotherms, the marine mammals, *are* seemingly able to achieve this coupling under the potentially hypoxic stress of diving, so we end this chapter by briefly examining this fascinating group of animals.

DIVING RESPONSE AS A FIRST LINE OF DEFENSE

In enforced breath-hold diving in aquatic animals, the two key provisions required by an O_2-limited cell, tissue, or organism (conserving fermentable substrate and minimizing end-product accumulation) are met, in part, by a set of physiological reflexes which, taken together, are termed the *diving response* and which may be taken as a first line of defense against potential O_2 shortages. In laboratory studies of simulated diving in aquatic animals, the diving response involves apnea, bradycardia, and peripheral vasoconstrictions. Metabolic consequences include: (1) a closely regulated release of (oxygenated) red blood cells from an enlarged spleen coupled with preferential redistribution of O_2 and blood-borne substrates to specific organs and tissues, (2) increased accumulation of anaerobic end products, such as lactate, in hypoperfused regions of the body, concomitant with declining plasma glucose levels, and (3) a distinct lactate washout profile during recovery with a concomitant hyperglycemia evident in the plasma.

For more than 40 years it has been known (1) that the amount of stored O_2 available at the beginning of diving is not adequate to maintain normoxic rates of aerobic metabolism during enforced breath-holding periods of near-maximum duration and (2) that not enough lactate is formed to account for the shortfall in energy produced by anaerobic glycolysis. That is why, as has been frequently observed since Scholander's initial studies, repayment of the O_2 debt generally equals only a modest fraction of the O_2 deficit incurred; recent evidence implies that the same process probably occurs during voluntary diving of Weddell seals at sea. In terms of the above analysis of hypoxia-tolerant animals, it means that, during enforced (and possibly during voluntary) diving, reversed Pasteur effects are sustained in hypoperfused tissues; therefore, lower metabolic rates are achievable than in pre- or postdive states, a process that accounts for both the missing lactate and the missing O_2 debt. Thus, of the two best defense strategies used by ectothermic anaerobes, at least one (metabolic arrest) also is seemingly utilizable during diving in aquatic animals. The question remains as to whether the second strategy of coupling of low-permeability membranes with metabolic arrest capacities is also harnessed.

Unfortunately this question cannot be answered rigorously. In the sense that hypoperfused organs and tissues may experience hundreds of dives per day with consequent partial metabolic arrest but with no apparent difficulties, it may be clear that the hypoxia-induced membrane failures, typical of terrestrial mammals, are somehow avoided in diving species. Unfortunately, no detailed data are available to assess this situation quantitatively for most hypoperfused tissues. However, the kidneys of the seal may be an exception, for here metabolic arrest capacities appear to be obviously coupled to low-permeability membrane functions, and the anoxia tolerance of the organ is predictably expanded toward the capacities typical of ectothermic anaerobes. Thus, in one mammalian organ in one group of endotherms, the same defense strategies against hypoxia are evidently utilizable as are widely used in ectothermic anaerobes. This is a hopeful insight for it raises the possibility, and may supply an initial experimental model, for refining and focusing a potentially effective intervention strategy to other mammals, including humans.

BIBLIOGRAPHY

Berridge MJ, Irvine RF: Inositol triphosphate, a novel second messenger in cellular signal transduction. Nature 312:315–321, 1984.
  An authoritative account of the historical background and biochemistry of inositol triphosphate.

Brezis M, Rosen S, Spokes K, Silva P, Epstein FH: Transport-dependent anoxic cell injury in the isolated perfused rat kidney. Am J Pathol 116:327–341, 1984.
  An interesting example of how arresting metabolism contributes to protecting against hypoxic injury.

Else PL: Studies in the evolution of endothermy: Mammals from reptiles. PhD thesis, University of Wollongong, Sydney, NSW, Australia, 1984.
  A most challenging account of the metabolic problems associated with this important step in evolution.

Elsner R, Gooden B: *Diving and Asphyxia. A Comparative Study of Animals and Man.* London, Cambridge, 1983, pp 1–168.
  A comprehensive but concise summary of diving physiology and metabolism.

Guppy M, Hill RD, Schneider RC, Qvist J, Liggins GC, Zapol WM, Hochachka PW: Microcomputer-assisted metabolic studies of voluntary diving of Weddell seals. Am J Physiol 250:R175–R187, 1986.
  The first metabolic data ever obtained on voluntarily diving animals at sea.

Halasz NA, Elsner R, Garvie RS, Grotke GT: Renal recovery from ischemia: A comparative study of harbor seal and dog kidneys. Am J Physiol 227:1331–1335, 1974.
  A classic study in biochemical adaptation for hypoxia tolerance.

Hansen AJ: Effect of anoxia on ion distribution in the brain. Physiol Rev 65:101–148, 1985.
  A comprehensive review of mammalian brain in O_2 lack, well illustrating the problems arising from decoupling metabolic and membrane functions.

Hillie B: Ionic Channels of Excitable Membranes. Sunderland, MA, Sinauer Assoc, 1984, pp 1–426.
  Accepted as an outstanding review of the physiology and biochemistry of ion channels.

Hochachka PW: Metabolic arrest as a mechanism of protection against hypoxia in Wauquier A, Borgers M, Amery WK (eds), *Protection of Tissues Against Hypoxia.* Amsterdam, Elsevier, 1982, pp 1–12.
  One of the first comprehensive attempts at ranking the effectiveness of metabolic arrest in defending against hypoxia.

Hochachka PW: Exercise limitations at high altitude: The metabolic problem and search for its solution in Gilles R (ed), *Circulation, Respiration, and Metabolism.* Berlin, Springer-Verlag, 1985, pp 240–249.
  A review of recent developments in biochemical and metabolic adaptations to chronic O_2 limitation.

Hochachka PW: Defense strategies against hypoxia and hypothermia. Science 231:234–241, 1986.
This review focuses on common problems of metabolic-membrane decoupling in hypoxia and hypothermia.

Hochachka PW, Guppy M: *Metabolic Arrest and the Control of Biological Time.* Cambridge, Massachusetts, Harvard, 1987, pp 1–227.
This new book analyzes the various biologic situations in which metabolic arrest is utilized in nature.

Hochachka PW, Mommsen TP: Protons and anaerobiosis. Science 219:1391–1397, 1983.
A simple but clear discussion of where in anaerobic metabolism protons are used and where they are produced.

Hochachka PW, Somero GN: *Biochemical Adaptation.* Princeton, NJ, Princeton, 1984, pp 1–537.
Emphasis is placed on the versatility of biochemical systems during animal adaptation to various parameters including low O_2.

Hulbert AJ, Else PL: Comparison of the "mammal machine" and the "reptile machine:" Energy use and thyroid activity. Am J Physiol 241:R350–R356, 1981.
A fascinating account of how the metabolic potential of endotherms is expanded over that of their ectothermic predecessors.

Jackson DC, Heisler N: Intracellular and extracellular acid-base and electrolyte status of submerged anoxic turtles at 3°C. Resp Physiol 53:187–201, 1983.
An authoritative analysis of a system in which metabolic and membrane functions remain coupled during hypoxia.

Matthys E, Patel Y, Kreisberg J, Stewart JH, Venkatachalam M: Lipid alterations induced by renal ischemia: Pathogenic factor in membrane damage. Kidney Intl 26:153–161, 1984.
Irreversible ischemic damage to the renal cortex and outer layers of the medulla correlates with persistent abnormalities of phosphatidylcholine metabolism and persistent elevations of free fatty acids, lysophosphatidylcholine, and diacylglycerol.

Palmer LG, Li JHY, Lindemann B, Edelman IS: Aldosterone control of the density of sodium channels in toad urinary bladder. J Membrane Biol 64:91–102, 1982.
In this study, particularly clear evidence is presented for hormonal control of functional channel density.

Qvist J, Hill RD, Schneider RC, Falke KJ, Liggins GC, Guppy M, Elliott RL, Hochachka PW, Zapol WM: Hemoglobin concentrations and blood gas tensions of free-diving Weddell seals. J Appl Physiol, 61:1560–1569, 1986.
Blood-gas and hemoglobin data obtained in voluntarily diving marine mammals.

Rubin RP, Weiss GB, Putney JW Jr (eds): *Calcium in Biological Fluids.* New York, Plenum, 1985, pp 391–490.
A comprehensive overview of where, how, and why calcium affects metabolism.

Scholander P: Experimental investigations on the respiratory function in diving mammals and birds. Hvalradets Skrifter, Norske Videnskap-Akad, Oslo 22:1–131, 1940.
This study is the first of its kind and sets the stage for diving physiology and biochemistry for the next 45 years!

Sick TJ, Rosenthal M, LaManna JC, Lutz PL: Brain K^+ homeostasis, anoxia, and metabolic inhibition in turtles and rats. Am J Physiol 243:R281–R288, 1982.
Some fascinating comparative data on ion gradient stability in a species highly tolerant to hypoxia.

Siesjo BK: Cell damage in the brain: A speculative synthesis. J Cereb Blood Flow Metab 1:115–185, 1981.
An interpretive analysis of the vast amount of data available on cell damage during hypoxia in the mammalian brain.

Srivastava DK, Bernhard SA: Enzyme-enzyme interactions and the regulation of metabolic reaction pathways. Curr Top Cell Regul 28:1–68, 1986.
Data are reviewed supporting concepts of channeling of substrates through metabolic pathways that show a great deal of structural or functional organization.

Stewart PW: How To Understand Acid-Base, in *A Quantitative Acid-Base Primer for Biology and Medicine.* New York, Elsevier-North Holland, 1981, pp 1–186.
A novel, albeit complex, way of looking at acid-base problems.

Surlykke A: Effect of anoxia on the nervous system of a facultative anaerobic invertebrate, *Arenicola marina*. Marine Biol Letters 4:117–126, 1983.

> *Striking evidence of stable ion gradients even after days of anoxia in this highly hypoxia-tolerant species.*

Theodore J, Robin ED, Jamieson SW, van Kessell A, Rubin D, Stinson EB, Shumway NE: Impact of profound reductions of Pa_{O_2} on O_2 transport and utilization in congenital heart disease. Chest 87:293–302, 1985.

> *In this highly provocative study, data are presented on biochemical adaptations in patients with congenital heart disease; the overall adaptational strategies show striking similarities to those utilized by high-altitude animals.*

Zapol WM, Liggins GC, Schneider RC, Qvist J, Snider MT, Creasy RK, Hochachka PW: Regional blood flow during simulated diving in the conscious Weddell seal. J Appl Physiol 47:968–973, 1979.

> *A comprehensive quantitative picture of the redistribution of cardiac output during activation of the diving response.*

Chapter 22

Regulation of Ventilation in Metabolic Acidosis and Alkalosis

Roberta M. Goldring / Homayoun Kazemi

Metabolic acidosis or alkalosis implies a change in $[H^+]$ in the blood. The immediate adjustment to a metabolic derangement in acid-base balance is effected by physicochemical buffering, which initially involves the extracellular fluids and, subsequently, the rest of the body. Respiratory and renal adjustments then come into play, operating to alter the diurnal balance of both CO_2 and H^+. The respiratory response influencing P_{CO_2} is immediate, whereas the renal response influencing $[H^+]$ comes into play minutes or hours later. The abnormality in blood pH that persists after the immediate buffering mechanisms have come into play controls, to a major degree, the respiratory and renal compensatory mechanisms to the acute upset. If the immediate buffer mechanisms are overwhelmed so that pH cannot be restored to the range of 6.8 to 7.8, survival is threatened.

IDENTIFICATION OF A METABOLIC ABNORMALITY

Acid-base disturbances influence whole-body buffering capacity in a predictable manner. Whole-body buffering capacity is composed of interacting buffer systems: the volatile bicarbonate system, HCO_3^-/H_2CO_3, and the nonbicarbonate buffers, $Buf^-/HBuf$, consisting predominantly of hemoglobin, proteins, and phosphates. The sum of the buffer anions, HCO_3^- and Buf^-, is the total buffer base and defines total-body buffering capacity.

Increase in $[H^+]$ indicates acidosis and is associated with a fall in total body buffer. Decrease in $[H^+]$ indicates alkalosis and is associated with a rise in total body buffer. Since all body buffer systems are in equilibrium, a change in the serum $[HCO_3^-]$ reflects concurrent changes in the other body buffer systems. $[HCO_3^-]$ is easily measured in serum and, therefore, is a useful clinical guide for detection of a metabolic acid-base disorder. Table 22-1 summarizes the pattern of abnormality of arterial blood acid-base parameters in the four classic acid-base disorders.

Serum $[HCO_3^-]$ is not a precise quantitative measure of the metabolic abnormality once respiratory adjustment has occurred, since alteration in P_{CO_2} also influences serum $[HCO_3^-]$ by changing the dissociation equilibrium of carbonic acid. The calculation of base excess or deficit, an estimate of the titratable acidity of blood or extracellular fluids, is independent of P_{CO_2} and provides an approach to quantifying the metabolic acid-base disturbance under standard ventilatory conditions. According to this approach, a base deficit marks the reduction of total body buffer in metabolic acidosis (Table 22-1). Conversely, a base excess designates a primary metabolic alkalosis. Since a base excess or deficit may also develop as a renal compensation for a primary respiratory acid-base disorder, clinical judgment must distinguish the compensatory change in total body buffer and serum $[HCO_3^-]$ from a primary metabolic acid-base disturbance.

RESTING VENTILATION IN METABOLIC ACID-BASE DISTURBANCES

In the absence of intrinsic lung disease, the level of alveolar or effective ventilation varies in accord with the total

TABLE 22-1
Primary Acid-Base Disturbances

Primary Disorder	Initial Abnormality	Compensatory Response
Metabolic acidosis	Decreased pH_a, decreased $[HCO_3^-]$ Base deficit	Decreased Pa_{CO_2}
Metabolic alkalosis	Increased pH_a, increased $[HCO_3^-]$ Base excess	Increased Pa_{CO_2}
Respiratory acidosis	Decreased pH_a, increased Pa_{CO_2}	Increased $[HCO_3^-]$ Base excess
Respiratory alkalosis	Increased pH_a, decreased Pa_{CO_2}	Decreased $[HCO_3^-]$ Base deficit

minute ventilation. Level of total ventilation changes as a function of metabolic demand. Under normal circumstances, Pa_{CO_2} is well controlled between 38 and 42 mmHg according to the relationship

$$Pa_{CO_2} = \frac{\dot{V}_{CO_2}}{\dot{V}_A}$$

where $\dot{V}_{CO_2}$ is CO_2 production (reflecting metabolic rate) and $\dot{V}_A$ is alveolar ventilation (reflecting CO_2 clearance).

In metabolic acid-base disturbances, the level and pattern of breathing undergoes considerable change. An elevation of Pa_{CO_2} above normal defines alveolar hypoventilation with respect to metabolism; a reduction of P_{CO_2} below normal defines alveolar hyperventilation. The magnitude of the change in Pa_{CO_2} in relation to change in plasma [HCO_3^-] determines the compensation in blood pH in accord with the Henderson-Hasselbalch equation:

$$pH = pK' + \log \frac{[HCO_3^-]}{Pa_{CO_2}}$$

In metabolic acidosis, alveolar hyperventilation reduces Pa_{CO_2}; in metabolic alkalosis, alveolar hypoventilation increases Pa_{CO_2}. The stereotype is Kussmaul's breathing in metabolic acidosis, in which tidal volume is characteristically large. Associated with this pattern is a fall in serum [HCO_3^-] reflecting the base deficit and low arterial P_{CO_2} as a marker of the respiratory compensation. In acute diabetic ketoacidosis, for example, ventilation increases moderately as arterial pH falls to 7.2. Below this level, minute ventilation increases sharply, and may approach levels as high as 35 L/min when pH is in the range of 7.1. Further intensification of the acidemia causes minute ventilation to diminish from the peak value, thereby blunting the effectiveness of the compensation when the underlying disorder is severe.

Depression of ventilation in metabolic alkalosis is more difficult to assess clinically. Part of the difficulty probably stems from an obscuring ventilatory drive arising either in the patient's anxiety or from the accompanying clinical disorder. Figure 22-1 illustrates data in a normal individual in steady-state metabolic acidosis and alkalosis. Acidosis was produced by ingestion of NH_4Cl and alkalosis by ingestion of $NaHCO_3$ and a diuretic. Plasma [HCO_3^-] ranged from 14 to 40 meq/L. There is a linear relationship between Pa_{CO_2} and [HCO_3^-] with a slope of approximately 0.7. However, the degree of respiratory compensation for a given level of extracellular alkalosis is controversial and may relate, in part, to differences in the manner in which the alkalosis was induced. In the studies of Goldring et al., metabolic alkalosis was induced in normal volunteers by a variety of agents. The respiratory compensation was maximal when alkalosis was induced by bicarbonate ingestion, tris buffer, or ethacrynic acid diuretic. Respiratory compensation was less, or ab-

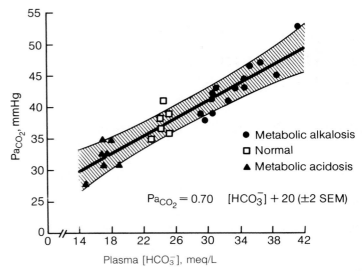

FIGURE 22-1 Relationship between arterial plasma [HCO_3^-] and Pa_{CO_2} in six healthy subjects prior to (normal) and during 14 episodes of steady-state metabolic alkalosis and 7 episodes of metabolic acidosis. The solid black line is the mean regression line, and the shaded area represents the 95 percent confidence interval. (*After Javaheri et al., 1982.*)

sent, when similar degrees of extracellular alkalosis were induced by aldosterone infusion or chlorothiazide. These observations underscore the fact that metabolic alkalosis is not a uniform entity and that, under certain circumstances, the initiating agents may inhibit or retard the respiratory adjustment by mechanisms not well understood.

In a given clinical situation, ventilation may be strongly affected by influences other than acid-base balance. Among these influences are body temperature, increase in circulating catecholamines or abnormal metabolites, changes in cerebral blood flow, changes in systemic blood pressure, and changes in the metabolic activities of different organs and tissues, as well as the physiological state of the lung itself.

The level of the minute ventilation in metabolic acid-base disturbances appears to vary inversely with the [HCO_3^-] as measured in extracellular fluid. This is depicted in Fig. 22-2. When the disorder is moderate, and serum [HCO_3^-] is in the range of 20 to 34 meq/L, respiratory adjustment of pH is virtually complete, and ventilation varies with the extracellular [HCO_3^-]. This relationship between ventilation and [HCO_3^-] appears to be mediated by adjustments in the tidal volume. When [HCO_3^-] in serum is outside the range of 20 to 34 meq/L depicted in Fig. 22-2, the slope of this relationship decreases. The extremes represent ranges of metabolic acidosis or alkalosis for which ventilatory compensation is incomplete, and the extracellular pH is not restored to normal range.

In general, ventilatory compensation is incomplete in sustained metabolic acid-base disorders, as judged by re-

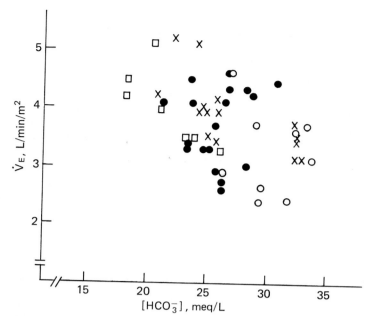

FIGURE 22-2 Relationship between minute ventilation and serum bicarbonate concentration [HCO_3^-] in patients especially selected for complete respiratory compensation of the metabolic acid-base disorder. When pH returns to normal (pH 7.37 to 7.44) by ventilatory adjustment, there is an inverse relationship between $\dot{V}E$ and [HCO_3^-]. ● = normal subjects with induced metabolic acidosis and alkalosis; ○ = patients with diuretic-induced metabolic alkalosis; □ = metabolic acidosis secondary to renal disease; × = observations selected from published reports. *(After Heinemann and Goldring, 1974.)*

turn of arterial blood pH toward, but not to, normal. The incomplete ventilatory adaptation to metabolic acid-base disturbances is not understood. It may reflect the inadequacy of the control system, a "compromise" solution imposed by an increase in the work of breathing in metabolic acidosis, disequilibrium between hydrogen ion activity in body fluids adjacent to, and remote from, the control site, or altered chemoresponsivity. Alternatively, the signal for correction of the acid-base disturbance may not be directed toward complete restoration of pH in arterial blood. Indeed, it may well be that the "control" system for H^+ homeostasis at some site other than blood is back to normal with incomplete pH compensation in blood. This control system for the central chemical drive of ventilation probably resides in the [H^+] of the brain extracellular fluid (ECF) and, as has more recently been suggested, maintains the protein charge state constant in the environment of respiratory neurons. This concept is further discussed below.

CARBON DIOXIDE VENTILATORY RESPONSE CURVES

The respiratory response to inhaled CO_2 is modified in chronic metabolic acidosis or alkalosis. When minute ventilation ($\dot{V}E$) is plotted as a function of arterial P_{CO_2} during CO_2 breathing or rebreathing, the resulting curve is shifted to the left in acidosis and to the right in alkalosis. This shift implies a change in the threshold of response of the chemosensitive structures to the P_{CO_2} stimulus when acid-base balance is disturbed. In addition, a change in the slope of $\dot{V}E$-P_{CO_2} response curves has been demonstrated in moderate to severe metabolic acid-base disturbances; the slope increases with acidosis and decreases with alkalosis. These observations suggest that the potency of CO_2 as a stimulus to ventilation varies according to the underlying acid-base status and is in keeping with a modulating effect of the level of [HCO_3^-] on the change in H^+ activity induced by a change in P_{CO_2}.

PERPETUATION OF SUSTAINED RESPIRATORY ADJUSTMENT

Respiratory compensation is immediately demonstrated by changes in Pa_{CO_2}, although it may not be complete for hours until body compartments reach equilibrium. Acute metabolic acidosis or alkalosis implies this transient state; chronic metabolic acidosis implies a steady state. Thus, the terms *acute* and *chronic* as applied to a metabolic or alkalosis acid-base disorder usually imply duration of the disorder.

Ventilation is sustained at high levels in chronic metabolic acidosis and at low levels in metabolic alkalosis, even though pH in arterial blood and cerebrospinal fluid (CSF) is virtually back to normal. Accordingly, perpetuation of the ventilatory compensation cannot be simply attributed to the degree of abnormality of pH in either compartment.

The [HCO_3^-] in body fluids could contribute importantly to regulation of ventilation by modifying the effectiveness of P_{CO_2} as a respiratory stimulus. In accord with the Henderson-Hasselbalch equation, the level of [HCO_3^-] determines the change in H^+ activity that a given alteration in P_{CO_2} induces. [HCO_3^-] at some chemosensitive control site could then act as a link in the control system that "sets" the P_{CO_2} of body fluids at about 40 mmHg and allows the system to "reset" in chronic acid-base disorders.

If this proposition is correct, the following relationships should be demonstrable: (1) inhalation of fixed concentrations of CO_2 will result in changes in H^+ activity that will be inversely proportional to the [HCO_3^-]; (2) changes in minute ventilation induced by the inhalation of CO_2 will be inversely proportional to the [HCO_3^-] of body fluid; and (3) the increment in ventilation will vary with the change in H^+ activity induced by inhaled CO_2 rather than with the change in P_{CO_2} that is induced.

Several observations indicate that the level of [HCO_3^-] in body fluid is related to the ventilatory adjustment to metabolic acid-base disorders. Figure 22-1 illustrates this relationship during the resting state in the chronic metabolic disorders. A consistent inverse relationship also exists between the level of serum [HCO$_3^-$] and the extent to which ventilation increases during CO$_2$ stimulation (Fig. 22-3A). When related to H$^+$ activity induced by the inhaled CO$_2$ (Fig. 22-3B), ventilatory responsiveness remains constant over the wide range of serum [HCO$_3^-$]. The demonstration that the size of the HCO$_3^-$ pool modifies the CO$_2$ stimulus to ventilation is in accord with the concept that H$^+$ activity within, or surrounding, respiratory neurons is an important stimulus for the central drive of ventilation. This is also consistent with the membrane charge hypothesis discussed below, which would dictate constancy of OH$^-$/H$^+$ ratio in the membranes of the chemoreceptors.

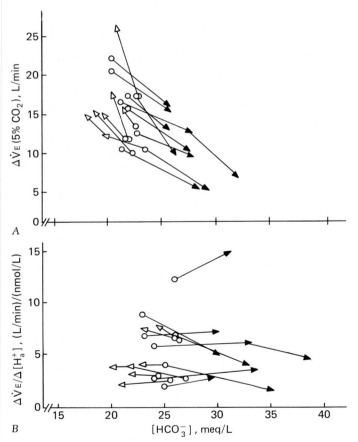

FIGURE 22-3 *A.* Increment in minute ventilation during 30 min of 5% CO$_2$-in-air breathing in 14 normal volunteers. In each individual, the increase in ventilation varied inversely with the serum [HCO$_3^-$]. ○ = control state; ▶ = induced metabolic alkalosis; ▷ = induced metabolic acidosis. *B.* Increment in minute ventilaton per unit change in blood [H$^+$] during 5% CO$_2$-in-air breathing. Ventilatory response expressed in this fashion did not vary with induced changes in serum [HCO$_3^-$]. Symbols same as in *A.* (*After Goldring, Heinemann, and Turino, 1975.*)

QUANTIFICATION OF RESPIRATORY COMPENSATION TO METABOLIC ACID-BASE DISTURBANCES

Haldane suggested that ventilation was mediated centrally by the acidity of the environment of the respiratory centers in the brain and that the fall in P$_{CO_2}$ in metabolic acidosis was an index of this central response. Peters subsequently described the relationship between alveolar P$_{CO_2}$ and CO$_2$ combining power, a measure of [HCO$_3^-$], in stable acid-base disturbances in humans.

Pierce and coworkers examined the time course of ventilatory compensation during the development and correction of severe uncomplicated metabolic acidosis in patients with cholera. They found that once the base deficit had been established, the ventilatory response, as estimated by stability of arterial P$_{CO_2}$, reached steady-state values within 24 h or less. However, transient disturbances, such as those arising from unsteady-state rapid development or correction of the base deficit, or an increase in CO$_2$ production, complicate distinctions between "simple" and "mixed" disturbances. These observations stress the importance of sequential determinations, as well as clinical correlation of arterial blood-gas composition, as a basis for identifying the nature of an acid-base disturbance.

Studies in humans and animals during induced or spontaneous acid-base disturbances have shown that the degree of compensation follows predictable patterns which vary with the magnitude as well as duration of the primary disturbance. Current approaches are directed toward relationship between body buffer as reflected in serum [HCO$_3^-$] or base excess, and the level of alveolar ventilation as reflected in arterial P$_{CO_2}$. Figure 22-4 demonstrates graphically the relationship between plasma [HCO$_3^-$], P$_{CO_2}$, and pH. The designated areas represent the variety of clinical acid-base disorders (see legend).

Computerized programs of clinical acid-base disorders have exploited this approach. These patterns are expressed graphically as nomograms, or mathematically as regression equations, and provide a framework for the evaluation of acid-base abnormality and adequacy of compensatory response. This approach serves as a guide to clinical interpretation of acid-base disorders from arterial blood-gas analysis to facilitate appropriate therapeutic intervention.

SITE OF CONTROL OF VENTILATION IN METABOLIC ACID-BASE DISORDERS

Control of breathing in metabolic acidosis and alkalosis cannot be entirely accounted for by changes in the acid-base balance of the blood. Fluids in other body compartments, especially those bathing respiratory chemosensitive neurons, must be taken into account. Indeed, a

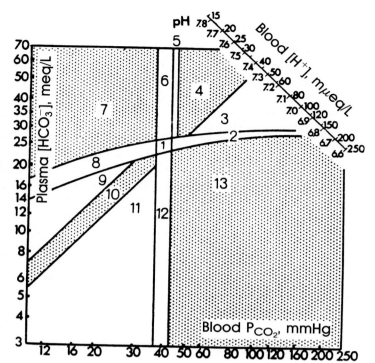

FIGURE 22-4 Interpretation of acid-base abnormalities from arterial blood-gas analysis: 1 = normal; 2 = respiratory acidosis; 3 = respiratory acidosis—compensated; 4 = respiratory acidosis and metabolic alkalosis (mixed); 5 = metabolic alkalosis—compensated; 6 = metabolic alkalosis; 7 = respiratory alkalosis and metabolic alkalosis (mixed); 8 = respiratory alkalosis; 9 = respiratory alkalosis—compensated; 10 = metabolic acidosis and respiratory alkalosis (mixed); 11 = metabolic acidosis—compensated; 12 = metabolic acidosis; 13 = metabolic acidosis and respiratory acidosis (mixed). (*Pulmonary Unit, Massachusetts General Hospital.*)

major determinant of the resting ventilation appears to be the pH of brain extracellular fluid. Relevant to this conclusion is the fact that for the same degree of blood acidosis, carbonic acid evokes a larger increment in minute ventilation than do organic acids, presumably because CO_2 has much more rapid access to the brain ECF than do fixed acids.

The peripheral chemoreceptors respond promptly to changes in the pH of arterial blood and account for the immediate adjustment in ventilation to a change in blood pH. Consistent with this fact is the observation that in chemodenervated animals, the initial increase or decrease in ventilation to an acid or alkali load is absent. After the first minutes the same degree of change in Pa_{CO_2} occurs with or without peripheral chemoreceptors, suggesting that respiratory drive is controlled at sites other than, and/or in addition to, peripheral chemoreceptors. The site of particular interest is the central chemoreceptors residing on or near the ventral surface of the medulla. The chemical environment of this site(s), particularly $[H^+]$, is relevant to the central drive of ventilation.

Under normal conditions, $[HCO_3^-]$ in CSF is about 0.9 that in plasma. The P_{CO_2} in CSF is close to that in cerebral venous blood, e.g., 6 to 10 mmHg higher than arterial P_{CO_2}. Thus, the pH of CSF is acid with respect to plasma, ranging from 7.26 to 7.36. Relationships between changes in $[HCO_3^-]$ and in P_{CO_2} during metabolic acid-base disturbances are less predictable in CSF than in blood. Changes in CSF pH are small relative to plasma and may even deviate in an opposite direction from plasma during transient clinical states. It is worth emphasizing that, with respect to control of breathing, meaningful samples of CSF are difficult to obtain in human beings. Resort to lumbar puncture is a practical expedient but always leaves uncertainty about how well the sample represents CSF that is in contact with chemosensitive areas of the brain.

It is now accepted that even the pH in the cisterna magna is not the key pH in the central ventilatory drive and that it may be at variance with the brain ECF pH both in the transient and steady states of acid-base imbalance. In acute metabolic acid-base disorders the change in CSF $[HCO_3^-]$ is approximately 0.4 of that in plasma. Thus, brain ECF acid-base status is well regulated, and these regulatory mechanisms do not allow for significant excursions in $[H^+]$.

The question remains as to what is being regulated in the brain ECF. Mitchell postulated that the ventilatory response to acute acidosis is tempered by a concomitant rise in the pH of CSF: as the increase in ventilation mediated by the peripheral chemoreceptors decreases arterial P_{CO_2}, CO_2 diffuses more rapidly than HCO_3^- from CSF to blood, thereby increasing CSF pH and decreasing ventilation. Thereafter, $[HCO_3^-]$ in CSF is adjusted toward normal even though the pH in extracellular fluid remains low; therefore, the drive from the central chemoreceptors no longer opposes the increased peripheral chemoreceptor drive. Fencl et al. take exception to this formulation. They propose, instead, that plasma acidosis leads to a decrease in the pH of cerebral interstitium which equilibrates readily with blood; accordingly, the hyperventilation of acute acidosis, as well as the hypoventilation of acute alkalosis, is elicited centrally.

Regulation of brain ECF $[H^+]$ and $[HCO_3^-]$ has been suggested to be both active and passive, possibly involving "pumps" at the brain-blood barrier. The concept of "dependent" and "independent" ions in weak salt solutions without inherent buffers such as brain ECF and CSF has been recently introduced to the understanding of acid-base balance. An independent variable is that which can be changed from outside the system, e.g., strongly dissociated cations and anions; a dependent variable, e.g., H^+, OH^-, and HCO_3^-, responds only to the change in the independent variables. The difference between the fully dissociated cations and anions is termed the *strong ion difference* (SID), which in turn determines the concentration of the "dependent" anion HCO_3^-. CSF $[HCO_3^-]$, then, equals the difference between completely dissociated anions and cations in this essentially protein-free fluid. Transport of HCO_3^- or H^+ across membranes does not occur unless accompanied by strong ions. It is the effect of the transport of these strong ions that determines SID which, in turn, defines the $[HCO_3^-]$ and $[H^+]$ in each body compartment.

The major anion and cation in the brain ECF are Cl^- and Na^+. Na^+ is well regulated in the central nervous system (CNS), most likely because it is the key ion in *osmoregulation*. Thus, regulation of $[Cl^-]$ in brain ECF becomes important in determining the SID and thus $[HCO_3^-]$. In metabolic and respiratory acid-base disorders, changes in CSF $[HCO_3^-]$ and $[Cl^-]$ are reciprocal and equimolar in accord with the above concept. Calculation of base excess or deficit is an estimate of the deviation of SID (or its equivalent "buffer base") from normal.

The relevance of this ionic regulation to respiratory drive remains to be fully clarified. In order to integrate acid-base regulation and receptor function, Reeves and Rahn have proposed the hypothesis that it is not arterial, ECF, or intracellular $[H^+]$ that is being regulated, but rather the constancy of fractional dissociation of γ-imidazole of histidine found in proteins of the entire animal kingdom. Regulation of γ-imidazole (alphastat regulation) would maintain cellular protein charge state constant, allow for enzymatic function to continue unimpeded, and also maintain the OH^-/H^+ ratio constant in all compartments. For alphastat regulation to be correct the central chemical drive of ventilation would also have to directly relate to alphastat regulation, a phenomenon which has been demonstrated experimentally. Thus, in terms of central drive of ventilation, there is evidence to support active regulation of Cl^- in the brain ECF, which then determines the concentration of dependent ions HCO_3^- and H^+. Change in Pa_{CO_2}, reflecting level of alveolar ventilation, is determined by alphastat regulation, which maintains the OH^-/H^+ ratio constant in membranes of the cells in the chemosensitive areas of the medulla.

The specific mechanisms of central control of breathing during metabolic acid-base disturbances remain controversial, as does the relative significance of peripheral chemoreceptors in the respiratory adjustments. Divergent observations still need to be reconciled.

MIXED ACID-BASE DISTURBANCES

Mixed acid-base disorders involve two or more underlying primary disturbances and are conceptually distinct from compensated simple disorders. The distinction between compensation and a second primary acid-base disorder is essential in defining therapeutic goals. Therapy directed to a primary disorder will result in spontaneous reversal of compensatory changes. Two distinct therapeutic approaches need to be considered if two primary disorders coexist.

In patients with respiratory failure and chronic respiratory acidosis (chronic hypercapnia), reduced ventilatory response to CO_2 stimulation is, in part, due to diseases of the lungs or chest bellows. Modification of chemical stimuli (Fig. 22-5) can also exert important influences on the control of breathing. Any disorder that predisposes to further retention of bicarbonate, such as the metabolic alkalosis of diuretic therapy or nasogastric suction, automatically enhances the prospect of promoting further CO_2 retention, particularly if the kidney is handicapped in its adjustments by hypochloremia or hypokalemia. The clinical sequelae of acute hypercapnia, e.g., personality disturbances, and loss of consciousness, as well as worsening hypoxemia, may then follow.

Conversely, the induction of metabolic acidosis to increase ventilatory drive has been advocated as a therapeutic measure in patients with chronic hypercapnia sec-

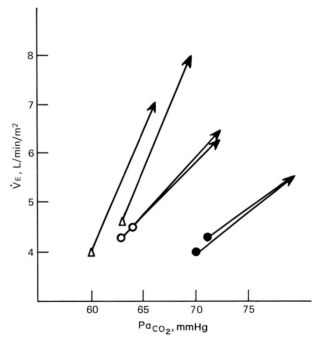

FIGURE 22-5 "Steady-state" ventilatory responses to inhalation of 5% CO_2-in-air in a patient with cardiorespiratory failure from kyphoscoliosis. Control values were obtained while patient was on diuretic therapy and sodium-restricted diet without electrolyte replacement therapy. The administration of KCl (100 mmol/day) upon cessation of diuretic therapy reduced resting P_{CO_2} of arterial blood and increased the slope of the ventilatory response curve. Addition of NH_4Cl (100 mmol/day) induced a further decrease in arterial P_{CO_2} and an increase in slope of the ventilatory response curve; discontinuation of NH_4Cl was associated with a return of the slope to KCl-treated values. ● = control; ○ = KCl; △ = NH_4Cl. *(From Goldring, Turino, and Heinemann, 1971.)*

ondary to respiratory failure. Acetazolamide (Diamox) has been used for this purpose. Although these agents do cause a transient increase in ventilatory drive, the combination of metabolic and respiratory acidosis may pose hazards of its own unless used in a setting of mechanical ventilatory support.

BIBLIOGRAPHY

Cohen JJ, Kassirer JP: *Acid-Base.* Boston, Little, Brown, 1982, chaps 7–9, 12.
Comprehensive review of acid-base physiology with emphasis on both pathophysiology and clinical evaluation.

Dempsey JA, Skatrud JB, Forster HA, Hanson PG, Chosy LW: Is brain ECF (H$^+$) an important drive to breathe in man? Chest 73(suppl):251–253, 1978.
The role of an intracranial H$^+$ receptor as a major determinant of ventilation is questioned and discussed.

Fencl V: Acid-base balance in cerebral fluids, in Fishman AP (ed), *Handbook of Physiology sect 3: Respiration, vol II: Control of Breathing.* Bethesda, MD, American Physiological Society, pp 115–140.
An in-depth review of current concepts, including divergent views, of mechanisms of central control of ventilation.

Fencl V, Miller TB, Pappenheimer JR: Studies on the respiratory response to disturbances of acid-base balance, with deduction concerning the ionic composition of cerebral interstitial fluid. Am J Physiol 210:459–472, 1966.
A classic article defining an important role for cerebral interstitial fluid composition in the central control of ventilation.

Goldring RM, Cannon PJ, Heinemann HO, Fishman AP: Respiratory adjustment to chronic metabolic alkalosis in man. J Clin Invest 47:188–202, 1968.
Respiratory adjustment for metabolic alkalosis induced in normal subjects varied with different methods of induction.

Goldring RM, Heinemann HO, Turino GM: Regulation of alveolar ventilation in respiratory failure. Am J Med Sci 269:160–170, 1975.
A review of the pathophysiology and physiological consequences of carbon dioxide retention.

Goldring RM, Turino GM, Heinemann HO: Respiratory-renal adjustments in chronic hypercapnia in man. Am J Med 51:772–784, 1971.
The role of electrolyte balance in the renal compensation for respiratory acidosis.

Heinemann HO, Goldring RM: Bicarbonate and the regulation of ventilation. Am J Med 57:361–370, 1974.
A review article exploring the concept that extracellular bicarbonate concentration is an important determinant of resting ventilation and ventilatory response to carbon dioxide by modulation of hydrogen ion activity.

Hornbein TF, Roos A: Specificity of H$^+$ ion concentration as a carotid chemoreceptor stimulus. J Appl Physiol 18:580–584, 1963.
A study designed to separate the quantitative contributions of [H$^+$] and P$_{CO_2}$ as chemoreceptor stimuli.

Javaheri S, Herrera L, Kazemi H: Ventilatory drive in acute metabolic acidosis. J Appl Physiol 46:913–918, 1979.
Comparison of the relative role of central and peripheral chemoreceptors in respiratory adjustment to metabolic acidosis.

Javaheri S, Shore NS, Rose B, Kazemi H: Compensatory hypoventilation in metabolic alkalosis. Chest 81:296–301, 1982.
Definition of linear relationship between Pa$_{CO_2}$ and [HCO$_3^-$] in metabolic acidosis and alkalosis induced in human subjects.

Kazemi H, Johnson DC: Regulation of CSF acid-base balance. Physiol Rev 66:953–1037, 1986.
A comprehensive and up-to-date review.

Kety SS, Polis DB, Nadler LS, Schmidt CFS: The blood flow and oxygen consumption of the human brain in diabetic acidosis and coma. J Clin Invest 27:500–509, 1948.
Cerebral blood flow as an important input to acid-base balance.

Leusen I: Aspects of the chemosensitivity of the respiratory centers, in Cunningham DJC, Lloyd BB (eds), *The Regulation of Human Respiration*. Oxford, Blackwell, 1961, pp 207–222.
Classic discussion of blood-cerebral fluid interplay in regulation of respiration.

Lloyd BB, Cunningham DJC: A quantitative approach to the regulation of human respiration, in Cunningham DJC, Lloyd BB (eds), *The Regulation of Human Respiration*. Oxford, Blackwell, 1961, pp 331–349.
Discussion of methods of quantitation of ventilatory response.

Marks CE, Goldring RM, Vecchione JJ, Gordon EE: Cerebrospinal acid-base relationships in ketoacidosis and lactic acidosis. J Appl Physiol 35:813–819, 1973.
Relationship of cerebrospinal fluid to plasma acid-base characteristics in metabolic acidosis.

Mitchell RA: The regulation of respiration in metabolic acidosis and alkalosis, in Brooks M, Kao FF, Lloyd BB (eds), *Cerebrospinal Fluid and the Regulation of Respiration*. Oxford, Blackwell, 1964, pp 109–131.
Discussion of pH dependence of HCO_3^- distribution.

Peters JP: The response of the respiratory mechanism to rapid changes in the reaction of the blood. Am J Physiol 48:84–108, 1917.
A classic study defining the role of blood acidity in respiratory control.

Pierce NF, Fedson DS, Brigham KL, Mutra RC, Sack RB, Mondal A: The ventilatory response to acute base deficit in humans. Ann Intern Med 72:633–640, 1970.
Sequential acid-base measurements in patients with cholera suggesting that failure of equilibration of body compartments with blood may influence apparent HCO_3^--PCO_3 relationships in unsteady or transient states.

Posner J, Plum F: Spinal fluid pH and neurologic symptoms in systemic acidosis. N Engl J Med 277:605–609, 1967.
Failure of cerebral fluid to accurately reflect blood acid-base parameters.

Reeves RB, Rahn H: Patterns in vertebrate acid-base regulation, in Wood S, Lenfant C (eds), *Evolution of the Respiratory Process: A Comparative Approach*. New York, Dekker, 1979, pp 225–252.
Defines a role for the protein charge state in determining distribution of OH^- and H^+ between body compartments.

Schuitmaker JJ, Berkenbosch A, DeGoede J, Olievier CN: Ventilatory responses to respiratory and metabolic acid-base disturbances in cats. Respir Physiol 67:69–83, 1987.
In the ventilatory response to an acute metabolic acid-base disturbance, both the peripheral and central chemoreceptors play a role. The sensitivity of the peripheral chemoreceptors to isocapnic changes in the arterial H^+ concentration is twice as large as the sensitivity of the central chemoreceptors.

Seisjo BK: The regulation of cerebrospinal fluid pH. Kidney Int 1:360–374, 1972.
A review of classic studies addressing the relationship of CSF to blood in clinical acid-base disorders.

Severinghaus JW: Acid-base balance nomogram: A Boston-Copenhagen detente. Anesthesiology 45:539–541, 1976.
Discusses concept of extracellular base excess as an index of metabolic component of acid-base disorder.

Siggaard-Andersen O: An acid-base chart for arterial blood with normal and pathophysiological reference areas. Scand J Clin Invest 27:239–245, 1971.
Presents a graphic display of acid-base parameters as a useful clinical tool.

Stewart PA: How to understand acid-base balance, in *A Quantitative Acid-Base Primer for Biology and Medicine*. New York, Elsevier, 1981.
Introduction of new concept and theory into clinical understanding of acid-base disorders.

Chapter 23

Adaptation to Respiratory Acidosis and Alkalosis

Nicolaos E. Madias / Jordan J. Cohen

From a physiological perspective, the hydrogen ion concentration of body fluids is determined, moment by moment, by the prevailing ratio between the partial pressure of carbon dioxide (P_{CO_2}) and the concentration of bicarbonate [HCO_3^-]. As a corollary, changes in the acidity of the body fluids can occur only through a change in the P_{CO_2} or [HCO_3^-] or both. This chapter is concerned with the abnormalities in acid-base equilibrium initiated by a change in arterial carbon dioxide tension (Pa_{CO_2}).

The level of Pa_{CO_2} in normal individuals is maintained within a narrow range around a mean value of approximately 40 mmHg. Regulation is accomplished by precise adjustments in CO_2 elimination by the lungs to balance CO_2 production by cellular metabolism. Disruption in this regulatory system leads to increases and decreases in Pa_{CO_2}, denoted by the terms *hypercapnia* and *hypocapnia*, respectively. Hypercapnia acidifies body fluids and initiates the acid-base disturbance known as *respiratory acidosis*. Hypocapnia alkalinizes body fluids and initiates the acid-base disturbance that is known as *respiratory alkalosis*.

Respiratory disturbances activate secondary physiological responses that lead to changes in the level of plasma bicarbonate concentration: primary hypercapnia is followed by a secondary increase in bicarbonate concentration; primary hypocapnia is attended by a secondary decrease in bicarbonate concentration. Thus, the degree to which plasma acidity is altered in response to primary changes in Pa_{CO_2} reflects not only the magnitude of the initiating change but also the magnitude of the secondary change in plasma bicarbonate concentration. Equally important for understanding the acid-base consequences of respiratory disorders is the recognition that the adaptive changes in plasma bicarbonate concentration

pursue a distinct time course and that they generate readjustments in acid-base equilibrium that are quantitatively related to the magnitude of the primary change in Pa_{CO_2}. In both respiratory acidosis and alkalosis, the secondary adjustments in bicarbonate concentration tend to restore the pH toward normal but fall short of returning hydrogen ion concentration to completely normal levels. As a result, some degree of acidemia or alkalemia persists as long as the initiating hypercapnia or hypocapnia, respectively, continues. In clinical medicine, respiratory acid-base disorders are not only common but often they coexist with other acid-base disturbances. Proper analysis of the disturbance in terms of a single or mixed derangement in acid-base balance depends on the appreciation of how plasma acid-base equilibrium responds to acute or chronic changes in Pa_{CO_2} of graded severity.

ADAPTATION TO RESPIRATORY ACIDOSIS

The time course of the changes in plasma acid-base equilibrium during adaptation of the intact organism to respiratory acidosis is shown schematically in Fig. 23-1. Throughout this chapter, hydrogen ion concentration is expressed as neq/L or 10^{-9} eq/L; when expressed in these units, hydrogen ion concentration is equal to antilog (9 − pH). Hypercapnia, by increasing the carbonic acid concentration of the body fluids, causes a prompt increase in hydrogen ion concentration. The acidemia is ameliorated

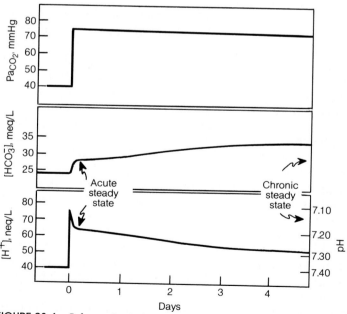

FIGURE 23-1 Schematic time-course of the changes in plasma acid-base equilibrium during the development of respiratory acidosis. In this scheme, Pa_{CO_2} is assumed to rise abruptly from 40 to 75 mmHg and to remain unchanged thereafter. *(From Cohen and Madias, 1978.)*

acutely by an increase in plasma bicarbonate concentration that stems from the titration of nonbicarbonate body buffers. If hypercapnia persists, renal adaptive mechanisms cause a much larger secondary increment in plasma bicarbonate that ameliorates the acidemia further. The two components of this biphasic response can be examined separately.

Acute Respiratory Acidosis

TIME COURSE

The concentration of bicarbonate in plasma increases within 5 to 10 min after the abrupt onset of hypercapnia. Barring further changes in Pa_{CO_2}, no further changes in acid-base equilibrium are detectable for a few hours. Consequently, this period has been designated an *acute steady state* (Fig. 23-1).

MECHANISMS

The increment in plasma bicarbonate elicited by acute hypercapnia results, almost exclusively, from the acidic titration of nonbicarbonate body buffers; such buffers generate bicarbonate by combining with free hydrogen ions derived from the dissociation of carbonic acid:

$$H_2O + CO_2 \rightleftharpoons H_2CO_3 \rightleftharpoons H^+ + HCO_3^-$$
$$H^+ + Buf^- \rightleftharpoons HBuf$$

The role of nonbicarbonate buffers in yielding the acute increase in plasma bicarbonate concentration is illustrated by the consequences of CO_2 titration in a pure bicarbonate solution with the same bicarbonate concentration as that normally found in plasma (i.e., 24 meq/L). In such a system, increasing P_{CO_2} from 40 to 80 mmHg proportionally increases the hydrogen ion concentration from 40 to 80 neq/L (a decrease in pH from 7.40 to 7.10). Because of the absence of nonbicarbonate hydrogen-ion acceptors, only a trivial amount of additional carbonic acid need dissociate before chemical equilibrium is reestablished; although in the process a number of new bicarbonate ions equivalent to the number of new hydrogen ions will be generated (each 40 neq/L), the new level of bicarbonate (24.00004 meq/L) will be negligibly, and unmeasurably, different from the original value of 24 meq/L.

In contrast, in the living organism the presence of nonbicarbonate buffers allows a much larger quantity of carbonic acid to dissociate because the hydrogen ions released are taken out of solution; as a result, a small but measurable change in bicarbonate concentration occurs before equilibrium is reestablished. In the above example, an acute increase in plasma bicarbonate of 3 meq/L in the living organism (a value consistent with experimental observations) limits the new level of plasma hydrogen ion concentration to 71 neq/L or pH 7.15 (rather than 80 neq/L, pH 7.10).

Fully 97 percent of the adaptive response to acute respiratory acidosis depends on cellular buffering, the remainder being accounted for by titration of plasma proteins. Approximately one-third of the cellular buffering is attributed to hemoglobin and is evidenced by the entry of chloride into erythrocytes in exchange for bicarbonate (the so-called chloride shift). Other cellular buffers abstract hydrogen ions from the extracellular fluid in exchange for sodium and potassium. A small fraction of the increment in extracellular bicarbonate can be attributed to net utilization of extracellular lactate, a process that generates an equivalent number of bicarbonate ions.

Although the increment in plasma bicarbonate during acute hypercapnia stems almost exclusively from body buffering, evidence exists that renal adaptation occurs even during this early phase of the disorder. Nonetheless, that this early renal response is not sufficient to make a measurable contribution to the acute increment in plasma bicarbonate elicited by body buffering is indicated both by the establishment of an acute steady state of several hours duration and by comparative observations in intact and nephrectomized animals.

ACUTE STEADY-STATE RELATIONSHIPS

Figures 23-2 and 23-3 depict the acute steady-state relationships among Pa_{CO_2}, plasma bicarbonate concentration, and plasma hydrogen ion concentration during graded degrees of acute hypercapnia. These observations were obtained by sequentially exposing unanesthetized, normal human volunteers to increasing concentrations of inspired carbon dioxide in a large environmental chamber. As shown in Fig. 23-2, increasing degrees of hypercapnia are associated with a curvilinear rise in plasma bicarbonate concentration, the successive increments diminishing in size at successively higher levels of Pa_{CO_2}.

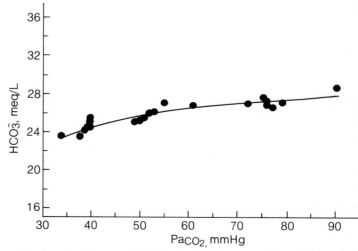

FIGURE 23-2 Relationship between plasma bicarbonate concentration and Pa_{CO_2} during acute hypercapnia in normal humans. (*Based on data from Brackett, Cohen, and Schwartz, 1965.*)

However, the cumulative increment in plasma bicarbonate over the entire range of hypercapnia is quite small, amounting to only 3 to 4 meq/L, even when Pa_{CO_2} is increased to 80 to 90 mmHg. In contrast, the relationship between plasma hydrogen ion concentration and Pa_{CO_2} is strikingly linear over a range of Pa_{CO_2} extending to 90 mmHg (Fig. 23-3). As a result of the modest increment in plasma bicarbonate concentration elicited by nonbicarbonate body buffers, the average rise in plasma hydrogen ion concentration is limited to about 0.75 neq/L for each millimeter of mercury acute rise in Pa_{CO_2}. This is in contrast with the predicted increase of 1.0 neq/L per mmHg increase in Pa_{CO_2} that would occur if acute hypercapnia caused no increase in plasma bicarbonate concentration above its normal value of 24 meq/L.

Figure 23-4 depicts the 95 percent confidence intervals for plasma bicarbonate and hydrogen ion concentrations in uncomplicated acute respiratory acidosis. They were calculated from data obtained in the same human subjects as in Figs. 23-2 and 23-3. These limits represent the range of responses within which acid-base equilibrium would be expected to fall if an acute increase in Pa_{CO_2} were the only factor disturbing plasma acidity.

The quantitative aspects of the adaptive response to acute hypercapnia are influenced markedly by the baseline acid-base status. Acute hypercapnia induces a larger increment in both plasma bicarbonate and hydrogen ion concentrations in animals with preexisting hypobicarbonatemia (whether from metabolic acidosis or from chronic respiratory alkalosis) than in animals with preexisting hyperbicarbonatemia (whether from metabolic alkalosis or from chronic respiratory acidosis). Clinical data are consistent with the experimental observations: in patients with chronic respiratory acidosis who experience acute increments in Pa_{CO_2}, the increments in both plasma bicarbonate concentration and hydrogen ion concentra-

tion per millimeter of mercury change in Pa_{CO_2} are smaller than in normals.

Hypoxemia per se does not alter the acid-base response to acute respiratory acidosis but, if sufficiently severe ($Pa_{O_2} < 40$ mmHg), it can induce a complicating lactic acidosis. Indeed, acute respiratory acidosis and lactic acidosis make up one of the most common mixed acid-base disorders.

The modest increase in plasma bicarbonate concentration observed during acute CO_2 equilibration in vivo contrasts sharply with the large increase obtained during in vitro CO_2 equilibration of whole blood over the same range of carbon dioxide tensions. This discrepancy can be explained largely by the differences in the volume of distribution of the newly generated bicarbonate. Bicarbonate generated by hemoglobin and other nonbicarbonate buffers of blood is, of course, confined to the plasma phase during in vitro CO_2 titration, whereas in vivo it diffuses freely into the large, poorly buffered interstitial compartment. Despite the participation of nonerythrocytic tissue buffers in the living organism, the total quantity of new

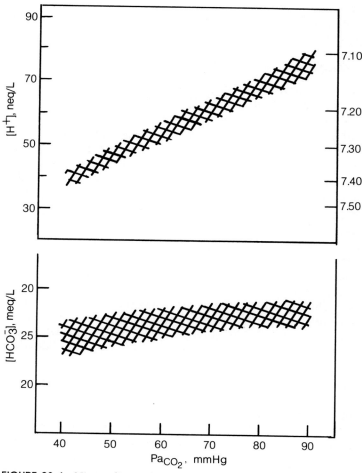

FIGURE 23-4 Ninety-five percent confidence bands for plasma hydrogen ion and bicarbonate concentrations during acute hypercapnia in normal humans. *(From Brackett, Cohen, and Schwartz, 1965.)*

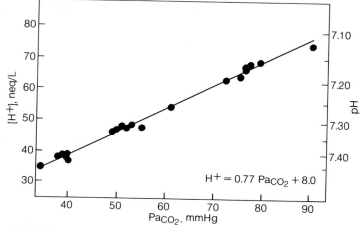

FIGURE 23-3 Relationship between plasma hydrogen ion concentration and Pa_{CO_2} during acute hypercapnia in normal humans. *(From Brackett, Cohen, and Schwartz, 1965.)*

bicarbonate generated during acute hypercapnia in vivo is insufficient to increase the extracellular bicarbonate concentration in the body to the same extent as the plasma bicarbonate concentration increases during in vitro titration.

Chronic Respiratory Acidosis

TIME COURSE

Several hours after the acute titration of body buffers, the renal response to persistent hypercapnia is manifested by a further, gradual increase in plasma bicarbonate concentration (Fig. 23-1). Studies in the dog indicate that 3 to 5 days elapse after the onset of a fixed increment in Pa_{CO_2} before this renal adaptation is fully expressed; at that point, plasma bicarbonate concentration no longer increases and a new steady state of acid-base equilibrium is established. Whether the same temporal pattern applies to the response of humans to a stepwise increase in Pa_{CO_2} is unknown. In patients, chronic hypercapnia often results from a gradual deterioration in pulmonary function rather than from an abrupt increase in Pa_{CO_2} to high levels that are subsequently sustained. Under these circumstances, full adaptation to hypercapnia may keep pace with the slowly rising Pa_{CO_2} without a perceptible time lag.

MECHANISMS

The "second wave" of plasma bicarbonate increment superimposed on that derived acutely from tissue buffering can be ascribed entirely to renal adaptive responses. This adaptation entails a persistent increase in the tubular hydrogen ion secretory rate and a decrease in the rate of chloride reabsorption. As a consequence of these changes in renal function, net acid excretion (largely in the form of ammonium) transiently exceeds endogenous acid production, leading to negative hydrogen ion balance and the generation of new bicarbonate ions for the body fluids. Conservation of these new bicarbonate ions is ensured by an augmented rate of bicarbonate reabsorption which, per se, is a reflection of the hypercapnia-induced, persistent increment in hydrogen ion secretory rate.

During the provision of exogenous alkali, this adaptive increase in the rate of renal bicarbonate reabsorption roughly parallels the spontaneous increase in plasma bicarbonate concentration. A new steady state emerges when the augmented filtered load of bicarbonate is precisely balanced by the accelerated rate of bicarbonate reabsorption and when net acid excretion returns to the level required to offset daily endogenous acid production. While bicarbonate stores are augmented by the transient increase in net acid excretion, chloride stores are correspondingly depleted by a transient rise in renal chloride excretion. Chloride excretion appears to outstrip acid excretion during the first 1 or 2 days of adaptation; the dif-

ference is accounted for by an increase in the excretion of sodium and potassium. Thus, some degree of sodium and potassium depletion typically accompanies adaptation to chronic hypercapnia. The resultant hypochloremia is, of course, sustained by a persistently depressed renal chloride reabsorption rate.

The specific segments of the nephron responsible for eliciting the adaptive response to chronic respiratory acidosis have not been characterized fully. But, given the marked increase in the rate of bicarbonate reabsorption that is characteristic of chronic hypercapnia, proximal tubule acidification almost certainly should be increased. This supposition is in accord with the recent micropuncture observations in the proximal tubule of the rat which suggest that absolute bicarbonate reabsorption rate is increased during chronic hypercapnia. Whether acidification sites of the cortical and medullary collecting tubules also are involved in the adaptation process is currently unclear. Although the signal that triggers the renal adaptation to persistent hypercapnia remains undefined, present evidence favors the increase in Pa_{CO_2}, per se, rather than the decrease in systemic pH (Fig. 23-5).

The renal response to chronic hypercapnia is not altered appreciably by the coexistence of such stresses as moderate hypoxemia (Pa_{O_2} of 45 to 55 mmHg), deprivation of sodium or chloride in the diet, moderate potassium depletion, alkali loading, or adrenalectomy. Clinical studies indicate that moderate hypoxemia also does not affect

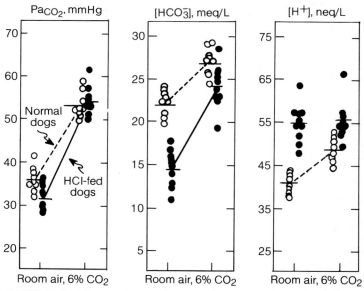

FIGURE 23-5 Changes in steady-state plasma acid-base parameters during prolonged exposure of normal (non-HCl-fed) dogs (open circles) and dogs with HCl acidosis (closed circles) to a 6% CO_2 atmosphere. The large increment in plasma bicarbonate concentration produced by chronic hypercapnia was associated with a substantial rise in plasma hydrogen ion concentration in normal animals but with no detectable change in the level of acidity in HCl-fed animals. (*From Madias, Wolf, and Cohen, 1985.*)

plasma acid-base equilibrium in patients with chronic pulmonary insufficiency. However, the return of body bicarbonate stores to normal during *recovery* from chronic hypercapnia is hampered by chloride deprivation; under such a circumstance, the chloride losses that accumulate during the adaptive process cannot be replenished following restoration of a normal Pa_{CO_2}, and plasma bicarbonate concentration remains abnormally high. As a result, a state of "post-hypercapnic" alkalosis is created. Moderate potassium depletion, on the other hand, does not interfere with full repair of acid-base equilibrium following the return to eucapnia.

STEADY-STATE RELATIONSHIPS

A highly predictable relationship exists between the degree of chronic hypercapnia and the levels at which plasma bicarbonate concentration and hydrogen ion concentration stabilize following full physiological adaptation (Fig. 23-6). In dogs, over the entire range of Pa_{CO_2}

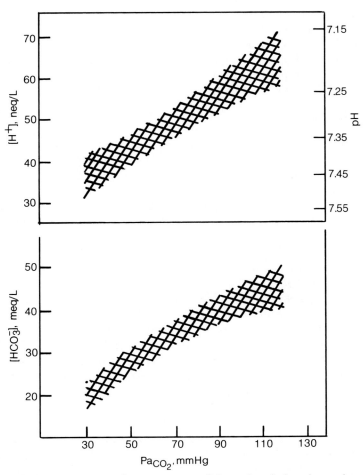

FIGURE 23-6 Ninety-five percent confidence bands for plasma hydrogen ion and bicarbonate concentrations during chronic hypercapnia in the dog. Using an environmental chamber, graded degrees of chronic hypercapnia were induced by stepwise increments in Pa_{CO_2}. *(From Schwartz, Brackett, and Cohen, 1965.)*

shown in Fig. 23-6, the relationship between bicarbonate and Pa_{CO_2} is curvilinear, successive increments in bicarbonate diminishing somewhat in magnitude at higher levels of Pa_{CO_2}. Between values of Pa_{CO_2} ranging from 40 to 90 mmHg, which encompasses most values encountered clinically, this curvilinear relationship between plasma bicarbonate and Pa_{CO_2} is closely approximated by a straight line with a slope of 0.3; hence, over this range, each millimeter of mercury chronic increment in Pa_{CO_2} is associated, on average, with an approximately 0.3-meq/L increment in steady-state plasma bicarbonate.

The magnitude of the change in plasma bicarbonate concentration at any level of Pa_{CO_2}, of course, substantially exceeds that observed during adaptation to acute hypercapnia; this difference between acute and chronic hypercapnia reflects the large renal contribution to the adaptive process that occurs in response to prolonged increase in Pa_{CO_2}. The corresponding relationship between plasma hydrogen ion concentration and Pa_{CO_2} is strikingly linear, hydrogen ion concentration increasing on the average by 0.32 neq/L for each millimeter of mercury chronic elevation in Pa_{CO_2}.

Efforts to examine this relationship experimentally in normal humans have been precluded by the severe discomfort produced by prolonged exposure to high levels of inspired carbon dioxide. However, systematic observations in patients with chronic, stable respiratory acidosis appear to confirm the presence of a predictable pattern of response when no complicating acid-base disturbances are present. These observations indicate that in humans, hydrogen ion concentration increases on average by some 0.24 to 0.30 neq/L for each millimeter of mercury chronic elevation in Pa_{CO_2}. However, as illustrated by one study in humans (Fig. 23-7), the statistical limits at all levels of

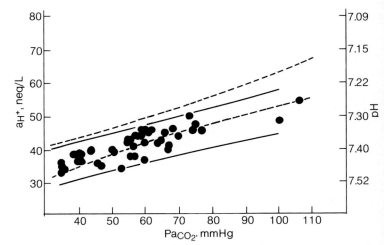

FIGURE 23-7 Ninety-five percent confidence band for plasma hydrogen ion activity during chronic uncomplicated hypercapnia in humans (solid line); a = estimated hydrogen ion activity. The dashed line represents the confidence band obtained in the dog (Fig. 23-6). *(From Brackett, Wingo, Muren, and Solano, 1969.)*

Pa$_{CO_2}$ are broader than in the dog because of the different experimental circumstances.

Clinical data for levels of Pa$_{CO_2}$ greater than 70 mmHg are scant and somewhat conflicting. Some observers contend that bicarbonate concentration increases so slightly over the higher ranges of Pa$_{CO_2}$ that plasma hydrogen ion concentration increases more briskly than it does over the more commonly encountered levels of hypercapnia. Unfortunately, this contention is difficult to evaluate because of the presence of complicating metabolic acid-base disturbances as well as of instability in the level of carbon dioxide tension in patients with such severe hypercapnia.

ADAPTATION TO RESPIRATORY ALKALOSIS

In the intact organism, primary decrements in Pa$_{CO_2}$ elicit certain physiological responses that lead to secondary reductions in plasma bicarbonate concentration. In close analogy with respiratory acidosis, the adaptive reductions in plasma bicarbonate concentration in respiratory alkalosis pursue a characteristic time course and occur in two distinct steps (Fig. 23-8). Hypocapnia reduces the carbonic acid concentration of the body fluids and causes a prompt fall in hydrogen ion concentration. Acutely, this alkalemia is ameliorated by a secondary, adaptive reduction in plasma bicarbonate concentration that stems principally from titration of nonbicarbonate body buffers. During protracted hypocapnia, renal adaptive mechanisms

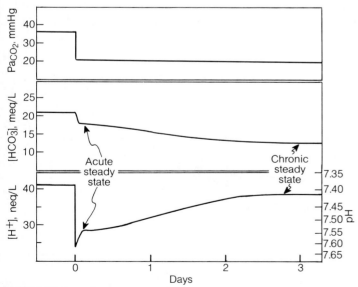

FIGURE 23-8 Schematic time course of the changes in plasma acid-base equilibrium during the development of respiratory alkalosis. In this scheme, it is assumed that a reduction in Pa$_{CO_2}$ of 15 mmHg occurs abruptly and is maintained unchanged thereafter. *(From Gennari and Kassirer, 1982.)*

yield a further and larger secondary reduction in plasma bicarbonate that results in still greater amelioration of the alkalemia.

The biologic importance of these secondary responses is underscored by noting how extreme would be the effect of even modest hyperventilation, and its resultant hypocapnia, on plasma hydrogen ion concentration if no change in bicarbonate concentration were to occur. Thus, an increase in alveolar ventilation sufficient to reduce Pa$_{CO_2}$ from 40 to 20 mmHg would, in the presence of a normal bicarbonate level, cause hydrogen ion concentration to fall to the dangerously low level of 20 neq/L (pH 7.70). In contrast, such alarming reductions in hydrogen ion concentration in metabolic alkalosis would require extreme increments in bicarbonate concentration even if secondary, adaptive hypercapnia were to fail to occur.

Acute Respiratory Alkalosis

TIME COURSE

The plasma bicarbonate concentration decreases within 5 to 10 min after the abrupt onset of hypocapnia. As shown in Fig. 23-8, assuming no further changes in Pa$_{CO_2}$, no additional detectable changes in acid-base equilibrium occur for a period of several hours. Therefore, this period can be considered as an operational acute steady state.

MECHANISMS

The adjustment in acid-base equilibrium following the induction of acute hypocapnia results totally from nonrenal mechanisms and appears to be accounted for principally by the alkaline titration of the nonbicarbonate buffers of the body. It has been estimated that approximately one-third of the total buffering response can be ascribed to hemoglobin and plasma protein buffering, the remainder being attributed to nonerythrocytic cellular buffering. The contribution of organic acids, notably lactic acid, to the reduction in plasma bicarbonate concentration during acute hypocapnia has been debated over the years. The consensus seems to be that even though an increase in lactate might reasonably be expected to occur, the increase would be modest, reflecting the net increase in lactic acid production that occurs when intracellular pH increases sufficiently to stimulate 6-phosphofructokinase activity.

Although a reduction in renal bicarbonate reabsorption and renal net acid excretion are detectable promptly after induction of acute respiratory alkalosis, the cumulative impact of these changes on plasma acid-base composition is negligible during the first few hours of hypocapnia. Therefore, as noted above, the acute steady-state response of acid-base equilibrium to hypocapnia may be regarded as originating exclusively from nonrenal mechanisms.

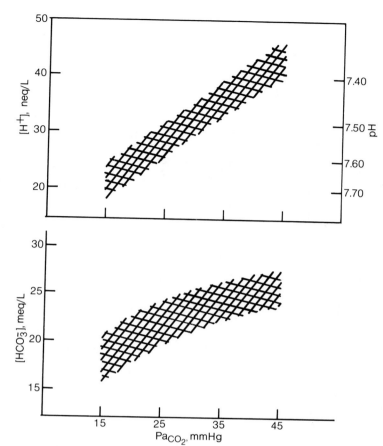

FIGURE 23-9 Ninety-five percent confidence bands for plasma hydrogen ion and bicarbonate concentrations during acute hypercapnia in humans. The data are based on acute, "whole-body" titration experiments involving passive hyperventilation of anesthetized human subjects undergoing minor surgical procedures. The limits represent the range of responses in acid-base equilibria that would be expected if an acute reduction in Pa_{CO_2} were the only factor disturbing the acidity of the plasma. *(From Arbus, Hebert, Levesque, Etsten, and Schwartz, 1969.)*

ACUTE STEADY-STATE RELATIONSHIPS

In acute uncomplicated respiratory alkalosis (Fig. 23-9), the acute secondary change in plasma bicarbonate concentration is substantially greater than that which occurs during acute hypercapnia of comparable degree, falling by approximately 0.2 meq/L for each millimeter of mercury acute decrement in Pa_{CO_2}; thus, a reduction in plasma bicarbonate of some 3 to 4 meq/L occurs within minutes after Pa_{CO_2} is lowered to 20 to 25 mmHg. However, the resulting change in plasma hydrogen ion concentration is strikingly similar to that observed during acute hypercapnia; on the average, plasma hydrogen ion concentration decreases by approximately 0.75 neq/L for each millimeter of mercury acute reduction in Pa_{CO_2}.

Chronic Respiratory Alkalosis

TIME COURSE

Approximately 2 to 3 days are required after the onset of a fixed decrement in Pa_{CO_2} before plasma bicarbonate concentration ceases to fall and a new steady state of acid-base equilibrium supervenes (Fig. 23-8).

MECHANISMS

When hypocapnia persists beyond the acute phase, the additional decrement in plasma bicarbonate concentration that occurs is a consequence of renal adaptive responses and reflects a dampening of hydrogen ion secretion by the renal tubule. As a result, a transient suppression of net acid excretion occurs, largely manifested by a fall in ammonium excretion and, early on, by an increase in bicarbonate excretion; these changes, in turn, lead to positive hydrogen ion balance and a reduction in the body's bicarbonate stores. Persistence of the resulting hypobicarbonatemia is explained by the continued inhibition of tubular hydrogen ion secretion and suppression of bicarbonate reabsorption.

Although micropuncture and microperfusion studies have shown that proximal and distal acidification is suppressed during acute hypocapnia, comparable studies have not been carried out during persistent hypocapnia. The adaptive retention of acid during sustained hypocapnia is normally accompanied by a loss of sodium into the urine; the resultant decrease in extracellular fluid causes the typical hyperchloremia of chronic respiratory alkalosis. Upon reaching a new steady state, the net excretion of acid by the kidneys returns to control levels, and the altered anionic picture of the extracellular fluid, namely, hypobicarbonatemia and hyperchloremia, is maintained by a reduced bicarbonate reabsorption and an enhanced chloride reabsorption. In the face of dietary sodium restriction, acid retention is accompanied by increased excretion of potassium rather than of sodium. If both sodium and potassium in the diet are restricted, phosphate retention rather than cation loss accompanies the renal acid retention during adaptation to hypocapnia. There is no appreciable change in plasma lactate during chronic hypocapnia, even in the presence of moderate hypoxemia.

The renal adaptation to persistent hypocapnia appears to be mediated, not by changes in plasma or "whole-body" intracellular pH, but by some direct effect of reduced Pa_{CO_2} itself. Thus, in animals in which plasma bicarbonate had been substantially reduced prior to adaptation to sustained hypocapnia (induced by means of the chronic administration of a large HCl load), the renal response to a primary reduction in Pa_{CO_2} was the same as in normal individuals, even though the net effect of this adaptation was an overt fall in plasma pH (Fig. 23-10).

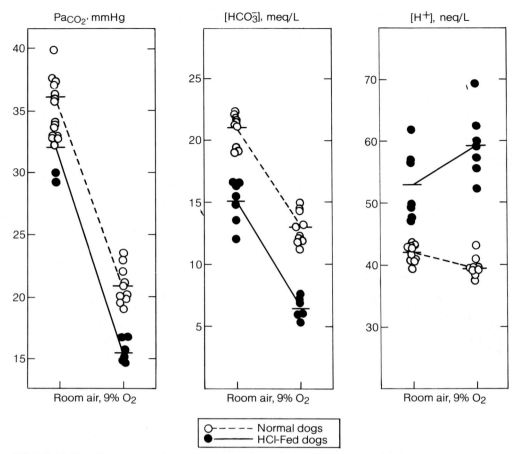

FIGURE 23-10 Changes in plasma bicarbonate concentration and hydrogen ion concentration during prolonged exposure to hypocapnia in normal dogs (dashed lines) and in dogs with chronic HCl acidosis (solid lines). Similar decrements in Pa$_{CO_2}$ in the two groups produced nearly equivalent reductions in plasma bicarbonate concentration, despite divergent effects on hydrogen ion concentration. *(From Cohen, Madias, Wolf, and Schwartz, 1976.)*

STEADY-STATE RELATIONSHIPS

The renal adaptive mechanisms described above result in a highly predictable relationship between the degree of chronic hypocapnia and the level at which plasma bicarbonate stabilizes. Studies in the dog have shown that each millimeter of mercury chronic reduction in Pa$_{CO_2}$ is associated with a fall in plasma bicarbonate concentration averaging 0.4 to 0.5 meq/L. Although only limited data are available in humans (patients subjected to chronic hypocapnia, high-altitude dwellers, volunteers at simulated altitude), it would appear that changes in plasma bicarbonate concentration are similar to those observed in the dog.

The impact of the secondary changes in plasma bicarbonate concentration on plasma hydrogen ion concentration depends strongly on the level of plasma bicarbonate prior to adaptation to hypocapnia. In the normal dog, the plasma bicarbonate concentration is about 21 meq/L, and the magnitude of the adaptive decrement in bicarbonate concentration during chronic hypocapnia suffices to limit the fall in hydrogen ion concentration dramatically (Fig. 23-11); indeed, plasma hydrogen ion concentration falls by only 0.17 neq/L for each millimeter of mercury chronic reduction in Pa$_{CO_2}$. In contrast, because the basal level of plasma bicarbonate in humans is higher (of the order of 24 to 25 meq/L), and even though the magnitude of the secondary response of bicarbonate is apparently similar, the degree of alkalemia that usually occurs during chronic respiratory alkalosis in humans is greater than that in the dog: in humans, the plasma hydrogen ion concentration decreases by 0.4 to 0.5 neq/L for each millimeter of mercury chronic decrement in Pa$_{CO_2}$.

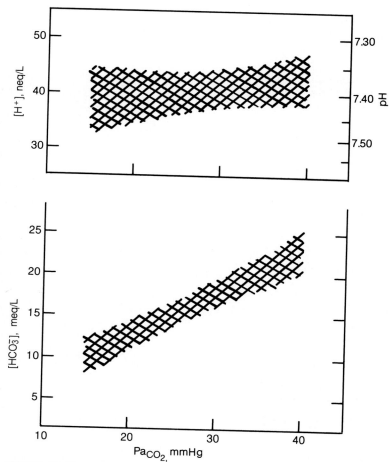

FIGURE 23-11 Ninety-five percent confidence bands for plasma hydrogen ion and bicarbonate concentrations during chronic hypocapnia in the dog. *(From Gennari, Goldstein, and Schwartz, 1972.)*

BIBLIOGRAPHY

Adrogué HJ, Madias NE: Influence of chronic respiratory acid-base disorders on acute CO_2 titration curve. J Appl Physiol 58:1231–1238, 1985.

  The background presence of a chronic respiratory acid-base disorder influences markedly the quantitative aspects of the adaptation to superimposed acute hypercapnia.

Al-Awqati Q: The cellular renal response to respiratory acid-base disorders. Kidney Int 28:845–855, 1985.

  A state-of-the-art exposition of the cellular acidification responses of urinary epithelia to altered CO_2 concentrations.

Anderson LE, Henrich WL: Alkalemia-associated morbidity and mortality in medical and surgical patients. South Med J 80:729–733, 1987.

  Alkalemia-associated illnesses are common in hospitalized patients and are associated with high mortality in both medical and surgical patients, though the death rate is higher among medical patients. Mixed respiratory and metabolic alkalosis appears to be associated with a particularly poor prognosis.

Arbus GS, Hebert LA, Levesque PR, Etsten BE, Schwartz WB: Characterization and clinical application of the "significance band" for acute respiratory alkalosis. N Engl J Med 280:117–123, 1969.
Quantitative description of the plasma acid-base response to acute respiratory alkalosis in humans.

Brackett NC Jr, Cohen JJ, Schwartz WB: Carbon dioxide titration curve of normal man: Effect of increasing degrees of acute hypercapnia on acid-base equilibrium. N Engl J Med 272:6–12, 1965.
Quantitative description of the plasma acid-base response to acute respiratory acidosis in humans.

Brackett NC Jr, Wingo CF, Muren O, Solano JT: Acid-base response to chronic hypercapnia in man. N Engl J Med 280:124–130, 1969.
Quantitative description of the plasma acid-base response to chronic respiratory acidosis in humans.

Clark DD, Chang BS, Garella SG, Cohen JJ, Madias NE: Secondary hypocapnia fails to protect "whole body" intracellular pH during chronic HCl-acidosis in the dog. Kidney Int 23:336–341, 1983.
Evidence that the renal response to chronic hypocapnia is not geared toward the defense of "whole body" intracellular pH.

Cogan MG: Chronic hypercapnia stimulates proximal bicarbonate reabsorption in the rat. J Clin Invest 74:1942–1947, 1984.
Micropuncture evidence for augmented bicarbonate reabsorption in the proximal nephron of the rat during chronic respiratory acidosis.

Cohen J, Madias NE: Acid-base disorders of respiratory origin, in Brenner BM, Stein JH (eds), Contemporary Issues in Nephrology, vol 2. Acid-Base and Potassium Homeostasis. New York, Churchill-Livingstone, 1978, pp 137–167.
The interplay between acid-base balance and the adaptive changes in potassium homeostasis.

Cohen JJ, Madias NE, Wolf CJ, Schwartz WB: Regulation of acid-base equilibrium in chronic hypocapnia. Evidence that the response of the kidney is not geared to the defense of extracellular [H$^+$]. J Clin Invest 57:1483–1489, 1976.
Evidence that the renal adaptation to chronic respiratory alkalosis is a direct consequence of the change in Pa$_{CO_2}$ itself, rather than of plasma pH.

Gennari FJ, Goldstein MB, Schwartz WB: The nature of the renal adaptation to chronic hypocapnia. J Clin Invest 51:1722–1730, 1972.
Quantitative description of the plasma and renal acid-base responses to chronic respiratory alkalosis in the dog.

Gennari FJ, Kassirer JP: Respiratory alkalosis, in Cohen JJ, Kassirer JP (eds), Acid-Base. Boston, Little, Brown, 1982, pp 349–376.
Comprehensive review of all aspects of respiratory alkalosis.

Madias NE, Adrogué HJ: Influence of chronic metabolic acid-base disorders on the acute CO_2 titration curve. J Appl Physiol 55:1187–1195, 1983.
The background presence of a chronic metabolic acid-base disorder influences markedly the quantitative aspects of the adaptation to superimposed acute hypercapnia.

Madias NE, Cohen JJ: Respiratory acidosis, in Cohen JJ, Kassirer JP (eds), Acid-Base. Boston, Little, Brown, 1982, pp 307–348.
Comprehensive review of all aspects of respiratory acidosis.

Madias NE, Wolf CJ, Cohen JJ: Regulation of acid-base equilibrium in chronic hypercapnia. Kidney Int 27:538–543, 1985.
Evidence that the change in Pa$_{CO_2}$ itself, rather than in plasma pH, is responsible for maintaining the secondary hyperbicarbonatemia characteristic of chronic respiratory acidosis.

Nattie EE: Gas exchange in acid-base disturbances, in Farhi LE, Tenney SM (eds), Handbook of Physiology, sec 3: Respiration, vol IV: Gas Exchange. Bethesda, American Physiological Society 1987, pp 421–438.
This chapter considers the effects of acid-base imbalance on the O_2 delivery system, from the outside air to within the cell.

Schwartz WB, Brackett NC Jr, Cohen JJ: The response of extracellular hydrogen ion concentration to graded degrees of chronic hypercapnia: The physiologic limits of defense of pH. J Clin Invest 44:291–301, 1965.
Quantitative description of the plasma and renal acid-base responses to chronic respiratory acidosis in the dog.

Chapter 24

Alveolar Ventilation and Its Disorders

Alfred P. Fishman

ALVEOLAR VENTILATION

The partial pressures (tensions) of O_2 and CO_2 in arterial blood are held almost constant by an elaborate regulatory system (Fig. 24-1). By way of negative feedback, the rate and depth of breathing are automatically adjusted in accord with the changing metabolic needs of the body. As a result, a normal sea-level dweller can be expected to have an arterial P_{O_2} of approximately 95 mmHg and an arterial P_{CO_2} of about 40 mmHg. For those who live at altitude, the system is geared to maintain arterial P_{O_2} and P_{CO_2} at lower levels; the higher the altitude, the more marked are hypoxemia and hypocapnia. Moderate exercise does not change arterial blood-gas levels appreciably from resting values. Therefore, abnormal blood-gas levels, either at rest or during moderate exercise, indicate the existence of either a disturbance in ventilation, imbalances between the distribution of inspired air and pulmonary capillary blood, or impaired diffusion of gases across the alveolar-capillary membrane.

The term alveolar ventilation refers to the part of the total ventilation which participates in gas exchange with pulmonary capillary blood. Because the conducting airways are interposed between the alveoli and the outside world, the rate of alveolar ventilation cannot be measured directly. Instead, it is determined indirectly, e.g., as the difference between the minute ventilation and the dead-space ventilation, or from the alveolar ventilation-metabolism equation [(Table 24-1, Eq. (1)].

Estimation

For clinical purposes, the absolute value for alveolar ventilation is usually unnecessary. Instead, an estimate of the adequacy of the alveolar ventilation suffices. This estimate is made from the CO_2 tension of alveolar gas or of arterial blood. Even a brief examination of Eq. (1) will suffice to demonstrate the pivotal role of the CO_2 tension (P_{CO_2}) in the assessment of alveolar ventilation.

The level of alveolar ventilation is a function of both the tidal volume and the respiratory frequency (Table 24-2). The contribution of the tidal volume to alveolar ventilation depends on how much of each breath is wasted in the dead space. The dog turns this interdependence to good advantage for the sake of heat loss: during panting, high levels of dead-space ventilation dissipate heat without inducing alveolar hyperventilation.

Calculation

Based on the assumption that the alveolar and arterial P_{CO_2} are about equal, both values have been used interchangeably to calculate the alveolar ventilation. However, even in normal individuals, it is difficult to obtain a reliable measure of mean alveolar P_{CO_2} by sampling expired

TABLE 24-1

Equations Used to Calculate Alveolar Ventilation

Calculation of alveolar ventilation from CO_2 production and arterial P_{CO_2}:

$$\dot{V}_A = k \times \frac{\dot{V}_{CO_2}}{Pa_{CO_2}} \qquad (1)$$

where

$\dot{V}_A$ = alveolar ventilation, ml/min (BTPS)
$\dot{V}_{CO_2}$ = CO_2 production, ml/min (STPD)
  k = 863; used for conversion of ml STPD to ml BTPS and for the fraction of CO_2 to the corresponding partial pressure

Calculation of alveolar ventilation from physiological dead space:

$$\dot{V}_A = \dot{V}_E - V_D \times f \qquad (2)$$

where

$\dot{V}_A$ = alveolar ventilation, ml/min (BTPS)
$\dot{V}_E$ = volume of expired gas, ml/min (BTPS)
V_D = volume of the physiological dead space, ml (BTPS)
  f = respiratory frequency, per minute

The Bohr equation, using CO_2 as the test gas, provides a measure of V_D:

$$V_D = V_T \left(\frac{Pa_{CO_2} - Pe_{CO_2}}{Pa_{CO_2}} \right) \qquad (3)$$

where

V_T = tidal volume, ml (BTPS)
Pa_{CO_2} = partial pressure of CO_2 in arterial blood, mmHg
Pe_{CO_2} = partial pressure of CO_2 in expired air, mmHg

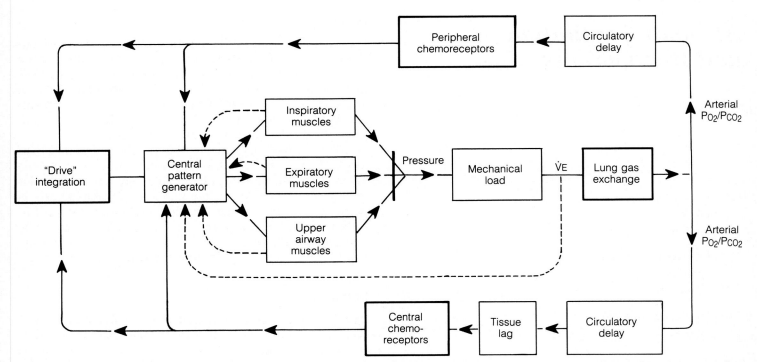

FIGURE 24-1 The control system for breathing. The coordinated behavior of the respiratory muscles relies heavily on feedback systems that adjust the level of ventilation to metabolic need. One pivotal feedback system includes the peripheral and central chemoreceptors which monitor the arterial P_{O_2} and P_{CO_2} so that alveolar ventilation is automatically adjusted to oxygen consumption over a wide range of activities. *(From Fig. 9-1.)*

TABLE 24-2
Effect of Changing Tidal Volume and Respiratory Frequency
on Alveolar Ventilation

Tidal Volume, ml	Dead-Space Volume, ml	Respiratory Frequency, per Minute	Total Ventilation, ml/min	Dead-Space Ventilation, ml/min	Alveolar Ventilation, ml/min
500	150	15	7500	2250	5250
375	150	20	7500	3000	4500
150	150	30	7500	4500	3000
150	150	50	7500	7500	0

gas because of differences in the composition of gas from the different parts of the lungs as well as the cyclic changes in alveolar air caused by the breathing cycle. These inhomogeneities and variations are usually greatly exaggerated in patients with diffuse lung disease. Therefore, arterial P_{CO_2} is widely used as a measure of mean alveolar P_{CO_2}.

The use of arterial P_{CO_2} as a measure of mean arterial P_{CO_2} is based on reasonable grounds: (1) CO_2 diffuses rapidly from blood to air, thus precluding a serious diffusional limitation to equilibrium between alveolar gas and pulmonary capillary blood; (2) the arteriovenous difference in P_{CO_2} across the lung is only about 6 mmHg so that, even if respiratory compensation did not occur, a large right-to-left shunt would not increase arterial P_{CO_2} by

more than a few millimeters of mercury; and (3) the CO_2 dissociation curve of blood is nearly linear between 30 and 80 mmHg so that the P_{CO_2} that results from mixing blood with different values for P_{CO_2} (i.e., from alveoli having different ventilation-perfusion ratios) is the simple algebraic sum of the P_{CO_2} from each component; i.e., each is weighted according to the proportion of the total volume that it contributes without undergoing the multiplying effect that is inherent in a curvilinear relationship, such as that of the O_2 dissociation curve. These assumptions have been repeatedly verified during the last few years. In practice, a value for arterial P_{CO_2} less than 35 mmHg or greater than 45 mmHg is abnormal, the low P_{CO_2} indicating alveolar hyperventilation, the high P_{CO_2} indicating hypoventilation.

ALVEOLAR HYPERVENTILATION

Alveolar hyperventilation can occur in the setting of normal or abnormal lungs. In patients with normal lungs, the increase in minute hyperventilation parallels the increase in alveolar ventilation so that minute ventilation provides a reliable index of the level of alveolar ventilation. In patients with abnormal lung mechanics, such as those with stiff lungs from diffuse interstitial disease, the pattern of rapid shallow breaths increases dead-space ventilation. Thus, the level of minute ventilation need not provide a reliable guide to the level of alveolar ventilation.

Clinical Causes

The most common cause of acute alveolar hyperventilation is anxiety (Table 24-3). Although these patients may be relatively asymptomatic, overbreathing can rapidly precipitate a syndrome of central nervous system and peripheral neuromuscular symptoms which include apprehension; a sensation of smothering; light-headedness; feelings of unreality; blurred vision; buzzing in the ears; muscle stiffness; paresthesias of the face, hands, and feet; and even tetany. In susceptible individuals, hyperventilation can cause syncope or seizure activity. The central nervous system manifestations seem to be due largely to diminished cerebral blood flow that is, in turn, secondary to cerebral vasoconstriction elicited by hypocapnia and alkalosis.

In contrast to the acute form of alveolar hyperventilation, there are usually no signs or symptoms associated with the more chronic forms of alveolar hyperventilation, such as that seen in altitude dwellers, in patients with diffuse interstitial fibrosis or cirrhosis, or in pregnant women.

Management

As noted above, it is the acute, rather than chronic, forms of hyperventilation that evoke clinical manifestations requiring medical attention. First, attention is directed toward uncovering and relieving initiating mechanisms. Acute alveolar hyperventilation caused by anxiety can usually be terminated by reassurance and by having the patient rebreathe expired air from a paper bag. Once the episode is over, further reassurance is generally needed to dispel the concern about organic disease as the basis for the clinical syndrome.

ALVEOLAR HYPOVENTILATION

The cardinal feature of alveolar hypoventilation—regardless of cause—is an abnormally high arterial P_{CO_2}. Invariably, a drop in arterial P_{O_2} accompanies the hypercapnia. However, arterial hypoxemia is far less distinctive as a sign of alveolar hypoventilation than is hypercapnia (see Chapter 82).

RESPIRATORY ACIDOSIS AND ALKALOSIS

Acute disturbances in alveolar ventilation affect acid-base balance promptly by changing arterial P_{CO_2} and pH; the latter unleash homeostatic mechanisms of their own that are directed at returning arterial P_{CO_2} and pH toward normal. In time, the body buffers and the kidneys can restore the acid-base balance virtually to normal levels but always falling a trifle short of full compensation unless the original insult is discontinued. The constellations of arterial P_{CO_2}, pH, and bicarbonate used for the recognition of acid-base disorders arising from primary alveolar hyper- or hypoventilation, acute or chronic, are considered elsewhere in this book (Chapters 72 and 163).

TABLE 24-3
Causes of Alveolar Hyperventilation

Increase in stimuli from the periphery
    Hypoxia (including high altitude)
    Diffuse interstitial edema or disease
    Pulmonary emboli
    Pain
    Circulatory collapse
    Cooling

Increase in central nervous system stimulation
    Anxiety
    Voluntary
    Fever
    Brain-stem lesions
    Salicylates, analeptics
    Intracranial hemorrhage
    Metabolic acidosis
    Descent from altitude

Unknown stimuli
    Cirrhosis of the liver
    Uremia
    Pregnancy (progesterone)

Assisted mechanical ventilation

BIBLIOGRAPHY

Anthonisen NR, Fleetham JA: Ventilation: total, alveolar, and dead space, in Farhi LE, Tenney SM (eds), *Handbook of Physiology, sect 3: The Respiratory System, vol IV: Gas Exchange.* Bethesda, MD, American Physiological Society, 1987, pp 113–129.
  A review of the diverse physiological approaches to distinguishing between the alveolar and dead-space components of the minute ventilation.

Cunningham DJC, Robbins PA, Wolff CB: Integration of respiratory responses to changes in alveolar partial pressures of CO_2 and O_2 and in arterial pH, in Cherniack NS, Widdicombe JG (eds), *Handbook of Physiology, sect 3: The Respiratory System, vol II: Control of Breathing.* Bethesda, MD, American Physiological Society, 1986, pp 475–528.
  A comprehensive and quantitative assessment of the chemical drive to breathing in the overall regulation of breathing. Particular emphasis is placed on feedback mechanisms which provide a stable background on which a variety of feedforward factors operate.

Euler C von, Lagercrantz H: *Neurology of the Control of Breathing.* New York, Raven, 1987.
  A series of papers relating to a symposium that brought together physiologists and neuroscientists. A fine overview of present understanding provided by workers in the field.

Fried R: *The Hyperventilation Syndrome.* Baltimore, Johns Hopkins University Press, 1987.
  A review of breathing disorders unrelated to organic disease focusing on hyperventilation as a manifestation of reactions to stress or of emotional disorders.

Nattie EE: Gas exchange in acid-base disturbances, in Farhi LE, Tenney SM (eds), *Handbook of Physiology, sect 3: The Respiratory System, vol IV: Gas Exchange.* Bethesda, MD, American Physiological Society, 1987, pp 421–438.
  This chapter in the Handbook of Physiology examines the effects of acid-base imbalance in many aspects of gas exchange, including alveolar ventilation.

West JB, Hackett PH, Maret KH, Milledge JS, Peters RM Jr, Pizzo CJ, Winslow RM: Pulmonary gas exchange on the summit of Mount Everest. J Appl Physiol 55:678–687, 1983.
  Samples of alveolar gas were taken from altitudes of 8050 m to the summit of Mt. Everest (alt 8848 m). When these were related to determinations of barometric pressure and venous blood samples (two taken at 8050 m), an integrated picture emerged of human gas exchange at the highest point on earth.

Whipp BJ: Ventilatory control during exercise in humans. Annu Rev Physiol 45:393–413, 1983.
  A consideration of the vast array of control mechanisms that presumably operate during the hyperpnea of exercise leaves unsettled why the ventilation increases only to a level commensurate with the CO_2 output.

Chapter 25

Abnormal Breathing Patterns

Neil S. Cherniack

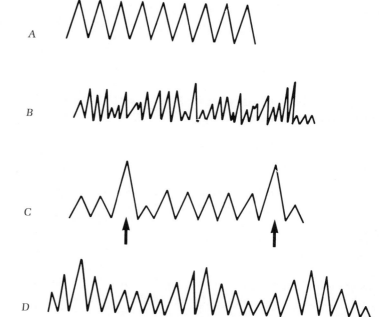

FIGURE 25-1 *A. Absolutely regular breathing. Completely regular breathing probably never occurs. A close approximation is sometimes seen in stages 3 and 4 of NREM sleep. B. Noisy breathing characterized by random fluctuations. Sometimes also called* ataxic breathing *if apneas occur. The extreme variability of breathing shown in this trace can sometimes be observed in an audience listening to a modern symphonic composition. C. Sighs (at arrows) may interrupt breathing. They are often followed by smaller than normal breaths. D. A rhythmic fluctuation in breathing when apneas occur instead of periods of low tidal volume. This kind of breathing has been termed* Cheyne-Stokes respiration.

Under constant environmental conditions and metabolic rate, tidal volume swings and the time of inspiration and expiration are nearly the same from breath to breath. This monotonous respiratory pattern depends on a complex web joining bulbopontine neuronal groups with mechanoreceptors and chemoreceptors, allows fine control of respiratory activity, and maintains nearly constant arterial blood-gas tensions.

But breathing is never absolutely regular. Three kinds of mechanisms disturb the constancy of normal breathing: (1) noise, (2) sighs, and (3) rhythmic oscillations (see Fig. 25-1).

Small random variations in ventilation (noise) originate in neuronal circuits so that motor output varies slightly with each breath, in minor changes in chest wall and lung mechanics which alter the effectiveness of motor signals, in the cardiovascular system as a result of small transient changes in the delivery of CO_2 to the lungs and the uptake of O_2, and in minute disturbances in the environment.

Sighs or augmented breaths appear at predictable intervals probably as a response to the slow decrease in lung compliance that occurs whenever constant ventilation is maintained.

Ventilation and blood-gas tensions vary rhythmically with the circadian cycle of wakefulness and sleep, but also over much shorter time intervals. Some of these swings seem to correspond to the circulation time between the lung and peripheral or central chemoreceptors, whereas other cycles are longer, having periods of minutes, and may be caused by physiological oscillators concerned with the release of hormones and neuromediators which have a respiratory action.

In certain abnormal states disturbances in the regularity of respiration are more obvious. Damage to the medulla can cause grossly irregular breathing, and severe cardiac failure can produce cyclic swings in ventilation called Cheyne-Stokes breathing.

But even in apparently normal people, grossly irregular breathing can occur in a tumultuous environment or during rapid eye movement (REM) sleep. Apneas are the most dramatic disturbance to regular breathing patterns, and although they can signal the presence of serious illness, they are sometimes seen even during health.

FEEDBACK CONTROL OF BREATHING

Ventilation is adjusted to meet changes in external conditions and internal demands by regulating systems which limit variations in arterial P_{CO_2} and P_{O_2} using feedback control. Although biologic control systems are much more complex than physical ones, design principles seem to be similar and some abnormalities in breathing resemble disturbances occurring in systems used to control machines. Ideally, biologic control systems minimize the effects of disturbances and rapidly restore steady-state conditions to prevent wide swings in the internal conditions and in addition operate with minimal use of energy. It may not be possible for the control system to meet all these objectives simultaneously. Fluctuations in arterial blood-gas tensions can arise if the system is excessively stressed or from destruction of key components in the control system which render it insensitive; but, less obviously, they may also occur if control is too rigorous.

Like physical control systems, the respiratory regulatory system can be considered to consist of a controller and controller elements linked by feedback loops. In this system the controller consists of sensors and neurons in the brain. The peripheral chemoreceptors which monitor arterial P_{CO_2} and P_{O_2}, and the central chemoreceptors which monitor hydrogen ion concentration in the interstitial fluid, communicate with groups of neurons in the brain (most heavily concentrated in the bulbopontine areas) which govern the activity of the muscles of breathing, allowing the lungs to be ventilated. The controlled system consists of these respiratory muscles and the O_2 and CO_2 chemically bound and physically dissolved in the body (the gas stores). Hypoxia and hypercapnia may affect the electrical activity and the forces generated by the upper airway and chest wall muscles dissimilarly so that coordination of the activity of these different muscles is crucial. Changes in ventilation alter the amount of CO_2 and O_2 stored in the lung, blood, and tissues and so adjusts the level of P_{CO_2} and O_2. Information on gas tension levels is transmitted to the sensors by the circulation. The bulbopontine neurons sense the difference between the input from the chemosensors and desired reference value levels and readjust the output to the respiratory muscles to reduce the discrepancy. State of alertness and sleep alter reference values.

While the function of feedback control systems is to maintain oxygen and acid-base homeostasis and not to regularize ventilation, in steady states they have this effect.

In feedback control systems, cyclic changes in output can result from rhythmic changes in input or instability in control system operation. Common mechanisms that produce instability include transport delays and increased loop gain (caused by greater controller sensitivity or changes in operating point which allow the controller to exert a larger effect on the controlled system). In linear control systems, the occurrence of instability and the characteristics of the cyclic changes can be predicted by graphic techniques, for example, by the Bode and Nyquist diagrams. However, the respiratory control system behaves alinearly, and the prediction of the effects of specific alterations in system components usually requires the use of mathematical models. While differing somewhat in details, models of the respiratory system show that unstable operations can occur with alterations in the activity of the components of the system or can be triggered by disturbances that are well within the range of physiological possibility.

Because the respiratory control system interacts with other systems that regulate circulation and body temperature, the stability of respiratory control can be affected by the operation of these systems.

THE REGULARITY OF BREATHING

The normal range of variability of breathing has been studied by only a few investigators. Tidal volume and inspiratory and expiratory times tend to fluctuate more than ventilation because breath duration is generally longer with larger tidal volumes and is shorter when tidal volume is smaller. This suggests that these fluctuations in pattern may sometimes arise from random changes in the threshold of bulbopontine neurons which determine inspiratory length or in vagal input from the lungs. Variability tends to be less with exercise and hypercapnia, but hypoxia has a less consistent effect, sometimes improving the constancy of breathing but at times causing cyclic fluctuations in ventilation level. Individuals with absent or poor ventilatory responses to hypercapnia and hypoxia frequently have irregular breathing patterns at rest.

While these random variations can be considered to be an unwanted feature of breathing, it is possible that these fluctuations in breathing patterns may serve a useful purpose allowing the controller to better detect changes in the mechanical characteristics of the respiratory muscles and lungs.

Irregularities in breathing depth may also help improve lung function. When patients are artificially ventilated at constant rates for prolonged periods of time, areas of atelectasis form and lung compliance decreases. This reduction in compliance can be reversed by intermittently causing the patient to sigh (allowing the ventilator to produce large tidal volumes). Sighs also occur during normal spontaneous breathing and seem to have the same purpose of reopening atelectatic lung regions. Sighs occur more frequently when breathing is stimulated, particularly when the stimulus is hypoxia. Irritant receptor stimulation also provokes sighs, but sighs can occur even after vagal traffic is eliminated surgically.

In addition to random disturbances and sighs, regularly recurring short-period oscillations in ventilation, gas exchange, and blood-gas tensions have been reported, but variations in arterial P_{O_2} rarely exceed 3 to 4 mmHg and in P_{CO_2} are even less. Techniques such as autocorrelation, power spectral density analysis, and more recently comb filtering have been used to uncover periodicities in ventilation and in blood pressure and heart rate that are not immediately obvious because of the masking effect of noise.

In addition to short ultradian oscillations in ventilation, circadian oscillations in ventilation and circulation have been described. These circadian oscillations are found in many biologic systems and seem to depend on the presence of internal clocks.

In higher animals it is believed that there is a multiplicity of such clocks arranged in a hierarchical order. Circadian changes seem to be under the control of at least two master clocks. One master clock seems to be located in the suprachiasmatic nucleus (SCN) of the hypothalamus and is responsible for the circadian variation in calcium secretion in the urine, growth hormone release, recurrence of non-rapid eye movement (NREM) sleep, and skin temperature. Destruction of the SCN produces sleep fragmentation. A retinohypothalamic projection between the SCN and the eye apparently accounts for the entrainment of the circadian activity cycle to the light-dark variation.

However, even when the SCN is destroyed, the circadian oscillation in core temperature persists. Hence there seems to be still another master clock with as yet undetermined location. In addition to temperature this clock also appears to control the circadian secretion of cortisols, the REM sleep pattern, and urinary excretion of potassium.

It is known that the amplitude of circadian oscillations in activity and temperature shows considerable interindividual differences. It is possible that similar variability occurs in circadian respiratory oscillations, depending on the relative sensitivity of ventilation to temperature and metabolic changes.

APNEAS

Probably apnea is the most frequent and striking abnormality in respiratory rhythm. Apneas are observed most often in the premature infant but can occur in healthy adults, especially during sleep, and can be isolated events or can be recurrent. Because apneas sometimes produce severe hypoxia and hypercapnia, they may cause clinically significant cardiac arrhythmias or have long-lasting effects such as pulmonary hypertension.

Several different mechanisms can potentially produce random apneas. These include (1) loss of nonspecific respiratory excitatory stimulation (noise, light, tactile stimuli) and (2) active suppression of breathing by respiratory inhibitory reflexes arising from the cardiovascular system, the lung and chest wall, or via somatic and visceral afferents. For example, excitation of receptors located in the upper airway can, via the superior laryngeal nerve, trigger an apnea. Stimulation of J receptors in the lungs by inhaled irritants may produce a temporary apnea. Apnea may also occur as a result of a stimulus which produces hypocapnia but represses mechanisms which normally help maintain breathing even when

chemical stimulation is minimal, such as the posthyperventilation hyperpnea described by Eldridge.

Recurrent apneas may appear as part of a pattern of grossly irregular ataxic breathing. Patients with this kind of breathing usually have functional or actual structural medullary damage. The breathing disturbance results from a kind of sputtering of damaged respiratory neuronal circuits. Breathing responds poorly to stimulants, and the patients with this disorder tend to hypoventilate.

In other types of abnormalities, such as Cheyne-Stokes breathing and Biot's breathing, apneas occur more predictably (as shown in Fig. 25-2). Apneas may be separated by periods of gradually increasing and decreasing breathing, as in Cheyne-Stokes breathing, and often in sleep apnea, or as in Biot's breathing by breaths with a fixed tidal volume. Recurrent apneas may be associated with either hypoventilation or hyperventilation.

Two different mechanisms may be involved in producing recurrent apneas: (1) an instability in the feedback control of respiration which produces periodic breathing by the same mechanisms that produce oscillatory output in physical control systems when they become unstable; and (2) an exaggeration of the mechanisms which may normally produce oscillations in ventilation.

Sleep Apneas

On the basis of EEG criteria, sleep has been divided into REM and NREM sleep. Sleep usually begins in the NREM stage, which has been divided in two substages on the basis of a progressive slowing in EEG frequencies. REM sleep (the stage in which dreaming tends to occur) usually follows NREM states. It is characterized by the occurrence of a dysynchronized EEG and periods of abrupt eye movements. REM sleep is also accompanied by inhibition of motor neurons, which leads to a profound loss of muscle tone that affects the diaphragm less than other respiratory muscles.

In both REM and NREM sleep, ventilatory responses to hypoxia and hypercapnia are reduced. Changes in lung mechanics occurring during sleep (increased upper air-

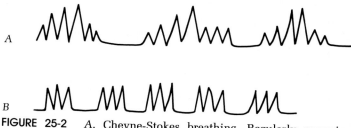

FIGURE 25-2 *A.* Cheyne-Stokes breathing. Regularly recurring swings in ventilation separated by periods of apnea. *B.* Biot's breathing. Unlike Cheyne-Stokes breathing, the tidal volumes between periods of apnea are uniform. It is unclear whether Cheyne-Stokes breathing and Biot's breathing are produced by the same mechanism.

way resistance and decreased compliance) may also contribute to depressed ventilatory responses.

Responses to stimulation of mechanoreceptors are also altered by sleep. For example, the compensatory response in motor activity which occurs during wakefulness when the airway is obstructed is reduced or eliminated during sleep.

Apneas occur occasionally during sleep in considerable numbers of healthy individuals. But in those who have the sleep apnea syndrome, apneas are frequent and prolonged so that much of the night is spent hypoxemic. These same individuals are frequently sleepy during the day and may have elevated levels of arterial P_{CO_2} and pulmonary artery pressure. Sleep apnea occurs most frequently in premature infants, adult males, and postmenopausal women. Apneas are often but not always associated with obesity, anatomic narrowing of the upper airway passages, and snoring. Sleep apneas generally occur in clusters, each of the apneas separated by a gradual increase and decrease in ventilation. Arousal terminates some of the periods of apnea. Apneas are most frequent in the lighter forms of NREM sleep and in REM sleep.

The interruptions in breathing that occur during the night have been divided into two types, central apneas and obstructive apneas. In *central apneas* there is no detectable respiratory activity, while during *obstructive apneas* respiratory efforts continue but there is no flow of air at either the nose or mouth. It is believed that a block in the upper airway occurs during obstructive apnea which prevents the movement of air into the lungs.

The distinction between obstructive and central apnea is not always clear. Frequently apneas are mixed in type, beginning with a central component followed by an obstructive period of ineffectual respiratory efforts. Many patients have both kinds of apnea even within the same night. Also, therapeutic interventions which are designed to prevent the occurrence of one or the other forms of apnea sometimes just substitute one type for the other.

Differences in the response of upper airway and chest wall muscles to chemical and mechanical stimuli could cause obstructive apnea. When the diaphragm contracts, a negative intrapharyngeal pressure is produced which tends to displace mobile upper airway structure and block airflow. Contraction of the upper airway muscles counterbalances this force to prevent obstruction during inspiration. According to this idea, maintenance of upper airway patency depends on fine coordination of the movements of upper airway and chest wall muscles. This coordination is more crucial when the airway is anatomically narrow.

Patterns of response of upper airway muscles may depend on which receptors are stimulated. For example, in anesthetized animals, hypercapnia inhibits the adductor muscles which close the larynx. But hypoxia, on the other hand, seems to exert an excitatory effect on laryngeal adductors narrowing the laryngeal aperture. CO_2 acting on peripheral chemoreceptors may affect the relative activity of the muscles of the tongue and diaphragm more than when it acts only on central chemoreceptors. Whether or not the same differences exist during sleep is unknown, but it is conceivable that they do.

The decrease in drive occurring during sleep may silence upper airway muscles before it stops the diaphragm, creating an imbalance of forces that promotes the collapse of the upper airway. Also, altered alignment of the respiratory muscles in the upper airway caused by changes in posture and the effects of gravity tend to increase the forces needed to maintain airway patency during sleep. Both mechanisms tend to produce an obstructive apnea.

Recent work has examined the idea that both sleep apnea and Cheyne-Stokes breathing are caused by an instability in feedback control.

Cheyne-Stokes Breathing

Cheyne-Stokes breathing is characterized by a cyclic rise and fall in ventilation with recurrent periods of apnea. It was initially observed in patients with cardiac or neurologic disease, but it has since been reported in seemingly normal humans. The appearance of Cheyne-Stokes breathing can be triggered by the administration of sedatives and opiates and is more common during sleep. The period of the oscillations in ventilation in Cheyne-Stokes breathing is related to the circulation time measured from the lung to a systemic artery. Cycle length increases when circulation time is prolonged. Arterial blood P_{CO_2} is highest during the phase of hyperpnea while arterial P_{O_2} is then at its minimum, but alveolar gas tensions cycle in the opposite way. Changes in the level of alertness occur coincidentally with the respiratory oscillations. Arousal tends to occur during the hyperpneic phase along with an increase in cerebral blood flow. The EEG shows greater fast-wave activity. The pupils dilate and muscle tone is increased. The sensorium seems more depressed during apnea, the pupils are constricted, and muscle tone is diminished. Cerebral blood flow is often less during apnea, and there is a higher percentage of slow-wave activity in the EEG. It is of interest that arousal also frequently seems to terminate an episode of apnea during sleep.

While the apneas occurring in Cheyne-Stokes breathing are more commonly central in type, Lyons et al. in 1958 reported recurrent obstructive apnea in patients with congestive heart failure and Cheyne-Stokes breathing.

Cheyne-Stokes breathing has not been consistently produced in animals by lesions in the central nervous system, but it has been shown to follow manipulations that are likely to produce unstable feedback control of breathing. For example, the steadiness of the output in a feedback control system depends on the ability of the control system to be adequately informed of the consequences of its actions. If delays in information transfer are sufficiently great, the controller action to correct the effects of a disturbance may result in cyclic output changes. Delays can occur in the respiratory system when circulation time is prolonged between the lungs and the respiratory chemoreceptors. Experiments have shown that artificial prolongation of the circulation time causes Cheyne-Stokes breathing in anesthetized dogs.

Increased controller gains also enhance tendencies for instability in physical control systems. One way to increase the gain of the respiratory controller is to produce hypoxia. Posthyperventilation apnea can be used as a device to produce hypoxia at subnormal levels of CO_2 drive. In anesthetized dogs with normal circulation times, periodic breathing can occur following a period of artificial hyperventilation.

Recent studies in humans have demonstrated that artificial hyperventilation during NREM sleep is frequently followed by a period of apnea and then Cheyne-Stokes-type breathing. Also, although Cheyne-Stokes breathing is common at high altitude, it occurs mainly in lowlanders who have much greater ventilatory responses to hypoxia than the native of high altitude who has much lower hypoxic sensitivity.

Periodic breathing has also been produced in anesthetized cats ventilated with a respirator governed by phrenic nerve output so that feedback loops remained intact. Periodic breathing could be elicited sometimes just by increasing the gain of the servorespirator, but at other times also required respiring the cat with hypoxic gas mixtures. Cooling the ventral medullary surface of the cat, which increased controller set point (the P_{CO_2} during resting breathing), also led to periodic breathing.

Instability as a Potential Cause of Sleep Apnea

The sequence of recurrent apneas (both central and obstructive) observed in humans during sleep often closely resembles the pattern of Cheyne-Stokes breathing. This suggests that the apneas occurring during sleep, whether they are obstructive or central, may have a common basis: an instability in the feedback regulation of breathing. The major inciting disturbance could be the sudden increase in set point of the controller during sleep onset, i.e., the elevation in resting P_{CO_2}.

In addition to gain, a major factor that affects the stability of breathing is the position of the ventilation-CO_2 response line (controller slope, as shown in Fig. 25-3). In general, the greater the displacement of this line to higher levels of CO_2, the less the damping action of the control system and the more likely it is for instability to occur. The cause of the instability is a greater ability of ventilation changes to alter Pa_{CO_2}. Respiratory depressants and

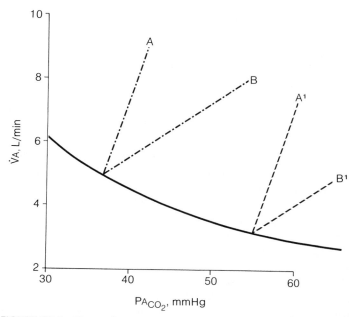

FIGURE 25-3 Heavy line shows the effect of ventilation ($\dot{V}_A$) and Pa_{CO_2}. Broken lines show the effect of changes in Pa_{CO_2} on ventilation (controller response). An increase in controller response from B to A decreases control system stability. A shift in controller responses from A to A^1, or B to B^1, also increases the possibility for oscillations in ventilation to occur as a result of instability in the respiratory feedback control system.

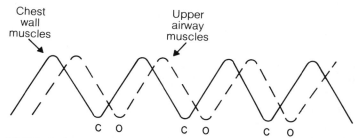

FIGURE 25-4 Diagram illustrating effect of possible out-of-phase oscillations in chest wall and upper airway muscle activity. When chest wall muscle activity reaches its nadir, central apnea (C) occurs; when upper airway muscle activity reaches its nadir, obstructive apnea (O) occurs.

sleep decrease the controller slope but also shift the position of the response line to the right, raising arterial P_{CO_2} as resting ventilation is reduced. In general, such rightward shifts, no matter how they are produced, increase tendencies for instability even when there is an associated decrease in ventilatory responses to chemical stimuli. Individuals who have the greatest increase in resting P_{CO_2} with sleep also seem to have the most central apneas.

It seems possible then that an instability in feedback control could cause the motor activity of both the chest wall muscles and the upper airway to cycle but with differences in amplitude and/or phase. The apneas would be central or obstructive depending on the differences in responses to chemical stimuli of the upper airway and chest wall muscles (Fig. 25-4).

Other changes in the operation of the control system might also cause instability. The responsivity of respiratory chemoreceptors to stimuli at or below the usual resting level has been little studied in anesthesia, wakefulness, or sleep. But these low-level responses are particularly important theoretically in determining the appearance of apnea, length of periodicities, and the amplitude of oscillations. It may be that as CO_2 is lowered below its usual arterial level of 40 mmHg, responsivity changes become greater. An increase in responsivity at subnormal levels of P_{CO_2} would be a potent mechanism for producing instability even if responses at hypercapnic levels were depressed.

Reflex responses to mechanical stimuli may also have an important effect on upper airway muscles. Since upper airway structures are mobile, displacement of these structures may mechanically excite receptors, triggering reflexes (e.g., from the superior laryngeal nerve) which could produce apnea or differential activity of upper airway and chest wall muscles.

Other Explanations for Sleep Apnea

It has been previously suggested that the oscillations that occur during sleep in breathing may just be an exaggerated form of normally occurring oscillations. Periodic breathing can be caused by oscillations in other physiological systems. For example, when cyclic changes in blood pressure are caused by hemorrhage, cyclic changes in breathing can occur simultaneously.

Preiss, Iscoe, and Polosa found cycles in blood pressure activity, sympathetic nerve activity, and phrenic nerve activity lasting 24 s in hemorrhaged cats after carotid clamping. The phrenic nerve cycles persisted even after artificial ventilation was instituted and blood pressure was stabilized. They suggested that cyclic changes were caused by oscillatory networks of neurons in the central nervous system which drove both respiratory and vasomotor neurons. These kinds of observations make it difficult to discount the idea that physiological oscillations contribute to periodic apneas.

Sleep may make the cyclic oscillations that are barely discernible during wakefulness more obvious by eliminating the random superimposed effects of environmental noise. Apneas rather than just swings in ventilation occur because sleep, in addition to reducing the respiratory stimulatory effects of hypoxia and hypercapnia, also depresses metabolic rate and the overall level of respiratory excitatory input.

Other causes of recurrent sleep apnea which have been suggested include exaggerated cerebral blood flow changes during sleep, which secondarily affect respiration, and severe depression of drive so that respiratory neurons are only intermittently stimulated sufficiently to fire.

A variety of sleep promoting factors have been identified. These include a number of monamines, polypeptides (such as substance S-delta sleep inducing peptide, muramyl depeptide, substance S, and interleukin 1), and prostaglandin D_2. While it is not clear whether any of these agents are responsible for natural sleep, it is possible that natural sleep varies in its cause, and sleep is not always the same even when EEG patterns appear identical. Sleep may be produced by different combinations of these substances in different individuals. It is even possible that only some sleep-inducing substances are capable of producing the changes in controller response that lead to apnea and that the cause of apnea depends ultimately on differences in the mix of the biochemical agents producing sleep. It is interesting that some of the putative sleep substances are pyrogens and that feverish patients often have disturbed sleep.

BIBLIOGRAPHY

Alex CG, Önal E, Lopata M: Upper airway occlusion during sleep in patients with Cheyne-Stokes respiration. Am Rev Respir Dis 133:42–45, 1986.
   Patients with Cheyne-Stokes respiration may develop upper airway occlusion during sleep, consistent with the contention that sleep-induced periodic breathing in patients with sleep apnea syndrome is primarily due to the development of occlusive apneas.

Brouillette RT, Thach BT: A neuromuscular mechanism maintaining extrathoracic airway patency. J Appl Physiol 46:772–779, 1979.
   Describes an important series of experiments indicating the importance of upper airway muscle in preventing obstruction.

Brown HW, Plum F: The neurologic basis of Cheyne-Stokes respiration. Am J Med 30:849–860, 1961.
   Description of the neurologic mechanisms involved in Cheyne-Stokes respiration based on case studies.

Brusil PJ, Waggener TB, Kronauer RE, Gulesian P Jr: Methods for identifying respiratory oscillations disclose altitude effects. J Appl Physiol 48:545–556, 1980.
   A description of some of the more sophisticated analytical methods that can be useful in detection of periodic variations in breathing.

Cherniack NS: Sleep apnea and its causes. J Clin Invest 73:1501–1506, 1984.
   A review of the pathophysiology and possible causes of sleep apnea.

Cherniack NS, Longobardo GS: Cheyne-Stokes breathing. An instability in physiologic control. N Engl J Med 288:952–957, 1973.

Review of the pathophysiology of Cheyne-Stokes breathing.

Cherniack NS, Longobardo GS: Abnormalities in respiratory rhythm, in Cherniack NS, Longobardo GS (eds), *Handbook of Physiology, sec 3: The Respiratory System, vol 2: The Control of Breathing.* Bethesda, MD, American Physiological Society, 1986, pp 729–749.

Detailed review of the mechanisms which cause variations in breathing pattern.

Cherniack NS, von Euler C, Glogowska M, Homma I: Characteristics and rate of occurrence of spontaneous and provoked augmented breaths. Acta Physiol Scand 111:349–360, 1981.

Experimental study in cats of the factors which produce sighing.

Dark DS, Pingleton SK, Kerby GR, Crabb JE, Gollub SB, Glatter TR, Dunn MI: Breathing pattern abnormalities and arterial oxygen desaturation during sleep in the congestive heart failure syndrome. Improvement following medical therapy. Chest 91:833–836, 1987.

Congestive heart failure is a contributing factor for breathing abnormalities and arterial oxygen desaturation during sleep.

Dempsey JA, Skatrud JB: A sleep-induced apneic threshold and its consequences. Am Rev Respir Dis 133:1163–1170, 1986.

In the absence of the stabilizing influences of wakefulness, ventilatory control becomes overwhelmingly dependent on CO_2 in maintaining a rhythmic breathing pattern.

Dowell AR, Buckley CE III, Cohen R, Whalen RE, Sieker HO: Cheyne-Stokes respiration. A review of clinical manifestations and critique of physiological mechanisms. Arch Intern Med 127:712–726, 1971.

One of the most complete reviews of the symptoms and signs of Cheyne-Stokes breathing. Also provides an excellent historical perspective on the theories of causes of Cheyne-Stokes breathing.

Eldridge FL, Gill-Kumar P: Central neural respiratory drive and afterdischarge. Respir Physiol 40:49–63, 1980.

Classic description of studies which demonstrate that ventilatory stimulation can persist at times even when the exciting stimulants have been removed.

Goodman L, Alexander DM, Fleming DG: Oscillatory behavior of respiratory gas exchange in resting man. IEEE Trans Biomed Engin 13:57–64, 1966.

Pioneering study describing spontaneously occurring oscillations in humans.

Khoo MC, Kronauer RE, Strohl KP, Slutsky AS: Factors inducing periodic breathing in humans: A general model. J Appl Physiol 53:644–659, 1982.

A description of a mathematical model simulating periodic breathing particularly at high altitude.

Lahiri S, Hsiao C, Zhang R, Mokashi A, Nishino T: Peripheral chemoreceptors in respiratory oscillation. J Appl Physiol 58:1901–1908, 1985.

An important examination of the relationship of ventilatory responses to hypoxia to the occurrence of periodic breathing.

Lange RL, Hecht HH: The mechanism of Cheyne-Stokes respiration. J Clin Invest 41:42–52, 1962.

An early theoretical and experimental analysis of Cheyne-Stokes breathing, emphasizing the importance of feedback instability in humans.

Lenfant C: Time-dependent variations of pulmonary gas exchange in normal man at rest. J Appl Physiol 22:675–684, 1967.

Study in humans at rest of variations in ventilation and pulmonary gas tensions.

Lyons HA, Burno F, Stone RW: Pulmonary compliance in patients with periodic breathing. Circulation 17:1056–1061, 1958.

One of the first studies demonstrating the existence of obstructive apnea.

Önal E, Lopata M, O'Connor T: Pathogenesis of apneas in hypersomnia-sleep apnea syndrome. Am Rev Respir Dis 125:167–174, 1982.

A description of studies in humans during sleep, suggesting the importance of reflex changes and muscle mechanics in sleep apnea.

Önal E, Burrows DL, Hart RH, Lopata M: Induction of periodic breathing during sleep causes upper airway obstruction in humans. J Appl Physiol 61:1438–1443, 1986.

Periodic breathing resulting in periodic diminution of upper airway muscle activity is associated with increased upper airway resistance that predisposes upper airways to collapse.

Phillipson EA: Control of breathing during sleep. Am Rev Respir Dis 118:909–939, 1978.
Comprehensive review of the subject.

Preiss G, Iscoe S, Polosa C: Analysis of a periodic breathing pattern associated with Mayer waves. Am J Physiol 228:768–774, 1975.
Describes a series of experiments which suggest that there are naturally occurring oscillations in blood pressure and breathing.

Skatrud JB, Dempsey JA: Interaction of sleep state and chemical stimuli in sustaining rhythmic ventilation. J Appl Physiol 55:813–822, 1983.
Demonstrates the importance of CO_2 in maintaining ventilation during sleep.

Telakivi T, Partinen M, Koskenvuo M, Salmi T, Kaprio J: Periodic breathing and hypoxia in snorers and controls: validation of snoring history and association with blood pressure and obesity. Acta Neurol Scand 76:69–75, 1987.
Self-reported habitual snoring is a reliable screening method for the obstructive sleep apnea syndrome.

Warner G, Skatrud JB, Dempsey JA: Effect of hypoxia-induced periodic breathing on upper airway obstruction during sleep. J Appl Physiol 62:2201–2211, 1987.
Hypoxia-induced instability in breathing pattern can cause obstructed breaths during sleep coincident with reduced motor output to inspiratory muscles. However, this obstruction is only manifest in subjects susceptible to upper airway atonicity and narrowing (such as snorers).

Webber CL Jr, Speck DF: Experimental Biot periodic breathing in cats: Effects of changes in $P_{I_{O_2}}$ and $P_{I_{CO_2}}$. Respir Physiol 46:327–344, 1981.
Excellent study of this form of periodic breathing.

Part 4

Approach to the Patient with Respiratory Signs or Symptoms

Chapter 26

Approach to the Pulmonary Patient with Respiratory Signs and Symptoms

J. Peter Szidon / Alfred P. Fishman

The approach to patients presenting with predominant respiratory symptoms is governed by the same logic that applies to the approach to any patient. The central cognitive task is the definition of the clinical problem. Clinical judgment is then used to weigh diagnostic possibilities, to guide the choice of additional studies, to balance the advantages, costs, and risks of treatments, to elicit accurate patient preferences for alternative therapies, and, finally,

to recommend and implement strategies of medical care. Investigations into the diagnostic thinking of experienced physicians suggest that they use the scientific method for this initial approach in a manner analogous to that of an investigator performing a laboratory experiment. As soon as the interview is initiated, the process of formulating hypotheses begins. Seasoned diagnosticians seem to be able to entertain several diagnostic hypotheses simultaneously. By a process of iterative testing, working diagnoses are successively generated as the interview proceeds, briefly analyzed, used to direct further questioning, sustained temporarily, or rejected.

Similarly, physical examination of the respiratory patient is more than a systematic screening method; it is also greatly influenced by the working hypotheses ("working diagnoses") generated during history taking. Because of these hypotheses, the attention of the physician is directed to performing a more meticulous evaluation of suspected areas or of presumed expressions of abnormal function expected to be associated with the tentative diagnosis. Nonetheless, although the physical examination is focused by the history, the habit of a comprehensive and meticulous physical examination often elicits unexpected abnormalities such as cyanosis, clubbing of the digits, edema, or distinctive skin lesions and may promote further refinement of the original hypotheses or the generation of new hypotheses. The diagnostic precision resulting from the synthesis of this early information depends critically on the medical knowledge of the clinician and on his or her ability to refer to an integrated system of pathophysiology. For example, enuresis, morning headaches, and diurnal somnolence, seemingly unrelated manifestations elicited as complaints from an obese patient, become logically integrated into the pathophysiological concepts of the sleep apnea syndrome as expressions of sleep deprivation and altered arterial blood gases during sleep.

Recent clinical applications of decision-making theory continue to enlarge our understanding of how to characterize diagnostic tests and how to interpret their results (see Chapter 29). This approach will contribute to refining the selection of diagnostic information, including the appropriate uses of probability and decision trees. Gottlieb et al. have recently provided an excellent example of the application of this approach to the diagnosis of sarcoidosis.

PREDISPOSING INFLUENCES

Without a clear picture of the patient's background, the physician is apt to be either adrift or on the wrong track. In a heavy smoker, the problem of a pneumonia that is reluctant to heal focuses sharply on the possibility of an inapparent carcinoma of the lungs. The sudden onset,

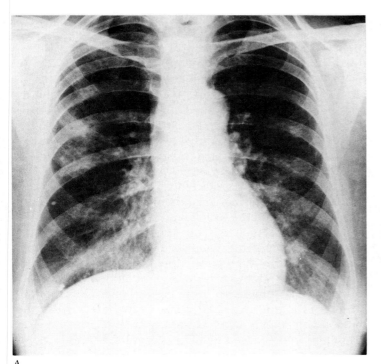

A

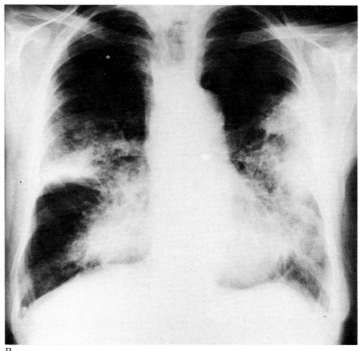

B

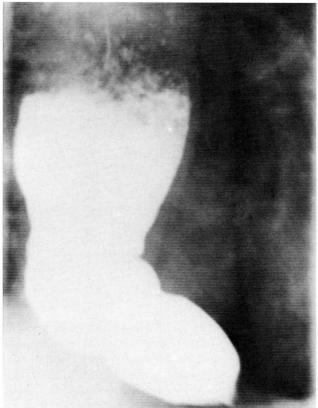

C

FIGURE 26-1 Chronic aspiration pneumonia in a 72-year-old man hospitalized for repair of hernia. *A*. Admission. Patchy infiltrates bilaterally. No pulmonary manifestations. *B*. Eighteen months later. Persistent cough and breathlessness. *C*. Upper gastrointestinal series showing achalasia of the esophagus to which the repeated aspiration was attributed.

without overt cause, of wheezing in a middle-aged or elderly person raises the prospect of left ventricular failure rather than allergy. The elderly are also prone to asymptomatic aspiration. Often the cause of the aspiration is unknown; sometimes it occurs without symptoms during sleep. In some instances, the fault proves to be either in muscles guarding the laryngeal aperture or in the upper gastrointestinal tract (Fig. 26-1).

Defense mechanisms are often seriously compromised in the patient with diabetes mellitus, or cancer, or a blood dyscrasia, predisposing these individuals to infection, not only with conventional organisms, particularly pneumococci, staphylococci, gram-negative bacilli, and the tubercle bacilli, but also to opportunistic microbes, particularly *Nocardia, Candida, Aspergillus, Pneumocystis,* and cytomegalovirus. The administration of corticosteroids, antibiotics, and immunosuppressive agents enlarges the prospects for infection with unusual organisms.

Personal habits and life-style often shape the course and nature of a pulmonary infection. Lipoid pneumonia caused by nose drops is currently uncommon, but does occur still (Fig. 26-2). Chronic alcoholics are prime candidates for pneumococcal and *Klebsiella* pneumonia; they also develop aspiration pneumonia. Recent contact with varicella or measles sometimes helps to explain a mysterious pneumonia. Patients receiving drugs are candidates for allergic reactions; among the most notorious in this regard are nitrofurantoin and busulfan (Fig. 26-3). Persistent use of these agents, after the pneumonic process has become manifest, causes protracted pulmonary disability.

The relationship between pulmonary infections, AIDS, and homosexual or intravenous drug abusers' life-styles illustrates how important is the characterization of life-styles in pulmonary diagnosis.

The geographic history of the patient sometimes is a clue to solving the mystery of a puzzling pneumonia. Histoplasmosis and North American blastomycosis are prevalent in the southern United States and are also found in old wood and soil; either an acute pneumonic or cavitary form of these diseases can be the reason for seeking medical help. South American blastomycosis is common in Brazil (Fig. 26-4).

The occupational and the epidemiologic histories are sometimes extraordinarily revealing. Some disorders, particularly asbestosis, evolve gradually over years (Fig. 26-5). Even brief exposure to asbestos fibers 30 years ago—by working as a plumber's helper in a navy yard or by washing clothes contaminated with asbestos fibers or by living downwind from a polluted environment—sometimes suffices to trigger clinical asbestosis or even mesothelioma. Usually easier to trace are contacts with birds; exposure to poultry and bird droppings alerts the examiner to the prospect of histoplasmosis, psittacosis, or cryptococcosis. Cave explorers are unique candidates for histoplasmosis.

Hereditary syndromes sometimes present distinctive clinical features. Among those of interest to pulmonary disease are cystic fibrosis of the pancreas, α_1-antitrypsin deficiency, Marfan's syndrome, von Recklinghausen's neurofibromatosis, and hereditary hemorrhagic telangiectasia.

Cystic fibrosis is a useful illustration of hereditary influences. Once its genetic aspects and pathogenesis are appreciated, it is difficult to overlook. The disease is a consequence of an autosomal recessive disorder that is produced by a gene with relatively high frequency. The gene frequency is higher in some ethnic groups than in others: in North Europeans it constitutes the most frequent lethal Mendelian disorder of childhood and adolescence, i.e., about 1 per 1600 births. In contrast to its prevalence in North Europeans, the disease is rare in Africans and Asians.

The clinical manifestations of cystic fibrosis are those of a generalized disorder of exocrine glands that causes them to elaborate abnormally viscid secretions. The disease generally makes its presence known in the first decade of life. In early childhood, malabsorption from deficiency of pancreatic enzymes is the leading problem. Later in childhood and during adolescence, pulmonary

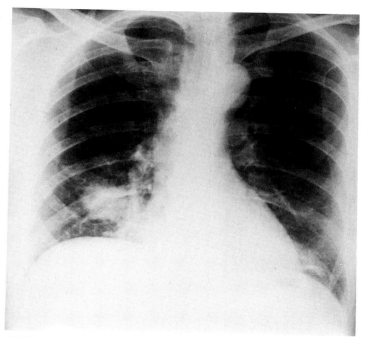

FIGURE 26-2 Lipoid pneumonia. Oily nose drops used for many years. Bilateral lesions of lung bases unchanged for 5 years. Lipoid material obtained in bronchial aspirate.

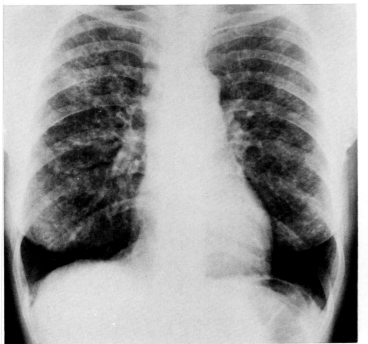

A

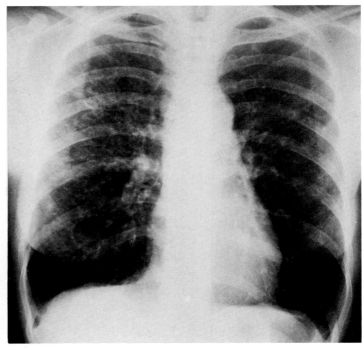

B

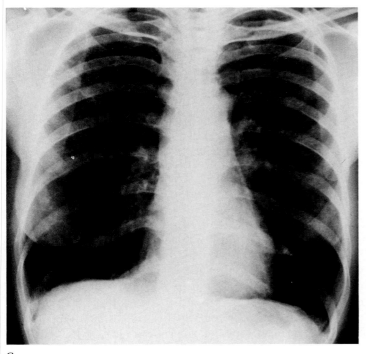

C

FIGURE 26-3 Hypersensitivity pneumonitis. The appearance of patchy interstitial and alveolar changes throughout both lungs was associated with ingestion of nitrofurantoin, 50 mg qid.   A. Initial chest radiographs, after 2 months of nitrofurantoin.   B. Taken 1 month after nitrofurantoin was stopped.   C. Taken 3 months after nitrofurantoin was stopped.

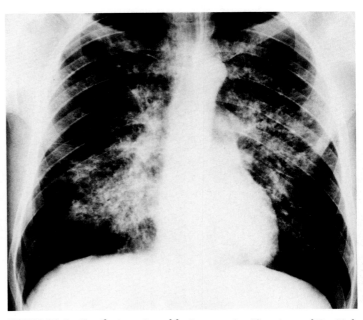

FIGURE 26-4 South American blastomycosis. *(Courtesy of Dr. Nelson Porto.)*

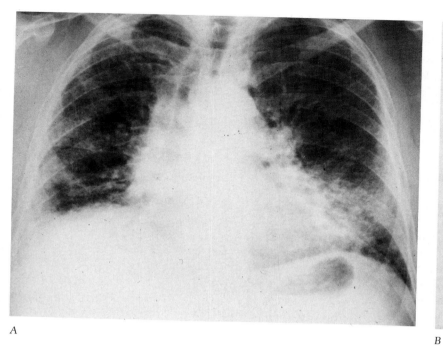

A

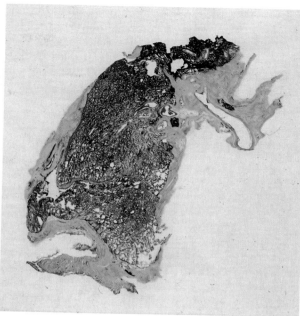

B

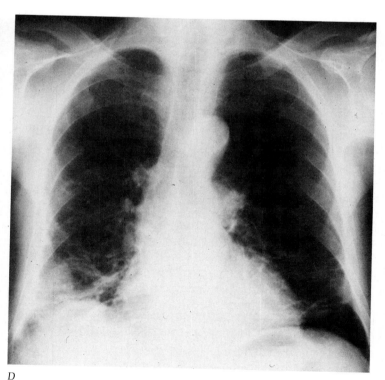

C

D

FIGURE 26-5 Restrictive lung disease. *A.* Asbestosis in 55-year-old man with no known history of exposure. At autopsy the lungs were encased by thickened pleura and interstitial fibrosis was widespread (see Fig. 26-10*B*). *B.* Sagittal section of lung. Asbestosis. Restrictive lung disease caused by encasement of right lung by pleural thickening and by interstitial fibrosis. *C.* Interstitial lung disease ("usual interstitial pneumonitis") in a 67-year-old man, before and after steroids. Before corticosteroids. Widespread interstitial lung disease, more marked on the right. The lung function tests were characteristic of severe restrictive lung disease. *D.* After corticosteroids. Pulmonary function tests improved dramatically along with clearing of the pulmonary lesions on the chest radiograph.

infection, emphysema, bronchiectasis, pulmonary fibrosis, and cor pulmonale become increasingly important. Some patients develop biliary cirrhosis. Excessive loss of sodium and chloride in sweat is a hallmark of the disease. The diagnosis of cystic fibrosis is made by demonstrating excess sodium and chloride in the sweat and a deficiency in the excretion of pancreatic enzymes.

BEDSIDE APPRAISAL

Physical findings had a greater importance in the past because respiratory diseases tended to present later in their course, with florid clinical manifestations, and also because sophisticated diagnostic techniques were not available. The advent of modern radiology and fiberoptic bronchoscopy has been associated with a rapid erosion of physicians' skills in eliciting and interpreting bedside findings and the relegation of these talents to a secondary role. This oversight sometimes sacrifices important leads in differential diagnosis. For example, clipped sentences in the course of the interview may call attention to breathlessness and raise the possibility of a low ventilatory reserve. Hoarseness or Horner's syndrome or body wasting provides a vital lead to the nature of a pulmonary lesion. The clinical clues often change the orientation from looking *at* a patient to looking *for* evidence of a particular disease.

The Physical Examination

Important clues are often available before the chest is reached. Neglected pyorrheal teeth are an important source of organisms for necrotizing pneumonia. A lacerated tongue suggests a convulsive episode that led to aspiration. Subtle changes in consciousness or coordination occasionally announce that metastasis has occurred to the brain from a primary carcinoma of the lung. A clouded sensorium or a disturbed personality sometimes signifies acute CO_2 retention in obstructive disease of the airways.

A variety of endocrine syndromes can accompany a carcinoma of the lungs. Clubbing of the digits is common in idiopathic pulmonary fibrosis; sometimes it directs attention to unsuspected bronchiectasis or to a carcinoma of the lung. Although a number of clinical disorders can be associated with clubbing (Table 26-1), its pathogenesis remains tantalizingly enigmatic. A minute skin abscess can be the source of multiple lung abscesses. Distinctive scars over the antecubital veins of a drug addict sometimes clarify the cause of old scars in the lungs as well as of fresh abscesses. Erythema nodosum and erythema multiforme occasionally complicate sarcoidosis, tuberculosis, histoplasmosis, and coccidioidomycosis; sometimes they are part of a drug reaction.

A puffy face, neck, and eyelids, coupled with dilated veins of the neck, shoulder, thorax, and upper arm, i.e.,

TABLE 26-1

Clinical Disorders Commonly Associated with Clubbing of Digits

Pulmonary and thoracic
    Primary lung cancer
    Metastatic lung cancer
    Bronchiectasis
    Cystic fibrosis
    Lung abscess
    Pulmonary fibrosis
    Pulmonary arteriovenous malformations
    Empyema
    Mesothelioma
    Neurogenic diaphragmatic tumors
Cardiac
    Congenital
    Subacute bacterial endocarditis
Gastrointestinal and hepatic
    Hepatic cirrhosis
    Chronic ulcerative colitis
    Regional enteritis (Crohn's disease)
Miscellaneous
    Hemiplegia

the "superior vena caval syndrome," occasionally is the first clinical evidence of extrinsic obstruction of the superior vena cava by a neoplasm of the lung. Although the causes of the superior vena caval syndrome are many and diverse, at least 80 percent of all instances are attributable to a primary carcinoma of the lung. In the patient in whom a neoplasm has evoked acute signs and symptoms of increased systemic venous pressure that progresses rapidly, e.g., to laryngeal edema, early diagnosis and prompt irradiation of the neoplasm may be lifesaving. Similarly, the detection of a Horner's syndrome—unilateral ptosis, miosis, and anhidrosis—in a heavy smoker who is a logical candidate for carcinoma of the lung, raises the possibility that the neoplasm is inoperable because of spread to the ipsilateral sympathetic pathway within the thorax.

The Breathing Pattern

Close attention to the vital signs was advocated by Hippocrates. In modern times, however, the rate and pattern of breathing are often treated perfunctorily. A respiratory rate of more than 12 to 15 per minute at rest is abnormal. In afebrile patients, rapid, shallow breathing accompanies the stiff lungs of interstitial fibrosis and granuloma, pulmonary congestion, and pulmonary emboli. Conversely, slow, deep breathing is often a feature of obstructive disease of the airways. In the patient with lobar pneumonia, both the rate and depth of breathing increase as body temperature increases.

Chest Movements

The movements of the chest are sometimes informative. Asymmetry often localizes the side of the pleural effusion, or of a pulmonary infection, or of a paralyzed diaphragm. The position of the trachea is a useful guide to atelectasis of one lobe or to obstruction of a major bronchus. Quiet inspection of the chest and abdomen during sleep may reveal paradoxical inward movement of the abdomen that is characteristic of episodes of obstructive sleep apnea. Thoracoabdominal discoordination in the supine position calls to mind the possibility of bilateral diaphragmatic paresis or paralysis.

Percussion

The response to percussion is impaired whenever something other than air-filled lung lies directly beneath the chest wall. Common causes are consolidation or atelectasis of the lung, fluid in the pleural space, pleural thickening, or a large mass at the surface of the lung. Unfortunately, distinction is not always made between dullness and flatness: dullness is characteristic of pneumonic consolidation or atelectasis, whereas a flat percussion note at the lung base generally signifies a large pleural effusion or a high diaphragm. Increased resonance to percussion is more difficult to detect than a decrease in resonance. Widespread hyperresonance can often be elicited in emphysema and circumscribed hyperresonance over a pneumothorax or large bulla. As a rule, a decrease in breath sounds, as over a large bulla, is more telling than an increase in resonance.

Lung Sounds

Recent technical advances in sound recording and analysis have revived interest in the origin, transmission properties, and clinical significance of lung sounds. Although this renaissance has not paid definite clinical dividends, it does seem likely that more precise and scientific understanding of these phenomena is destined to have considerable diagnostic impact.

A widespread decrease in the intensity of breath sounds occurs because air movement is impaired, as in emphysema, or because a diaphragm is paralyzed, or a bronchus is completely obstructed, or transmission of sound to the chest wall is impaired, as in pleural effusion, pleural thickening, and pneumothorax. Regional distribution of ventilation, assessed by xenon equilibration scintigrams, correlates well with the distribution of breath sound intensity. An abnormal increase in intensity of breath sounds is accompanied by a change in their character; because of abnormal transmission of breath sounds from the larger airways, the sounds become either harsh or bronchial in nature. The abnormal sounds are heard over consolidated, atelectic, or compressed lung as long as the airway to the affected portion of the lung remains patent. Consolidated lung is presumed to act as an acoustic conducting medium that, unlike normal lung, does not attenuate transmission of tracheal sound to the periphery.

Changes in voice sounds are often easier to appreciate than changes in breath sounds. Distant or inaudible sounds are produced by large pleural effusions, pneumothorax, and bronchial occlusion. Transmission of voice sounds is enhanced by consolidation, infarction, atelectasis, or compressions of lung tissue. Accompanying the increased transmission is a change in the character of the voice sounds that causes them to be heard as higher-pitched and less-muffled than normal (*bronchophony*). When bronchophony is extreme, spoken words assume a nasal, or bleating, quality (*egophony*) and the sound "ee" is heard through the stethoscope as "ay." Egophony is most common when consolidated lung and pleural fluid coexist; sometimes it is heard over an uncomplicated lobar pneumonia or pulmonary infarction. Transmission of whispered voice sounds with abnormal clarity (whispered pectoriloquy) has the same significance as bronchophony.

A pleural friction rub is a coarse, grating, or leathery sound that is usually heard late in inspiration and early in expiration, most often low in the axilla or over the lung base posteriorly. It sounds close to the ear and usually is not altered by coughing.

The classic nomenclature of lung sounds and their presumed clinical significance has always been somewhat confusing and of limited usefulness. A preliminary attempt at a more rational formulation based on acoustical analysis of tape recordings was proposed by the American Thoracic Society (Table 26-2) using terms introduced by Forgacs. The lung sounds were separated into *continuous* (wheezes and ronchi) and *discontinuous* (crackles). Crackles (or rales) were further subdivided into *fine* and *coarse* based on the observation that the characteristics of individual crackles in time-expanded waveforms correlated well with their subjective distinction by ear. Continuous adventitious sounds are attributed to narrowing of airways, either by spasm, edema, or thickening of the mucosa, or by luminal obstruction, such as by tumors or secretions.

Despite this welcome initiative in categorizing lung sounds according to pathophysiological principles, the exact mechanisms responsible for production of lung sounds are still speculative. Crackles are believed to be generated by the sudden popping open, in rapid succession, of small airways causing a sequence of "miniexplosions" and resembling the noise made by crumpling cellophane.

Although the mechanisms responsible for crackles (or rales) is still uncertain—a recent concept implicating local tissue forces in their genesis—their diagnostic value is on firmer footing. Early inspiratory rales, usually few in

TABLE 26-2
Classification of Common Lung Sounds

Acoustic Characteristics	American Thoracic Society Nomenclature	Common Synonyms	Laennec's Original Terms
Discontinuous, interrupted explosive sounds Loud, low in pitch; average values: IDW = 1.25, 2CD = 9.32	Coarse crackle	Coarse rale	Rale muquex ou gargouillement
Discontinuous, interrupted explosive sounds Less loud than above and of shorter duration; higher in pitch than course crackles or rales; average values, IDW = 0.92, 2CD = 6.02	Fine crackle	Fine rale, crepitation	Rale humide ou crepitation
Continuous sounds longer than 250 ms, high-pitched; dominant frequency of 400 Hz or more, a hissing sound	Wheeze	Sibilant rhonchus	Rale sibilant sec ou sifflement
Continuous sounds longer than 250 ms, low-pitched; dominant frequency about 200 Hz or less, a snoring sound	Rhonchus	Sonorous rhonchus	Rale sec sonore ou ronflement

SOURCE: After Loudon R, Murphy RLH, 1984.

NOTE: IDW = initial deflection width; 2CD = two cycle duration.

number and best heard at the lung bases, generally represent the opening of small airways that have closed prematurely during the previous expiration, particularly if abetted by a decrease in elastic recoil (emphysema) or secretions in the airways (bronchitis). Persistence of early inspiratory rales is common in obstructive airways disease. Rales that clear after a cough or two have a different meaning since they probably represent secretions in the upper airways.

Rales that occur late in inspiration have a different diagnostic value. In the upright position, they are heard best at the lung bases and they shift toward the dependent parts of the lungs when posture is changed. They occur in interstitial lung disease, e.g., fibrosing alveolitis, asbestosis, and pulmonary edema, and in pneumonia. These rales run the course of the disease. In contrast, late inspiratory rales at the lung bases in the elderly or bedridden generally disappear after a few deep breaths.

MANIFESTATIONS OF RESPIRATORY DISORDERS

The most common clinical manifestations of a respiratory disorder are dyspnea and cough; the latter is usually associated with the production of sputum. Far less common are hemoptysis, thoracic pain, cyanosis, or an abnormal breathing pattern.

Some of these manifestations usually signify local disease, e.g., hemoptysis; others are characteristic of a generalized derangement, e.g., dyspnea. But these distinctions are far from invariable: hemoptysis also occurs in

Goodpasture's syndrome, which inflicts widespread damage on the lungs; conversely, terrifying breathlessness sometimes characterizes the lodging of a foreign body in the upper airways. Therefore, the clinical context, the sequence, and the constellation of signs and symptoms generally determine the importance and significance that is attached to individual manifestations.

A vast majority of respiratory illnesses are in the lungs, but derangement in any part of the control mechanism or of the thoracic cage can also cause clinical disease. The hallmark of these extrapulmonary disorders are cyanosis and disturbances in breathing pattern.

Localized lesions, such as a bronchogenic carcinoma, are sometimes so circumscribed and confined to quiet zones of the lung that they cause no clinical disturbance until they are too far gone for effective therapy (Fig. 26-6). In contrast, other local disorders, such as a pneumonia, generally begin explosively with clinical disability that cannot be ignored.

The likelihood of clinical manifestations increases if the pulmonary lesion affects the airways, large structures at the hilus, or the pleura. This circumstance is typified by carcinoma of the lung in which involvement of the large airways generally evokes cough, sputum, and sometimes hemoptysis. Once a lesion has invaded the hilus (Fig. 26-7A),

FIGURE 26-6 Sagittal (Gough) sections of lung. Normal lungs (*A* and *B*) are included for reference. *A.* Normal lung from a 50-year-old man. *B.* Normal lung from a 76-year-old man. This large lung, once called "senile emphysema," causes no functional abnormality. *C.* Squamous cell carcinoma of the lung. Metastases were present in the brain and spleen. (*Courtesy of Dr. S. Moolten.*)

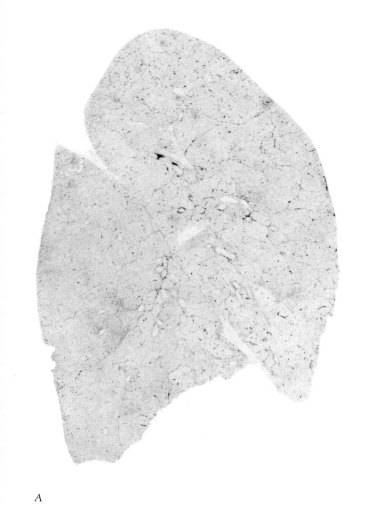

A

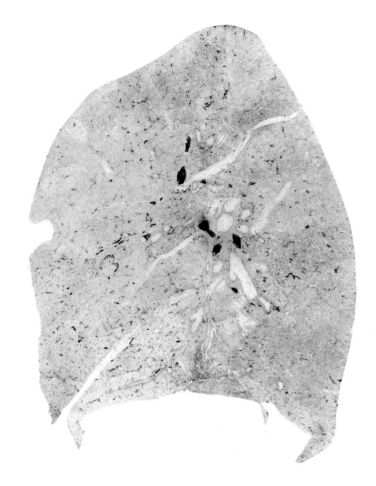

B

C

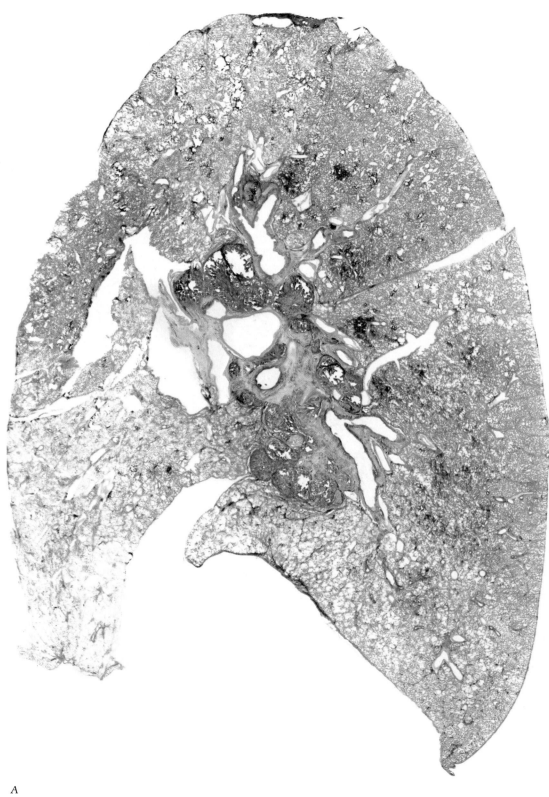

A

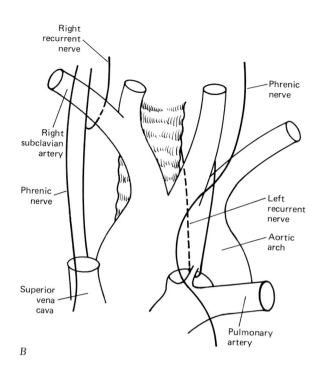

Right
recurrent
nerve

Phrenic
nerve

Right
subclavian
artery

Phrenic
nerve

Left
recurrent
nerve

Aortic
arch

Superior
vena
cava

Pulmonary
artery

B

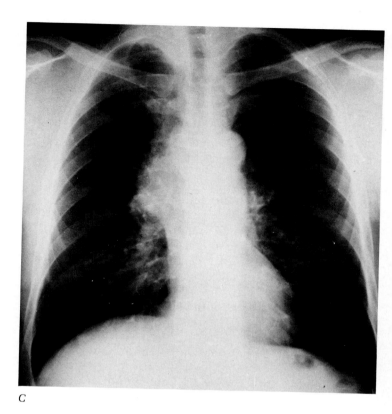

C

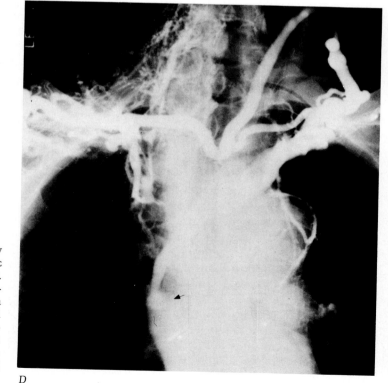

D

FIGURE 26-7 Some features of carcinoma of the lung in the vicinity of the hilus. *A (opposite).* Sagittal section illustrating anaplastic carcinoma (blue) in the vicinity of the hilus. H & E. *(Courtesy of Dr. S. Moolten.)* *B.* Course of the recurrent laryngeal nerves, illustrating relationships to adjacent structures. Invasion of a nerve by a carcinoma of the lung results in paralysis of the ipsilateral vocal cord. *C.* Patient with poorly differentiated squamous cell carcinoma of the lung at the right hilus. The presenting complaint was a "puffy, red" face due to superior vena caval obstruction. *D.* Angiogram in the same patient showing site of obstruction (arrow) and extensive collateral circulation.

a variety of signs can be evoked depending on the structures that it reaches: hoarseness (Fig. 26-7B), plethora (Fig. 26-7C and D), Horner's syndrome, or paralysis of one leaf of the diaphragm. Should the neoplasm gain access to the bloodstream, the stage is set for manifestations of malfunctioning in remote organs, i.e., brain or liver.

Generalized pulmonary disorders are usually chronic, start insidiously, and progress slowly. Not infrequently, progressive infirmity is compensated for by a subconscious circumscription of physical activity supplemented by a natural inclination to ignore early disability. Thus, breathlessness is often attributed to advancing age, obesity, and "poor condition," and some of the more strenuous activities of the day are either avoided or performed at a slower pace. Also, an increase in ventilatory effort is ignored until it becomes incapacitating. Because of this human propensity for self-denial of illness, many individuals with diffuse pulmonary disease do not seek medical help until the respiratory ailment is almost beyond repair.

For convenience, the individual manifestations of respiratory diseases will be considered separately. This approach should not obscure the interrelationships among signs and symptoms that characterize distinctive clinical syndromes. For example, hemoptysis that is recent in origin probably has one cause if it occurs in a middle-aged heavy smoker who has had cough, sputum, and weight loss for a few months and another if it occurs in a breathless patient with the murmur of mitral stenosis. Indeed, to interpret any single manifestation of pulmonary disease, it is essential to take full inventory of the physical and mental state of the patient as well as to place the manifestations in the full perspective of the onset of the circumstances that predisposed to the illness, the pattern of evolution of the disorders, and the other disorders that have to be discounted in arriving at a diagnosis.

Dyspnea

Dyspnea is a professional, or scientific, term for a respiratory sensation that laypersons usually describe as breathlessness or shortness of breath. Unfortunately, the correspondence is not very precise, since each of these terms has its own shades of meaning. In order to stave off semantic confusion, in relating experimental to clinical observations, it is important to bear in mind that when a physician says dyspnea, it almost invariably implies respiratory distress, whereas when the physiologist uses the term, it means only that breathing, which is ordinarily effortless and conducted at subconscious levels, has reached the level of awareness.

No matter how defined, communication about dyspnea is handicapped further on two accounts: (1) it is a subjective experience that is difficult to describe, and probably refers to multiple respiratory sensations; and (2) unlike the sensations of vision or pain, it has proved diffi-

cult to quantify. It is also inherently a complex experience that includes at least two separate elements: (1) the processing of sensory information that is converging upon integrating centers in the brain, not only from the respiratory apparatus, but also from elsewhere in the body and brain; and (2) the interpretation of the sensation. Finally, as noted above, meaningful exchange between patient and examiner has to surmount language difficulties: the patient speaks in terms of "shortness of breath" which the physician has to translate into dyspnea. For example, the normal person uses shortness of breath to describe the breathlessness that follows running for the bus; the asthmatic patient uses the same term for the episode of a tightness of the chest that characterizes a paroxysm of asthma.

Richards described dyspnea as "a strange phenomenon of life, caught midway between the conscious and unconscious, and particularly sensitive to both." It is not difficult to substantiate this view. The everyday example noted above is that of the normal person's dashing for the bus: during the first burst of effort, the individual is too preoccupied with achieving the goal to sense respiratory discomfort. But, once on board, while fumbling for the coin to deposit, the individual suddenly becomes aware of overbreathing: breathing has reached the level of consciousness. In contrast, the asthmatic person caught in an attack is unremittingly preoccupied with breathing; it is impossible for this person to escape the impression that life depends on the next breath. This difference between "awareness of breathing" by the normal individual and respiratory distress of the asthmatic patient who is concerned about the next breath underscores the possible role of emotional factors in altering the sensation of breathlessness. Blunting of the sensorium by narcotics or by acute hypercapnia often eliminates the sensation of breathlessness without modifying the breathing pattern. During Kussmaul's breathing, "air hunger" is obvious, but the patient is often unaware of breathlessness. The subjective experience of breathlessness is very likely to be modified by affective or cognitive influences and by the clinical context in which it is experienced.

Dyspnea due to anxiety is generally described by the patient as "a feeling of smothering" or an "inability to take a satisfying deep breath." These ill-defined sensations have been designated as *psychogenic dyspnea*: the breathing pattern is irregular, the deep sighs feature prominently. Occasionally, the full-blown syndrome of hyperventilation ensues with light-headedness, tingling of the hands and feet, tachycardia, inversion of T waves on the electrocardiogram, and even syncope.

Usually, psychogenic dyspnea poses no diagnostic problem. However, the sensations involved in psychogenic dyspnea are probably entirely different from the "awareness" of breathing described by the normal subject or the tight-chested discomfort of the asthmatic. Psychogenic dyspnea demonstrates that cortical influences can play an important pathogenic role in the sensation of respiratory discomfort.

Not yet readily related to clinical dyspnea are the recent advances in delineating the physiological and psychological basis for the sensations generated during breathing. For example, the pioneering studies of Campbell, which dealt initially with the ability of normal subjects to detect small respiratory mechanical loads, resulted in the formulation of a *length-tension inappropriateness theory* to explain the mechanisms involved in load sensation. Since then, considerable experimental evidence indicates that the intensity of breathlessness increases along with the fraction of the maximum force-generating capacity of the respiratory muscles used in breathing. Deformation could be elicited by pulmonary congestion or edema on the one hand or by interstitial (and peribronchiolar) fibrosis on the other (Fig. 26-8). Because the basic abnormalities in the mechanics of the lungs and airways are virtually irreversible in chronic obstructive airways disease and in widespread interstitial lung disease, the load on the respiratory muscles cannot be appreciably alleviated by medical management. Accordingly, therapeutic interest in these disorders has turned to ways by which the performance of the respiratory muscles can be improved. These have taken the form of training exercises to facilitate adaptive changes and to increase both muscle strength and endurance.

CLINICAL CORRELATES

The closest correlate with dyspnea (sensation of breathlessness) is an excessive ventilation for the level of activity (generally measured as O_2 uptake). Usually, but not invariably, an increase in respiratory rate accounts for most of the increase in ventilation, particularly in patients with stiff lungs, e.g., due to acute or chronic pulmonary congestion and edema. However, worthy of note is the common dissociation of tachypnea and dyspnea: in the patient with chronic mitral stenosis, marked tachypnea is often unassociated with breathlessness. This discrepancy between sensation and objective evidence of excess ventilation indicates that adaptation has occurred to the sensation of breathlessness when the stimulus is sustained.

DYSPNEA AND VENTILATORY PERFORMANCE

Over the years, a variety of indices have been used as physiological guideposts to mechanisms involved in the genesis of dyspnea. Among these have been the level of minute ventilation, the portion of the maximum breathing capacity used for breathing (*breathing reserve*), the work of breathing, and the force exerted upon the lungs by the chest bellows during breathing. Although none of these can explain all instances of dyspnea, they have reinforced the idea that the major causes of dyspnea are to be found in the ventilatory apparatus per se.

Measurements of Ventilation

The level of minute ventilation at rest and during exercise correlates well with the sensation of dyspnea in many patients with diffuse interstitial fibrosis or with chronic bronchitis and emphysema. The correlation is improved by relating minute ventilation to maximum ventilation: the closer the minute ventilation to the maximum breathing capacity, the more likely is the subject to complain of breathlessness. When the actual level of ventilation reaches 30 to 40 percent of the maximum breathing capacity, dyspnea is inevitable.

Unfortunately, the breathing reserve [maximal voluntary ventilation (MVV) minus actual $\dot{V}_E$] correlates better with the dyspnea of normal subjects during exertion than with the dyspnea of chronic bronchitis and emphysema or of left ventricular failure. In chronic bronchitis and emphysema, the actual minute ventilation may be a very large fraction of the MVV (greater than 50 percent) without eliciting dyspnea. In acute left ventricular failure, a mild increase in ventilation and a near-normal MVV may be associated with considerable breathlessness.

Another time-honored correlate of dyspnea is the maximum breathing capacity. It is decreased by diseases of the lungs, airways, or chest cage. The smaller the maximum breathing capacity, the more apt is dyspnea to occur.

Mechanics of Breathing

One teleologic way to regard dyspnea is as a sensation that prompts an unconscious effort to minimize the work, energy cost, or force of breathing (Fig. 26-9). Thus, it protects the respiratory apparatus from overwork and inefficient operation. This approach has led to exploration of the relationships between the work of breathing and dyspnea, and close correlations have been found in various pulmonary and chest wall disorders. Although it has not been possible to identify a critical level for the work of breathing at which dyspnea will occur, fractionation of work of breathing into its elastic, resistive, and inertial components has helped to relate physiological disturbances to particular diseases. For example, in chronic mitral stenosis with pulmonary congestion, the elastic work is greatly increased, whereas in obstructive airways disease, resistive work predominates. Moreover, the concept has emerged that patterns of breathing are automatically adjusted so as to achieve least work for the respiratory muscles.

A related approach has been the determination of the O_2 cost of breathing. The relationship between ventilation and O_2 consumption by the respiratory muscles is curvilinear (Fig. 26-10). The O_2 cost of breathing increases extraordinarily in patients with stiff lungs, obstructive airways disease, and abnormalities of the chest wall. Indeed, the O_2 consumption occasioned by the large ventilatory effort may fail to provide sufficient O_2 for the aerobic needs of the respiratory muscles, leading to anaerobic

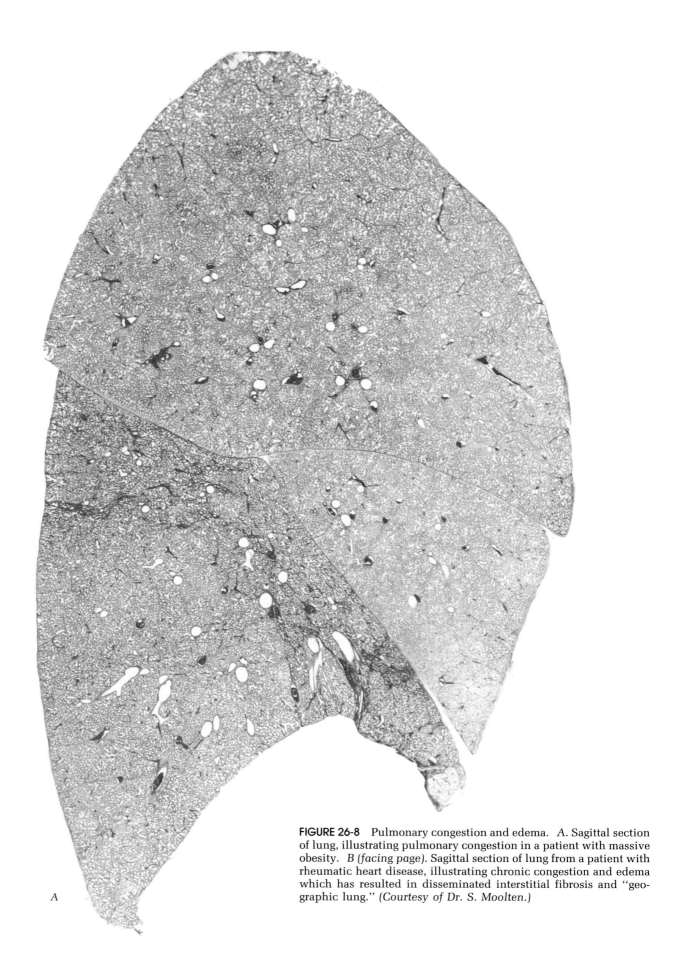

FIGURE 26-8 Pulmonary congestion and edema. A. Sagittal section of lung, illustrating pulmonary congestion in a patient with massive obesity. B (facing page). Sagittal section of lung from a patient with rheumatic heart disease, illustrating chronic congestion and edema which has resulted in disseminated interstitial fibrosis and "geographic lung." (Courtesy of Dr. S. Moolten.)

A

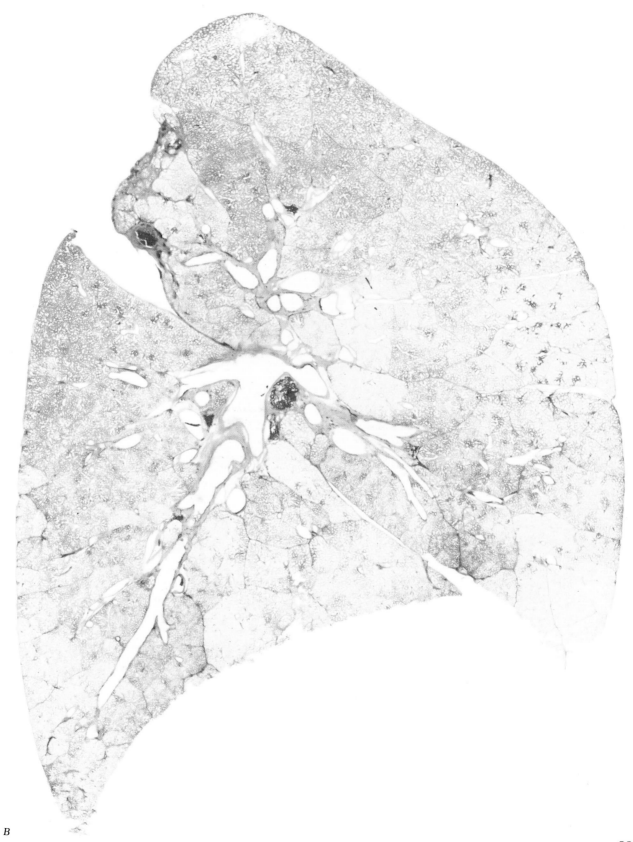

B

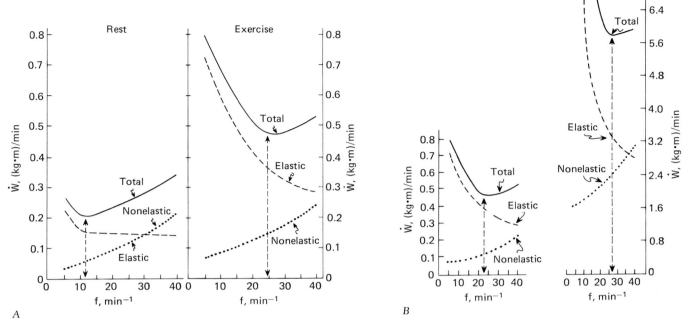

FIGURE 26-9 Calculated work of ventilating the lungs at rest and during exercise. The dashed vertical line (capped by arrowheads) in each frame indicates the respiratory frequency at which respiratory work was minimal. *A.* Normal. The minimal work of breathing at rest was at a respiratory frequency of 12 breaths per minute; during exercise, the minimal work was done at a higher frequency, i.e., 25 breaths per minute. *B.* Mitral stenosis. At rest, the frequency for least respiratory work was abnormally high, i.e., 22 breaths per minute; during exercise it increased further, i.e., to 28 breaths per minute. *(After Christie, 1953, with permission.)*

metabolism and lactic acidosis. Although clearly the greater the abnormality, the greater the O_2 cost and the likelihood of dyspnea, the determination of O_2 cost provides no more useful insight into the mechanism of dyspnea than does the work of breathing; nor is the situation improved by determination of the efficiency of breathing in which the work of breathing is related to its energy cost.

These shortcomings have encouraged the search for other indices. Many years ago, Marshall, Stone, and Christie called attention to the fact that, during exercise, the onset of breathlessness is related to the maximal force exerted by the respiratory muscles, measured as peak intrapleural pressure during inspiration. Subsequently, Mead proposed that the force exerted on the lungs, rather than the mechanical work of breathing, is responsible for the sensation of dyspnea.

At present, dyspnea can be expected to occur whenever a disproportionately large ventilation exists for the level of activity, i.e., when the "breathing reserve" is small. When the lungs and chest bellows are abnormal, the high level of ventilation is associated with other abnormalities, i.e., an inordinate work and energy cost of breathing, and an inordinate force applied to mobilize the lungs. In summary, the intensity of the sensation of breathlessness for any given ventilatory task seems to be related to the fraction of the maximum respiratory-force generating capacity that is utilized.

Exercise Testing

Breathing that is effortless at rest often reaches the level of consciousness during exercise; awareness gives way to intolerable discomfort at low levels of exercise in patients with cardiac or pulmonary disease. By appropriate tests, the overall performance of the cardiopulmonary apparatus in gas exchange and in satisfying the metabolic needs of the body can be tested; often the particular component at fault—cardiac, pulmonary or metabolic—can be identified or surmised (see Chapters 18 and 66).

DYSPNEA IN PULMONARY DISEASE

Acute and chronic diseases of the lungs are common causes of dyspnea. Only three of the most common are considered here.

Chronic Bronchitis and Emphysema

The disturbances in the ventilatory apparatus that result from obstructive disease of the airways are frequently severe (Fig. 26-11). In chronic bronchitis and emphysema, the maximum breathing capacity is consistently impaired. Generally, it correlates well with the severity of the dyspnea, and, as the disease progresses, increasing disability due to dyspnea accompanied by a decreasing maximum breathing capacity is the rule in the "pink puffer." In the "blue bloater" with similar pulmonary disability, dyspnea is less troublesome, presumably because of the

(Text continues on page 336.)

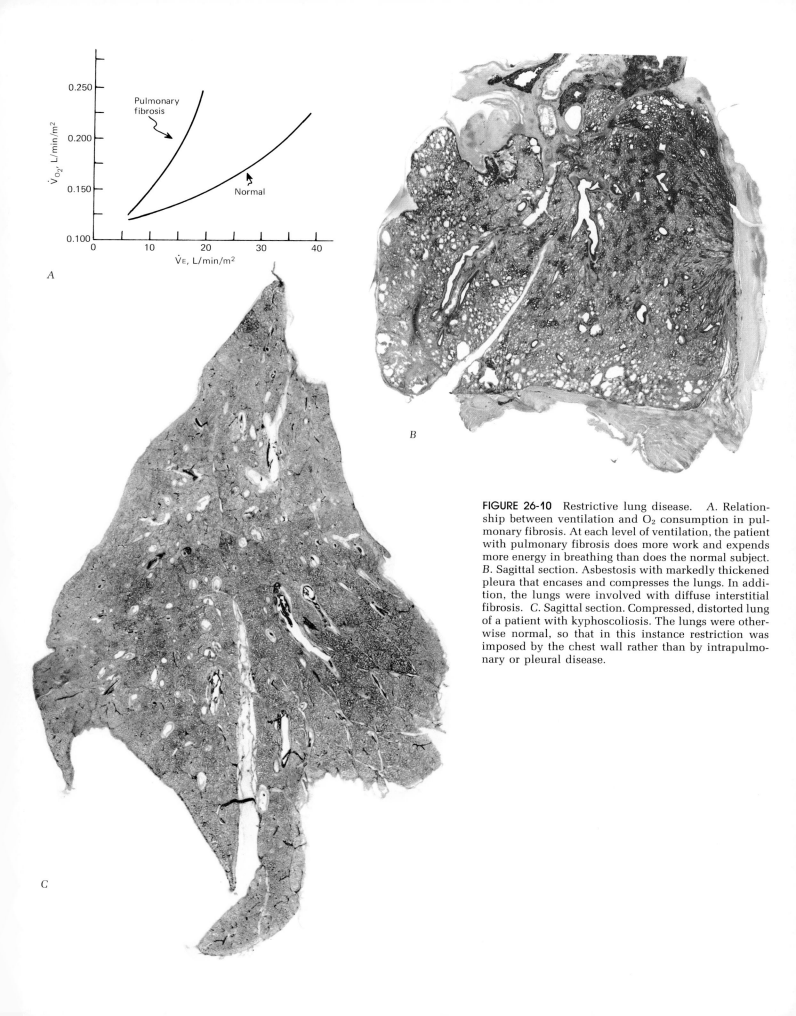

FIGURE 26-10 Restrictive lung disease. *A*. Relationship between ventilation and O_2 consumption in pulmonary fibrosis. At each level of ventilation, the patient with pulmonary fibrosis does more work and expends more energy in breathing than does the normal subject. *B*. Sagittal section. Asbestosis with markedly thickened pleura that encases and compresses the lungs. In addition, the lungs were involved with diffuse interstitial fibrosis. *C*. Sagittal section. Compressed, distorted lung of a patient with kyphoscoliosis. The lungs were otherwise normal, so that in this instance restriction was imposed by the chest wall rather than by intrapulmonary or pleural disease.

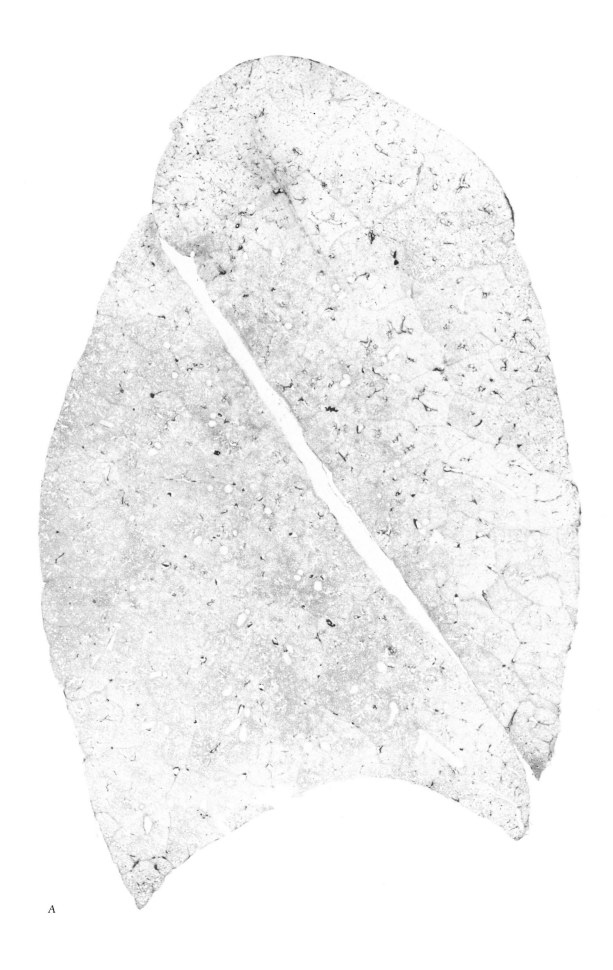

A

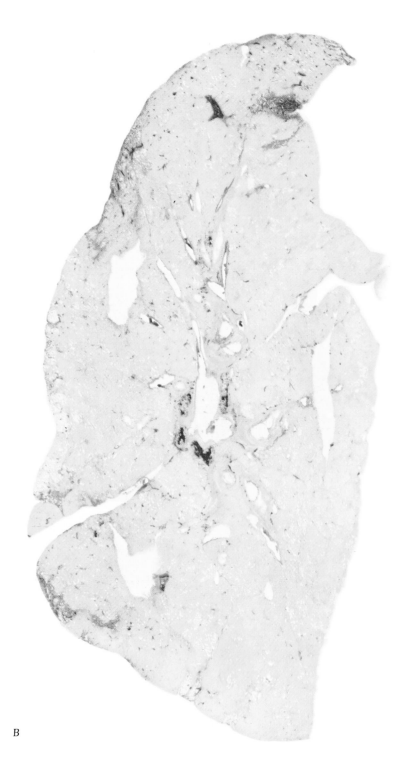

B

◀FIGURE 26-11 Obstructive disease of the airways. Sagittal sections. The first two patients (A and B) are included for reference; the last four (C to F) died with cor pulmonale. A. Normal lung in a patient who died of unrelated disease. The lobular pattern of the gas-exchanging surface of the lung is apparent. B. Alveolar proteinosis. The normal pattern shown in A is obscured by proteinaceous fluid that gives the lung a waxy appearance. (*Courtesy of Dr. S. Moolten.*)

(*Continued on next page*)

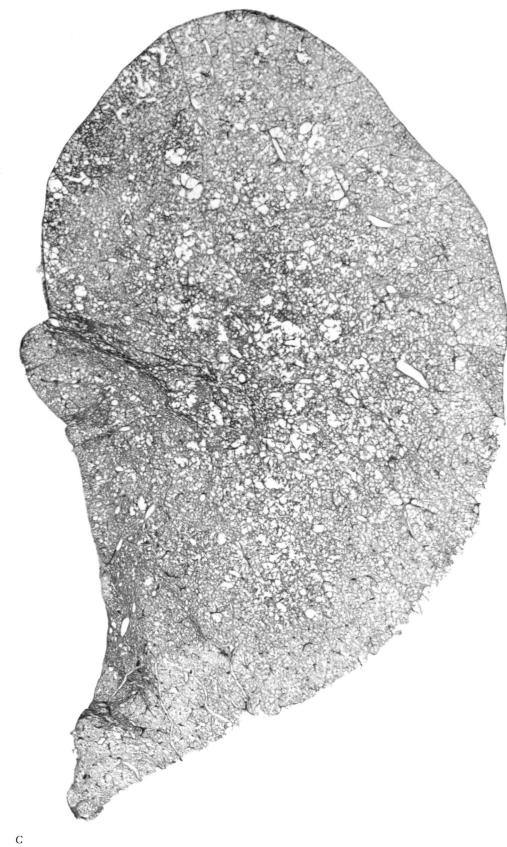

C

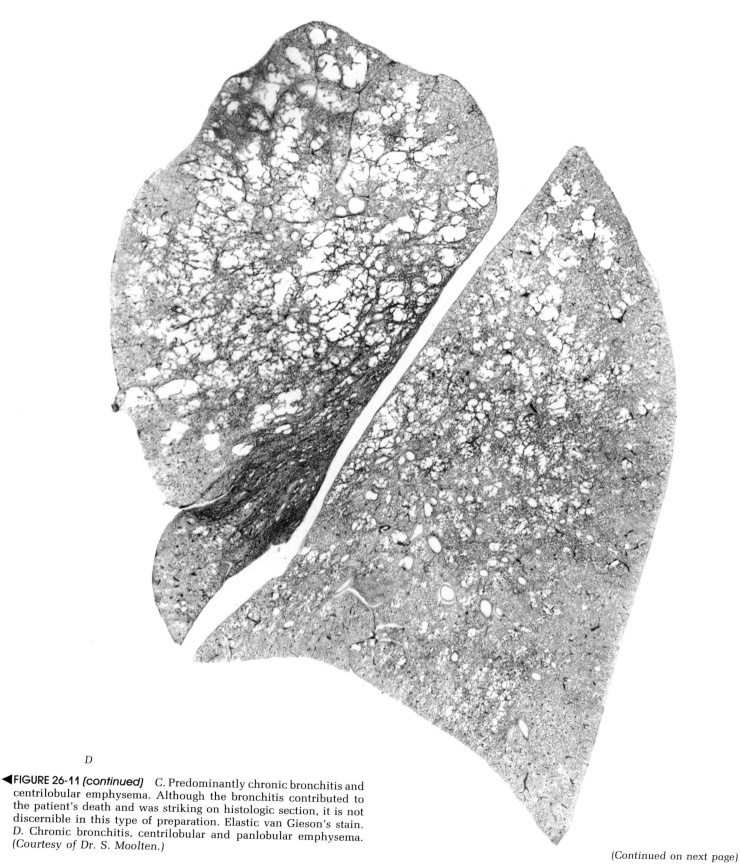

D

◀FIGURE 26-11 *(continued)* C. Predominantly chronic bronchitis and centrilobular emphysema. Although the bronchitis contributed to the patient's death and was striking on histologic section, it is not discernible in this type of preparation. Elastic van Gieson's stain. D. Chronic bronchitis, centrilobular and panlobular emphysema. *(Courtesy of Dr. S. Moolten.)*

(Continued on next page)

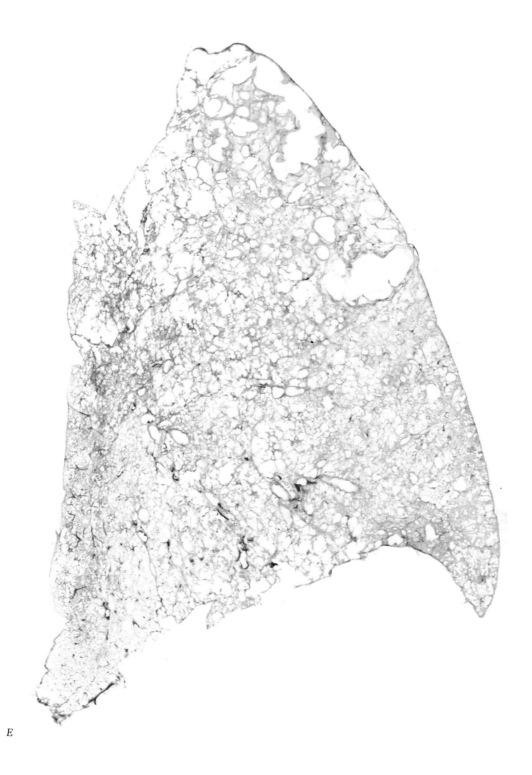

E

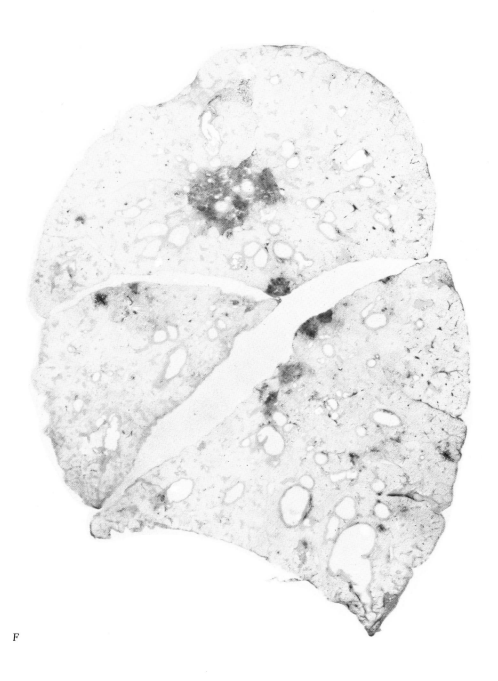

F

◀FIGURE 26-11 *(continued)*   *E.* Predominant panlobular emphysema. Centrilobular emphysema is less marked.   *F.* Cystic fibrosis of the pancreas. The large bronchi are widely dilated and were full of in- spissated mucoid material, whereas the parenchymal architecture is well preserved. *(Courtesy of Dr. S. Moolten.)*

chronic hypercapnia, the diminished urge to breathe, and the lesser increase in resting minute ventilation.

The work of breathing is also increased. At rest, it often is only slightly greater than normal, but on exercise, it increases greatly. The patient with bronchitis and emphysema often does more work in breathing at rest than the normal individual during moderate exercise. The greatest part of this work is spent on overcoming resistance to airflow in the airways, an act requiring active participation of the expiratory muscles.

The O_2 cost of breathing is correspondingly high. Dramatic increments in O_2 consumption have been recorded in resting patients with chronic bronchitis and emphysema as they increased their ventilation: instead of the normal increase of about 1 ml of O_2 uptake per liter of ventilation per minute, the O_2 uptake increases enormously, e.g., up to 25 ml/min. Relief of bronchitis causes the O_2 consumption to decrease, but generally not to normal, e.g., to 6 ml/L of ventilation per minute.

Total ventilation at rest in chronic bronchitis and emphysema is often only slightly larger than normal, but it occupies an abnormally large fraction of the maximum breathing capacity. The swings in intrapleural pressure (a measure of force applied to the lungs) are large, and a considerable muscular effort is expended in breathing.

The increased resistances that have to be overcome during breathing, the augmented O_2 costs of breathing, and the increased forces applied to the lungs during breathing are all likely sources of stimuli that converge upon the brain. In addition, abnormalities in arterial blood-gas composition provide chemical stimuli that may both excite and depress the brain. Finally, should O_2 delivery to the overworked respiratory muscles be insufficient, fatigue and exhaustion may add nervous and chemical signals of their own. In those patients who develop heart failure, the accumulation of excess water in the lungs provides additional stimulation from "J-like receptors."

One intriguing enigma is why some patients with chronic bronchitis and emphysema settle for a lower ventilation than others. For example, despite equal abnormalities in conventional pulmonary function tests, the blue bloater, who has powerful ventilatory stimuli in the form of respiratory acidosis and arterial hypoxemia, often breathes less than does the pink puffer, who has near-normal blood-gas levels. One reward of this adaptation for the blue bloater is less dyspnea, presumably due, directly or indirectly, to the lower ventilation.

Recently, Gottfried has shown evidence of blunting of the ability of patients with chronic obstructive airways disease both in detecting small resistive loads and in scaling the magnitude of added loads; the blunting of respiratory sensations was proportional to their ability to respond to loading by increasing their ventilation. These abnormalities in detecting and scaling resistive loads may

be an expression of adaptation to the chronic loading imposed by the airways disease.

Pulmonary Fibrosis

In widespread fibrosis, the maximum breathing capacity is generally well preserved (Fig. 26-12). Both at rest and during exercise, patients with pulmonary fibrosis breathe faster and more than do normal subjects (Fig. 26-10). The work of ventilating the stiff lungs is increased. Tachypnea is the rule. Often, the tachypnea appears inordinate for the degree of parenchymal involvement that can be seen on the chest radiograph. In these patients, it seems likely that the considerable muscular effort associated with ventilating the abnormal lungs and the sustained tachypnea are involved in the sensation of dyspnea. During exercise, when both the mechanical and nervous stimuli are driving the ventilation, the sensation of dyspnea may become oppressive.

Asthma

This disorder evokes several different respiratory sensations. Paramount is the "tightness" in the chest that is quite different from the ordinary breathlessness that identifies dyspnea in normal individuals. Emotional factors can strongly affect the sensation of dyspnea in asthma. Also, part of the variability encountered between the degree of dyspnea and the severity of airways obstruction may be attributable to adaptation over time to the airways obstruction. The possibility also exists that behavioral conditioning occurs in these patients, leading to the adoption of breathing patterns that minimize dyspnea.

DYSPNEA IN CARDIAC DISEASE

The mechanisms responsible for dyspnea in cardiac disease differ depending on the stiffness of the lungs.

Cardiac Disease with Stiff Lungs

In cardiac disease associated with chronic pulmonary venous hypertension, a variety of anatomic changes can stiffen the lungs, stimulate the ventilation, and contribute to an increase in the work of breathing. Among these are congestion, edema, and pulmonary fibrosis (Fig. 26-8). Swings in pleural pressure are large, and resistance to airflow in the intrapulmonary airways may also be greater than normal, thereby adding to the work and energy cost of breathing. Arterial hypoxemia is modest, but probably augments the ventilatory drive. Exercise exaggerates the pulmonary congestion and edema, promotes arterial and mixed venous hypoxemia and increases the dyspnea.

In patients with pulmonary congestion and edema, tachypnea is a regular feature at rest, and increases during exercise. Although tachypnea is consistent, its degree is generally modest and probably not entirely responsible for the dyspnea. Fatigue is a common concomitant of low cardiac output and may stem from diminishing O_2 deliv-

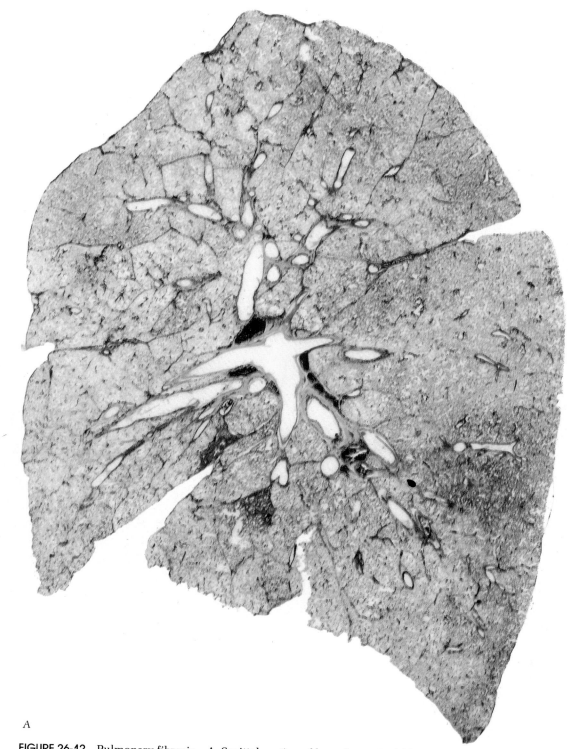

A

FIGURE 26-12 Pulmonary fibrosis. A. Sagittal section of lung. Interstitial fibrosis with areas of focal pneumonia (dark areas).

(Continued on next page)

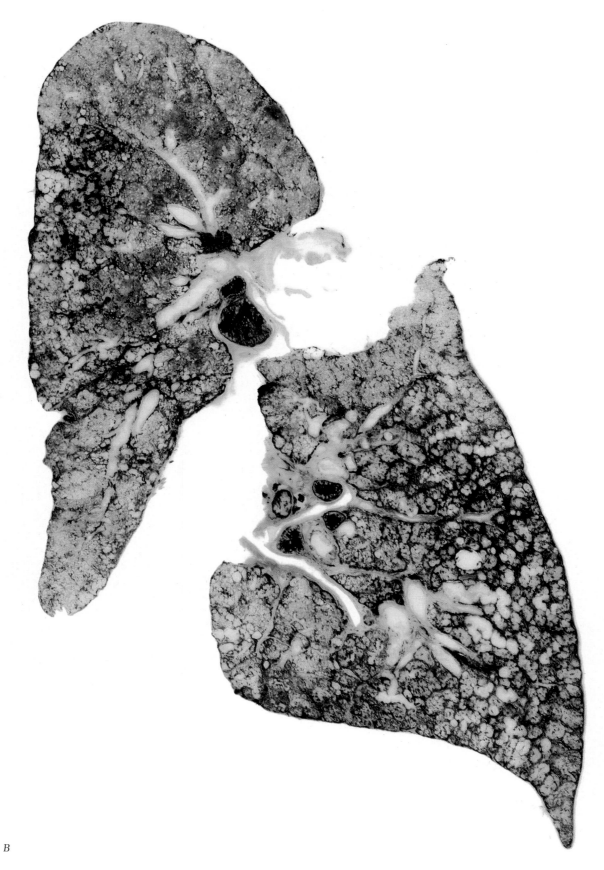

ery to the respiratory muscles, thereby contributing to respiratory discomfort.

Cardiac Disease without Stiff Lungs

Dyspnea occurs in many forms of heart disease that are not associated with congestion of the lungs. Uncomplicated pulmonic stenosis is an excellent example. Probably the symptom is related to an inadequate cardiac output during exercise. In tetralogy of Fallot, dyspnea is sometimes severe and often relieved by assuming a squatting position. In this and other forms of cyanotic heart disease, both dyspnea and fatigue appear during exertion when the arterial oxyhemoglobin saturation has fallen appreciably below the resting level.

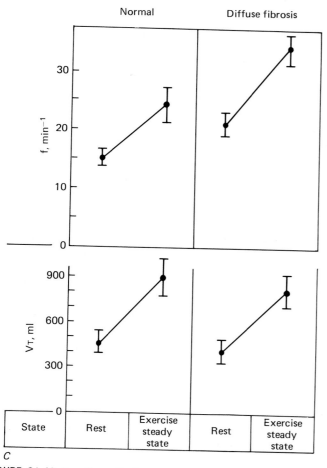

Anemia

Exertional dyspnea is a common symptom of anemia and is particularly marked in the more acute and the severe forms. Its pathogenesis is not completely understood, but may reflect inadequate O_2 delivery to the contracting respiratory muscles.

DYSPNEA: A SYNTHESIS

Dyspnea is a medical translation of the patient's complaint of difficult breathing. It encompasses several different respiratory sensations. In medicine, distinction is rarely made between respiratory discomfort and the normal sensation of breathlessness that healthy individuals experience immediately after exercise. Physiologists have focused on the relationship between breathlessness and the effort of breathing. They have concluded that the sensation generally originates in the ventilatory apparatus. Although the stimuli, the sensory receptors, and the nerve pathways that participate in its appreciation are unknown, it is known that a wide variety of receptors, both within and without the lungs, can convey information to the brain, thereby bringing breathing to the level of consciousness. In the brain, this sensory information is modulated and integrated and is either brought to the level of consciousness or suppressed at a subconscious level. Awareness is a prerequisite for the perception of dyspnea. Distraction or blunting of consciousness affects the awareness of dyspnea.

Because dyspnea is a subjective sensation and involves consciousness and communication between patient and physician, its analysis depends heavily on observations of human beings. Numerous acute and chronic lung diseases affect the various components of the ventilatory apparatus. Such disturbances, if sufficiently severe, decrease the capacity of the apparatus to ventilate and exaggerate the effort that is necessary for it to function. In many conditions, the levels of ventilation required at rest and especially during exercise are greater than normal and serve to overtax a disabled ventilatory apparatus.

To appraise dyspnea clinically, it is necessary to relate the level of ventilation and the pattern of breathing to the clinical and physiological disorders. By use of history and physical examination, insights have to be sought into the disability of the ventilatory apparatus, and factors that increase the demands for ventilation must be sought. Detailed studies of pulmonary and cardiac function are often helpful. However, until some way is developed to quantify dyspnea as a sensation, correlations in the clinic and in the laboratory are destined to remain empirical.

Orthopnea

Orthopnea is a common symptom of pulmonary congestion. It is the term applied to dyspnea at rest while in the recumbent, but not in the upright or semivertical, posi-

◀FIGURE 26-12 *(continued)* *B.* Sagittal section of lung. Interstitial fibrosis associated with honeycomb lung and alveolar cell carcinoma (bottom right). *(Courtesy of Dr. S. Moolten.)* *C.* Restrictive lung disease. Ventilatory patterns at rest and during exercise. At rest, patients with pulmonary fibrosis have a higher respiratory rate and a slightly lower tidal volume than the normal subjects. During exercise, the respiratory rate increases much more than the tidal volume (49 normal subjects and 19 patients with diffuse interstitial fibrosis.) *(After Lourenco, Turino, Davidson, Fishman, 1965.)*

tion. It is usually relieved by two or three pillows under the head and back. Marshall and coworkers observed in patients with mitral stenosis considerable decrease in pulmonary compliance in the flat as compared to the upright position. The swings in intrapleural pressure during the respiratory cycle were consequently greater (over 50 cmH$_2$O) and the work of breathing was two to three times greater in recumbency than in the upright position. The respiratory rate also increased to a frequency that corresponded strikingly to the frequency at which the work of ventilating the more rigid lungs was at a minimum.

The decrease in compliance on lying flat probably is related to the fact that more of the lung lies at or below the level of the heart. Thus, the increased vascular pressures are distributed throughout a greater portion of the lungs and are augmented in the most dependent regions by the overlying column of blood. In the upright position, a greater portion of the lungs lies above the heart. In these regions, pulmonary venous and capillary pressures are lowered by hydrostatic effects.

Vigorous movements of the chest bellows are effected more readily in the upright position. This probably explains why some patients with chronic lung disease or bronchial asthma are intolerant of the recumbent position.

Paroxysmal Nocturnal Dyspnea

Paroxysmal nocturnal dyspnea occurs in mitral stenosis or in any condition that taxes the left ventricle sufficiently to cause it to fail (such as hypertension or aortic insufficiency). The attack may be severe, dramatic, and terrifying.

The patient is aroused from sleep gasping for air and must sit up or stand to catch his or her breath; sweating may be profuse. Sometimes the patient throws a window open wide in an attempt to relieve the oppressive sensation of suffocation. The chest tends to become fixed in the position of forced inspiration. Both inspiratory and expiratory wheezes, often simulating typical asthma, are heard. In some instances, overt pulmonary edema occurs, accompanied by many rales at end-inspiration; the acute pulmonary edema rarely terminates fatally. Occasionally, the attacks recur several times a night, necessitating that the patient sleep upright in a chair.

Responsible for these attacks are the factors that produce orthopnea (see above) as well as the pulmonary hypervolemia that follows mobilization of peripheral edema fluid toward the lungs when body position is changed from vertical to horizontal upon retiring. The acute pulmonary hypervolemia increases pulmonary venous and capillary pressures and imposes a barely tolerable burden on the left ventricle. The actual attack is often "triggered" by coughing, abdominal distention, the hyperpneic phase of Cheyne-Stokes respiration, a startling noise, or anything causing a sudden increase in heart rate and further

acute increase in pulmonary venous and capillary pressures. Usually, the attack is terminated by assumption of the erect position and a few deep breaths of air. Cough, an important manifestation of pulmonary congestion, frequently occurs during the attack.

Cardiac Asthma

The asthmatic wheezes often heard in patients with pulmonary congestion have given rise to the term *cardiac asthma*. The wheezes are a manifestation of pulmonary edema, and often are accompanied by other signs of this disorder. An important element in the production of cardiac asthma is the reduction in the lumen of the airways and thickening of bronchial walls by edema. In addition, the high intrathoracic pressures that are required to overcome the obstruction during expiration tend to narrow the airways further and even to collapse them. The resistance to airflow is increased somewhat during both inspiration and expiration in pulmonary congestion, but becomes much more abnormal in frank pulmonary edema. The compliance of the lungs is reduced greatly in pulmonary edema, and values as low as one-tenth normal are sometimes reached. Upon recovery from edema, airway resistance and pulmonary compliance return toward normal.

Abnormal Breathing Patterns

An important clue to the nature of a clinical problem in pulmonary disease is sometimes provided by bedside observation of a patient's respiratory pattern. The pertinent features are the rate, regularity, depth, and apparent effort involved. A normal person at rest breathes from 8 to 16 times per minute, with a tidal volume of 400 to 800 ml. The pattern is quite regular except for an occasional slow, deep breath, and the respiratory movements appear effortless. Normally there is a brief end-expiratory phase that is abolished during sleep.

Limited and paradoxical ventilatory excursions provide important, often telltale, insight into the nature of the underlying disorder. Central depression, due to narcotic overdosage, sometimes slows breathing to the point of complete arrest. Restriction in the depth of breathing, and a corresponding increase in frequency, is characteristic of restrictive lung disease due to interstitial fibrosis and of acute pulmonary edema. Labored breathing at the top of the lung volume, abetted by pursed lips to enlarge the caliber of the airways, is characteristic of severe obstructive airways disease. Involvement of a pleural space by pneumothorax, effusion, or fibrothorax limits excursions on the affected side. Severe skeletal deformity may limit chest excursions to the point of alveolar hypoventilation; massive obesity can do the same. Neuromuscular weakness, from any cause, can not only diminish ventilatory excursions due to general involvement of the respiratory muscles (e.g., myasthenia gravis, Guillain-Barré syndrome) but may, by paralyzing certain respiratory muscles, impose added demands upon the unaffected muscles (e.g., residua of poliomyelitis). Massive chest trauma can impair chest movements by causing flail chest, often in association with the consequences of injury to the diaphragm. Weaning from mechanical ventilators relies heavily on the coordinated motions of the chest and abdomen for success.

KUSSMAUL'S BREATHING

This form of breathing is characterized by a regular pattern, a moderate or slightly rapid rate, an abnormally large tidal volume, and usually little apparent effort. The end-expiratory pause is abolished. Despite the apparent increase in ventilation, the arterial blood gases are virtually normal, i.e., the patient is hyperpneic rather than hyperventilating. This is the pattern adopted automatically by normal individuals during exercise; in patients with metabolic acidosis it occurs at rest.

OBSTRUCTED BREATHING

In the presence of airway obstruction, the work of breathing is minimized by maintaining a slow rate and increased tidal volume. Depending on the site of obstruction, either inspiration or expiration may be relatively prolonged and labored and is often associated with audible wheezing or stridor.

RESTRICTED BREATHING

This type of breathing is characterized by a small tidal volume and a rapid rate, often with little apparent effort. It is seen in patients with a decrease in distensibility of the lung or chest wall or with reduction of the vital capacity from any other cause. During exercise, minute ventilation increases inordinately with respect to the level of O_2 uptake, and frequency increases more than tidal volume (Fig. 26-8).

GASPING RESPIRATIONS

This pattern is characteristic of severe cerebral hypoxia. It consists of irregular, quick inspirations associated with extension of the neck and followed by a long expiratory pause. It is commonly seen in shock or in other conditions associated with severe reduction in cardiac output.

CHEYNE-STOKES RESPIRATION

One distinctive pattern of periodic breathing is Cheyne-Stokes breathing. It is characterized by alternating periods of hypoventilation and hyperventilation (Fig. 26-13). In its typical form, an apneic phase that lasts for 15 to 60 s is followed by a phase during which tidal volume increases with each breath to a peak level and then decreases in a progressive fashion to the apneic phase. At the onset of

apnea, CO_2 tension in brachial or femoral arterial blood is at its lowest. As apnea persists, CO_2 tension gradually increases, and respiration is simulated. Carbon dioxide tension continues to increase until maximum hyperventilation is attained, after which it and ventilation decrease until apnea again occurs. The arterial oxyhemoglobin saturation varies in an inverse manner, being highest at onset of apnea and lower during midhyperpnea. During the cycle, CO_2 tension varies by as much as 14 mmHg and oxyhemoglobin saturation by as much as 18 percent.

One of the factors fundamental to the production of the respiratory oscillations is the circulatory-induced delay in the feedback of information to the brain regarding the effects of ventilation on the pulmonary capillary blood. The circulation time from lung to peripheral artery has been shown to be one-half of the length of the Cheyne-Stokes cycle. Thus, the oscillating ventilatory pattern produces cyclic variations in the concentrations of respiratory gases in blood passing through the lungs; these cyclic variations eventually reach the respiratory control system, but with a temporal phase shift of 180°. Cheyne-Stokes breathing has been produced in dogs by prolonging the circulation time from heart to brain using an external circuit.

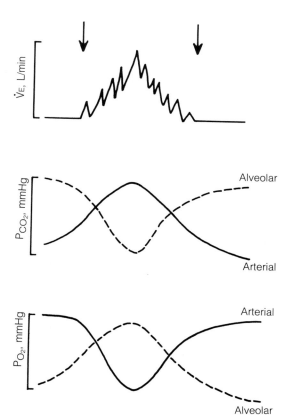

FIGURE 26-13 Cheyne-Stokes breathing, illustrating the relationship between the ventilation and the blood and alveolar gas tensions during the periods of apnea and hyperpnea. (*After Cherniack and Fishman with permission.*)

At one time, the respiratory center was believed to be depressed in Cheyne-Stokes respiration. This hypothesis was in error, since it has been shown that the respiratory response to inhalation of CO_2 is greater than normal. Respiratory alkalosis is frequently present, and the arterial P_{CO_2} remains subnormal in both the apneic and hyperpneic phases.

Plum and Brown have called attention to supramedullary dysfunction of the brain in the pathogenesis of Cheyne-Stokes respiration: in most of their patients who had destructive lesions of the central portion of the tegmentum of the pons, a stage of typical Cheyne-Stokes respirations anteceded the development of an absolutely regular hyperpnea (central neurogenic hyperventilation).

Cheyne-Stokes respiration is sometimes seen in normal infants, in healthy elderly persons, and in normal individuals at high altitude. It also follows the administration of respiratory depressants (e.g., morphine) and often accompanies an increase in intracranial pressure, uremia, or coma.

Cyclic changes in cerebral blood flow during Cheyne-Stokes respiration (flow being greater during hyperpnea) probably account for any fluctuations in mental state, electroencephalographic pattern, and signs of nervous system dysfunction during the cycle.

SIGHING RESPIRATIONS

A strikingly irregular pattern of breathing with frequent, deep, sighing inspirations is seen in anxious patients, but is rarely associated with structural disease of the lungs.

Hypoventilation

Clinical recognition or suspicion of inadequate ventilation is of considerable therapeutic, as well as diagnostic, importance, but it is surprising how frequently even a grossly reduced minute volume is apt to be overlooked if breathing is not labored. Minute ventilation can be estimated at the bedside as the product of respiratory rate and tidal volume. Normally, it exceeds 5 L/min. The adequacy of the tidal volume can be assessed roughly from the extent of thoracic excursions, by listening for the intensity and duration of breath sounds, and by feeling the rate at which air is expired using a hand in front of the patient's mouth. It should be emphasized that an adequate minute ventilation is associated with alveolar hypoventilation during shallow breathing or when lung disease causes an inordinate dead-space ventilation. Alveolar hypoventilation is usually the result of severe alterations in the mechanics of breathing, such as marked airway obstruction, or of abnormalities in the control of breathing caused by a cerebrovascular accident, head trauma, or oversedation.

Cough

An important element in the self-cleansing and protective mechanisms of the lungs is an explosive expiration, i.e., a cough; it protects the lungs against aspiration and helps the movement of secretions and other airway constituents upward to the mouth. It is a complex reflex act that usually arises from stimulation of the bronchial mucosa somewhere between the larynx and the second-order bronchi. The stimuli are diverse: inhaled particles, mucus that has been elaborated by the lining of the airways, inflammatory exudate in airways or parenchyma, a new growth or foreign body in an airway, or pressure on the external wall of the bronchus. On rare occasions the cause is remote: impacted cerumen in an external ear or an inflammatory process of the pleura.

A cough that is hardly noticed by the patient is sometimes important as an early manifestation of disease. An acute, nonproductive cough often heralds the start of an acute bronchitis or a viral pneumonia. An inhaled foreign body elicits a dry cough that persists until it is removed. Irritating fumes also elicit a dry cough.

Much more worrisome clinically is a persistent dry cough of uncertain etiology. Most often, a persistent dry cough is caused by an endobronchial tumor (Fig. 26-14) or pulmonary congestion. Occasionally, it is caused by extraluminal pressure on the trachea or bronchus. When persistent cough is not associated with abnormal chest radiographs, lung cancer is infrequent. In this type of patient, fiberoptic bronchoscopy is usually of little help. Conversely, in some instances, spirometry or bronchial challenge with methacholine reveals unsuspected asthma, i.e., cough is a clinical wheeze equivalent.

A dry cough has different implications from a productive cough. Before accepting a cough as nonproductive, it should be auditioned with particular reference to the possibility that sputum has been produced but swallowed. Much confusion about the productivity of cough in British versus American patients with chronic bronchitis was dispelled by careful analysis of the cough that both American patients and examiners had originally discounted as nonproductive, finding it to be productive.

A cough that is productive of purulent sputum is generally a reliable indication of infection in the tracheobronchial tree or lung. When this symptom is associated with an acute illness, the characteristics of the sputum may be of considerable diagnostic help. Rust-colored sputum, which obtains its distinctive coloration from the even dispersion of blood in yellow, purulent sputum, occurs most often in pneumococcal pneumonia. The sputum in Friedländer pneumonia often resembles currant jelly: it also contains blood, but its appearance is bright red and more translucent and viscid than the sputum of pneumococcal pneumonia. Purulent sputum with a foul odor usually

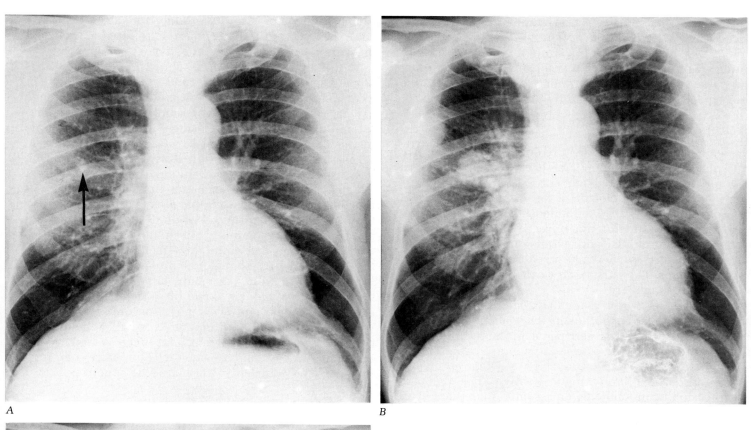

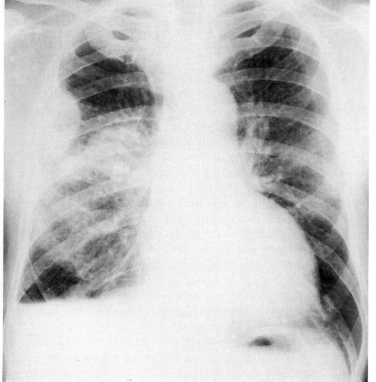

A

B

C

FIGURE 26-14   Carcinoma of the lung in a 70-year-old man. It was first manifested by a cough that persisted for several weeks and by recurrent slight hemoptysis. *A.* Chest radiograph when first seen. A small nodule is in the right midlung (arrow). *B.* Fourteen months later. The nodule has grown into a large mass with metastases to the pleura and hilar lymph nodes. *C.* Three months after *B.* Further growth of masses in the right lung with metastases to the hilar and peribronchial lymph nodes, pleura, and fourth and fifth ribs on the right. The patient died 2 months later of severe pneumonia on the right upper lobe and of left lobar pneumonia.

indicates an anaerobic infection, commonly due to streptococci or *Bacteroides* in a lung abscess. A persistent cough that is productive of purulent sputum occurs in chronic bronchitis, bronchiectasis, and a variety of other suppurative conditions. Sputum which is mucoid is a consequence of any long-standing bronchial irritant.

MECHANISM

A cough can be voluntary or involuntary. Often the two interplay as the patient deliberately attempts to control an involuntary cough. A cough consists of the following steps: an inspiration; closure of the glottis; contraction of the expiratory muscles (abdominal and thoracic) to develop high pressure in the lungs (Fig. 26-15); sudden opening of the glottis; and expulsion of a burst of air through airways that were narrowed by the high intrathoracic pressures. The burst of air carries with it the offending particulate matter.

Attempts have been made to explain the efficiency of the cough in bulk transport using the concepts of dynamic compression of airways and equal pressure points (see Chapters 13 and 163). In essence, dynamic compression of intrathoracic airways occurs during a cough as pleural pressures become increasingly positive. The dynamic compression is undoubtedly an essential ingredient of an effective cough since airway cross section decreases without decreasing flow; in this way, the linear velocity of gas molecules in the airstream is increased, thereby enhancing the movement of offending particles at the wall of the airway. The lung volume at which the cough occurs influences the effectiveness of the cough: cough is only effective in removing particles downstream (toward the mouth) from the "equal pressure points." In healthy individuals at high lung volumes, the equal pressure points are located in the larger airways; they move upstream (toward the alveoli) as lung volume decreases. A series of coughs without an intervening inspiration moves the equal pressure points closer and closer to the small airways, thereby helping to clear the depths of the lungs.

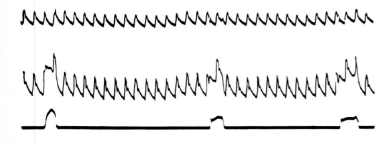

FIGURE 26-15 Circulatory consequences of a cough. The upper tracing was obtained using a differential manometer which subtracted the intrathoracic pressure *(bottom trace)* from systemic arterial pressures recorded directly via an indwelling needle *(middle trace).* *(After Hamilton, Woodbury, Harper, 1944, with permission.)*

Changes in compressibility produced by airways disease could be expected to have important effects on the equal pressure points and on the effectiveness of cough.

Although the concept of "equal pressure points" is beyond cavil, translating the concept into the anatomy of a cough is difficult. For example, although it is possible to generalize about how equal pressure points move as pleural and alveolar pressures change, it is neither a simple matter to define the anatomic sites at which the equal pressure points occur nor to differentiate compressed, from patent, airways. Also, although it seems clear that lengths of compressed segments change with lung volume, the lengths of airways that are compressed is uncertain. At present, theories based on dynamic compression and equal pressure points are useful in picturing events in the airways that determine the effectiveness of cough in the bulk transport of material predominantly from the large, but also from the small, airways. However, the translation from models to real life is largely hypothetical in normal people and even more speculative when airways are mechanically abnormal, except that one can recognize that when airflow rates and linear velocity of gas molecules are low, and airways are abnormally compressible, cough is inevitably destined to be effective.

SITES OF STIMULATION

It is natural for physical examination directed toward finding the reason for a cough to focus on the respiratory tract. However, continuing alert has to be maintained to avoid overlooking not only the upper airways, i.e., the larynx and the nasal sinus, but also remote areas, such as the ears and the heart.

In the lungs, receptors in the epithelium of the mucosal lining of the airways are the sites of stimulation leading to cough. These "irritant" receptors in the large airways are histologically indistinguishable from those in the distal ramifications of the tracheobronchial tree, but they are more consistent in eliciting a cough.

Three categories of stimuli are commonly involved: mechanical, inflammatory, and psychogenic. A familiar cause of cough is the inhalation of smoke or dust. In cigarette smokers, the acute irritation of inhaled particles and fumes is compounded by residual pharyngitis, laryngitis, and tracheobronchitis. Another cause is distortion of airways by pulmonary fibrosis or atelectasis. Less common, but diagnostically important, are the distortions produced by extrabronchial masses, particularly mediastinal tumor or aortic aneurysm.

Most often cough reflects tracheobronchial inflammation and its sequelae. The site of predominant irritation can sometimes be localized by accompanying symptoms. The cough of acute tracheitis is often associated with retrosternal "burning." Acute laryngitis is usually associated with hoarseness and sore throat as well as cough. Tuberculosis of the larynx is associated not only with painful swallowing but also with unequivocal evidence of pulmonary tuberculosis.

As a general rule, cough represents organic disease. On occasion, psychogenic cough occurs in troubled individuals; this cough is generally dry and can be related to nervous tension. An organic cough is often aggravated by psychogenic stress.

SPECIFIC ETIOLOGIES

Occasionally, as in chronic bronchitis or in bronchiectasis, a cough is distinctive and points to etiology (Table 26-3).

TABLE 26-3
Some Causes and Characteristics of Coughs

Cause	Characteristics
Acute infections of lungs	
Tracheobronchitis	Cough associated with sore throat, running nose and eyes.
Lobar pneumonia	Cough often preceded by symptoms of upper respiratory infection; cough dry, painful at first; later becomes productive.
Bronchopneumonia	Usually begins as acute bronchitis; dry or productive cough.
Mycoplasma and viral pneumonia	Paroxysmal cough, productive of mucoid or blood-stained sputum associated with flulike syndrome.
Exacerbation of chronic bronchitis	Cough productive of mucoid sputum becomes purulent.
Chronic infections of lungs	
Bronchitis	Cough productive of sputum on most days for more than 3 consecutive months and for more than 2 successive years. Sputum mucoid until acute exacerbation, when it becomes mucopurulent.
Bronchiectasis	Cough copious, foul, purulent, often since childhood. Forms layer upon standing.
Tuberculosis or fungus	Persistent cough for weeks to months often with blood-tinging of sputum.
Parenchymal inflammatory processes	
Interstitial fibrosis and infiltrations	Cough nonproductive, persistent, depends on etiology.
Smoking	Cough usually associated with injected pharynx; persistent, most marked in morning, usually only slightly productive unless succeeded by chronic bronchitis.
Tumors	
Bronchogenic carcinoma	Nonproductive to productive cough for weeks to months; recurrent small hemoptysis common.
Alveolar cell carcinoma	Cough similar to bronchogenic carcinoma except in occasional instance when large quantities of watery, mucoid sputum are produced.
Benign tumors in airways	Cough nonproductive, occasionally hemoptysis.
Mediastinal tumors	Cough, often with breathlessness, caused by compression of trachea and bronchi.
Aortic aneurysm	Brassy cough.
Foreign body	
Immediate, while still in upper airway	Cough associated with progressive evidence of asphyxiation.
Later, when lodged in lower airway	Nonproductive cough, persistent, associated with localizing wheeze.
Cardiovascular	
Left ventricular failure	Cough intensifies while supine along with aggravation of dyspnea.
Pulmonary infarction	Cough associated with hemoptysis, usually with pleural effusion.

Sometimes, as in asthma, the cough is part of a constellation of manifestations of airway obstruction. When the pathologic process is changing, as in pneumonia or a neoplasm, the cough undergoes parallel change, reflecting the evolution of the disorder.

CIRCULATORY CONSEQUENCES

A spontaneous cough by a normal adult increases intrathoracic pressure by 50 to 100 mmHg; this increase is evident in a direct record of systemic arterial pressure (Fig. 26-15). Powerful adults can generate intrathoracic pressures of the order of 300 to 400 mmHg. The increment in intrathoracic pressure is matched by an equal rise in cerebrospinal pressure as well as in arterial pressure, implying that distending pressure (transmural pressure) in the vessels of the brain, as well as that in the heart and lungs, is not altered by the cough. Thus, vessels to vital organs are not torn even during violent coughing.

The increase in intrathoracic pressure is accompanied by reflex vasodilatation of systemic arteries and veins, both effects contributing to a decrease in cardiac output that sometimes lowers arterial pressure to syncopal levels. In right ventricular heart failure, the impediment to right ventricular filling produced by a cough decreases the cardiac overload and often improves stroke output.

POSTTUSSIVE SYNCOPE

This type of syncope is defined as a faint that occurs in the course of a cough. Charcot recognized this syndrome 100 years ago. Once considered a rarity, it is now recognized more frequently. Originally conceived of as a form of epilepsy or a consequence of a laryngeal reflex, it is now attributed to the same circulatory consequences of raised intrathoracic pressure that coughing evokes in a normal individual. However, the patient with cough syncope probably coughs more forcefully and longer than do normal persons.

The syncope usually develops within a few seconds after the onset of a paroxysm of coughing and ends quickly once the coughing has stopped. Return to consciousness is without sequelae unless the subject falls and is injured during the faint. Posttussive syncope nearly always occurs in men, presumably because they can generate higher intrathoracic pressures, and thereby decrease cardiac output more, than women. Not clear is why this type of fainting occurs in the supine as well as the upright position. This occurrence suggests that the reduction in cerebral blood flow during posttussive syncope involves more than interference with cardiac output. The extent to which intense reflex vasodilatation contributes to posttussive syncope is unclear. In this regard, patients in severe heart failure, who do not experience a posttussive drop in systemic arterial blood pressure, also do not experience

posttussive syncope; i.e., posttussive syncope is presumptive evidence of a good circulation with intact reflexes.

Hemoptysis

The coughing up of blood is defined as *hemoptysis*. The material that is produced varies from blood-tinged sputum to virtually all blood. The first decision faced by the physician who is told that blood has been "coughed up" is whether to conclude that the blood is coming from the respiratory tract. Although any portion of the respiratory tract can be the source, bleeding more often comes from a main bronchus or the lungs than from the nose or throat. On occasion, blood from the nose and throat is inhaled and then expectorated. As long as this possibility is kept in mind, bleeding that originates in the nose, throat, or larynx is not apt to be overlooked.

There is usually no problem in distinguishing hemoptysis from hematemesis (vomited blood). Even if the blood is aspirated and then coughed up, the patient can usually tell if the blood originated in the respiratory or alimentary tract. The appearance of the bloody material also helps to distinguish between hemoptysis and hematemesis: blood that originates in the airways is usually bright red, mixed with frothy sputum, has an alkaline pH, and contains alveolar macrophages that are laden with hemosiderin; in contrast, blood from the stomach usually is dark, has an acid pH, contains food particles, and occurs in a patient with a long history of gastric complaints.

Once it has been settled that the blood comes from the lungs, a determined effort is made to localize the intrapulmonary site of bleeding. The patient can be exceedingly helpful in this regard, particularly if the chest radiograph discloses any abnormality or shows bilateral pulmonary lesions. Occasionally, the detection of rales or rhonchi over one side or area of the lung directs the search. Sputum is zealously collected and examined: venous blood comes from the pulmonary arterial tree; bright red blood stems either from a bronchial vein (as in mitral stenosis) or from a bronchial artery (as in bronchiectasis). Expectorated blood clots indicate that blood has been sitting in the lung for a while.

Because hunting for the cause and the source of bleeding is generally uncomfortable and expensive, the intensity of the search depends on the circumstances. For example, rarely is a search for the bleeding site needed in a patient with acute bronchitis, or pneumonia, or bronchopulmonary suppuration. But, as a general rule, unless the cause is evident, a full-scale investigation is mandatory, particularly if this is not the first episode.

The list of causes of hemoptysis is long and diverse (Table 26-4). The clinical setting is usually helpful in identifying etiology. As a general rule, hemoptysis before middle age brings to mind mitral stenosis, tuberculosis, pneumonia, or bronchiectasis; after 40 to 45 years of age,

TABLE 26-4

Some Common Causes of Hemoptysis

Infections
  Bronchitis
  Tuberculosis
  Fungus infections
  Pneumonia
  Lung abscess
  Bronchiectasis
Neoplasms
  Bronchogenic carcinoma
  Bronchial adenoma
Cardiovascular disorders
  Pulmonary infarction
  Mitral stenosis
Trauma
Miscellaneous
  Foreign body
  Blood dyscrasia
  Goodpasture's syndrome

bronchogenic carcinoma and tuberculosis head the list. In patients left with a pulmonary cavity after pulmonary disease, e.g., tuberculosis, has healed and in regions of the country where pulmonary fungal diseases are prevalent, a bout of hemoptysis is occasionally the first sign of the disease. In patients who have a predisposing cause, such as oral contraceptives or chronic heart failure, pulmonary embolism is a likely etiology.

INFECTIONS

Hemoptysis can accompany a severe infection anywhere from the top to the bottom of the respiratory tract. It is uncommon in the usual viral or bacterial pneumonia. Conversely, it is not uncommon in the pneumonia that complicates bronchogenic carcinoma or in the pneumonia that is caused by staphylococci, influenza virus, or *Klebsiella.*

The organism determines the appearance and composition of the material that is expectorated with the blood. As indicated above, in pneumococcal lobar pneumonia, the sputum at the outset is characteristically rusty in appearance; but sometimes is faintly, or grossly, bloody. In staphylococcal pneumonia, the blood is admixed with pus. In *Klebsiella* pneumonia, the bloody sputum often resembles currant jelly. Brisk bleeding is common in lung abscess; the blood is mixed with copious amounts of foul-smelling pus. In lung gangrene, blood is associated with necrotic lung tissue.

Bleeding is common in bronchiectasis. Because it usually originates in a bronchial artery, bleeding is often brisk. It is rarely life-threatening, tends to recur, and, almost invariably, each episode stops spontaneously.

Should pneumonia complicate bronchiectasis, blood-stained sputum will be obtained.

The common source for hemoptysis used to be an active tuberculous cavity. But now tuberculous pneumonia is a more common cause of hemoptysis than is active cavitation, and, because of effective antituberculous therapy, both are unusual. If tuberculosis is allowed to progress to the point of extensive fibrosis and caseation, or becomes complicated by bronchiectasis, hemoptysis can be troublesome and persistent (Fig. 26-16).

The right middle lobe syndrome is frequently associated with hemoptysis. It is due to a partial or complete obstruction of the right middle lobe bronchus, resulting in atelectasis, pneumonitis, or both in the right middle lobe. The obstruction is more often caused by scarring and/or inflammation than by physical compression of the lumen by an enlarged lymph node. The cause is usually infectious, and the infection can be tuberculous.

Fungal infections of the lungs also produce hemoptysis (Fig. 26-17). As in tuberculosis, hemoptysis is generally a consequence of a continuing necrotizing and ulcerating inflammation process or of bronchiectasis. The most common fungal disorder that is associated with hemoptysis is a "fungus ball" that occupies either a healed tuberculous area (Fig. 26-16) or a cystic residue of sarcoidosis.

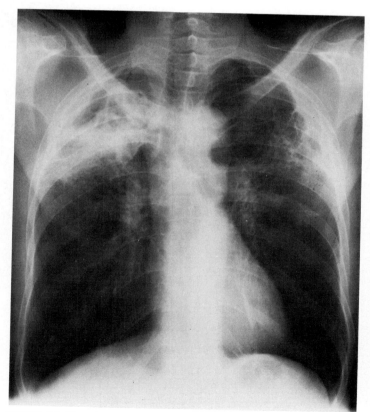

FIGURE 26-16 Old tuberculous cavities in right apex. They were removed surgically to control hemoptysis.

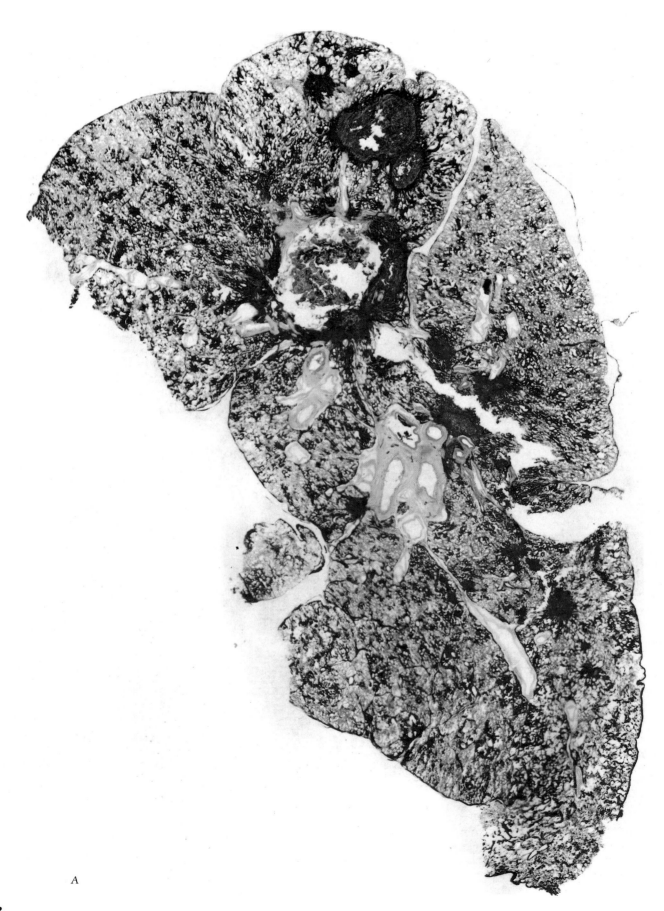

A

Usually *Aspergillus* is the cause; sometimes *Nocardia* or other fungi are the etiologic agents.

In parts of the world where amebiasis is endemic, hemoptysis follows perforation into the airways of a lung abscess that is continuous with a hepatic abscess. The sputum resembles anchovy sauce.

NEOPLASMS

Hemoptysis is so common in bronchogenic carcinoma that it should be regarded as the likeliest possibility in patients between 40 and 60 years of age. The likelihood is greatly increased if there is a history of cigarette smoking for years. Usually a troublesome cough and a vague chest pain precedes and accompanies the hemoptysis. For hemoptysis to occur, the lesion must communicate with the airways. Most often, the bleeding is a consequence of ulceration caused by the expanding tumor; sometimes it is due to a pneumonic process or an abscess in the lung behind the obstruction. With few exceptions, hemoptysis

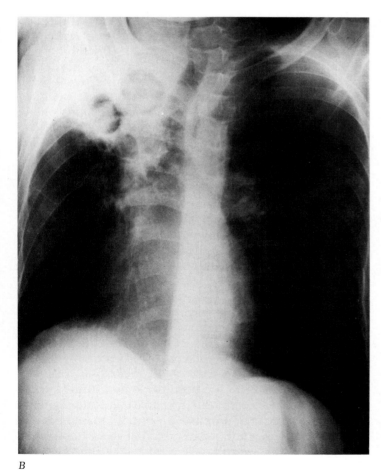

B

FIGURE 26-17 Fungous balls (mycetoma) due to aspergillosis. *A (opposite).* Sagittal section of lung. Fungous ball in coal miner's pneumoconiosis. *(Courtesy of J. Gough.)* *B.* Fungous ball due to aspergillosis in old tuberculous cavity. Recurrent hemoptysis was arrested by surgical removal of right upper lobe.

rarely complicates metastatic tumors of the lungs since few, particularly renal and colon carcinomas, intrude on the airways until preterminally.

Not only malignant, but also benign, tumors of the lung cause bleeding. The classic example is bronchial carcinoid which often causes bleeding that is generally difficult to arrest.

CARDIOVASCULAR DISORDERS

Tight mitral stenosis is sometimes first manifested by a bout of brisk, bright-red hemoptysis that is difficult to control. The source of the bleeding is the submucosal bronchial veins, which proliferate considerably in this disorder. A large hemoptysis is a medical emergency and is an indication for surgical intervention to relieve the obstruction at the mitral valve.

Pulmonary congestion and alveolar edema sometimes produce blood-tinged sputum. In chronic pulmonary congestion secondary to left ventricular failure or to mitral valvular disease, alveolar macrophages are often laden with hemosiderin ("heart failure cells"). In severe congestion and edema, the sputum is often pink and frothy. Usually there is no difficulty in recognizing that inadequate performance of the left ventricle is the cause of the bloody sputum.

Pulmonary embolism and, less often, pulmonary thrombosis produce hemoptysis only when associated with infarction. The hemoptysis of pulmonary infarction is usually associated with pleuritic pain and often with a small pleural effusion because of the peripheral location of the infarct.

Hemoptysis from other circulatory disorders is much less common. Occasionally, an aortic aneurysm penetrates into the tracheobronchial tree causing death by exsanguination and asphyxiation. An extraordinary event is the communication of an arteriovenous fistula with a small airway, causing bleeding that is exceedingly difficult to arrest.

TRAUMA

Hemoptysis follows a variety of chest injuries: puncture of a lung by a fractured rib; contusions of a lung by severe blunt trauma to the chest; or necrosis of the lining of the tracheobronchial tree by inhaled fumes or smoke. Blunt trauma from the steering wheel during an automobile collision sometimes lacerates or fractures the tracheobronchial tree. Stab or gunshot wounds often tear the lungs or airways. On occasion, mucosal lacerations in the course of severe coughing evoke hemoptysis.

After pneumonectomy or lobectomy, a large hemothorax sometimes empties into the airways. This is an alarming and ominous event. Its imminent occurrence is often heralded by the expectoration of blood-stained sputum after a paroxysm of coughing. Either the hemothorax must be promptly evacuated, or the bronchus must be surgically repaired. Hemoptysis within a few weeks to months after pneumonectomy has different implications: either recurrence of tumor, or granulation tissue, or bronchial sutures. Prompt bronchoscopy is necessary for accurate appraisal of the situation.

MISCELLANEOUS

Other causes of hemoptysis are indicated in Table 26-4. They vary enormously in etiology, severity, urgency, and prognosis. Sometimes the cause is obscure, as in the occasional instances of hemoptysis that accompany menstruation ("vicarious menstruation"). An aspirated foreign body produces bleeding by damaging the mucosa where it impacts; if allowed to remain in place, it sometimes causes bronchiectasis which, in turn, may cause bleeding. Pulmonary calcific foci, either in the pulmonary parenchyma or in lymph nodes, sometimes cause hemoptysis by ulcerating into a bronchus.

Blood dyscrasias, notably thrombocytopenic purpura and hemophilia, and the therapeutic use of anticoagulants, are occasional causes of hemoptysis. In areas where scurvy is endemic, vitamin C deficiency becomes an important etiology.

Hemoptysis in Goodpasture's syndrome (Fig. 26-18) or in idiopathic hemosiderosis is life-threatening. This grim prospect has led to drastic therapeutic interventions, including the combination of plasmapheresis plus immunosuppression.

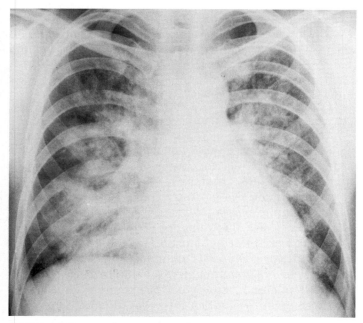

FIGURE 26-18 Goodpasture's syndrome.

APPROACH TO MANAGEMENT

An important first step is to assess the amount and nature of the blood that is being expectorated. Often the patient's impression is exaggerated. Slight, but persistent, bleeding is common in bronchogenic carcinoma. Recurrent, small bouts of brisk bleeding are more characteristic of bronchiectasis and endobronchial tuberculosis. A large hemoptysis is sometimes a feature of dry bronchiectasis, hemorrhage into a cavity, and pulmonary infarction.

In most patients, a detailed history and physical examination, followed promptly by standard chest radiography (posteroanterior and lateral), suffice to establish the cause of bleeding. Standard laboratory tests are useful in excluding a bleeding diathesis, a blood dyscrasia, or an active infection. The combination of history, physical examination, chest radiographs, and standard laboratory tests usually also excludes mitral stenosis and pulmonary infarction.

Should the cause and site of bleeding remain obscure, bronchoscopy is in order. The fiberoptic bronchoscope has greatly enlarged the diagnostic potential with respect to hemoptysis. But, as indicated in Chapter 32, the construction of the instrument has enhanced flexibility and versatility at the expense of capability to control large hemorrhage. Despite all diagnostic efforts, hemoptysis remains unexplained in 5 to 10 percent of patients.

Handling a pulmonary hemorrhage depends on the cause and the quantity of blood that is expectorated. Most spontaneous bleeding stops of its own accord, but the production of 400 to 500 ml of blood in a few hours creates an urgent situation. Depending on etiology, asphyxia caused by aspiration of blood into the unaffected lung is the usual cause of death. The critical decision in large hemorrhages from the airways is whether surgery is needed: in a few situations, such as an acute laceration of the lung or an aneurysm that has penetrated the airways, the need for surgery is evident; the situation is less clear when a lung abscess causes a large hemoptysis, because even though most abscesses stop bleeding spontaneously and respond to antibiotic therapy, in a few, hemorrhage is uncontrollable without surgery. Sometimes aspiration of blood can be prevented by inflating a Fogarty balloon catheter proximal to the bleeding site or by placing a special double lumen endotracheal tube.

Once the decision has been made that surgical intervention is not mandatory, an intensive medical program is begun: the patient is propped up in bed, reassured, and sedated cautiously until anxiety is relieved without compromising cough. Morphine and related antitussives pose the hazard of favoring the retention of blood in the lungs. Tilting the patient toward the side of bleeding affords the prospect of sparing the good lung. Selective catheterization of bronchial arteries, with the injection of coagulants, has been used with success in some instances and should be considered as a realistic therapeutic alternative to surgery.

Cyanosis

A bluish discoloration of the skin that is caused by increased amounts of reduced hemoglobin in the subpapillary venous plexus is designated as *cyanosis*. The discoloration is most apparent in the lobes of the ears, the cutaneous surfaces of the lips, and the nail beds. In patients with dark skin, the mucous membranes and the retina are important sites to examine for cyanosis. Unless flow through the skin is slowed, as in heart failure, cyanosis implies arterial hypoxemia. Cyanosis does not appear in carbon monoxide poisoning or in severe anemia in which the arterial O_2 content is extremely low. The presence of abnormal pigments in blood, such as methemoglobin or bilirubin, complicates the detection of cyanosis.

CAPILLARY O_2 CONTENT

An increase in the amount of reduced hemoglobin in the capillaries of the skin, as elsewhere, results from either inadequate oxygenation of arterial blood, excessive removal of O_2 from capillary blood (as when the circulation through a region is slowed by vasoconstriction), or a combination of the two. The concentration of reduced hemoglobin in the skin capillaries must reach about 5 g per 100 ml before cyanosis becomes discernible. The combination of intense vasoconstriction and excess of reduced hemoglobin is responsible for the distinctive gray, or heliotrope, color that is frequently seen in patients with circulatory collapse and severe pulmonary edema.

In severe pernicious anemia, in which hemoglobin concentrations are exceedingly low, i.e., of the order of 3 to 4 g per 100 ml, virtually all the hemoglobin can be reduced in traversing the skin capillaries without causing cyanosis. Oppositely, the polycythemic patient develops cyanosis at a higher arterial O_2 saturation than does the normal subject.

CAUSES

Several types of cyanosis are usually identified according to initiating mechanisms. They include peripherally induced cyanosis, cyanosis arising from pulmonary disease, cyanosis due to venous admixture, and cyanosis due to abnormal pigments in the blood.

Peripheral Cyanosis

This type is secondary to abnormally large extraction of O_2 as blood flows through peripheral capillaries. The most common cause is diminished cardiac output associated with peripheral vasoconstriction. Peripheral vaso-constriction per se, as in Raynaud's disease, also produces cyanosis of the nail beds. Not only the hands and feet, but also the tip of the nose becomes blue in severe heart failure. Indeed, in an occasional patient with intractable heart failure, necrosis develops at the tip of the nose.

Pulmonary Disease

Patients with chronic bronchitis and emphysema characteristically manifest derangements in ventilation-perfusion relationships. In some, arterial hypoxemia results. In patients with diffuse interstitial fibrosis, normal arterial oxygenation at rest is succeeded by arterial hypoxemia, and sometimes by cyanosis, during exercise. Less common as a cause of arterial hypoxemia are the syndromes of alveolar hypoventilation in patients with normal lungs. In any of these situations, cyanosis is intensified by heart failure that slows blood flow through the skin, i.e., decreases O_2 delivery.

Venous Admixture

In patients with intracardiac right-to-left shunts, cyanosis arises from admixture of venous and arterial blood. The effect of venous admixture is particularly striking if the O_2 content of mixed venous blood is inordinately low, as in some types of congenital heart disease and in severe heart failure. Often secondary polycythemia contributes to the cyanosis. On occasion, regional cyanosis is diagnostic. For example, in patent ductus arteriosus with reversal of blood flow, the lower extremities are deeply cyanotic, whereas the upper extremities are virtually normal in color.

Abnormal Pigments

Methemoglobinemia is an occasional cause for cyanosis. The causes may be either hereditary, i.e., due to the presence of hemoglobin M or a deficiency in methemoglobin reductase, or more often, acquired, e.g., by chemical agents such as analine dyes, chlorates, nitrates, and nitrites, or by drugs, such as acetanilide, nitroglycerin, phenacetin, and primaquine.

In methemoglobinemia, the ferrous iron has been oxidized to ferric iron, rendering the hemoglobin molecule incapable of binding O_2 or CO_2. Methemoglobin is formed continuously in the normal erythrocyte, but its level within the cell is kept low (less than 2 percent) by intracellular reductive mechanisms. High levels of methemoglobin result from hereditary abnormalities (e.g., a deficiency in methemoglobin reductase) or from exposure to drugs or chemicals that increase the rate of oxidation beyond the reductive capacity of the erythrocytes. Clinical manifestations of methemoglobinemia vary with the blood levels. Concentrations of methemoglobin between 10 and 25 percent usually cause asymptomatic cyanosis. When these levels are exceeded, dizziness, fatigue, and headache appear.

Nitrates are a common cause of methemoglobinemia. Nitrates are reduced to nitrites by bacteria in the intestinal tract. Excessive use of nitroglycerin, an organic nitrate, leads to methemoglobinemia. However, the effects of the abnormal blood pigment are complicated by the cardiovascular effects of the agent.

Methemoglobinemic blood is chocolate brown in color, and spectrophotometric examination of blood reveals the characteristic pigment. Arterial blood examination discloses a normal P_{O_2}.

Because of the normal methemoglobin reductase and NADH that is generated during anaerobic glycosis, treatment is unnecessary unless serious manifestations occur, i.e., angina, stupor, or coma. Then, methylene blue is given intravenously (1 to 2 mg/kg as a 1 percent solution) over 5 to 10 min. Cyanosis should disappear within 1 h, or the dose should be repeated. Larger doses of methylene blue engender the risk of aggravating the methemoglobinemia.

Clubbing

Clubbing is a classic enigma in medicine that dates back to Hippocrates' awareness of the association between characteristic changes in the fingertips and empyema. Occasionally it constitutes a valuable clue to clinically inapparent disease of the lungs and pleura. Clubbing of the fingers designates the selective bulbous enlargement of the distal segments of the digits due to an increase in soft tissue (Fig. 26-19). Most often it is painless. When full blown, clubbing is easy to recognize: (1) the nails, particularly the index finger, become abnormally curved in the longitudinal and coronal planes; (2) the hyponychial angle, viewed in profile, becomes blunted, as a rule in conjunction with softening and sponginess of the base of the nail; and (3) the undersurface of the terminal digit becomes large and bulbous. Early stages of clubbing are subtle and generally difficult to diagnose. Clubbing often has to be distinguished from simple curvature of the nails and occasionally from chronic paronychia and Heberden's nodes. A variety of methods have been proposed for quantifying clubbing, i.e., measures on casts of the fingertips, but none has become popular.

Clubbing is generally acquired but may be hereditary. Acquired clubbing is seen in a wide variety of disorders, extrathoracic as well as thoracic (Table 26-1). As a rule, clubbing is bilaterally symmetric, involving hands and feet; on occasion, local factors, such as injury of a finger or of the median nerve, may cause clubbing that is confined to a single finger. Clubbing confined to the digits of one hand is seen rarely in an ipsilateral Pancoast tumor that has invaded the brachial plexus or after hemiplegia. In certain types of congenital heart disease, telltale patterns of clubbing are of considerable diagnostic value. For example, in patent ductus arteriosus associated with reversal of shunt through the ductus, clubbing affects only the toes.

INTRATHORACIC DISEASE AND CLUBBING

Symmetric acquired clubbing occurs in approximately one-quarter of patients with carcinoma of the lung; in some of these, hypertrophic osteoarthropathy accompanies the clubbing. In pulmonary tuberculosis, clubbing occurs only when the lung is severely distorted by fibrosis, or when a complication, such as bronchiectasis or empyema, exists. Clubbing is uncommon in chronic obstructive disease of the airways unless suppurative complications, particularly bronchiectasis, develop. Two pulmonary diseases that are commonly associated with clubbing are cystic fibrosis and idiopathic pulmonary fibrosis. Although clubbing is sometimes a helpful lead to the presence of bronchiectasis, the coincidence of clubbing and bronchiectasis is only of the order of 10 percent. Mesothelioma is also associated with clubbing.

A strong correlation exists between the occurrence of digital clubbing and the number and size of bronchial arterioles and arteries. Proliferation of this collateral circulation is a prominent feature of bronchiectasis, chronic pulmonary suppuration of any kind, pulmonary fibrosis, pulmonic stenosis, and congenital cyanotic heart failure. However, proliferation of the collateral circulation of the lungs is not always a prerequisite for clubbing. Two important exceptions are carcinoma of the lung and subacute bacterial endocarditis, neither of which have a remarkable proliferation of the bronchial circulation, although clubbing is sometimes prominent.

PATHOGENESIS OF CLUBBING

The pathogenesis of clubbing is unknown, and no suitable animal model of clubbed fingers has as yet been developed, largely because so few species, other than primates, have fingers. A common denominator in the pathogenesis of clubbing appears to be vasodilatation of vessels in the fingertip, including the arteriovenous connections. As a result, hydrostatic pressures increase in the capillaries and venules, promoting the transudation of fluid into the interstitium. The reason for this preferential vasodilatation is unclear. A popular notion is that a humoral substance escapes normal deactivation by pulmonary capillaries. This theory could account for clubbing in cyanotic congenital heart disease, in various pulmonary diseases in which proliferation of the bronchial circulation occurs, and in hepatic cirrhosis in which pulmonary arteriovenous anastomoses and right-to-left shunts are common. However, it is difficult to relate this theory to the high incidence of clubbing in subacute bacterial endocarditis.

At present, a single hypothesis that would account for the clubbing that occurs in such diverse disorders as subacute bacterial endocarditis, carcinoma of the lungs, hemiplegia, chronic mountain sickness, and purgative abuse is not possible. Indeed, it seems likely that clubbing of the

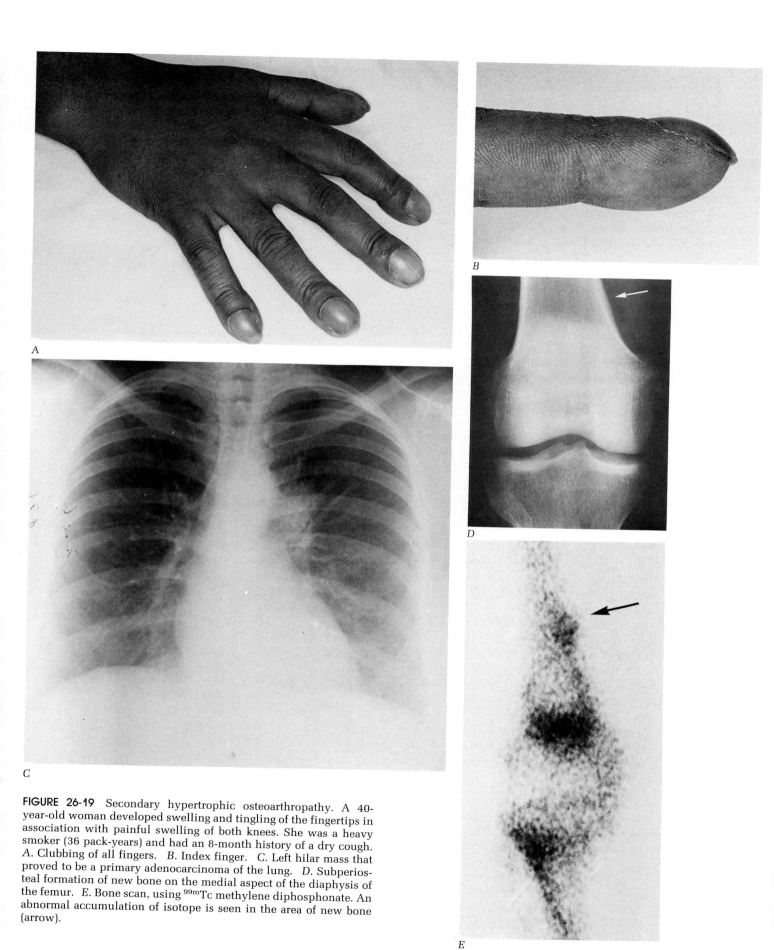

FIGURE 26-19 Secondary hypertrophic osteoarthropathy. A 40-year-old woman developed swelling and tingling of the fingertips in association with painful swelling of both knees. She was a heavy smoker (36 pack-years) and had an 8-month history of a dry cough. *A.* Clubbing of all fingers. *B.* Index finger. *C.* Left hilar mass that proved to be a primary adenocarcinoma of the lung. *D.* Subperiosteal formation of new bone on the medial aspect of the diaphysis of the femur. *E.* Bone scan, using ^{99m}Tc methylene diphosphonate. An abnormal accumulation of isotope is seen in the area of new bone (arrow).

digits is a stereotyped consequence of diverse influences that have in common the capacity to induce marked digital vasodilatation and interstitial edema.

HYPERTROPHIC OSTEOARTHROPATHY

Occasionally clubbing of the digits is accompanied by hypertrophic osteoarthropathy, a separate entity both clinically and radiographically: clinically, hypertrophic osteoarthropathy is manifested by pain and swelling of the soft tissues over the distal ends of the long and tubular bones; radiographically, the distinctive feature of hypertrophic osteoarthropathy is the formation of new bone beneath the periosteum of the distal diaphyses of the long bones of the extremities (Fig. 26-19).

The most common disorder associated with hypertrophic osteoarthropathy is carcinoma of the lung. The incidence is about 5 percent and is unrelated to the cell type of the cancer except that oat cell carcinoma is rarely implicated. A peripheral carcinoma of the lung is slightly more common than a central location. Joint symptoms precede the local signs of tumor in about one-third of the cases; the interval is sometimes as long as 2 years.

Pulmonary tuberculosis is rarely, if ever, associated with hypertrophic osteoarthropathy. Pulmonary metastases also rarely cause hypertrophic osteoarthropathy.

As in the case of clubbing of the digits, theories about pathogenesis tend to focus on humoral factors generated elsewhere. However, a neurogenic theory has also been advanced based on two types of observations: (1) in a few patients, vagotomy relieved the symptoms of inoperable carcinoma of the lung and led to regression of the bony lesions, and (2) in keeping with the observations on the few patients, in dogs, vagotomy was usually followed by a decrease in blood flow to the limbs. At present, neither theory has much convincing support, but both suggest future directions for exploration.

In contrast to clubbing of the digits, which is rarely painful, hypertrophic osteoarthritis associated with carcinoma of the lung often causes severe rheumatic symptoms. These symptoms vanish after resection of the carcinoma—even though clubbing usually remains. In patients who are treated with radiotherapy for unresectable carcinoma, pains in the vicinity of the joints usually decrease greatly and as a rule do not recur even if metastases develop to the lungs or elsewhere.

Effects of P_{CO_2}

The blood vessels of the skin depend for their normal state of dilatation upon a normal CO_2 tension. A decrease in the partial pressure of CO_2 in blood causes vasoconstriction. Oppositely, an increase in arterial P_{CO_2} elicits vasodilatation: one characteristic manifestation of acute hypercapnia is a pounding headache due to cerebral vasodilatation; in chronic hypercapnia, conjunctival and retinal vessels are visibly dilated. Along with these vasomotor changes, disturbances are induced by chronic hypercapnia in the central and sympathetic nervous systems, the ventilatory response to increments in arterial P_{CO_2} is blunted, and the renal reabsorption of bicarbonate is increased.

Thoracic Pain

First thoughts about chest pain almost invariably turn to the pain of myocardial ischemia. However, cardiac pain is generally distinguishable from other types of chest pain because of its vicelike nature, its characteristic radiation to the left arm, shoulder, or neck, and its lack of relation to breathing.

PLEURITIC PAIN

The most characteristic pain associated with the respiratory apparatus is pleural pain. It originates in the parietal pleural and endothoracic fascia; the visceral pleura is insensitive to pain. In contrast to deep, substernal pain and oppression of myocardial infarction, the pain is identified as being close to the thoracic cage. It is predominantly an inspiratory pain reflecting the stretching of inflamed parietal pleura during movement of the thorax; coughing or laughing are exceedingly distressing, and the patient often clutches the chest to minimize its excursion. The pain is usually local, but sometimes spreads along the course of the intercostal nerves that supply the affected area.

As a rule, pleural pain is part of a syndrome of pleural infection that includes malaise and fever; an important exception to this generalization is the pleural pain of pulmonary infarction, which is often unassociated with any premonitory signs. Irritation of the diaphragmatic pleura by an inflammatory process either below or above the diaphragm often causes ipsilateral shoulder pain; sometimes the pain is referred to the abdomen.

PULMONARY PAIN

A second distinctive type of respiratory chest pain accompanies a tracheitis or tracheobronchitis. The pain is searing and is most pronounced after cough. Invariably this central chest pain is associated with evidence of upper respiratory infection, generally a flulike syndrome.

An uncommon type of respiratory pain is due to pulmonary hypertension. It is usually absent at rest and appears during exertion. The pain is substernal and is invariably associated with dyspnea; it subsides promptly when exercise stops. It is often mistaken for angina until the presence of pulmonary hypertension is uncovered.

CHEST WALL PAIN

Pain in the chest is a common clinical problem. It may arise from within the thorax, i.e., the heart, pericardium, lungs, pleura, chest wall, or be referred from elsewhere, e.g., from below the diaphragm. As a rule, characteristic patterns and associations help to clarify the source of the pain.

Pleural pain is generally associated with fever or dyspnea. Most often, it is abrupt in onset, unilateral, and incapacitating. As a rule, it affects the lower part of the chest but occasionally is referred to the shoulder or abdomen. Almost invariably, it is aggravated by deep breathing or coughing. The patient tends to splint the chest on the affected side. Tachypnea, using small tidal volumes, is a consistent pattern.

Musculoskeletal pain arising in the chest, that is also aggravated by breathing, may be confused with pleuritic pain. But, it is rarely severe and incapacitating, often bilateral, and generally is intensified by changes in body position or flexing the thorax. The affected muscles are often tender to gentle pressure. A fractured rib is usually identified as the source of pain by a history of fall, injury, or trauma; point tenderness and crepitus of the affected area; reproduction of the pain upon manual compression of the chest; and radiographic evidence of the broken rib.

Pain arising from the large airways is usually burning in nature and retrosternal in location and is disturbing rather than incapacitating. It is aggravated by cough and is commonly accompanied by evidence of a bronchitis.

Quite distinctive is the pain of a Pancoast tumor (Fig. 26-20). This unusual tumor was originally described in 1932 as a "superior pulmonary sulcus tumor," characterized by pain along the distribution of the eighth cervical and the first and second thoracic nerves, Horner's syndrome, local destruction of bone by the tumor, and atrophy of hand muscles. The chest radiograph is distinctive in showing a small, sharply defined shadow at one apex (Fig. 26-20) and destruction of one or more of the upper three ribs posteriorly and of their adjacent transverse processes.

CARDIAC PAIN

Attention was called above to the pain of myocardial ischemia. Another type of cardiac pain is that of pericarditis. Pericardial pain is often aggravated by deep breathing and, almost invariably, is accompanied by a telltale rub that is synchronous with the heartbeat.

The postcommissurotomy (postpericardiotomy) syndrome is characterized by chest pain that usually develops within a few days to weeks after surgery on the heart or after pericardiotomy. The pain is usually sudden in onset and substernal, with radiation to the left side of the neck; often it is aggravated by deep breathing. Low grade fever and a high sedimentation rate are regular concomitants. The diagnosis is usually clear when account is taken of the antecedent history of cardiac surgery. Indeed, confusion is more apt to arise with the pain of myocardial infarction than with respiratory causes of chest pain.

MISCELLANEOUS PAIN

Other structures in the mediastinum can be the source of chest pain. Noteworthy are the types of pain arising from the esophagus (peptic esophagitis) and dissection of the aorta. Their patterns and intensity serve to distinguish them from respiratory pain.

Arthritis of the cervical spine is a common cause of thoracic pain. Usually the cause is quite clear because of the characteristic distribution of the pain. Cervical spondylosis occasionally causes severe pain in the chest and arms but is more apt to mimic myocardial infarction than respiratory pain. A metastatic tumor to the thoracic spine often causes bilateral, symmetric pain, whereas unilateral pain, along with distribution of an intercostal nerve, is characteristic of herpes zoster before the appearance of the skin eruption.

Anxiety can produce, or intensify, chest pain. Usually, pain originating in nervousness is accompanied by dyspnea and hyperventilation. Not infrequently, manifestations of vasomotor instability, such as excessive palmar sweating, flushing, and tachycardia, accompany the complaint of chest pain. Rarely does the pain conform to a characteristic or consistent pattern. Anxiety also interferes with the quantification of pain originating in a somatic lesion and also with its management using analgesics.

Fever

In the patient with lung disease, fever generally signifies infection. When the lung disease is chronic, as in bronchitis and emphysema, a bout of acute bronchitis usually elicits only a modest fever even though the sputum turns purulent. In contrast, an acute pneumonia or lung abscess causes high fever.

The presence of fever lends urgency to the situation. Elsewhere in this book, the patterns of acute pulmonary infection are considered with particular attention to systemic effects, chest radiography, white blood cell count, sedimentation rate, and sputum examination. Often overlooked at the outset is miliary tuberculosis, which occasionally escapes detection on the initial chest radiograph. Favoring this diagnosis is a history of recent contact with active tuberculosis, general malaise, easy fatigability, and anorexia during the previous few weeks. This insidious onset differs strikingly from the more explosive onset of acute pneumonia. A therapeutic trial of antituberculosis therapy is warranted while concrete evidence of disseminated tuberculosis is sought in a biopsy of liver and bone marrow.

Neoplasms are also associated with fever. In certain neoplasms, such as carcinoma of the bronchus, the fever is generally a secondary effect attributable to infection distal to obstruction; necrosis within the tumor is a less common cause. In others, such as hypernephroma, fever

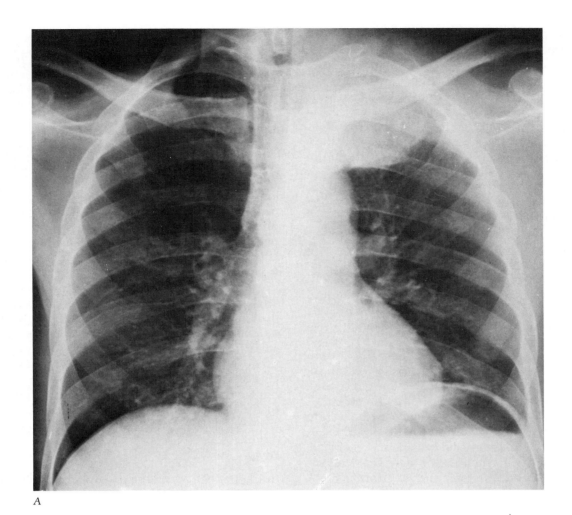

A

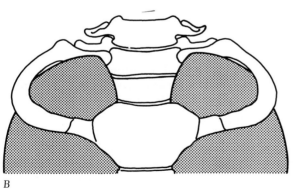

B

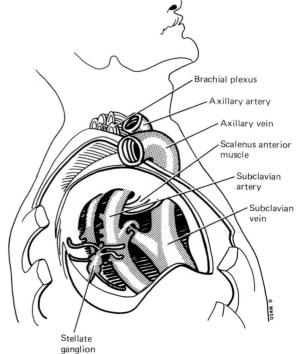

Brachial plexus

Axillary artery

Axillary vein

Scalenus anterior muscle

Subclavian artery

Subclavian vein

Stellate ganglion

C

FIGURE 26-20 Anatomic bases for pain in Pancoast tumor. *A.* Chest radiograph. Superior sulcus (Pancoast) tumor. *B.* Relationships of apex of the lung to adjacent bony structures. *C.* Lateral view of area occupied by apex of lung, showing proximity not only to nerves of brachial plexus but also to sympathetic chain and to blood vessels. A mass that grows posteriorly and laterally can encounter sympathetic chain and bony structures; superiorly, the axillary vessels, brachial plexus, and bony structures; anteriorly, the subclavian vein and its tributaries. *(C After Pernkopf E: Atlas of Topographical and Applied Human Anatomy, Philadelphia, Saunders, 1964, p 22, with permission.)*

356

and chills are striking even though evidence of infection is absent. A mesothelioma of the pleura is often associated with fever; removal of the tumor is generally followed by defervescence. Presumably, in patients with neoplasms who have no evidence of infection, necrosis within the tumor leads to the elaboration of pyogenic substances within, and around, the tumor.

Extrinsic allergic alveolitis sometimes is followed by fever as well as by pulmonary disability after exposure to the offending antigen. Usually the etiologic diagnosis poses no problem once the nature of the illness is suspected.

In contrast to the pulmonary disorders in which fever is a characteristic feature, pulmonary sarcoidosis rarely is associated with fever unless widespread extrapulmonary involvement, or erythema nodosum, coexists. Nor is pneumoconiosis associated with fever unless complicated by necrosis in the midst of conglomerate fibrosis or by superimposed tuberculosis. Among the other extensive disorders of the lungs that cause no fever (and few systemic complaints) are idiopathic pulmonary fibrosis, lymphangitic carcinomatosis, multiple pulmonary metastases, alveolar proteinosis, idiopathic pulmonary hemosiderosis, and alveolar microlithiasis.

RADIOLOGIC EVALUATION

The radiologic evaluation of the patient presenting with respiratory symptoms is dealt with in considerable detail elsewhere in this book (see Chapter 35). The value of routine screening films in asymptomatic subjects, e.g., as part of annual physicals, or in chronic cigarette smokers to detect cancer, is still a matter of debate. As a rule, the diagnostic yield of such studies has not been impressive. In contrast, the chest radiograph is an integral component of the initial evaluation of the patient with new respiratory symptoms. Fraser and Pare have shown how the differential diagnosis of respiratory diseases can be approached and structured using the chest radiograph as the initial step.

CHOOSING PULMONARY FUNCTION TESTS

Elsewhere in this book, considerable attention is paid to individual pulmonary function tests. Often a combination of pulmonary function tests is needed to characterize a patient's abnormalities. Some of the tests are simple; others require special facilities and personnel. A few are still experimental. For example, closing volume and closing capacity have become popular as "sensitive" tests for obstruction of small airways. They are regularly abnormal in heavy smokers. However, their relation to clinically important disease of the airways is unknown. Nor is there any value to these sensitive tests once the FEV_1 is abnor-

mal. Therefore, closing volume and closing capacity currently have no meaning for clinical disease even though they may prove useful in screening for obstruction of small airways in occupational disease. Because they only measure physiological derangements, the tests generally provide no information about etiology or pathology.

However, the battery of tests that is necessary to portray the full length and breadth of the patient's pulmonary disorder is rarely needed to categorize the disorder for the sake of management. This fortunate circumstance stems from the relatively few abnormal physiological patterns that result from a wide variety of etiologies. As may be seen in Table 26-5, virtually all diseases that compromise pulmonary performance can be categorized into a few distinctive patterns: (1) obstructive disease of the airways, (2) restrictive lung disease, (3) obliterative vascular disease, and (4) alveolar hypoventilation due to malfunctioning of the chest bellows or control mechanisms.

Chronic Obstructive Airways Disease

Pulmonary function tests are particularly important in obstructive diseases of the airways because chest radiographs are often normal. Obstruction of the airways generally occurs during expiration. Because most pulmonary function tests are based on expiratory maneuvers, this type of obstruction has been categorized by a wide variety of tests. But it is remarkable how much information about the obstruction can be obtained from two traditional tests: (1) the FEV_1, determined serially and before and after administering a bronchodilator, and (2) arterial blood-gas analyses, performed periodically.

Preoccupation with expiration tended for a while to obscure disorders that were characterized primarily by inspiratory obstruction. These were commonly overlooked because of the failure to elicit stridor on the physical examination. But more and more instances of inspiratory obstruction are being uncovered, particularly in patients who have undergone prolonged tracheal intubation. Once alerted to this prospect by detecting a wheeze over the trachea—usually but not invariably during inspiration—a comparison of maximum inspiratory and expiratory flow rates generally points to the upper airways as the site of obstruction (Fig. 26-21). Not infrequently, other tests, particularly tomography, bronchography, or aortography, are needed to complete the appraisal of the affected area.

Chronic obstructive (primarily expiratory) disease of the lower airways constitutes a more familiar clinical picture than does chronic inspiratory obstruction. To appreciate the abnormalities in pulmonary performance that these expiratory disorders produce, it must be recalled that even in the normal lung, bronchial and bronchiolar calibers decrease, and resistance to airflow increases, during expiration; this normal pattern is exaggerated by a

TABLE 26-5
Practical Initial Aproaches to Assessing Pulmonary Disorders*

Clinical State	First-Order Tests	Comments
Obstructive disease of airways		
Expiration		
Asthma	FEV$_1$; before and after bronchodilator	Detect bronchospasm
	Arterial blood-gas levels	Increasing P$_{CO_2}$ requires assisted ventilation
Chronic bronchitis	FEV$_1$; before and after bronchodilator	Degree of obstruction; reversibility
	Arterial blood-gas levels	Magnitude of ventilation-perfusion abnormalitites
Emphysema	FEV$_1$	Degree of obstruction; reversibility
	Arterial blood-gas levels	Extent of ventilation-perfusion abnormalities
	Elastic recoil pressure	Abnormally low if emphysema predominates over bronchitis
Inspiration	FEV$_1$	Normal
	Maximal inspiratory and expiratory flow curves	Characteristic configurations of curves (Figs. 26–1 to 26–16)
Restrictive lung disease		
Diffuse interstitial inflammation, infiltration, fibrosis; thickened pleura	Chest radiograph	Characteristic patterns
	Lung volumes	Concentric reduction
	Arterial P$_{O_2}$ at rest and exercise	Arterial hypoxemia during exercise
	Diffusing capacity	Conformity
Alveolar hypoventilation		
Secondary to obstructive disease of airways ("net")	Same as obstructive diseases of airways	Seriously abnormal lungs
	Arterial blood-gas levels	Hypoxemia, hypercapnia, respiratory acidosis
Primary mechanism outside lungs; respiratory centers, chest bellows; coordinating mechanisms	FEV$_1$; spirometry	Normal
	Arterial blood-gas levels	Hypoxemia, hypercapnia, respiratory acidosis
	Response to assisted ventilation	Normalization of blood-gas levels
	Maximum inspiratory and expiratory pressures	Assess muscle weakness
Obliterative pulmonary vascular disease	Chest radiograph	Characteristic
	Electrocardiogram	Right ventricular hypertrophy
	Spirometry; FEV$_1$	Normal
	Right-sided heart catheterization	Pulmonary hypertension
Complications of sources of ambiguity		
Respiratory failure	Arterial blood-gas levels; identify etiology	Guide to therapy
Pulmonary congestion and edema	Chest radiograph	Enlarged heart; vascular and interstitial pattern
	Vital capicity	Response to diuretics and cardiotonic agents
Cyanosis		
Polycythemia vera	Spirometry; FEV$_1$; arterial blood-gas levels	All near-normal
Anatomic right-to-left shunt	Same	Severe hypoxemia without hypercapnia
Abnormal pigment	Arterial P$_{O_2}$; spectrophotometry	Normal; identify pigments

*Emphasizing simplicity of tests as well as their specificity in substantiating clinical diagnosis. The more elaborate tests that are used for further discrimination are discussed elsewhere.

forced expiration and is perpetuated by disease. Because decrease in airway calibers is produced clinically by different mechanisms and etiologic agents, pulmonary function tests in these disorders lack specificity. The common denominator is an increased resistance to airflow in the bronchi and bronchioles. In chronic obstructive disease of the airways, notably chronic bronchitis, at least three separate elements generally contribute to an increase in airway resistance: bronchoconstriction, inflammation or edema of small airways (bronchioles), and "secretions" in

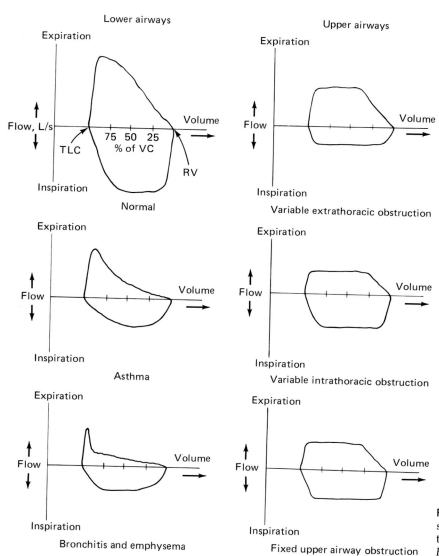

FIGURE 26-21 Schematic flow-volume tracings. Obstructive patterns of the lower airways *(left)* are contrasted with those of the upper airways *(right)*. *(After Harrison, 1939.)*

the airways, often consisting of mucus and inflammatory exudate. The importance of these mechanisms is that they are all potentially reversible by medical management.

In contrast to involvement of the medium-sized bronchi in chronic bronchitis, airway resistance in emphysema is increased primarily because of diminished calibers of small airways (bronchioles) resulting from a decrease in the elastic recoil of the pulmonary parenchyma. Unfortunately, the decrease in elastic recoil is a result of destruction of alveolar walls and is, therefore, not reversible.

Chronic bronchitis and emphysema consist of a mixture of these reversible and irreversible components: to the extent that bronchitis predominates, there is some basis for optimism in therapy, particularly during an acute exacerbation; however, chronic bronchitis is also generally more life-threatening because it produces altered ventilation-perfusion relationships and abnormal arterial blood-gas levels, whereas emphysema amputates

ventilation and perfusion symmetrically leaving arterial blood gases at near-normal levels.

Asthma is a syndrome characterized by generalized wheezing during inspiration and expiration. Although etiologies vary, they are generally categorized as intrinsic and extrinsic. Except for those patients who can relate attacks to specific antigens, two common mechanisms often precipitate an episode: a respiratory infection, usually viral rather than bacterial, or an emotional upset. Between episodes, most asthmatics, even those who are symptom-free, can be shown to have heightened bronchomotor tone (Fig. 26-22). In a latent asthmatic, a brief period of hyperventilation generally suffices to induce a bout of asthma. In patients with left ventricular disease, a paroxysm of wheezing ("cardiac asthma") occasionally heralds acute pulmonary congestion and edema. Accordingly, because a cardiotonic program is so effective in cardiac asthma, fresh-onset asthma in older persons should be carefully assessed with respect to the state of the left

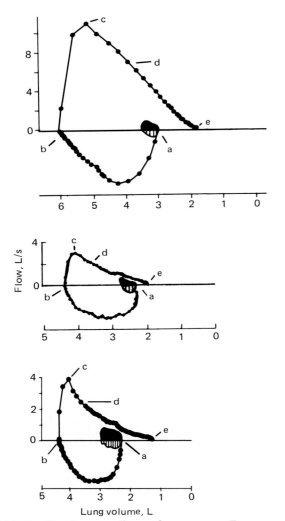

FIGURE 26-22 Simultaneous flow-volume curves. *Top*, normal subject. Beginning at the end of a quiet expiration, a, the curves were recorded during a normal tidal breath (small, shaded loops) and during a forced expiration from peak lung inflation, b, to full expiration, e. Peak flow rates were reached at c. Expiration then continued along segment cde. In the record of the tidal breath, inspiration is hatched, and expiration is solid black. The interval between each dot is 0.04 s. *Center*, asthmatic subject. The vital capacity (be) is abnormally small, and flow rates along cde are diminished. *Bottom*, same asthmatic subject, 2 weeks after clinical recovery. Although flow rates are considerably higher than during the acute attack, the slope of segment de is still abnormally low, indicating that the resistance to airflow as lung volume decreases is still inordinately high. *(After Mellins, Lord, Fishman, 1967.)*

ventricle before vigorous bronchodilator therapy using sympathomimetic substances is begun.

Restrictive Lung Disease

The diagnosis of restrictive lung disease usually begins with a complaint of dyspnea reinforced by a telltale chest radiograph. Indeed, without abnormalities on the chest radiograph, detection of interstitial disease by pulmonary function testing is uncommon. The combination of tachypnea, the typical chest radiography, concentric reduction in lung volumes, and the appearance of arterial hypoxemia during exercise almost invariably clinches the diagnosis; a low value for the diffusing capacity of the lungs is final proof and is useful in following the course of the disease. Much more troublesome is the identification of the cause (Table 26-5).

An important distinction at the outset is whether the disease is acute or chronic (Table 26-6). Some types of interstitial disease, such as asbestosis, take years to become symptomatic. Others, such as the Hamman-Rich syndrome, run a fulminating course from start of symptoms to death within weeks.

Another help in categorization is the presence of systemic complaints. Sometimes, particularly in immunosuppressed patients undergoing renal dialysis, distinction between interstitial infection and interstitial edema may be difficult to make (Fig. 26-23). Persistent fever suggests infection. That lungs are sharing in a systemic disease, such as scleroderma, is often suggested by telltale stigmata in extrapulmonary sites (Fig. 26-24). In some instances, the cause is self-evident. This relationship is striking in some occupational disorders, e.g., silo-filler's disease that occurs after exposure to moldy hay. Also, the chest radiograph in sarcoidosis or silicosis is sometimes so characteristic as to be virtually diagnostic (Fig. 26-25). But, not infrequently, the cause remains enigmatic or idiopathic despite elaborate laboratory investigations, including lung biopsy.

In essence, the uncovering of etiology in many instances of diffuse interstitial fibrosis is often a matter of painstaking and discriminating medical detection. The flash of brilliant insight, in the tradition of Sherlock Holmes or Lord Peter Wimsey, is apt to be less revealing about etiology than is a meticulous, systematic account of life-style, habits, occupation, and background. This historical chart and compass begins with a consideration of familial tendencies (e.g., cystic fibrosis of the pancreas) and proceeds to relevant personal history (e.g., exposure to a patient with overt tuberculosis or to an area in which histoplasmosis or coccidioidomycosis is endemic), previous medical history (e.g., chronic mitral stenosis or scleroderma or a stroke that has impaired the swallowing mechanism), and history of recent ingestion of medications [e.g., hexamethonium or hydralazine (Apresoline) for hypertension, immunosuppressive agents for cancer (Fig. 26-23), or nitrofurantoin for urinary infection]. Sometimes the identification of abnormal constituents in sputum is diagnostically helpful (e.g., blood or blood products in the macrophages of the patient with Goodpasture's syndrome or eosinophils in the patient with a hypersensitivity disorder). But, in many instances, etiologic diagnosis rests on lung biopsy. Unfortunately, bi-

TABLE 26-6

Common Prototypes of Diffuse Interstitial Disease according to Etiology

Etiology	Example	Common Features
Acute		
Infections	Miliary tuberculosis, histoplasmosis	Opportunities for exposure
	Pneumocystis, cytomegalic inclusion virus, fungi	Immunosuppresion
Radiation therapy	After mastectomy	Shortly after treatment
Pulmonary edema	Narcotic overdosage; nitrogen dioxide (silo-filler's disease); uremia	Distinctive history
Inhalation	Bysssinosis	Monday morning asthma and fever
Aspiration	After loss of consciousness	History of alcoholism or epilepsy
Immunologic	Goodpasture's syndrome	Renal and pulmonary involvement
Carcinoma of lung	Alveolar cell carcinoma	
Idiopathic	Hamman-Rich syndrome	
Chronic		
Inhalation	Pneumoconioses	History of exposure
Radiation therapy	After mastectomy	Gradual evolution after treatment
Lymphangitic spread	Carcinoma of breast, lung, stomach, pancreas	Evidence of primary carcinoma
Medications	Hexamethonium; hydralazine; bleomycin; busulfan; nitrofurantoin	History; suggestive chest radiograph
Systemic disorders	Boeck's sarcoid, collagen disorders, histiocytosis X, amyloidosis; tuberous sclerosis	Multiorgan involvement; biopsy
Idiopathic	Diffuse interstitial fibrosis	Exclusion of known etiologies

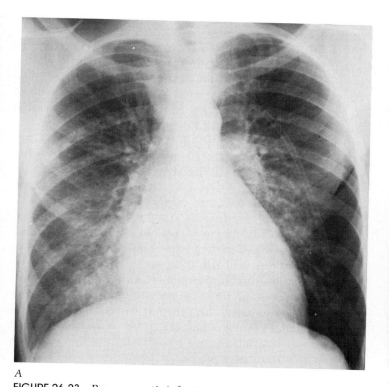

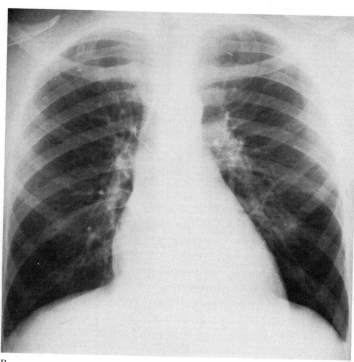

A

B

FIGURE 26-23 *Pneumocystis* infection in an immunosuppressed patient in uremia. A. Bilateral interstitial and alveolar pattern and enlarged cardiac silhouette suggestive of pulmonary edema. *Pneumocystis carinii* obtained by bronchial lavage. B. Three weeks later. Reduction in size of cardiac silhouette and clearing of infiltrates after diuresis of 10 lb and treatment with pentamidine isethionate.

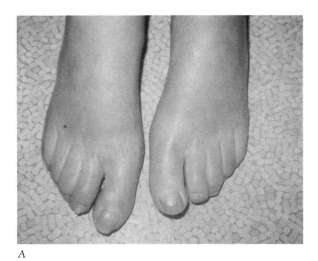

A

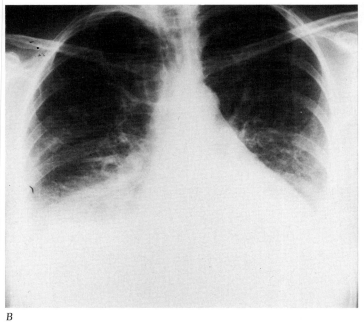

B

FIGURE 26-24 Scleroderma. *A.* Raynaud's phenomenon of the toes. *B.* Diffuse bibasilar interstitial infiltrates on chest radiograph.

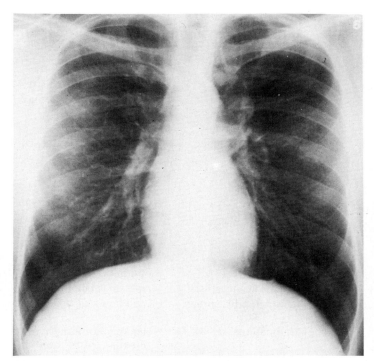

FIGURE 26-25 Unilateral hilar adenopathy due to sarcoidosis. Twenty-seven-year-old asymptomatic male with left hilar adenopathy and interstitial lung disease of upper lobes. Bronchoscopic biopsy disclosed widespread noncaseating granulomas.

opsy is often deferred to the stage of nonspecific interstitial fibrosis when scarring is indiscriminate so that neither etiology nor pathogenic mechanisms are decipherable. Also, even when biopsy is done, an irrelevant part of the lung is sometimes sampled, e.g., a bronchoscopic biopsy may provide tissue from a part of the lung that does not reflect a subpleural process; and open biopsy of the lingula, once a popular site of biopsy by thoracic surgeons, may represent an inflammatory process that is unrelated to disease elsewhere in the lungs.

The physiological hallmarks of diffuse interstitial disease are those of restrictive lung disease, i.e., stiffening of the lung (low compliance) and concentric reduction in

lung volumes (decrease in vital capacity, residual volume, and total lung capacity). Accompanying the decrease in compliance is an increase in the work of breathing and a breathing pattern of rapid, shallow tidal volumes. The chest radiograph demonstrates the inability of the patient to expand fully the stiffened lungs. Dyspnea is evoked at first by mild exercise and later persists at rest.

One prototype of chronic interstitial disease is sarcoidosis. At one time, the disorder was pictured as a homogeneous thickening of the alveolar-capillary interfaces. Now it is appreciated that the pathologic process is usually very nonhomogeneous, so that areas of diffuse alveolar-capillary thickening are interspersed with nodules, amputated alveoli, and adjacent areas of overdistended alveoli. Also, small airways are generally distorted not only by peribronchial filtration and fibrosis, but also by intraluminal lesions. Consequently, instead of a pure diffusion disorder, sarcoidosis, particularly as the disease progresses, is usually complicated by ventilation-perfusion imbalances that are manifested by an increase in both dead-space ventilation and venous admixture, particularly late in the disorder. Nonetheless, because of widespread involvement of alveolar-capillary interfaces by the granulomatous disease, the diffusing capacity is low and arterial hypoxemia develops promptly whenever metabolic activity is increased by exercise.

Finally, the once-popular picture of widespread disease confined to the alveolar-capillary interstitium in sarcoidosis has been modified by the frequent involvement of alveoli in the underlying process. In interstitial pulmonary edema, groups of alveoli often are flooded. In inflammatory processes, such as sarcoidosis or desquamative interstitial pneumonia, alveoli, as well as the interstitial space, are commonly caught up in the process. In pneumonia caused by *Pneumocystis carinii*, the organisms are found in alveoli as well as in the interstitial spaces. Therefore, the designation of diffuse interstitial disease should not be misconstrued as being confined solely to the interstitium of the lungs even though it generally does identify the predominant seat of the disease.

Syndromes of Alveolar Hypoventilation

The common denominator in disorders characterized by alveolar hypoventilation is an abnormally high value for arterial (and alveolar) P_{CO_2}. The most common cause is chronic bronchitis and emphysema which produces hypercapnia by deranging ventilation-perfusion relationships. This "net" alveolar hypoventilation is conceptionally different from the "generalized" alveolar hypoventilation that results from a disorder of respiratory control or of the chest bellows. The usual manifestation of generalized alveolar hypoventilation is the combination of normal lung volumes and FEV_1, normal chest radiograph in conjunction with arterial hypoxemia, hypercapnia, and respiratory acidosis.

Obliterative Vascular Disease

Pulmonary thromboemboli usually affect large as well as small vessels. Occlusive vascular disease confined to small ("resistance") pulmonary vessels is uncommon. More often, the pulmonary resistance vessels are involved as part of diffuse interstitial disease. In pulmonary vascular disease that compromises the area available for gas exchange, the diffusing capacity becomes subnormal. Occlusive vascular diseases of the lung are usually recognized when the extent of the disease is sufficient to cause considerable pulmonary hypertension. At that time, a characteristic constellation of findings usually prevails: (1) the chest radiograph shows central pulmonary arteries that are unduly large, in conjunction with pruning of the peripheral pulmonary vessels, (2) the electrocardiogram reveals right ventricular enlargement, and (3) pulmonary function tests show normal lung volumes and arterial blood-gas composition. Right-sided heart catheterization settles the diagnosis by revealing pulmonary arterial hypertension without evidence of pulmonary venous hypertension.

Complications and Ambiguities

Also listed in Table 26-5 are complicating or confusing states. Respiratory failure is a complication of the first three categories or of unrelated disorders, such as supervening adult respiratory distress syndrome. Pulmonary congestion and edema sometimes simulates, and often complicates, primary pulmonary disorders. Dyspnea is the usual trigger for pulmonary function tests; however, on occasion, unexplained cyanosis launches the search. Unless the lungs are implicated on clinical grounds, cyanosis generally proves to be extrapulmonary in origin. Most valuable in excluding the lungs as the cause for unexplained cyanosis is the demonstration that arterial blood oxygenation is normal.

BIBLIOGRAPHY

Altose M, Cherniack NS, Fishman AP: Respiratory sensations and dyspnea. Perspective. J Appl Physiol 58:1051–1054, 1985.
> *Editorial summary of a recent National Heart, Lung and Blood Institute workshop on respiratory sensations and dyspnea. It describes succinctly the current state of progress in the area.*

Braman SS: Pulmonary signs and symptoms. Clin Chest Med 8:177–337, 1987.
> *A wide-ranging collection of papers that deal first with cough, hemoptysis, dyspnea, wheezing and stridor, chest pain, snoring, and then with the physical examination and clinical signs.*

Brobowitz ID, Ramakrishna S, Shim YS: Comparison of medical vs. surgical treatment of major hemoptysis. Arch Intern Med 143:1343–1346, 1983.
> *In contrast to the Crocco article (see below), these authors favor conservative management.*

Burdon JGW, Juniper EF, Killian KJ, Hargreave FE, Campbell EJM: The perception of breathlessness in asthma. Am Rev Respir Dis 125:825–828, 1982.
> *A consistent relationship was found between induced changes in FEV_1 and degrees of breathlessness in asthmatics. However, a great deal of variability in the relationship requires additional contributing factors to play a significant role.*

Campbell EJM, Freedman S, Smith PS, Taylor ME: The ability of man to detect added elastic loads to breathing. Clin Sci 20:223–231, 1961.
> *Pioneering experiments dealing with mechanisms of breathing sensations.*

Cherniack NS, Altose MD: Mechanisms of dyspnea. Clin Chest Med 8:207–214, 1987.
  Although dyspnea, in large part, is an expression of the sense of the effort of breathing, the intensity and quality of the subjective experiences during breathing also depend on afferent feedback primarily from receptors in the respiratory muscles.

Cherniack NS, Fishman AP: Abnormal breathing patterns. Dis Month July 1975, pp 3–45.
  A review article that focuses on the chemical control of breathing and the disturbances that lead to characteristic clinical patterns.

Christie RV: Dyspnea in relation to the visco-elastic properties of the lung. Proc R Soc Med 46:381–386, 1953.
  Splendid review and an early hypothesis on the possible mechanism of dyspnea.

Comroe JH Jr: Some theories of the mechanism of dyspnea, in Howell JBL, Campbell EJM (eds), Breathlessness. Oxford, Blackwell, 1966, pp 1–7.
  Provocative review on the mechanism of dyspnea. (See also Richards, below.)

Cournand A, Richards DW Jr, Bader ME: The oxygen cost of breathing. Trans Assoc Am Physicians 67:162–165, 1954.
  One of the earliest discussions of this concept. Careful studies on humans showed relationships between level of ventilation and the oxygen cost of breathing.

Crocco JA, Rooney JJ, Fankushen DS, DiBenedetto RJ, Lyons HA: Massive hemoptysis. Arch Intern Med 121:495–498, 1968.
  A much quoted article which proposes early surgical intervention based on the quantity of blood expectorated (600 ml). High mortality with conservative management in their experience may have been due to bias in the selection of patient population.

Diamond MA, Genovese RD: Life-threatening hemoptysis in mitral stenosis. Emergency mitral valve replacement resulting in rapid, sustained cessation of pulmonary bleeding. J Am Med Assoc 215:441–444, 1971.
  Even though hemoptysis tends to subside spontaneously, cessation of hemorrhage in the cases reported above appeared to have been influenced by surgery.

Enarson DA, Vedal S, Schulzer M, Dybuncio A, Chan-Yeung M: Asthma, asthmalike symptoms, chronic bronchitis, and the degree of bronchial hyperresponsiveness in epidemiologic surveys. Am Rev Respir Dis 136:613–617, 1987.
  The results of a methacholine test for bronchial hyperresponsiveness were more closely associated with asthma than with any asthmalike symptoms elicited by a questionnaire developed for the study of chronic bronchitis.

Forgacs P: The functional basis of pulmonary sounds. Chest 73:398–405, 1978.
  An impressive review of current understanding of the origins and characteristics of pulmonary sounds.

Fraser RG, Pare JAP: Diagnosis of Diseases of the Chest, 2d ed. Philadelphia, Saunders, 1978.
  The differential diagnosis of chest diseases is approached and structured using the chest radiograph as the initial step.

Freundlich IM, Israel HL: Pulmonary aspergillosis. Clin Radiol 24:248–253, 1973.
  Approximately 70 percent of patients with opportunistic Aspergillus infection in chronic cavitary disease presented with hemoptysis.

Gavriely N, Kelly KB, Grotberg JB, Loring SH: Forced expiratory wheezes are a manifestation of airway flow limitation. J Appl Physiol 62:2398–2403, 1987.
  A study of the mechanism of generation of respiratory wheezes.

Gottfried SB, Altose MD, Kelsen SG, Cherniack NS: Perception of changes in airflow resistance in obstructive pulmonary disorders. Am Rev Respir Dis 124:566–570, 1981.
  Abnormalities in the perception of changes in ventilatory loading may relate causally to impairments in ventilatory responses to increases in airways resistance.

Gottlieb JE, Fanburg BL, Pauker SG: A decision analytic view of the diagnosis of sarcoidosis, in Fanburg BL (ed), Sarcoidosis and Other Granulomatous Diseases of the Lung. New York, Dekker, 1983, pp 349–380.
  Excellent example of application of decision analytical methods to diagnosis.

Hamilton WF, Woodbury RA, Harper HT Jr: Arterial, cerebrospinal and venous pressures in man during cough and strain. Am J Physiol 141:42–50, 1944.
  Intrathoracic pressures are shown to be transmitted to intraaortic and cerebrospinal fluid pressures in humans during respiratory maneuvers.

Harrison DW. Upper airway obstruction. A report on 16 patients. Q J Med 45:625–645, 1976.
Characteristic patterns can be seen in flow-volume plots of the forced vital capacity maneuver which have diagnostic value.

Harrison TR: *Failure of the Circulation*, 2d ed. Baltimore, Williams & Wilkins, 1939, pp 186–226.
Almost one-helf century ago, the mechanisms of dyspnea began to be explored systematically.

Kalia M: Visceral and somatic reflexes produced by pulmonary receptors in newborn kittens. J Appl Physiol 41:1–6, 1976.
Experimental study of the consequences of stimulating pulmonary vagal afferents.

Killian KJ, Bucens DD, Campbell EJM: Effect of breathing patterns on the perceived magnitude of added loads to breathing. J Appl Physiol 52:578–584, 1982.
The perceived magnitude of added resistive or elastic loads is shown to depend both on the magnitude of inspiratory force and its duration.

Kraman SS. Lung sounds. Sem Respir Med 6:157–241, 1985.
A series of separate papers tells all that the reader might want to know about lung sounds: their history, transmission, classification, nature, implications, practical applications, and future directions.

Lane, R, Cockcroft A, Adams L, Guz A: Arterial oxygen saturation and breathlessness in patients with chronic obstructive airways disease. Clin Sci 72:693–698, 1987.
In patients with chronic obstructive airways disease, the reduction in breathlessness produced by preventing exercise desaturation using supplemental oxygen cannot be explained entirely by the decrease in ventilation, suggesting that hypoxia, per se, may be a stimulus for breathlessness.

Lanken PN, Fishman AP: Clubbing and hypertrophic osteoarthropathy, in Fishman AP (ed), *Pulmonary Diseases and Disorders*. New York, McGraw-Hill, 1980, pp 84–91.
A comprehensive overview of the subject that emphasizes the practical utility of detecting and assessing clubbing and hypertrophic osteoarthropathy, the quantitative approaches used for assessing clubbing, and the open questions about pathogenesis.

Leblanc P, Bowie DM, Summers E, Jones NL, Killian KJ: Breathlessness and exercise in patients with cardiorespiratory disease. Am Rev Respir Dis 133:21–25, 1986.
Experimental reaffirmation in humans of the hypothesis that breathlessness is the perception of respiratory muscle effort and is present when the tension developed by muscles increases, when the muscles are weak, or when both conditions are present simultaneously.

Leith DE. Cough. Phys Ther 5:439–445, 1968.
Review of lung mechanics relevant to efficiency of cough mechanisms.

Loudon RG: The lung exam. Clin Chest Med 8:265–272, 1987.
Reemphasizes the value of the stethoscope as a diagnostic medical instrument.

Loudon R, Murphy RLH: Lung sounds. Am Rev Respir Dis 130:663–673, 1984.
Summarizes current knowledge on production, transmission, and clinical significance of lung sounds.

Lourenco RV, Turino GM, Davidson LAG, Fishman AP: The regulation of ventilation in diffuse fibrosis. Am J Med 38:199–216, 1965.
The ventilatory response to carbon dioxide and to exercise in patients with diffuse pulmonary fibrosis is described.

Mahler DA, Rosiello RA, Harver A, Lentine T, McGovern JF, Daubenspeck JA: Comparison of clinical dyspnea ratings and psychophysical measurements of respiratory sensation in obstructive airway disease. Am Rev Respir Dis 135:1229–2133, 1987.
Clinical methods and psychophysical testing provide different information about breathlessness.

Marshall R, Stone PW, Christie RV: The relationship of dyspnea to respiratory effort in normal subjects. Mitral stenosis and emphysema. Clin Sci 13:625–631, 1954.
A classic paper that focuses on optimization of the breathing pattern for the sake of minimal work.

McIntosh HD, Estes EH, Warren JV: The mechanism of cough syncope. Am Heart J 52:70–82, 1956.
The transmission of changes in intrathoracic pressures to the cerebrospinal fluid is postulated to decrease cerebral perfusion.

Mead J: Control of respiratory frequency. J Appl Physiol 15:325–336, 1960.
Classic observations showing that the respiratory frequency adopted at rest and in exercise appears to minimize the average force exerted by respiratory muscles.

Mellins RB, Lord GP, Fishman AP: Dynamic behavior of the lung in acute asthma. Med Thorac 24:81–98, 1967.

An early attempt to examine the dynamic properties of the airways in patients with severe airway obstruction.

Narbed PG, Marcer D, Howell JBL: The contribution of the accelerating phase of inspiratory flow to resistive load detection in man. Clin Sci 62:367–372, 1982.

Using techniques from signal detection theory, the authors find that information used for detection of small resistive loads is generated early in inspiration and probably consists of rate changes in airflow and pressure.

Nath AR, Capel LH: Inspiratory crackles and mechanical events of breathing. Thorax 29:695–698, 1974.

Acoustic recordings of successive breaths show that individual crackles recur at the same lung volume and transpulmonary pressure.

Noble MIM, Eisele JH, Trenchard D, Guz A: Effect of selective peripheral nerve blocks on respiratory sensations, in Porter R (ed), *Breathing: Hering-Breuer Centenary Symposium.* London, J. & A. Churchill, 1970, pp 233–245.

Experiments are reported on the effects of vagal blockade on respiratory sensations in human volunteers.

Paintal AS: Vagal sensory receptors and their reflex effects. Physiol Rev 53:159–227, 1973.

A comprehensive review of pioneering experiments that led to the concept of J receptors. Although the localization of these receptors in the alveolar-capillary barrier has been cast into doubt since then, the idea still seems valid.

Ploysonsan Y, Pare JAP, Macklau PT: Correlation of regional breath sounds with regional ventilation in emphysema. Am Rev Respir Dis 126:526–533, 1982.

The existence of this correlation supports the theory of regional (versus central) production of breath sounds.

Plum F, Brown HW: The effect on respiration of central nervous system disease. Ann NY Acad Sci 109:915–931, 1963.

A report of the commoner forms of neurologic respiratory abnormalities with particular reference to correlations among clinical observations, pathophysiology, and neuroanatomic defects. Among the disorders considered are posthyperventilation apnea, Cheyne-Stokes breathing, central neurogenic hyperventilation, and ataxic breathing.

Poe RH, Israel RH, Utell MJ, Hale WJ: Chronic cough: Bronchoscopy or pulmonary function testing? Am Rev Respir Dis 126:160–162, 1982.

Bronchoscopy was of little value if the chest radiograph was normal. Bronchial inhalation challenge or spirometry discovered several cases of unsuspected asthma.

Richards DW Jr: The nature of cardiac and pulmonary dyspnea. Circulation 7:15–29, 1953.

This article and the one by Comroe (see above) are masterful introductions to the conceptual and experimental difficulties of investigating mechanisms of dyspnea. Even though the emphasis has evolved since their writing, some of the formulations are still insightful.

Robertson AJ. Rales, ronchi and Laennec. Lancet 2:417–423, 1957.

An amusing historical account of the evolution of the terminology of lung sounds.

Rosenheim SH, Schwartz J: Cavitary pulmonary cryptococcosis complicated by aspergilloma. Am Rev Respir Dis 111:549–553, 1975.

Case report illustrating lung disease caused by two fungal organisms acting by two different mechanisms.

Smith R, Olson M: Drug-induced methemoglobinemia. Semin Hematol 10:253–268, 1973.

Good review of the subject.

Thomas NW, Wilson RF, Puro HE, Arbulu A: Life-threatening hemoptysis in primary lung abscess. Ann Thorac Surg 14:347–358, 1972.

In lung abscess, hemorrhage can be severe.

Tucker AK, Pemberton J, Guyer PB: Pulmonary fungal infection complicating treated malignant disease. Clin Radiol 26:129–136, 1975.

This article and those of Murray and Freundlich cited above describe case reports of various forms of pulmonary mycosis in which hemoptysis was a prominent manifestation.

Chapter 27

Pulmonary Cutaneous Disorders

Brian V. Jegasothy / Elizabeth F. Sherertz

Types of Skin Lesions
White Macules
Brown Macules
Red Macules
Diffuse Erythema
Flesh-Colored Papules and Nodules
Red Papules and Nodules
Blue Papules and Nodules
Brown Papules
Scaling Papules
Vesiculobullous Lesions
Pustules
Purpura
Nails
Skin Texture Change

Skin Lesions in Pulmonary-Systemic Disorders
Atopic Dermatitis
Infectious Disorders
Cutaneous Sarcoidosis
Congenital and Developmental Disorders
Pulmonary Vasculitis
Neoplastic Disorders
Collagen Vascular Disorders
Complications of Medications

Examination of the skin can provide important clues in the diagnosis and treatment of individuals with pulmonary disease: some skin lesions either accompany pulmonary disease or complicate its treatment; occasionally, systemic diseases that affect both skin and lung first manifest themselves in the skin; certain primary diseases of the skin, such as mucosal erythema multiforme, are associated with important pulmonary complications. In addition, common skin lesions, many of which are unrelated to lung disease, have to be taken into account in patients being examined for pulmonary disease.

TYPES OF SKIN LESIONS

The pattern of the skin lesion, i.e., macule, nodule, vesicles, and coloration, can be useful in sorting the type of process that is occurring in the skin and its relevance to the pulmonary disease in question.

White Macules

Macules are areas of whitish or hypopigmented color change that are not palpable. For example, in young adults or in patients taking steroids, tinea versicolor is a common eruption of white or red-brown macules over the upper torso (Fig. 27-1A). In infants, nonscaling macules or ash-leaf spots concurrent with adenoma sebaceum (pink, smooth papules over the central face) may be an early sign of tuberous sclerosis. Vitiligo occurs in patients with thyroid disease, Addison's disease, pernicious anemia, diabetes, and polyglandular failure. It is characterized by white macules that are usually symmetrically disposed over the extremities and around body orifices; occasionally, vitiligo is segmental over a dermatome.

Brown Macules

Brown macules occur as a consequence of sun exposure (freckles) or at the site of previously inflamed lesions, such as acne. Pigment cell nevi are brown macules that usually develop in childhood or young adulthood; as a rule they are symmetric and uniform in color (Fig. 27-1B); suspicion of melanoma should be aroused when the lesions are either irregular in border, or blue, red, brown or black in color (Fig. 27-1C), or rapidly growing, or bleeding. In older adults, seborrheic keratosis may first appear as oval brown macules before becoming papules.

Larger (2 to 20 cm), circumscribed brown macules, i.e., café au lait spots, occur in 10 percent of the population. The presence of 6 or more of such lesions larger than 1.5 cm raises the prospect of neurofibromatosis.

Diffuse flat hyperpigmentation occurs after sun exposure (tanning). The skin of patients with scleroderma occasionally develops a pattern of mottled "salt and pepper" hyperpigmentation. In obese individuals, flexural pigmentation about the neck and under the axillae, at times associated with flesh-colored skin tags, is called pseudoacanthosis nigricans; in the nonobese adult, these lesions raise the question of acanthosis nigricans, a potential marker of internal malignancy. Although acanthosis nigricans is generally associated with adenocarcinoma of the gastrointestinal tract, it occasionally accompanies carcinoma of the lung.

Red Macules

Telangiectasias are red macules or papules that are usually vascular in appearance. Scattered telangiectasias are common in sun-exposed areas of the skin such as the V of the anterior neck and the upper back. In patients with obstructive airways disease, linear telangiectasia is sometimes seen along the anterior costal margins; this pattern is known as *costal fringe*. Well-formed spider telangiectasias, common on the upper chest, occur in chronic liver disease or in states of hyperestrogenism. Spider telangiec-

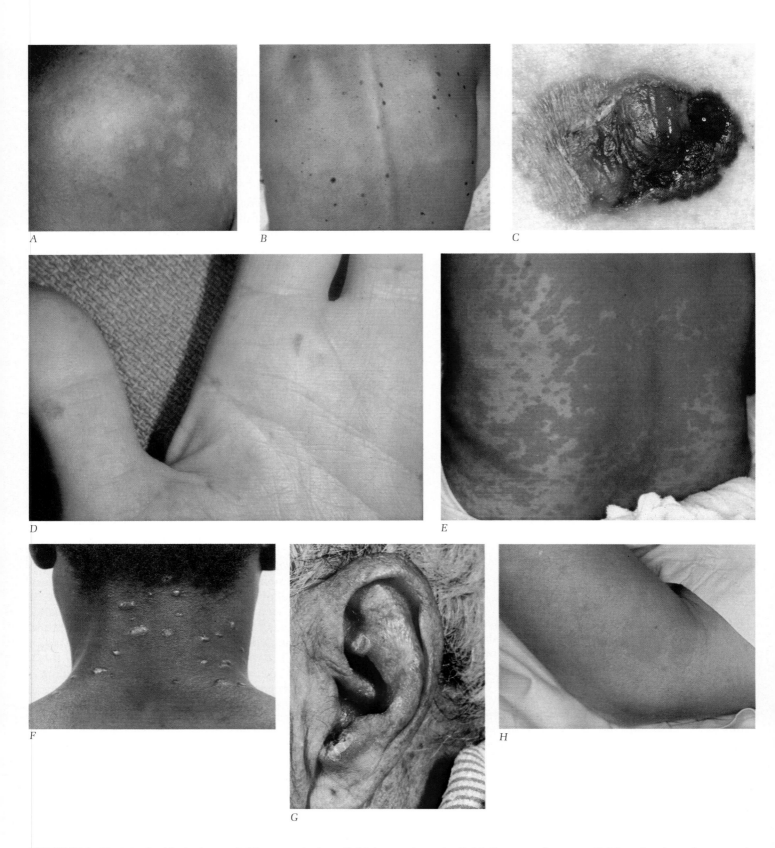

FIGURE 27-1 Prototypic skin lesions. *A.* Tinea versicolor. *B.* Melanocytic nevi. *C.* Malignant melanoma. *D.* Mat telangiectasia as seen in scleroderma or Osler-Weber-Rendu disease. *E.* Exanthematous eruption. *F.* Sarcoid. Flesh-colored papules of upper eyelid and inner canthus. *G.* Metastatic nodule from primary lung carcinoma. *H.* Urticaria.

tasia of the trunk, mucosa, fingers, and hands is seen in Osler-Weber-Rendu disease, whereas larger "mat" telangiectasias distributed in the same areas are seen in scleroderma (Fig. 27-1D). Telangiectasia and persistent edema of the face sometimes occur after repeated bouts of flushing in the carcinoid syndrome. On rare occasions, telangiectasia with mottled hyperpigmentation occurs in systemic mastocytosis.

Diffuse Erythema

This type of erythema may be acute or chronic in onset.

ACUTE

A maculopapular, or exanthematous, eruption is characterized by the acute appearance of multiple red macules that become confluent to form a diffuse erythema (Fig. 27-1E). The pattern is nonspecific and, in adults, is due either to a drug reaction or to an infectious, especially viral, process. The drugs most often responsible for this type of reaction are antibiotics, especially trimethoprimsulfamethoxasole and the penicillins, phenytoin, allopurinol, blood products, isoniazid, and carbamazepine. Aminophylline sometimes elicits this type of eruption, especially in a patient who has been previously sensitized to ethylenediamine, a common stabilizer in some topical products, such as Mycolog cream.

Viral and bacterial systemic infections can also cause an exanthematous eruption. In classic measles (rubeola) and rubella, fever and upper respiratory symptoms sometimes precede the exanthem, which usually starts on the face. In atypical measles, which occasionally occurs in adults who have developed partial immunity after receiving killed measles vaccine, the onset is generally more insidious and the skin eruption ranges from urticarial to petechial, favors the extremities, and is associated with pneumonia and high fever. Other respiratory viral infections are sometimes accompanied by nonspecific exanthems that are usually truncal; usually the eruption lasts for only a few days and is followed by superficial scaling. In the immunocompromised host, an exanthem sometimes accompanies a fulminant cytomegaloviral infection; in some of these patients, cytomegalic inclusions have been seen in a skin biopsy.

Among the bacterial infections, streptococcal scarlet fever and the staphylococcal scaled skin syndrome are most often associated with a diffuse erythematous eruption. The toxic shock syndrome, a systemic illness induced by staphylococcal toxin, may be associated with bright red truncal erythema and, subsequently, with desquamation of palmar and digital skin. Systemic bacterial sepsis due to a variety of organisms, e.g., the meningococcus or *Pseudomonas*, occasionally elicits a generalized, nonspecific erythematous eruption; Legionnaires' disease can do the same. As a rule, biopsy or culture of the eruption is unrewarding.

CHRONIC

This category is characterized by the subacute or insidious development (over weeks to months) of a generalized or diffuse erythema (erythroderma). One example is atopic dermatitis which, in adults, often represents an irritant or allergic reaction to a topical product, such as soap or occupational exposure. Exposed areas show erythema, evidence of scratching, and secondary scaling and thickening of the skin. Usually there is a history of childhood eczema or sensitive skin, and a personal or family history of asthma, hay fever, or environmental allergies. In some patients with atopic dermatitis, increased itching of the skin appears to be a prodrome to asthma attacks.

In dermatomyositis, a red violaceous hue commonly appears around the eyes (heliotrope) accompanied by fine scaling; the upper trunk and extensor surfaces of the extremities may be similarly involved. Gottron's papules—red, atrophic papules over the finger joints—are present in about one-third of patients. In lupus erythematosus, erythema, telangiectasia, and atrophy tend to affect the sun-exposed areas of the face and arms; sometimes the upper trunk is similarly involved.

A chronic insidious onset of generalized erythroderma may be secondary to drugs, or to infiltrative skin disease, such as cutaneous lymphoma or leukemia, or to mastocytosis, or it may be a reaction to an internal malignancy, including carcinoma of the lung.

Flesh-Colored Papules and Nodules

In neurofibromatosis, flat, pigmented, café au lait patches that appear in childhood are often accompanied in adulthood by flesh-colored, soft papules and nodules. The lesions of basal cell carcinoma are flesh-colored or translucent papules with telangiectasia and erosion, and they occur particularly in sun-exposed areas of fair-skinned individuals (Fig. 27-1D).

In sarcoidosis, distinctive lesions in the form of firm, flesh-colored papules of the face and upper trunk occur in 20 to 25 percent of affected individuals (Fig. 27-1F). Environmental exposure to beryllium can also reproduce the lesions clinically and histologically. However, much more common now than beryllium-induced lesions from the atmosphere are beryllium-induced lesions that develop in cuts from broken fluorescent bulbs.

Neoplastic or metastatic lesions (Fig. 27-1G) are noninflamed, asymptomatic, firm-to-rock-hard, flesh-colored or red nodules of the skin. Metastases from a carcinoma of the lung or breast, or cutaneous infiltrates due to B-cell lymphomas, are particularly likely to involve the anterior upper trunk. In men, carcinoma of the lung is a most common cause of cutaneous metastases; the skin metastases usually involve the scalp, the anterior chest, and the abdomen.

Red Papules and Nodules

Cherry angiomas are typically persistent, cherry-red papules, 1 to 8 mm in diameter; they commonly affect the trunk and proximal extremities in the elderly, in pregnant women, and in individuals who are in a state of hyperestrogenism. They occur in Osler-Weber-Rendu disease, occasionally in association with pulmonary arteriovenous fistulas. Dermatomal hemangiomas are congenital vascular patches that may be associated with underlying spinal vascular malformations.

Urticarial lesions take the form of scattered, *transient,* red papules, plaques and wheals that may be annular or serpiginous in shape and edematous-pink to dusky in color (Fig. 27-1*H*). The wheals may occur anywhere on the body. Pruritus is generally a prominent feature. The individual lesions usually last for only 24 to 48 h.

Urticaria is common and generally nonspecific: on the one hand, it may herald a life-threatening anaphylactic reaction; on the other, it may be a fleeting localized reaction of no great moment. Among the potential causes of urticaria are topical or systemic medications, food inhalant allergens, infections, and psychological factors.

Dermographism is a type of urticaria in which wheals develop in response to stroking the skin; it occurs in up to 5 percent of normal individuals but may also develop transiently after upper respiratory tract illness and some medications. *White dermographism* is a vasoconstrictive response to skin stroking that may be quite prominent in individuals with atopic dermatitis. Cholinergic urticaria (Fig. 27-2*A*) is characterized by small (1 to 3 mm) pruritic wheals with surrounding red flare reactions; they occur in response to heat, cold, exercise, and emotional stress. Transient symptoms of wheezing or shortness of breath may accompany the onset of cholinergic urticaria, and pulmonary function tests may provide evidence of bronchospasm. The process seems to be mast cell-mediated; treatment with antihistamines, such as hydroxyzine, is usually of benefit.

In erythema multiforme, annular erythematous papules sometimes progress to target lesions with overlying blisters (Fig. 27-2*B*). The lesions can occur anywhere on the body but may be limited to the hands and feet. When erythema multiforme is accompanied by fever, skin lesions, and mucosal involvement of the mouth and/or eyes, it is called the *Stevens-Johnson syndrome* (Fig. 27-2*C*). Erythema multiforme may occur as a reaction to drugs, including penicillin, sulfa derivatives, gold, and barbiturates. A long list of infections may also elicit erythema multiforme: herpes simplex I and II, influenza A, adenovirus, psittacosis, β-hemolytic streptococcus, *Pseudomonas,* tularemia, histoplasmosis, coccidioidomycosis, and tuberculosis.

Several types of large (>1 cm) erythematous nodules occur in patients with pulmonary disease. One type that has no bearing on the pulmonary process is a simple infected epidermal cyst that develops suddenly as a tender, red nodule at the site of a preexisting lesion, commonly on the posterior neck and back. Oppositely, red nodules may represent vascular, inflammatory, or neoplastic processes that cannot be distinguished without excisional biopsy. The nodular vasculitides, including allergic, Wegener's, and lymphomatoid granulomatosis, are discussed later in this chapter.

Multiple tender red nodules over the anterior surfaces of the lower extremities suggest erythema nodosum (Fig. 27-2*D*), a reactive inflammation of the subcutaneous fat that may be associated with a number of infections, drugs, and underlying inflammatory diseases. In the patient undergoing treatment for acute or subacute pulmonary disease, a medication may be the cause, especially oral contraceptives, sulfonamides, other antibiotics, iodides or bromides. In up to 16 percent of patients with erythema nodosum, sarcoidosis is the cause. Occasionally, sarcoidosis is first manifested as an acute febrile illness with erythema nodosum, hilar adenopathy, malaise, and arthritis (Lofgren's syndrome). As a rule, sarcoidosis that begins with erythema nodosum is a self-limited disease. Erythema nodosum also occurs in some individuals with tuberculosis, psittacosis, histoplasmosis, blastomycosis, and coccidioidomycosis.

A variety of pulmonary infections (blastomycosis, coccidioidomycosis, histoplasmosis, cryptococcosis, tuberculosis, actinomycosis, and nocardiosis) may be accompanied by skin lesions in the form of crusted, erythematous nodules and plaques (Fig. 27-2*E* and *F*). They may occur anywhere on the skin; as a rule, they are nonspecific in appearance and asymptomatic. The development of this type of crusted plaque or nodule in a patient with a chronic pulmonary infection calls for biopsy and histopathologic examination using special stains and cultures for suspected organisms.

Blue Papules and Nodules

Blue color is generally transmitted from vascular structures or melanin pigment deep in the dermis. Blue nevi are benign dermal melanocytic neoplasms that are uniform in shape; they may occur over the head or the paraspinal area of the trunk. A blue-black, irregular, or friable lesion raises the possibility of a melanoma. A vascular lesion is generally partially compressible or palpable. Venous angiomas occur over the lips, ears, and upper trunk of older individuals. Kaposi's sarcoma, particularly in patients with acquired immunodeficiency syndrome, may present as asymptomatic bluish papules or plaques on the mucosa, upper trunk, and extremities (Fig. 27-3*A*); these lesions may become quite extensive.

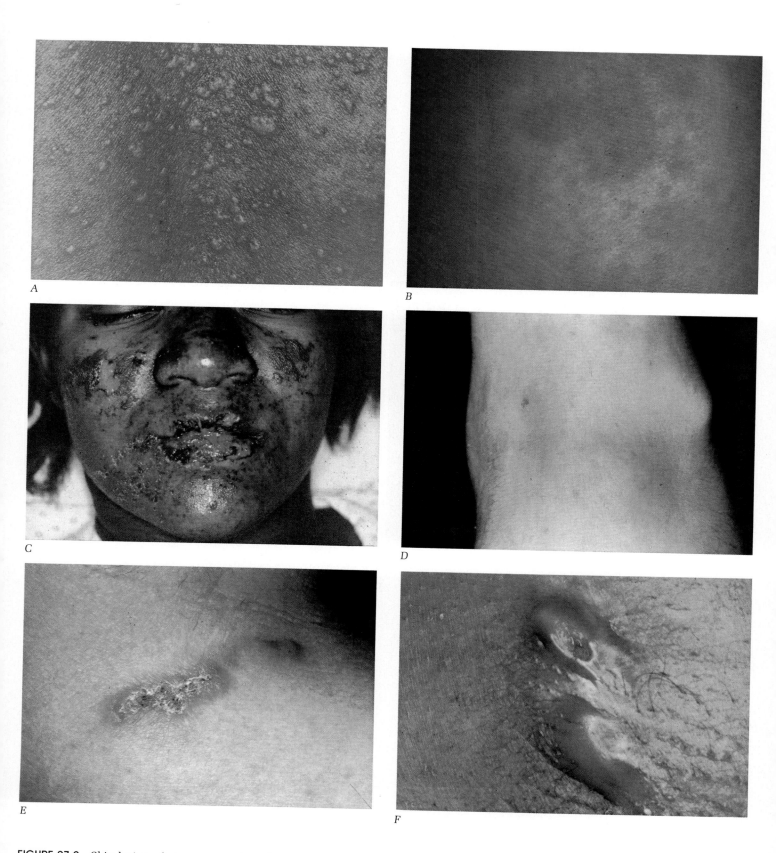

FIGURE 27-2 Skin lesions that may occur in pulmonary patients. *A.* Cholinergic urticaria. *B.* Erythema multiforme. *C.* Stevens-Johnson syndrome. *D.* Erythema nodosum. *E.* Blastomycosis. *F.* Tuberculous abscess.

Brown Papules

Melanocytic nevi (Fig. 27-1B) and seborrheic keratoses (Fig. 27-3B) are the most common lesions of this type. Pigmented nevi are usually uniform, both in brown color and shape. Dysplastic nevi are atypical lesions that are irregular and red-brown in color; they may give rise to malignant melanoma. As indicated above, irregular borders or surface, or blue-black or red colors to the lesions should raise concern about malignant melanoma (Fig. 27-1C). Seborrheic keratoses are waxy or rough-shaped superficial brown papules usually found in elderly adults, particularly over the back, neck, and face.

Scaling Papules

A number of skin disorders can present as multiple scaling red papules or plaques; among these are psoriasis, pityriasis rosea, secondary syphilis, and fungal infections. Sarcoid may also have scaling plaques and papules that resemble psoriasis.

Certain scaling lesions are common over the neck and back. Among these are actinic keratoses, which are small, rough lesions on sun-exposed areas of the face, neck, back and arms. They are most prominent in fair-skinned individuals with outdoor occupations. Bowen's disease (in situ squamous cell carcinoma) is usually a single scaling

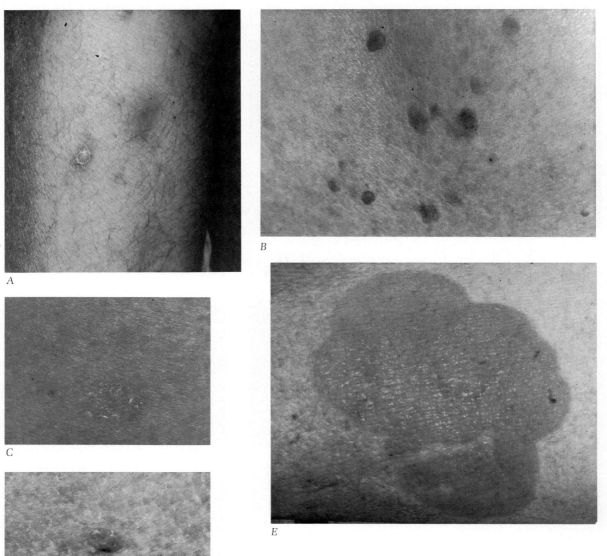

FIGURE 27-3   Skin lesions that may be encountered in patients with pulmonary disease.   *A.* Kaposi's sarcoma in a patient with acquired immunodeficiency syndrome.   *B.* Seborrheic keratoses (brown) and cherry (red) angiomata.   *C.* Basal cell carcinoma, superficial type. *D.* Basal cell carcinoma.   *E.* Mycosis fungoides.

or eczematous plaque that may occur anywhere on the body; this type of persistent solitary lesion requires biopsy to establish the diagnosis. The occurrence of Bowen's disease in non-sun-exposed areas raises the possibility of an internal neoplasm, including a carcinoma of the respiratory tract; a latent period of 8 years may intervene between the onset of Bowen's disease and detection of the internal neoplasm. Superficial basal cell carcinoma is a variant of this common sun-induced tumor; it presents as a single patch or as several scaling red patches, often on the trunk (Fig. 27-3*C* and *D*).

Mycosis fungoides is a malignant lymphoma of the skin that progresses through three stages. The first, or pre-*mycotic*, phase is characterized by lesions that resemble either psoriasis, seborrheic dermatitis, or eczema; characteristically, the lesions are very pruritic (Fig. 27-3*E*). In the second phase which may be long-delayed, the lesions become infiltrative, forming indurated red-to-purple plaques in conjunction with exfoliative dermatitis and erythroderma (Figs. 27-3*F* and *G*). The final stage is characterized by the formation of tumors that usually become necrotic. This sequence may take 8 to 12 years to evolve. However, on occasion, mycosis fungoides blossoms de novo as a mushroomlike growth on normal skin (d'emblée form). The final stage is often accompanied by systemic manifestations, including Sézary's syndrome.

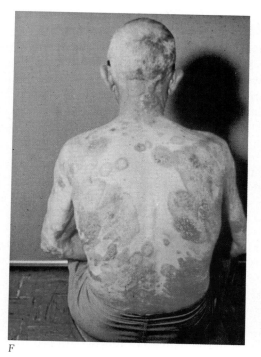

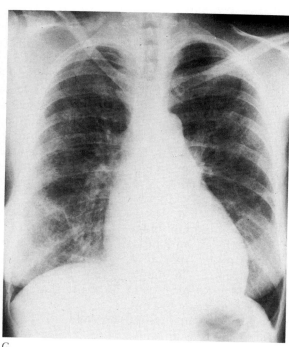

F   G

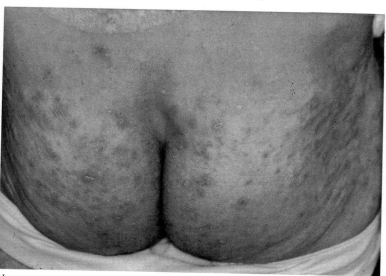

H

FIGURE 27-3 *(continued)* *F.* Mycosis fungoides. Asymmetric diffuse, superficial, gyrate plaques of dermatitis. *G.* Chest radiograph shows diffuse reticular nodular density, proved by open lung biopsy to be mycosis fungoides. *H.* Larva migrans in a patient with Loeffler's syndrome. *(From Katz and Beerman, Pulmonary-cutaneous disorders, in Pulmonary Diseases and Disorders, Fishman AP (ed). New York, McGraw-Hill, 1980.)*

The lungs are frequently involved in mycosis fungoides. Two-thirds of patients who die of disseminated mycosis fungoides have pulmonary involvement at autopsy: usually the lesions are in the form of multiple nodules; few have diffuse patchy or confluent infiltrates. Histologically, tumor cells are seen infiltrating alveolar walls. The neoplasm spreads via the bloodstream leaving uninvolved contiguous or regional lymph nodes. Chest radiographs usually show mediastinal and hilar adenopathy, reticulonodular parenchymal lesions, and, occasionally, pleural effusions.

The extracutaneous sites that are most often involved by cutaneous T-cell lymphoma are blood, lymph nodes (in 75 percent of patients at autopsy), and lungs (in 66 percent at autopsy). This visceral involvement is often asymptomatic but is important in clinical staging and survival. When the lungs are affected, the chest radiograph may show hilar and mediastinal adenopathy (Fig 27-3G) and a reticulonodular pattern of pulmonary infiltration. Lung biopsy shows the tumor lymphocytes infiltrating alveolar walls.

Vesiculobullous Lesions

Of the skin lesions that present as fluid-filled blisters, the herpes virus group of diseases is the most relevant to pulmonary disease. These are discussed subsequently.

Primary blistering disorders may also involve the respiratory mucosa. Stevens-Johnson syndrome has already been mentioned. Pemphigus vulgaris, an immunologically mediated bullous disease in which IgG antibodies develop against the epidermal intercellular substance, presents as multiple flaccid bullous lesions. The mouth and oropharynx may be the initial and most prominent sites of involvement. Certain variants of a congenital bullous disorder, epidermolysis bullosa, may also involve the pharyngeal and respiratory mucosa, leading to erosions, scarring, and stricture.

Pustules

Skin lesions that present as pustules should raise the possibility of bacterial infection. The most common of these is probably a folliculitis in which pustules develop around hair follicles. Most often a folliculitis is due to *Staphylococcus aureus* infection, and the lesions may progress to furuncles or to deep cutaneous abscesses. Manipulation of such lesions can lead to bacteremia and multiple septic pulmonary abscesses. Parenteral drug users are at risk for developing multiple cutaneous abscesses at needle sites. Patients with underlying deep fungal disease, actinomycosis, or nocardiosis may develop indurated, pustular plaques or cutaneous abscesses. For identification of the causative organism, the lesions may have to be incised or biopsied for staining and culture.

Drug-induced acne presents as multiple small pustules, often over the upper chest. Steroids in high doses, bromides, or iodides are common causes. In areas and societies where larvae of nematodes can gain access to the skin, secondary pyoderma caused by scratching of the pruritic lesions is often superimposed on the linear tracts or papules produced by the entering larvae. The skin pattern is often a bizarre combination of lesions, and larva migrans should be considered in a patient who presents with a compatible history and skin lesions, especially over the buttocks and back (Fig. 27-3H). *Strongyloides stercoralis*, and some other nematodes, can cause these skin lesions (larva currens) in association with acute fever, asthma, and eosinophilia (Loeffler's syndrome).

Purpura

Purpura results from disruption or extravasation of blood from cutaneous vessels; it is a nonspecific finding. It occurs commonly over traumatized sites in older patients, particularly in sun-exposed areas. Patients receiving steroid or anticoagulant therapy, or with defects in collagen, e.g., the Ehlers-Danlos syndrome or amyloidosis, are prone to traumatic purpura. Punctate petechiae may develop on the palate, face, and upper chest of patients with severe coughing spasms. Raised or palpable purpuric lesions should suggest a vasculitis. Because the etiologies of vasculitis are diverse, e.g., infections, medications, hypersensitivity reactions, and small-vessel disease, examination of the skin has to be followed by more elaborate diagnostic studies, including biopsy. Involvement of medium or large cutaneous vessels with vasculitis causes painful red to purpuric nodules with secondary ulceration; once again, the clinical appearance is nonspecific.

Nails

A number of changes in the nails may suggest underlying systemic disease. Clubbing and hypertrophic osteoarthropathy are discussed elsewhere (see Chapter 26). Yellow-brown staining of the nails where cigarettes are held is very common in individuals with obstructive airways disease who have not stopped smoking. The designation *yellow nail syndrome* refers to thickening, yellowing, and curvature of all the nails in association with lymphedema; it may be associated with pleural effusions, chronic pulmonary infections, and bronchiectasis.

Periungual telangiectasia and digital infarcts are seen in patients with lupus erythematosus, scleroderma, dermatomyositis, and overlap syndromes. Splinter hemorrhages are often due to trauma and are generally nonspecific despite their historical link to bacterial endocarditis. Sarcoidosis in the form of lupus pernio may involve the nails and underlying bones, leading to dystrophic, ridged nails and distal swelling.

Skin Texture Change

Thickening or sclerosis of the skin is most often associated with scleroderma; this disorder may present as distal digital sclerosis or it may be diffuse, most prominently over the trunk, and cause the typical drawn facies of scleroderma. The pulmonary changes are discussed in Chapter 43. Scleredema adultorum is a rare cutaneous disorder with striking mucopolysaccharide infiltration of the face, neck, and trunk; it may be confused clinically with scleroderma.

Increased elasticity of the skin is associated with certain types of Ehlers-Danlos syndrome; it is associated with defects in collagen synthesis. Conversely, in cutis laxa, the skin loses its elasticity because of a defect in the formation of elastin. Both disorders are considered below (see "Disorders of Collagen and Elastin").

SKIN LESIONS IN PULMONARY-SYSTEMIC DISORDERS

Atopic Dermatitis

Atopy refers to a group of conditions, including asthma, hay fever, and atopic dermatitis, in which immune and pharmacologic responses are characteristically abnormal. The atopic individual usually has a family history of one or more of these conditions. Atopic dermatitis is a common disorder, affecting 1 to 3 percent of the population in the United States. In 85 percent of affected individuals, the skin lesions appear before 5 years of age. The dermatitis generally improves as the patient reaches adulthood; in the adult, either the skin lesions or respiratory systems may predominate.

In infants, the skin lesions often begin as dry, erythematous plaques on the cheeks; excoriations and scaling may be prominent. In older children, the lesions localize in flexures; lichenification and excoriated papules are prominent features (Fig. 27-4A). In adults, the lesions favor the hands and extremities (nummular dermatitis) (Fig. 27-4B). Atopic individuals also manifest prominent folds of the lower eyelids, periorbital hyperpigmentation with facial pallor, generalized dry skin, and white dermographism. At any age, pruritus may be prominent and become secondarily infected, leading to bacterial impetigo within the lesions. In some patients, increased itching may be a prodrome to exacerbation of asthma.

The cause of atopic dermatitis is unknown. In all likelihood, the pathogenesis is multifactorial, probably including disordered immune regulation as a causative factor. In individuals with atopic dermatitis, abnormalities in cell-mediated immunity and in lymphocyte function increase the risk of disseminated viral and fungal skin lesions. The role of food or environmental antigenic challenge in flares of atopic dermatitis is unsettled, but it is known that asthma can be precipitated by such challenges. Treatment of atopic dermatitis in adults is aimed at eliminating possible environmental irritants and allergens.

Infectious Disorders

The skin and lungs are sometimes involved simultaneously in infectious disorders, including viral, bacterial, mycoplasma, and fungal diseases.

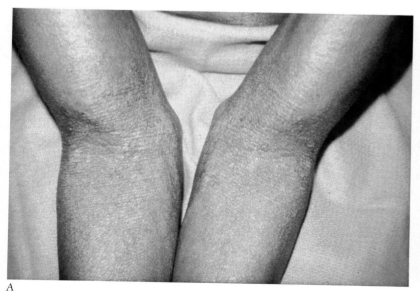

A

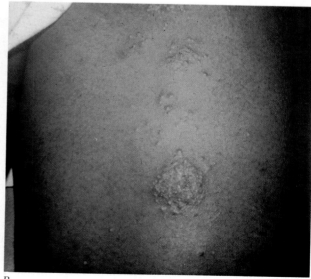

B

FIGURE 27-4 Skin lesions in pulmonary-systemic disorders. *A.* Atopic dermatitis—flexural lichenification. *B.* Atopic dermatitis—nummular lesions.

VIRAL

Three types of viral infection are often involved in pulmonary cutaneous syndromes: herpes simplex, herpes zoster-varicella, and measles.

Herpes Simplex

The lesions of herpes simplex appear as groups of small vesicles (1 to 5 mm) on an erythematous base; they may occur anywhere on the body surface, but the most common sites are around the lips or genital area. Recurrence of the lesions can be triggered by fever, upper respiratory infection, trauma, or exposure to sunlight. Patients with underlying skin diseases such as atopic dermatitis may be at risk for developing generalized herpes simplex, i.e., eczema herpeticum. In immunocompromised patients, the lesions may be atypical and take the form of persistent crusted ulcers or erosions. This should be kept in mind when doing bronchoscopy, suctioning or other procedures on patients with perioral ulcerations. Medical personnel are at risk for acquiring herpes simplex infection of the fingers, i.e., the herpetic whitlow, a tender vesicular cellulitis of the digit.

Herpes Zoster and Varicella

Herpes zoster and varicella have potential pulmonary complications. Varicella often starts with a prodromal fever, malaise, headache, and sore throat, followed by onset of small (1 to 3 mm) distinct vesicles on a red base that rapidly progress to umbilicated and crusted lesions. Lesions appear in crops over the body and may also involve the mucous membranes. The major complication of adult varicella is pneumonia, and the extent of pulmonary involvement tends to correlate with the extent of the cutaneous eruption. Radiographic findings may be more prominent than symptoms: infiltrates are seen in up to 16 percent of adult patients with varicella, whereas respiratory symptoms occur in only about 5 percent of adults.

In more than two-thirds of patients with herpes zoster, the lesions affect the thoracic region. Prodromal symptoms of localized pain prior to the eruption may mimic pleuritic pain, angina, or an acute abdomen; local itching, tenderness, or hyperesthesia may be followed by erythematous papules or urticarial plaques over the distribution of one or two sensory ganglia. Within 12 to 24 h the lesions develop into vesicles; crusting occurs within 7 to 10 days. Overlapping dermatomes may be involved, and a few isolated vesicles may lie outside these dermatomes. The associated pain is usually most severe early in the course and may lead to respiratory splinting. Involvement of the cervical roots may lead to diaphragmatic paralysis on the same side. The lesions cluster on the face, scalp, chest, and abdomen; the palms and soles are spared. The hard palate, tonsillar pillars, and larynx also develop vesicles which rupture, leaving white ulcers with an erythematous halo. Histologically, zoster and varicella lesions contain intraepidermal bullae. Infected cells contain eosinophilic, intranuclear inclusions surrounded by a clear halo and a circle of dark-staining chromatin. Multinucleated giant "balloon" cells are often present.

Pneumonia is the most common pulmonary complication of active infection with the varicella-zoster virus; pulmonary infarction has also been described. Although the cutaneous form of the disease is common in children, 90 percent of those developing pneumonia are more than 20 years old; most of these are in the third to fifth decade. The most frequent symptoms of varicella pneumonia develop 1 to 6 days following the onset of rash; they consist of cough, fever, cyanosis, dyspnea, and hemoptysis. Chest radiographs show a nodular or reticulonodular infiltrate throughout all lung fields, with a tendency toward coalescence at the base. Pleural effusions and hilar adenopathy have also been reported. Radiographic changes correlate well with cutaneous lesions: the chest radiograph clears rapidly as the skin manifestations resolve, leaving only minor abnormalities as residue; these often persist for months. Small calcifications in both lungs, especially at the bases, are common sequelae of varicella pneumonia.

Measles

Measles, a myxoviral infection, characteristically develops cutaneous manifestations after an incubation period of about 10 days. The initial phase of cutaneous manifestations, which lasts 4 to 7 days, consists of an erythematous or petechial eruption in the soft palate followed by the appearance of blue-white lesions surrounded by a bright red halo on the buccal mucosa (Koplik's spots). The buccal lesions proliferate, become confluent, and resolve within 72 h of their appearance. The characteristic macular eruption in the scalp then develops and rapidly spreads to the upper part of the neck, extremities, and trunk. This exanthema progresses to soft papules and becomes confluent over the face before beginning to scale. Systemic manifestations include high fever, chills, conjunctivitis, coryza, and a dry, hacking cough. This cough is a common symptom in the initial invasion phase, and it sometimes recurs as the disease progresses.

Segmental pneumonia and atelectasis are common in patients with measles. In most instances, these are complications of superinfection with bacteria. However, the virus per se sometimes causes a giant cell pneumonia, especially in children. Giant cell pneumonia occurs before, or coincident with, the peak of the measles exanthema. In these children, the chest radiograph shows a diffuse reticular pattern, usually accompanied by hilar adenopathy.

MYCOPLASMA

Pneumonia caused by *M. pneumoniae* is associated with a wide variety of mucocutaneous lesions. Approximately 25 percent of those with pneumonia have dermatologic manifestations, including erythema nodosum, pityriasis rosea, scaly erythema, and urticara, as well as petechia, macular, papulovesicular, and morbilliform rashes. Occasionally, patients with *M. pneumoniae* infection develop the Stevens-Johnson syndrome. Erythema multiforme also occurs as vesicles or bullae in the oropharynx which appear within 2 weeks of the onset of respiratory illness and frequently persist despite resolution of pulmonary signs and symptoms.

FUNGAL

Fungal infections of the lungs in individuals with normal immune mechanisms are not often accompanied by skin lesions. However, in the immunocompromised host, a disseminated fungemia often evokes striking and distinctive manifestations in the lungs and skin.

Blastomycosis

In blastomycosis, skin lesions are as common as pulmonary lesions: cutaneous, localized blastomycosis usually arises from a pulmonary focus that is often small and inapparent. Its typical presentation is as a solitary papule or nodule on the face, wrists, hands, or feet, which subsequently ulcerates and discharges pus. The lesions grow eccentrically at the periphery and atrophy centrally over a period of months, eventually forming an acriform or serpiginous contour with sharply elevated and verrucous borders. Miliary abscesses are seen along the borders of the lesions. In disseminated blastomycosis, multiple subcutaneous nodules are common, generally in association with osteolytic lesions: the skin lesions tend to ulcerate.

Actinomycosis

The thoracic form of this disease presents as a pulmonary parenchymal process that sometimes forms multiple draining sinus tracts. The draining exudate contains the characteristic sulfur granules.

Coccidioidomycosis

This fungal disease sometimes produces acute or chronic cutaneous manifestations. During the initial primary pulmonary infection, approximately one-fifth of patients develop an erythema nodosum, often accompanied by arthropathy and eosinophilia. As the pulmonary disease progresses, the skin is one of the organs most likely to be affected. Subcutaneous granulomatous eruptions form and undergo necrosis and ulceration. After several months they tend to become verrucous. Disseminated disease has a poor prognosis.

Sporotrichosis

Almost invariably, this is strictly a dermatologic disorder. Following injury to the skin by an object contaminated with the spores of *Sporotrichum schenckii*, the affected individual develops the primary cutaneous eruption. These lesions, often mistaken for boils or luetic chancres, usually remain localized, but on rare occasions disseminate via lymphatics to other organs, including the lungs.

Aspergillosis

The invasive form of this disease is occasionally associated with skin lesions. In most cases, the cutaneous eruptions are multiple and scattered, suggesting hematogenous spread from a primary pulmonary focus. It is uncertain whether direct cutaneous inoculation with *Aspergillus* can lead to disseminated disease. The dermatologic manifestations of systemic aspergillosis are nonspecific and include solitary necrotizing plaques, subcutaneous granulomas and abscesses, suppurative maculopapules, and a variety of other lesions. *Aspergillus fumigatus* is the species most frequently cultured from skin lesions in patients with systemic aspergillosis.

Candidiasis

Patients with disseminated candidiasis sometimes develop diffuse, macronodular, erythematous skin lesions. Biopsy of the skin lesions demonstrates pseudohyphae in the dermis and blood vessels, whereas the dermis is intact. Blood cultures are as often positive for *Candida* species as are cultures of cutaneous lesions in this disseminated form of the disease.

TUBERCULOUS

Cutaneous involvement results from direct inoculation with the tubercle bacillus, either via the skin or mucous membranes or as a consequence of widespread organ involvement that begins in the respiratory tract. The skin lesion occurs either as a primary infection or as a result of reactivation of infection with *Mycobacterium tuberculosis*.

When the tubercle is introduced via the skin or mucous membranes by a contaminated syringe or a wound in a previously unexposed host, a nodule usually develops at the site of injury. Within several weeks, the nodule evolves into a chancre, i.e., a well-circumscribed ulcer. Particularly if host defenses are impaired, these chancreform lesions, which are typically located on the extremities, develop associated regional lymphadenitis, followed by systemic dissemination of the organism.

A person who was previously infected with *M. tuberculosis* is apt to develop *tuberculosis verrucosa cutis* after receiving a cutaneous inoculation. The characteristic lesion in a sensitized individual is a papule or a pustule which becomes verrucous. On occasion, this disorder produces plaquelike lesions of the extremities, consisting of verrucoid, indurated papules surrounded by an erythematous halo.

Lupus vulgaris is the most common form of cutaneous postprimary tuberculosis that follows inoculation or lymphatic or hematogenous spread of *M. tuberculosis*.

Patients with this disorder typically present with reddish brown plaques surrounded peripherally by yellowish nodules, especially on the hand, neck, or extremities. The skin lesions tend to spread centrifugally as the center of the cutaneous disorder atrophies. Papillary growths also occur in the nasal, buccal, and conjunctival mucosa. Histologically, lupus vulgaris generally shows epithelioid tubercles without caseation necrosis. Tubercle bacilli are rarely observed or cultured from skin biopsy specimens. Chronic cutaneous eruptions tend to involute, leaving considerable residual scarring. Chemotherapy using the usual antituberculosis drugs is effective in treating these skin manifestations.

Disseminated miliary tuberculosis can result in macules, papules, or vesicles. In children, especially those who are debilitated, subcutaneous nodules or gummas appear, ulcerate, and eventually develop draining sinus tracts, especially in the extremities and trunk. *Scrofuloderma*, which occurs following the necrosis of cervical nodules, is associated with fistula and sinus tract formation in the overlying cutaneous tissues.

Tuberculids are skin lesions that are considered to represent either hypersensitivity reactions to *M. tuberculosis* or an embolic response to atypical *Mycobacteria*. Erythema nodosum also occurs in association with primary tuberculosis (Fig. 27-5).

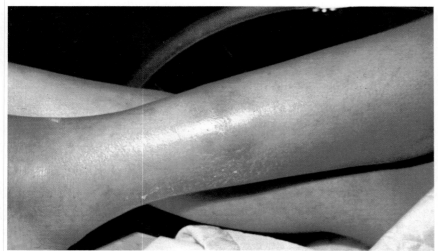

A

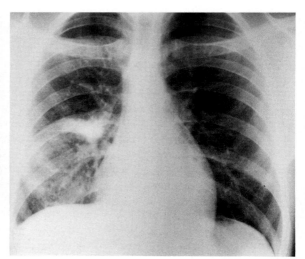

B

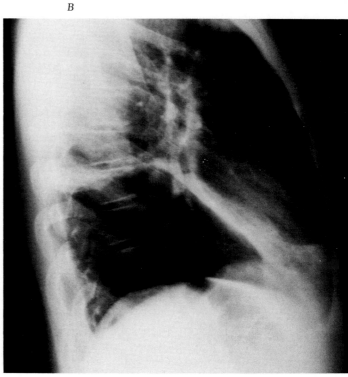

C

FIGURE 27-5   Erythema nodosum and primary tuberculosis. *A.* Discrete, tender, erythematous nodules over the pretibial region. *B.* and *C.* Infiltrates in the right middle lobe and the superior segment of the right lower lobe. Sputum smears and cultures were positive for *M. tuberculosis*. (*From Katz and Beerman, 1980.*)

Cutaneous Sarcoidosis

CLINICAL

Twenty to thirty-five percent of patients with systemic sarcoidosis develop cutaneous lesions at some time; in up to 10 percent, skin lesions are the initial complaint (Fig. 27-6). Some of the skin lesions are specific histologically, i.e., they show noncaseating granulomatous lesions on histologic examination, whereas others, notably erythema nodosum, are nonspecific, i.e., they do not show the characteristic (but not unique) granulomas of sarcoidosis. Erythema nodosum (Fig. 27-2D) occurs in 3 to 25 percent of patients with sarcoidosis and, as noted previously, is often associated with the acute onset of self-limited pulmonary disease. Other nonspecific skin lesions, such as generalized pruritus and erythema multiforme, are uncommon and may be coincidental.

The specific lesions of cutaneous sarcoid are commonly flesh-colored to violaceous papules that have a predilection for the face, neck, and upper trunk (Fig. 27-1F and 27-6A to C) and are firm, sometimes annular or serpiginous; "angiolupoid" lesions are large violaceous plaques in which telangiectasia features prominently. Most papular and plaque forms of cutaneous sarcoid resolve without scarring. However, the violaceous plaques of lupus pernio, that occur over the nose, ears, and digits

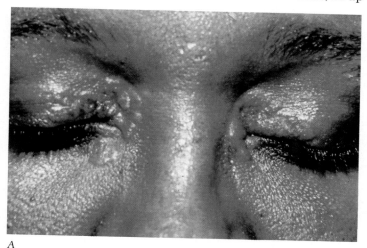

A

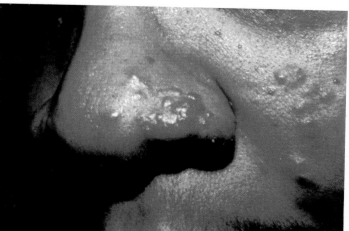

B

FIGURE 27-6 Sarcoidosis. *A* and *B*. Grouped papular lesion on the medial aspects of the eyelids, alae nasi, and cheek. *C*. Bilateral hilar adenopathy and reticular nodular lung infiltrates. Skin and lung biopsies demonstrated noncaseating granulomas consistent with sarcoidosis. *D*. Sarcoid lupus pernio involving fingers. (*A* to *C* from Katz and Beerman, 1980.)

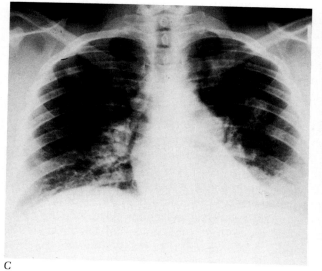

C

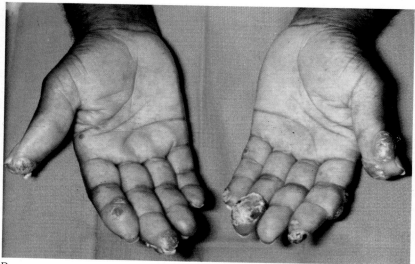

D

and involve underlying bone, do scar and are both permanent and disfiguring (Fig. 27-6D). Lupus pernio accompanies involvement of multiple systems by sarcoidosis, including the upper respiratory tract.

Other lesions which prove to be sarcoid on histologic examination may be nonspecific in appearance; among these are alopecia, ichthyosislike involvement of the lower legs, psoriasiform, and erythrodermic, follicular, and hypopigmented lesions. Deep subcutaneous nodules also occur. Sarcoidal lesions sometimes develop at sites of previous trauma or surgical scars. However, unless accompanied by systemic findings, skin biopsy of a scar cannot be used as the basis for a diagnosis of systemic sarcoidosis.

COURSE

Patients with systemic sarcoidosis who have specific cutaneous lesions tend to have a chronic course that often includes pulmonary fibrosis and uveitis.

THERAPY

The management of cutaneous lesions depends on the type and extent of skin involvement as well as on the need to treat systemic lesions. In acute sarcoidosis, nonsteroidal anti-inflammatory agents, such as indomethacin, may be adequate for the symptoms of erythema nodosum and the arthralgias. Lupus pernio is treated more aggressively, e.g., using systemic steroids, antimalarials such as hydroxychloroquine, weekly low-dose systemic methotrexate, or, more recently, oral retinoids. In patients with localized lesions, e.g., cutaneous papules or plaques, but in whom there is no evidence of systemic involvement, treatment of the local lesions using topical or intralesional steroids is often helpful.

Congenital and Developmental Disorders

A wide variety of heredocongenital anomalies as well as developmental disorders affect both the skin and the lung. Among these are: (1) disorders of collagen and elastin, (2) vascular malformations, (3) neurocutaneous syndromes, and (4) miscellaneous processes.

DISORDERS OF COLLAGEN AND ELASTIN

The most important disorder of collagen affecting the skin and the lungs is the Ehlers-Danlos (cutis hyperelastica) syndrome, a hereditary disorder of collagen in which the skin and blood vessels are unduly elastic and fragile and the joints are hyperextensible. The skin is smooth, rubbery, and bruisable; the joints are hypermobile. Associated systemic abnormalities include megaesophagus, megacolon, dissecting aortic aneurysm, and diaphragmatic and inguinal hernias. Among the pulmonary disorders are spontaneous pneumothorax, arteriovenous fistulas, megatrachea, and bronchial ectasia.

Cutis laxa is due to a disorder in the formation of elastin that is transmitted as a dominant hereditary trait. In children with this disorder, skin folds of the abdomen and face are large and pendulous. The pulmonary manifestations of cutis laxa are emphysema and pulmonary artery stenosis.

VASCULAR MALFORMATIONS

The most common congenital vascular malformation involving the skin and the lungs is hereditary hemorrhagic telangiectasia (Osler-Rendu-Weber syndrome). This is an autosomal dominant disorder that is manifested by hemangiomas in various organs, including the skin, where it may affect the lips, tongue, nasal mucosa, palate, and palms; on rare occasions, it is accompanied by arteriovenous fistulas in the lungs (Fig. 27-7). Epistaxis, melena, and hemoptysis are common in adults. The typical cutaneous lesion is slightly raised with an ill-defined border and one or more branching "legs" radiating from an eccentrically placed punctum; it is easily overlooked if it is located under the nails or on the soles of the feet. Large pulmonary arteriovenous communications are accompanied by clubbing, cyanosis, and polycythemia.

NEUROCUTANEOUS SYNDROMES

These disorders are characterized by dysplasia of ectodermally derived tissues, such as the skin and brain, as well as by disruption of organs formed from mesoderm, including the lungs. This group includes neurofibromatosis, tuberous sclerosis, and ataxia-telangiectasia. Pulmonary disease in these disorders may be either a manifestation of the systemic involvement by the disease process or an indirect consequence of neuromuscular weakness that causes aspiration pneumonia and lung abscess.

Neurofibromatosis (von Recklinghausen's disease) (Fig. 27-8) is a hereditary disorder, transmitted as a dominant trait, which is characterized by cutaneous neurofibromas, café au lait spots, and axillary freckles. The cutaneous tumors derive from the nerve sheaths of the Schwann cells. A feature of these lesions that is virtually pathognomonic is the ability to invaginate small lesions by digital pressure. The café au lait spots represent giant pigmented granules in the melanocytes and epidermal cells; they are specific for neurofibromatosis only if they are larger (greater than 1.5 cm) and numerous, i.e., more than five spots. Approximately 15 percent of patients with cutaneous lesions have intrathoracic neurofibromas. In some patients with neurofibromatosis, the lungs are the seat of interstitial fibrosis, leiomyomas, and bullae.

Tuberous sclerosis is a hereditary disorder that is characterized by mental retardation, epilepsy and, as indicated previously, adenoma sebaceum. Also seen as part of this disorder are retinal phacomas, calcification of the basal ganglia, and ungual fibromas. Shagreen patches occur in approximately one-fifth of patients; they consist of soft plaques, with a pebbly appearance, in the lumbosacral region. Approximately 9 percent of those with visceral tuberous sclerosis have pulmonary manifestations; some of the pulmonary lesions are cystic and may be associated with recurrent spontaneous pneumothorax and hamartomas. Certain poorly understood diseases, such as fibrocystic pulmonary dysplasia, may represent forme fruste of tuberous sclerosis.

Ataxia-telangiectasia is a recessively transmitted disorder that is characterized by choreoathetosis, ocular apraxia, and progressive cerebellar ataxia. These manifestations appear in early childhood; subsequently, telangiectasia of the conjunctiva and skin develops. Many of the affected children suffer from chronic sinopulmonary infections in association with an abnormality in delayed hypersensitivity and a decrease in the production of the immunoglobulin IgA.

MISCELLANEOUS DISORDERS

Histiocytosis X often begins with dermatologic manifestations. The characteristic lesions, most often seen in infants and young children with the Letterer-Siwe and Hand-Schüller-Christian forms of this disorder, consist of seborrheiclike scaling and erythema in the scalp, behind the ears, and in the groin, surrounded by reddish brown and yellowish brown papules, which frequently ulcerate. Purpura as well as ulcerations of the buccal mucosa and gingiva also occur. Eosinophilic granuloma rarely has cutaneous manifestations.

Pulmonary Vasculitis

This category includes three entities: systemic vasculitis with asthma and eosinophilia, lymphomatoid granulomatosis, and Wegener's granulomatosis. Here, only the skin manifestations of these disorders are considered.

CHURG-STRAUSS SYNDROME (SYSTEMIC VASCULITIS WITH ASTHMA AND EOSINOPHILIA)

The clinical picture of allergic rhinitis, asthma, peripheral eosinophilia, and pulmonary infiltrates concomitant with systemic vasculitis has been designated the *Churg-Strauss syndrome* (see Chapter 69). However, the histologic finding of necrotizing granulomas and tissue eosinophilia is not unique to this clinical syndrome. Indeed, the same histologic appearance may be seen in a wide variety of systemic diseases, including allergic granulomatosis, Wegener's granulomatosis, rheumatoid arthritis, and lymphoproliferative disease.

One or more types of skin lesions develop in 70 percent of patients with the Churg-Strauss syndrome. Most common is palpable purpura of the extremities; histologically, these lesions show necrotizing vasculitis without granuloma formation. In one-third of the patients, the cutaneous lesions are nonspecific, i.e., erythematous and

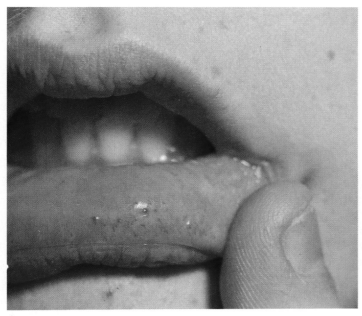

A

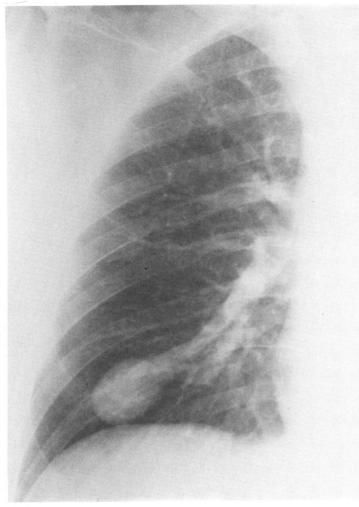

B

FIGURE 27-7   Osler-Rendu-Weber syndrome.   *A.* Punctate hemangiomas of the lower lip.   *B.* Arteriovenous fistulas of right lower lobe shown by angiography. *(From Katz and Beerman, 1980.)*

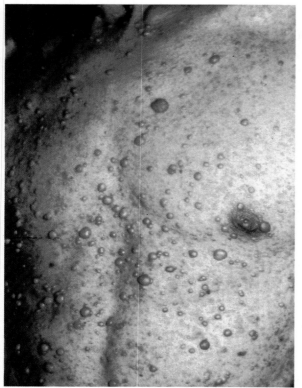

A

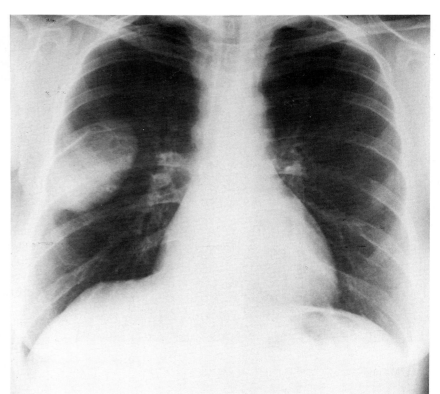

B

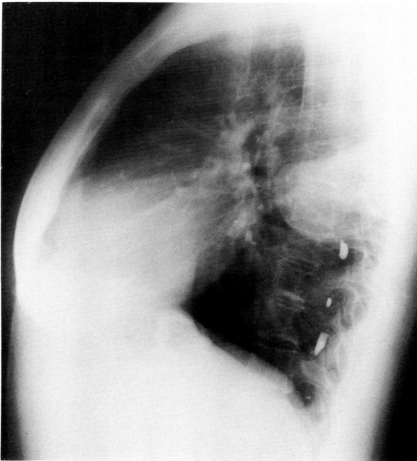

C

FIGURE 27-8 Von Recklinghausen's disease. *A.* Multiple soft, subcutaneous neurofibromas over the chest and abdomen. *B.* Chest radiograph shows a soft-tissue, extrapleural mass eroding the right sixth rib as well as bilateral apical masses and a widened mediastinum. These lesions are caused by neurofibromas. *C.* Lateral film demonstrates scalloping of the posterior bodies of the lower thoracic vertebrae as a consequence of dural ectasia. *(From Katz and Beerman, 1980.)*

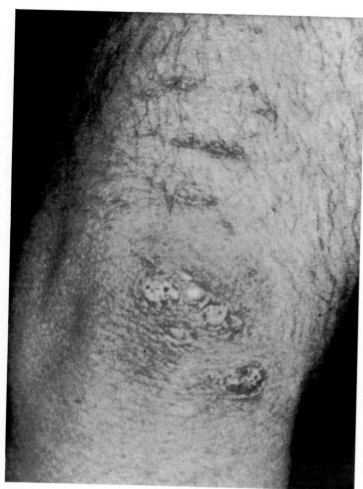

FIGURE 27-9   Churg-Strauss granulomatous vasculitis.

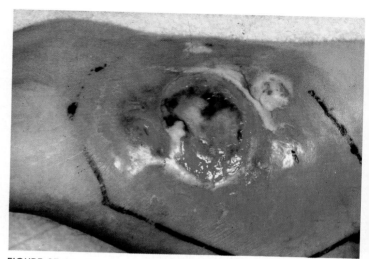

FIGURE 27-10   Lymphomatoid granulomatosis.

urticarial. However, in another third, the skin lesions are distinctive, i.e., tender red to violaceous, indurated nodules, measuring 0.5 to 2 cm, which develop central crusting or become infarcted (Fig. 27-9). These nodules occur most often over the scalp or symmetrically over the extensor surfaces of the extremities. It is these nodules which are most likely to have the histologic picture of necrotizing granulomatous vasculitis and eosinophilic infiltration; immunofluorescence staining may show vascular deposition of fibrin and complement. The skin lesions in the Churg-Strauss syndrome generally respond to systemic corticosteroids or to adjuvant cytotoxic therapy.

LYMPHOMATOID GRANULOMATOSIS

The skin is the most commonly involved extrapulmonary site in lymphomatoid granulomatosis, cutaneous lesions occurring in 40 to 50 percent of patients. In 10 to 25 percent of patients with this disorder, the skin lesions are the first clinical evidence of the disorder; the skin lesions sometimes precede involvement of the lungs by 2 weeks to 9 years. Because of the frequent occurrence of skin lesions, the ease of biopsying the skin, and the characteristic histology of this disease, careful dermatologic examination should be carried out in patients suspected of having lymphomatoid granulomatosis.

The characteristic cutaneous lesions in lymphomatoid granulomatosis are 1- to 4-cm erythematous-to-purplish macules, papules, or subcutaneous nodules that sometimes ulcerate; the lesions generally occur over the buttocks, thighs, and lower extremities (Fig. 27-10) but may occur anywhere. Healing is often accompanied by scarring and hyperpigmentation. Other cutaneous lesions are nonspecific, i.e., small vesicles, generalized ichthyosis, patchy alopecia, localized lack of sweating, and annular plaques.

This histopathology of the skin lesions is similar to that of the lesions in the lungs: a mild to deep dermal angiocentric and angiodestructive vasculitis with a mixed-cell granulomatous infiltrate; some atypical lymphoreticular cells are seen, but eosinophils are sparse. Secondary inflammation and destruction of skin appendages, such as sweat glands and nerves, may be present; should deep vessels be involved, adjacent fat necrosis evokes a panniculitis. Ultrastructurally, the histocytosis shows certain distinctive features, including ruffling of the cell membrane, a well-developed Golgi apparatus, and collections of microfilaments and microtubules in the cytoplasm.

The papules or nodules in lymphomatoid granulomatosis sometimes clear spontaneously; more often, they recur. The skin lesions do seem to respond to therapy with systemic corticosteroids and cyclophosphamide. Localized radiation therapy has been used for some refractory skin lesions.

WEGENER'S GRANULOMATOSIS

Although skin lesions do occur in approximately 45 percent of patients with Wegener's granulomatosis, as a rule they are nonspecific, both clinically and histologically. Thus, biopsy of skin lesions is not apt to either make or refute a diagnosis of Wegener's granulomatosis.

Attention has been called above to the nonspecific nature of cutaneous involvement in this disorder. Subcutaneous nodules, papules, and vesicles are common, often accompanied by purpura and petechiae. Bleeding, crusty, nonhealing lesions form at the nostrils or nasal septum and sometimes progress to severe paranasal sinusitis and to nasopharyngeal ulceration; the end result may be perforation of the nasal septum and saddlenose deformity. Involvement of the middle ear is signaled by a purulent otitis; in the mouth, the process leads to extensive gingivitis with necrosis of the alveolar ridge, palatal ulcers, and perforation and ulceration of the tongue. Except for infarcts or gangrenous lesions, the skin involvement generally improves in response to the systemic administration of corticosteroids and cyclophosphamide; the recurrence of cutaneous lesions often presages systemic relapse.

Neoplastic Disorders

In some patients, carcinoma of the lung metastasizes to the skin; in others, nonspecific cutaneous lesions are part of the systemic effects of a pulmonary neoplasm. Neoplasms of the skin sometimes metastasize to the lung and pleura.

Although the skin is an uncommon site for metastases, carcinoma of the lung is the third most common source; the breast and the stomach are more common primary sites. Neoplastic lesions of the skin are rock-hard, subcutaneous, or intradermal nodules; in color, they range from flesh to purple to brown-black; often they are localized to the chest wall. Occasionally, a cutaneous metastasis is first discovered in the scalp. Except for those in the scalp, skin lesions rarely ulcerate; sometimes the scalp lesions are associated with alopecia.

ECTOPIC HORMONES

Various systemic syndromes that include cutaneous manifestations occur in conjunction with malignant neoplasms of the lungs. The most common systemic manifestations of a primary carcinoma of the lungs are due to ectopic production of hormones. Hyperpigmentation is part of the Cushing's syndrome produced by ACTH-like and/or melanin stimulating hormone (MSH)-like peptides arising in the pulmonary neoplasm; most often, the pulmonary neoplasm is a small cell carcinoma. Cushing's syndrome is a harbinger of death in pulmonary neoplasm: most affected individuals die within weeks of the appearance of the hyperpigmentation. Gynecomastia, often painful, complicates carcinoma of the lung, especially the undifferentiated variety that elaborates gonadotropins.

The carcinoid syndrome, usually secondary to appendiceal or intestinal tumors, is occasionally produced by bronchial adenomas. Occasionally, the repeated vasomotor episodes are followed by a lingering cyanotic flush of the face and telangiectasia.

NONSPECIFIC DERMATOLOGIC SYNDROMES

Cutaneous abnormalities associated with carcinoma of the lungs (and with other visceral carcinomas as well) include dermatomyositis, scleroderma, pachydermoperiostosis, acanthosis nigricans, and pruritis.

In 15 to 34 percent of patients with dermatomyositis, a carcinoma of the lung is present. The dermatomyositis sometimes precedes, and other times follows, the discovery of the internal malignancy. Moreover, about three quarters of patients older than 50 years who present with late-onset myopathy prove to have an internal neoplasm.

Scleroderma occasionally accompanies a pulmonary neoplasm, particularly a bronchoalveolar carcinoma or an adenocarcinoma. Conversely, patients with the extensive pulmonary fibrosis of chronic scleroderma are at high risk of developing carcinoma of the lung.

Pachydermoperiostosis is a syndrome in which hypertrophic osteoarthropathy is associated with cutaneous changes of the face and extremities that are similar to those that occur in acromegaly. Although this disorder is generally benign, occasionally it is associated with bronchogenic carcinoma.

Acanthosis nigricans is a frequent concomitant of internal neoplasia. Approximately 80 to 90 percent of malignant acanthosis is associated with abdominal cancer. But neoplasms of the lungs have also been associated with this skin disorder. The characteristic skin lesion is a brown-to-black area of pigmentation which is extensively folded and appears dirty; later on, the lesion becomes papillomatous, verrucous, and shaggy in appearance. The skin lesions favor sites of flexion, including the neck, axillae, groin, and anticubital spaces; they also occur on the areolae and around the perineal and umbilical regions. The average survival time between the onset of acanthosis nigricans and death is 12 months.

LYMPHOMAS AND LEUKEMIAS

About half of all patients with lymphomas develop dermatologic manifestations during the course of the disease. Among the nonspecific markers of lymphomas and leukemias are pruritus exfoliative dermatitis, ichthyosis, mycosis fungoides, and bullous eruptions. The nonspecific dermatoses include nodules, papules, and skin tumors that originate from the epidermis or subcutaneous regions. These lesions vary in size and pigmentation and occur anywhere on the body surface. Dermatologic manifestations of malignant lymphomas often antedate systemic disease by months to years. Bluefarb has identified "11 p's" as characterizing the cutaneous lesions of Hodgkin's disease: pallor, pruritus, prurigolike papules, pigmentation, pyoderma, purpura, pemphigoid, postspinal root ganglionitis (herpes zoster), pityriasis rubra, phlebitis, poikilodermatomyositis. Pruritis is particularly common; the 11 manifestations are found in 25 to 35 percent of patients with this type of lymphoma.

BOWEN'S DISEASE

Epidermoid carcinoma in situ of the skin (Bowen's disease) is commonly associated with neoplasms of any organ, including the lungs. The lesions are asymptomatic, slow-growing, psoriasiform, or eczematoid.

ARSENICALS AND CHROMATES

Inorganic arsenicals are carcinogens that cause neoplasms of both skin and viscera. The skin lesions may occur years after chronic exposure to inorganic arsenicals, as in drinking water. They are characterized by hyperpigmentation and palmar and plantar dermatoses; frequently, they are confused with Bowen's disease (squamous cell carcinoma of the skin in situ). Like Bowen's disease, arsenical toxicity is associated with a high incidence of visceral neoplasms (respiratory, gastrointestinal, and genitourinary).

Exposure to chromate dusts or vapors is associated with a frequency of pulmonary neoplasms that is about 29 times greater than that of the unexposed population. Chromate workers also develop perforations of the nasal septum as well as ulcerations of the hands, forearms, and feet.

PRIMARY CUTANEOUS NEOPLASMS

Certain primary neoplasms of the skin involve the lungs. Paramount in this group are malignant melanoma and mycosis fungoides. The latter has been noted above (see "Scaling Papules").

Malignant melanomas constitute approximately 1 to 2 percent of all neoplasms. They occur most often in the fifth to seventh decade, particularly in fair complected individuals of North European descent. The typical lesion is a deeply pigmented nodule with irregular borders (Fig. 27-11). The usual course is one of progressive enlargement of the skin lesion, metastasis to regional lymph nodes, and hematogenous dissemination to the lungs and liver. Widespread metastasis is associated with diffuse hyperpigmentation of the skin and mucous membranes. Among the pulmonary manifestations of melanoma are nodules in the lungs (solitary, multiple, or miliary), hilar and mediastinal lymphadenopathy, and exudative pleural effusions caused by pleural metastases. Primary melanomas of the lungs are exceedingly rare. When they do occur, they usually masquerade as carcinoma, lymphoma, or sarcoma, often causing bronchial obstruction and distal atelectasis.

KAPOSI'S SARCOMA

Until the recent outbreak of AIDS, Kaposi's sarcoma encountered in the United States was a rare disorder seen predominantly in middle-aged men. Its usual course was indolent and confined primarily to the lower extremities. At the outset, the lesions were dark blue, purplish, or reddish papules, macules, and nodules; after months to years, plaques evolved in association with thickening of the skin from midtibia to ankle, and lymphedema.

The epidemic of AIDS brought to light an aggressive form of the disease that is widespread in its cutaneous manifestations. In the AIDS patient, the respiratory tract is second only to the gastrointestinal tract in frequency of involvement. Tumors sometimes involve the larynx, trachea, bronchi, pulmonary parenchyma, and pleura. Accordingly, local manifestations of involvement of the respiratory tract range from hoarseness, signs of airway obstruction, cough, and hemoptysis, to dyspnea. When the parenchyma of the lung is affected, chest radiographs usually show multiple, small nodules; occasionally, parenchymal infiltration of the lung is massive. On bronchoscopic examination, bronchial and tracheal lesions appear as small, bluish nodules. Bloody pleural effusions are rare.

Collagen Vascular Disorders

Many of the collagen vascular diseases either begin clinically with cutaneous lesions or develop them in the course of the illness.

LUPUS ERYTHEMATOSUS

Cutaneous lupus erythematosus usually takes the form of well-circumscribed discoid lesions that are raised, firm, and red to violaceous in color. Often the lesions are accompanied by telangiectasia, atrophy, and scarring. Silvery white discolorations of the lips and of the mucosa of the mouth and lips are characteristic. A butterfly configuration over the bridge of the nose and on the cheeks is both less common and less specific. Subcutaneous nodules develop underneath the typical discoid lesions of lupus (lupus profundus). In addition to the discoid type of plaque and telangiectasia, patients sometimes exhibit urticarial plaques and alopecia. Discoid and systemic forms of lupus are believed to be different expressions of the same disorder. About 10 percent of patients who present only with cutaneous disease eventually develop generalized manifestations; on the other hand, 50 to 90 percent of those with systemic disease eventually develop some cutaneous abnormalities.

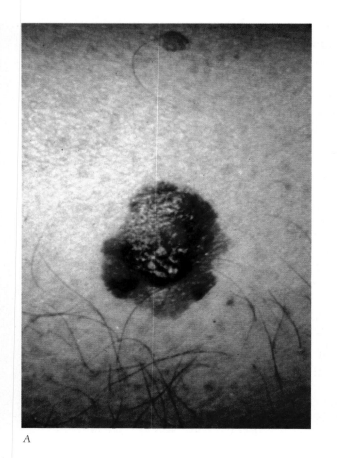

A

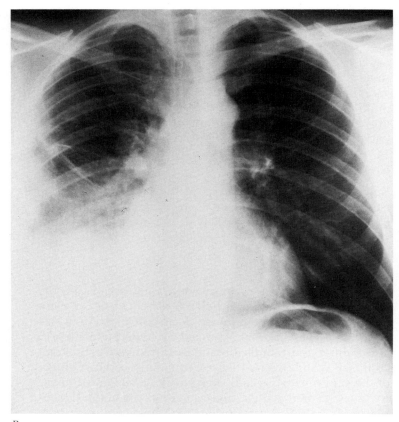

B

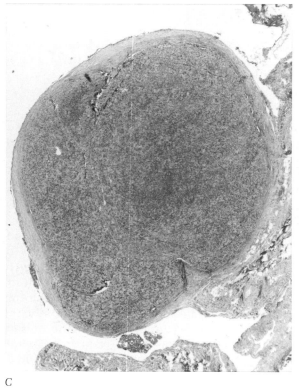

C

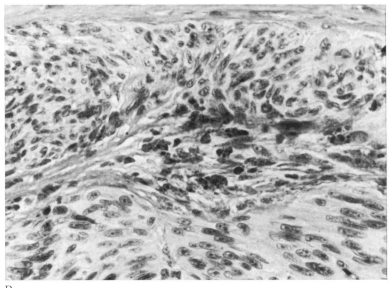

D

FIGURE 27-11   Metastatic melanoma.   *A.* Deeply pigmented, raised facial lesion with irregular surface.   *B.* Chest radiograph shows right pleural effusion with nodulation.   *C.* Biopsy of the lung (×27) reveals a large nodule on pleural surface.   *D.* Spindle-shaped cells, some of which are filled with melanin pigment (×400). *(From Katz and Beerman, 1980.)*

RHEUMATOID ARTHRITIS

A wide variety of dermatologic manifestations occur in rheumatoid arthritis, often together with pulmonary disease. Subcutaneous nodules occur in about 20 percent of patients with systemic rheumatoid disease. The lesions are generally located around the elbows, hands, ankles, and feet. Similar nodules also occur in the pulmonary parenchyma, heart, sclera, and dura mater and within the visceral pleura. Histologically, fibrinoid necrosis in vascular walls is surrounded by palisading histiocytic and mononuclear cells. Other dermatologic manifestations of rheumatoid arthritis are secondary to widespread angiitis and include necrotic leg ulcers, gangrene of the extremities, hemorrhagic infarcts along the finger pulp or nail fold, and generalized erythematous macules and papules. Involvement of the lungs is often associated with characteristic abnormalities of the hands (Fig. 27-12).

DERMATOMYOSITIS

The characteristic skin lesions of dermatomyositis are blotchy, purplish macules located on the extensor surfaces of the elbows, knuckles and knees, anterior chest, and malar area of the face. Periorbital and eyelid edema are common in association with a heliotrope discoloration of the affected skin. Raynaud's phenomenon occurs in about 10 to 20 percent of patients with this disorder. A fine, scaly erythema sometimes appears over the extensor surfaces of the large and interphalangeal joints as well as on the plantar and palmar surfaces of the hands. Periun-

gual and linear telangiectasia occurs at the cuticle. As the disease progresses, bullous lesions and poikiloderma—a speckled pattern of hypopigmented and hyperpigmented small macules—are sometimes interspersed with telangiectasia and cutaneous atrophy. Another late and specific manifestation of dermatomyositis is the Gottron papule, a purplish rash which appears on the dorsal interphalangeal joints.

The cutaneous manifestations of dermatomyositis usually precede muscle involvement by several months; but, on occasion, the skin is affected after muscle disease is extensive and quite evident. Biopsy of the skin lesions in dermatomyositis usually reveals a nonspecific inflammatory reaction. If the myositis is prolonged and severe, widespread calcification of skin and muscle sometimes occurs, as early as 2 years after the onset of the disease.

SCLERODERMA

The two principal forms of systemic scleroderma are acrosclerosis and diffuse scleroderma. Acrosclerosis, by far the more common of the two, is characterized by sclerosis of the skin of the fingers (sclerodactyly) and Raynaud's phenomenon. In contrast, diffuse scleroderma presents with tightening of the skin, especially over the chest, without Raynaud's phenomenon; the prognosis for diffuse scleroderma is much worse than for acrosclerosis. Acrosclerosis is often preceded by diffuse arthralgias or arthritis resembling rheumatoid arthritis. The skin manifestations begin with transient, recurrent swelling of the

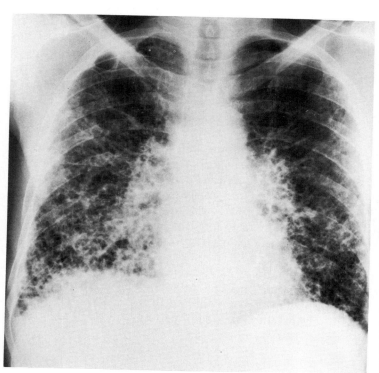

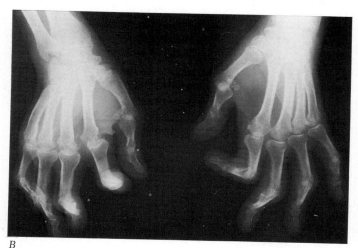

B

FIGURE 27-12 Rheumatoid arthritis. *A.* Chest radiograph shows a course, reticulonodular, honeycomb pattern, most prominent at the bases consistent with rheumatoid arthritis. *B.* Hand radiographs show typical rheumatoid changes consisting of: (1) synovitis, with erosions of the metacarpal heads; (2) soft-tissue swelling around multiple joints (intercarpal, metaphalangeal, proximal interphalangeal); (3) periarticular demineralization secondary to hyperemia; (4) fusion of carpal bones; (5) early ulnar deviation. *(From Katz and Beerman, 1980.)*

A

hands that progresses to tapered fingers with shiny, hide-bound skin (sclerodactyly). The feet, chest, face, and scalp are often involved in the sclerotic process. In time, the skin becomes taut, leading to contractures of the large and small joints that culminate in a clawlike deformity of the hand. A variety of pigmentary disturbances have been described in scleroderma including generalized hyperpigmentation that resembles adrenal insufficiency, focal hyperpigmentation and hypopigmentation, and areas of perifollicular pigmentation that resemble vitiligo (Fig. 27-13). Raynaud's phenomenon leads to small, pitted scars at the fingertips or frank ulceration with or without gangrene of the fingertips, toes, knuckles, and ankles, especially the malleoli. Calcium is sometimes deposited in the major joints; fingers become involved late in the course of scleroderma (Thibierge-Weissenbach syndrome).

The face often undergoes distinctive changes leading to a fixed stare, wrinkled forebrow, and inability to wrinkle the forehead. As facial tissues shrink, the nose becomes pinched, the cheeks sunken, and the mouth small with thin lips. In diffuse scleroderma, cutaneous sclerosis, accompanied by a yellowish-brownish hue, spreads from the chest to the head and extremities. Sharply delineated, broad telangiectatic macules appear on the face, buccal mucosa, lips, and hands. The constellation of calcinosis cutis, Raynaud's phenomenon, sclerodactyly, and telangiectasia is known as the CRST syndrome. This form of scleroderma is usually benign but is occasionally associated with pulmonary hypertension.

Complications of Medications

Medications used to treat respiratory disorders sometimes cause cutaneous reactions. Major offenders are antibiotics, particularly the penicillins, ampicillin, and trimethoprim-sulfamethoxasole, all of which can cause exanthematous, urticarial, or erythema multiforme-type reactions. The continued administration of corticosteroids systemically can elicit the cutaneous manifestations of Cushing's syndrome. In addition, chronic corticosteroid therapy may predispose to poor wound healing and to fungal infections of the skin, such as tinea versicolor and dermatophytes.

Aminophylline administered parenterally occasionally causes a generalized papulovesicular eruption. The usual setting for this reaction is the patient who has been previously sensitized to ethylenediamine by using a topical preparation of Mycolog cream or certain antihistamines (promethazine or tripelennamine). Since the delayed hypersensitivity reactions to aminophylline are due in this setting to the ethylenediamine component, theophylline preparations can be substituted. Immediate hypersensitivity reactions, i.e., urticarial, are uncommon for theophylline or aminophylline.

Codeine also can cause a number of cutaneous reactions, including generalized exanthematous eruptions, pruritus with or without skin lesions, and urticaria. The last may occur because of a nonimmunologic release of histamine owing to a direct effect of codeine on mast cells. Potassium iodide, previously frequently used as an expectorant, may cause urticaria, an acneiform eruption, erythema nodosum, or iododerma. Heparin and warfarin anticoagulants can cause a temporary hair thinning; hair loss begins 6 weeks to 4 months after the start of therapy. Other medications used in pulmonary therapy have a fairly low incidence of cutaneous reactions, but drug eruption should be considered in the differential diagnosis of almost any cutaneous pattern.

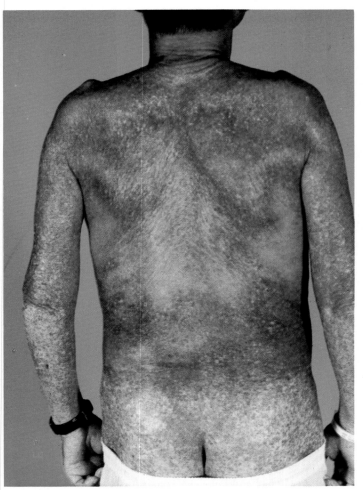

FIGURE 27-13   Scleroderma. Mottled hyperpigmentation.

BIBLIOGRAPHY

Callen JP: Cardiopulmonary disorders, in Callen JP (ed), *Cutaneous Aspects of Internal Disease.* Chicago, Yearbook, 1981, pp. 311–414.
  This textbook section reviews cutaneous aspects of pulmonary-systemic conditions including sarcoidosis, vasculitides, tuberculosis, and deep fungal infections with extensive references.

Epstein EH, Levin DL, Croft JD Jr, Lutaner MA: Mycosis fungoides: Survival, prognostic features, response to therapy and autopsy findings. Medicine 51:61–72, 1982.
  Evidence of pulmonary involvement occurs in 66 percent of patients at autopsy.

Fauci AS, Haynes BF, Katz P, Wolff SM: Wegener's granulomatosis: Prospective clinical and therapeutic experience with 85 patients for 21 years. Ann Intern Med 98:76–85, 1983.
  Review of 85 patients followed at the National Institutes of Health. Thirteen percent of patients had skin rash as a presenting sign of Wegener's granulomatosis, and overall 45 percent of the patients developed skin involvement at some time during the course.

Foley JF, Linder J, Koh J, Severson G, Purtilo DT: Cutaneous necrotizing granulomatous vasculitis with evolution to T-cell lymphoma. Am J Med 82:839–844, 1987.
  The evolution of cutaneous lymphomatoid granulomatosis in a patient with systemic T-cell lymphoma was followed over a 12-year period. The case history illustrates the difficulty of classifying the skin biopsy lesions.

Fria MD, Winkelmann RK: The cutaneous extravascular necrotizing granuloma (Churg-Strauss granuloma) and systemic disease: A review of 27 cases. Medicine 62:142–158, 1983.
  A review of 27 patients with cutaneous Churg-Strauss granuloma reveals that 26 had underlying systemic disease; 14 of 26 had some type of systemic vasculitis, and the remainder had some type of immunoreactive or inflammatory disease.

Gibson LE, Winkelmann RK: Cutaneous granulomatous vasculitis: its relationship to systemic disease. J Am Acad Dermatol 14:492–501, 1986.
  A review of the microscopic and medical findings in twenty-six patients with skin biopsy specimens that showed granulomatous vasculitis demonstrated vascular histocytic granulomas with fibrinoid destruction of blood vessels in the dermis and panniculus.

Guillevin L, Guittard T, Bletry O, Godeau P, Rosenthal P: Systemic necrotizing angiitis with asthma: causes and precipitating factors in 43 cases. Lung 165:165–172, 1987.
  Causes and precipitating factors of systemic necrotizing angiitis with asthma are described in 43 patients, focusing on a history of vaccination and desensitization. Mean age of patients was 43.2 years.

Hanafin JM: Atopic dermatitis. J Am Acad Dermatol 6:1–13, 1982.
  Well-referenced review of information on pathophysiological mechanisms in atopic dermatitis.

Hanno R, Needelman A, Eiferman RA, Callen JP: Cutaneous sarcoidal granulomas and the development of systemic sarcoidosis. Arch Dermatol 117:203–207, 1981.
  Follow-up of outpatients presenting with cutaneous sarcoid suggests that a poorer prognosis of systemic disease in such patients may not occur in this population.

Harris RB, Heaphy MR, Perry HO: Generalized elastolysis (cutis laxa). Am J Med 65:815–822, 1978.
  Generalized elastolysis is a rare systemic disorder of defective elastase fibers resulting in cutis laxa, emphysema, aneurysms, and diverticula. A discussion of possible etiologic aspects is presented along with a review of 17 cases.

James WD, Odom RB, Katzenstein ALA: Cutaneous manifestations of lymphomatoid granulomatosis. Arch Dermatol 117:196–202, 1981.
  Forty-four cases with cutaneous involvement are reviewed, indicating most common types of skin lesions and occurrence in the course of the systemic disease.

Katzenstein ALA, Carrington CB, Leibow AA: Lymphomatoid granulomatosis: A clinicopathologic study of 152 cases. Cancer 43:360–373, 1979.
  This classic retrospective review summarizes the presenting signs and systemic sites of involvement of 152 cases of lymphomatoid granulomatosis and presents the typical histologic features in the lung.

Lanham JG, Elkon KG, Pusey CD, Hughes GR: Systemic vasculitis with asthma and eosinophilia: A clinical approach to Churg-Strauss syndrome. Medicine 63:65–81, 1984.
  This review suggests that a diagnosis of Churg-Strauss syndrome should be considered with compatible clinical features of allergic rhinitis, asthma, and eosinophilia. The classic histologic picture is found in a minority of cases.

Leavitt RY, Fauci AS: Pulmonary vasculitis. Am Rev Respir Dis 134:149–166, 1986.
A review of granulomatous vasculitides that involve the lung, including Wegener's granulomatosis, allergic angiitis and granulomatosis, the polyangiitis overlap syndrome, and necrotizing sarcoid granulomatosis.

Martin AG, Kleinhenz ME, Elmets CA: Immunohistologic identification of antigen-presenting cells in cutaneous sarcoidosis. J Invest Dermatol 86:625–629, 1986.
Considerable evidence exists to show that activated T lymphocytes preferentially accumulate at sites of disease activity in sarcoidosis. OKT6-reactive Langerhans cells play a primary role in T-lymphocyte activation by the skin and in granuloma formation.

Mathews KP: Urticaria and angioedema. J Allergy Clin Immunol 72:1–14, 1983.
General review of types, mechanisms, associated causes, and treatment of urticaria and angioedema.

Neville E, Mills RGS, Jash DK, MacKinnon DM, Carstairs LS, James DG: Sarcoidosis of the upper respiratory tract and its association with lupus pernio. Thorax 31:660–664, 1976.
Lupus pernio occurred in 26 out of 34 patients presenting with sarcoidosis of the upper respiratory tract and nose.

Olive KE, Kataria YP: Cutaneous manifestations of sarcoidosis: Relationships to other organ system involvement, abnormal laboratory measurements, and disease course. Arch Intern Med 145:1811–1814, 1985.
This chart review of 329 patients with sarcoidosis showed that patients with nonerythema nodosum skin lesions were more likely to have hepato- or splenomegaly than those without skin lesions. Improved prognosis of systemic sarcoidosis was seen in white patients with erythema nodosum.

Pavlidakey GP, Hashimoto K, Blum D: Yellow nail syndrome. J Am Acad Dermatol 11:509–512, 1984.
Features of this clinical "pearl" syndrome are summarized and include the triad of yellow nails, lymphedema, and pleural effusions with associated respiratory tract involvement.

Robin JB, Schanzlin DJ, Meisler DM, deLuise VP, Clough JD: Ocular involvement in the respiratory vasculitides. Surv Ophthalmol 30:127–140, 1985.
Three separate respiratory vasculitides, Wegener's granulomatosis, Churg-Strauss syndrome (allergic granulomatosis and angiitis), and lymphomatoid granulomatosis may have ophthalmic manifestations; indeed, ocular involvement may be the presenting sign.

Sontheimer RD, Garibaldi RA, Krueger GG: Stevens-Johnson syndrome associated with *Mycoplasma pneumoniae* infections. Arch Dermatol 114:241–244, 1978.
This report reviews 24 documented literature cases of Stevens-Johnson syndrome associated with mycoplasma infection. It also offers a brief review of pulmonary involvement in Stevens-Johnson syndrome.

Soter NA, Wasserman SI, Austen KF, McFadden ER: Release of mast cell mediators and alterations in lung function in patients with cholinergic urticaria. N Engl J Med 302:604–608, 1980.
Exercise-induced cholinergic urticaria is associated with pulmonary symptoms, decreased 1-s forced-expiratory volumes, maximal mid-expiratory flow rates, and systemic release of mast cell mediators.

Thompson PJ, Gibb WRG, Cole P, Citron KM: Generalized allergic reactions to aminophylline. Thorax 39:600–603, 1984.
Forty-five of 147 reactions of aminophylline were dermatologic-allergic and may be due to the ethylenediamine component. Reaction rate is higher with parenteral use. Skin reactions to theophylline are rare.

Veien NK, Stahl D, Brodthagen H: Cutaneous sarcoidosis in Caucasians. J Am Acad Dermatol 16:534–540, 1987.
One hundred eighty-eight Caucasian patients with cutaneous sarcoid lesions were studied prospectively. Twenty-five had erythema nodosum, while 163 had infiltrative cutaneous lesions.

Chapter 28

Systemic Manifestations of Pulmonary Disease

Alfred P. Fishman

Endothelium as a Metabolic Organ

Injury by Oxygen-Derived Products

General Systemic Effects of Pulmonary Disease
  Fever, Chills, and Sweating
  Body Wasting

Particular Systemic Effects of Pulmonary Disease
  Clubbing of the Digits and Hypertrophic Osteoarthropathy
  Remote Organ Failure

Aside from gas exchange, the lungs lead a life of their own as a metabolic organ. And, since their enormous endothelial surface is washed uninterruptedly by the entire cardiac output, an injury or metabolic upset of the lungs has the potential for exerting effects on remote vessels and organs. The manifestations of injury or of deranged metabolism can be considered under two headings: (1) *general*, which the lungs have in common with other organs, and (2) *specific*, which although rarely unique are more specifically related to the lungs.

The mine of diverse cells that make up the airways and parenchyma of the lungs is described in Chapter 2. Each of these, ranging from the chloride-secreting cells that line the airways to the sporadic enterochromaffin cell, can go wrong and cause serious systemic derangements. The same can be said of the alveolar lining cells that are responsible for generating and handling surfactant. In this chapter, a few words are said about the endothelium to underscore certain aspects of the lining of the pulmonary blood vessels relevant to systemic disorders.

ENDOTHELIUM AS A METABOLIC ORGAN

The various functions served by pulmonary capillary endothelium are described in Chapter 15 and summarized in Table 28-1. Instead of serving as the passive lining of blood vessels, the endothelium turns out to be a distributed organ that differs from other viscera in that it is spread throughout the body as the lining of blood vessels. In different locales, it assumes specialized functions. Its functions relate to the clotting of the blood, to the generation, uptake, and processing of biologically active materials, to interplay with adjacent muscle cells in vasomotor regulation, and to its participation in certain vital homeostatic mechanisms such as the regulation of systemic blood pressure via the renin-angiotensin-aldosterone system.

Injury to the endothelium unleashes a flood of local regulatory mechanisms. Circulating white blood cells and platelets are drawn to the injured site, undergo activation, and release factors that contribute to the response. If the injury is on the abluminal side, all cells and humors must traverse endothelium to arrive at the site of disturbance. Many of the interplays between endothelium and circulating cells and humors are exceedingly complex: thrombin can serve as a procoagulant molecule that activates platelets, cleaves fibrinogen, stimulates the endothelial release of tissue factors, and releases von Willebrand factor from Weibel-Palade bodies; alternatively, it can serve as an anticoagulant molecule that stimulates protein C activity, promotes prostacyclin secretion, and causes the liberation of tissue plasminogen activators. Fibronectin, which contributes importantly to the integrity of endothelium, is not only generated locally but is also brought to the site of injury from afar by the plasma.

Two prevalent disorders of humankind illustrate the role of endothelium in systemic disease: (1) the preferential lodging of bloodborne metastases at various sites

TABLE 28-1
The Processing of Certain Vasoactive Substances by the Lungs

Metabolized at the luminal surface
  Angiotensin I
  Bradykinin
  Adenine nucleotides
Uptake by endothelium and then metabolized
  Serotonin
  Norepinephrine
  Prostaglandins E and F
Released by Endothelium
  Lipoprotein lipase
  Heparin
  Prostacyclin
  Kallikrein
  Leukotrienes
Unaffected in traversing the lungs
  Angiotensin II
  Epinephrine
  Dopamine
  Vasopressin
  Prostaglandin A
  Vasoactive intestinal polypeptide
  Oxytocin

throughout the body is clearly a function of endothelium, and (2) the occurrence of atherosclerosis in systemic arteries is a response to subtle and prolonged endothelial injury. The nature of the injury is unclear. But, the level of blood pressure seems to be involved since the low-pressure pulmonary circulation is generally unaffected by atherosclerosis while systemic arteries are being corroded by the disorder.

INJURY BY OXYGEN-DERIVED PRODUCTS

Phenomena such as atherosclerosis have focused attention on the meaning of biologic injury. During the last few years, the concept of biologic injury has been revised downward from gross insult to minor perturbation. For example, metabolic dislocations that are continued over years, such as hypercholesterolemia, are now envisaged as acting in concert with other stresses, such as prolonged hypertension, to evoke atherosclerosis. But some types of biologic injury are so subtle that they leave no morphologic trace until the damage is far advanced. One of these is the injury attributed to oxygen-derived products.

Most of molecular oxygen entering the body is reduced sequentially to water via the respiratory chain. However, in the course of the serial reductions that are part of normal intermediary metabolism, superoxide anion (O_2^-) and hydrogen peroxide (H_2O_2) are generated as undesirable by-products. In turn, these products can generate other reactive oxygen species, including the hydroxyl radical (OH^-) (Fig. 28-1). A chain reaction then ensues which leads to the formation of lipid hydroperoxides; these, together with their own breakdown products, can damage biologic membranes and macromolecules. Currently, the role of reactive oxygen species is being investigated in a wide range of injuries that range on the one hand from the acute upsets in function caused by hyperoxia, drugs and toxins, inflammatory cells, radiation, and reperfusion to the chronic biologic processes of aging and carcinogenesis on the other.

$$O_2 \xrightarrow{1e^-} O_2^{\cdot-} \underset{pK\ 4.7}{\rightleftharpoons} HO_2^{\cdot}$$

$$O_2 \xrightarrow[2H^+]{2e^-} H_2O_2$$

$$2O_2^{\cdot-} + 2H^+ \xrightarrow{SOD} H_2O + O_2$$

$$2H_2O_2 \xrightarrow{Catalase} 2H_2O + O_2$$

$$H_2O_2 + O_2^{\cdot-} \xrightarrow{Fe^{3+} / Fe^{2+}} OH^- + \cdot OH + {}^1O_2$$

(Metal catalyzed Haber-Weiss)

$$H_2O_2 + Fe^{2+} \longrightarrow OH^{\cdot} + OH^- + Fe^{3+}$$

(Fenton reaction)

FIGURE 28-1   The generation of oxygen-free radicals by the addition of electrons. (*From Glass, Karnovsky and Fishman, in press.*)

The lungs are natural targets of study as a model of oxidant injury since they are continuously exposed to high concentrations of O_2 and they are rich in inhaled oxidants. However, study of injury produced by oxygen-derived products in the lungs is complicated by the presence of polymorphonuclear leukocytes that can generate not only O_2-derived products but also proteases that amplify the injury.

The best studied model of injury produced by O_2-derived products is O_2 toxicity. While breathing 100% O_2, metabolic derangements of the endothelium generally become manifest within 24 h; by 48 h, the lungs are full of inflammatory cells and edema that overflow from interstitium into alveoli and culminate in the adult respiratory distress syndrome. Three other clinical areas in which oxidant-produced injury features prominently are (1) the inhalation or ingestion of oxidants, e.g., paraquat; (2) chronic injury, such as that caused by smoking, which predisposes to low-level inflammation, pulmonary damage, and neoplasm; and (3) reperfusion injury of the heart, brain, and intestine that follows a bout of ischemia. In each of these instances, the role of antioxidants such as superoxide dismutase (SOD) in mitigating the injury is being explored.

GENERAL SYSTEMIC EFFECTS OF PULMONARY DISEASE

Pulmonary infections and neoplasms are notorious for the systemic effects that they can elicit (Table 28-2). Pneumonias caused by bacteria, mycoplasma, viruses, or fungi can cause a spectrum of disturbances that range from mild fever to bacteremia and circulatory collapse. Viral infections are notorious for inducing leukopenia, anemia, and thrombocytopenia. Metabolic derangements are also the rule in these acute disorders; abnormal hepatic, and bone marrow function are the bases for common abnormalities, e.g., the high erythrocyte sedimentation rate and leukocytosis. The span of disturbances is just as great for neoplasms not only because they encroach on adjacent structures and functions but also because of derangements of remote bodily functions that they cause by releasing biologically active materials (see Chapter 125). The impact of

TABLE 28-2

General Systemic Effects of Nonrespiratory Diseases of the Lung

Disturbances in the control of body temperature (Fever, chills, sweating)

Central nervous abnormalities (Euphoria, irritability, confusion, delerium)

Faintness reduced alertness, syncope (Postural hypotension, arrhythmias, decreased blood flow to the brain)

Anorexia, asthenia, cachexia

Remote organ failure

pulmonary disease on the rest of the body rises exponentially when infectious organisms or neoplastic cells escape the confines of the lungs to enter the bloodstream.

Bacteremia is a serious complication of a pneumonia. Bacteremia becomes more virulent with increasing age and with increasing numbers of organisms in the bloodstream. Mortality from bacteremia is high at all ages but jumps in the elderly. A wide variety of organs can be influenced detrimentally by bacteremia: the brain by meningitis or abscess; the joints by septic arthritis; the heart by endocarditis, myocarditis, or pericarditis; the gallbladder by empyema. Disseminated intravascular coagulation as a complication of pneumonia and bacteremia portends a grim prognosis. Different organisms have different propensities for bacteremia. In addition to bacteria, viral or fungal infections of the lungs may invade the bloodstream to exert profound, and sometimes lethal, derangements.

Particular systemic consequences of pulmonary infections and neoplasms are dealt with individually throughout this book as manifestations of the different diseases and disorders. Here attention focuses on two disturbances that are common and of considerable theoretical and practical importance: (1) fever and associated phenomena, and (2) body wasting.

Fever, Chills, and Sweating

Chills, fever, and sweating are familiar elements of the syndrome of pneumococcal pneumonia and of its complications. Pneumonia caused by different infecting organisms tends to be associated with distinctive diurnal fever patterns that were once highly esteemed for their diagnostic value. Although not as much clinical attention is now paid to patterns, sometimes the peaks and valleys in temperature suggest clues to etiology and undue persistence often signals a complication.

The body is constructed to maintain internal core temperature stable at about 37.1°C (corresponding to a rectal temperature of about 37.6°C) and equipped with automatic feedback devices that minimize fluctuations in the core temperature. Regulation of the core temperature is accomplished almost entirely by neural feedback mechanisms, virtually all of which are controlled by temperature-regulating mechanisms in the hypothalamus. Fever represents an upward shift in the thermostatic set point. The automatic attempt by the body to restore body temperature to normal includes cutaneous vasodilatation, sweating, decreased chemical thermogenesis, and a widespread decrease in muscle tone due to reflex inhibition of the "primary motor center for shivering."

Chills are a response to an abrupt disparity between the set point of the thermostat in the hypothalamus and the temperature of the blood. Certain substances, notably pyrogens or products of tissue destruction (see next paragraph), can suddenly raise the hypothalamic set point

without raising body temperature. Until the body temperature catches up, mechanisms to raise body temperature are turned on, and the individual feels cold and experiences chills—even while the body temperature is increasing to match the hypothalamus set point: the cold sensation is a consequence of cutaneous vasoconstriction, whereas shivering causes the "shakes." When the body temperature reaches the higher set point, chills cease and the individual feels neither cold nor hot. Until the factor responsible for increasing the set point stops, the febrile state is maintained by the usual mechanisms. Precipitous discontinuance of the initiating factor results in widespread cutaneous dilatation and flushing and intense sweating, i.e., "the crisis."

Pyrogens feature prominently in causing clinical fevers. They do so directly or indirectly by raising the thermostatic set point in the hypothalamus. Particularly effective in this regard are endotoxins produced by gram-negative bacteria. Leukocytes and macrophages act as intermediaries in this process: these phagocytic cells, after digesting the bacterial products, release leukocyte or endogenous pyrogen which, in minute amounts, stimulates the hypothalamus to raise its set point; prostaglandin E_1 is presumably the intermediary within the cells of the hypothalamus that effects the febrile response. Blockage of prostaglandin formation, as by aspirin, can prevent or reduce the febrile response.

Body Wasting

Progressive infection or the growth of a neoplasm often elicits anorexia, weight loss, and cachexia. The negative caloric and nitrogen balance that characterizes the cachectic state often culminates in death. These systemic effects are attributable to humoral substances liberated by the infection or neoplasm; in turn, the cachectic state disturbs the body defenses against the insult and its by-products.

Anorexia is a common antecedent of weight loss. It is a lack of the desire to eat. The start of anorexia appears to be related to the infection or neoplasm; but, in time, psychological factors supervene, other physical ailments and body rest compound the problem, and often anorexigenic therapeutic agents add to dulling of the appetite.

Normally, the intake of food is regulated by two centers in the hypothalamus, a feeding center and a satiety center. Cholecystokinin (CCK), a ubiquitous brain-intestinal peptide, has been implicated as a regulator of feeding behavior. The mechanisms responsible for the dulling of appetite by disease are not well understood. Anorexigenic peptides released by the infection or neoplasm have been postulated. Anorexia is so common that it is of little diagnostic value.

Frequent concomitants of anorexia are weakness, easy fatigability, and impaired mentation. The nature of the substances responsible for this syndrome of asthenia

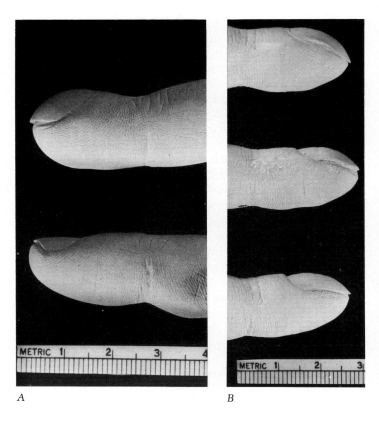

FIGURE 28-2 Casts of clubbed fingers. A. The third right finger of a 40-year-old woman with digital clubbing (*above*), compared with that of a normal 36-year-old woman (*below*). B. The second right finger of an 18-year-old girl with tetralogy of Fallot, before and after operation. *Upper*, preoperatively, showing marked clubbing. *Middle*, 2 months later, showing partial reversal of changes. *Lower*, regression of the clubbing. (*From Mellins, Fishman: Circulation 33:143–145, 1966.*)

A

B

are unclear. However, one consequence of anorexia and the asthenic syndrome is loss of weight. Any continuing loss of weight that is not the result of voluntary change in diet or exercise or of an inordinate loss of calories in stool or urine must be regarded as a signal of uncontrolled organic disease.

Cachexia is a wasting illness characterized primarily by an inexorable loss of weight that is inordinate for the degree of anorexia and the resultant decrease in food intake.

A search for the mechanisms responsible for the cachexia of chronic disease has recently led to the detection of a macrophage hormone, cachectin, that suppresses lipoprotein lipase, thereby evoking hypertriglyceridemia. This substance, in turn, has proved to be identical with "tumor necrosis factor" as well as the mediator of endotoxin shock, a common antecedent of the adult respiratory distress syndrome. Among the other effects of cachectin are its direct toxicity for endothelium, its role as a pyrogen, its capability for suppressing adipose-specific enzymes, and its effects as an important mediator of the inflammatory process. Clinical trials are now exploring the value of cachectin (tumor necrosis factor) as an antineoplastic agent.

Of special interest to the critical care physician is the relationship between the toxic effects of endotoxin and cachectin. Endotoxin is the most potent stimulus known for the production of cachectin. Instead of acting directly to cause injury, endotoxin (or its lipopolysaccharide) prompts the formation of host factors (including cachectin) that cause the damage. The macrophage is deeply involved in generating the host factors responsible for the injurious effects of endotoxin. Infusion of cachectin into experimental animals virtually duplicates the pathologic effects of administering endotoxin. Thus, although the role of cachectin in the pathogenesis of the cachexia of chronic disease is still unclear, the substance has emerged as a common denominator in a variety of other disease processes.

PARTICULAR SYSTEMIC EFFECTS OF PULMONARY DISEASE

Certain systemic manifestations, although not unique for pulmonary disease, occur often enough to warrant special mention. The extrapulmonary syndromes associated with neoplasms of the lungs are considered elsewhere (Chapter

125). Here clubbing of the digits is examined (see also Chapter 26).

Clubbing of the Digits and Hypertrophic Osteoarthropathy

The characteristic and preferential bulbous enlargement of the distal segment of the digits (Fig. 28-2) and the distinctive bony lesions of secondary hypertrophic osteoarthropathy are generally explained in terms of humoral mediators that cause selective vasodilatation of the digital precapillary vessels. As has been noted in Chapter 26, this explanation seems to suffice in certain disorders, e.g., the clubbing of the digits and the hypertrophic osteoarthropathy that accompanies carcinoma of the lungs, but not in others, e.g., subacute bacterial endocarditis. One other intriguing aspect of clubbing is its association both with chronic bronchiectasis, in which the adjacent collateral circulation of the lungs undergoes remarkable proliferation, and with carcinoma of the lung, in which the collateral blood supply is modest.

Remote Organ Failure

In the adult respiratory distress syndrome, successful treatment of the lungs does not always ensure recovery of the patient. Not infrequently, other organs appear to be mortally affected. The effects of a pulmonary disorder that result in systemic organ failure are considered elsewhere (see Chapters 140 and 141).

BIBLIOGRAPHY

Becker KL, Gazdar AF: *The Endocrine Lung in Health and Disease.* New York, Saunders, 1984.
  A sweeping attempt to view the lung as an endocrine organ because of its role in degrading, transforming, and activating substances derived locally and brought to it from afar.

Bell RC, Coalson JJ, Smith JD, Johanson WG Jr: Multiple organ system failure and infection in adult respiratory distress syndrome. Ann Intern Med 99:293–298, 1983.
  Underscores malfunction of the central nervous coagulation, endocrine, gastrointestinal, and renal systems in determining morbidity and shaping outcome in the adult respiratory distress syndrome. In patients with bacteremia, identification and drainage of site of infection was a sine qua non for survival.

Beutler B, Cerami A: Cachectin: More than a tumor necrosis factor. N Engl J Med 316:379–385, 1987.
  A review of the diverse biologic effects of this molecule and its potential role in a wide range of human diseases.

Cross CE, Halliwell B, Borish ET, Pryor WA, Ames BN, Saul RL, McCord JM, Harman D: Oxygen radicals and human disease. Ann Intern Med 107:526–545, 1987.
  A series of presentations dealing with oxygen-free radicals as pathologic mediators in a variety of clinical disorders.

Fisher A, Forman HJ: Oxygen utilization and toxicity in the lungs, in Fishman AP, Fisher AB (eds), *Handbook of Physiology, Sec 3: The Respiratory System, vol I, Circulation and Nonrespiratory Functions.* Bethesda, American Physiological Society, 1985, pp 231–254.
  A review of oxygen utilization at a cellular level, with emphasis on ATP generation, nonmitochondrial pathways for O_2 utilization, and the toxic effects of O_2-reduction products.

Fishman AP (ed): *Endothelium.* New York, The New York Academy of Sciences, 1982.
  An overview of the structure and function of vascular endothelium as a barrier to the exchange of substances across its walls and as a nonrespiratory organ.

Glass M, Karnovsky MJ, Fishman AP: Oxygen free radicals. J Appl Physiol. In press.
  A brief review of the types of biologic injury produced by O_2 free radicals and their clinical implications.

Hansen-Flaschen J, Nordberg J: Clubbing and hypertrophic osteoarthropathy. Clin Chest Med 8:287–298, 1987.
  A current and comprehensive review of the literature that focuses on the clinical recognition of clubbing and hypertrophic osteoarthropathy, including schematics for quantification.

Holroyde CP, Reichard GA Jr: General metabolic abnormalities in cancer patients: Anorexia and cachexia. Surg Clin North Am 66:947–956, 1986.
  The focus of this paper on general metabolic abnormalities is sharpened by succeeding papers in the same volume devoted to nutrition and cancer.

Lanken PN, Fishman AP: Clubbing and hypertrophic osteoarthropathy, in Fishman AP (ed), *Pulmonary Diseases and Disorders,* New York, McGraw-Hill, 1980, pp 84–91.
  A comprehensive overview of somewhat neglected signs that focuses on pathogenetic mechanisms.

Part **5**

Diagnostic Procedures

Chapter 29

Diagnostic Reasoning

Randall D. Cebul

The Patient as Starting Point
   Pretest Probability (Prior Probability)
   Perceived Importance

Information Inherent in Diagnostic Tests
   Test Sensitivity and Specificity
   Evaluating Nonbinary Tests

Measures of Test Performance in Practice
   The Prediction of Disease
   Test Accuracy

Return to the Patient: Pretest Probability

The Threshold Approach to Clinical Decision Making

The clinician generally uses diagnostic tests for one or more of four purposes: (1) to exclude a clinical diagnosis from further consideration; (2) to provide support for a suspected diagnosis; (3) to determine the extent of illness in order to guide stage-specific therapy, or to establish prognosis; or (4) to monitor the course of disease or the response to treatment. Occasionally diagnostic tests are done for the sake of reassurance—for either the patient or the clinician.

THE PATIENT AS STARTING POINT

The process of diagnostic reasoning begins during the earliest moments of the patient-physician encounter. Indeed, usually the process is well on its way before "definitive" testing is considered. Two patients suspected of having deep venous thrombosis in the legs may help to illustrate this point (Table 29-1).

The first patient (PC) is an 80-year-old man who came to the emergency room because of the acute onset of a heavy, swollen, and painful right lower extremity and a low-grade temperature. His medical history is notable for a recent radical prostatectomy for prostatic cancer, mild renal insufficiency from long-standing outlet obstruction, varicose veins, and prior deep venous thrombosis (DVT). On physical examination, he was found to have normal vital signs (except for an oral temperature of 100°F), normal cardiac findings, clear lungs, marked swelling of his right thigh and leg, tenderness without lymphadenopathy in his right groin and thigh, and dilatation of the dorsal veins of his right foot. His stool and urine were negative for occult blood. All blood studies were normal except for a urea nitrogen of 28 and a creatinine of 2.5 mg/dl.

The second patient (BC) is a 20-year-old college football player with no significant past medical history except a 3-month swelling in the area of his left popliteal fossa. He presented with the sudden onset of severe left calf pain, which occurred during football practice. On examination, his left calf was swollen, warm, and tender; Homan's sign was present; there was trace ankle edema, and no venous cords were felt. All blood and urine studies were normal.

In these cases, as in most clinical situations, the clinician typically generates diagnostic hypotheses in the first minutes of the interview, prepares a mental list of possibilities, and then expands and pares the list in response to focused questions and particular physical findings. Diagnostic possibilities for further evaluation are usually selected for one of two reasons: (1) the perceived likelihood or (2) their perceived importance.

TABLE 29-1

Two Patients Suspected of Deep Venous Thrombosis When First Seen by Clinician

	Patient PC	Patient BC
Age	80 years, retired	20 years, football player
Chief complaint	Heavy, swollen, painful right lower leg, acute onset; low grade fever	Swelling behind left knee, 3 weeks; onset of severe left calf pain during football practice
Past history	Radical prostatectomy for prostatic cancer; mild renal insufficiency secondary to outlet obstruction of bladder; several episodes of deep venous thrombosis	Normal
Physical findings	Right leg and thigh markedly swollen and tender; no regional lymphadenopathy; markedly swollen veins on dorsum of right foot	Swollen tender, warm left calf; positive Homan's sign; trace ankle edema, left
Laboratory data	Blood urea nitrogen: 28 mg/dl; Blood creatinine: 2.5 mg/dl	Normal

Pretest Probability (Prior Probability)

The perceived likelihood of a diagnosis—the pretest probability, or prior probability—is a quantitative measure of the evidence in favor of a particular diagnosis; its scale ranges from 0 percent when the disease is unequivocally absent to 100 percent when the disease is definitely present.

The two patients listed in Table 29-1 have markedly different pretest probabilities for DVT; in the first patient, PC, the prior probability of having ileofemoral thrombosis is very high; in the second patient, BC, probability is very low. As shown below, these differences markedly influence the yield and the clinical significance of the results of the diagnostic tests performed in the two patients.

Perceived Importance

Quantitative approaches to decision making distinguish sharply between the concept of *importance* and measures of disease likelihood: importance has to do more with the *consequences* of diagnostic classifications (or misclassifications) than with diagnosis per se. In Fig. 29-1 is shown, in general terms, the four possible consequences of diagnostic classifications, and Fig. 29-2 uses a simple decision tree to illustrate how they apply to the two patients in Table 29-1.

The adverse consequences of diagnostic misclassification may be worse in one direction than the other, depending on the patient, problem, and treatment under consideration. For example, it is much more important to avoid missing the diagnosis of a serious and treatable disease than to mistakenly start treatment for it in a patient who does not have the disease. This is especially true if the treatment is not risky or expensive. In this example, the principal reason for diagnostic testing is to avoid missing an opportunity for treatment and depends less on the pretest probability of disease.

Once the diagnostic hypotheses are formulated, i.e., early in the interview of the patient, and as data are accumulated in an increasingly focused manner, certain diagnoses begin to appear as the more likely, and others, perhaps entirely different, as the more important. A decision is then made about whether the additional information from diagnostic testing will be worth its cost and risk.

Several factors enter into this decision. Among them are the benefits and risks of the alternatives for treatment and the quality of information in the tests being considered.

INFORMATION INHERENT IN DIAGNOSTIC TESTS

The most commonly used quantitative measures of diagnostic test performance can be determined by using a *two-by-two* table (Fig. 29-3). Two of these measures, test sensitivity and test specificity, generally are considered to be stable properties of the test itself.

Test Sensitivity and Specificity

The *sensitivity* of a diagnostic test refers to its ability to identify patients who have the disease being considered; it provides a quantitative measure of the pick-up rate of a test. Since it is calculated by determining the proportion of patients with a particular disease in whom the test is positive (Fig. 29-3), sensitivity is also referred to as the *true positive* (or TP) rate for a test. A popular acronym for sensitivity is PID rate, signifying "positivity in disease" (not "pelvic inflammatory disease"!). A very sensitive diagnostic test usually detects the disease in patients, whereas an insensitive diagnostic test provides a relatively high proportion of false-negative diagnostic classifications.

Specificity refers to the ability of a diagnostic test to categorize correctly those patients who appear to have a certain disease but who, in reality, do not have it. Since it

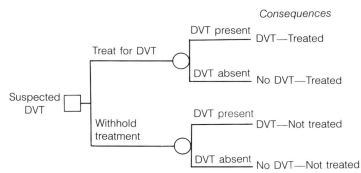

FIGURE 29-2 Decision tree illustrating treatment options for patients with suspected DVT. The consequences of diagnostic and therapeutic misadventure will depend heavily on the particular clinical setting: in some settings, the inappropriate withholding of anticoagulation will be the worst possible error, whereas in others, erroneous anticoagulation is the error to be avoided most. Diagnostic testing (not shown in this tree) will reduce the uncertainty inherent in this treatment decision, enabling the clinician to determine the likelihood of each possible outcome. □ = Decision node. Branches following this node represent alternative actions which may be taken by the decision maker. ○ = Chance (probability) node. Branches following these nodes represent probabilistic "events" which are not explicitly under the decision maker's control, e.g., underlying disease states, or the sequelae of treatment.

Diagnostic classification	Actual disease status	
	Present	Absent
"Diseased"	Treated disease	Unnecessary label Unnecessary treatment
"Not diseased"	False reassurance Untreated disease	Reassurance

FIGURE 29-1 The consequences of diagnostic classifications.

is calculated as the proportion of suspected but nondiseased patients in whom the diagnostic test is negative (Fig. 29-3), specificity is also called the *true negative* (or TN) rate for a test.

Impedance plethysmography is a noninvasive test that is being widely applied for the diagnosis of DVT. Illustrative values for the sensitivity and specificity of impedance plethysmography for DVT are shown in Fig. 29-4 using the two-by-two table format. The results indicate that the discriminating value of impedance plethysmography in patients with DVT is excellent: positive results using impedance plethysmography occur in approximately 95 percent of patients with proximal DVT, i.e., thrombosis that extends proximal to the popliteal vein, and in only 7 percent of patients who do not have proximal DVT.

Evaluating Nonbinary Tests

Intrinsically, most results of diagnostic tests are neither simply "normal" nor "abnormal." Instead, they provide finer grades of information. This generalization applies to *nonbinary* tests, e.g., to most of the findings from the history and physical examination and virtually all laboratory data.

For these nonbinary tests, a *positive result* is usually defined in terms of a particular cutoff for normality, e.g., for fever, a temperature greater than 38°C, for arterial P_{O_2}, a value less than about 90 mmHg. This popular practice entails the selection of a specific level beyond which abnormality begins. Moreover, it raises the possibility of choosing alternative criteria for defining the test as "positive."

For most clinical laboratory tests, a *normal range* of values is established in diagnostic laboratories by performing the test on a group of apparently healthy individuals; positive results are then arbitrarily defined as those values which fall beyond two standard deviations from the average result for the group. Clearly, other positivity criteria (or *cutoff values*) might be chosen.

The diagnostic implications of choosing alternative cutoff values for a diagnostic test are illustrated in Fig. 29-5. Importantly, changes in the cutoff value, in either direction, produce predictable trade-offs in test sensitivity and specificity: making the cutoff value more stringent enhances the specificity of the test at the cost of decreased

Test result	Disease status		
	Present	Absent	
Positive	(TP) True Positive	(FP) False Positive	TP + FP
Negative	(FN) False negative	(TN) True negative	FN + TN
	Total with disease (TP + FN)	Total without disease (FP + TN)	

Term	Synonyms	Calculation
Disease prevalence	Pretest probability Prior probability	(TP+FN)/(TP+FN+FP+TN) x 100
Sensitivity	True positive rate	TP/(TP+FN) x 100
Specificity	True negative rate	TN/(FP+TN) x 100
Accuracy	Efficiency	(TP+TN)/(TP+TN+FP+FN) x 100
Predictive value of a positive test	Predictive value positive Posttest probability of disease given a positive test	TP/(TP+FP) x 100
Predictive value of a negative test	Predictive value negative Posttest probability of no disease given a negative test	TN/(TN+FN) x 100

FIGURE 29-3 Common measures of test performance using a two-by-two table.

Results of impedance plethysmography	Proximal DVT	
	Present	Absent
Positive	74	13
Negative	4	183
	78	196

$$\text{Sensitivity (percent)} = \frac{\text{true-positive results}}{\text{all patients with proximal DVT}} \times 100$$

$$= \frac{74}{78} \times 100 = 94.9 \text{ percent}$$

$$\text{Specificity (percent)} = \frac{\text{true-negative results}}{\text{all patients without proximal DVT}} \times 100$$

$$= \frac{183}{196} \times 100 = 93.4 \text{ percent}$$

FIGURE 29-4 Test characteristics of impedance plethysmography for proximal DVT. In a series of 274 patients, 78 had venogram-documented proximal DVT, whereas 196 had either distal disease only (36 patients) or no DVT (160 patients). The results of impedance plethysmography in these two groups of patients are displayed here using a two-by-two table format, allowing simple calculation of the test's sensitivity and specificity.

TEST RESULTS OF THE POPULATION

Disease status of the population

Nondiseased — TN — FP

Cutoff value of test

← Increased sensitivity | Increased specificity →

Diseased — FN — TP

FIGURE 29-5 Effect of changing the cutoff value of a test on its sensitivity and specificity.

sensitivity (increased false-negative classifications); choosing a less restrictive cutoff value enhances the sensitivity at the cost of decreased specificity (increased false-positive classifications).

RECEIVER OPERATING CHARACTERISTIC CURVES

Receiver operating characteristic (ROC) curves and likelihood ratios are two expedients for determining the informational properties of nonbinary tests and for enabling

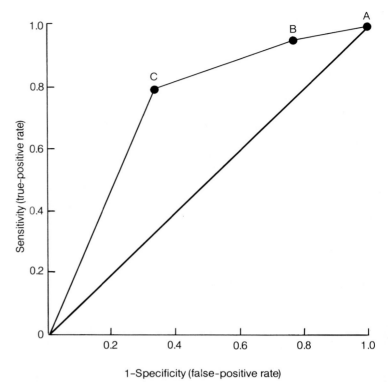

FIGURE 29-6 ROC curve for three results of the perfusion lung scan for pulmonary embolism. At point A, all results greater than or equal to "indeterminate" are called positive. At point B, all results with at least one or more subsegmental defect are called positive. At point C, all results with at least one or more segmental defect are called positive. The solid diagonal line reflects a hypothetical test with no discriminating ability; its true-positive rate is equal to its false-positive rate at all cutoff values for the test.

the selection of the proper cutoff value in a particular clinical setting. An ROC curve is a plot of a test's sensitivity (true-positive rate) against its false-positive rate (100 percent minus specificity) at different cutoff values. Importantly, the curve shows the quantitative trade-off between sensitivity and specificity produced by using different criteria for positivity.

Figure 29-6 displays an ROC curve constructed from recently published data for three findings of the perfusion lung scan. In 89 patients with clinical findings suggestive of pulmonary embolism, pulmonary angiograms were positive in 45 and negative in 44; the corresponding results of the perfusion scans were classified as *indeterminate, subsegmental,* or *segmental.* As shown in Fig. 29-6, using indeterminate results as the basis for further evaluation or treatment would properly classify all 45 pulmonary embolism patients (sensitivity = 100 percent). However, this excellent sensitivity would be at the expense of misclassifying all 44 nondiseased patients (false-positive rate = 100 percent). At the other extreme, the choice of the segmental value as the cutoff would reduce the false-positive classifications to 34 percent, but this also would reduce the sensitivity to 80 percent.

TABLE 29-2

Likelihood Ratios Calculated for Selected Findings on Lung Scan

| | Pulmonary Embolism | | | | |
| | Present | | Absent | | |
Finding	Number	Proportion	Number	Proportion	Likelihood Ratio
One or more segmental perfusion defects	36	36/45 = 0.80	15	15/44 = 0.34	0.80/0.34 = 2.35
One or more subsegmental perfusion defects	7	7/45 = 0.16	19	10/44 = 0.43	0.16/0.43 = 0.37
Indeterminate	2	2/45 = 0.04	10	10/44 = 0.23	0.04/0.23 = 0.17
	45	45/45 = 1.00	44	44/44 = 1.00	

Choosing the proper cutoff value as the basis for further evaluation or treatment depends on the particular patient, the disease, and the treatment under consideration. According to the principles of decision analysis, relatively lenient criteria for positivity should be chosen when the pretest probability of disease is high; more stringent criteria for positivity should be used when the pretest probability of disease is low. For example, in a patient in whom the clinical findings strongly suggest pulmonary embolism, it would be reasonable to start anticoagulation on the basis of one or more subsegmental perfusion defects; in contrast, in a patient in whom the clinical probability is low, further evaluation would be in order to establish the diagnosis, and treatment for pulmonary embolism should be withheld unless more definitive evidence of pulmonary embolism can be adduced, e.g., by a definitely abnormal perfusion scan or angiography.

The principles of decision making also state that the choice of cutoff value for a test should be guided by the benefit-to-risk ratio of management: relatively lenient criteria should be used when the expected benefits of treatment are high; more stringent criteria should be used when the expected benefit-to-risk ratio is low. For example, a patient with strong relative contraindications to anticoagulation should not be treated unless the evidence for pulmonary embolism is definite, whereas a patient who is clinically similar but lacks such contraindications could be treated on the basis of the lung scan results alone.

LIKELIHOOD RATIOS

The *likelihood ratio* is a second method for evaluating the informational properties of a nonbinary test. Instead of defining the test's sensitivity and specificity at a single, arbitrarily defined, cutoff value, the likelihood ratio expresses the *odds* that a *given level* of test abnormality would be expected in a patient who has the disease being considered. In particular, the likelihood ratio contrasts the proportion of patients with and without the disease who have a particular test result; it can also be calculated for one or more levels of test abnormality:

$$\begin{pmatrix} \text{Likelihood} \\ \text{ratio for} \\ \text{a given} \\ \text{test result} \end{pmatrix} = \frac{\begin{pmatrix} \text{proportion of diseased} \\ \text{patients with the result} \end{pmatrix}}{\begin{pmatrix} \text{proportion of nondiseased} \\ \text{patients with the result} \end{pmatrix}} \quad (1)$$

Table 29-2 displays the likelihood ratios for the same data on perfusion lung scans as those used for the ROC curve in Fig. 29-6. The likelihood ratios for varying degrees of abnormality in the lung scans range from 0.17 for an "indeterminate" scan to 2.35 for a scan that contains one or more segmental perfusion defects. The value of 2.35 is calculated by dividing the proportion of patients with pulmonary embolism who have this finding (36 of 45, or 0.80) by the proportion of patients *without* pulmonary embolism who have this finding (15 of 44, or 0.34); the likelihood ratio of 2.35 indicates that segmental perfusion defects are more than twice as likely to occur in patients with pulmonary embolism as in patients without pulmonary embolism. Similarly, the likelihood ratio of 0.17 for an indeterminate scan result indicates that results of this sort are only 17 percent as likely to come from patients with pulmonary embolism as from patients without pulmonary embolism. Appropriately, subsegmental perfusion defects (an "intermediate" grade of abnormality) are associated with an intermediate likelihood ratio value (although still less than 1.0).

The clinical implications of likelihood ratios are discussed in the next section. Here it is useful to emphasize that likelihood ratios generally are considered to be stable test properties (like test sensitivity, specificity, and the measures obtainable from ROC curves). Most importantly, values of likelihood ratios are not affected by differences in pretest probability. This feature is in marked contrast to the highly variable performance measures of test accuracy and predictive value considered in the next section.

MEASURES OF TEST PERFORMANCE IN PRACTICE

It was noted above that the *sensitivity* of a diagnostic test is the probability that a diseased patient will have a positive result and that the specificity of a test is the probability that a nondiseased patient will have a negative result. However, a diagnostic test is ordered because the clinician does *not* know whether a particular disease is present or absent; since the calculations of sensitivity and specificity are based on patients whose disease status is known with certainty, the quantitative determination of sensitivity and specificity has not solved the right clinical problem. Indeed, although knowledge of these values is necessary for predicting the presence or absence of disease, it is not sufficient.

The Prediction of Disease

The most pressing clinical question about the results of a diagnostic test has to do with its *predictive value*, i.e., how well the results predict the presence or absence of disease in a particular patient. The *predictive value of a positive test*, or the *positive predictive value*, is the probability that a patient with a positive test result has the suspected disease; values for this measure range from 0 to 100 percent. The predictive value of a positive test is calculated by determining the proportion of clinically simi-

lar patients with positive test results who have the specified disease. The *predictive value of a negative test* (or *negative predictive value*) is the probability that a patient with a negative test result does *not* have the disease in question (Fig. 29-3).

Predictive values can be calculated in several ways, e.g., by using two-by-two tables or Bayes' formula or by quantitatively manipulating likelihood ratios. Importantly, their calculation by any method requires estimates of three values: the sensitivity and specificity of the diagnostic test (or a measure, such as the likelihood ratio, which relates the two values) and the pretest probability of disease.

Because the pretest probability of disease varies considerably from patient to patient, predictive values also depend heavily on the clinical features of a given patient; the same test result will have different predictive values and clinical significance in different patients. For example, Fig. 29-7A illustrates the use of the two-by-two table method for calculating predictive values for impedance plethysmography in patient PC. For the sake of this analysis, patient PC was assumed to have an 80 percent pretest

Assumptions of Analysis

A. Pretest probability = 80 percent
    Sensitivity = 95 percent
    Specificity = 93 percent

IPG Results	Proximal DVT Present	Proximal DVT Absent	
Positive	760	14	774
Negative	40	186	226
	800	200	1000

Predictive Value Calculations

Positive predictive value (%) $= \dfrac{760}{774} \times 100 = 98.2$ percent

Negative predictive value (%) $= \dfrac{186}{226} \times 100 = 82.3$ percent

B. Pretest probability = 10 percent
    Sensitivity = 95 percent
    Specificity = 93 percent

IPG Results	Proximal DVT Present	Proximal DVT Absent	
Positive	95	63	158
Negative	5	837	842
	100	900	1000

Positive predictive value (%) $= \dfrac{95}{158} \times 100 = 60.1$ percent

Negative predictive value (%) $= \dfrac{837}{842} \times 100 = 99.4$ percent

FIGURE 29-7 Two patients suspected of having DVT. Calculations of predictive value using two-by-two tables. The tables display the predictive values of the positive and negative results of impedance plethysmography (IPG) for patients PC (*A*) and BC (*B*), who are assumed to have pretest probabilities of 80 percent and 10 percent, respectively. *A*. Of 1000 patients like patient PC, 800 will have proximal DVT and 200 will not. Given the known sensitivity and specificity of IPG, 760 diseased patients will have positive results (95 percent of 800) and 186 nondiseased patients will have negative results (93 percent of 200). The predictive value calculations proceed across the two *rows* of the table. *B*. Of 1000 patients like patient BC, 100 will have proximal DVT and 900 will not. The calculations of predictive values for BC are similar in all other respects to those for patient PC.

probability of having DVT. It may be inferred from Fig. 29-7A that in patient PC, positive results are more than 98 percent likely to represent proximal DVT, whereas negative results leave an almost 18 percent chance that DVT is present, despite the disconforming (albeit imperfect) evidence.

Similar calculations are shown in Fig. 29-7B for patient BC. For the sake of this analysis, the patient was assumed to have a 10 percent pretest probability of having proximal DVT. In contrast to patient PC, positive results in BC indicate a probability of almost 40 percent that proximal DVT is absent, despite the supportive (albeit imperfect) evidence. In this patient, the negative test results virtually exclude the diagnosis of DVT from further consideration.

The results of these *probability revisions* (revising the pretest probability to its corresponding posttest value) indicate that the predictive values of impedance plethysmography depend considerably on the likelihood that the patient has proximal DVT *before* the test is performed. As shown in Table 29-3, *positive* results of impedance plethysmography in patients in whom the probability of DVT is very low are as likely to represent some other cause for the presenting complaints as they are to reflect proximal DVT; similarly, *negative* results in patients with clinically obvious proximal DVT should be looked upon with skepticism since they do not allow exclusion of the diagnosis with confidence.

The process of probability revision also illustrates that impedance plethysmography is most useful for diagnostic purposes when applied to patients in whom the probabilities of the disease are midrange, i.e., for patients in whom the diagnosis is most uncertain before the test is performed. Indeed, regardless of the test and disease under consideration, diagnostic certainty increases most

TABLE 29-3
The Predictive Values of Impedance Plethysmography for Proximal DVT at Different Pretest Probabilities of Disease*

| Pretest Probability of Proximal DVT Percent | Impedance Plethysmography | |
	Predictive Value Positive, %	Predictive Value Negative, %
5	42	100
10	60	99
20	77	99
50	93	95
80	98	82
90	99	67
95	100	50

* All calculations assume a sensitivity of 95 percent and a specificity of 93 percent for impedance plethysmography; predictive values in table are rounded to the nearest integer.

when the test is used in patients for whom the presence is a probabilistic coin toss before the test is done. When the pretest disease probability of the disease is close to 100 percent, "good" tests will usually be positive (adding little to the clinician's pretest certainty); if negative, the tests will not rule out the suspected disease. When the pretest probability of disease is close to 0 percent, good tests are usually negative; if positive, they do not rule in the disease in question.

As mentioned above, likelihood ratios can also be used to determine the posttest probability of disease. It was noted above that likelihood ratios reflect the odds that a given level of test abnormality would be expected in a patient with the disease. The predictive power of likelihood ratios relates to their ability to determine the odds favoring disease *after* a given test result is known, according to the following equation:

$$\begin{pmatrix} \text{Pretest odds} \\ \text{for disease} \end{pmatrix} \times \begin{pmatrix} \text{likelihood ratio for} \\ \text{the test results} \end{pmatrix}$$
$$= \begin{pmatrix} \text{posttest odds} \\ \text{for disease} \end{pmatrix} \quad (2)$$

Instead of calculating the odds by (2), to determine posttest probability of a disease, a simple nomogram, based on the likelihood ratio for a particular diagnostic test result, can be used (Fig. 29-8).

Test Accuracy

The designation *accuracy* is commonly used to mean the "goodness" of a diagnostic test. The accuracy of a diagnostic test is defined as the proportion of all diagnostic classifications made by the test, which are correct (Fig. 29-3). However, unlike test sensitivity and specificity, accuracy is not a stable measure of diagnostic test performance since its value varies with changes in pretest probability. Therefore, even though the concept of accuracy does have limited usefulness as an overall measure of diagnostic test performance, it has little predictive power for making decisions about patient care.

RETURN TO THE PATIENT: PRETEST PROBABILITY

Largely unanswered by the considerations above is the question of how to assign pretest estimates of the probability of a disease to patients who have unique combinations of signs, symptoms, and results of prior tests. In certain clinical settings, these estimates can be made with reasonable confidence on the basis of published data, statistical prediction rules, or computerized data bases.

In most clinical settings, however, clinical judgment must guide the assessment of prior probability. Clinicians routinely use some form of quantification in assessing the likelihood of disease, often designated as

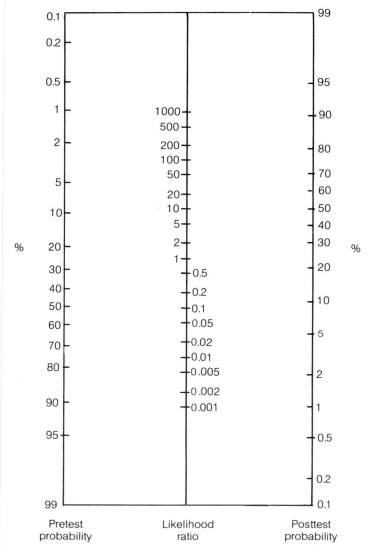

| Pretest probability | Likelihood ratio | Posttest probability |

FIGURE 29-8 A nomogram for using likelihood ratios to calculate the posttest probability of disease. To use the nomogram, a ruler or other straight edge is anchored at the estimated pretest probability of disease on the left. The straight edge is then pivoted on this anchor until it lines up with the likelihood ratio for the test's results in the middle of the nomogram. Finally, the posttest probability of disease is determined by sighting along the straight edge in the right-hand column. The likelihood ratios for positive and negative impedance plethysmography results can be determined from Fig. 29-4 to be about 14 and 0.05, respectively. As an exercise, the nomogram can be used to estimate posttest probabilities of proximal DVT at a variety of pretest probabilities, and the results compared with the values in Table 29-20. (NOTE: the posttest probability of disease after a *negative* result is equal to 100 percent minus its predictive value negative). *(From Sackett DL, Hayness RB, Tugwell P: Clinical Epidemiology. Toronto, Little, Brown, 1985, p 112.)*

their *index of suspicion* and quantified loosely as "highly likely," "a 50:50 chance," or "highly unlikely." For example, the patient who presents with obvious phlegmasia cerulea dolens would be categorized as highly likely with respect to having proximal DVT; in this instance, positive

results using impedance plethysmography would merely confirm the clinician's high index of suspicion of DVT. Appropriately, indeterminate or negative results of impedance plethysmography would be regarded with skepticism in this patient. Quantitative methods in diagnosis, such as those described in this chapter, certify the validity and importance of such pretest diagnostic stratification.

THE THRESHOLD APPROACH TO CLINICAL DECISION MAKING

Using decision analysis, a threshold approach to patient management decisions has been described (Fig. 29-9), in which judgments about the desirability of performing a diagnostic test are based, first and foremost, on the pretest probability of disease in an individual patient. The *test threshold* is defined as the pretest probability of disease *below* which treatment should be withheld without further testing. The *treatment threshold* is defined as the pretest probability of disease *above* which specific treatment should be initiated without further testing. The *testing zone* is the range of pretest probabilities within which testing is warranted because of its potential for guiding a decision about treatment. Importantly, the precise values for the test and treatment thresholds depend entirely on factors that are unique both to the patient and problem being evaluated. These factors include: (1) the characteristics of the test (its informational value, cost, and risk), and (2) the characteristics of the disease and treatment being considered (specifically, the relative risks, costs, and benefits of alternative treatment decisions).

Principles for selecting diagnostic tests based on the threshold approach are illustrated graphically in Fig. 29-9. Starting with a typically "good" test and "reasonably effective" treatment for a particular disease, Fig. 29-9A illustrates that there is a pretest probability of disease below which the clinician should forgo testing and treatment for that disease—and perhaps pursue other diagnostic possibilities; similarly, there is a level of pretest certainty above which the clinician should treat the patient as diseased—even without perfect certainty. Because the typically good test provides imperfect information and has definable risks and costs, the clinician should use it only when he or she is fairly uncertain about the presence of disease, i.e., in the hypothetical baseline case, from pretest probabilities of 30 to 70 percent.

As compared with the typically good test, a better test is indicated in a larger range of situations. The better test may provide more information, or the same information at lower cost or risk. The better test is represented in Fig. 29-9B as a broader testing zone; the test threshold in this situation is lower than in the baseline case, and the treatment threshold is higher.

CLINICAL SETTING

MANAGEMENT THRESHOLDS

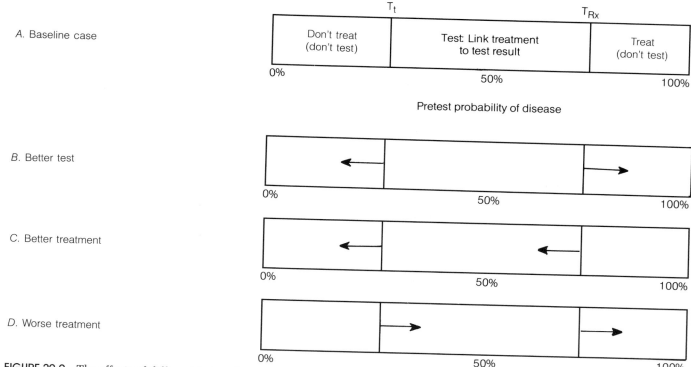

FIGURE 29-9   The effects of different test and treatment attributes on management thresholds. T_t = test threshold; T_{Rx} = treatment threshold.

If more effective treatment were available, the "no testing and no treatment" option rarely would be the optimal choice. In the setting of more effective therapy, both management thresholds decrease (Fig. 29-9C as compared with 29-9A). This has the effect of minimizing the incidence of false-negative management decisions, or missed opportunities for treatment. In contrast, both management thresholds *increase* if treatment is relatively ineffective, risky, or costly (Fig. 29-9D as compared with 29-9A). In these situations, the clinician intuitively wants to avoid false-positive management decisions, and testing and/or treatment should be withheld unless there is a reasonably high pretest probability of disease.

Although the quantitative application of the threshold approach is elaborate and requires the assignment of numerical values to clinical factors that are difficult to assess, the principles are useful in deriving the greatest benefit from imperfect diagnostic tests and therapies. This approach encourages the clinician to look ahead to the potential consequences of performing diagnostic tests, to select *particular* tests for *specific* reasons, and to individualize interpretations based on the unique features of the patient and problem at hand.

BIBLIOGRAPHY

Diagnostic Testing, Clinical Epidemiology, and Decision Analysis

Cebul RD, Beck LH: Teaching Clinical Decision Making. New York, Praeger, 1985.
  Written primarily for clinical educators, this book provides a structured approach to learning and teaching the principles of diagnostic test evaluation, decision analysis, and cost-effectiveness analysis. Easy to read and use as a reference, it includes a variety of clinical illustrations and an extensive annotated bibliography.

Fletcher RH, Fletcher SW, Wagner EH: *Clinical Epidemiology—The Essentials.* Baltimore, Williams and Wilkins, 1982.
>   Chapters 2 to 4 introduce diagnostic test properties from the perspective of the clinical epidemiologist, including discussions of the sources of variation in clinical measurements, bias in test evaluation, and guidelines for screening for disease.

Galen RS, Gambino SR: *Beyond Normality: The Predictive Value and Efficiency of Medical Diagnoses.* New York, Wiley, 1975.
>   Already a classic, this simple and readable text covers the fundamental properties of diagnostic tests and their performance characteristics in practice: sensitivity, specificity, and predictive value. A variety of tests and clinical problems are used for illustration.

Sackett DL, Haynes RB, Tugwell P: *Clinical Epidemiology. A Basic Science for Clinical Medicine.* Toronto, Little, Brown, 1985.
>   An oftentimes entertaining and always informative textbook of clinical epidemiology for inquisitive clinicians. The first section (chaps. 1 to 5) covers principles of diagnosis, including the selection and interpretation of diagnostic tests and the definitive word on test likelihood ratios. The second ("Management") and third ("Keeping Up to Date") sections also are worthwhile reading, designed to enhance the clinician's skills in appraising published evidence.

Weinstein MC, Fineberg HV: *Clinical Decision Analysis.* Philadelphia, Saunders, 1980.
>   The definitive textbook on the subject. Diagnostic testing principles are introduced in a decision-oriented context; i.e., how should a diagnostic test result influence decisions in patient management? Includes material on multiple testing, receiver operating characteristic curve analysis, the valuation of clinical outcomes, and the means by which uncertain probability values should be examined.

Diagnostic Testing

Griner PF, Panzer RJ, Greenland P: *Clinical Diagnosis and the Laboratory: Logical Strategies for Common Medical Problems.* Chicago, Year Book, 1986.
>   The basics, applied to many common clinical settings, including the evaluation of tests for several pulmonary problems.

Hershey JC, Cebul RD, Williams SV: Clinical guidelines for using two dichotomous tests. Med Decis Making 6:68–78, 1986.
>   Expands on the threshold model for management to include clinical situations in which two binary tests are being considered, addressing questions such as whether one or both tests should be performed, whether the tests should be performed sequentially or together, and how to make the treatment decision when the test results disagree.

McNeil BJ, Keeler E, Adelstein SJ: Primer on certain elements of medical decision making. N Engl J Med 293:211–215, 1975.
>   Includes discussion of ROC curves and the formula for selecting the optimal cutoff point for a nonbinary diagnostic test.

Metz CE: Basic principles of receiver operating characteristic (ROC) curve analysis. Semin Nuc Med 8:283–293, 1978.
>   An excellent discussion of ROC curves and their applications to diagnostic test evaluation.

Pauker SG, Kassirer JP: The threshold approach to clinical decision making. N Engl J Med 302:1109–1117, 1980.
>   A classic article outlining the principles of management thresholds and illustrating how these thresholds should guide the use of diagnostic tests.

Poses RM, Cebul RD, Collins M, Fager SS: The importance of disease prevalence in transporting clinical prediction rules: The case of streptococcal pharyngitis. Ann Intern Med 105:586–591, 1986.
>   Caveats to using statistical approaches for estimating the pretest probability of disease.

Ransohoff DF, Feinstein AR: Problems of spectrum and bias in evaluating the efficacy of diagnostic tests. N Engl J Med 299:926–930, 1978.
>   A short but very important paper illustrating common pitfalls in diagnostic test evaluation.

Sox HC Jr: *Common Diagnostic Tests: Use and Interpretation.* Philadelphia, American College of Physicians, 1987.
>   Probability theory applied in reviews of a large variety of common diagnostic tests; peer-reviewed chapters originally appearing in the Annals of Internal Medicine, with guidelines for use endorsed by Blue Cross and Blue Shield.

Wasson JH, Sox HC, Neff RK, Goldman L: Clinical prediction rules: Applications and methodological standards. N Engl J Med 313:793–799, 1985.

Standards for statistical approaches to prediction of disease probability or prognosis.

Diagnostic Tests for Thromboembolic Disease

Hull RD, Hirsh J, Carter CJ, Jay RM, Dodd PE, Ockelford PA, Coates G, Gill GJ, Turpie AG, Doyle DJ, Buller HR: Pulmonary angiography, ventilation lung scanning, and venography for clinically suspected pulmonary embolism with abnormal perfusion lung scan. Ann Intern Med 98:891–899, 1983.

An important paper documenting diagnostic test results for 139 patients evaluated prospectively because of signs and symptoms of venous thromboembolism. Data from table 3 (p. 895) were used to illustrate various points in the current chapter.

Hull R, Hirsh J, Sackett DL, Taylor DW, Carter C, Turpie AG, Zielinsky A, Powers P, Gent M: Replacement of venography in suspected venous thrombosis by impedance plethysmography and ^{125}I-fibrinogen leg scanning. Ann Intern Med 94:12–15, 1981.

One of several papers by investigators from the Hamilton District Thromboembolism Programme which has influenced the more widespread adoption of noninvasive diagnostic tests for the evaluation of suspected deep vein thrombosis. Data from the text related to table 1 (p. 13) were abstracted to illustrate various points in the current chapter.

Chapter 30

Sputum Examination

Sanford Chodosh

Constituents and Characteristics of Sputum

Sputum Collection Methods
    Expectoration
    Gastric Aspiration
    Tracheobronchial Aspiration
    Bronchoscopy
    Transtracheal Aspiration
    Percutaneous Needle Aspiration

Methods for Sputum Examination
    Physical Characteristics
    Microscopic Evaluation
    Gram Stains and Bacteriologic Cultures
    Identification of Mycobacteria
    Cancer Cytology

Application of Sputum Data to Clinical Situations
    Infectious Processes
    Chronic Bronchial Diseases

Sputum coughed up by a patient is indicative of an ongoing pathologic process in the bronchopulmonary system. It is frequently the neglected "biopsy" material which is usually repetitively available without requiring invasive procedures. Sputum can be evaluated for its physical characteristics, infectious microorganisms, malignant cells, the nature of inflammatory processes, and pathologic changes in the bronchial mucosa. Gross observation, microscopic assessment of a wet preparation, and Gram stain of the specimen are simple and well within the ability of clinicians or the scope of their laboratory services. In addition, selection of true sputum—true, as opposed to oral secretions, e.g., saliva—improves the reliability of specimens sent for more sophisticated examinations.

The interpretation of the data obtained from sputum evaluations is usually direct and uncomplicated. The clinician can determine the microorganisms responsible for an infectious process, differentiate allergic from nonallergic bronchopulmonary disease, diagnose malignancy, follow the efficacy of specific therapy, differentiate between necrotizing and nonnecrotizing pulmonary infections, and determine the likely etiology of acute exacerbations of chronic bronchial disease. As with all laboratory data, the information obtained must be considered within the framework of the total clinical picture.

CONSTITUENTS AND CHARACTERISTICS OF SPUTUM

Sputum may be defined as any abnormal secretion produced in, or expectorated from, the bronchopulmonary system. It is not saliva, and it is not nasopharyngeal in origin. It is a variable mixture of cellular, noncellular, and nonpulmonary material dependent on the underlying pathologic process (Fig. 30-1). The cellular elements may be inflammatory or red blood cells from the airways, exfoliated bronchial and alveolar cells, or malignant cells shed from tumors. Nonpulmonary cells such as oropharyngeal squamous cells, vegetable cells, and animal cells may become part of the sputum if they have been aspirated into the lung and subsequently coughed up. The noncellular constituents have their origin from mucus-producing cells of the lung, alveolar and bronchial exudate or transudate, aspirated material, and cellular breakdown products. Water is the major constituent of sputum, usually accounting for over 90 percent of the weight, with proteins, enzymes, carbohydrates, fats, and glycoproteins making up the balance. The clinician may also find various microorganisms which may be etiologic to the disease process.

The volume of sputum expectorated usually reflects the severity of the disease process. Poorly understood but complex interactions among the various constituents determine the physical properties of the material which relate to the patient's ability to clear the secretions. The thickness and stickiness of sputum are partly related to the amounts of extracellular mucopolysaccharide and deoxyribonucleic acid molecules present. The purulence of sputum is due to the green peroxidases released from degenerated neutrophils or eosinophils. Rather than providing a reliable index for infection, it is an excellent indicator of the speed of clearing secretions. Mucoid sputum indicates prompt clearance and may contain as many inflammatory cells as a purulent specimen.

SPUTUM COLLECTION METHODS

Virtually all methods of collection inherently allow the bronchopulmonary sputum to become contaminated with nonbronchopulmonary material. The choice of method(s) should be dictated by clinical judgment in each case. The factors to be considered include the seriousness of the disease, the need to establish a definitive diagnosis, the risks of the procedure, and the ability of a given technique to provide the needed information.

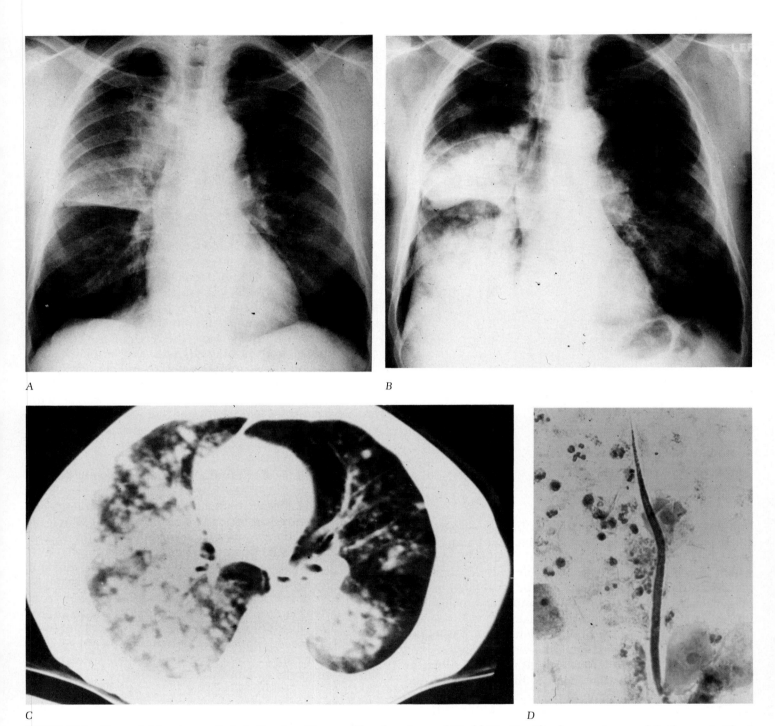

A

B

C

D

FIGURE 30-1 *Strongyloides stercoralis* infection in a 65-year-old male veteran of World War II with adenocarcinoma of the lung. *A.* Chest radiograph on admission. Obstructive lesion of bronchus to right upper lobe. *B.* Chest radiograph 16 months later, after needle biopsy. Pneumothorax on right. Histology revealed adenocarcinoma. *C.* Computed tomography at same time as *B*. Nodular lesions are clearly seen in the lower lobes. *D.* Sputum cytology. Larva of *Strongyloides stercoralis* suggesting a parasitic, rather than neoplastic, etiology for the nodules despite proven adenocarcinoma of right upper lobe. *(Courtesy of Dr. R. A. Panettieri, Jr.)*

Expectoration

Expectorated sputum requires no invasive procedure, and it is repetitively available for following the course of the disease process. Sputum collected over a set period of time permits quantitative assessment of the severity of the inflammatory response and the extent of the bronchial mucosal damage. The 24-h sputum collection is particularly useful in patients whose expectoration is variable over the day. Material produced by deep cough usually originates from the chest, but secretions produced by throat clearing may have come from the bronchopulmonary system. Microscopic examination will determine the true origin.

Patients not expectorating sputum when clinical circumstances suggest the presence of secretions may be induced to be productive. Urging the patient to utilize more efficient cough maneuvers, repetitive chest percussion with cupped hands or externally applied vibrators, and appropriate postural drainage maneuvers are useful methods. Dyspneic or fragile patients may not be able to tolerate the discomfort of such physical procedures. The utilization of inhaled aerosols of bronchodilator and normal or even mildly hypertonic saline often stimulates a more productive cough. Ultrasonic nebulization may be more effective than standard nebulizers. Success is more likely if the inhaled aerosol stimulus is followed by mechanical induction maneuvers. More invasive methods should not be used unless this approach to the induction of sputum is unsuccessful. Although without risk, the common pediatric practice of swabbing secretions on the posterior pharynx when sputum cannot be readily obtained rarely provides useful information concerning the pathology in the bronchopulmonary system. There may be considerable risk in making clinical decisions based on such specimens.

Gastric Aspiration

Aspiration of gastric contents via a gastric tube may be used to obtain bronchopulmonary secretions swallowed during the night. The procedure must be carried out in the early morning before the patient rises, since gastric emptying occurs rapidly once the patient has become active. Cultures of the material obtained can be important in determining the presence of tuberculosis infection. However, acid-fast smears can be falsely positive due to ingested saprophytic acid-fast microorganisms. Gastric contents containing mucous plugs obtained through aspiration or in vomitus are worth examining if no better material is available from the patient.

Tracheobronchial Aspiration

This method is practical when the patient cannot cooperate because of depressed mental status or inability to develop an effective cough. Passing the catheter in alert patients requires their understanding and cooperation. The catheter is passed through the nose or mouth and secretions obtained with gentle and intermittent suctioning. Catheter placement usually induces cough which can move secretions closer to the catheter tip. A few milliliters of sterile saline introduced as a bolus may loosen secretions and induce productive cough. Advantages are that secretion removal may be therapeutically indicated anyway, more invasive procedures can be avoided, specially

trained professionals are not required, thicker secretions are more likely obtained through the large bore of the catheter, and the procedure can be readily repeated. Dangers include damage to the epithelium, mucosal bleeding, induction of vomiting with aspiration, apnea secondary to neural reflex stimulation, and hypoxemia unless the inspired air is oxygen-enriched during the procedure. Aspiration is the obvious method in patients with an endotracheal tube or tracheostomy. Contamination of these specimens by aspiration of upper respiratory material into the tracheobronchial tree is often observed.

Bronchoscopy

The flexible fiberoptic bronchoscope has made bronchoscopy a practical means of obtaining secretions from abnormal areas of the lung under direct visualization. This is particularly pertinent when other bronchopulmonary disease is present. When secretions are insufficient for aspiration, localized lavage brushing or biopsy may provide useful material for diagnostic evaluation.

Transtracheal Aspiration

Transtracheal aspiration via direct, percutaneous cricothyroid puncture has been associated with serious complications. Although relatively safe in the hands of experienced individuals, it should not be a routine procedure for obtaining secretions. Experimentally it has provided important information concerning the bacteriology of the lower respiratory tract. The major advantage of transtracheal aspiration is that less-contaminated secretions can be obtained by avoiding the upper airways, but bronchoscopy that includes special provision for obtaining shielded samples can achieve similar results. Transtracheal aspiration is contraindicated if the patient has a bleeding diathesis or a severe cough; active hemoptysis is a lesser contraindication. The advantage of avoiding contaminants from above the cricothyroid entrance site is lost if the catheter tip is inadvertently directed toward the larynx or is coughed into that position by the patient. Aspiration of thick secretions through the small bore catheter that is used in this procedure is difficult. Lavage using sterile saline to dislodge secretions decreases the bacterial selectivity.

Percutaneous Needle Aspiration

As described in Chapter 33, transthoracic needle aspiration can be used to obtain material from areas of pneumonitis or from pulmonary lesions. This technique has been used for decades by pediatricians to determine the etiology of pneumonias. The complications are similar to those caused by transtracheal aspirations. Among the indications for percutaneous needle aspiration are pneumonia in an immunocompromised host when early and specific etiologic diagnosis is critical for proper management, and failure of a pneumonia to respond to treatment. The obvious advantage of this approach is obtaining pathologic material directly from the lesion. Potential complications are pneumothorax and hemoptysis. The material obtained will be small, so the plan for diagnostic studies should be clear.

METHODS FOR SPUTUM EXAMINATION

Appropriate handling of the specimen during and after collection is just as important as the method used to collect it. Secretions may be obtained under conditions that thwart efforts to identify etiology. Inadequate examination of the specimen can lead to incomplete and/or misleading information. These faulty methods may be the accepted routine of the institution so that errors are often not recognized. Results must be interpreted with these limitations in mind. Other problems to consider are the inhibiting effect of local anesthetics on the growth of cultured microorganisms, inadvertent contamination during the procedure by secretions in the upper airways, lavage using sterile saline that contains bacteriostatic additives, and the selective attraction of mycobacteria in watery secretions to some of the hydrophobic surfaces of the materials used to collect the specimen. Specimens being aspirated should be directed into a sterile Lukens trap without the use of any solution. When anaerobic or other fastidious microorganisms are suspected, cultures should be made as soon as possible after collection. Prompt fixation of specimens to be examined for malignant cells should be routine.

Physical Characteristics

The first step in sputum examination should be description of its gross physical appearance.

VOLUME

When a timed sputum collection has been obtained, the volume should be recorded. Daily sputum volume provides a useful parameter for following the course of a number of chronic sputum-producing pulmonary diseases and of acute lung abscess. Weighing the specimen or using graduated collecting containers makes the measurement simple. An adjustment of the volume should be made after the percentage of the specimen which is actually sputum has been more specifically determined by microscopic evaluation.

PHYSICAL PROPERTIES

The thickness and stickiness of the sputum should be estimated, since this can be important information in diseases where secretions may be a significant factor in blocking airways. Estimates of thickness can be easily determined by inverting the sample in the collection container. The thinnest specimens flow like water, and the thickest do not change shape with this maneuver. The stickiness of the sputum can be simultaneously described as the degree to which the specimen sticks to the wall of the container. Grades of thickness between the extremes can be estimated by how the specimen holds together when a wooden applicator stick is horizontally pulled out of the specimen.

MUCOPURULENCE AND COLOR

Mucopurulence is an estimation of how much of the specimen is mucoid and how much is purulent. Used alone, this characteristic is often undependable since contaminating saliva may look mucoid and expectorated sinonasal drainage may look purulent. It is more useful to describe the translucency and color of the sputum areas of the specimen.

Mucoid sputum has the clear transparency of fresh egg white, but it takes on a whitish or opalescent appearance as more cells are concentrated in the specimen. This appearance is characteristic of secretions which are cleared quickly from the airways. Yellow to green coloration of the sputum is indicative of "purulence." This coloration implies stasis of the secretions in the airways, thereby allowing time for polymorphonuclear cells, either neutrophils or eosinophils, to break down and release their peroxidases which impart their color to the sputum; the more peroxidases released, the greener the specimen. Expectorated mucoid sputum can show this same change to purulence with time. A gray or brownish color of the sputum usually suggests excessive dust or tobacco smoke in the specimen, although distinctly brown sputum may be the result of red blood cell breakdown products. Evidence of red blood should be noted and quantitated.

Microscopic Evaluation

Microscopic examination is essential to ascertain that the specimen originated in the bronchopulmonary system, since most collected specimens are contaminated with variable amounts of oropharyngeal material.

SELECTION OF MATERIAL

Inspection of the sample usually reveals strands or flecks of denser material suspended in a clearer mucoid matrix. Strands vary in size from barely visible to grossly apparent plugs, likely dependent on the size of the bronchi from which they were coughed up. In exudate from necrotizing infections, the secretions lack these strands and are often thin and puslike. These characteristics can be best appreciated if the specimen is poured out into half of a petri

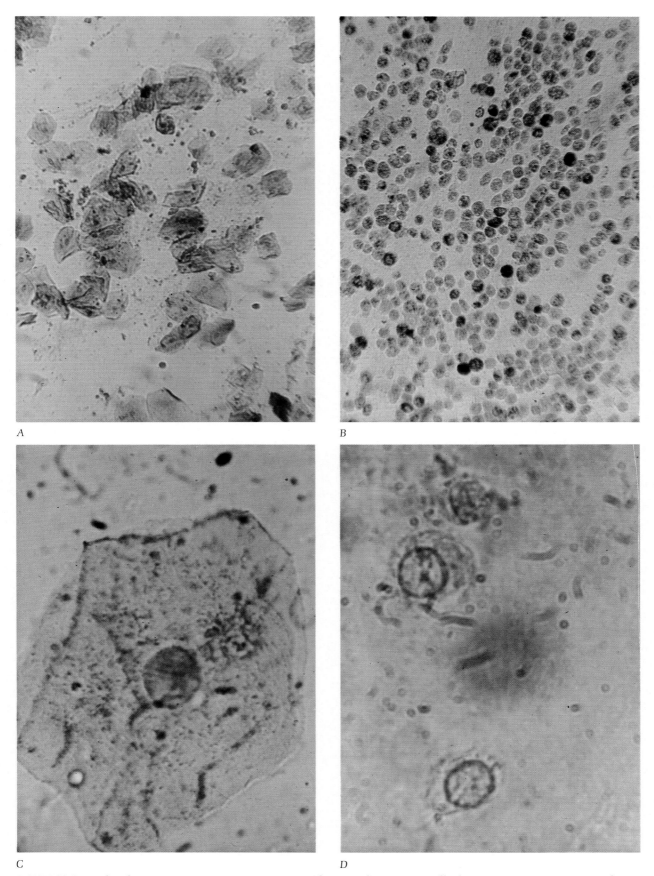

A

B

C

D

FIGURE 30-2   Unfixed, wet sputum preparations.   A. Oropharyngeal squamous cells, low power (×90).   B. Macrophages and other inflammatory cells, low power (×90).   C. Oropharyngeal squamous cell (×900).   D. Bronchial epithelial cells from basal layer (×900). *(From Chodosh S: Current Topics in the Management of Respiratory Diseases, vol. 2. New York, Churchill-Livingstone, 1985.)*

dish and viewed in a good light against a dark background. A likely portion is separated from the rest of the specimen using the pointed ends of a broken wooden applicator stick, placed intact on a microscope slide, and gently spread out.

This thick wet preparation should be scanned using the lower power ($\times 10$) objective of the microscope with the light reduced by lowering the condenser. Contaminated large oropharyngeal squamous cells are easily identified, and if predominant, the aliquot should be discarded and a different portion selected for examination (Fig. 30-2). Mucous strands in which inflammatory polymorphonuclear cells, macrophages, and bronchial epithelial cells are embedded indicate a pulmonary origin (Fig. 30-2). The presence of macrophages assures the specimen's bronchopulmonary origin. A good area can be teased away, even from surrounding contaminating material, for subsequent examinations. Experience will improve the ability to select representative aliquots. The tiny (approximately 5 mm in diameter) aliquot is transferred to a clean slide. Although staining is not essential, gentle mixing with a small amount of aqueous metachromatic stain such as crystal violet may facilitate cell identification. The wet preparation must be covered with a gently pressed-down coverslip. Good areas can now be selected by scanning the slide under low power. Cell identification requires the use of the oil immersion objective.

OBSERVATIONS ON THE CELLULAR POPULATIONS

Qualitative and Quantitative Evaluation

The relative frequency of each of the major cell types can be determined from the wet preparation for the qualitative description of the cellular population. These rough estimates usually suffice for most clinical applications. Qualitative descriptions can also be made from a Papanicolaou stained smear which may have been prepared for cancer detection. Epithelial cell types and some intracellular inclusions are more readily identified, but mast cells and noncellular elements are not easily distinguished. The staining procedure precludes the ability to examine the preparation immediately.

For quantitation, an estimate of the cell concentration should be made in areas of the slide where the preparation is only one or two cells in depth. A low concentration represents about 3 to 15 cells per oil immersion field, moderate about 25 to 50 cells per oil immersion field, and high more than 75 cells per oil immersion field. The cell concentration can be determined more precisely by counting undiluted sputum in a standard hemocytometer. With the measurements of the daily sputum volume, the estimated cell concentration, and the qualitative description of the major cell types, an approximation of the quantitative levels of each cell type excreted per day by the individual patient can be made. This is useful as a measure of the severity of the disease and can be used to observe changes over time in individual patients.

Identification of Cellular Constituents

The cells that originate from lung tissue are mainly bronchial epithelial cells. Other cells in this group which could be considered to be of pulmonary origin are plasma cells, tissue mast cells, alveolar macrophages, and tissue lymphocytes. The inflammatory cells include the neutrophil, eosinophil, monocyte, nonalveolar macrophage, and lymphocyte. Noncellular elements include crystals, Curschmann's spirals, elastic fibers, myelin, and corpora amylacea. Some fungi and parasites can also be observed in these preparations.

Contaminating oropharyngeal cells The hallmark of oropharyngeal secretions is the large, flat, irregularly shaped squamous cells that are exfoliated from the nonrespiratory epithelium of the oropharynx and upper esophagus. These cells vary in diameter from 20 to 80 m and have crinkled cell surfaces, and the ovoid nucleus is small compared with the cytoplasmic area (Fig. 30-2). Basal cells from the squamous epithelium may also be seen. These have a more even ovoid shape without the crinkly cell surface. Neutrophils and lymphocytes may also be present in oropharyngeal secretions, but their proximity to squamous cells is indicative of their nonpulmonary origin. Macrophages never occur in oropharyngeal secretions.

Bronchial epithelial cells Exfoliated bronchial epithelial cells (BEC) originate in the mucosal epithelium lining the bronchial lumen and are of four types. The nuclei of all BEC types are ovoid to round with distinct chromatin structure, whereas the cytoplasmic structures change with differentiation. The basal BEC is the stem cell originating from next to the basement membrane and is about the size of a lymphocyte (Fig. 30-2). The cytoplasm usually has a fine granular-reticular texture. BECs from the intermediate layer have more cytoplasm than basal BECs, which have a somewhat polygonal shape, and are less frequently recognized. Ciliated columnar BECs are roughly rectangular with the nonciliated end often tapering to a long tail (Fig 30-3). Goblet BECs often have a rough, triangular shape, lack cilia, and may have vacuoles that contain their mucopolysaccharide products. These normal-appearing BECs often occur in aspirated specimens or postbronchoscopy sputum. The sputum of patients with bronchial disease rarely contains normal-appearing BECs because of degenerative changes caused by the disease process. Loss of cilia and a rounding of the normally straight lumenal border are the usual changes in nonallergic bronchial disease. Progressive changes of this pyknotic degeneration lead to a shrinking of the cell and nucleus (Fig. 30-3). Metaplastic BECs have a crinkly appearance of their cell structures. Swollen BECs are characteristic of allergic and viral bronchial involvement,

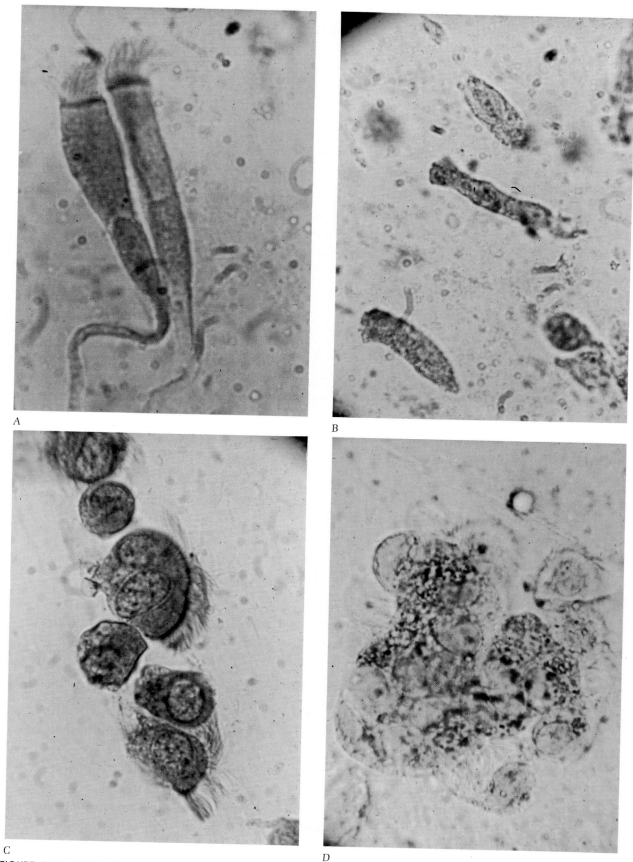

FIGURE 30-3 Unfixed, wet sputum preparations. *A.* Normal ciliated columnar bronchial epithelial cells (×900). *B.* Pyknotic degeneration of columnar bronchial epithelial cells (×900). *C.* Swollen bronchial epithelial cells (×900). *D.* Cluster of swollen bronchial epithelial cells or Creola body (×900). *(From Chodosh S: Current Topics in the Management of Respiratory Diseases, vol. 2. New York, Churchill-Livingstone, 1985.)*

with cells often retaining their cilia in this hydropic degeneration (Fig. 30-3). Such swollen cells may be exfoliated in clusters, "Creola bodies," that may be mistaken for neoplastic cells except that ciliary borders are often observed (Fig. 30-3). Ciliocytophthoria is a peculiar fragmentation of ciliated BECs leaving intact cilia.

Mast cells   Tissue mast cells are easily identified in wet preparations when they contain more than 50 percent of their large granules. Otherwise, they may be difficult to differentiate from macrophages. They are usually about 15 to 25 m in diameter but may be considerably larger. Large granules typically pack the cytoplasm so that their ovoid nucleus is usually obscured (Fig. 30-4). Mast cells may be prominent in asthma but are frequently noted in chronic bronchitis.

Plasma cells   Plasma cells also occur in sputum but are not common. They have a round, eccentric nucleus with characteristically dense chromatin which, in wet preparation, lack the spoke-wheel appearance seen in hematoxylin-stained smears. A lacelike cytoplasm is typical. Their significance in sputum is not known, but they may reflect immunologic stimulation.

Inflammatory cells   The elements of this group of cells develop in bone marrow, are carried in the circulating blood, and selectively collect in areas of inflammation. The neutrophil is the most prevalent of these cells in nonallergic, bronchopulmonary diseases, but may be prominent in allergic diseases as well (Fig. 30-4). Their numbers generally reflect the level of the inflammatory reaction in the lung. Their diameters range from 10 to 15 m. The nucleus is usually multilobed and, in wet preparations, may appear to be multinucleated, as the interlobar bridges are not easily seen. Their cytoplasmic granules appear as fine specks that may manifest Brownian movement. Conglomeration of granules (toxic granulation) and phagocytized materials may be evident in their cytoplasm. When surrounded by mucus, neutrophils are generally round or ovoid. In watery specimens, amoeboidlike shapes may be seen. The eosinophil is usually seen in significant numbers in allergic bronchopulmonary diseases (Fig. 30-4). Similar to neutrophils in size, they differ in that the nucleus is rarely more than bi-lobed, and the cytoplasm is uniformly filled with large granules. Even in unstained wet preparations, there is a distinctive pale hemoglobinlike hue to the granules.

Monocytes are commonly seen in sputum. They are easily identified by their typical horseshoe-shaped nucleus with fine reticular chromatin and indentations. The cytoplasm is characteristically clear. Monocytes vary in size from 10 to 20 m. The macrophage, or histiocyte, varies in size from 10 to 40 m. The nucleus is ellipsoid and located eccentrically in the cell, although more than one nucleus may be present (Fig. 30-4). The macrophage appears to develop commonly from the blood monocyte since transitional forms are often seen. Alveolar macrophages cannot be easily differentiated from other macrophages. The cytoplasm varies from a finely reticulated appearance to being completely filled with vacuoles and ingested materials such as dust, microorganisms, cells, and lipids. Clues to the pathologic process may be deduced from the types of phagocytized materials. The numbers of macrophages and monocytes appear to reflect the adequacy of the cellular host defenses.

Lymphocytes are seen in all chronic bronchial diseases in small numbers. Easily confused with basal BECs, they are distinguishable by their relatively clear cytoplasm in which a few scattered small granules may be seen. The nucleus is round and somewhat eccentrically placed. The specific significance of lymphocytes in sputum has not been deduced.

Noncellular elements   A number of noncellular elements, which provide useful information, can be identified in wet preparations of sputum. Charcot-Leyden crystals are extracellular structures formed from granules and cytoplasmic components of eosinophils and basophils or mast cells. They can be intrepreted as eosinophil equivalents. They characteristically appear as elongated rhomboids varying in length from 2 to 50 m (Fig. 30-5). They are difficult to find in fixed preparations. Curschmann's spirals may be seen in the sputum in any bronchial disease in which inspissation of secretions occurs. Their size is dependent on the size of the airway in which they are formed. Usually detected microscopically, they can rarely be noted macroscopically. They appear as spirally twisted mucinous material around a central thread (Fig. 30-5). Larger ones may have trapped cells and crystals; these components are dependent on the nature of the associated inflammatory process. Myelin degeneration can be seen intracellularly and extracellularly, but it is most common extracellularly. Phospholipid in composition, it usually assumes round and ovoid formations with smooth, convoluted, and often concentric contours (Fig. 30-5) and is distinctly different from the more refractile lipid droplets. Myelin forms are most easily identified in wet preparations. Their presence suggests that the disease is stable or mild. Elastic fibers originate from parenchymal tissue, and presence in sputum is indicative of a destructive process. They are wavy, double-contoured, highly refractile fibers with curled ends. When they appear in bundles, they likely arise from lung parenchyma, whereas single strands usually come from the bronchial wall.

Gram Stains and Bacteriologic Cultures

Gram staining of the sputum is essential whenever bacterial infection is suspected and the outcome should determine the need for bacteriologic cultures and antibiotic sensitivity testing. Antimicrobial therapy should be instituted promptly based on the presumptive identification of bacteria in a Gram-stained smear. Results of culture

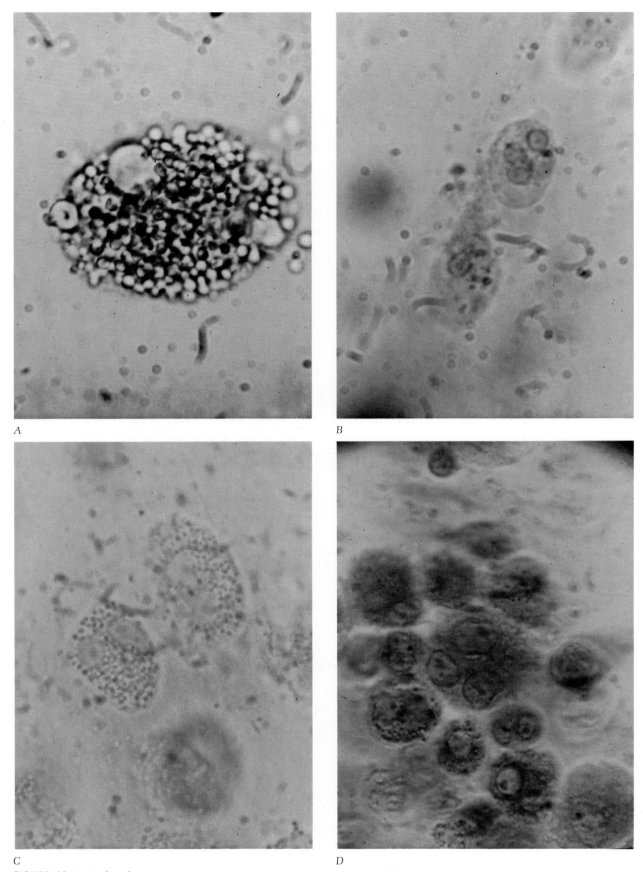

FIGURE 30-4 Unfixed, wet sputum preparations. *A.* Tissue mast cell (×900). *B.* Polymorphonuclear neutrophils (×900). *C.* Polymorphonuclear eosinophils (×900). *D.* Macrophages, some multinucleated (×360). *(From Chodosh S: Current Topics in the Management of Respiratory Diseases, vol. 2. New York, Churchill-Livingstone, 1985.)*

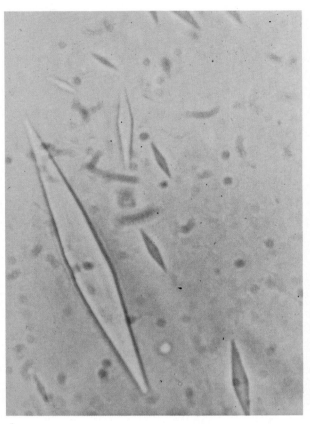

A

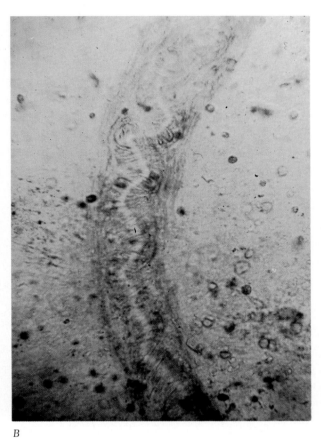

B

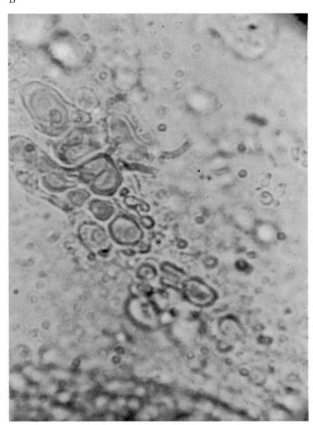

C

FIGURE 30-5 Unfixed, wet sputum preparations. *A.* Charcot-Leyden crystals (×900). *B.* Curschmann's spiral (×90). *C.* Myelin degeneration (×900). *(From Chodosh S: Current Topics in the Management of Respiratory Diseases, vol. 2. New York, Churchill-Livingstone, 1985.)*

should be interpreted with the data from the Gram stain in mind. The absence of bacteria or the predominance of oropharyngeal squamous cells renders culture unnecessary or clinically misleading. In the outpatient management of acute exacerbations of chronic bronchitis, increased numbers of the usual causative bacteria on Gram stain suffice as a basis for treatment so that cultures are not necessary. Conversely, the presence of gram-negative bacilli or staphylococci on the Gram stain, or persistent bacteria while the patient is on antibiotics, is an indication for cultures and sensitivities. When lung abscess or necrotizing pneumonitis is suspected, and Gram staining reveals large numbers of a variety of microorganisms, anaerobic cultures may be helpful in directing antibiotic therapy. Only aliquots that are confirmed microscopically as being bronchopulmonary in origin are used for smears and cultures. Gentle spreading of the specimen on the microscopic slide generally preserves the integrity of the mucous strands, thereby enabling the assessment of the morphologic types and numbers of bacteria in areas that are identifiable as originating in the lung while avoiding other areas that are contaminated with oropharyngeal secretions. Under oil immersion, there should be at least 5 to 10 inflammatory cells in the field being evaluated; areas containing multilayered cells are avoided. When more than one inflammatory process is present in the lung, i.e., lung abscess superimposed on chronic bronchitis, it may be possible to determine from which lesion the aliquot originated by assessing cytologic characteristics along with the microbiologic evaluation.

Using the wet preparation, the presence of bacterial infection can be inferred when significant (see "Infectious Processes") numbers of bacteria are associated with an increase in the neutrophilic inflammatory response; the Gram stain cannot be used since eosinophils cannot be distinguished from neutrophils. When cultures are indicated, plating the material within 10 to 15 min gives the best results, particularly for fastidious bacteria. When a longer delay is necessary, the use of holding, or transport, media may maintain the viability of the microorganisms. As a last resort, keeping the specimen at low temperatures may decrease the overgrowth of the less fastidious bacteria in the specimen.

Other methods have been suggested to improve the quality of cultured material. Using the Gram stain, the ratio of the number of oropharyngeal squamous cells to the number of neutrophils has been advocated as a basis for deciding whether a specimen should be cultured. This approach is not recommended since it allows too many bacteria-laden squamous cells to be cultured. As a strategy for decreasing the number of contaminating microorganisms originating from supralaryngeal secretions, washing of macroscopically selected plugs using sterile saline has been proposed. However, this is too cumbersome for routine use; it also lacks the selectivity of the microscopic method, which makes it possible for the clinician to supervise the selection of material to be sent to the microbiologic laboratory.

Identification of Mycobacteria

Although a number of mycobacterial species can be found in sputum, the major pathogen remains *Mycobacterium tuberculosis hominis*. It can be presumptively identified in acid-fast prepared smears of sputum, but the definitive identification requires growth on culture. In acid-fast smears the tubercle bacillus can be confused with a number of other pathogenic and some saprophytic mycobacteria as well as *Nocardia* species (Chapters 99 and 114). Reports of acid-fast smears should be available within 24 h, whereas cultures take from 3 to 12 weeks to be reported. At least three specimens should be sent as soon as possible after the suspicion of tuberculous infection is raised.

Examination of sputum for fungi, parasites, and other less common microorganisms requires expertise beyond the capability of most clinicians and many microbiology laboratories (Chapters 31, 104, and 110).

Cancer Cytology

Sputum or secretions obtained from the bronchopulmonary system frequently contain malignant cells exfoliated from cancers in the lung (Chapter 31). Examination of five separate specimens using the Papanicolaou staining of fixed sputum smears can detect 70 to 80 percent of all primary lung tumors and 50 percent of metastatic tumors. The yield is better for centrally located tumors. Laboratories vary in the methods for preparing specimens. Whatever the preparatory method, the overall yield is best if microscopically ascertained sputum is sent for examination. Specimens are usually either smears that have been fixed or whole sputum that has been dropped or expectorated into a fixative solution. The more productive times to collect specimens are in the immediate postbronchoscopy period or when the patient is raising blood-streaked sputum. If the specimen proves to be inadequate, or if it is judged to be suspicious for malignancy, then more than the customary five should be sent.

APPLICATION OF SPUTUM DATA TO CLINICAL SITUATIONS

Which of the many examinations that have been described should be applied in individual clinical situations rests with the clinician and the facilities available to do the tests. However, a number of procedures are simple and can be performed with a minimum of equipment, space, and time.

Infectious Processes

Sputum is most commonly used for the diagnosis of infectious diseases of the lung. To confirm the suspicion of a bacterial bronchopulmonary infection, two criteria should be met: the number of microorganisms should be abnormally high, and the exudate should reflect an inflammatory cell response. Increased numbers of bacteria without an increase of neutrophils suggest colonization. A nonbacterial etiology, such as viral or chemical, is suggested when an increase in the number is unaccompanied by an abnormally high number of bacteria. Bacteria seen in close proximity to, or within, neutrophils or macrophages support a bacterial etiology. Swollen bronchial epithelial cells, both single and in clusters, which may show intracytoplasmic or intranuclear inclusion vacuoles, suggest a viral etiology, particularly when associated with a neutrophilic response. A predominantly eosinophilic response, in association with swollen bronchial epithelial cells without an increase in the number of bacteria, indicates an allergic etiology. Chemical irritants are associated with increases of neutrophils or macrophages while bacteria are absent or minimal in number.

Even with objective microbiologic data in hand, the results require care in interpretation. Results noted on Gram stain do not always correlate with the culture results: either microorganisms seen on the Gram stain fail to grow or the species reported on culture are not seen on the Gram stain. These discrepancies make it difficult to attribute an etiologic role to an identified microorganism. This situation arises typically in chronic bronchitics or in hospitalized patients in whom an artificial airway has been installed. The Gram stain then provides the best means of estimating the numbers and morphologic types of bacteria, whereas the culture identifies the specific microorganism.

The number of microorganisms that is considered to be abnormal depends on the disease. A few tubercle bacilli may be sufficient for the diagnosis of tuberculosis, but a few pneumococci per oil immersion field are meaningless in the bronchitic patient. In the patient who normally produces no sputum and develops an acute bronchopulmonary infection, finding even a few neutrophils in the sputum is abnormal. In the patient with chronic bronchopulmonary inflammation, it can be inferred that the number of neutrophils is increased when the production of sputum increases and the sputum cytology shows a predominance of neutrophils. More convincing is a comparison of the pre- and postacute inflammatory number of neutrophils. In essence, interpretation of numbers of cells and microorganisms with respect to the diagnosis of pulmonary infection must be weighed individually for each specific type of infection. Failure of infection to respond to specific therapy requires a new sputum evaluation.

SPECIFIC INFECTIONS

Pneumonia

The predominant inflammatory cell in bacterial and viral pneumonias is the neutrophil. The number of BECs seen depends on the extent of bronchial involvement. Sputum volume in lobar pneumonia is scanty. The color of the sputum cannot be counted on to determine the etiology of the infection. The Gram stain usually provides the presumptive bacterial etiology. The characteristic appearance of *Streptococcus pneumoniae* is a gram-positive, encapsulated lancet-shaped diplococcus, but not infrequently it is a gram-positive, encapsulated diplococcus. In pneumococcal pneumonia, the Gram stain is generally believed to be more reliable than cultures in identifying this bacterium as the etiologic agent. *Hemophilus influenzae* is characteristically a small, gram-negative pleomorphic coccobacillary form. *Klebsiella*, *Pseudomonas*, and other large gram-negative bacilli are not easily identified morphologically as specific species and require cultures and antibiotic sensitivity testing. Staphylococci are gram-positive cocci that cluster together irregularly (grapelike).

Acute Bronchitis

The etiology is usually viral. When symptoms persist beyond 5 to 7 days, another etiology is likely. The sputum changes are identical to those seen in pneumonia. The differentiation of viral from bacterial infections can be readily made using the wet sputum preparation and the Gram stain.

Bronchiectasis

Bronchiectasis during active infection usually demonstrates distinctive sputum findings (Chapter 97). The sputum consists almost entirely of the exudate originating from deformed and dilated bronchi; it contains little mucus. The copious sputum is usually thin or pus-like with a dirty green color. The smell may or may not be foul, depending on the responsible microorganisms. Composed almost entirely of neutrophils mixed with cellular debris, the concentration of cells is often less than would be suspected from the gross appearance of the sputum. The types of bacteria vary considerably. Cultures and sensitivities are usually indicated, although most exacerbations respond to broad-spectrum antimicrobial therapy so that sputum production sometimes ceases completely. When sputum production persists, its characteristics are those seen in chronic bronchitis. A useful way to monitor these patients is by following the daily volume of sputum.

Lung Abscess and Necrotizing Pneumonia

These are usually associated with anaerobic microorganisms. Although the clinical presentation is usually distinctive, the putrid-smelling exudate is often absent. Expectorated sputum is inadequate for anaerobic culture because of oropharyngeal contamination by anaerobic microorganisms. However, the Gram stain of the sputum and cytologic evaluation is virtually diagnostic of anaerobic infection, showing large numbers of bacteria that differ in morphology in association with cytologic features that resemble those of bronchiectasis.

Cultures are rarely needed when these microscopic findings are encountered in the appropriate clinical setting. Failure of large-dose penicillin therapy, or the presence of atypical clinical features, may necessitate anaerobic cultures. Transtracheal aspiration, or the use of a telescoping plugged catheter with brush that is passed via a bronchoscope, is the proper way to collect material for anaerobic culture. Monitoring the volume of the sputum provides useful information. With proper drainage, sputum production should be commensurate with the size of the abscess; a small volume of sputum during active infection suggests that the desired drainage is not occurring. During successful therapy, cultures may continue to grow pathogens, but the Gram stain generally shows a marked reduction of bacteria.

Tuberculosis

The sputum characteristics of pulmonary tuberculosis vary, depending on the nature and extent of the pathologic process. When tuberculosis is first diagnosed, there is often an associated bacterial infection. The sputum then reflects the superimposed pathology. In noncavitary tuberculosis, sputum may not be expectorated. The cytologic characteristics of the sputum are usually similar to those of chronic bronchitis. In cavitary tuberculosis, the sputum sometimes appears caseous; under the microscope, few cells and much debris are seen. The multinucleated giant cells typical of tuberculous lesions are rarely observed in sputum. The Gram stain is usually negative; only special acid-fast stains and cultures can definitively establish the diagnosis.

Mycotic Infections

In most mycotic infections of the lung, sputum is either absent or scant. In general, the diagnosis depends on special cultures and staining procedures. Occasionally, wet preparation reveals fungal cells, particularly if an aqueous buffered stain such as crystal violet is used. *Cryptococcus, Blastomyces,* and *Candida* can be strongly suggested by their typical morphology. *Candida* and the delicate branching gram-positive *Nocardia* can be identified in the Gram stain. When fungal infection is suspected, special cultures should be requested.

Chronic Bronchial Diseases

Chronic bronchitis and bronchial asthma are the common sputum-producing chronic bronchial diseases; bronchiectasis and cystic fibrosis are less common. The gross physical properties, wet preparation, cytology, and Gram stain provide information that can be clinically useful in differential diagnosis, in determining the etiology of acute exacerbations, in objectively documenting the course of the patient's chronic bronchial disease, and in following the effects of therapy. As with all laboratory tests, interpretation must be considered in the perspective of the clinical findings.

DIFFERENTIAL DIAGNOSIS

Each specific chronic bronchial disease usually presents with distinctive diagnostic features. However, there is overlap. For example, presenting symptoms may fail to distinguish between chronic bronchitis and bronchial asthma. The difficulties are compounded in patients having both chronic bronchitis and asthma. The sputum cytologic profile can be of help in identifying the pathologic process affecting the airways.

Chronic Bronchitis

The cellular composition of the sputum reflects the nonallergic inflammation of the bronchi which characterizes the disease. The epithelial cells seen in the sputum are exfoliated as individual cells and demonstrate various degrees of pyknotic degeneration. Cilia are lost from the ciliated columnar bronchial epithelial cells (BECs) and rarely do goblet BECs contain mucopolysaccharide vacuoles. Intracytoplasmic bacteria are occasionally seen; metaplastic changes are usually present. In clinically stable patients, although the number of individual cells in the sputum may vary considerably, about 7 to 21 percent of the cells are BECs, 60 to 85 percent neutrophils, and 5 to 25 percent macrophages. Some mast cells usually are seen. Eosinophils range up to 3 percent; the persistent finding of more should suggest another disease. In chronic bronchitis, the number of BECs excreted per day reflects the level of the ongoing damage to the bronchial epithelium, the number of neutrophils reflects the level of acute inflammation, and the number of macrophages is a measure of the balance between acute and chronic inflammatory activity.

Bronchial Asthma

The cellular composition of the sputum reflects the underlying allergic inflammation. BECs are swollen and may be four times their normal size. The ciliated columnar BECs retain their cilia. In the wet preparation, because of hydropic degeneration, the morphology of the BEC may appear indistinct. Clusters of BECs (Creola bodies) may be seen and are more frequent during acute attacks of asthma. Ciliocytophthoria is common. In stable, sputum-producing asthma, BECs represent 18 to 35 percent of all cells. The number of eosinophils varies from 5 to 8 percent; lower values are typical of asthmatic patients who are either receiving steroid therapy or are at the crisis of an acute attack. Charcot-Leyden crystals are variably present; in some specimens they may be the only evidence of allergic inflammatory response. The number of macrophages is similar to that in chronic bronchitis. An increased number of macrophages suggests a more stable clinical state. The number of mast cells varies considerably from patient to patient, but these cells are consistently sparse during acute attacks of asthma. Neutrophils are often more numerous than eosinophils in the stable asthmatic. Indeed, they may represent as much as 80 percent of all cell types. As in the bronchitic patient, the numbers of BECs reflect the extent of epithelial damage.

Combined Disease

The patient who has a mixture of both stable chronic bronchitis and asthma has a cytologic picture that combines features of both diseases. However, during an exacerbation of either the bronchitis or asthma, the cytologic and Gram stain findings reflect the specific inflammatory response. Conversely, effective specific therapy that suppresses one or the other of the two diseases results in a cellular distribution that reflects the disease that has not been treated.

DETERMINING THE ETIOLOGY OF ACUTE EXACERBATIONS

Patients with chronic bronchitis, or asthma, or both, often have periods of acute or subacute worsening of their pulmonary symptoms that represent acute exacerbations. Among the pulmonary symptoms that are common to the exacerbations are cough, sputum production, dyspnea, wheezing, and pulmonary congestion. Table 30-1 lists various clinical circumstances in which sputum examination

TABLE 30-1
Sputum Cytologic and Bacteriologic Patterns of Various Exacerbations in Chronic Bronchial Diseases

Type of Exacerbation	Clinical State						
	Acute Bacterial Infection	Subclinical Bacterial Infection	Bacterial Colonization	Acute Viral Infection	Acute Secretion Problems	Acute Irritant Exposure	Acute Allergic
Bacteria on Gram stain	INCREASED	INCREASED	INCREASED	NO CHANGE	NO CHANGE	NO CHANGE	NO CHANGE
Sputum volume	INCREASED	USUALLY INCREASED	No change	Increased	USUALLY DECREASED	Increased	Usually increased
Sputum cell concentration	INCREASED	USUALLY INCREASED	No change	Increased	Usually increased or no change	Usually increased	INCREASED
Neutrophils: %	Usually increased	Increased or no change	NO CHANGE	Usually increased	Usually no change	Usually no change or increased	Usually no change or decreased
no. per day	INCREASED	INCREASED	NO CHANGE	INCREASED	Usually no change or decreased	INCREASED	Usually increased or no change
Macrophages: %	Usually decreased	Increased or no change	NO CHANGE	Usually decreased	Usually no change	Usually decreased or no change	Usually decreased
no. per day	Variable	USUALLY INCREASED	NO CHANGE	USUALLY DECREASED	Usually no change or decreased	Usually no change	Variable
Bronchial epithelial cells: %	Usually decreased	Usually decreased	NO CHANGE	Usually increased	Usually no change	USUALLY INCREASED	Usually increased
no. per day	INCREASED	INCREASED	NO CHANGE	INCREASED (swollen and in clusters)	Usually no change or decreased	INCREASED	INCREASED (swollen and in clusters)
Eosinophils or Charcot-Leyden crystals: % and no. per day	Usually decreased	Usually decreased	No change	Usually decreased	No change	Decreased	INCREASED

NOTE: Comments in capital letters are considered to be the key factors in establishing the exacerbation etiology.

is likely to be helpful. Exacerbations can be caused by viral or bacterial infection, troublesome secretions, excessive exposure to inhaled irritants, or allergy. Changes in the sputum findings are best assessed by reference to sputum obtained while the patient is clinically stable. Absolute changes in cellular populations are the critical criterion, since changes in the percentage of the less common cell types can be misleading because of the large increases of the predominant inflammatory polymorphonuclear cell.

Establishing the cause of acute exacerbations in chronic bronchial disease has immediate value in making therapeutic decisions. In addition, detecting environmental changes which induce exacerbations, e.g., increased smoking or decreased humidity, often provides long-range benefits for the patient.

COURSE OF DISEASE

These same simple sputum examinations provide objective criteria for following the course of the chronic bronchial diseases. Daily sputum volume is a rough index of the level of activity. Improvement usually results in a decrease of volume produced per day. Periodic determinations of the numbers of neutrophils, eosinophils, and macrophages excreted per day provide a good estimate of the level and nature of the inflammation; a decrease in the polymorphonuclear types should be observed if therapy is successful. The ideal goal is to eliminate sputum production. This goal can be achieved in some bronchitics and in many asthmatics.

MONITORING EFFECTS OF THERAPY

Measurements of the gross physical characteristics, wet preparation, and Gram stain provide simple means of monitoring the efficacy of various therapies. In chronic bronchitis and bronchiectasis, the response to antimicrobial therapy of an acute bacterial exacerbation can be observed in the daily sputum volume, the numbers of neutrophils, and the numbers of bacteria on Gram stain. Appropriate therapy should reduce these back to at least the levels noted before the acute infection. In both chronic bronchitis and asthma, the effects of hydration, expectorants, and mucolytic therapy can be monitored by assessing the thickness, stickiness, and color of the sputum. In asthmatics, the sputum volume and numbers of eosinophils should be effectively reduced by antiasthma therapy, e.g., corticosteroids or removal of the offending antigen. These reliable objective measurements are easily repeated whenever clinically indicated.

SECRETION PROBLEMS

Detecting difficulty in clearing secretions from the bronchial tree depends on observations of the thickness and stickiness of sputum. However, the hallmark of stasis of secretion is a change in the color of the sputum to yellow or green. Although usually suspected from the patient's complaints, severely ill, hospitalized patients, particularly those who are intubated, may not be able to communicate their problem. Changes in the sputum properties should alert the care team that a secretion problem is present.

BIBLIOGRAPHY

Baigelman W, Chodosh S, Pizzuto D: Quantitative sputum Gram stains in chronic bronchial disease. Lung 156:265–270, 1979.
A useful methodology for assessing the bacterial flora in sputum in chronic bronchitis and chronic asthma.

Barrett-Connor E: The nonvalue of sputum culture in the diagnosis of pneumococcal pneumonia. Am Rev Respir Dis 103:845–848, 1974.
A practical evaluation of the use of sputum Gram stains and cultures in pneumococcal pneumonia.

Bartlett JG: Diagnostic accuracy of transtracheal aspiration bacteriologic studies. Am Rev Respir Dis 115:777–782, 1977.
One of the classic evaluations of the bacteriologic capability of transtracheal-aspiration-obtained secretions.

Bartlett JG: Diagnosis of bacterial infections of the lung. Clin Chest Med 8:119–134, 1987.
This report reviews basic principles in collecting, processing, and staining sputum for the accurate identification of respiratory bacterial pathogens.

Chodosh S: Examination of sputum cells. N Engl J Med 282:854–857, 1970.
A simple description of the methods and value of the assessment of sputum, nonmalignant cytology.

Chodosh S: Sputum cytology in chronic bronchial disease. Advan Asthma Allergy 4:8–27, 1977.
A review of the diagnostic guidelines for the differential diagnosis of specific chronic bronchial disease and for determining the etiology of acute exacerbations in these diseases.

Chodosh S: Sputum observations in status asthmaticus and therapeutic considerations, in Weiss EB (ed), *Status Asthmaticus.* Baltimore, University Park Press, 1978, pp 173–200.
Observations of sputum cytology and physical properties during status asthmaticus and following corticosteroid therapy.

Chodosh S, Fred HL: Sputum examination in bronchopulmonary infections. The Medical Journal, St. Joseph Hospital, Houston, TX 14:5–10, 1979.
A review of the methods and value of various means of obtaining specimens of bronchial secretions.

Erozan YS: Cytopathologic diagnosis of pulmonary neoplasms in sputum and bronchoscopic specimens. Semin Diagn Pathol 3:188–195, 1986.
Cytopathologic examination of sputum is effective for the detection of early squamous cell carcinoma, but not for diagnosing early peripheral neoplasms such as adenocarcinomas. Advanced neoplasms of any type, however, can be diagnosed in sputum.

Faling LJ, Medici TC, Chodosh S: Sputum cell population measurements in bronchial injury. Observations in acute smoke inhalation. Chest 65:56S–59S, 1974.
A description of the sputum cellular dynamics of acute bronchitis following smoke inhalation injury.

Frost JK, Ball WC Jr, Levin ML, Tockman MS, Erozan YS, Gupta PK, Eggleston JC, Pressman NJ, Donithan MP, Kimball AW Jr: Sputum cytopathology: use and potential in monitoring the workplace environment by screening for biological effects of exposure. J Occup Med 28:692–703, 1986.
Sputum cytopathologic monitoring detects squamous cell lung cancers at an extremely early stage (x-ray negative). It holds further potential for detecting epithelial alterations that reflect environmental hazards and for reducing mortality from squamous cell carcinoma.

Goldman AL, Light L: Anterior cervical infections: Complications of transtracheal aspirations. Am Rev Respir Dis 111:707–708, 1975.
An example of the many types of complications of transtracheal aspiration.

Joyce SM: Sputum analysis and culture. Ann Emerg Med 15:325–328, 1986.
When properly performed and interpreted, sputum analysis and culture are valuable tools in the diagnosis and treatment of lower respiratory tract infection.

Lee SH, Barnes WG, Schaetzel WP: Pulmonary aspergillosis and the importance of oxalate crystal recognition in cytology specimens. Arch Pathol Lab Med 110:1176–1179, 1986.
The presence of calcium oxalate crystals in pulmonary biopsy and cytology specimens can be regarded as an important diagnostic aid in the diagnosis of pulmonary aspergillosis due to A. niger.

Medici TC, Chodosh S: Sputum cell dynamics in bacterial exacerbations of chronic bronchial disease. Arch Intern Med 129:597–603, 1972.
A description of the sputum cellular dynamics of acute bronchitis associated with bacterial infection in chronic bronchitis.

Medici TC, Chodosh S: Non-malignant sputum cytology. in Dulfano MJ (ed), *Sputum.* Springfield, IL, Charles C. Thomas, 1973, pp 332–381.
A comprehensive review of the inflammatory response of the bronchial system in diseases affecting the bronchi.

Pereira W, Kovnat DM, Snider GL: A prospective cooperative study of complications following flexible fiberoptic bronchoscopy. Chest 73:813–816, 1978.
A prospective assessment and review of the complications following flexible fiberoptic bronchoscopy.

Pitchenik AE, Ganjei P, Torres A, Evans DA, Rubin E, Baier H: Sputum examination for the diagnosis of Pneumocystis carinii pneumonia in the acquired immunodeficiency syndrome. Am Rev Respir Dis 133:226–229, 1986.
Pneumocystis carinii pneumonia was diagnosed by sputum examination and/or by a bronchoscopic procedure in 20 patients; of these, sputum samples were positive for Pneumocystis organisms in 11 (55%). Sputum examination for P. carinii organisms, employed as a first diagnostic step in patients with AIDS with pulmonary infiltrates, often obviates the need for bronchoscopy.

Chapter *31*

Pulmonary Cytology

Muhammad B. Zaman / Myron R. Melamed

Sputum Cytology
  Specimen Collection
  Criteria for Adequate Sputum
  Inflammatory Process
  Neoplastic Disease
  Early Detection of Carcinoma of the Lung

Bronchial Cytology
  Brushing and Washing
  Bronchoalveolar Lavage

Pleural Effusion

Percutaneous Fine-Needle Aspiration Cytology

Cytologic examinations of pulmonary specimens are often successful in diagnosing primary and metastatic neoplasms of the lungs. They are often equally effective in diagnosing the nature of acute infiltrative lesions of the lungs due to viral, fungal, and parasitic infections. However, with few exceptions, the etiologic diagnosis of chronic diffuse infiltrative lung diseases requires histologic examination after lung biopsy. Cytologic techniques are now widely used for the diagnosis of pulmonary lesions. Each technique has its own indications and its own limitations; frequently they complement one another. Thus, carcinoma presenting as a peripheral coin lesion of the lung will not usually yield a diagnosis by sputum or bronchial cytology, whereas percutaneous needle aspiration will almost always provide the diagnosis of neoplasm; conversely, carcinoma of a lobar or segmental bronchus is more readily diagnosed by sputum or bronchial cytology than by percutaneous needle aspiration.

SPUTUM CYTOLOGY

Specimen Collection

Because of the increasing incidence of pulmonary carcinoma and the interest in early detection, sputum cytologic examination is indicated in the adult patient who is suspected of having a pulmonary carcinoma or manifests a persistent, unexplained abnormality of the lungs. Moreover, it should be repeated as often as practical until the problem is resolved. The best type of specimen is produced by a deep spontaneous cough. Since there is often a delay before the specimen is brought to the laboratory, the cough specimens are collected directly in 50% ethyl alcohol with 2% Carbowax; in this fixative, cellular material remains well preserved for days to weeks.

If it is not possible to obtain a good sputum specimen at the time of initial examination, the patient is provided with a wide-mouthed, screw-cap jar containing fixative and is instructed to collect sputum at home. Sometimes a good cough specimen can be obtained on arising in the morning or after the first cigarette of the day. It is essential to point out that saliva from the mouth and mucus "hawked up" from the throat are of no diagnostic value; written instructions that accompany the sputum jar help to emphasize this point. For the occasional patient with a dry, hacking cough that is nonproductive, mucorrheic agents such as iodides are sometimes helpful.

Various techniques are used in different clinics to induce a productive cough in the patient who has no cough at all. These include using irritating inhalants (e.g., SO_2) and aerosols of water or saline salt solutions, which some clinics prefer to be heated. In our clinic, slightly irritating mucorrheic vapor is produced by nebulizing a solution containing 15% saline and 20% propylene glycol heated to 115°F. The patient breathes this vapor for 1 min through a mouthpiece while the nose is pinched shut, then takes a deep breath, and repeats the procedure once or twice more. If a productive cough is not evoked in 3 to 5 min, the patient is instructed to rest for 1 min and then to attempt a deep cough again; if still unsuccessful, the inhalation procedure is repeated. Most patients, particularly those who smoke cigarettes, are able to produce a good sputum specimen. Those who are unsuccessful after two or three tries are given a sputum bottle to take with them in anticipation that a productive cough will occur later in the day. Side effects of the nebulization procedure are few, predominantly dizziness from the hyperventilation or nausea from the hypertonic salt solution. In an asthmatic individual, the procedure occasionally induces bronchospasm. For patients with asthma, severe bronchitis, or dietary salt restriction, heated water vapor is apt to be better tolerated than the nebulized saline solution.

The sample obtained in a single cough specimen is not likely to represent the complete bronchial tree. For example, cancer cells are found in the initial sputum specimen of only about one-half of patients with lung carcinoma, whereas three or more good specimens will yield cancer cells in over 80 percent of patients. As a compromise between the need for multiple specimens and the cost of multiple examinations, several cough specimens are collected in a single container over 3 to 5 days, then blended and processed as a single specimen. This approach affords better opportunity for sampling multiple divisions of the bronchial tree. If a lesion can be localized on the chest radiograph, it is often helpful to position the patient so that the affected bronchus drains downward and to promote the dislodging of mucous plugs by thumping the chest and urging deep respiration and cough. The total number of specimens that is needed for adequate sampling varies from patient to patient. A single positive specimen suffices to clinch the diagnosis of a malignant tumor; a single negative finding is of limited value, though repeated negative specimens assume increasing diagnostic importance.

Criteria for Adequate Sputum

Under normal conditions, the epithelium that lines the tracheobronchial tree is tightly coherent and does not exfoliate easily into the sputum. Thus, the best indication of a deep cough is the presence of alveolar phagocytes. Less often, metaplastic bronchial cells (Fig. 31-1A), indicating chronic irritation of the respiratory tract, or a mucous cast of a bronchiole known as Curschmann's spiral (Fig. 31-1B), are present and also indicate that a deep cough specimen has been provided. In contrast, saliva is characterized by the presence of superficial squamous cells from the mouth, often with particles of food and cellular and acellular debris. Some saliva inevitably accompanies and is mixed with the sputum; a good technician is able to identify and separate sputum from saliva before processing (see Chapter 30).

Inflammatory Process

Acute pyogenic reactions that accompany pneumonia, lung abscess, and acute bronchitis are characterized by an abundance of polymorphonuclear leukocytes that tend to form small clusters and to undergo degeneration. Broken nuclei are streaked out into hematoxylin-staining, fibrin-like strands. Bacteria are common in most sputum specimens but are without diagnostic value unless a particular organism is predominant and abundant.

Chronic bronchitis and bronchiectasis are characterized by epithelial necrosis, regeneration, and atypia, as well as an inflammatory cellular reaction consisting of lymphocytes, monocytes, plasma cells, and polymorphonuclear leukocytes. Some bronchial cells show striking nuclear enlargement, hyperchromasia, and nucleolar prominence as a result of inflammatory or irritant processes. As a rule of thumb, these changes are regarded as benign as long as the cells retain cilia or a terminal bar (Fig. 31-1C). Chronic bronchitis also elicits an increase in the number of mucus-secreting goblet cells within the respiratory epithelium and hyperplasia of basal or reserve cells; squamous metaplasia of the bronchial epithelium is common and is sometimes extensive (Fig. 31-1A).

The sputum in chronic bronchitis is characterized by an increase in mucus, condensed mucous "casts" of small bronchioles (Curschmann's spirals) (Fig. 31-1B), fragments of normal or regenerating and hyperplastic epithelium that have been dislodged by forceful coughing (Creola bodies) (Fig. 31-1C), and groups of hyperplastic reserve cells that are either undifferentiated or are undergoing squamous metaplasia (Fig. 31-1A). Eosinophilic leukocytes and Charcot-Leyden crystals suggest asthmatic bronchitis. These components of sputum are considered elsewhere in this book (Chapter 30).

Some inflammatory processes have cytologic features that are of specific diagnostic value. For example, the viral cytopathic effects of herpes simplex are quite characteristic: homogenization of nuclear chromatin, margination and beading of nuclei, multinucleation and nuclear molding, and sometimes well-formed nuclear inclusions. Cytomegalic inclusion disease is identifiable by the large size of affected cells containing a single large nucleus and an intranuclear inclusion; sometimes several small cytoplasmic inclusions are also present (Fig. 31-1D). Although cytopathic effects of other viruses are less distinctive, they are nonetheless helpful diagnostically. For example, the degenerative change in bronchial epithelium that Papanicolaou termed *ciliocytophthoria* is probably not specific but has been associated with influenzal viral pneumonia; the tufted end of the ciliated bronchial cell is pinched away from the rest of the cell, and one or more small eosinophilic inclusions are found in the cytoplasm of either fragment.

Fungi in the sputum do not always signify clinical disease. Actinomycotic granules, for example, are a common inhabitant of tonsillar crypts and are frequently dislodged by coughing. *Monilia*, present in the mouth of many individuals with poor oral hygiene, is also a frequent finding in sputum specimens. *Aspergillus* and mucormycosis are more unusual and generally indicate pulmonary disease. But, in a survey for detection of lung cancer, these fungi have been found occasionally in sputum from subjects who are apparently healthy (Fig. 31-1E). Other fungus infections of the lung that have been diagnosed by cytologic examinations of sputum include blastomycosis, cryptococcosis, and coccidioidomycosis.

Pneumocystis carinii is rarely identifiable in the sputum of patients with *P. carinii* pneumonia. It is better diagnosed in bronchoalveolar lavage using Gram-Weigert stain (Fig. 31-1F). The advantage of the technique is described in greater detail later in this chapter. On rare occasions, *Strongyloides* has been identified in fixed sputum, but this is better demonstrated in fresh, unstained preparations of sputum (Fig. 31-2A).

Granulomatous reactions usually imprint no distinctive cytologic features on the sputum. One exception is the lipid pneumonia that occurs in reaction to aspirated oil. The sputum contains distinctive single, or multinucleated histiocytes with cytoplasmic bubbles of fat that are diagnostic; they can be recognized even after the fat has been dissolved in the alcohol fixatives. To confirm

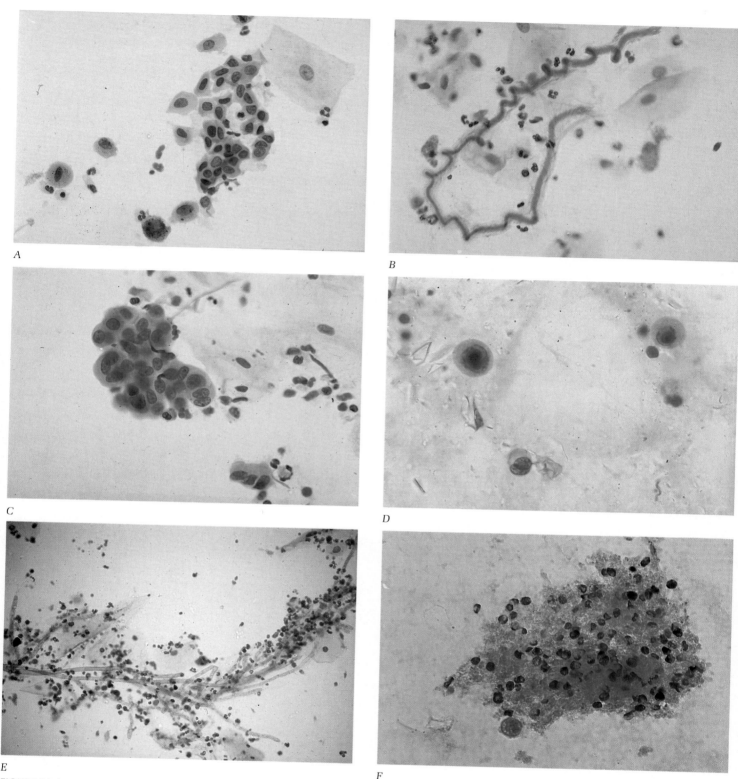

FIGURE 31-1 *A.* Metaplastic bronchial cells (squamous metaplasia) in sputum. Note flat uniform cells in mosaic pattern and the amphophilic pink and blue cytoplasm. Several alveolar phagocytes or dust cells in lower left corner indicate that a good, deep cough specimen has been produced. (This and all subsequent photomicrographs are taken at ×570 magnification and except when indicated to the contrary, they were stained by the Papanicolaou technique.) *B.* Curschmann's spiral, a mucous cast of bronchiole. A central condensed core is typical. Squamous cells in the background are oral contamination. *C.* Marked bronchial atypia, simulating bronchial adenocarcinoma. Compare with Fig. 31-3*A*. Also note three bronchial cells below with intact cilia. *D.* Large intranuclear inclusions of cytomegalovirus in infected alveolar phagocytes. *E.* Branching septate hyphae of aspergillus in the sputum of an apparently healthy smoker. Similar finding in an immunosuppressed patient with pulmonary infiltrates would be indicative of disease. (×140.) *F. Pneumocystis carinii* in bronchoalveolar lavage. The minute cysts contain a clear area giving them a crescent- or disk-shape. The amorphous pink granular background in the Gram-Weigert stain is commonly seen and represents alveolar cast washed out by lavage.

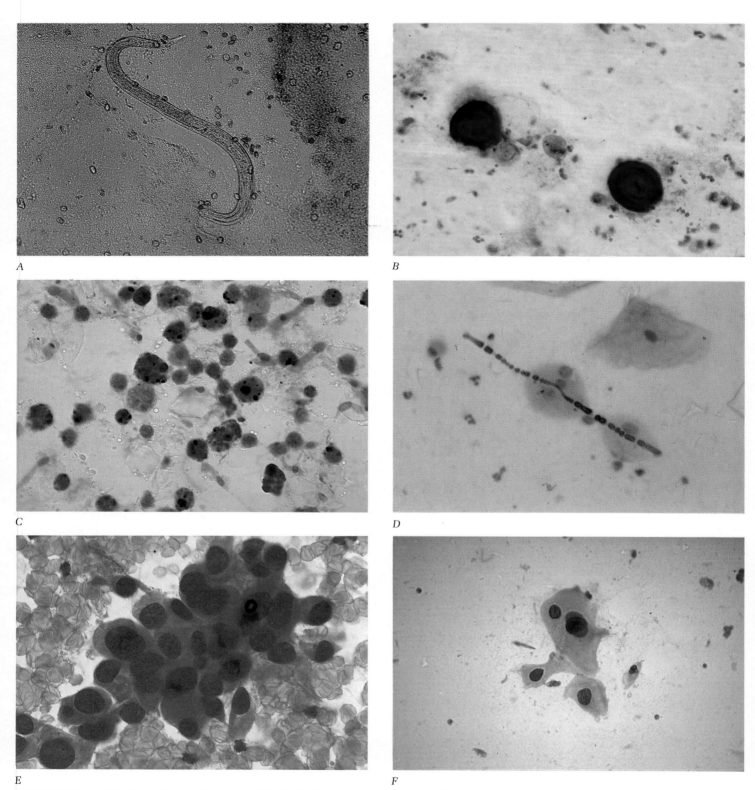

FIGURE 31-2 *A.* Filariform larvae of strongyloides in fresh sputum stained by a drop of iodine. *B.* Calcific concretions, appearing as dark lamillated round structures in the sputum of a man with alveolar microlithiasis. *C.* Ferrocyanide stain showing many hemosiderin-laden macrophages in bronchoalveolar lavage fluid. *D.* Asbestos body. The thin, central asbestos fiber is sheathed by a bright gold protein-iron coat. Note two alveolar macrophages attempting to engulf the foreign body. *E.* A 2-cm peripheral epidermoid carcinoma in asymptomatic smoker detected by a screening chest radiograph and confirmed by needle aspiration. The patient is now 10 years postlobectomy and doing well. (H & E stain.) *F.* Squamous carcinoma cells in sputum. Note cellular enlargement and pleomorphism. Compare with Fig. 31-1A.

the diagnosis, fat stains can be carried out on a fresh, unfixed specimen. Multinucleated histiocytes (or multinucleated epithelial cells) per se are of no diagnostic significance. Occasional calcific concretions may be seen in sputum of patients with chronic pulmonary diseases. When present in abundance, the possibility of alveolar microlithiasis (Fig. 31-2B) should be explored.

Fresh blood in a sputum specimen sometimes follows a paroxysm of coughing or bleeding from the gums or elsewhere in the upper respiratory tract. More meaningful is the presence of hemosiderin in histiocytes, so-called heart failure cells. These indicate intrapulmonary hemorrhage and are seen in chronic congestive heart failure and in pulmonary infarction. Diffuse hemorrhage can occur in immunosuppressed patients with low platelet count. Sputum and bronchoalveolar lavage then may show numerous hemosiderin-laden macrophages (Fig. 31-2C). Occasionally, hemosiderin is phagocytized by bronchial epithelial cells. But, more often, the bronchial cells in older patients contain a yellow-brown cytoplasmic lipochrome that resembles hemosiderin.

Foreign particles are also found in the sputum. Most are contaminants and can be discounted; pollen is introduced in the respired air; other contaminants are introduced from air or tap water in the course of processing the preparation. Food particles coming from the mouth are also very common and also can be ignored. The most important foreign particulate that is apt to be encountered in sputum is the ferruginous or asbestos body (Fig. 31-2D). Although the asbestos body does indicate exposure to asbestos, usually neither its presence nor its number in a single cough specimen is helpful in estimating either the degree of exposure or the existence of clinical disease.

Neoplastic Disease

Sputum cytology is the only noninvasive technique that is currently available to confirm the diagnosis of lung cancer. About 80 percent or more of primary carcinomas and 50 percent of metastatic cancers in the lungs can be diagnosed by a series of three or more good sputum specimens. In addition, the histologic classification of most carcinomas can be determined with considerable reliability from exfoliated epithelium.

Nearly all carcinomas of lung can be classified according to four histologic and cytologic patterns: (1) *epidermoid or squamous carcinoma*, (2) *bronchiolar or adenocarcinoma*, (3) *small cell or oat cell carcinoma*, and (4) *undifferentiated large cell carcinoma*. Most *epidermoid* carcinomas, which now account for about 31 percent of pulmonary primary neoplasms, arise from segmental bronchi and extend to the proximal lobar and distal subsegmental branches. These carcinomas shed flattened, platelike cancer cells that are usually large and pleomorphic (20 to 50 μm) with abundant eosinophilic cytoplasm

and angular, hyperchromatic, coarsely textured nuclei (Fig. 31-2E). Sometimes they form concentric whorled "pearls." The well-differentiated keratinizing epidermoid carcinomas are subclassified as *squamous*; they yield cells that contain densely staining, eosinophilic or orangophilic cytoplasm and pyknotic, hyperchromatic nuclei (Fig. 31-2F). Keratinizing squamous carcinomas of lung tend to grow to considerable size locally before metastasizing to regional lymph nodes and beyond. Sputum cytology affords the prospect of early recognition and enhances the prospects for operability.

Adenocarcinoma and bronchiolar carcinomas of lung constitute the largest group, about 48 percent. Exfoliated cells from these cancers are round rather than flat, and tend to form small groups or clusters. Individually, the cells are medium-sized (15 to 30 μm); often they contain large, smoothly contoured nuclei with finely structured chromatin and a prominent nucleolus (Fig. 31-3A). Less often, the nuclear chromatin is coarsely textured and hyperchromatic, as in epidermoid carcinoma. The cytoplasm is moderate in amount, amphophilic, less abundant, and less deeply stained than that in epidermoid carcinoma. On occasion, cytoplasmic mucin gives some of the cells a signet-ring appearance. These carcinomas tend to arise from small peripheral bronchi or bronchioles, but about 15 percent are central in location and seem to arise from major bronchi. Those neoplasms that grow distinctively and resemble adenocarcinomas of other organs are generally subclassified as adenocarcinoma; those that grow diffusely within the alveolar framework of pulmonary parenchyma and resemble mucus- or non-mucus-secreting bronchial epithelium are classified as bronchiolar. However, only occasionally is it possible to distinguish between these two types of carcinomas on the basis of exfoliative cytology.

Oat cell (small cell) carcinomas constitute about 14 percent of pulmonary primary carcinomas. They are made up of small cells (10 to 12 μm) that have given the neoplasm its name because of their ovoid nuclei and very scanty cytoplasm. Nuclear staining varies from moderate to densely hyperchromatic; nucleoli are sometimes visible within the nuclei that stain less intensely. On casual examination, oat cell carcinoma in the sputum can be mistaken for groups of lymphocytes or for hyperplastic reserve cells. However, the tumor cells are slightly larger and, in contrast with the noncoherent lymphocytes and tightly clustered reserve cells, they tend to form loosely coherent clusters. In sputum and bronchial specimens, a characteristic molding artifact of nuclei can be seen (Fig. 31-3B). Cytologic diagnosis of this tumor type is critical because the tumor is almost always inoperable, whereas irradiation and chemotherapy are often helpful in palliation.

About 6 percent of pulmonary primary carcinomas are made up of large cells reminiscent of the epidermoid,

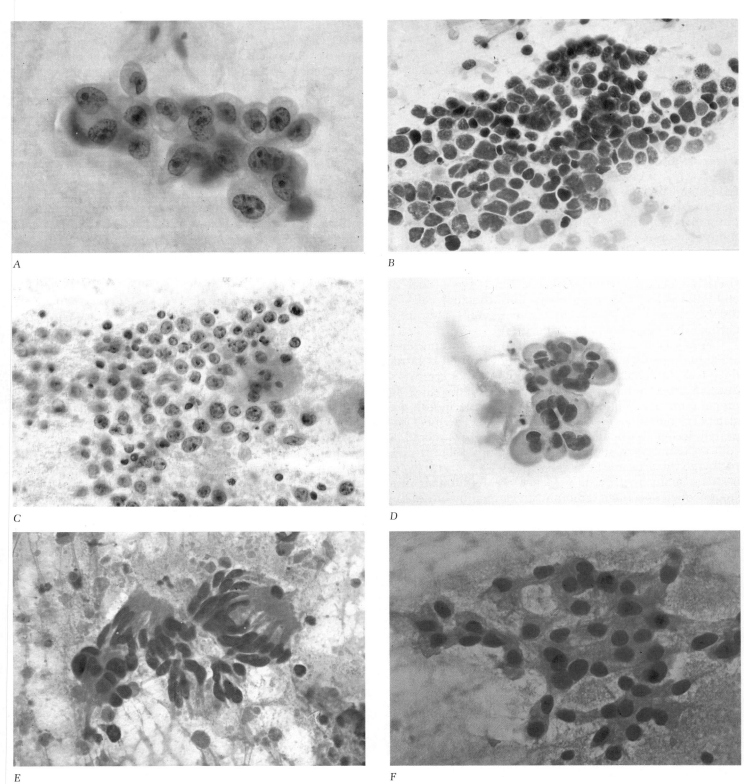

FIGURE 31-3 *A.* Adenocarcinoma in bronchial wash. Three-dimensional cluster and mucinlike vacuole in cytoplasm are characteristic. *B.* Oat cell carcinoma in bronchial brushing. Molding artifact is pronounced in air dried cells. Compare cell size with a bronchial cell nucleus. *C.* Histiocytic lymphoma in sputum. Isolated cells with nuclear lobulation and prominent nucleoli differentiate it from oat cell carcinoma. *D.* Epithelial mesothelioma in pleural effusion. *E.* Percutaneous aspiration of colonic adenocarcinoma metastatic to the lung. Tall columnar cells with straight border in a necrotic background is characteristic. (H & E stain.) *F.* Metastatic adenocarcinoma from the contralateral side was diagnosed by needle aspiration in this patient treated 2 months before by lobectomy. Note microacini formation. (H & E stain.)

bronchiolar, or adenocarcinomas but otherwise too poorly differentiated to be classified. These are separately categorized as *large cell undifferentiated carcinomas*. The exfoliated cancer cells that appear in the sputum come from parts of the tumor that communicate with bronchi. In these areas, differentiation is often more pronounced than elsewhere in the tumor. Therefore, sputum cytology sometimes erroneously categorizes a tumor of this kind as *epidermoid or adenocarcinoma* instead of *large cell undifferentiated* carcinoma.

A small number of carcinomas of other types—bronchial carcinoids, adenoid cystic carcinomas, sarcomas, and mixed tumors—either arise or are first detected in the lungs. Most of these do not exfoliate well in sputum. But, on occasion, a lymphoma, a sarcoma, and a melanoma have been sufficiently distinctive to be diagnosed by sputum cytology (Fig. 31-3C).

Early Detection of Carcinoma of the Lung

Three cooperative studies sponsored by the National Cancer Institute were undertaken in the past decade to test the efficacy of periodic sputum cytology in detecting early lung cancer in high-risk groups. The results suggest that epidermoid or squamous carcinomas arising in lobar or segmental bronchi can be recognized by exfoliative cytology while still in situ or while superficially invasive and before radiologic abnormalities appear. In contrast, only a handful of carcinomas of other cell types were detected by cytology, and these were in advanced stages. Ironically, in the control population, epidermoid carcinomas detected later by annual chest radiographic examinations, albeit more advanced, were still localized and still could be treated as effectively by surgery. Thus sputum cytology did not offer any advantage over the annual chest radiograph alone in the compliant individual. But, for the individual who is not apt to submit to annual chest radiographic examinations, it has been shown that a single cytologic examination of sputum for screening in conjunction with a chest radiograph will uncover more primary carcinomas of the lungs than will the chest radiograph per se.

BRONCHIAL CYTOLOGY

Brushing and Washing

Cytologic specimens are generally collected as a routine part of the bronchoscopic examination. In some clinics, this part of the procedure has been systematized to include mucus aspirated from each bronchus as well as washings of saline irrigation. Material obtained at bronchoscopy is useful not only in confirming a diagnosis of carcinoma that is based on examination of sputum, but even more valuable in localizing the source of the cancer

cells. If the bronchus draining a carcinoma is occluded by mucus or completely blocked by tumor, exfoliated cancer cells may not be carried out in a cough specimen of sputum. In that case, the first cytologic diagnosis of cancer is sometimes made on material obtained by aspiration or irrigation at the time of bronchoscopy.

One of the most important advances in bronchoscopy has been the development of flexible fiberoptic bronchoscopes that are capable of entering segmental and subsegmental bronchial branches. Using the rigid bronchoscope, only 20 to 30 percent of lung carcinomas can be reached for biopsy; an additional 10 percent can be diagnosed by bronchial aspiration and irrigation cytology. On the other hand, using the flexible fiber bronchoscope, only the most peripheral bronchiolar carcinomas remain out of reach; biopsy or cytologic diagnoses can be made on more than 80 percent of lung carcinomas. Moreover, if necessary each lobar and segmental bronchus can be systematically brushed for cytologic samples in order to localize a pulmonary carcinoma that has been disclosed by sputum cytology but remains invisible on chest radiography. This technique has proved successful in identifying some carcinomas either in situ or very superficially invading the bronchus (so-called stage O carcinoma of lung).

Bronchoalveolar Lavage

This technique has proved to be exceedingly effective in the diagnosis of diffuse pulmonary infiltrates in immunosuppressed patients. More than 80 percent of infections caused by *P. carinii*, fungi, and viruses can be diagnosed in this way (Figs. 31-1D and 31-1F). The yield is somewhat lower in patients with infiltrates due to neoplasms or drug toxicity. As previously noted, intrapulmonary hemorrhage is easily diagnosed by the presence of hemosiderin-laden macrophages (Fig. 31-2C). The lavage technique is more sensitive than transbronchial biopsy, bronchial washing, or brushing for evaluation of acute diffuse pulmonary infiltrates, and has virtually replaced open lung biopsy for the diagnosis of infectious disease. Complications from using this technique are rare.

More recently, bronchoalveolar lavage has been employed in the diagnosis of pulmonary lesions of patients with AIDS. Although it has been very useful in identifying infectious agents, it has proved to be of little use in detecting pulmonary involvement by Kaposi's sarcoma.

PLEURAL EFFUSION

Neoplastic pleural effusions are due to metastatic tumor, to carcinoma of the lung, or to mesothelioma. In most cases the effusion is a late manifestation of a clinically obvious carcinoma. However, in peripheral bronchiolar carcinomas of the lung, a pleural effusion is sometimes the first sign of disease. Thus, the detection of cancer cells in pleural fluid from a patient without evidence of neoplasm elsewhere raises the strong prospect of an underlying bronchiolar carcinoma.

The first evidence of diffuse epithelial mesothelioma (see Chapter 135) is almost invariably a pleural effusion. The cytologic diagnosis depends on a careful interpretation of the usually abundant and atypical mesothelial cells in the fluid (Fig. 31-3D). An important caveat in the interpretation of these specimens is the fact that long-standing effusions, whatever the cause, are likely to have similarly abundant and often atypical reactive mesothelial cells. Features of particular diagnostic value are: the presence of mucicarminophilic droplets within cytoplasm of suspected cancer cells, an indication of metastatic mucin-secreting adenocarcinoma; tumor "cell balls," strongly suggesting papillary epithelial mesothelioma; hyaluronidase-sensitive mucopolysaccharides, which suggest mesothelioma; and CEA immunoperoxidase positive reaction, which strongly suggests carcinoma. Immunohistologic reactions for cytokeratin have not proved to be of value since they simply reflect stages in the differentiation of a mesothelioma.

PERCUTANEOUS FINE-NEEDLE ASPIRATION CYTOLOGY

This technique is particularly useful for a suspected carcinoma that arises in the periphery of the lung and is not well represented in sputum or bronchial secretions. It was made possible by technical advances in biplane fluoroscopy and image amplification which make it feasible to locate and aspirate intrathoracic lesions that are as small as 2 cm in diameter. Aspirations can be done under computed tomographic control, if necessary, although this technique is more time-consuming and impractical in very obese patients. The cytologic diagnosis of carcinoma using percutaneous fine-needle aspirates is highly reliable when positive; a negative aspirate can be due to poor sampling. In a study of 1558 aspirations performed over an 8-year period on patients with intrathoracic lesions radiographically suggestive of malignant tumors, 1007 (65 percent) contained malignant cells. Follow-up on 979 of the 1007 patients yielded only two (0.2 percent) false-positive diagnoses. Complications of the percutaneous fine-needle aspiration are few, the most common being pneumothorax and hemoptysis.

Percutaneous fine-needle aspiration biopsy has proved most helpful in confirming the diagnosis of carcinoma in the lungs of patients with intrathoracic recurrences or metastases (Fig. 31-3E), in patients with presumed lung carcinoma who have negative sputum and bronchial cytology and are candidates for treatment by chemotherapy and irradiation (Fig. 31-3F), and in the occasional patient who is reluctant to undergo thoracotomy for the diagnosis of a solitary, peripheral lung lesion (Fig. 31-2E). A number of benign diseases have been correctly diagnosed by needle aspirates, including tuberculosis, fungus infections, *P. carinii* pneumonia, and hamartomas. Hamartomas are better diagnosed by microscopy, that is by using a larger-bore needle (#18) and processing the aspirate plug by histologic section rather than by smearing on slides. Similarly, large-bore-needle biopsies can be used for the diagnosis of granulomas and other benign lesions of the lung. Needle microbiopsies of this kind afford the prospect of sparing some patients from thoracotomy for peripheral coin lesions that are not carcinomas. Unfortunately, the larger needles required for microbiopsies also are apt to cause more complications.

BIBLIOGRAPHY

Broaddus C, Dake MD, Stulbarg MS, Blumenfeld W, Hadley WK, Golden JA, Hopewell PC: Bronchoalveolar lavage and transbronchial biopsy for the diagnosis of pulmonary infections in the acquired immunodeficiency syndrome. Ann Intern Med 102:747–752, 1985.

By combining these two techniques, the yield for all pathogens was 98 percent and the sensitivity for Pneumocystis carinii infections was 100 percent.

Burke MD, Melamed MR: Exfoliate cytology of metastatic cancer in lung. Acta Cytol 12:61–74, 1968.

Up to 50 percent of malignant tumors metastatic to the lung yield exfoliated cancer cells in sputum or in bronchial aspirate specimens. In most cases a classification by cell type is possible, and occasionally the cytology is unique.

Gal AA, Koss MN, Hawkins J, Evans S, Einstein H: The pathology of pulmonary cryptococcal infections in the acquired immunodeficiency syndrome. Arch Pathol Lab Med 110:502–507, 1986.

Specimens from premortem pulmonary cytology, transbronchial biopsy, and autopsy were studied in patients with acquired immunodeficiency syndrome who developed pulmonary cryptococcal disease. Overall, bronchoscopy yielded a diagnosis in seven of eight patients.

Johnston WW, Frable WJ: The cytopathology of the respiratory tract: a review. Am J Pathol 84:372–414, 1976.
A comprehensive review of pulmonary neoplastic and nonneoplastic conditions diagnosed by cytology.

Khouri NF, Stitik FP, Erozan YS, Gupta PK, Kim WS, Scott Jr WW, Hamper WM, Mann RB, Eggleston JC, Baker RR: Transthoracic needle aspiration biopsy of benign and malignant lung lesions. Am J Radiol 144:281–288, 1985.
Combined cytologic and histologic processing of specimens yields diagnosis in 88 percent of patients with benign lung lesions.

Koss LG: *Diagnostic Cytology and Its Histopathologic Basis*, 3d ed. Philadelphia, Lippincott, 1979.
The standard text.

Koss LG, Melamed MR, Goodner JT: Pulmonary cytology: A brief survey of diagnostic results from July 1, 1952, until December 31, 1960. Acta Cytol 8:104–113, 1964.
A review of the effectiveness of sputum and bronchial aspirate cytology for the diagnosis of pulmonary carcinoma before the advent of fiberoptic bronchoscopy.

Melamed MR, Flehinger BJ, Zaman MB, Heelan RT, Perchick WA, Martini N: Screening for early lung cancer. Results of the Memorial Sloan-Kettering Study in New York. Chest 86:44–53, 1984.
Early diagnosis of epidermoid carcinoma is possible by periodic sputum cytology. Confirming earlier reports of changing histology in lung cancer, 138 of 288 cancers in this study of male smokers were adenocarcinomas.

Melamed MR, Zaman MB: Pathogenesis of epidermoid carcinoma of lung, in Shimosato Y, Melamed M, Nettischaim P (eds), *Morphogenesis of Lung Cancer* vol 1, Florida, CRC Press, 1982.
Epidermoid carcinomas, like other lung cancers, arise primarily in the upper lobe. Approximately two-thirds are central in origin and can be detected in the asymptomatic stage by sputum cytology.

Melamed MR, Zaman MB, Martini N, Flehinger BJ: Radiologically occult in situ and incipient invasive epidermoid lung cancer. Am J Surg Pathol 1:5–16, 1977.
Detailed histopathologic study of seven early epidermoid carcinomas detected by sputum cytology.

Nagasaki F, Martini N: Flexible fiberoptic bronchoscopy without fluoroscopy in the diagnosis of lung carcinoma. Transactions of the American Broncho-Esophagological Association, 159–162, 1983.
Cytologic material from 109 consecutive patients with carcinoma of the lung gave 81 percent positive diagnosis.

Naib ZM, Stewart JA, Dowdle WR, Casey HL, Marine WM, Nahmias AJ: Cytologic features of viral respiratory tract infections. Acta Cytol 12:162–171, 1968.
Morphologic cellular changes observed in cells exfoliated from the respiratory tract of children with suspected viral respiratory infections are described.

Papanicolaou GN: Degenerative changes in ciliated cells exfoliating from the bronchial epithelium as a cytologic criterion in the diagnosis of diseases of the lung. NY State J Med 56:2647–2650, 1956.
See text under "Inflammatory Process."

Rosen PP, Melamed MR, Savino A: The ferruginous body content of lung tissue: a quantitative study of eighty-six patients. Acta Cytol 16:207–211, 1972.
All but nine patients had ferruginous bodies in 5-g samples of lung tissue. These were unrelated to age, sex, place of residence, or underlying disease.

Selvaggi SM, Gerber M: Pulmonary cytology in patients with the acquired immunodeficiency syndrome (AIDS). Diagn Cytopathol 2:187–193, 1986.
Awareness of the wide range of AIDS-associated pulmonary cell atypias is required to rule out a diagnosis of malignancy.

Stover DE, Zaman MB, Hajdu SI, Lange M, Gold J, Armstrong D: Bronchoalveolar lavage in the diagnosis of diffuse pulmonary infiltrates in the immunosuppressed host. Ann Intern Med 101:1–7, 1984.
Cytologic and microbiologic examination of bronchoalveolar lavage fluid was diagnostic for infectious pathogens in 38 of 46 patients with pulmonary infections.

Zaman MB, Hajdu SI, Melamed MR, Watson RC: Transthoracic aspiration cytology of pulmonary lesions. Semin Diagn Pathol 3:176–187, 1986.
An overview of the topic, this contains up-to-date information and discussion of controversial areas.

Chapter 32

Bronchoscopy and Related Procedures

Edward F. Haponik / Paul Kvale / Ko-Pen Wang

Since Killian introduced the bronchoscope in 1897, the roles of this instrument, and the uses to which it has been put by the chest physician, have evolved dramatically. The widening applications have paralleled major technical innovations. Chevalier Jackson perfected the therapeutic applications of the bronchoscope for retrieval of foreign bodies and advanced its diagnostic use in patients with neoplastic and inflammatory conditions. His addition of a series of telescopes permitted visualization of more distant airways, and bronchology became a major discipline. Ikeda's introduction of the fiberoptic instrument in 1966 extended not only the visible range and diagnostic potential of bronchoscopy, but also the use of the procedure to a broader group of patients.

At present, bronchoscopy is performed regularly by internists, surgeons, and anesthesiologists in a wide variety of settings, and it is accomplished safely in children, critically ill, immunocompromised, and elderly patients. Recently, advances in laser technology have returned bronchoscopy to its original therapeutic objectives. Appraisal of the current roles of bronchoscopy requires a thorough understanding of the technical aspects of the procedure, the breadth and limitations of the information that it can provide, and the appreciation of indications and contraindications for its use.

TECHNICAL CONSIDERATIONS

Instruments

The simple concept of examining the airways through a hollow tube has yielded to sophisticated, technologic improvements that provide a high-resolution image, allow precise, safe instrumentation of endobronchial abnormalities, and permit evaluation of conditions in the periphery of the lung, beyond the range of direct vision. The rigid and fiberoptic bronchoscopes are complementary tools that are well suited for a variety of clinical and research applications.

RIGID BRONCHOSCOPE

The modern rigid bronchoscope is a specialized, open metal tube. A blunted, beveled distal tip allows insertion of the instrument, with minimal trauma, into the airway; the proximal end of the bronchoscope is adapted for observation of the airways, maintenance of gas exchange, and introduction of accessory instruments. A proximal side arm is for the administration of oxygen, and a Venturi attachment enables mechanical ventilation during bronchoscopy. A light carrier channel and an aspirating tube incorporated within the wall of the instrument provide for illumination and suction without compromising the lumen of the airways. These channels are diversely situated in different instruments, thereby increasing options for matching the instrument to the diagnostic or therapeutic goals of the procedure. The standard Jackson (rigid) bronchoscope has a 7-mm-diameter lumen and 40-cm length; the pediatric instrument (3 mm in diameter, 20 cm in length) is still in common use despite the increasing availability of small fiberoptic bronchoscopes. The immediate detection range of the rigid instrument is limited to abnormalities within the lobar, segmental, or subsegmental bronchi in the middle and lower lobes. The segmental and subsegmental bronchi of both upper lobes cannot be visualized consistently, but a selection of telescopes (right angle, retrograde, oblique) permit bronchoscopic visualization of these otherwise inaccessible airways.

FIBEROPTIC BRONCHOSCOPE

The flexible, fiberoptic bronchoscope contains a cluster of glass fibers, strategically disposed, that serves to illuminate and transmit the image. A hollow channel is incorporated for suctioning, instillation of medications or lavage fluid, introduction of accessory instruments, and retrieval of diagnostic specimens. In the newer instruments, the suction channel ranges in size from 1.8 to 2.6 mm, leaving the quality of the image virtually unaffected. Movement of the tip of the bronchoscope through a wide range (approximately 190 to 270°) is controlled by a cable so that the flexible instrument may be directed into all segments of the tracheobronchial tree (Fig. 32-1). Several other recent modifications in design have contributed to the ease of bronchoscopy: an increased angle of view (from 70 to 90°) permits better visualization of more peripheral endobronchial sites and requires less movement of the tip of the bronchoscope by the operator; valve systems allow simultaneous suctioning and insertion of accessory instruments. Also, the total waterproofing of the newer bronchoscopes has enhanced cleaning and maintenance, thereby increasing the availability of a single instrument for multiple procedures.

Using a standard 5.2-mm-external-diameter bronchoscope, all third-order and approximately half of sixth-order bronchi can be entered, and the orifices of nearly all fifth- and most sixth-order orifices can be visualized. Therefore, the principal levels at which bronchogenic carcinomas originate are accessible to the bronchoscope for inspection and biopsy. Smaller-diameter, ultrathin fiberoptic instruments have been developed for use in children and for examination of more peripheral airways in adults. A 1.8-mm prototype flexible instrument that is inserted through the channel of a fiberoptic bronchoscope can provide access to tenth-generation bronchi. In addition, shorter fiberoptic instruments, i.e., nasopharyngoscopes, have played increasing roles in examining the upper airway and in facilitating endotracheal intubation. Most fiberoptic instruments are comparable in quality and well suited for diverse situations. However, subtle differences in instrument size, weight, rigidity, angulation of the tip, and caliber or position of the suction channel may make particular models advantageous in certain patients.

ACCESSORY TOOLS

An array of forceps, brushes, probes, hooks, curettes, aspirating and irrigating catheters, and needles may be introduced through either the rigid bronchoscope or the working channel of the fiberoptic instrument. Their usage varies considerably, depending on the objectives of the procedure and the preferences of the operator. For example, although the curette has achieved considerable popularity abroad as a biopsy instrument, it is not used as much in the United States. Forceps that have had their cups modified are specially suited for grasping foreign bodies or for cutting biopsy specimens. Serrations on the jaws of alligator forceps make it easier to "tear" tissue. Viewing forceps and deflector forceps, which permit biopsies of the lateral wall of the airway, promote the ease and quality of endobronchial biopsy, whereas steerable brushes and curettes aid sampling of more peripheral abnormalities. The relatively large size of the rigid bronchoscope permits insertion of sponge carriers, bougies, snares, knives, scissors, electrodes, diathermic coagulators, magnets, and other specialized devices. Lasers can be introduced through both rigid and fiberoptic bronchoscopes. Proper choice of instruments requires understanding of and familiarity with these accessory instruments and appreciation of their applicability to a variety of conditions encountered during bronchoscopy and their potential for airway trauma or other complications.

INSTRUMENT SELECTION

Selection of the bronchoscope that is optimum for a situation is usually straightforward. Although the use of the flexible bronchoscope has supplanted that of the rigid instrument in many circumstances, the two instruments are properly viewed as complementary. Their merits are compared in Table 32-1. Improved tolerance by patients, increased safety, access to more peripheral airways, use in conjunction with local anesthesia in settings outside the operating room, and lower cost of the procedure have contributed to the widespread use of fiberoptic bronchoscopy. In addition, the flexible instrument permits bronchoscopy under conditions in which rigid bronchoscopy is contraindicated. Among these are disorders that limit extension of the neck, such as severe cervical osteoarthritis, and others, such as thoracic aneurysm and cerebrovascular disease.

Although the fiberoptic bronchoscope has been used safely by experienced operators in certain patients to clear an obstruction from the central airway, the rigid bronchoscope remains preferable in this setting because it ensures a patent airway. In addition, the rigid bronchoscope can

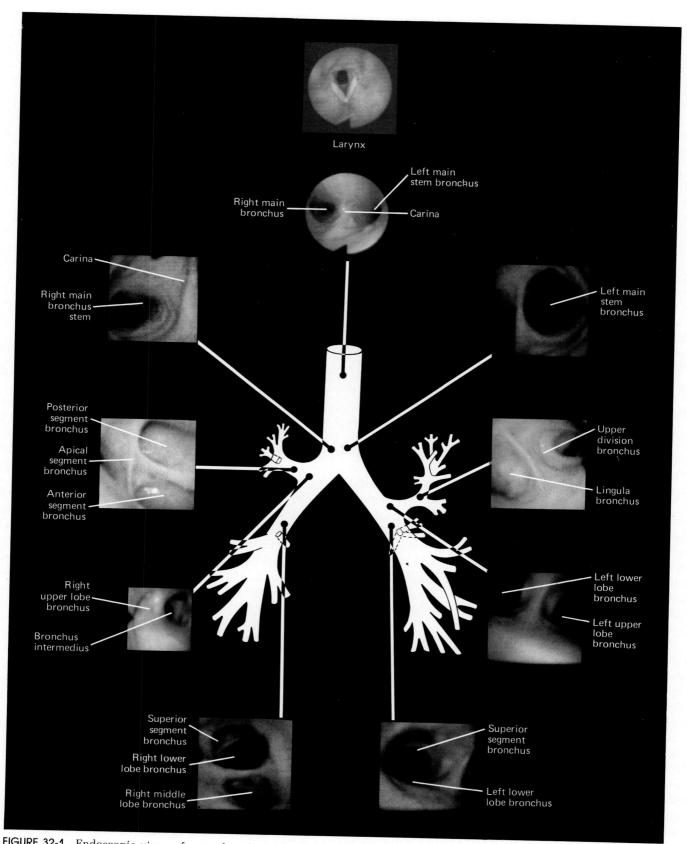

FIGURE 32-1 Endoscopic views of normal tracheobronchial tree. (*Courtesy of M. Altose.*)

TABLE 32-1
Relative Merits of Rigid and Fiberoptic Instruments

	Rigid Bronchoscopy	Fiberoptic Bronchoscopy
Range of direct airway visibility	++	++++
Peripheral range for biopsy	++	++++
Suction capability	++++	+
Airway control	++++	+
Biopsy specimen size	++++	++
Risk, endobronchial survey only	+	−−
Risk with biopsy	+	+
Operator convenience	++	++++
Patient tolerance	+	++++
Anesthesia	General preferable	Local
Setting	Operating room, inpatient, usual	Variable, outpatient, usual
Financial cost of procedure	+++	+
Resolution, clarity of image	++++	+++
Instrument durability, ease of maintenance	++++	++

accommodate larger instruments for retrieval of a foreign body for performing biopsies, for resecting endobronchial tumors, or for tamponading bleeding sites; it also permits the introduction of large suction catheters or of bronchial tampons.

Even large-channel fiberoptic instruments can be overwhelmed by large volumes of blood or secretions and easily obstructed by inspissated clot or mucus. If a fiberoptic instrument is chosen for use in a patient in whom a major airway is obstructed by stricture or neoplasm, the choice must be made with full understanding that there is little room for error on the part of the operator: edema caused by inadvertent mechanical trauma, relatively minor bleeding, or even minimal secretions can readily convert a narrowed airway to critical (or even complete) obstruction. The rigid instrument must be on hand, and familiarity with its use is mandatory. As a rule, when the rigid instrument is needed, the situation is desperate and it must be used immediately.

The rigid bronchoscope has certain major advantages in evaluating and managing most patients with tracheal tumors or strictures; in removing foreign bodies or broncholiths; in performing most bronchoscopic procedures in children; in suctioning large volumes of blood or secretions; and in the therapeutic lavage of patients with alveolar proteinosis. In addition, the rigid instrument provides important backup for the management of pulmonary hemorrhage that occasionally complicates fiberoptic procedures; it also complements the use of the fiberoptic instrument for the diagnosis of mediastinal disease and the staging of bronchogenic carcinoma using transbronchial needle aspiration. Finally, the rigid instrument is more durable, more economically maintained, and less susceptible to breakage than is the fiberoptic bronchoscope.

Setting for Bronchoscopy

The optimum setting for performing a bronchoscopy is determined by the needs and state of a given patient. Among the factors to be taken into account are the patient's overall clinical status, e.g., the presence and severity of intrinsic pulmonary or cardiac disease, the technical proficiency and the ability of the endoscopist to respond promptly to contingencies during bronchoscopy, and the immediate availability of personnel and equipment to deal with complications.

When bronchoscopy is performed at the patient's bedside, the minimum supportive environment must include facilities for cardiopulmonary resuscitation, airway maintenance, oxygen delivery, and cardiac monitoring. Additional requirements are dictated by the demands of a specialized procedure, e.g., foreign body removal, fluoroscopically guided biopsy, and laser photocoagulation. For high-risk patients, a prepared operating room or intensive care area provides the necessary support. In stable outpatients, diagnostic bronchoscopy can be performed safely and expeditiously in the ambulatory setting. However, the in-hospital setting remains prudent in patients with underlying cardiopulmonary disease or other complicating medical illnesses in order to assure optimum preoperative preparation and postoperative observation. Perhaps the most important aspect of the environment in which bronchoscopy is performed relates to the personnel assisting the qualified endoscopist: availability of the same, well-trained and experienced nurse or technical staff is a key factor in the success and safety of the procedure.

Anesthesia and Patient Preparation

General anesthesia is preferred for rigid bronchoscopy in most patients and may be necessary in anxious patients, in those in whom difficult foreign body extraction is anticipated, and in those whose anatomic features hamper use of this instrument, e.g., short muscular neck, prominent upper teeth, widened maxilla, and narrow, shortened mandible. Recently, high-frequency ventilation has proved to be an effective adjunct during rigid bronchoscopy. Most fiberoptic procedures are performed under local anesthesia; but, general anesthesia is often used for children or anxious or uncooperative adults, or when a technically complex and prolonged procedure is necessary.

Preoperative preparation of patients for elective bronchoscopy is generally simple. One illustrative regimen is as follows: The patient is given nothing by mouth during the night before most procedures. Thirty to sixty minutes before bronchoscopy, a narcotic and drying agent are administered subcutaneously. Meperidine and atropine are often used; occasionally, diazepam or morphine are administered intravenously during the procedure via an intravenous line or a heparin lock placed prior to bronchoscopy. However, preoperative agents and protocol vary considerably from institution to institution.

Local anesthesia of the upper airway is usually achieved preoperatively using lidocaine administered by either a hand-held nebulizer or aerosolizer, followed by direct, topical application of lidocaine to the glottis and the tracheobronchial tree via the bronchoscope. Topical cocaine is sometimes substituted if nasopharyngeal edema is present; viscous lidocaine is often used for its anesthetic and lubricant effects. Occasionally, local anesthesia is achieved by transtracheal administration and/or by superior laryngeal nerve block. Effective anesthesia of the upper airway is the key to a safe, well-tolerated procedure. Interestingly, patients consistently characterize passage of the bronchoscope through the larynx as the most uncomfortable aspect of their bronchoscopy experience.

Operative Approach

Rigid bronchoscopy is performed by the oral route, whereas the fiberoptic instrument may be introduced directly through the nose or through a naso- or oropharyngeal airway, endotracheal tube, tracheostomy tube, or rigid bronchoscope. The approach selected should be the least hazardous and the most comfortable for the patient. Most fiberoptic procedures are performed transnasally, without an endotracheal tube. The need for intubation during elective fiberoptic bronchoscopy depends on the likelihood of a major airway complication, the ventilatory reserve of the patient, and the extent of instrumentation that is planned. For example, patients with massive hemoptysis or copious secretions may require intubation prior to the procedure. The advisability of preoperative intubation is increased if the patient has an ineffective cough, abnormal mentation, or severe underlying pulmonary disease. Should endotracheal intubation be needed

for fiberoptic bronchoscopy, it can be accomplished easily using direct laryngoscopy in the awake, communicative patient. Alternatively, the airway is anesthetized via the fiberoptic instrument, and intubation is performed using the bronchoscope as a stylette. When an endotracheal tube is necessary, a minimum tube diameter of 8.5 mm is desirable; a smaller airway with a standard fiberoptic instrument is associated with a marked increase in airway resistance and entails a greater risk of barotrauma if the patient is to be mechanically ventilated. Although the fiberoptic instrument can be used effectively through a nasotracheal tube, the degree of obstruction caused by the instrument often makes the procedure technically difficult.

The position of the bronchoscopist relative to the patient is usually a matter of personal preference. All rigid bronchoscopies and most fiberoptic procedures are performed while the patient is supine and with the operator standing behind the patient's head. However, the operator should be capable of doing complete fiberoptic bronchoscopy while the patient is in other positions. Some endoscopists prefer to perform the study with the patient seated upright: this position is sometimes advantageous because it facilitates the basal distribution of local anesthetic or because it minimizes closure of dependent airways and resultant hypoxemia.

Preoperative Planning

Knowledge of the relationships of bronchial anatomy to characteristic radiographic presentations of segmental disease is fundamental to preoperative planning of bronchoscopy in patients with abnormal radiographs. Biopsy procedures are often directed by additional radiologic studies performed either before, or during, bronchoscopy. Fluoroscopic guidance is essential for accurate sampling of most peripheral nodules and masses or of localized parenchymal infiltrates, and it can assist in the forceps biopsy of patients with diffuse disease. In some instances, information from bronchography or computed tomography helps to identify a preferred route to a localized lesion (Fig. 32-2) or to clarify a mediastinal abnormality. But, as a rule, neither computed tomography nor bronchography are prerequisite for bronchoscopic biopsy. Occasionally, radionuclide studies, e.g., a gallium scan to localize sites of active inflammation or a technetium sulfur colloid scan to localize sites of active inflammation or a technetium sulfur colloid scan to localize sites of occult bleeding, increase the diagnostic yield. It cannot be overemphasized that safe application of diagnostic bronchoscopic needle aspiration and therapeutic laser procedures requires thorough appreciation of the anatomy of extrabronchial structures, their normal relationships to endobronchial landmarks, and the ways in which these relationships may be altered by disease.

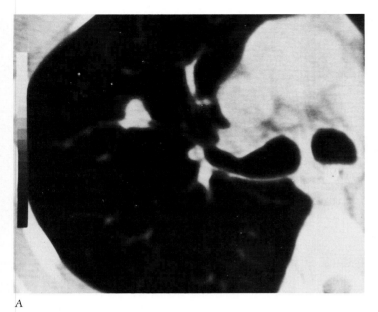

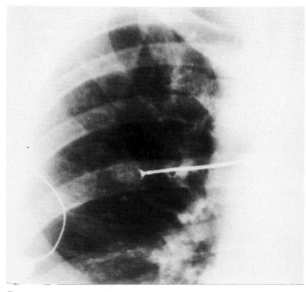

A   B

FIGURE 32-2 *A.* Preoperative computed chest tomography demonstrates a direct path into a small, solitary pulmonary nodule. *B.* Intraoperative fluoroscopy confirms placement of biopsy forceps within the tumor.

Evaluation of the Airway

During rigid bronchoscopy the patient is placed in the supine posture with the head fully extended, and the instrument is then either passed directly through the glottis or is introduced via a laryngoscope. Access to all tracheobronchial segments is achieved by the combined use of telescopes and appropriate movements of the patient's head, e.g., turning the head rightward to evaluate the left tracheobronchial tree. These maneuvers contrast with those used during flexible bronchoscopy, in which the simple deflection of the tip of the fiberoptic instrument, together with rotation of the endoscopist's wrist, usually permits visualization and entry of all segmental orifices. When anatomic variations hinder access to all segments, coordinated movements of the patient's head, changes in the operator's position, or adjustment of the grasp of the bronchoscope to take advantage of maximum angulation of the tip often aid examination.

The bronchoscopist sequentially anesthetizes the upper airway, trachea, main-stem bronchi, and more peripheral airways before examining these consecutive areas. A systematic review is aided by the recognition of "landmark" appearances at several levels of the tracheobronchial tree. Because the dichotomous branches of more peripheral airways do not have a characteristic endobronchial appearance, the bronchoscopist must always bear in mind the route taken to a given site: whenever the precise location is unclear, withdrawal of the instrument to a more proximal, familiar landmark area is necessary to reaffirm the current location. The bronchoscope is always advanced while the airway lumen is directly visible; it should not be passed blindly. When the view is obscured by blood or secretions, these must be cleared.

Common technical errors relate to inadequate anesthesia of the supraglottic and immediate subglottic areas, premature entry of nondependent, i.e., unanesthetized airway segments, and failure to keep the bronchoscope in a central position within the bronchial lumen. In these situations, mechanical trauma by the instrument may result in laryngospasm, bronchospasm, or paroxysms of coughing that limit the procedure and increase its risk. Other common problems occur if an attempt at biopsy is made while the view is obscured by blood or secretions.

INFORMATION OBTAINED FROM BRONCHOSCOPY

Information that bronchoscopy can provide is summarized in Table 32-2. The overall yield represents the combined information obtained from inspection of the airway, cytopathologic examination and microbiologic studies of lung fluids, and bronchoscopic biopsies. Because institutional preferences dictate how specimens must be handled, close communication between the bronchoscopist and laboratory personnel is essential. For example, in the immunocompromised host who has unexplained pulmonary infiltrates, the nature of the primary disease, the prospect of opportunistic infection, the possible effects of drug therapy, or a combination of all three calls for economic use of the diagnostic material obtained during bronchoscopy; the pace of the patient's illness also requires timely processing and review. If proper support

TABLE 32-2

Information Obtained from Diagnostic Bronchoscopy

A. Upper airway evaluation

B. Tracheobronchial inspection

    1. Mucosal abnormalities

        Indistinct bronchial cartilages
        Inflammation: edema, erythema
        Telangiectasis
        Vascular tortuosity, engorgement
        Neoplasm
        Polyp
        Sutures, staples
        Laceration
        Suction trauma
        Atrophy
        Mucosal irregularity
        Enlarged gland orifices (pitting)
        Necrosis
        Pronounced longitudinal striations, corrugations

    2. Extramucosal abnormalities

        Blood
        Foreign body
        Secretions
        Broncholith
        Carbonaceous material

    3. Airway patency

        Endobronchial obstruction
          Tumor
          Broncholith
          Clot
          Foreign body
        Extrinsic compression, bulging
          Stenosis, stricture
          Ectasia

    4. Airway position
        Rotation, displacement by atelectasis, effusion

    5. Airway branching pattern
        Normal segmental distribution
        Anomalous branching

    6. Dynamic relationships
        Normal tracheobronchial movement during breathing, cough
        Fixation
        Accentuated collapse

C. Secretion collection for cytopathology and microbiologic studies

    Washings (selective and nonselective)
    Bronchoalveolar lavage

D. Biopsy (forceps, brush, curette, transbronchial needle)
    Apparent normal mucosa
    (e.g., diffuse parenchymal disease)
    Visible endobronchial lesions
    (e.g., tumor)
    Beyond visible range
        Transbronchial forceps biopsy
        (e.g., diffuse parenchymal disease)
        Peripheral mass, nodule
        Transbronchial needle aspiration
        (e.g., mediastinal lymphadenopathy)

E. Special studies
    Hematoporphyrin staining
    Endobronchial temperature, pH
    Physiological measurements
    Biochemical mediators, markers
    Mineralogic studies
    Electron microscopy

SOURCE: Modified after Ikeda, 1974, and Stradling, 1980.

---

cannot be provided by the laboratory, certain bronchoscopic procedures should not even be attempted. For example, transbronchial needle aspiration that provides scant cytopathologic material cannot be used reliably for diagnosis or staging unless a high-quality and cooperative cytopathology laboratory is available.

Endobronchial Inspection

Examples of endobronchial pathology (Fig. 32-3) are available in texts by Stradling, by Ikeda, and by Tsuboi. In some instances, the findings are non-specific and bear little relationship to the patient's primary problem; in others, subtle abnormalities have diagnostic importance. During the systematic review of the airways, the endoscopist must confirm airway patency—at least to the segmental and subsegmental levels—and also note the presence of alterations in airway placement or mobility. Ectasia of subsegmental bronchi sometimes makes it possible to visualize several branching generations far in the periphery, suggesting bronchiectasis. Blunting of airway branch points ("spurs") calls attention to the possibility of underlying inflammation, infiltration, or distortion by peribronchial disease. Displacement of the tracheobronchial tree, either because of a decrease in lung volume or by extrinsic compression, is an alert to abnormality. Pronounced airway collapse during forced expiration, cough, or even tidal breathing occurs in patients with obstructive lung disease, tracheomalacia, or achondroplasia. Fixation of the carina is associated with mediastinal tumor, previous surgery, or radiation therapy; a rigid, noncompliant airway is the result of neoplastic infiltration, amyloidosis, or inflammatory stricture. Accentuation of the normal mucosal corrugations of the posterior wall of the trachea or main-stem bronchi suggests neoplastic infiltration. Similarly, granular cobblestoning of mucosa is consistent with sarcoidosis or submucosal telangiectasis. Recently, hemorrhagic, inflammatory changes of endobronchial Kaposi's sarcoma have been identified in patients with the acquired immunodeficiency syndrome (AIDS).

Extramucosal abnormalities such as blood and secretions, or endobronchial obstructions by masses, foreign bodies, or broncholiths are usually obvious. Bronchogenic carcinoma is the most likely cause of an obstructing, en-

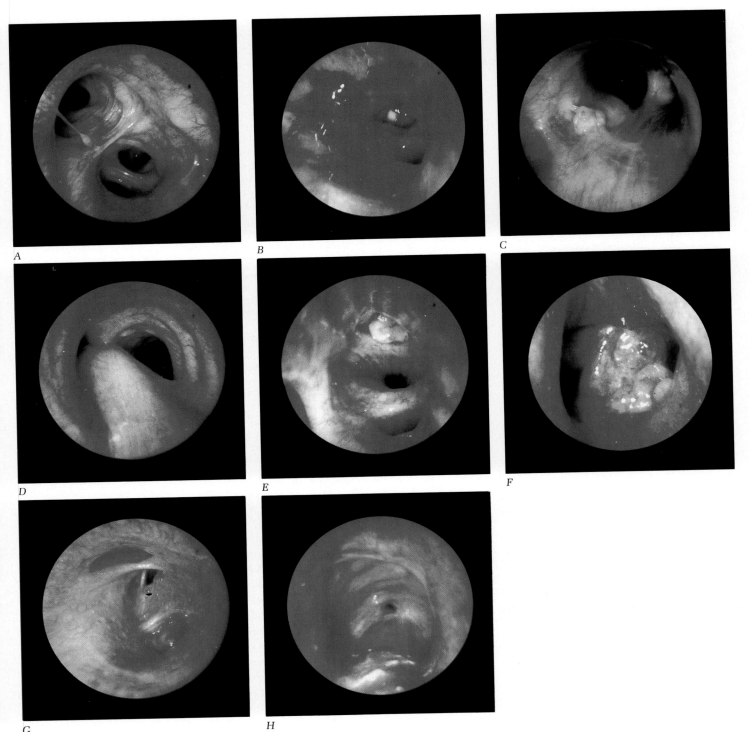

FIGURE 32-3 A. Chronic bronchitis. Primary division of left main bronchus. The vessels are dilated and prominent, producing general reddening of the mucosa. The surface is moist and glistening because of increased secretion, much of which has already been removed by suction. A residual string of mucus remains across the upper bronchus, to the left of the picture. B. Left basal and lingular bronchiectasis. Primary division of left main bronchus. The blood-obscured secondary carina and upper bronchus occupy most of the left half of the figure. On the right the left lower bronchus is seen, obstructed by pus and blood arising in the bronchiectatic basal system. C. Active tuberculous lymphadenitis. The widened carina is on the far left; the normal right upper orifice is on the far right. The medial and posteromedial walls of the right main bronchus are thrust into the lumen by subcarinal lymph node enlargement. To the right of the carina granulation tissue is erupting through the mucosa. The biopsy led to a diagnosis of active tuberculosis. D. Tracheal distortion by enlarged lymph nodes. An elongated, rigid, forward protrusion occupies the posterior wall of the trachea and continues into the left main bronchus, obscuring most of the carina from view. The right main bronchus is little affected. There are bronchitic changes in the mucosa. The findings are due to invasion of posterior tracheal lymph nodes by bronchial carcinoma. E. Intraluminal

dobronchial mass; other potential etiologies to be considered include benign airway tumors and metastatic neoplasms. Although the appearance of a smooth, glistening polypoid, pedunculated bronchial adenoma may be "classic," the gross characteristics of airway tumors generally do not permit distinction among them; in most instances, histologic confirmation is necessary. The appearances of fibrin and old blood clot, or of endobronchial obstruction by granulomatous disease, occasionally mimics a neoplastic process. Intrabronchial obstruction is occasionally due to the contents of ruptured lymph nodes, an aspirated foreign body, or to gastric material.

Lung Fluid Analysis

Bronchoscopy provides ready access to tracheobronchial secretions; these are usually collected in a trap attached to the suction line. The identification of neoplastic cells or pathogenic microorganisms may be definitive. Washings obtained over the surface of endobronchial tumors are often diagnostic and selective; segmental washings from peripheral airways occasionally disclose occult malignancy. The handling of cytopathologic smears varies considerably from clinic to clinic: material may be collected and transported in either Hank's balanced salt solution or in normal saline, and processed subsequently using a millipore filter technique; alternatively, cytopathologic smears may be prepared at the time of bronchoscopy by applying brushings directly to slides and then immersing the slides promptly into alcohol. Premature drying of cytopathologic specimens before placing the slides into fixative is a common technical error that renders them useless for diagnostic purposes. At some institutions, fixative is added to bronchial washings for subsequent processing. Because blood and inflammatory exudate hinders the examination of cytopathologic specimens, clean, uncontaminated specimens should be sought: separate collection of some material early in the course of bronchoscopy, before biopsy procedures, or deferring an elective bronchoscopy until a bout of acute bronchitis or pneumonia has resolved helps to minimize these problems.

During bronchoalveolar lavage, a large area of lung can be sampled by using large volumes of fluid for washing. Specimens collected in this way have proved useful in the diagnosis of opportunistic infection in immunocompromised hosts; they may also prove useful in dealing with patients who have interstitial lung disease. To perform this procedure, the fiberoptic bronchoscope is wedged into a subsegmental airway (usually in the middle or lower lobe), fluid is instilled incrementally, and the fluid is subsequently recovered by suctioning or by drainage under the influence of gravity. The total volume used generally varies from 60 to 200 ml; about half of the instillate is recovered for evaluation. Information from this "cellular biopsy" has contributed to the understanding of pulmonary host defenses, of acute lung injury, and of the pathogenesis of a wide range of conditions, including idiopathic pulmonary fibrosis, sarcoidosis, histiocytosis X, asthma, asbestosis, and the adult respiratory distress syndrome. Its value as a practical clinical tool, e.g., as a guide to therapy in these disorders, is currently under investigation.

◀ spread of bronchial carcinoma. Right basal system. Part of the medial basal orifice can be seen to the far left; a subapical orifice lies in the foreground, and the common origin for posterior and lateral basal bronchi is in the center of the figure. A small, mobile, fleshy tumor can be seen above center, protruding from the anterior basal orifice. This intraluminal extension had its distal origin in a large spherical carcinoma in the anterior basal segment. *F.* Intrabronchial eruption of carcinomatous lymph nodes. Bifurcation of trachea. The edge of the carina can still be seen to left of center, but the subcarinal area is clearly widened. From the right of the carina, exuberant tumor tissue has erupted and is spreading in the anterior wall of the right main bronchus, the lumen of which is greatly diminished. Paratracheal node enlargement also narrowed the trachea, which can be seen in the right foreground of the picture. *G.* Carcinoid adenoma. The right middle orifice is at the top of the picture; the origins of the basal system are in the distance with some secretion present. In the foreground the apical lower orifice is seen obstructed by a cherry red, smooth, round, carcinoid tumor. This appearance is typical, but such tumors may also be lobulated. *H.* Tracheal stricture. This followed removal of a tracheostomy tube 6 weeks previously. It was a rigid, tubular narrowing at the site of the inflatable cuff. Dilatation was repeatedly followed by restricture, and therefore cuff resection was successfully undertaken. Inflammatory changes, due to secondary infection, are seen in the mucosa with increased secretion in the foreground. *(A and D, courtesy of P. Stradling; B, C, and E to H, from Stradling, 1980, with permission.)*

Bronchoscopic Biopsies

The diagnostic yield of bronchoscopic biopsy varies with the experience and skill of the operator, the potential error in sampling that is inherent in the small samples provided by fiberoptic bronchoscopic biopsies, the pathologist who interprets the material, and the practices of the institution. At some institutions, the amount of tissue required for an "adequate" biopsy is less than at others. Pathologists are reluctant to offer definitive diagnoses on the basis of either cytopathologic or microbiopsy material alone. Although the handling of specimens varies among institutions, as a rule, hematoxylin and eosin stains, Masson's stains for collagen, and special stains for mycobacteria, fungi, or other pathogenic microorganisms are performed. Multiple, thin sections of specimens are generally obtained in order to maximize the use of the diagnostic material; loci of cancer or opportunistic pathogens, missed during routine processing of specimens, are sometimes detected in this way. In a few institutions, frozen sections are obtained at the time of endobronchial or transbronchial biopsy; although this practice may expedite diagnosis, the loss of histologic detail is an important disadvantage if, as usual, the total amount of tissue available for conventional processing is limited. Less often, specialized studies of bronchoscopic biopsies with immunofluorescent stains, electron microscopy, or mineralogic studies are done.

Accurate classification of certain neoplasms, particularly bronchogenic carcinomas of mixed cell types, metastatic tumors, or tumors with unusual histology, may be difficult. Thus, even an endobronchial biopsy that is diagnostic for malignancy may not be specific enough to guide therapy. Another common and challenging problem is the differentiation of lymphoma from small cell carcinoma. Although the presence of crush artifact may strongly suggest small cell carcinoma, this nonspecific finding often poses major uncertainties in evaluating the specimen (Chapters 119 and 126). A variety of biopsy specimens can be obtained from beyond the visible range of the bronchoscope: popular applications of this technique include transbronchial forceps biopsy in patients with unexplained, diffuse parenchymal disease and the sampling of peripheral pulmonary nodules and masses using brushes, curettes, forceps, or needles. Recently, proximal, extrabronchial disease within the mediastinum has been assessed using transtracheal, and transbronchial, needle aspiration.

ENDOBRONCHIAL BIOPSY

Endobronchial lesions can be biopsied with brushes, forceps, needles, or curettes. Brushes and curettes sample a larger but more superficial surface area, whereas forceps and aspirating needles provide more localized, deeper specimens. The sizes of most forceps biopsies vary from 2 to 5 mm; the larger forceps accommodated by the rigid bronchoscope permit deep, submucosal sampling. Directly visualized tumors account for most endobronchial biopsies, but "blind" biopsies of apparently normal mucosa are often useful. For example, a spur that is apparently normal is often biopsied in order to exclude the presence of submucosal, infiltrative carcinoma, thereby enhancing prospects for establishing clear margins for surgical resection.

Occasionally, pathologic examination is nondiagnostic despite unequivocal radiographic and bronchoscopic evidence of endobronchial disease. In large measure, this is due to inappropriate sampling. In selecting a site for biopsy, grossly necrotic and hypervascular areas of the tumor surface should be avoided: mucosal debris and a diagnostically useless specimen are apt to result in the former situation and a blood-filled field in the latter. The diagnostic yield is also less in patients in whom tumors are encapsulated or in whom endobronchial abnormalities are caused either by submucosal infiltration or by tumors extrinsic to the airways, without erosion into its lumen. Since forceps biopsy and bronchial brushing have

often proved to be insufficient in these circumstances, interest has been rekindled in the use of needle aspiration. When forceps biopsy or brushing is impractical because of the likelihood of inordinate bleeding, needle aspiration of the lesion can sometimes be done safely: it has been used to establish the diagnosis of necrotic tumor masses and for sampling vascular, carcinoid tumors.

TRANSBRONCHIAL FORCEPS BIOPSY

Transbronchial lung biopsy is a sampling technique that has proved useful for the bronchoscopic diagnosis of diffuse parenchymal disease and of focal nodules, masses, and infiltrates. The flexible instrument allows passage of forceps to the periphery of the lung where avulsion of small fragments of tissue is done easily. If a disease produces abnormalities that are located in the peribronchial spaces, then transbronchial lung biopsy often provides a definitive histologic diagnosis. Salient examples of this are sarcoidosis, metastatic carcinoma, and miliary tuberculosis, conditions which have characteristic histologic features. Microorganisms such as *Pneumocystis carinii*, cytomegalovirus, and some fungi, can be found in the lung tissue obtained by transbronchial biopsy; obtaining diagnostic material in this way can be of value in dealing with the pulmonary complications of the immunocompromised host. Oppositely, some disorders either have no distinguishing histologic features or are irregularly distributed throughout the pulmonary parenchyma; these are less amenable to diagnosis by transbronchial biopsy. This is particularly true for interstitial pulmonary fibrosis and for collagen vascular diseases involving the lung.

Operative techniques used for transbronchial forceps biopsy vary, but the basic approaches are similar. The closed biopsy forceps is passed into the lung periphery. When the appropriate site (visualized fluoroscopically) is reached, the forceps is withdrawn slightly, opened, and then readvanced until resistance is met. The forceps is closed and then removed with the specimen inside. A characteristic "tug" of parenchyma is felt by the operator and is usually visualized at fluoroscopy. Although the biopsy maneuvers are sometimes synchronized with expiration or breath-holding, this coordinated effort is not essential to successful biopsy in the cooperative patient. Immediately after biopsy, the bronchoscope is maintained in the wedged position in order to monitor for bleeding and to confine bleeding to the biopsied segment. There are few guidelines for positioning the forceps in patients with diffuse infiltrates, but the midzones of the lung are usually sampled; biopsies obtained further out increase the risk of pneumothorax, whereas more proximal "bites" make bleeding more likely. Although it seems reasonable that fresh areas of acutely evolving infiltrates, or bronchopulmonary segments in which densities are more confluent, would provide a greater diagnostic yield than other parts of the lung, this belief has not been tested systematically.

Larger pieces of lung tissue (approximately 5 mm) can be obtained with the forceps that are used in conjunction with a rigid bronchoscope; but the tissue obtained in this way is inevitably more centrally located, near the major carinal spurs. Forceps accommodated by large-channel fiberoptic instruments, "backloading" or retrograde forceps, and large "alligator" forceps have been devised in the attempt to increase the size and quality of biopsy specimens. Some of these intruments are more difficult to open in the periphery and can increase bleeding. Although a larger alveolar specimen may be obtained using these sampling methods, thereby facilitating diagnosis in individual patients, the overall diagnostic yield has not been substantially increased.

TRANSBRONCHIAL NEEDLE ASPIRATION

The needle aspiration of cytopathologic material using a specially adapted needle passed through the tracheal or bronchial wall has been used for diagnostic and staging purposes. Until recently, the rigid needles were inserted through a rigid bronchoscope; now this type of sampling is possible with the fiberoptic instrument. An intraluminal stylette within a flexible, polyethylene catheter tipped with a 1.3-cm, 23 gauge needle, imparts the rigidity needed to puncture the airway wall. Usually aspirates are obtained from the right paratracheal, subcarinal, and left paratracheal sites; endobronchial landmarks of these areas are easily identified. The cytopathology specimens must be obtained before the primary tumor is approached in order to avoid contamination. The presence of clusters of malignant cells and lymphocytes, together with the absence of epithelial cells, helps to confirm the nodal origin of this material.

Reporting of Results

With an increasingly multidisciplinary approach to patient management, accurate and timely communication of the information derived from bronchoscopy is essential. When mucosal or extramucosal abnormalities are identified, they must be described completely and their character and precise trancheobronchial locations specified. In addition, the number and exact sites of biopsies or aspirates must be recorded in detail. These data are central for assessing resectability in bronchogenic carcinoma or suitability with respect to palliative treatment of endobronchial disease using radiation or laser therapy. Finally, operators must not only outline their impressions at the time of the procedure but must also provide addenda as results from diagnostic specimens become available. A sine qua non is that the bronchoscopist should review all diagnostic material personally with the pathologist to enhance decisions about patient management and also to promote the understanding of anatomic and pathologic relationships.

In many instances effective reporting is enhanced by the photographic recording of the procedure or, alternatively, by detailed diagrams and systematic use of nomenclature. Jackson's original drawings of his bronchoscopic observations provide a model for the modern endoscopist. More recently, Polaroid photography has been used effectively for documentation, and both motion picture and videotape bronchoscopy records have proved useful in teaching and research. Although the use of increased numbers of fiberoptic bundles and improved illumination systems has improved the resolving power of fexible bronchoscopes so that excellent photographs can be obtained, the rigid instrument does afford a superior image because of better light transmission and sharper detail.

DIAGNOSTIC BRONCHOSCOPY

Common indications for diagnostic bronchoscopy are summarized in Table 32-3. Their relative frequencies are difficult to quantify because of variations in reporting and institutional differences in patient selection. Nonetheless, the most common indications for diagnostic bronchoscopy at both community hospitals and referral centers are radiographic abnormalities, symptoms that suggest bronchogenic carcinoma, and unexplained infiltrative lung disease.

Diagnosis of Lung Cancer

CENTRAL TUMORS

Most squamous cell carcinomas are located in segmental (second-order), subsegmental (third-order), and sub-subsegmental (fourth-order) bronchi. These sites are well within the visible range of fiberoptic instruments. Radiographic evidence of either major atelectasis, or a distinct proximal mass, or postobstructive pneumonia, or all three suggest endobronchial obstruction and a strong likelihood of making the diagnosis by bronchoscopy. Localized wheeze is often cited as an indication for bronchoscopy, but the predictive value of this physical sign without radiographic abnormality is unknown. Among patients with bronchogenic carcinoma who present with central or hilar masses, bronchoscopy is diagnostic in 68 to 98 percent. These tumors are usually within the visible range and directly accessible to biopsy. Ordinarily, diagnosis is achieved with few specimens and should approximate 100 percent in patients with exophytic masses. The combination of cytology and a single forceps biopsy of central

TABLE 32-3
Indications for Bronchoscopy

Diagnostic	Therapeutic
Unexplained roentgenographic abnormalities*	Foreign body removal*,†
1. Central/hilar masses (x)	Difficult endotracheal intubation*
2. Peripheral masses and nodules	Airway maintenance, massive hemoptysis†
3. Atelectasis (x)	Tracheobronchial toilet
4. Unresolved or recurrent pneumonia	(e.g., lobar atelectasis)*
5. Localized air trapping (x)	Bronchoalveolar lavage†
6. Diffuse infiltrative lung disease	(Pulmonary alveolar proteinosis)
(e.g., immunocompromised host)*	Laser photocoagulation
7. Pleural effusion	Brachytherapy
Staging known bronchogenic carcinoma*	Hematoporphyrin therapy
Cough	Local chemotherapy
Hemoptysis* (x)	Immunotherapy (BCG)
Bronchography, other contrast procedures	Electrocautery†
Unexplained positive sputum cytology	Bouginage†
Known head or neck malignancy	Transbronchial aspiration of cysts, abscesses
Diaphragmatic paralysis	Local antimicrobial administration
Hoarseness	Drainage of abscesses†
Localized wheeze	
Biopsy, manipulation of tracheal tumors, vascular tumors†	
Followup, antineoplastic therapy	
Inhalation injury	
Tracheobronchial trauma	
Evaluation of endotracheal tube-related injury	
Postoperative assessment (e.g., integrity of anastomosis)	
Confirmation of endotracheal tube position	

*Common indications.

†Rigid instrument preferred.

NOTE: x = visible endobronchial obstruction likely.

endobronchial lesions has afforded a 92 percent yield; three to four biopsies offer maximum yields, and washings and brushings add little to forceps biopsies. When the neoplasm is not directly accessible to either forceps or brush biopsy because of extrinsic compression of the airway, either by tumor or mediastinal lymphadenopathy, transbronchial needle aspiration is often diagnostic.

Superior vena caval obstruction can be an important problem in the management of mediastinal tumors, particularly lymphoma and small cell carcinoma. Diagnostic bronchoscopy is often performed early as a preliminary to the prompt initiation of radiation and/or chemotherapy. However, great caution is advised in electing to perform bronchoscopy because of the possibility of supraglottic and laryngeal edema that may accompany superior vena caval obstruction and of increased bleeding, either from airway trauma or biopsy sites.

PERIPHERAL NODULES AND MASSES

Fiberoptic bronchoscopy is diagnostic in approximately half of patients with peripheral nodules or masses. Percu-

taneous needle biopsy usually has a higher yield but, because bronchoscopy has a lower morbidity, it is often given priority either to establish the diagnosis before thoracotomy is performed or if histologic information is needed as a guide to palliative therapy in a nonsurgical candidate. Several factors influence the yield from bronchoscopy. First, the accessibility of a localized lesion to the sampling instrument is most important and depends on the anatomic relationship of a tumor to a patent bronchus (Fig. 32-2); the use of preoperative bronchographic mapping to define this relationship has resulted in diagnostic yields greater than 90 percent. When the neoplasm either originates within an airway or engulfs it and invades the bronchial lumen, diagnosis is usually feasible using any bronchoscopic instrument (forceps, brush, needle, or curette). In contrast, when the airway is compressed extrinsically and deviated by an enlarging tumor, or is obstructed proximally by associated lymphadenopathy, a direct path into the tumor may not be available. In Tsuboi's experience with patients in whom transbronchial biopsy was negative, the most important technical factor accounting for the negative result was obstruction of the affected bronchus by advanced neoplasm that prohibited the entry of instruments into the lesion. Flexible transbronchial needle aspiration increases the diagnostic yield in these situations because puncture of the airway permits sampling of extrabronchial sites.

A second factor influencing bronchoscopic diagnostic yield is the size of the lesion: the yield approximates 80 percent for tumors that exceed 2 cm in diameter and 20 to 40 percent for those smaller than 2 cm. This result is probably related to the availability of more routes to larger tumors and the better visibility of large tumors by fluoroscopy; the yield decreases when massive tumors displace feeding bronchi.

As with patients with peripheral infiltrates, another factor influencing yield is the number of biopsy specimens: maximum yields have been obtained by taking four to six specimens, but occasionally as many as 10 biopsies may be necessary. Also, the degree of inflammation surrounding a tumor or the presence of central necrosis are additional, but less easily quantifiable, factors that affect diagnosis.

Finally, yield is usually lower for tumors located in the outer third of the lung than for those in the mid-lung fields: more branch points, and possible false routes, must be negotiated in order to reach the more peripheral lesions. Cytopathology done on postbronchoscopy sputums which is generally not needed in patients with visible, central lesions, may increase the yield in patients with tumors that are not visualized bronchoscopically. Similarly, washings and brushings are more helpful in patients with peripheral rather than central tumors. Because some lesions in the mid-lung arise from bronchi which have a 90° orientation to the major airways, forceps or brush biopsies are not always possible; such bronchi can be entered with flexible needles. Occasionally, abnormalities in the lung apices and the superior basal segments of the lower lobes may be difficult to approach even by small fiberoptic instruments. Similar technical limitations may be encountered in the evaluation of patients with superior sulcus tumors; in these patients, percutaneous needle aspiration biopsy is preferable.

Nonneoplastic causes of peripheral nodules, e.g., mycobacteria, fungi, and amyloid, can be diagnosed bronchoscopically, thereby often obviating the need for surgery while enabling specific treatment. In patients with benign tumors, the sampling error associated with the small size of the histologic specimen often precludes a definite diagnosis of benignity; even larger biopsies obtained via the rigid instrument may not resolve the problem. The absence of malignant tissue in the bronchoscopic biopsy of a solitary pulmonary nodule does not prove that the lesion is benign. But when it is certain that the lesion has been entered by the forceps and that an adequate specimen has been obtained, the negative result by biopsy, coupled with clinical and radiographic signs that favor benignity, occasionally, make it possible to recommend nonsurgical management using serial radiography to monitor changes in size or behavior of the lesion. But, as a rule, failure to make the diagnosis by bronchoscopic biopsy leads to further diagnostic workup, e.g., percutaneous needle aspiration or thoracotomy.

Lung Cancer Staging

When bronchoscopy reveals an endobronchial tumor, the usual emphasis, quite appropriately, is on diagnosis. However, careful description of the extent of endobronchial disease is useful in identifying candidates for surgery, in prognosis, and in clarifying the role to be played by palliative therapy. This information is an essential component of the TNM staging classification of lung cancer: The T1 category requires the absence of airway involvement by tumor invasion proximal to a lobar bronchus; the T2 category requires that the most proximal extent of tumor be at least 2 cm away from the carina. Visualization of a tumor mass in a main-stem bronchus is rarely (<2 percent) associated with 5-year survival. The T3 category includes endobronchial lesions within 2 cm of the carina; curative resection is generally impractical.

Fixation of the carina, or extrinsic compression of the tracheobronchial tree, also provides important information about the severity of local disease. The mobility of the airway can be evaluated not only visually, but also by slight pressure applied with the rigid bronchoscope. Carinal fixation, blunting, or broadening suggests extensive involvement by mediastinal tumor and decreases the prospect of resectability. Paracarinal biopsy affords the opportunity for detecting microscopic, proximal extension of tumor through submucosal lymphatics which sometimes occurs even though no endobronchial abnormality is visible; this inapparent disease detected by paracarinal biopsy may provide exclusive evidence of unresectability: using either the rigid or fiberoptic instruments, forceps biopsy of apparently normal carinal mucosa has demonstrated otherwise unsuspected proximal submucosal spread of tumor in nearly 10 percent of patients. This finding has been associated with large mediastinal masses, major atelectasis, and lymphangitic carcinomatosis; it occurs less often in patients with peripheral masses.

Recent technical innovations in flexible transbronchial needle aspiration permit the safe evaluation of the extrabronchial, mediastinal extent of nodal disease (Fig. 32-4). Positive aspirates for malignancy have been obtained in approximately 40 percent of patients; they have correlated closely with the demonstration of tumor involvement by mediastinal exploration and with unresectable status. The yield of transbronchial needle aspiration is higher in patients who have radiographic evidence of an abnormal mediastinum (75 percent) than in those in

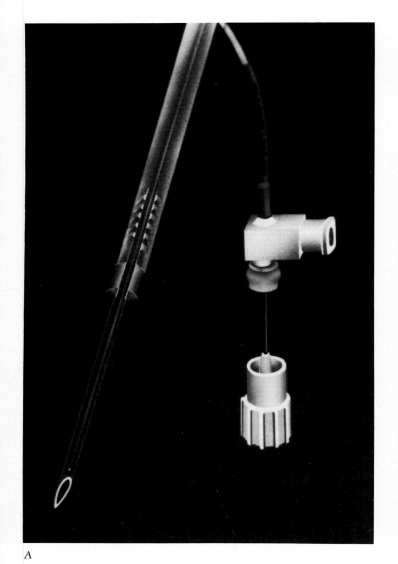

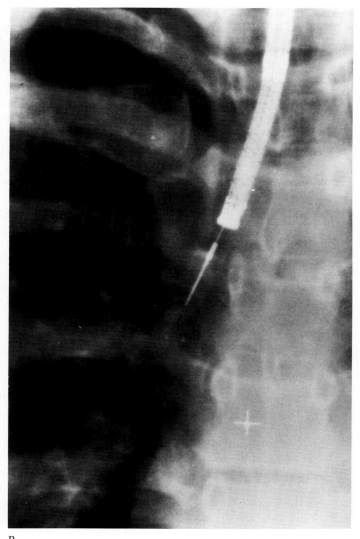

A   B

FIGURE 32-4 *A.* A flexible needle supported by an intraluminal stylette permits precise transtracheal puncture and aspiration of (*B*) a minimally enlarged right paratracheal node.

whom chest radiographs are normal (15 to 23 percent). The yield of this procedure is also greater in patients with endobronchial tumors, undifferentiated neoplasms, a grossly abnormal main carina, or evidence of extrinsic airway compression. However, a normal appearing airway does not assure a negative aspirate. Transbronchial needle aspiration can provide evidence of mediastinal lymph node involvement at sites that might preclude attempts at surgical cure; this technique also has clear advantages over staging maneuvers that do not provide material for histologic examination. When related to radiographic evidence of mediastinal disease, the results of transbronchial needle aspiration may not only complement mediastinoscopy, mediastinotomy, or thoracotomy, but also may obviate the need for these procedures. Because of the clinical implications of a positive result, great care must be taken

to avoid contamination of the aspirate with tracheobronchial secretions. Specimens must be obtained before an endobronchial tumor is approached and from a definite mediastinal, rather than a paratracheal, intrapulmonary, location. Needle aspiration is performed at the same time as diagnostic bronchoscopy and can be done safely in outpatients. Larger cores of tissue can be obtained using the rigid bronchoscope; a new prototype needle now permits biopsies with the flexible instrument as well.

Staging bronchoscopy sometimes provides other, clinically important information. Because of the multicentricity of lung cancer, bronchoscopy occasionally demonstrates a second, unexpected endobronchial tumor, a finding that strongly influences the approach to therapy. Identification of vocal cord paralysis may confirm mediastinal metastasis and unresectability. Finally, patients who are not surgical candidates may benefit from the procedure; the severity of luminal obstruction and the proximal extent of disease may be helpful with respect to choosing between radiation therapy and laser photocoagulation, or aid in timing when these modes of therapy are to be used.

Unexplained Positive Sputum Cytopathology

When sputum cytopathology is interpreted as suspicious or positive for neoplasm even though the chest radiograph is normal, bronchoscopy is sometimes helpful in identifying its origin. Although few patients with lung cancer present in this manner, the potential for early intervention is great. The bronchoscopic examination has to be thorough and done by an experienced bronchoscopist since the mucosal manifestations of early lung cancer are subtle. On occasion, repeated, extensive procedures have been done under general anesthesia, in order to obtain selective washings of all bronchopulmonary segments. Either diagnostic biopsy of a visible endobronchial lesion or consistent localization of diagnostic cytopathologic findings to the same anatomic site in the course of two separate procedures is required before surgical therapy is undertaken. Hematoporphyrin derivatives are currently being used in some clinics to help in localizing bronchoscopically occult tumors.

Because they share a similar pathogenesis, epidermoid malignancies, bronchogenic carcinoma, and upper airway tumors often coexist; synchronous (4 to 14 percent) and metachronous (12 to 19 percent) tumors of the aerodigestive tract have been associated with epidermoid neoplasms of the head and neck. Therefore, thorough examination of the nasopharynx, oral cavity, and larynx are an integral part of bronchoscopy performed for a diagnosis of an obvious abnormality on the chest radiograph. Patients with known esophageal carcinoma commonly undergo bronchoscopy in order to exclude local extension to the tracheobronchial tree.

Other Manifestations of Lung Cancer

Either vocal cord or diaphragmatic paralysis, secondary to involvement by lung cancer of the recurrent laryngeal or phrenic nerves, is often included as an indication for bronchoscopy. Although an endobronchial tumor that was not suggested by radiographic changes is found occasionally, more often, mucosal infiltration, or extrinsic compression of the tracheobronchial tree, is seen. The use of forceps, brush, and curette biopsies generally has a low yield; but transbronchial needle aspiration may provide access to the unresectable neoplasm.

The diagnostic yield from bronchoscopy in patients with unexplained pleural effusion is low unless an obvious mass or atelectasis coexists. Extrinsic compression and displacement of the tracheobronchial tree by the mass effect of the fluid is common but is nondiagnostic.

Cough

Bronchoscopy is an important diagnostic tool in patients with cough who have risk factors for carcinoma of the lung or radiographic abnormalities that suggest bronchial obstruction. In the absence of these clinical features, bronchoscopy is of questionable value in assessing patients with cough. Before embarking on bronchoscopy, common causes of cough should be painstakingly excluded, reserving bronchoscopy for those with radiographic abnormalities, advanced age, a history of cigarette smoking, and other risk factors for cancer.

Hemoptysis

Hemoptysis remains unexplained in approximately one-fourth of patients who undergo fiberoptic bronchoscopy. In many instances, complete evaluation is performed easily and with negligible risk. At the other extreme, safe and satisfactory examination becomes a major technical accomplishment because visibility is marginal and blood is aspirated into other areas of the tracheobronchial tree. In a few patients, bronchoscopy is a harrowing, hazardous procedure performed as part of an urgent, combined diagnostic and supportive approach to life-threatening hemorrhage.

Lung cancer is found in approximately one-third of patients who undergo bronchoscopic evaluation for hemoptysis, and particularly in those who are more than 40 years of age, who have an abnormal chest radiograph, and who have been bleeding for more than 1 week; anemia, weight loss, and cigarette smoking have also correlated with malignancy. In patients in whom lung cancer proves not to be the cause of the hemoptysis, a cause of bleeding is usually not found, i.e., the bleeding is "essential," "idiopathic," or "cryptogenic."

The etiologic diagnoses most commonly invoked to explain hemoptysis are bronchitis or bronchiectasis. As a rule, these are diagnoses of exclusion, since proof that these conditions are the cause is difficult to obtain by bronchoscopy. Occasionally the diagnosis of bronchiectasis is suggested by airway branching, inflamed mucosa, and purulent secretions seen far beyond the subsegmental level. To verify the diagnosis, radiographic contrast material (either oily Dionosil or water-soluble agents) can be administered either directly through the channel of the fiberoptic bronchoscope or, preferably, via a bronchoscopically introduced catheter. However, bronchiectasis is an uncommon cause of hemoptysis (from 4 to 10 percent) in patients in whom the chest radiograph fails to identify an abnormal area and in whom bronchoscopy is not diagnostic. With respect to bronchiectasis, the principal uses of bronchoscopic bronchography are either to establish the diagnosis or to define the extent of the localized disease that is to be surgically resected.

The optimum timing for bronchoscopy in patients with hemoptysis is unknown. Although prompt localization of the source of bleeding is generally considered to be essential for proper management, it has not been shown that early bronchoscopy either improves morbidity or decreases mortality. It is true that active bleeding and a discrete anatomic cause can often be visualized when bronchoscopy is performed during the initial 24 h. Conversely, acute hemorrhage may obscure vision sufficiently to preclude complete examination, and bleeding may be exacerbated by either removal of formed clot or by paroxysms of coughing evoked by the procedure. Manipulation of endobronchial blood clot is generally ill-advised unless it is causing obstruction of the central airway or inducing life-threatening abnormalities in gas exchange; instead, bronchoscopy should be repeated later, i.e., after the clot has undergone spontaneous resolution. In essence, neither the final diagnosis, overall management, nor clinical outcome of patients may be different in those who undergo early bronchoscopy from those in whom the procedure is delayed until active bleeding has subsided.

In patients with massive or life-threatening hemoptysis the ideal time for bronchoscopy is also debatable except for the consensus that bronchoscopic localization of the bleeding site is mandatory immediately before surgical resection or angiography is undertaken. Unless these interventions are called for, bronchoscopy should probably be deferred. On occasion, this conservative approach may cause a bleeding site to be overlooked. But, as a rule, thorough examination at a later time will identify the source of the massive bleeding. Bronchoscopy in patients with massive bleeding is best done using the rigid instrument since suctioning through the flexible bronchoscope is inadequate. Furthermore, the rigid instrument ensures a patent airway and allows more options for acute management. Using the rigid bronchoscope, the bleeding site can be isolated by a balloon-tipped catheter or a specially designed bronchial blocker by tamponade achieved with gauze or Gelfoam, or by lavage with iced saline. Fiberoptic techniques are sometimes used as temporizing measures. For example, to cope with intraoperative bleeding, endobronchial instillation of epinephrine (1:20,000 dilution) or Gelfoam and occlusion of the affected segment with an inflated balloon-tipped catheter have been used. Although these measures may buy time, particularly when hemorrhage complicates diagnostic bronchoscopy, they do not represent primary therapy for hemoptysis. Recently, laser photocoagulation has been used in selected patients to control hemoptysis.

In approximately 10 percent (from 0 to 27 percent) of patients in whom hemoptysis is associated with either a normal or nonlocalizing chest radiograph, bronchogenic carcinoma is the cause of the hemoptysis; in many of the others, a benign cause of the bleeding can be identified bronchoscopically. Because of the high diagnostic yield of bronchoscopy and its low morbidity, bronchoscopic examination is widely used in the examination of most pa-

tients with hemoptysis in whom symptoms cannot otherwise be explained satisfactorily. Another value of bronchoscopy derives from its negative predictive value when the diagnosis is made of essential, idiopathic, or cryptogenic hemoptysis; long-term follow-up indicates that this diagnosis implies a benign prognosis. Therefore, even a bronchoscopy that fails to pinpoint a cause for hemoptysis may be reassuring.

Bronchoscopy can probably be deferred in young patients (<40 years) with normal chest radiographs in whom the episodes of bleeding have been brief (<1 week in duration) and sporadic, or in patients in whom nonneoplastic causes of bleeding are obviously responsible, e.g., uncomplicated pneumonia and pulmonary embolus with infarction. In patients in whom bleeding is associated with diffuse parenchymal disease or pulmonary-renal syndromes, or in whom hemoptysis is secondary to a coagulopathy, the diagnostic yield of bronchoscopy is low. The demonstration of diffuse tracheobronchial bleeding, gross blood, or hemosiderin-laden macrophages is usually of little value in this setting, and alternative diagnostic procedures provide more useful information.

Unexplained Pulmonary Infiltrates

The evaluation of patients with either acute or chronic infiltrative disease has been strongly abetted by fiberoptic bronchoscopy and transbronchial forceps biopsy. Overall diagnostic yields cited for this procedure vary from clinic to clinic, ranging from 10 percent to 100 percent, and depend on the patient population, the radiographic pattern of the disease, and interpretation of nonspecific histologic findings of inflammation or fibrosis. Some of the conditions in which transbronchial biopsy may establish the diagnosis are listed in Table 32-4. Specific biopsy findings that are diagnostic of tumor, pathogenic microorganisms, or granulomatous inflammation are obtained more frequently by forceps biopsy in patients who have diffuse, multilobar infiltrates. A much lower yield is obtained by forceps biopsy in patients with localized infiltrates, probably because they are commonly caused by pneumonias that are responsible for the nonspecific histologic manifestations. Not surprisingly, the diagnostic yield from biopsies and washings is higher in patients with radiographic patterns and clinical courses suggestive of either tuberculosis or lung cancer than in patients with bacterial pneumonia.

The results of transbronchial forceps biopsy also depend on the prevalence of the specific diseases under consideration, the distribution of the lesions within the lung, i.e., homogeneous versus heterogeneous, the amenability of the lesions to diagnosis from a small histologic specimen, and the proficiency and interest of the pathologist. Multiple biopsies are required because of the minute size of most specimens, but the optimum number of transbron-

TABLE 32-4

Parenchymal Conditions Diagnosed with Transbronchial Forceps Biopsy

Specific Histology*	Nonspecific Histology†
Granulomatous pneumonitis (sarcoidosis, mycobacterial, fungal, foreign body)‡	Bacterial pneumonia
Metastatic, lymphangitic carcinoma‡	Idiopathic interstitial pneumonitis/fibrosis
Opportunistic infection (e.g., pneumocystis)‡	Collagen vascular disease
Viral pneumonia (e.g., cytomegalovirus)	Pneumoconiosis
Lymphoproliferative disease (e.g., lymphoma, lymphocytic interstitial pneumonia)	Allergic alveolitis
Vasculitis (e.g., Wegener's granulomatosis)	Hemosiderosis
Alveolar cell carcinoma	Lipoid pneumonitis
Eosinophilic pneumonia	Drug-induced pneumonitis
Histiocytosis X	Radiation pneumonitis
Pulmonary alveolar proteinosis	Bronchiolitis obliterans
Goodpasture's syndrome	

*Biopsy provides definitive information; impact on patient management usually high.

†Definitive pathologic findings are present occasionally, but diagnoses are often inferred from accompanying clinical information.

‡Common indications for transbronchial biopsy, high diagnostic yield.

chial biopsies is unsettled. In patients with diffuse granulomatous involvement by sarcoidosis, a plateau in the yield from transbronchial forceps biopsy occurs when six specimens have been obtained; at this level, 95 percent of the patients are diagnosed. In contrast, the diagnostic yield is small in patients with interstitial fibrosis that is either primary and idiopathic, or secondary either to systemic disease or drug administration; when one of these disorders is suspected by clinical and radiographic presentation, open lung biopsy is preferable to transbronchial biopsy. Finally, in normal and immunocompromised hosts who manifest either acute or chronic pulmonary infiltrates on the chest radiograph, open lung biopsies have disclosed treatable conditions missed by forceps biopsy.

GRANULOMATOUS DISEASE

Of the granulomatous diseases, sarcoidosis and, to a lesser extent, tuberculosis account for most of the bronchoscopic diagnoses; experience with fungal infections, hypersensitivity pneumonitis, and berylliosis has been much less rewarding.

The diagnostic yield of transbronchial forceps biopsy in sarcoidosis is particularly high, ranging from 50 to 100 percent among clinics. One factor influencing the yield is the "stage" of disease identified radiographically: in stage 1, 50 percent; in stage 2, 90 percent; and in stage 3, 75 percent. Symptoms and pulmonary function tests are less closely correlated. Bronchial biopsy, of either obviously inflamed airways or of apparently normal mucosa, often increases the yield by displaying submucosal granulomata. Transbronchial needle aspiration of a mediastinal lymph node can further improve the yield. The findings of

a mononuclear alveolitis or increased levels of angiotensin converting enzyme in bronchoalveolar lavage fluid are far less specific for sarcoidosis. Finally, bronchoscopy is occasionally useful in detecting upper airway involvement by sarcoidosis or chronic tracheobronchial obstruction related to peribronchial cicatrization, and in the evaluation of a complicating hemoptysis (that in sarcoidosis is usually caused by a mycetoma in a cyst resulting from fibrosis of adjacent parenchyma).

Fiberoptic bronchoscopy and transbronchial forceps biopsy provide diagnostic material in approximately half of patients who are suspected of having tuberculosis on clinical and radiographic grounds but who either lack a productive cough or whose sputum is nondiagnostic. Often bronchoscopy affords the only source of diagnostic material that includes smears, biopsies, brushings, and washings; culture of transbronchial biopsy specimens does not augment the yield appreciably. Bronchoscopy is particularly useful in assessing patients with cavitary or miliary patterns of tuberculous disease.

Nontuberculous mycobacterial infection can also be diagnosed bronchoscopically. Advantage has been taken of this capability in patients with AIDS in whom *Mycobacterium avium-intracellulare* is a devastating pathogen. However, the poorly formed granulomata that occur in AIDS may be more difficult to detect by transbronchial biopsy. Also, interpretation of "atypicals" isolated from bronchoscopic cultures requires close correlation with the patient's clinical course. Routine examination and culture of bronchial washings for mycobacteria are not indicated unless tuberculosis is suspected clinically because of the prevalence of nontuberculous mycobacteria and the likelihood of false-positive isolates.

OPPORTUNISTIC INFECTION

Bronchoscopy has proved useful in the evaluation of non-bacterial pneumonia in immunocompromised hosts by identifying one or more infectious agents either in forceps biopsies, lavage fluid, cytopathology specimens, or culture; the combined yields of forceps biopsy and brushing in immunocompromised patients approximates 50 percent. The detection of *Pneumocystis*, viruses (cytomegalovirus, herpes simplex), mycobacteria, *Nocardia*, and invasive fungi (*Aspergillus*, *Cryptococcus*, *Candida*, *Histoplasma*, *Blastomyces*) has been particularly noteworthy; polymicrobial infections have also been identified. Less often, newly recognized bacterial pathogens have been identified, e.g., *Legionella* species, *Toxoplasma gondii*, *Schistosoma mansoni*, and other parasites. Fifty to one hundred percent of patients with *Pneumocystis* pneumonia can be diagnosed bronchoscopically. This high yield is especially important in oncology and transplant centers where the organism is endemic as well as in patients with AIDS; in the latter, bronchoscopic biopsy and/or lavage is highly diagnostic, often disclosing the organism despite normal chest radiographs.

METASTATIC CARCINOMA

In 50 to 75 percent of patients with metastatic neoplasm presenting with diffuse pulmonary infiltrates, bronchoscopy provides diagnostic information; transbronchial forceps biopsy is more often diagnostic than is bronchial brushing. The diagnostic yield in patients with linear opacities is similar to that of patients with nodular patterns of interstitial disease. Unexpected, endobronchial metastases may be visible even when there is no radiographic evidence of major airway disease; endobronchial metastases are observed with the following frequency: carcinoma of the breast > carcinoma of the colon > carcinoma from a urogenital site > melanoma. When the principal manifestations of metastatic carcinoma are either solitary metastases, multiple nodules and masses, or mediastinal involvement, transbronchial needle aspiration increases the yield. In patients with large metastatic nodules, the diagnostic yield from forceps, brush, and cytopathology is very low (about 5 percent), probably because of the extrabronchial origin of the metastases and the distortion of the tracheobronchial tree by their growth.

INTERSTITIAL PULMONARY FIBROSIS

Transbronchial forceps biopsy is unlikely to provide useful information in patients with interstitial fibrosis. However, it has been found that bronchoalveolar lavage may provide insight into the activity of certain interstitial disorders, e.g., abundant leukocytes signal alveolitis in idiopathic pulmonary fibrosis (Chapter 48) and mononuclear cells indicate activity in sarcoidosis and in hypersensitivity pneumonitis (Chapters 42 and 44). Also, lavage may be useful prognostically: evidence of active alveolitis by lavage correlates with increased cellularity demonstrated by open lung biopsy; lymphocytosis correlates with steroid responsiveness. However, it must be cautioned that, per se, the results of bronchoalveolar lavage do not constitute grounds for either corticosteroid or cytotoxic therapy. Also, further experience is needed to learn if the results of serial lavage will be useful in monitoring the activity of alveolitis in patients with sarcoidosis or interstitial pulmonary fibrosis.

VASCULITIS

Although the diagnoses of Wegener's granulomatosis, lymphomatoid granulomatosis, allergic angiitis (Churg-Strauss syndrome) and nonspecific vasculitis have occasionally been made from transbronchial biopsies, the yield is usually low because of the small size and number of distal vessels that are sampled, and the nonspecificity of the finding of necrosis.

Bacterial Pneumonia

Bronchoscopy has little role in the evaluation and management of most patients with bacterial pneumonia: the endobronchial appearance is nonspecific, and routine bacteriology of specimens obtained through fiberoptic instruments is useless because the bronchoscope has to pass through the contaminated upper airway. Plugged telescoping catheters and protected brushes are being used in a few clinics, but their use requires a dedicated effort not only on the part of the bronchoscopist but also on the part of related services, e.g., microbiology laboratory.

Aspiration Pneumonia and Lung Abscess

Bronchoscopy has little role in aspiration pneumonia unless it is desirable to evaluate the extent of airway injury following aspiration of gastric contents or if the chest radiograph suggests that airway obstruction has occurred. "Therapeutic lavage" is useless, and bronchoscopy to remove food particles is generally unnecessary.

In lung abscess, as in bacterial pneumonia, bronchoscopy usually has little to offer. On occasion, however, it may be useful, e.g., when distinguishing a putrid lung abscess from other cavitary lung disorders (particularly bronchogenic carcinoma or tuberculosis), when an abscess is in an unusual site (e.g., a nondependent location), if there is no apparent predisposition to abscess, or if the course is complicated by hemoptysis. The usual endobronchial findings of edema, erythema, and purulent secretions are nonspecific. Morever, the need for reliable anaerobic cultures constitutes an inordinate demand on some bacteriologic laboratories.

Bronchoscopy may occasionally play a role in identifying a proximal, endobronchial mass or an aspirated foreign body that may be responsible for the localization of the abscess at a given anatomic site. Although rigid bronchoscopy has been done in the therapeutic attempt to drain a cavity or to instill antimicrobials, the efficacy of efforts along this line is questionable, particularly if an air-fluid level is present, indicating that communication with the tracheobronchial tree already exists and that no further benefit is to be expected from the procedure. If conversion to a closed cavity should occur spontaneously, then rigid bronchoscopy might become necessary to effect drainage or to look for hemorrhage, a complication that engenders a particularly high risk. Otherwise, even a carefully performed bronchoscopic examination entails the danger of mechanical trauma to the inflamed airway; worsening of local edema might then convert a draining cavity into a nondraining, "closed" cavity. Also, if an abscess cavity is entered, there is a major risk of "drowning" the patient in his or her own pus.

Acute Airway Injury

Bronchoscopy has a major role in the early assessment of patients with thoracic trauma and acute injury to the trachea or larynx. For example, fracture of the tracheobronchial tree has to be considered in the presence of posttraumatic hemoptysis, mediastinal emphysema, pneumothorax, and/or major atelectasis; bronchoscopy establishes and localizes the site of damage to the airway. Bronchoscopy is also helpful in defining the location and extent of respiratory tract injury in patients who have inhaled smoke and other irritant gases; at burn centers, fiberoptic bronchoscopy and nasopharyngoscopy have become central procedures in the evaluation of thermal and inhalation injury; because clinical criteria are often inaccurate, per se, in deciding if the upper airway has been seriously injured, visualization of the upper airway is essential for assessing the need for endotracheal intubation. Carbonaceous secretions are a nonspecific finding, but the detection of tracheobronchial inflammation promotes the recognition of patients who are at risk for delayed-onset pulmonary complications of smoke. After airway injury, fiberoptic bronchoscopy is also useful in evaluating late sequelae of intubation or tracheostomy.

Other Diagnostic Applications

Fiberoptic bronchoscopy performed during sleep has helped to clarify the nature of the repetitive upper airway occlusions of patients with obstructive sleep apnea. The procedure has been well tolerated and, together with fiberoptic nasopharyngoscopy, is sometimes useful clinically in the preoperative evaluation of candidates for surgical treatment.

Other Endoscopic Procedures

Both fiberoptic and rigid instruments have been introduced into the pleural space, and thoracoscopy is an important diagnostic option for assessment of patients with unexplained exudative pleural effusions. During thoracoscopy, the visceral and parietal pleural surfaces can be examined directly. Pleural nodules or other localized abnormalities can be biopsied with forceps, adhesions lysed, and bleeding sites cauterized. A chest tube and a controlled degree of pneumothorax are part of the procedure, but both are well tolerated by most patients, and complications are uncommon. In addition to evaluation and biopsy of pleural abnormalities, large-forceps biopsies of the lung have been performed via thoracoscopy, with little morbidity, both in adults and in children with unexplained pulmonary infiltrates. The avoidance of airway manipulation, the larger forceps accommodated by the thoracoscope, and the direct selection of grossly abnormal appearing lung for a biopsy site have been cited as advantages of this technique. Angioscopy is another fiberoptic procedure that has been used recently in a few patients with chronic pulmonary vascular disease. A clinical role for this procedure has not yet been established.

THERAPEUTIC INDICATIONS

Most therapeutic bronchoscopies (Table 32-3) involve treatment of acute and chronic obstruction of major airways and are managed optimally by using a ventilating bronchoscope. Among the indications are removing foreign bodies, maintaining patency of the airways during massive hemoptysis or overwhelming retention of secretions, and clearing of benign and malignant central tumors. Discrete, well localized, benign neoplasms can occasionally be removed in their entirety. The rigid instrument may also be used to dilate tracheal strictures. Subglottic stenosis has been treated bronchoscopically by surgical removal of granulation tissue and/or injection of corticosteroids. These traditional roles of bronchoscopy in the surgical treatment of endobronchial disease have recently been greatly enlarged by advances in laser technology. In addition, but far less commonly, bronchoscopy is used to administer antimicrobial agents or chemotherapeutic drugs, or to drain a peribronchial fluid collection.

Foreign Body Removal

Removal of foreign bodies remains the most important therapeutic application of bronchoscopy. Although grasping forceps, snares, and baskets have been designed for use with the fiberoptic bronchoscope, as a rule the rigid instrument is preferred for foreign body removal because of the control of the airways that it allows. The bronchoscopist must be familiar with the safest approaches to handling a variety of foreign bodies if certain risks are to be avoided: complete airway occlusion, particularly at the glottic or subglottic levels; migration or fragmentation of objects to more peripheral and inaccessible sites; direct airway trauma, e.g., laceration by an aspirated pin. In anticipation of removing foreign bodies, the bronchoscopist must be aware of the diverse accessories and grasping techniques and how their use is influenced by the shape of the object, its presenting position, and the "forceps space" available for instrument insertion. When the size or shape of an object is particularly unusual, rehearsal of the procedure by retrieving similar foreign bodies from models of the tracheobronchial tree and from animals may be essential for success in the patient. Not infrequently, removal of a foreign body is complicated by its association with edematous, friable, granulation tissue, a problem that is especially common with organic foreign bodies, or with sharp objects that have penetrated the tracheobronchial wall. Specialized grasping forceps, snares, balloon-tipped catheters, and magnets may be essential, and particular attention must be paid to the orientation of the foreign body with respect to the largest diameter of the airway. In general, the approach includes grasping the presenting part of the foreign body, moving it into the trachea, and rotating it so that its greater diameter is in a sagittal plane. By using the rigid bronchoscope as a sheath, the wall of the airway can be protected from injury by pointed objects.

Pulmonary Toilet

The most common therapeutic indication for fiberoptic bronchoscopy is for pulmonary toilet. In the intensive-care setting, bronchoscopy is commonly used to clear inspissated secretions in patients with atelectasis; indeed, it may be overused for this indication. In the intubated, postoperative patient, bronchoscopy is technically easy and elicits little morbidity, but it has not been shown that bronchoscopy has advantage over conventional respiratory therapy. Therapeutic bronchoscopy should be reserved for patients with lobar atelectasis in whom either conservative measures have been ineffective, or gas-exchange abnormalities or overall fragility require immediate clearing of the airway. Occasionally, reexpansion of atelectatic lung has been effected by insufflating air through balloon catheters introduced via a bronchoscope. When atelectasis follows lung resection, bronchoscopy provides both therapy and assessment of the integrity of a surgical anastomosis or bronchial stump.

Bronchoscopic removal of secretions may be facilitated by saline lavage or local instillation of mucolytic agents; N-acetylcysteine (Mucomyst) is most popular. Bronchoscopy coupled with lavage was once used routinely for removal of inspissated secretions in patients with chronic obstructive airways diseases; at present, this procedure is reserved for selected patients who require mechanical ventilation for acute exacerbations of airways disease. Bronchoalveolar lavage has been performed safely for investigative purposes in patients with asthma; also, selected patients with asthma and cystic fibrosis have undergone uncomplicated therapeutic lavage.

Endotracheal Intubation

Fiberoptic bronchoscopy has another important therapeutic application in the management of patients in the intensive-care setting. Intubation that is technically difficult, in patients who have cervical spine injuries, severe facial trauma, trismus, massive upper airway edema, cerebrovascular disease that might limit cervical extension, or aneurysms of the thoracic aorta, can be facilitated by the fiberoptic bronchoscope. On occasion, intubation is performed while the glottis is visualized through the bronchoscope; more often, the bronchoscope is used as a stylet over which the endotracheal tube is guided into the trachea. Use of this technique has averted tracheostomy in patients with upper airway obstruction. Bronchoscopy is also useful in ensuring that an endotracheal tube is properly positioned, in determining if a tube is working properly, e.g., to detect obstruction by encrusted secretions or overinflation of a balloon cuff, or in looking for complications of chronic intubation, e.g., tracheoesophageal fistula, tracheomalacia, or subglottic stenosis, after the patient has been extubated.

Laser Bronchoscopy

The most common usage of lasers with respect to the airways is to relieve obstruction of a central airway by a neoplasm. Because some lasers emit light energy that has both cutting and coagulating properties, it has become possible, via a bronchoscope, to resect portions of a tumor from a central airway more safely than could be done before lasers were introduced for this purpose. Moreover, benign lesions that obstruct the subglottic larynx or trachea, e.g., stenosis and granulomas, can be removed through the bronchoscope using a laser, thereby avoiding the need for an extensive surgical procedure to improve patency of the airway.

Several different types of lasers are available for bronchoscopic use. Each has a unique interaction with tissue and is applied under different circumstances. The major characteristics of each type of laser are outlined in Table 32-5. The carbon dioxide laser is the most precise cutting instrument. Because its wavelength is absorbed almost completely by water, this laser does not penetrate more than 0.1 mm into tissue. At present there are no fiberoptic delivery systems that can transmit carbon dioxide laser light through flexible bronchoscopes. Thus, resection of

TABLE 32-5
Lasers Used with Bronchoscopes

Type	Wavelength, nm	Depth of Penetration, mm	Principle Action	Bronchoscope System
CO_2	10,600	0.1	Cutting	Rigid
YAG	1,600	4	Coagulation; vaporization and shrinkage of tissue	Rigid or flexible
Tunable dye	630	1–2	Excites hematoporphyrin; causes cell necrosis	Flexible
Argon	405	1	Coagulation; causes fluorescence of hematoporphyrins for detection of small neoplasms	Flexible

airway lesions with these lasers requires rigid bronchoscopy. A special coupler for the carbon dioxide is attached to the ventilating bronchoscope and a helium-neon aiming laser is used to direct the carbon dioxide laser accurately to its target. The coupler has a joystick that is used to manipulate the mirrors and to pinpoint the laser light. The tumor mass or fibrous, stenotic lesions can be cut away from the tracheobronchial wall and large pieces of tissue removed with forceps. Although the rapid resection of such abnormal tissue is possible, the requirement that a rigid bronchoscope be used limits carbon dioxide laser application to the larynx, trachea, and main-stem bronchi. Furthermore, since the carbon dioxide laser photocoagulates only the smallest of blood vessels, there remains a moderate chance of bleeding during resection of vascular tumors.

Early in the 1980s the neodymium-yttrium-aluminum-garnet laser (YAG laser) was introduced for the management of obstructing lesions of the central airways. For most tissues, this instrument has the deepest penetrating power; it is also a more effective photocoagulating tool than the carbon dioxide laser. The YAG laser wavelength is delivered routinely through a flexible quartz fiber. Because it can be used in conjunction with a flexible bronchoscope, the YAG laser has become the most popular wavelength for pulmonary endoscopists, many of whom have not been trained to use an open, ventilating (rigid) bronchoscope. As experience accumulates with the use of the YAG laser worldwide, most bronchoscopists are turning to the rigid bronchoscopic approach because obstructing lesions are more readily removed. Furthermore, even though the YAG laser has better coagulation properties than does the carbon dioxide laser, the possibility of bleeding complications is not negligible.

Criteria for treatment with the carbon dioxide and YAG lasers vary somewhat from clinic to clinic. Dyspnea is the cardinal symptom for which laser photoresection is offered. Also, on occasion, a YAG laser can be useful in controlling bleeding from superficial vessels of an intraluminal tumor. The response of malignant tumors to laser treatment appears to be more favorable in patients with intraluminal lesions that involve a fairly short axial segment of the airway; ideally, at least a portion of the airway lumen should be visible beyond the site of obstruction. Conversely, patients who have predominantly extrinsic compression, long obstructed segments, or complete airway occlusion are less suitable candidates for laser therapy. Superficially bleeding vessels of an intraluminal tumor may be controlled in some instances with a YAG laser.

The use of hematoporphyrins in conjunction with lasers for the early diagnosis and treatment of some patients with malignancies is being investigated in a few medical centers. Hematoporphyrin derivative, a crude chemical made from the laboratory processing of ordinary hemoglobin, is distributed widely throughout the body after intravenous administration. Although much of this material is cleared quickly, it is cleared more slowly, and may even be concentrated, in rapidly proliferating tissues, including neoplasms. An argon laser that emits blue-green light can be used to excite hematoporphyrin and cause it to fluoresce. Special detection systems used with a bronchoscope can detect one peak of fluorescence at 630 nm (in the red spectrum), and this signal can be amplified, either as a visual or as an auditory signal. This system permits detection of occult carcinomas that cannot be recognized grossly. Brushings and biopsies directed at areas of enhanced signals can help to localize a malignancy at a very early stage, increasing the possibility of curative treatment.

Another aspect of laser bronchoscopy under investigation involves the induction of photosensitization for the sake of therapy: if the same hematoporphyrins are excited by light that is synchronous with its 630-nm peak, toxic oxygen radicals, especially singlet oxygen, are produced within the cytoplasm and can lead to cell necrosis. A tunable dye laser that is pumped by an argon laser has proved to be capable of emitting light of the proper wavelength for this purpose. But problems remain in adapting this type of therapy for the treatment of carcinoma: photosensitization therapy does not ablate neoplastic cells in peribronchial lymph nodes, and it may also cause tissue to slough to the point of producing serious airway hemorrhage and asphyxia. Moreover, the hematoporphyrins produce skin photosensitization so that exposure to direct sunlight must usually be avoided for approximately 1 month after therapy.

Although few patients have been treated with these new approaches, symptomatic benefit and improved functional status have been dramatic in some instances. Despite these encouraging results, the ultimate role of this therapy is still to be defined. Currently these bronchoscopic procedures are used primarily for palliation in patients with critical airway obstruction, in most of whom carcinoma has recurred following radiation therapy, e.g., as temporizing maneuvers to buy time for subsequent radiation in conjunction with brachytherapy (implanted radioactive sources). In addition, laser therapy offers a therapeutic alternative in certain patients who do not qualify for surgical resection. Whether this modality represents a realistic alternative to surgery for the patient who has a small, well-localized endobronchial neoplasm requires further study. For benign, obstructing lesions that are less than 1 to 2 cm long, laser photoresection may be a suitable alternative to conventional surgical methods.

Future Directions

Other therapeutic uses of bronchoscopy are being explored patient by patient. For example, the direct, endobronchial instillation of chemotherapeutic agents or immunologic modulators, e.g., Bacille bilié de Calmette-Guérin (BCG), is being used for the local treatment of carcinoma of the lung. In major tumors of the airway, radioactive sources, e.g., encapsulated radium, radon seeds, have been introduced into predetermined sites via the rigid bronchoscope to target local radiotherapy; more recently, flexible injection systems and specially adapted needles have been used to implant gold 198 or iodine 125 seeds into such lesions using large-channel fiberoptic instruments. The combined use of this brachytherapy and laser photocoagulation is being evaluated at several medical centers. Another form of bronchoscopic radiation therapy of bronchogenic carcinoma entails temporary placement of another radioisotope, iridium 192, into catheters that have been slipped through airways that are markedly narrowed.

COMPLICATIONS OF BRONCHOSCOPY

Jackson observed that "The watchword of the bronchoscopist should be 'If I can do no good, I will at least do no harm.'" This dictum remains the guidepost for the modern endoscopist. The relative risks of bronchoscopy must be appraised thoroughly in each patient, and weighted in the balance with the goals of the procedure

and the manner in which information that is obtained will influence management. There are few absolute contraindications to bronchoscopy. However, one noteworthy contraindication is the performance of bronchoscopy under local anesthesia in an uncooperative patient: in this circumstance, the likelihood of mechanical airway trauma is strong, comprehensive examination is not feasible, and risks of biopsy are prohibitive. Also, hazards of therapeutic bronchoscopy are usually increased. Adequate preoperative preparation is prerequisite for safe bronchoscopy.

Major complications occur in only 0.08 to 1.7 percent of fiberoptic bronchoscopy procedures. The patterns and frequencies of problems are similar in referral centers and community hospitals; most often they relate to preoperative medications and anesthesia, cardiopulmonary dysfunction, technical difficulties during bronchoscopy, and biopsy procedures (Table 32-6). Air embolism, fatal pneumonia, meningitis, and sepsis are unusual. High-risk subgroups of patients are readily identifiable, and potential hazards of bronchoscopy are usually obvious preoperatively. Fatalities are rare, occurring in 0.01 to 0.1 percent of fiberoptic bronchoscopies. As a rule, they relate to underlying cardiopulmonary disease, hypoxemia, and the overall debilitated status of the patient. Accordingly, elective bronchoscopy should be avoided until reversible risk factors have been eliminated or minimized. In high-risk patients, the study should be modified to obtain only information that is essential for management.

If bronchoscopy must be performed in a high-risk patient, the duration of the procedure should be limited, the

TABLE 32-6
Complications of Bronchoscopy

Premedication and anesthetics	Respiratory depression*
	Hyperexcitement
	Laryngospasm,* bronchospasm
	Seizures
	Hypotension, syncope
	Cardiorespiratory arrest
Technical problems	Airway or vascular trauma (e.g., perforation, bleeding)
	Instrument breakage
	Fire
Adverse effects of procedure	Upper airway (edema, laryngospasm)*
	Bronchospasm*
	Hypoxemia*
	Cardiac arrhythmia
	Fever
	Pneumonia (bacterial, mycobacterial)
	Bacteremia
Effects of instrumentation or biopsy	Hemorrhage*
	Mediastinal emphysema
	Pneumothorax*
	Pulmonary infiltrates*
	Air embolism

*Commonly encountered.

degree of instrumentation should be minimized, and the supportive environment should be adjusted to the patient's clinical status. Should bronchoscopy be poorly tolerated or a complication develop, it is usually advisable to discontinue the procedure unless completion is essential to urgent management. Following stabilization of the patient, the indications for bronchoscopy are reappraised and the specific problems encountered are reviewed. If bronchoscopy remains necessary, preoperative preparations and the operative approach are modified insofar as possible to minimize the likelihood of a recurrence.

Complications of Premedications and Anesthetics

The risks and complications of general anesthesia are similar to those associated with other surgical procedures. Most problems with local anesthesia can be avoided by observing a few basic principles. All medications must be administered cautiously, and their dosages individualized. The use of short-acting preparations that can be reversed readily in the event of adverse effects is preferable. Possible interactions with other medications that the patient may receive must be kept in mind and studiously avoided. Furthermore, in fragile individuals, the potential for respiratory depression or hemodynamic collapse makes it prudent to use minimal doses of medication. Often, the patient can be readily titrated with the agent during the procedure. Seizures related to lidocaine have occurred in elderly patients or in those with hepatic dysfunction, but they are unusual when the agent is prepared just before the procedure, the total dosage is less than 300 mg, and its administration during the procedure is closely monitored. Tetracaine for local anesthesia is avoided by most bronchoscopists because of the threat of arrhythmias.

Technical Problems

Technical difficulties during bronchoscopy relate to trauma of a major airway, lung injury, and instrument breakage; they can usually be minimized by sound operative methods. Central airway perforation that leads to pneumomediastinum, pneumothorax, and/or hemorrhage from vascular injury can complicate forceful use of the rigid bronchoscope. Breakage of forceps, brushes, and needles can be lessened by careful handling of these instruments, avoidance of force during their passage into the bronchoscope and airway, and observation of manufacturers' guidelines regarding the numbers of procedures advised for nondisposable accessories. Skill in removing foreign bodies is helpful in dealing with unexpected breakage of a brush or needle. Routine examination and maintenance of instruments, and prompt repair or disposal of damaged instruments are important preventive measures.

Newer applications of bronchoscopy entail potential problems that must be anticipated and avoided. Fever, bronchospasm, bleeding, transient pulmonary infiltrates, and pneumonia have followed bronchoalveolar lavage in healthy volunteers, but these complications are unusual (<5 percent). Laser procedures have been complicated by massive hemorrhage and asphyxiation, local edema that causes life-threatening airway occlusion and, occasionally, endobronchial fires caused by pyrolysis of endotracheal tubes and outer sheaths of fiberoptic instruments. The incidence of these problems has decreased as understanding of laser technique has improved, and patients have been selected more carefully. Ignition of the tips of quartz laser fibers has occurred due to accumulations of blood or mucus; cleaning of the instrument and monitoring of the inspired oxygen concentration have helped to avoid this problem.

Complications of Biopsy

BLEEDING

Bleeding from endobronchial biopsy is usually minor, i.e., <50 ml, and self-limited, neither requiring specific therapy nor limiting the procedure. However, the possibility always exists of severe hemorrhage and of associated aspiration or major airway obstruction. Hemorrhage may be life-threatening in patients with quantitative or qualitative coagulation disorders. Caution along these lines must be even greater if severe underlying airways disease compromises the ability of the patient to clear the airways of blood or if the anatomy of a lesion increases the prospect that bleeding will occur. The selection of a biopsy technique should depend not only on the apparent vascularity of a lesion but also on its anatomic position and the likelihood that major airway obstruction will follow even a minor hemorrhage. In fragile patients with large, proximal tumors, it is sometimes advisable to defer biopsy until other results of bronchoscopy become available. Fine-needle aspiration of endobronchial lesions provides diagnostic information with little risk; moreover, transbronchial needle aspiration of mediastinal tumors has not been complicated by bleeding. Indeed, inadvertent puncture of the aorta or pulmonary artery has not caused imposing endobronchial or mediastinal hemorrhage, probably because of the elasticity of these structures and the small size of the needles.

About 20 percent of patients who either have hematologic disorders or are receiving cytotoxic chemotherapy bleed inordinately after transbronchial biopsy; this complication is far less common in patients with normal coagulation status. Based on experience with other biopsy procedures, relative contraindications for forceps biopsy have been established arbitrarily. Among the reasonable criteria for exclusion that have been adopted are a prolonged prothrombin time, e.g., 60 percent of the control value, thrombocytopenia, i.e., a platelet count of <50,000 to 100,000 per cubic millimeter, and a prolonged bleeding time, i.e., >15 s. In thrombocytopenic patients, bronchial biopsy and brushing have been associated recently with a low (4 percent) incidence of bleeding; the extent to which the administration of platelets immediately before, and during, bronchoscopy can decrease this low incidence further is unsettled. When thrombocytopenia is pronounced, i.e., of the order of 10,000 to 20,000 platelets per cubic millimeter, careful brushing rather than forceps biopsy is advisable; only lavage should be performed if the platelet count is below this range. Fatal hemorrhage has followed transbronchial biopsy in patients with uremia and associated coagulopathy; these patients seem to present unique hazards so that bleeding occurs in almost half of those subjected to biopsy. When biopsy is required in this population, timing of bronchoscopy should be coordinated with dialysis in the attempt to reduce qualitative coagulation abnormalities.

When transbronchial lung biopsy is planned in a patient with an underlying coagulopathy, it is often worthwhile to insert an endotracheal tube prophylactically, i.e., before bronchoscopy, rather than to attempt a transnasal approach. For unknown reasons, bleeding after transbronchial biopsy occurs more often (20 percent) in elderly patients. The risk of hemorrhage also seems to be increased in patients with pulmonary hypertension.

PNEUMOTHORAX

Pneumothorax complicates approximately 5 percent of transbronchial forceps biopsy procedures, whereas pneumothorax or pneumomediastinum rarely (<1 percent) follows transbronchial needle aspiration. Although up to half of patients who develop a pneumothorax require a chest tube, many can be managed conservatively. In patients with widespread disease, transbronchial biopsy has been performed safely, without fluoroscopy, by experienced bronchoscopists. But, as a rule, fluoroscopic guidance seems advisable to direct the forceps away from the visceral pleura. Fluoroscopic guidance is mandatory for accurate positioning of biopsy forceps within focal, peripheral infiltrates and nodules: biplane fluoroscopy units are best suited for this purpose.

The periphery of the lung and zones that border on fissures should be avoided during transbronchial biopsy because of their proximity to the pleural surface. Similarly, the middle lobe is generally avoided in patients with diffuse disease because of the added risk presented by the minor fissure. Although the risk of pneumothorax would be expected to increase as the number of forceps biopsies increased, up to a dozen specimens have been obtained in some patients without adverse sequelae. The

presence of pleuritic chest pain during biopsy sometimes signals a pneumothorax, but this symptom is not invariable. Fluoroscopy immediately after biopsy is useful to exclude pneumothorax or local bleeding. Most pneumothoraxes are evident at the time of the procedure, but occasionally this complication may be delayed in onset. A chest radiograph is generally taken after transbronchial forceps biopsy. Other postbronchoscopy studies have a low yield and are not done routinely.

It is reasonable to expect, but it has not been proved, that the status of the pulmonary parenchyma influences the likelihood of pneumothorax. The relative risk of pneumothorax is probably increased in patients with emphysema, localized cystic diseases, or interstitial fibrosis associated with honeycombing. When cavitary lesions are approached, biopsy of the wall rather than the center of the lesion not only promises a higher yield, but also entails less risk of pneumothorax; in our experience, pneumothorax more often follows biopsy in patients with infiltrative disease than in those with peripheral nodules; abnormal pulmonary parenchyma probably predisposes to this complication. As a rule, transbronchial biopsy should not be performed bilaterally during the same procedure; moreover, it should be avoided, if possible, in patients treated with mechanical ventilation and/or positive end-expiratory pressure. In the latter groups, useful information may be obtained safely from bronchial brushings and washings.

Upper Airway Injury

Glottic and subglottic edema may follow rigid bronchoscopy, particularly if the procedure is prolonged. It is usually evident immediately after bronchoscopy. The problem can be avoided by selecting an instrument that is appropriate in size for the patient, by keeping the bronchoscopic examination brief, and by manipulating the airway gently.

The same principles apply to fiberoptic bronchoscopy. Should evidence of upper airway obstruction develop during local anesthesia or after the flexible bronchoscope has been introduced, the procedure should be promptly discontinued. If symptoms do not resolve, aerosolized racemic epinephrine, humidification and, on occasion, topical corticosteroids can be helpful. If the obstruction gets worse, prompt intubation is necessary; it may be achievable only with the aid of the bronchoscope.

Endoscopy in patients with known upper airway disease demands caution and experience. Bronchoscopy, including the use of the fiberoptic instrument, can be performed safely in evaluating and maintaining an open airway in patients with either epiglottis, upper airway, and tracheobronchial injuries secondary to thermal injury or superior vena caval obstruction. But, as a rule, the fiberoptic bronchoscope should not be used to traverse an obstruction in the proximal airway even if it means missing opportunity to diagnose obvious distal airway disease.

Pulmonary Dysfunction

Airway manipulation is apt to be hazardous in patients with unstable obstructive pulmonary disease: mechanical stimulation of airway receptors by either the topical anesthetic or the bronchoscope can induce laryngospasm and/or bronchospasm. An increase in the functional residual capacity during fiberoptic bronchoscopy implies an increase in airway resistance during the procedure. Should this situation arise, the administration pre- and postoperatively of bronchodilators, including atropine, parenterally and by aerosol, appears to lessen the likelihood of acute ventilatory failure; these agents and corticosteroids can be added to lavage fluid. Should bronchoscopy become mandatory in the hypercarbic patient, prophylactic endotracheal intubation and the immediate availability of mechanical ventilation are essential preoperative preparations.

Introduction of the bronchoscope, per se, into the airway causes arterial P_{O_2} to fall by 10 to 20 mmHg. In the course of an uneventful procedure, this drop in arterial P_{O_2} may be worsened considerably by the suctioning or washing that is part of the regular bronchoscopic examination. As a result, arterial hypoxemia is often more severe *after* bronchoscopy than it is during the procedure. In patients with normal cardiopulmonary function, the hypoxemia is usually tolerated well. But, even an abbreviated procedure may jeopardize those in whom pulmonary function is marginal. Moreover, patients with limited pulmonary reserve would be expected to tolerate poorly the other complications of bronchoscopy. Supplemental oxygen can be administered during, and after, bronchoscopy via nasal prongs or a variety of mask systems; it is advisable during most elective procedures and mandatory if the baseline arterial P_{O_2} is less than 70 mmHg or if extensive or prolonged instrumentation of the airway is planned. In high-risk patients, the level of arterial oxygenation can be monitored noninvasively during bronchoscopy by using ear or finger pulse oximetry to determine arterial O_2 saturation. When bronchoscopy is performed in the mechanically ventilated patient, 100 percent oxygen is administered during the procedure via a T-tube adaptor.

In the critically ill, intubated patient, the untoward effects of suctioning and airway obstruction by the bronchoscope can be minimized by brief, "in and out" procedures; the fiberoptic instrument is alternately inserted to achieve part of the examination and removed for a brief rest interval that enables the patient to be better oxygenated and ventilated. This process is repeated several times until the diagnostic or therapeutic maneuvers are completed.

Cardiovascular Complications

Atrial and ventricular cardiac arrhythmias sometimes complicate bronchoscopy; they are usually transient and occur in approximately 5 percent of elderly patients. It appears that the major risk factor for arrhythmia in these patients is unrecognized hypoxemia that is due either to premedication or passage of the instrument. Although bronchoscopy usually does not exacerbate preexisting rhythm disturbances, routine cardiac monitoring is advisable in the elderly or in patients with previously recognized cardiovascular disease. The major hemodynamic effects of bronchoscopy occur during administration of topical anesthesia, passage through the larynx, and suctioning. Invasive monitoring has confirmed that heart rate, mean arterial and pulmonary capillary wedge pressures, and cardiac index increase during these periods. In patients who have experienced recent myocardial infarction, there is no particular "safe" period beyond which fiberoptic bronchoscopy can be safely performed using local anesthesia. In these patients, the goals of the procedure and the therapeutic implications of its results are the major determinants of whether the risk of bronchoscopy is excessive.

Infection

Low-grade fever occurs in up to 16 percent of bronchoscopies; the manipulation of endobronchial tumors seems to predispose to fever. How often bacterial pneumonia occurs after bronchoscopy is uncertain, but it seems to be uncommon except in the elderly. Ambiguity in interpreting postbronchoscopic radiographic infiltrates is introduced by the possibility that they may represent atelectasis, aspiration, or bleeding that occurred during the procedure, as well as pneumonia. Immunocompromised patients do not appear to be at increased risk for postbronchoscopic infection.

Rigid bronchoscopy is not uncommonly associated with bacteremia (of the order of 33 percent); in contrast, bacteremia occurs infrequently (<2 percent) during fiberoptic bronchoscopy. Patients with valvular heart disease or prosthetic heart valves should probably receive antibiotic prophylaxis for bronchoscopy.

On occasion, inadequate cleansing of bronchoscopy equipment has resulted in outbreaks of nosocomial pneumonia caused by aerobic gram-negative bacilli. The use of iodophor compounds for the disinfection of fiberoptic instruments was responsible for some of these outbreaks; glutaraldehyde (Cidex) has proved more effective for sterilization. The rigid instrument can be sterilized readily, whereas fiberoptic instruments can be damaged by heat or gas sterilization using ethylene oxide at temperatures exceeding 55° C. On occasion, instruments and local anesthetics have been contaminated by nontuberculous mycobacteria; transmission of tuberculosis by bronchoscopy has also occurred.

Repeat Bronchoscopy

Because of the low morbidity of bronchoscopy, repetition of diagnostic and therapeutic procedures is well tolerated. Serial examination of patients who have undergone local treatment to the airway, e.g., laser photocoagulation, is often essential to management; "cleanup" bronchoscopies are sometimes required to remove necrotic material after laser surgery. In occasional instances, therapeutic procedures are "staged," using several sessions. Serial fiberoptic bronchoscopy has also been used to monitor the effectiveness of therapy, i.e., of combined chemotherapeutic and radiotherapeutic regimens in small cell carcinoma of the lung and radiation therapy in non-small cell neoplasms. Mucosal desquamation occurs after rigid bronchoscopy, but no residual damage has been found after fiberoptic bronchoscopy. Sites of mucosal biopsy generally heal within days.

Operator Risks

There is little information about the risks of bronchoscopy to the endoscopist. Patients with tuberculosis that has been treated with antimycobacterial agents should pose little hazard. The possibility of transmission of infectious hepatitis or AIDS has led to the recommendation that masks, gowns, and protective goggles be used in performing bronchoscopy on these patients. In addition, extra caution has been advised in the labeling, packaging, and handling of diagnostic specimens and in the sterilization of bronchoscopes and accessory instruments. Other safeguards for bronchoscopists include the monitoring of radiation exposure for those who perform fluoroscopically guided biopsies or apply brachytherapy, the wearing of appropriate shielding during these procedures, the use of eye protection during laser studies, and the avoidance of possible electrical hazards during laser and electrocautery procedures.

DECISION-MAKING WITH BRONCHOSCOPY

Bronchoscopy is a clinically important, relatively noninvasive procedure that is used widely in patients with respiratory disease. Bronchoscopy can be performed even in potentially high risk situations with an acceptably low morbidity; its diagnostic and therapeutic benefits are often immediate. However, neither the procedure nor the

information it may provide represent ends in themselves. Decisions concerning the use of bronchoscopy should take into account the risks and benefits of the procedure; this type of analysis is even more important for those in whom relative contraindications exist for the procedure. Some considerations, including the recognition of low-yield and high-risk situations, are summarized in Table 32-7.

Each study must be tailored to the needs of the individual patient. The objectives of bronchoscopy in the child who has aspirated a peanut differ considerably from those in an adult with postoperative atelectasis, hemoptysis despite normal chest radiographs, or an obvious mediastinal mass. One element of a complete diagnostic procedure might be contraindicated, whereas other aspects of bronchoscopy might be performed quite safely. For example, although transbronchial forceps biopsy in an immunocompromised patient with infiltrative disease might be precluded because of coagulopathy, it still might be safe

TABLE 32-7
Considerations in Clinical Use of Bronchoscopy

High-yield situations*
  Hemoptysis, abnormal chest radiographs
  Central tumors
  Major atelectasis
  Large peripheral nodules
  Diffuse infiltrates, suspected sarcoidosis, or pneumocystis
  Foreign body aspiration
Low-yield situations†
  Cough/hemoptysis, normal chest radiograph
  Small peripheral nodule
  Diffuse infiltrates, suspected interstitial fibrosis
  Localized infiltrates, suspected bacterial pneumonia
  Isolated pleural effusion
High-risk situations
  Major airway disease (e.g., foreign body, massive hemoptysis, proximal tumor)
  Endobronchial therapeutic procedures
  Relative contraindications present:

A. General	B. Biopsy procedures
Uncooperative patient	Coagulopathy (secondary
Uncontrolled obstructive	to hepatic, hematologic,
airways disease	or neoplastic disease,
Hypoxemia	uremia, drugs)
Alveolar hypoventilation	Emphysema, severe
Cardiovascular in-	cystic disease
stability:	Pulmonary fibrosis
cardiac arrhythmia,	Pulmonary hypertension
coronary artery disease,	Mechanical ventilation
recent myocardial	Positive end-expiratory
infarction, systemic	pressure (PEEP)
hypotension, severe	
anemia	
Obtunded patient	

*Benefits of bronchoscopy and impact on patient management usually high.

†Bronchoscopy potentially helpful, but yield low, and both benefit and impact of procedure usually low.

to perform the bronchoscopy and to obtain potentially valuable information by careful bronchoalveolar lavage and brushing. The extent of bronchoscopic examination should be limited according to the clinical status of the patient; its duration should be abbreviated in particularly fragile individuals. A brief, but complete survey of the tracheobronchial tree is possible in most patients. However, on occasion, it may be advisable to settle for a unilateral examination that emphasizes previously identified, local abnormalities.

BIBLIOGRAPHY

Anderson HA, Faber LP (eds): Diagnostic and therapeutic applications of the bronchoscope. Chest 73(suppl):685–778, 1978.
Collected papers from a symposium on bronchoscopy provide an overview of applications of the fiberoptic instrument.

Brutinel WM, Cortese DA, McDougall JC, Gillio RG, Bergstralh EJ: A two-year experience with the neodymium-YAG laser in endobronchial obstruction. Chest 91:159–165, 1987.
Using the flexible fiberoptic bronchoscope with lower laser power settings, neodymium-yttrium-aluminum-garnet (Nd:YAG) therapy proved to be a safe and effective means of relieving airway obstruction in the great majority of patients with obstructive lung cancer.

Fulmer JD: Bronchoalveolar lavage. Am Rev Respir Dis 126:961–963, 1982.
An objective appraisal of the research application of this technique and its current clinical limitations.

Golden JA, Hollander H, Stulbarg MS, Gamsu G: Bronchoalveolar lavage as the exclusive diagnostic modality for *Pneumocystis carinii* pneumonia. A prospective study among patients with acquired immunodeficiency syndrome. Chest 90:18–22, 1986.
Bronchoalveolar lavage detected Pneumocystis carinii pneumonia in 36 of 37 patients with AIDS and cytomegalovirus in 15 of 38 patients.

Ikeda S: *Atlas of Bronchofiberoscopy.* Baltimore, University Park Press, 1974.
A classic text summarizing the author's pioneering work with the fiberoptic bronchoscopes.

Jackson C: Bronchoscopy: Past, present, and future. N Engl J Med 199:759–763, 1928.
A concise review of the development of bronchology that is applicable to current progress.

Jackson C, Jackson CL: *Bronchoesophagology.* Philadelphia, Saunders, 1950.
A classic text, summarizing the principles of rigid bronchoscopy.

Kvale PA, Eichenhorn MS, Radke JR, Miks V: YAG laser photoresection of lesions obstructing the central airways. Chest 87:283–288, 1985.
The YAG laser effectively relieved benign and malignant central airway obstruction in symptomatic patients.

Lukomsky GI: *Bronchology.* St. Louis, Mosby, 1979.
An excellent review of rigid bronchoscopy and its use in the Soviet Union.

Reynolds HY: Bronchoalveolar lavage. Am Rev Respir Dis 135:250–263, 1987.
A critical appraisal of the clinical use of BAL that deals with uncertainties as well as diagnostic value.

Schenk DA, Bower JH, Bryan CL, Currie RB, Spence TH, Duncan CA, Myers DL, Sullivan WT: Transbronchial needle aspiration staging of bronchogenic carcinoma. Am Rev Respir Dis 134:146–148, 1986.
CT scanning is a useful adjunct in the staging of patients with bronchogenic carcinoma, and transbronchial needle aspiration is a sensitive and highly specific staging technique that may negate the need for surgical staging in a large number of patients with bronchogenic carcinoma.

Stradling P: *Diagnostic Bronchoscopy.* London, Churchill-Livingstone, 1980.
The best available atlas of bronchoscopic anatomy.

Tsuboi E: *Atlas of Transbronchial Biopsy.* Baltimore, Williams & Wilkins, 1970.
Summary of an extensive experience with curettes, brush, and needle biopsy of peripheral neoplasms.

Wall CP, Gaensler EA, Carrington CB, Hayes JA: Comparison of transbronchial and open biopsies of chronic infiltrative lung disease. Am Rev Respir Dis 123:280–285, 1981.
Critical analysis of transbronchial forceps biopsy, demonstrating the unreliability of a nonspecific specimen.

Wang KP, Terry PB: Transbronchial needle aspiration in the diagnosis and staging of bronchogenic carcinoma. Am Rev Respir Dis 127:344–347, 1983.
Description of the adaptation of a flexible needle to the fiberoptic instrument.

Chapter 33

Pulmonary Biopsy and Aspiration Procedures

Milton D. Rossman

In evaluating invasive procedures, the benefits of the procedure with respect to the care and management of the patient must be weighed against its potential risks. Certain considerations enter into the evaluation of each candidate for an invasive procedure.

1. Invasive procedures should be used only when the information cannot be obtained by a noninvasive method.
2. If the pulmonary involvement is apt to be part of a systemic disease, an accessible extrapulmonary site is usually preferable to a pulmonary biopsy (i.e., a peripheral lymph node in sarcoidosis or lung cancer).
3. The general condition of the patient must be taken into account. Is there an unmanageable systemic disorder that threatens undue morbidity or even mortality, e.g., a bleeding diathesis, or a recent myocardial infarction? Will the patient tolerate resection of a portion of the lung? Will the patient tolerate a small pneumothorax (a common complication)? Is the patient likely to develop upper airway obstruction after intubation?
4. The skills of the operator should strongly influence the choice of procedure.
5. The suspected nature of the pulmonary disorder should strongly influence the choice of procedure. Taken into account are the following: history of exposure to allergens and fibrogenic and carcinogenic agents, the type and severity of the symptoms, the nature and severity of pulmonary function impairment, arterial blood-gas tensions, and the radiographic appearance.
6. Finally, timing the invasive procedure is an important consideration. Some patients will allow only one invasive attempt at diagnosis. Clinical judgment is also required to establish the optimal time for the procedure: although early diagnosis may enhance the prospect for effective intervention, a prematurely invasive procedure can (1) miss the opportunity for an inflammatory process to declare itself noninvasively, e.g., by sputum culture, or (2) provide samples that are not yet diagnostic. Finally, inordinate delay may allow the disease to progress to the stage of irreversibility before the diagnosis is confirmed.

EXTRATHORACIC BIOPSY

As a rule, if histologic diagnosis of a pulmonary process is likely to be afforded by biopsying an extrapulmonary site, the extrapulmonary biopsy is preferable to thoracotomy for obtaining a sample of involved tissue. The skin, conjunctiva, peripheral lymph nodes, bone marrow, liver, and kidney frequently afford this opportunity. Thus, apparently involved skin or enlarged peripheral lymph nodes may be diagnostic of sarcoidosis, tuberculosis, histoplasmosis, or coccidioidomycosis. Peripheral lymph nodes and bone marrow biopsy may establish the diagnosis of lymphoma, thereby sparing the patient thoracotomy or mediastinoscopy. That pulmonary lesions are metastatic in nature can often be confirmed by uncovering the primary tumor or identifying other metastatic sites. Goodpasture's syndrome is more easily diagnosed by renal biopsy than by pulmonary biopsy.

TRANSTHORACIC NEEDLE ASPIRATION BIOPSY

Indications

Aspiration biopsy of the lung is useful in providing material for cytologic examination or microbiologic studies. It has proved to be valuable in identifying, and in distinguishing between, malignant and infectious lesions. Its greatest yield is from persistent, localized lesions that are larger than 0.5 mm in diameter and that can be localized radiographically. Accessible lesions, virtually anywhere in the lungs, can be sampled by this approach.

MALIGNANCY

Aspiration biopsy serves the following purposes for patients with malignancy:

1. Establishing that a small peripheral pulmonary lesion, not easily accessible to bronchoscopic biopsy or aspiration, is a carcinoma of the lung
2. Distinguishing between an oat cell carcinoma and a non-oat-cell carcinoma, thereby directing treatment
3. Identifying that a pulmonary lesion(s) is a metastasis from an extrapulmonary site that has been shown to be the seat of malignancy
4. Establishing that a pulmonary lesion in a patient with inaccessible carcinoma elsewhere (e.g., the brain) is either primary in the lung or the seat of generalized metastatic disease

INFECTION

Aspiration biopsy serves the following purposes for patients with infection:

1. Distinguishing between infection and neoplasm as the nature of a pulmonary lesion
2. Establishing that the etiology of a chronic pulmonary lesion(s) is infectious (e.g., tuberculous, fungal, or caused by aerobic bacteria)
3. Identifying the etiologic agents responsible for confluent or solitary pulmonary lesions in an immunocompromised host, especially in children

Techniques

Three types of direct aspiration or biopsy have been employed: (1) Vim-Silverman type of needle; (2) a high-speed drill or trephine biopsy; and (3) a long, spinal type, 18-25 gauge needle. Since the use of the Vim-Silverman type of needle and of the trephine biopsy has been shown to run an inordinate risk of mortality, their current use is confined to established experts who have acquired a large experience with these techniques (Table 33-1). Most clinics now perform the aspiration technique using the long, thin needle.

The screening of each patient based on clinical and pulmonary function criteria has been noted above. Before the procedure is undertaken, the prothrombin time and the platelet count are determined to ensure that no coagulopathy is present. Premedication is usually not necessary; nor is fasting. The attempt at direct aspiration or biopsy begins with clear localization of the lesion using fluoroscopy. Not infrequently, computed tomography is a valuable adjunct in localizing the lesion precisely. Only occasionally is the aspiration or biopsy performed entirely under computed tomography.

After appropriate preparation of the overlying skin site, the chest wall is anesthetized using 2 percent lidocaine. As a rule, a short guide needle (not long enough to penetrate the pleura) is introduced into the chest wall; the aspirating needle is then passed through the guide needle. As the aspirating needle is about to traverse the pleura, the patient is instructed to breath-hold. After the needle is advanced into the pulmonary parenchyma, the patient is

TABLE 33-1

Comparison of Various Techniques for Sampling Pulmonary Tissue

	Cutting Biopsy*	Transthoracic Trephine Biopsy†	Aspiration	Open Thoracotomy
Type of lesion	Nodules; pneumonia	Diffuse Large Nodules (>4 cm)	Nodules; pneumonia	All
Anesthesia	Local	Local	Local	General
Type of specimen	Tissue	Tissue	Cytology	Tissue
Time in hospital	24 h	24 h	3–24 h	3–5 days
Discomfort	Minimal	Minimal	Minimal	Moderate to severe
Yield, percent	70–80	70–90	70–90	85–95
Pneumothorax, percent	20–40	20–40	10–20	Controlled
Major hemorrhage, percent	8–30	4–16	< 1	Controlled
Decreased oxygen	Minimal	Minimal	Minimal	10–30 mmHg
Air embolus	Rare	Rare	Very rare	Extremely rare
Mortality, percent	− 1	− 1	0.1–0.3	− 1

* Vim-Silverman needle.

† Trephine.

instructed to breathe quietly. Once biplane fluoroscopy shows that the needle is in the lesion, 2 to 3 cm³ of sterile saline is injected before the attempt at aspiration; during aspiration, the needle is vibrated and rotated. Immediately after aspiration, the needle is withdrawn. The aspirate is either smeared on a slide, mixed in carbowax for cytologic examination, or sent to the microbiology laboratory for smears and cultures. A chest radiograph is obtained after the procedure to determine if a pneumothorax has been caused.

Results

Transthoracic needle aspiration has been shown to be diagnostic in more than 95 percent of patients with carcinoma of the lung who have been subjected to this procedure. This yield applies to patients with pulmonary parenchymal, hilar, or mediastinal lesions. However, when lymphoma, rather than carcinoma, is the cause of the lesion, this technique has yielded a correct diagnosis in only 50 percent of tested patients. Bronchogenic and

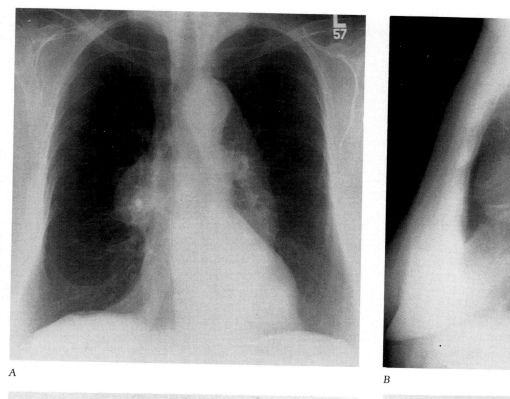

A

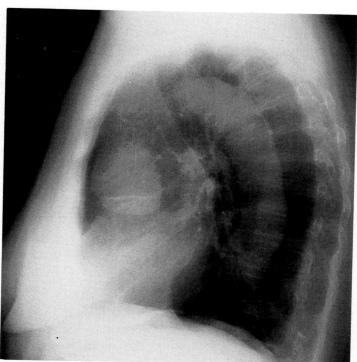

B

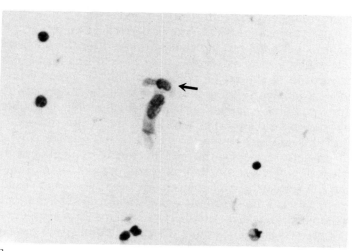

C

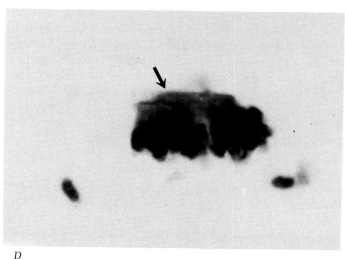

D

FIGURE 33-1 Bronchogenic cyst diagnosed by transthoracic needle aspiration. *A.* Posteroanterior chest radiograph demonstrating a large, sharply circumscribed right hilar mass. *B.* Lateral chest radiograph indicates that the lesion was anterior. *C* and *D.* Cytology of clear cyst fluid aspirated from the lesion. Individual cells and groups of benign bronchial epithelial cells are clearly identified in the cyst fluid (arrow) (×400).

mediastinal cysts can also be correctly identified and aspirated (Fig. 33-1). Benign neoplasms are more difficult to identify by aspiration. Hamartomas and bronchial adenomas have been correctly identified using aspirated materials. Infections caused by bacteria, mycoplasma, mycobacteria, fungi, parasites, and viruses can frequently be identified. The major limitation with the aspiration technique is that the small specimen may be insufficient for cytologic and microbiologic examination.

Complications

The most common complication of transthoracic needle aspiration is pneumothorax. Although this does occur in 20 percent of patients, in only 5 percent is a chest tube necessary to evacuate the air. Since the pulmonary leak usually seals off spontaneously within 24 h, a thin-bore chest tube usually suffices to keep the lung expanded until the perforation closes. As indicated above, all patients having a transthoracic needle aspiration should have a chest radiograph after the procedure to check for a pneumothorax. Major hemorrhage after transthoracic needle aspiration is extremely rare. A slight amount of hemoptysis (5 to 20 cm³) occurs in up to 5 percent of cases. Although air embolism is a possibility, the use of the small gauge needles has virtually eliminated this complication.

MEDIASTINOSCOPY AND MEDIASTINOTOMY

Indications

Cervical mediastinoscopy, anterior mediastinoscopy, and anterior mediastinotomy are surgical procedures used to gain direct access to mediastinal structures for visualization and biopsy. The ability of computed tomography to identify abnormal mediastinal structures has decreased the use of these surgical interventions to detect invasion of the mediastinum by neoplasms. As will be described later, the choice among these approaches depends on the location of the targeted nodes or mass in the mediastinum. These surgical approaches are generally used to explore the mediastinum for invasion by neoplasm. Mediastinoscopy is also useful for the diagnosis of sarcoidosis, tuberculosis, and histoplasmosis. Indications for mediastinoscopy or mediastinotomy include:

1. A widened mediastinum of unknown cause.
2. Staging of carcinoma of the lung. As a rule, but not invariably, the cell type of this carcinoma of the lung has been established by other diagnostic procedures before mediastinoscopy or mediastinotomy is contemplated. If the cell type remains unsettled, mediastinoscopy or mediastinotomy may provide histologically diagnostic tissue. But more often this approach affords information that pertains more to staging than to diagnosis. Familiar examples for which histologic confirmation of mediastinal spread of carcinoma of the lung would indicate inoperability are:

    a. When a small peripheral oat cell carcinoma is present and surgery is contemplated
    b. When a central or large (greater than 4 cm) peripheral adenocarcinoma of the lung is present
    c. Whenever a large cell carcinoma of the lung is present
    d. When a squamous cell carcinoma of the lung is present in a patient who is a poor risk for surgery (i.e., elderly, debilitated, or poor pulmonary reserve)

3. Confirmation of sarcoidosis or tuberculosis.
4. Diagnosis of mediastinal fibrosis.

Techniques

General anesthesia and endotracheal intubation are usually required.

Cervical mediastinoscopy is used to investigate the right paratracheal and subcarinal lymph nodes. A short transverse incision is made through the skin at the suprasternal notch. After clearing the way by blunt dissection to the trachea—behind the innominate artery and the aortic arch to the level of the carina—the mediastinoscope is introduced and biopsies are carefully taken.

Anterior mediastinoscopy is used to investigate the left mediastinum, especially when left upper lobe lesions are present. A vertical skin incision is made overlying the second intercostal space at the lateral edge of the sternum. Blunt dissection is carried out medial to the pleura and down to the aorticopulmonary window, exposing anterior and subaortic lymph nodes. The mediastinoscope is then introduced, and biopsies are taken. This procedure causes the patient less discomfort than a mediastinotomy since no cartilage is removed.

Anterior mediastinotomy is performed on either the right or left side, but is usually reserved for the left side where cervical mediastinoscopy is more difficult and less rewarding. It should be noted that mediastinotomy is a more extensive surgical procedure than mediastinoscopy and should be reserved for lesions that are not accessible by mediastinoscopy. On the right side, lymph nodes in the hilus, along the superior vena cava and trachea, can be readily visualized. On the left side, the hilar, paratracheal, subaortic, and anterior lymph nodes are available for biopsy. A transverse incision is made over the second costal cartilage, and the entire cartilage is removed. The internal mammary vessels are divided, and the mediastinal pleura is deflected laterally so that the extrapleural space can be entered. The incision can be extended so that both a pulmonary parenchymal and mediastinal biopsy can be performed simultaneously.

TABLE 33-2
Metastatic Involvement of the Mediastinum Disclosed by Mediastinoscopy or Mediastinotomy

Cell	Number of Patients	Percent Positive
Cell type		
Squamous	67	7
Adenocarcinoma	87	34
Undifferentiated	65	60
Location		
Peripheral	121	22
Central	92	55

SOURCE: Based on data from Jolly et al., 1980, and from Whitcomb et al., Am Rev Respir Dis 113:189–195, 1976.

Results

In more than 90 percent of patients with carcinoma of the lung in whom mediastinoscopy fails to disclose tumor, the carcinoma of the lung is resectable. Conversely, in about 40 percent of patients in whom the carcinoma of the lung is otherwise operable (without evidence of extrathoracic metastases), mediastinoscopy or mediastinotomy proves the patient to be inoperable (Table 33-2). In sarcoidosis, mediastinal lymph nodes contain noncaseating granulomas in more than 90 percent of patients who have stage I and stage II disease by radiographic criteria. In stage III sarcoidosis, the yield may be as low as 50 percent.

Complications

The morbidity of mediastinoscopy/mediastinotomy is low (less than 3 percent), and the mortality is extremely low (less than 0.01 percent). The major complication is bleeding. Occasionally, a thoracotomy is required for hemostasis. Because of this complication, sites to be biopsied are all aspirated with a needle before the biopsy to ensure that a major blood vessel is not present. Occasionally, the left vocal cord is paralyzed because of injury of the recurrent laryngeal nerve on that side. Pneumothorax and perforation of the esophagus are rare. Mediastinoscopy should not be done if a thymoma is anticipated because of the prevalent belief that biopsy of a benign thymoma can convert it to a malignant thymoma.

THORACOTOMY

Indications

Thoracotomy for diagnosis is usually undertaken as a last resort, i.e., after less traumatic procedures have proved to be of no avail. It affords the advantage of providing a large sample for examination. Special staining using immunologic techniques, electron microscopy, and chemical analysis can be applied to the specimens obtained by open lung biopsy. But, when certain rapidly progressive pulmonary disorders are expected, such as Wegener's granulomatosis, thoracotomy is the procedure of choice early in the evaluation.

Open lung biopsy is also useful in staging a pulmonary disease. In carcinoma of the lung, observations and tissue samples during thoracotomy determine the extent of operability and resectability. Staging of disease is often helpful in guiding medical therapy for interstitial lung disease since the cellularity of the biopsy and the amount of fibrosis may guide the choice of drugs.

Techniques

General anesthesia and endotracheal intubation are prerequisite for thoracotomy and open lung biopsy. The size of the incision depends on the nature of the procedure. If the lesion is circumscribed or if it is extensive and homogeneous so that a small piece of lung will suffice for histologic diagnosis, then a relatively small incision will do. However, a larger, standard incision allows the inspection and biopsy of pleural and mediastinal structures. Consultation with the thoracic surgeon is essential to ensure proper sampling, handling, fixation, and transport to the diagnostic laboratory for processing and interpretation.

Results

Open lung biopsy is the only procedure for sampling lung tissue that provides lung tissue all the time. It is also the most dependable way to obtain a histologic diagnosis. But, even open lung biopsy may fail to yield a histologic diagnosis if sampling is inadequate or nonrepresentative or if the tissue is not fixed or stained appropriately. Sometimes the lesions are consistent with a diagnosis but not, per se, conclusive, as in berylliosis or hypersensitivity pneumonitis. Occasionally, a characteristic lesion is nonspecific with respect to etiology, e.g., granulomas or fibrosis. Nonetheless, with proper skills and precautions, open lung biopsy is the gold standard against which all other approaches have to be judged.

Complications

Most postoperative complications can be avoided by careful selection of patients, coupled with meticulous operative technique and postoperative patient care. The mortality of a thoracotomy for open lung biopsy ranges from 0.9 to 3 percent. The skill of the surgeon and the choice of patients heavily influences the mortality: mortality is low in young patients who have pulmonary coin lesions; it is higher in the immunocompromised host in whom a pulmonary infiltrate is progressing rapidly. Complications of thoracotomy include pneumothorax, a persistent bronchopleural fistula, hemothorax, hemoptysis, atelectasis, pneumonia, and respiratory failure. Each of these complications is handled in the standard way as described elsewhere in this book.

BIBLIOGRAPHY

Brantigan JW, Brantigan CO, Brantigan OC: Biopsy of nonpalpable scalene lymph nodes in carcinoma of the lung. Am Rev Respir Dis 107:962–974, 1973.
> *An excellent review of the literature on scalene node biopsy in carcinoma of the lung. The authors make a strong argument for routine blind bilateral scalene node biopsies as a staging procedure in carcinoma of the lung.*

Carlens E: Mediastinoscopy: A method for inspection and tissue biopsy in the superior mediastinum. Dis Chest 36:343–352, 1959.
> *Carlens' original description of mediastinoscopy with the results of 100 procedures.*

Cucin RL, Coleman M, Eckardt JJ, Silver RT: The diagnosis of miliary tuberculosis: Utility of peripheral blood abnormalities, bone marrow and liver biopsy. J Chronic Dis 26:355–361, 1973.
> *Retrospective review of bone marrow and liver biopsy in 36 patients with miliary tuberculosis. Granulomas were seen in 52 percent of bone marrow biopsies and 91 percent of liver biopsies, but acid-fast bacilli were seen in only 24 percent of bone marrow biopsies and 43 percent of liver biopsies.*

Gaensler EA, Carrington CB: Open lung biopsy for chronic diffuse lung disease: Clinical, roentgenographic, and physiological correlations in 502 patients. Ann Thorac Surg 30:411–426, 1980.
> *A diagnostic yield of 92.2 percent was achieved with only a 0.3 percent mortality and 2.5 percent morbidity. The authors stress the need to biopsy average lung rather than the most abnormal region.*

Jolly PC, Li W, Anderson RP: Anterior and cervical mediastinoscopy for determining operability and predicting resectability in lung cancer. J Thorac Cardiovasc Surg 79:366–371, 1980.
> *The technique of anterior and cervical mediastinoscopy is described. Anterior mediastinoscopy appears to be a useful and safe procedure for the exploration of the left mediastinum.*

Johnston WW: Cytologic diagnosis of lung cancer. Principles and problems. Pathol Res Pract 181:1–36, 1986.
> *A comprehensive review of the current status of the principles and problems of cytology as applied to the diagnosis of lung cancer.*

Khouri NF, Stitik FP, Erozan YS, Gupta PK, Kim WS, Scott WW Jr, Hamper UM, Mann RB, Eggleston JC, Baker RR: Transthoracic needle aspiration biopsy of benign and malignant lung lesions. Am J Roentgenol 144:281–288, 1985.
> *The authors' experience with 650 patients suggests that transthoracic needle aspiration is useful for diagnosing benign and malignant lesions.*

Kline TS: Handbook of Fine Needle Aspiration Biopsy Cytology. St. Louis, Mosby, 1981.
> *Chapter 7 is devoted to the lung and has excellent examples of cytology specimens from a variety of benign and malignant disorders.*

Schenk DA, Bryan CL, Bower JH, Myers DL: Transbronchial needle aspiration in the diagnosis of bronchogenic carcinoma. Chest 92:83–85, 1987.
> *Transbronchial needle aspiration is particularly valuable diagnostically in patients with extratracheal and extrabronchial lesions. In contrast, it fails to contribute significantly to the diagnosis of cancer in patients with lesions readily accessible by conventional bronchoscopic techniques.*

Westcott JL: Needle aspiration biopsy of pulmonary, hilar, and mediastinal masses. Clin Chest Med 5:365–377, 1984.
> *The author's extensive experience with needle aspiration for the diagnosis of pulmonary parenchymal and mediastinal lesions.*

Winning AJ, McIvor J, Seed WA, Husain OA, Metaxas N: Interpretation of negative results in fine needle aspiration of discrete pulmonary lesions. Thorax 41:875–879, 1986.
> *A retrospective analysis of a consecutive series of 181 percutaneous fine needle aspiration biopsies of discrete pulmonary lesions, in which the outcome was established in 95%. Needle aspiration biopsy seems particularly appropriate for inoperable patients with probable bronchial carcinoma in whom sputum cytology and bronchoscopy do not yield a diagnosis.*

Chapter 34

The Electrocardiogram in Pulmonary Disease

Fred D. Holford

Asthma

Chronic Cor Pulmonale
    P-Wave Changes
    The QRS Complex
    Associated Left Ventricular Disease

Acute Cor Pulmonale
    Pulmonary Embolism
    Acute Respiratory Failure

Cardiac Arrhythmias

The diagnostic value of the electrocardiogram in pulmonary disease depends to a large degree on the underlying pulmonary or ventilatory disorder, its severity, or its duration. As a general rule, the electrocardiogram (ECG) is a reliable guide to cor pulmonale in those disorders that are not associated with obstructive disease of the airways, i.e., pulmonary vascular disease, interstitial disease, or alveolar hypoventilation with normal lungs. It becomes an uncertain index of pulmonary hypertension and cor pulmonale in chronic bronchitis and emphysema because of the hyperinflated lungs and the episodic nature of the pulmonary hypertension and right ventricular volume overload in these disorders.

In the patient with pulmonary disease, ECG changes are often absent. But, when present, they are very helpful, i.e., specificity is high. The lack of sensitivity of the ECG in pulmonary disease probably reflects the dominance of the left ventricle in the adult and the confounding effects of left-sided heart disease and pulmonary abnormalities.

Since the right ventricle is the cardiac chamber that is affected in cor pulmonale, it is customary to relate the ECG patterns in cor pulmonale to the right ventricular hypertrophy patterns that are seen in some types of congenital heart disease, i.e., pulmonic stenosis. But telling differences exist between acquired and congenital bases for right ventricular enlargement, mainly because of the higher systolic pressures in the right ventricle, the greater pulmonary vascular resistance, and the greater degree of right ventricular hypertrophy in congenital heart disease. In addition, ventricular balance is different in the two groups. In congenital heart disease, the extra right ventric-

ular hypertrophy caused by the disease state is added to the normal right ventricular dominance that is present at birth; consequently, the left ventricle is never dominant unless an independent pressure or volume overload exists to tax it. In contrast, in the right ventricular enlargement that characterizes cor pulmonale the left ventricle is dominant for years, so that the right ventricular enlargement must be considerable before it is apparent on the ECG.

ASTHMA

The electrocardiogram in asthma is usually normal except for sinus tachycardia. However, in status asthmaticus it is not uncommon to find right axis deviation of the QRS complex; P pulmonale in leads II, III, and aVR; a dominant R wave in aVR; and clockwise rotation of the electrical axis (Fig. 34-1A). After recovery from the attack (Fig. 34-1B), right axis deviation of the QRS often persists, but P waves become normal, the R wave in aVR becomes smaller, and the clockwise rotation disappears.

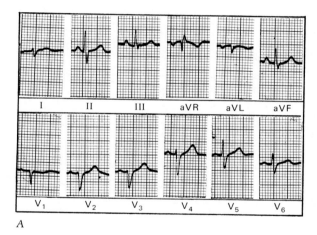

FIGURE 34-1   Changes in the ECG in a patient with chronic asthma. A. Acute exacerbation. B. After relief of bronchospasm, 3 days later.

CHRONIC COR PULMONALE

Depending on the level of the pulmonary artery pressure, the electrocardiogram in cor pulmonale secondary to pulmonary vascular disease, interstitial disease, or alveolar hypoventilation with normal lungs (Fig. 34-2) ranges from normal to the full-blown picture of right ventricular hypertrophy (Table 34-1). The electrocardiogram of the patient with cor pulmonale caused by obstructive disease of the airways has a number of distinctive features. These are listed in Table 34-2. Since clinical evidence of right ventricular enlargement is rarely conclusive in chronic bronchitis or emphysema, the ECG in these patients may be helpful in settling the diagnosis (Fig. 34-3).

The complexity of the electrocardiographic changes of cor pulmonale rests, in part at least, with the fact that the electric potentials may be altered by structural changes outside the heart as well as by those within the right ventricle. Electric potentials from the right ventricle

TABLE 34-2
*ECG Changes in Chronic Cor Pulmonale with Obstructive Disease of the Airways**

1. Isoelectric P waves in lead I or right axis deviation of the P vector
2. P-pulmonale pattern (an increase in P-wave amplitude in II, III, aVF)
3. Tendency for right axis deviation of the QRS vector
4. R/S amplitude ratio in $V_6 < 1$
5. Low-voltage QRS
6. S_1Q_3 or $S_1S_2S_3$ pattern
7. Incomplete (and rarely complete) right bundle branch block
8. R/S amplitude ratio in $V_1 > 1$
9. Marked clockwise rotation of the electrical axis
10. Occasional large Q wave or QS in the inferior or midprecordial leads suggesting healed myocardial infarction

*The first seven criteria are suggestive but nonspecific; the last three are more characteristic of cor pulmonale in obstructive disease of the airways.

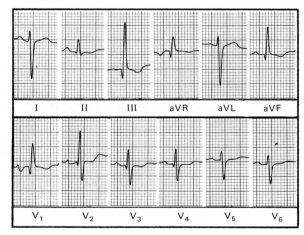

FIGURE 34-2 The ECG from a patient with interstitial pulmonary fibrosis showing marked right axis deviation, the S_1Q_3 pattern, tall r wave in V_1 and V_2, and marked clockwise rotation.

TABLE 34-1
*ECG Criteria for Cor Pulmonale without Obstructive Disease of the Airways**

1. Right axis deviation with a mean QRS axis to the right of +110°
2. R/S amplitude ratio in $V_1 > 1$
3. R/S amplitude ratio in $V_6 < 1$
4. Clockwise rotation of the electrical axis
5. P-pulmonale pattern
6. S_1Q_3 or $S_1S_2S_3$ pattern
7. Normal-voltage QRS

*Any one of the first three criteria suffices to raise suspicion of right ventricular hypertrophy. The diagnosis becomes more certain if two or more of these findings are present. The last four criteria commonly occur in cor pulmonale secondary to primary alveolar hypoventilation, interstitial disease of the lung, or pulmonary vascular disease.

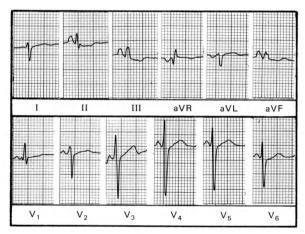

FIGURE 34-3 The ECG from a patient with obstructive disease of the airways. The low-voltage, right axis deviation, prominent P waves in II, III, and aVF, P pulmonale, R/S amplitude ratio <1 in V_1, clockwise rotation, and R/S amplitude <1 in V_6 are characteristic of cor pulmonale secondary to bronchitis and emphysema.

may be modified by (1) changes in the spatial orientation of the right ventricle, (2) changes in the anatomic structures around the heart, (3) changes in the right ventricular myocardium, and (4) changes in the time course of ventricular depolarization.

Although the exact mechanisms for the ECG changes seen in cor pulmonale secondary to chronic bronchitis and emphysema are unclear, it is believed that the following factors are important:

1. In chronic obstructive disease of the airways the diaphragm is flattened, and the anteroposterior diameter of the chest is enlarged. The flattened diaphragm and the enlarged chest cause the heart to become more vertical and to rotate leftward on its longitudinal axis. The right atrium and ventricle rotate anteriorly, and the apex is displaced posteriorly. As a result, the anterior surface is occupied by the right atrium and ventricle, whereas the left ventricle lies more posteriorly than normal.

2. In emphysema, the electric conductivity of the lungs is reduced so that the magnitude of electric forces reaching the body surface is subnormal. The resistance of the deflated lung (at residual volume) is about 400 Ω, but that of the overinflated lung is 1200 to 1350 Ω. In addition, the increase in the anteroposterior diameter of the chest increases the distance between the electrodes and the myocardium.

3. The changes in the heart secondary to pulmonary disease are complex. ECG evidence of early pulmonary heart disease is usually absent or nonspecific, and only suggestive evidence of right-sided heart involvement is usually present, particularly P pulmonale in leads II, III, and aVF; an S_1Q_3 pattern; an $S_1S_2S_3$ pattern; right axis deviation; or an R/S ratio in leads V_5 and V_6 that is less than 1. Only late in the disease do more characteristic changes occur. These include right axis deviation to the right of $+110°$, an R/S ratio in V_1 greater than 1, and marked clockwise rotation of the electrical axis. In obstructive disease of the airways, low-voltage QRS complexes in the limb leads and occasionally large Q waves or QS in the inferior or midprecordial leads suggest healed myocardial infarction.

One of the earliest anatomic changes in the heart in patients with chronic lung disease and pulmonary hypertension is hypertrophy of the crista supraventricularis, a muscular ridge located on the posterior wall of the right ventricular outflow tract. Hypertrophy of the crista supraventricularis is associated with an increase in the magnitude of the vectors produced during electric depolarization. Because of the anatomic location of the crista, the electric forces produced by it during depolarization are directed superiorly and to the right. Thus, prominent S waves are commonly seen in the standard leads and in leads V_5 and V_6 in patients with lung disease. S waves also occur in people with normal but ptotic hearts, but these S waves are usually narrow, whereas they are often wide, slurred, or notched in patients with early cor pulmonale and hypertrophy of the crista supraventricularis (Fig. 34-4).

As the lung disease progresses and pulmonary vascular resistance increases, the right ventricle performs increased amounts of pressure work, resulting in hypertrophy of the right ventricular free wall and dilatation and hypertrophy of the right atrium. The ECG and vectorcardiogram begin to exhibit the conventional signs of the right ventricular hypertrophy. The progressive hypertrophy and dilatation of the right ventricle cause further clockwise rotation of the heart so that the mean QRS vector becomes oriented anteriorly to the right and inferiorly. Similar changes are seen in subjects who live at high altitudes (greater than 10,000 ft) who have neither vertical hearts nor emphysema that may influence the conduction of electric activity. In addition, patients with normal lungs who develop pulmonary hypertension from alveolar hypoventilation, primary pulmonary hypertension, or recurrent pulmonary emboli, exhibit the same changes.

4. Incomplete and complete right bundle branch block have been described in chronic lung disease. However, the pattern of incomplete right bundle branch block reflects late depolarization of the crista supraventricularis or depolarization of a hypertrophied crista rather than an abnormal course of depolarization in the myocardium. Therefore, the r′ in V_1 and the wide S waves in the standard leads ($S_1S_2S_3$ pattern) reflect unopposed, or inadequately opposed, late and usually slow depolarization of the crista supraventricularis. The r′ has a smooth and sharp downstroke in normal subjects, whereas in patients with hypertrophy of the crista supraventricularis, the downstroke of the r′ tends to be slurred (Fig. 34-1B). Complete right bundle branch block is not uncommon in patients with chronic obstructive pulmonary disease, but it is more commonly due to coronary artery disease than to lung disease.

P-Wave Changes

One of the earliest and most consistent ECG changes associated with chronic bronchitis and emphysema is a shift to the right of the depolarization forces of the atria. As a

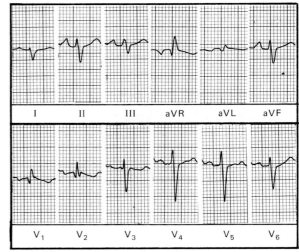

FIGURE 34-4 The ECG from a patient with chronic bronchitis and emphysema illustrates the deep, wide S waves in standard leads and in V_5 and V_6 resulting from hypertrophy at the crista supraventricularis.

result, the P waves become more vertically oriented in the frontal plane. The P wave that is normally upright in lead I first becomes diphasic and then isoelectric as the P vector begins to shift vertically downward (Fig. 34-5). The vertical shift in P vector occurs relatively early in this disease, progresses to +90°, but does not shift further to the right even though the disease progresses. In patients over middle age, a diphasic P wave in lead I or aVL should bring to mind the possibility of underlying obstructive lung disease. In younger patients, such P waves are occasionally seen as a normal variant.

The vertical orientation of the P vector in the frontal plane produces inverted P waves in aVL and peaked, symmetric P waves in leads II, III, and aVF (P pulmonale). Their amplitude is often large (over 2.5 mm), but it is their characteristic configuration rather than their height that identifies them; the duration of the P wave in chronic lung disease with cor pulmonale usually is not prolonged. When the P vector reaches +90° in the frontal plane, the P waves in the right precordial leads frequently become characteristic of right atrial enlargement; they become either entirely upright or diphasic, with sharp deflections.

The QRS Complex

In the ventricles, as in the atria, hyperinflation from chronic obstructive disease of the airways causes the QRS vector in the frontal plane to become more vertical; these changes reflect shift in the position of the heart rather than increase in pulmonary artery pressure. As the vector changes, the amplitude of the R wave in lead I diminishes and eventually becomes isoelectric, approaching +90°.

The combination of an isoelectric P wave and an isoelectic QRS complex in lead I strongly suggests the presence of underlying bronchitis and emphysema, particularly if the patient is middle-aged or older. The tallest R waves are seen in leads II, III, and aVF, associated with a tendency toward decreased amplitude of the QRS complex in all the limb leads (Fig. 34-6).

The QRS vector in the frontal plane often does not shift further than +90°. However, as the disease progresses, the terminal portion of the QRS (S wave) frequently manifests itself in the frontal plane as a vector that is directed upward and to the right. In the bipolar leads, this vector produces an S wave in leads I, I, and III (Fig. 34-4). Although this pattern superficially resembles left axis deviation, the mean QRS axis is really indeterminate since the initial and terminal forces of the QRS complex are approximately 180° apart (RS in all standard leads) (Fig. 34-5). When the $S_1S_2S_3$ pattern is present, aVL and aVR resemble each other, both having late upward deflections. Accordingly, aVF has a late downward deflection (S wave). The S wave is frequently somewhat slurred on the upstroke in some or all leads; this is probably due to hypertrophy of the crista supraventricularis. This pattern with a terminal vector directed upward, posteriorly, and near the midline is rarely seen except in underlying lung disease, most often chronic bronchitis and emphysema.

The precordial leads reflect the posterior orientation of the mean QRS vector by showing a prominent S wave across the precordium as the terminal electric activity moves away from the exploring electrode on the anterior chest. The R/S ratio is usually 1 or less as far to the left as lead V_5 (Fig. 34-6). As the heart rotates clockwise, the transitional zone moves to produce the pattern that is usu-

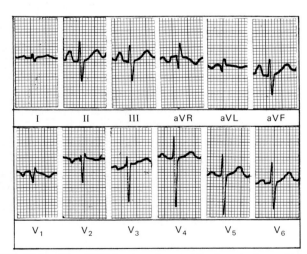

FIGURE 34-5 The ECG in a patient with chronic bronchitis and emphysema exhibiting the indeterminate QRS vector in the standard and unipolar limb leads. The R/S ratio in the standard leads I, II, and III is near unity, aVR and aVL are similar in morphology, and a deep S wave is present in aVF. An rSr pattern is present in the precordial leads associated with marked clockwise rotation of the electrical axis.

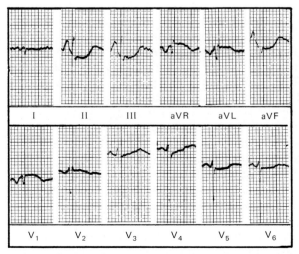

FIGURE 34-6 The ECG from a patient with emphysema illustrating the nearly isoelectric P wave and QRS in lead I together with incomplete right bundle branch block in V_1 and V_2.

ally designated as *clockwise rotation of the electrical axis.* The terminal vector occasionally has a late anterior component as it swings to the right and causes an r′ in the right precordial lead.

Occasionally, this upward terminal vector completely overshadows the initial downward forces of the QRS complex in the frontal plane. When this occurs, leads II, III, and aVF assume a predominantly QS configuration that often simulates that of inferior myocardial infarction (Fig. 34-7A). Indeed, the similarity is often so great that it is impossible to exclude an inferior myocardial infarction unless the evolutionary pattern of the infarction is available or if other stigmata of infarction can be perceived. For example, if the deflection in lead II is neither entirely downward (QS) nor predominantly downward (small r′ deep S), but instead is W-shaped or QR in configuration, it is probable that the ECG changes are due to myocardial

infarction regardless of the presence or absence of emphysema.

The characteristic terminal vector of underlying lung disease, which is directed superiorly and posteriorly, frequently causes a QS deflection in the right and/or midprecordial leads, suggestive of septal or anterior wall myocardial infarction. In order to elucidate the meaning of QS deflections in the right precordial leads (V_1 and V_2), recording the precordial leads one or two interspaces lower than at conventional sites usually demonstrates the initial r waves if the changes are due to bronchitis and emphysema. In contrast, the ECG recorded using such leads in myocardial infarction is identical with that obtained from the conventional sites of recording.

Associated Left Ventricular Disease

The ECG abnormalities produced by chronic obstructive disease of the airways are sometimes obscured by changes related to left ventricular disease. For example, the ECG of a patient with both lung disease and hypertensive cardiovascular disease is likely to be dominated by the strain of the left ventricle and to show only the pattern of left ventricular hypertrophy. The ECG of a patient with underlying coronary disease in addition to lung disease often exhibits conduction disturbances (such as left bundle branch block or an extensive old myocardial infarction) that mask ECG evidence of pulmonary disease. As mentioned above, complete right bundle branch block (RBBB) is not uncommonly seen in patients with chronic obstructive disease of the airways. This pattern (complete RBBB) should be attributed to cor pulmonale only if the P vector and the initial QRS vector are vertically oriented.

ACUTE COR PULMONALE

Pulmonary Embolism

The classic description of the electrocardiographic changes associated with acute cor pulmonale secondary to pulmonary embolism was made in 1935 by McGinn and White (see Fig. 34-6). The changes consisted of a prominent S wave in lead I, a Q wave in lead III, and later T-wave inversion in lead III. A depressed ST segment with a staircase ascent may be seen in leads I and II. This description of the $S_1Q_3T_3$ complex has since been associated with acute cor pulmonale (Fig. 34-8).

Since that time it has become clear that this distinctive combination occurs only in the minority of patients with acute pulmonary emboli. In submassive emboli, patterns are much less distinctive. Indeed, in approximately one-quarter of these patients, the electrocardiogram is normal. Another 25 percent show either the $S_1Q_3T_3$ pattern, RBBB, P pulmonale, or right axis deviation. Most common are nonspecific T-wave changes and nonspecific

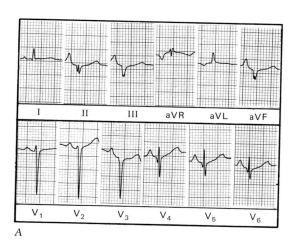

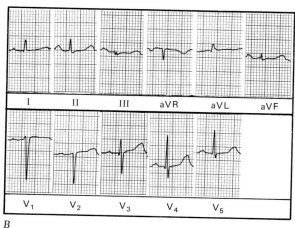

FIGURE 34-7 The ECG in a patient with chronic bronchitis and emphysema showing the pattern of inferior myocardial infarction and the loss of anterior forces in the midprecordial leads. *A.* During a respiratory infection both patterns occurred. *B.* The patient was improved and the ECG returned toward normal 2 days later. V_6 was not recorded.

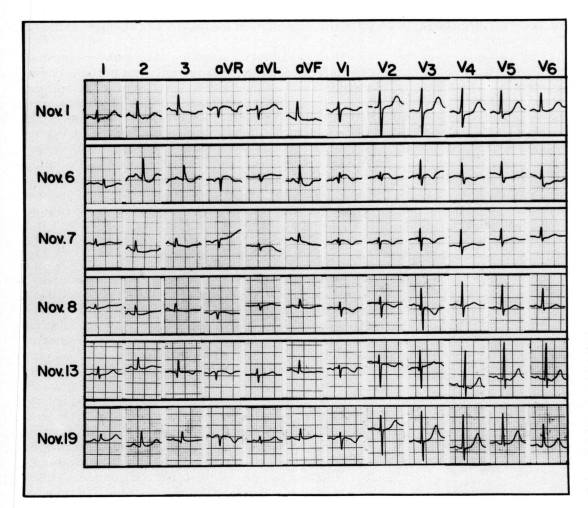

FIGURE 34-8 Serial ECGs from a patient with acute thrombophlebitis. Baseline ECG (November 1) followed by serial tracings subsequent to an acute pulmonary embolism proved by pulmonary angiogram and V/Q scan. The serial changes in the ECG subsequent to the pulmonary embolism occurring on November 5 are classic as they evolve and return to normal.

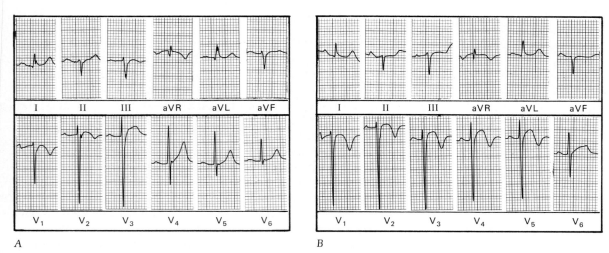

A   *B*

FIGURE 34-9   The ECG from a patient with emphysema and systemic hypertension.   A. The left axis deviation and deep S waves in V_2 and V_3 are consistent with left ventricular hypertrophy.   B. During a bout of respiratory failure, the P wave in leads II, III, and VF became more prominent, the T waves became inverted in V_1 to V_5, and clockwise rotation of the electrical axis occurred.

abnormalities—either elevation or depression—of the RST segments. Most of the electrocardiographic abnormalities are gone within 2 weeks; inversion of the T wave is the most persistent abnormality. Atrial arrhythmias are not uncommon, particularly in patients with antecedent cardiac disease.

The mechanism responsible for the electrocardiographic changes is unknown. However, the consensus favors acute dilation of the right ventricle, possibly in combination with arterial hypoxemia.

It should be noted that electrocardiographic changes are most apt to occur with massive or submassive emboli. Small emboli that lodge in peripheral pulmonary arterial vessels are apt to be entirely without effect on the electrocardiogram.

Acute Respiratory Failure

An episode of respiratory failure is a common precipitating mechanism for acute cor pulmonale in the patient with chronic pulmonary disease. Sinus tachycardia is common. Often the axis of the P wave is +70° or more. Clockwise rotation, upright T waves in the precordial leads, deep S waves in leads I and II, and a dominant R wave in aVR are common but transient. Q waves are infrequent. As the patient improves, the ECG changes gradually resolve (Fig. 34-9).

CARDIAC ARRHYTHMIAS

Cardiac arrhythmias are common in patients with chronic bronchitis and emphysema. These arrhythmias adversely affect the clinical course and sometimes are life-threatening. Arterial hypoxemia and respiratory acidosis are commonly associated. Occasional ECGs underestimate the incidence of these transient disturbances of rhythm. Long-term ECGs show a wide variety of arrhythmias of both supraventricular and ventricular origin.

BIBLIOGRAPHY

Burch GE, De Pasquale NP: The electrocardiographic and vectorcardiographic diagnosis of pulmonary heart disease. Acad Med NJ 9:239–260, 1963.
A review of the ECG in chronic pulmonary disease is fairly characteristic when present and may be explained on the basis of changes in spacial orientation of the heart and the insulating effect of the overinflated lungs.

Caird FI, Standfield CA: The electrocardiogram in asphyxial and in acute cor pulmonale. Br Heart J 24:313–323, 1962.
The ECG in acute asphyxial cor pulmonale as may be seen in an exacerbation of chronic bronchitis or asthma is compared with that of acute embolic cor pulmonale.

Cutforth RH, Oram S: The electrocardiogram in pulmonary embolism. Br Heart J 20:41–60, 1958.
Ninety-four patients diagnosed as having pulmonary embolism; in 50 the diagnosis was considered certain based on autopsy or by clinical and radiologic material.

Eiriksson CE Jr, Writer SL, Vestal RE: Theophylline-induced alterations in cardiac electrophysiology in patients with chronic obstructive pulmonary disease. Am Rev Respir Dis 135:322–326, 1987.
Electrophysiologic testing was performed before and during aminophylline (theophylline ethylenediamine) infusions in 10 male patients with stable chronic obstructive airways disease. The mean plasma theophylline concentration was 15.6 ± 0.9 μg/ml and plasma catecholamine concentrations increased. No arrhythmias were induced but in 5 patients symptoms occurred during rapid atrial pacing and aminophylline infusion.

Goodwin J, Abdin ZH: The cardiogram of congenital and acquired right ventricular hypertrophy. Br Heart J 20:523–544, 1958.
The clarification of the ECG changes in congenital and acquired right ventricular hypertrophy that aids in the assessment of severity which facilitates diagnosis.

Holford FD, Mithoefer JC: Cardiac arrhythmias in hospitalized patients with chronic obstructive pulmonary disease. Am Rev Respir Dis 108:879–885, 1973.
Seventy-two-hour continuous ECG recording on tape revealed that cardiac arrhythmias are common in patients with chronic bronchitis and emphysema and may adversely affect the clinical course, including causing sudden death.

Hudson LD, Kurt TL, Petty TL, Genton E: Arrhythmias associated with acute respiratory failure with chronic airway obstruction. Chest 63:661–665, 1973.
Patients with acute respiratory failure are commonly found to have cardiac arrhythmias. Ventricular arrhythmias are associated with a high mortality. The importance of continuous ECG monitoring in acute respiratory failure is emphasized.

Krowka MJ, Pairolero PC, Trastek VF, Payne WS, Bernatz PE: Cardiac dysrhythmia following pneumonectomy. Clinical correlates and prognostic significance. Chest 91:490–495, 1987.

Cardiac tachydysrhythmias occurred in 53 (22 percent) of 236 consecutive patients undergoing pneumonectomy. Atrial fibrillation was the most common dysrhythmia (64 percent), followed by supraventricular tachycardia (23 percent) and atrial flutter (13 percent). No episodes of ventricular tachycardia were documented.

Littman D: The electrocardiographic findings in pulmonary emphysema. Am J Cardiol 5:339–348, 1960.

Emphysema may cause curious ECG patterns, probably owing to extraordinary position of the heart and altered conduction pathways which may simulate myocardial infarction.

McGinn S, White PD: Acute cor pulmonale resulting from pulmonary embolism. Its clinical recognition. JAMA 104:1473–1480, 1935.

Presentation of case histories of nine patients with acute cor pulmonale secondary to pulmonary embolism accompanied by ECG changes.

Meyers GB: QRS-T patterns in multiple precordial leads that may be mistaken for myocardial infarction. II. Right ventricular hypertrophy and dilatation. Circulation 1:860–877, 1950.

Abnormal ECG patterns consistent with anterior, anterolateral, or inferior infarction have been recorded in well-documented cases of chronic cor pulmonale. The mechanism for these changes is unknown but may be due to right ventricular hypertrophy with or without dilatation and changes in spacial orientation and posterior displacement of the apex.

Mounsey JPD, Ritzman LW, Siverstone MJ: Cardiographic studies in severe pulmonary emphysema. Br Heart J 14:442–450, 1952.

ECG findings of right ventricular hypertrophy, if present, are related directly to right heart pressures by cardiac catheterization. This study confirmed that the value of the ECG appeared to be more confirming the nature of the heart disease present rather than diagnosing its inception.

Murphy ML, Hutchinson F: The electrocardiographic diagnosis of right ventricular hypertrophy in chronic obstructive lung disease. Chest 65:622–627, 1974.

Seventy patients with unequivocal clinical and pathologic evidence of severe obstructive pulmonary disease were studied using right ventricular mass rather than wall thickness alone. Only 30 patients had a definite increase in right ventricular mass. Four ECG criteria were found to be the most reliable in making the correct diagnosis.

Roman GT, Walsh TJ, Massie E: Right ventricular hypertrophy; correlation of EKG and anatomic findings. Am J Cardiol 7:481–487, 1961.

A review of the ECG criteria necessary to make the diagnosis of right ventricular hypertrophy.

Scott RC: The electrocardiogram in pulmonary emphysema and chronic cor pulmonale. Am Heart J 61:843–845, 1961.

The relationship of the heart assuming a more vertical position, a tendency toward clockwise rotation electrical axis on a longitudinal plane, plus the effects of the overinflated lungs and the spatial QRS vector being posteriorly directed results in a characteristic ECG pattern.

Stein PD, Dalen JE, McIntyre KM, Sussaharu AA, Wenger MK, Willis PW III: The electrocardiogram in acute pulmonary embolism. Prog Cardiovasc Dis 17:247–257, 1975.

A broader spectrum of ECG abnormalities associated with pulmonary embolism is now possible because of pulmonary angiography and ventilation-perfusion scanning of the lung.

Sullivan MM, Moss RB, Hindi RD, Lewiston NJ: Supraventricular tachycardia in patients with cystic fibrosis. Chest 90:239–242, 1986.

In four patients with cystic fibrosis who developed supraventricular tachycardia (SVT), three had cor pulmonale, as evidenced by echocardiogram, and all had baseline tachycardia. Because of bronchospasm, all were taking theophylline, prednisone, and beta-2 adrenergic agonists.

Wadler S, Chahinian P, Slater W, Goldman M, Mendelson D, Holland JF: Cardiac abnormalities in patients with diffuse malignant pleural mesothelioma. Cancer 58:2744–2750, 1986.

The electrocardiographic (EKG) and echocardiographic findings in 64 patients with biopsy-proven malignant pleural mesothelioma were reviewed. The EKG and echocardiogram are helpful in differentiating cardiac involvement from progressive pulmonary disease in patients with pleural mesothelioma.

Chapter 35

Radiographic Evaluation of the Chest

Wallace T. Miller

GENERAL ASPECTS

In recent years, fresh concepts and new techniques have greatly expanded the diagnostic armamentarium of chest radiology. As a rule, the new approaches have strengthened the underpinnings of conventional chest radiography as well as extending its diagnostic capabilities. The diagnostic appraisal from the perspective of chest radiography invariably begins with conventional radiographs and is supplemented, as indicated, by supplementary radiographs.

The Routine Examination

In young individuals or in asymptomatic patients a posteroanterior (PA) projection alone is generally used as a screening procedure. This projection is the easiest to interpret since the anatomy is quite familiar, and most pathologic conditions in the chest will appear in this view. Ideally, a lateral view should also be part of the routine examination. The lateral view adds valuable information about certain areas that are not well seen on the PA view. This is particularly true of the anterior part of the lung close to the mediastinum, which may be obscured by overlying heart and aortic shadows (Fig. 35-1). The vertebral column is another high yield area on the lateral view since it is not well seen on the PA view. A small pleural effusion is best seen, and often only seen, as blunting of a costophrenic sulcus posteriorly (Fig. 35-2).

In determining which costophrenic angle is blunted, certain characteristics of the lateral view are useful. Correctly identifying each hemidiaphragm on the lateral view may be difficult. If the lateral radiograph is taken in the left lateral position, as is usual, the magnified ribs are on the right side, and the unmagnified ribs are on the left side and will be associated with the appropriate hemidiaphragm (Fig. 35-2). Moreover, the outline of the left hemidiaphragm is often obscured anteriorly because it merges with the shadow of the heart. Finally, the left hemidiaphragm may be recognized by its proximity to the stomach bubble.

Supplementary Plain Radiographs

In addition to the PA and lateral chest radiographs, other projections serve special purposes.

Oblique views are sometimes invaluable in delineating a pulmonary mass or infiltrate from structures that overlie it on the PA and lateral views. Barium in the esophagus serves as a useful adjunct in clarifying the location of mediastinal lesions on oblique films.

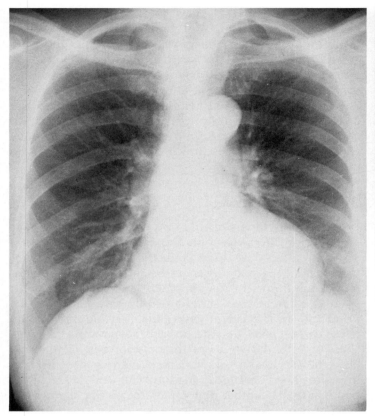

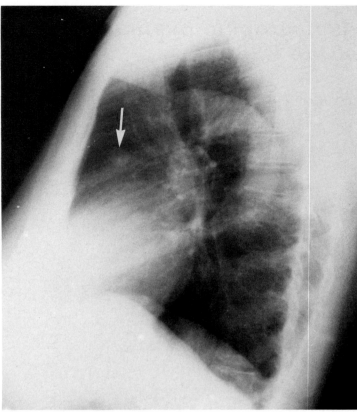

A

B

FIGURE 35-1 The lateral view in uncovering a solitary nodule. *A.* PA view. No nodule is discernible. *B.* Lateral view. A small nodule (arrow) overlies the left hilus. The nodule proved to be a granuloma.

In interpreting oblique films, it is helpful to keep in mind that a pulmonary lesion that maintains a fairly constant relationship to the heart as the patient is rotated lies in the anterior portion of the chest; a lesion that does the same with respect to the spine is posterior.

The *lateral decubitus* projection (Fig. 35-3C) is often used to identify the presence of a pleural effusion. As little as 25 to 50 ml of pleural fluid can be visualized, even though 300 ml may be required to blunt the costophrenic sulcus on PA view. The decubitus view is particularly useful in determining if blunting of a costophrenic sulcus is due to pleural effusion or to pleural thickening. While a pleural effusion is often an important finding, pleural thickening usually follows an exudate or blood in the pleural space and is usually unimportant.

The *lordotic* projection (Fig. 35-4B) enables the evaluation of the apical portions of the lungs by displacing shadows of the first rib and the clavicle, which may be confusing on the PA projection (Fig. 35-4A).

The *lordotic* view may also be useful in demonstrating collapse of the right middle lobe.

The *overpenetrated grid* radiograph (Fig. 35-5A) is useful for evaluating densities that lie behind the heart or

diaphragm and are poorly seen on routine radiographs. *Expiratory* films often disclose air trapping or demonstrate a pneumothorax that is poorly shown on the routine radiograph. *Stereoscopic* views can be helpful in localizing any pulmonary lesion but are particularly useful in apical lesions where they can separate pulmonary lesions from the overlying clavicle and first rib.

Magnification radiographs are occasionally used in diffuse lung disease to clarify minute details of the pulmonary parenchyma. *Supravoltage* radiographs (1000 kV or more) are occasionally helpful in evaluating pulmonary or mediastinal lesions.

Laminography

The technique of laminography (tomography, body section radiography, planigraphy) utilizes the reciprocal movement of the x-ray tube and film about a fixed fulcrum to generate a radiograph of a plane that is several millimeters thick, which is in focus while other anatomic details are blurred. Essentially, this technique provides a view of

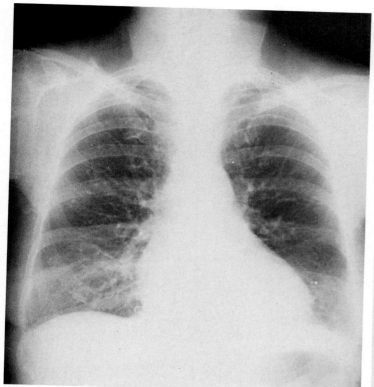

A

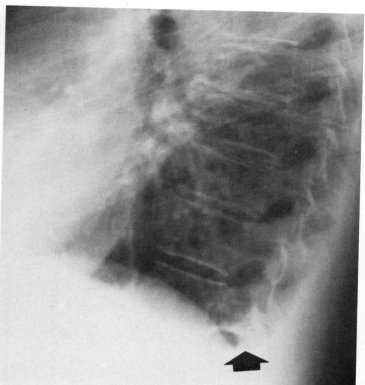

B

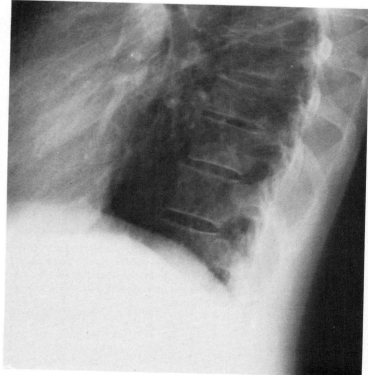

C

FIGURE 35-2 The lateral view in uncovering a small pleural effusion. *A.* PA view. No evidence of a pleural effusion. *B.* Lateral view. The right costophrenic sulcus is blunted (arrow). *C.* Lateral view. After treatment for heart failure, the effusion is gone. Note the magnification of the posterior (right) ribs.

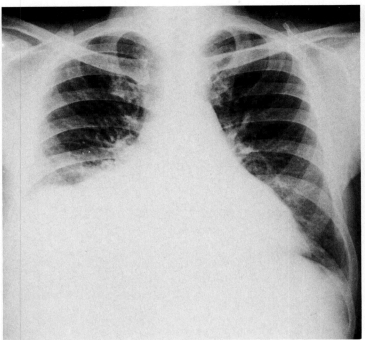

A

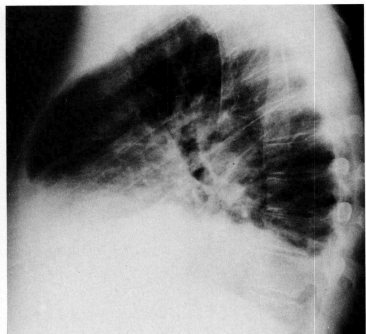

B

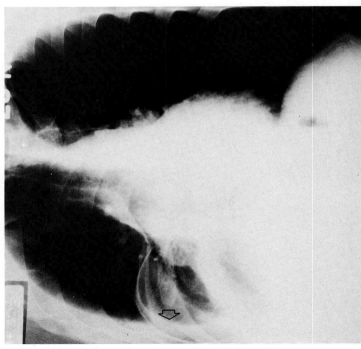

C

FIGURE 35-3   Infrapulmonary effusion. Neither the PA view *(A)* nor the lateral view *(B)* shows blunting of the costophrenic sulcus. However, elevation of the right hemidiaphragm suggests the presence of an infrapulmonary effusion. A right lateral decubitus film *(C)* shows the presence of a free pleural effusion on the right. The effusion was secondary to congestive heart failure.

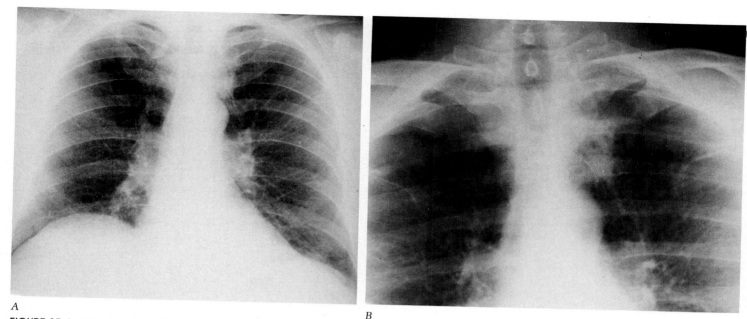

A

B

FIGURE 35-4   Carcinoma of the left upper lobe.   *A.* PA view. A small nodule is present in the left upper lobe adjacent to the mediastinum, just above the aortic knob.   *B.* Lordotic view. This nodule is much more apparent. It proved to be a primary adenocarcinoma of the lung.

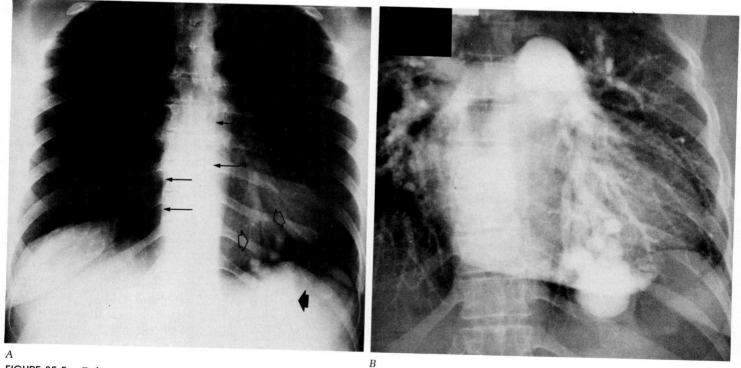

A

B

FIGURE 35-5   Pulmonary arteriovenous malformation.   *A.* Overpenetrated grid (Bucky) radiograph shows a nodule behind the diaphragm (closed arrow).   *B.* Pulmonary angiogram confirmed the diagnosis of arteriovenous malformation. Also visible bilaterally on the over-penetrated Bucky film are the posterior paraspinal lines (small arrows). The left posterior paraspinal line is medial to the aorta. The right paraspinal line is ordinarily not discernible but can be seen in this patient because of small osteophytes that arise from the vertebral bodies and displace laterally the pleura on the right.

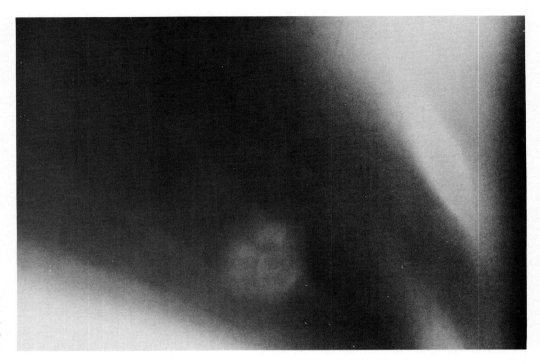

FIGURE 35-6 Hamartoma. A tomogram of a pulmonary nodule shows that the nodule contains several calcifications within its center. This nodule proved to be a hamartoma.

a thin slice of lung and affords a close look at a suspected abnormality. It is useful in demonstrating the presence of calcification within a pulmonary nodule (Fig. 35-6) and occasionally in providing insight into the nature of the lesion. For example, scattered "popcorn" calcifications indicate benign disease. The different implications of various types of calcifications are considered subsequently.

Laminography occasionally discloses cavitation within a pulmonary lesion, particularly in pulmonary tuberculosis, that is not evident on the routine radiograph. Laminography is seldom useful in searching blindly for a clinically suspected lesion that cannot be seen on the routine radiograph. It is also apt to be unrewarding with respect to supplying additional information when a routine chest film has clearly depicted the lesion. But laminography of both lung fields is occasionally useful in uncovering multiple lesions when only a solitary nodule is visible on routine films. Also, when the likelihood of pulmonary metastasis is strong, laminography may be useful in uncovering a pulmonary metastasis that is not apparent on the routine radiograph. Computed tomography is even more sensitive in this regard.

Fluoroscopy

Fluoroscopy of the chest is useful for examining the movement of pulmonary and cardiac structures and for localizing a pulmonary lesion that is visible in only one of the two conventional radiographic projections. It is particularly helpful for examining diaphragmatic motion. When searching for diaphragmatic paralysis, the patient is best fluoroscoped in the lateral projection so that the motion of both hemidiaphragms can be observed simultaneously. A paralyzed hemidiaphragm moves paradoxically. This paradoxical motion may be difficult to see during quiet breathing but usually becomes readily apparent during a quick, short "sniff" (*sniff test*). Localized weakness in part of one hemidiaphragm (eventration) (Fig. 35-7) is often misinterpreted as diaphragmatic paralysis. This error can be avoided by fluoroscopy in the lateral projection; partial eventration is then manifested by paradoxical motion of one portion of the hemidiaphragm, whereas the remainder moves normally. Eventration of an entire hemidiaphragm is impossible to distinguish from paralysis since, in both instances, the entire hemidiaphragm moves paradoxically.

Fluoroscopy of the heart is useful in demonstrating calcifications in cardiac valves or in coronary arteries. It often suggests the presence of pericardial effusion much more convincingly than do chest radiographs. But fluoroscopy is rarely definitive for pericardial effusion, and other procedures, particularly ultrasound [but also CT or MRI (magnetic resonance imaging)], are generally used to confirm a suspected pericardial effusion.

Fluoroscopy often helps to identify the nature of a mediastinal lesion. When coupled with a barium swallow, lesions within the esophagus can be seen. Moreover, the pattern of displacement of the esophagus by a mass in the middle mediastinum often helps to determine the nature of the mass. Respiratory maneuvers affect the size of

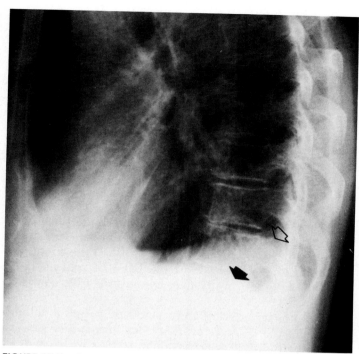

FIGURE 35-7 Partial eventration of the diaphragm. The lateral view shows elevation of the posterior portion of the right hemidiaphragm (open arrow). The normal contour of the left hemidiaphragm (closed arrow) appears immediately beneath. This partial eventration is due to a localized weakness in the posterior aspect of the right hemidiaphragm.

large venous structures in the chest: they become smaller during the Valsalva maneuver and larger during the Mueller maneuver. These maneuvers leave unchanged the size of solid masses. Pulsation of a mediastinal mass raises the prospect that it is vascular. However, pulsation has to be interpreted with care: masses that are adjacent to the aorta often transmit its pulsations and appear to be pulsating; conversely, large aortic aneurysms often pulsate poorly.

In years gone by, fluoroscopy of the chest was used as a screening procedure for routine examination of the chest. This is no longer acceptable for several reasons: the patient's x-ray exposure is much greater during a short fluoroscopic examination than during standard radiographs; small lesions in the lung fields are easily overlooked at fluoroscopy; and no permanent record of the fluoroscopic examination is available. Indeed, unless some specific information is being sought, fluoroscopy of the chest is not warranted.

Computed Tomography

Computed tomography is a radiologic technique for scanning cross sections of the entire body. The underlying principle is the production of x-ray absorption profiles that are made at different angles in the same cross-sectional plane. A pencil-thin beam of x-rays passes through the body as the radiographic tube rotates around the patient, and the transmitted radiation is detected by a sodium iodide crystal. By means of electronic transformation, the signals are fed into a computer which synthesizes them into a picture that displays the relative absorption coefficients of each small area in the plane of the scan. This instrument is highly accurate, and its sensitivity to differences in density is considerably greater than is standard radiographic film. This technique is discussed in greater detail in Chapter 36.

Nuclear Magnetic Resonance

Magnetic resonance (MR), or nuclear magnetic resonance (NMR), is a technique which uses radiowaves modified by a strong magnetic field to produce a diagnostic image. The images produced are somewhat similar to CT, but differ in that vascular structures are usually well seen without contrast material and that various differing images can be obtained by manipulation of the radio-wave frequency and timing of the impulses delivered. This technique is discussed in greater detail in Chapter 36.

Contrast Examinations

Air in the bronchi and alveoli is a superb contrast medium, outlining the pulmonary vasculature, the heart, the aorta and other mediastinal structures, the diaphragm, and the chest wall. In addition, pathologic processes in the lung often produce characteristic changes in the pattern of the pulmonary vessels or the air-filled alveoli. Thus the plain film of the chest is a very useful tool in diagnosis of disease states, and further manipulation is usually not necessary.

However, supplementary information may be gained by introducing extraneous contrast material into different components of the chest. Positive contrast material, such as barium sulfate suspension, is commonly introduced into the esophagus: other suitable media are used to visualize cardiac chambers, trachea and bronchi, pulmonary vessels, aorta, bronchial and mediastinal arteries, superior vena cava and mediastinal veins, and the mediastinal lymphatics. For negative contrast, air or other gases are introduced into the pleural cavity, the peritoneal cavity, and the mediastinum. Carbon dioxide or nitrous oxide has been used to outline the cardiac chambers on the right side of the heart.

Of all the contrast examinations, the barium swallow, generally carried out under fluoroscopic guidance, is the simplest to perform. The thick mixture of barium sulfate outlining the esophageal contour makes it easy to detect displacement of the esophagus by adjacent mediastinal structures, such as tumor-containing lymph nodes, or by a

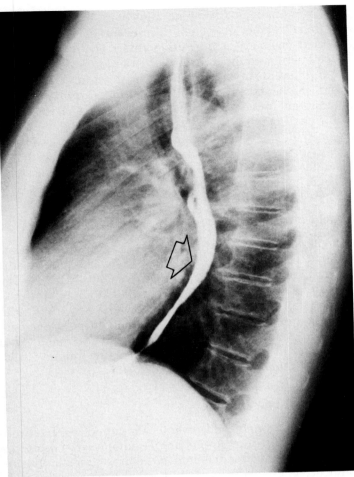

FIGURE 35-8   Enlarged left atrium. The esophagus is displaced posteriorly by an enlarged left atrium (arrow).

Pulmonary Angiography

Pulmonary angiography involves the rapid injection of a radiopaque dye into the pulmonary circulation by introducing a catheter into the pulmonary arterial tree or into a large systemic vein leading into the right atrium. Angiography is the gold standard in investigating thromboembolic disease of the lungs (Figs. 35-11 and 35-12). Ventilation and perfusion scans of the lung using radioactive isotopes are valuable screening procedures in detecting pulmonary embolism, but if doubt exists about the true diagnosis, pulmonary angiography is indicated.

Congenital abnormalities of the pulmonary vascular tree, such as hypoplasia or agenesis of the pulmonary artery, arteriovenous malformation, pulmonary varix, or anomalous pulmonary venous return, are also identified by pulmonary angiography (Fig. 35-5B). These abnormalities are often suspected on the basis of routine radiographs, but angiography may be necessary for confirmation.

Pulmonary arteriography can also be used in a therapeutic fashion. Arteriovenous malformations can be treated by pulmonary artery embolization with appropriate embolic material. Bleeding from the pulmonary arteries, as from bronchial vessels, can also be treated by embolism.

Aortography and Systemic Arteriography

Puzzling shadows in the vicinity of the middle (visceral) compartment of the mediastinum can be explored by aortography which takes advantage of the fact that the aorta is contained primarily within the middle compartment.

Opacification of the aorta using contrast material usually involves retrograde catheterization of the aorta for direct injection. Middle mediastinal masses frequently prove to be vascular in nature, i.e., dissecting aneurysms of the aorta, saccular or fusiform aneurysms of the aorta (Fig. 35-13), or an anomaly or unusual tortuosity of the aorta or great vessels. CT or MR often makes arteriography unnecessary.

The great vessels or the coronary arteries are also selectively catheterized and studied for specific indications, e.g., arterial stenosis. Coronary arteriography has tremendous value in identifying those patients with angina who may be successfully treated by angioplasty or coronary artery bypass.

Due to the dual blood supply of the lung, pulmonary arteriography may not be rewarding with certain pulmonary lesions in which bronchial arteriography is of major value. In patients with massive hemoptysis due to tumor or infection (tuberculosis, bronchiectasis, or aspergillosis), the major blood supply is usually from the bronchial circuit. Embolization of feeding bronchial arteries can yield temporary or even permanent control of bleeding.

large left atrium (Fig. 35-8). Abnormalities of the esophagus itself, such as achalasia or tumor, are also easily seen.

Although the trachea and major bronchi are readily seen in the mediastinum and hili, bronchography is necessary to demonstrate abnormalities in peripheral bronchi, the thin walls of which are not sharply delineated from the alveolar portions of the lungs.

Bronchography is performed using one of several different contrast media. Figure 35-9 is a bronchogram obtained by using oily Dionosil as the contrast medium.

Since the advent of fiberoptic bronchoscopy, bronchography has fallen into disuse as a technique for exploring the tracheobronchial tree for tumor. Bronchoscopy yields much more information without additional discomfort. Therefore, the bronchogram is now reserved primarily for investigating bronchiectasis (Fig. 35-10) and has become a seldom used procedure.

(Text continued on page 490.)

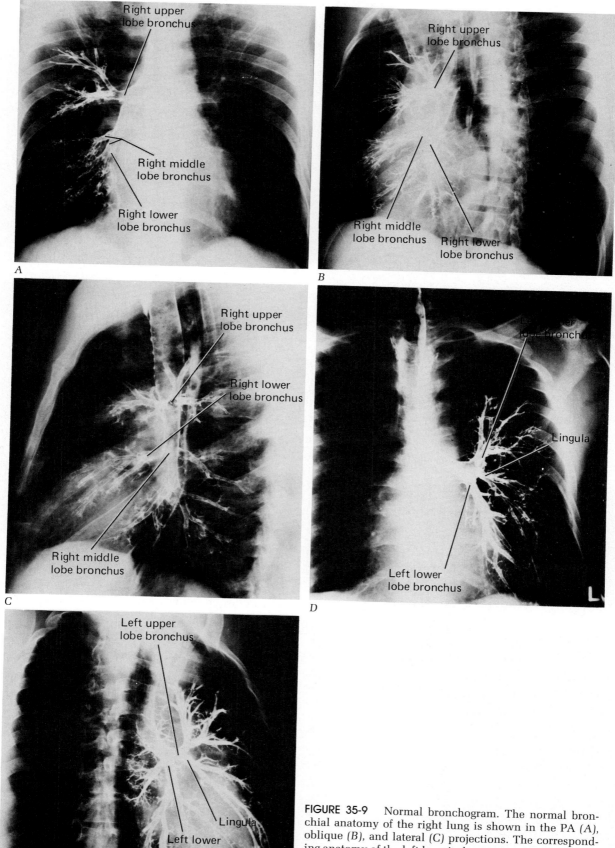

FIGURE 35-9 Normal bronchogram. The normal bronchial anatomy of the right lung is shown in the PA (A), oblique (B), and lateral (C) projections. The corresponding anatomy of the left lung is demonstrated in the PA (D) and oblique (E) projections. The lateral projection for the left lung appears in Fig. 35-10, which also illustrates bronchiectasis. A schematic representation of the bronchial tree in the PA projection appears in Fig. 35-27.

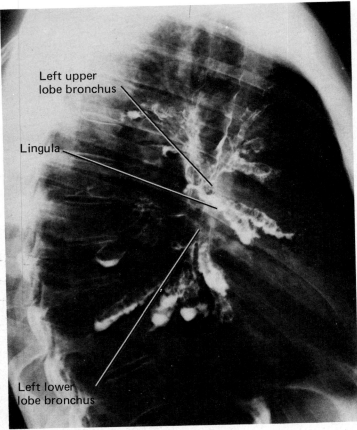

FIGURE 35-10 Bronchiectasis. The lateral view shows extensive bronchiectasis of the left lung. All the bronchi that contain contrast medium show saccular dilatation of their segments.

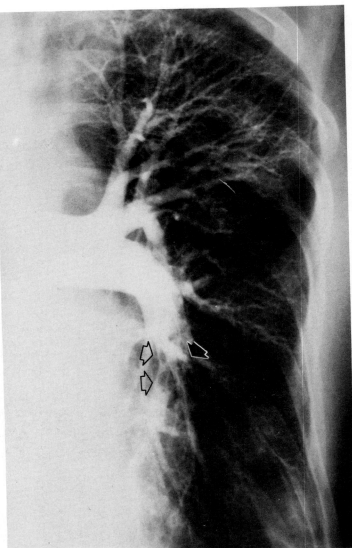

FIGURE 35-12 Small pulmonary emboli. Angiography shows small filling defects in the posterior basal artery (open arrows). Several of the other basal divisions are cut off (closed arrow). Blood flow to the left upper lobe is well preserved. Angiography was helpful diagnostically in this patient because the lung scan was equivocal.

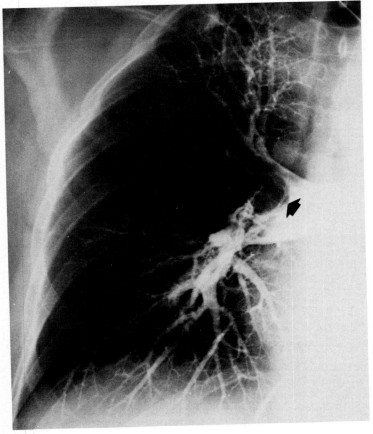

FIGURE 35-11 Large pulmonary embolus. A large pulmonary embolus is lodged in the right main pulmonary artery and has compromised blood flow primarily to the arteries of the right upper lobe (arrow). The peripheral vessels in the right mid-lung zone are not filled.

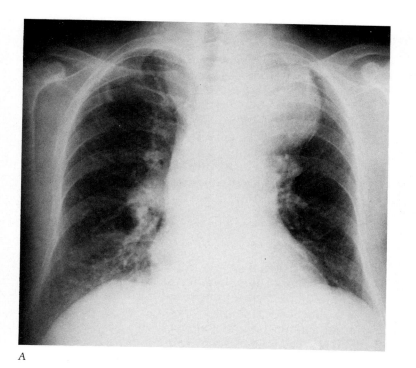

A

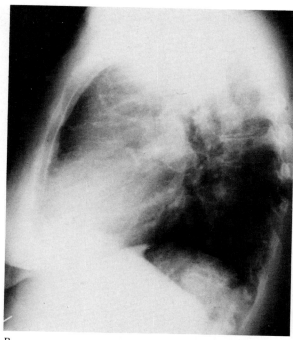

B

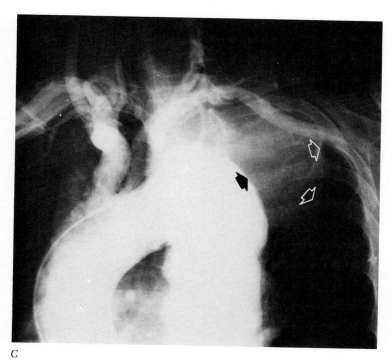

C

FIGURE 35-13 Aortic aneurysm. *A.* PA view. A large mass is in the left upper mediastinum. *B.* Lateral view. This mass appears to be within the middle mediastinal (visceral) compartment. *C.* Aortogram. The dye column is irregular at the site of the aortic aneurysm (closed arrow), most of which is filled with clot (open arrows).

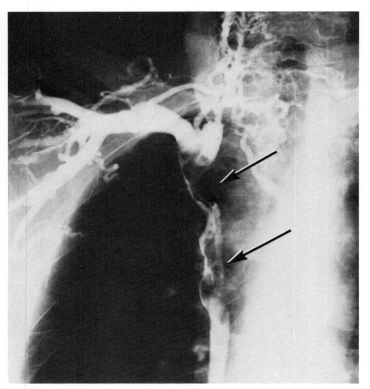

FIGURE 35-14   Superior vena caval invasion by metastatic tumor. A superior vena cavogram shows invasion of the superior vena cava in several places (arrows) by metastatic tumor involving the mediastinal lymph nodes.

Bronchial arteries supply most lung tumors. Perfusion of these tumors via the bronchial circuit with various chemotherapeutic agents has been attempted for palliative control of nonresectable malignancy. At this date, this has not been a very fruitful approach.

Venography can also be helpful. After injection of radiopaque material into a large vein of one or both upper extremities, displacement or obstruction of the superior vena cava by mediastinal masses or scarring after inflammatory process can be identified (Fig. 35-14). The azygos vein can also be opacified and is occasionally helpful in evaluating mediastinal lesions or bronchogenic carcinoma.

Air Contrast Studies

Air has occasionally been introduced into the various compartments of the chest for diagnostic purposes. For example, deliberate introduction of air into the pleural space (diagnostic pneumothorax) has been used to demonstrate pleural lesions. Pneumothorax has fallen out of vogue because other diagnostic measures, such as pleural biopsy, yield much more definitive and reliable information. Diagnostic pneumothorax or diagnostic pneumoperitoneum are still useful, on occasion, in investigating masses in the vicinity of the diaphragm. Air in the peritoneal cavity is particularly useful in demonstrating a subphrenic abscess. Diagnostic pneumomediastinum has been used in clarifying the nature of a mediastinal mass.

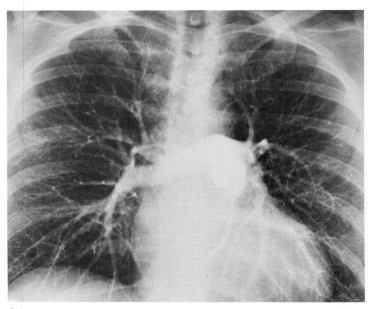
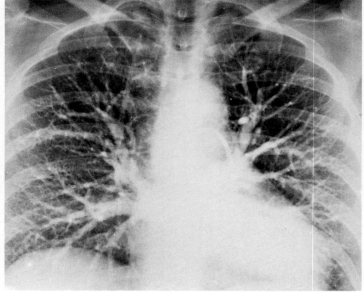

A

B

FIGURE 35-15   Pulmonary arteries and veins.   A. The early phase of the pulmonary angiogram depicts the normal course of the pulmonary arteries.   B. The late phase shows the normal course of the pulmonary veins. The veins have a more horizontal course than the arteries and enter the hilus below the arteries.

For example, in a patient with myasthenia gravis, it occasionally discloses a thymoma that has escaped detection by more conventional techniques. Computed tomography has largely eliminated this technique.

PULMONARY ARTERIES AND VEINS

The pulmonary arteries follow the course of the bronchial tree much more clearly than do pulmonary veins (Fig. 35-15) and can be recognized accompanying the bronchi and branching in a similar fashion. The pulmonary veins take a somewhat different course.

In the lower lobes, the veins are considerably lower than the corresponding arteries; the veins are situated at the level of the eighth to tenth ribs posteriorly, whereas the arteries are at the level of the seventh and eighth ribs. In the upper lobes, the pulmonary veins are lateral to the arteries.

The direction taken by a pulmonary vessel is the most useful basis for establishing its identity. Near the hili, particularly in the lower lobes, the pulmonary veins are more horizontal than the pulmonary arteries. At the hili, the pulmonary veins lie below and lateral to the arteries (Fig. 35-15). Although it is often possible to distinguish arteries from veins, this distinction is seldom useful; most often they are collectively referred to as pulmonary *vessels* or *vasculature*. Laminography enhances distinctions between pulmonary arteries and veins; angiography is currently the last word; NMR holds great promise for the future.

Distribution of Pulmonary Blood Flow

Blood flow is not uniform in the normal upright human lung. Moreover, the pattern shifts with changes in posture and exercise, as well as in different types of heart and lung disease. In a normal pulmonary circulation, gravity is the predominant determinant of the pattern of blood flow (and blood volume). Under the influence of gravity, hydrostatic pressure in pulmonary arteries, capillaries, and veins decreases at a rate of approximately 1 cmH$_2$O per centimeter of distance from the bottom to the top of the lung. Accordingly, in the upright position, blood flow is minimal at the apex and maximal at the base. In the supine position, blood flow becomes much more uniform. If the lung is inverted, the normal pattern is reversed so that the flow to the apex (now dependent) increases considerably and exceeds basal blood flow (Fig. 35-16). During walking (mild exercise in the upright position), total pulmonary flow increases, but blood flow to the upper part of the lung increases more than to the lower, so that the topographic distribution of blood flow becomes more uniform.

Should pulmonary arterial pressure at the top of the lung fail to exceed alveolar pressure, the capillaries will collapse. In a normal lung, pulsatile pulmonary blood flow suffices to perfuse the apexes, but when pulmonary arterial pressure falls, as in hemorrhagic hypotension, the normal marginal perfusion of the apexes may give way to cessation of blood flow. Gravity plays less of a role in determining the distribution of pulmonary blood flow once an increase in pulmonary vascular resistance has raised pulmonary arterial pressure to hypertensive levels.

Lung disease often modifies the pattern of pulmonary blood flow mechanically and by pulmonary vasoconstriction (Fig. 35-17). Heart disease may also affect the pattern of distribution. For example, in left-to-right intracardiac shunts, pulmonary blood flow not only increases but becomes more uniform than normal. The pattern is quite similar to that of exercise. In heart disease associated with high pulmonary venous pressures, as in chronic left ventricular failure or mitral stenosis, the distribution of blood flow tends to become more uniform early in the disease. In time, the apexes become relatively hyperperfused as a result of interstitial edema and fibrosis and hypoxic vasoconstriction at the lung bases, which increases pulmonary vascular resistance there (pulmonary venous hypertension) (Fig. 35-18). In prolonged severe pulmonary venous hypertension, further constriction of the pulmonary vasculature occurs diffusely through the lungs resulting in the pruned tree appearance of pulmonary arterial hypertension. Chronic lung disease or idiopathic pulmonary hypertension (Fig. 35-19) may also exhibit the pruned tree appearance of pulmonary arterial hypertension. In general, the diagnostic accuracy of the radiologist is much greater for pulmonary venous hypertension than for pulmonary arterial hypertension.

The influence of gravity on the distribution of blood flow bears on the interpretation of the chest radiograph. The mainstay of the concept illustrated in Fig. 35-20 is that in the upright lung, even though gravity causes pulmonary arterial and pulmonary venous pressures to increase from the top to the bottom of the normal lung, alveolar pressure remains virtually constant everywhere (see Chapter 13). Upsets in the normal relationships between pulmonary arterial, venous, and alveolar pressures from the top to the bottom of the upright lung cause derangements in the pattern of flow. For example, a regional change in alveolar pressure, due to bronchoconstriction or to obstruction of a bronchus by a foreign body or a mucous plug, raises alveolar pressures locally because of air trapping. In chronic obstructive airways disease, this mechanism contributes to rearrangement of blood flow, adding a functional component to the anatomic obliteration of parts of the vascular bed by disease.

The change in the patterns of pulmonary blood flow caused by heart disease has been previously discussed. Other disease processes also cause characteristic patterns of redistribution of pulmonary blood flow. For example, uncommon, but of great diagnostic value, is the oligemic

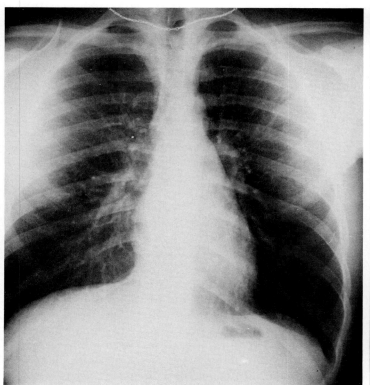

A

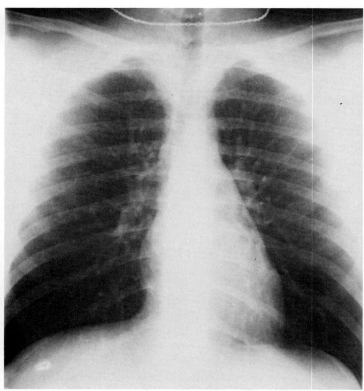

B

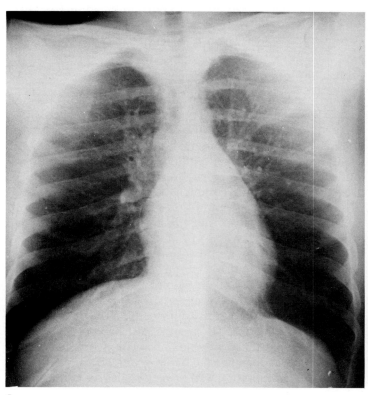

C

FIGURE 35-16 Effect of gravity on the pulmonary vasculature. Vascular patterns are compared in a normal subject in the erect, supine, and upside-down positions. *A.* Erect posture. The vascular pattern is more prominent at the bases. *B.* Supine position. The vascular pattern is more uniform. *C.* Upside-down position. The vascular pattern is more marked at the apexes.

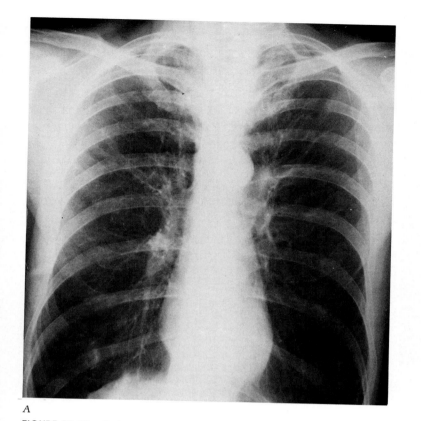

A

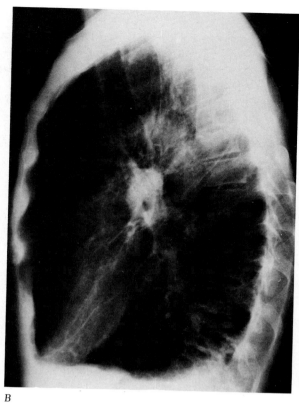

B

FIGURE 35-17   Pulmonary emphysema.   *A.* PA view. Both lungs appear to be hyperradiolucent. Blood flow to the left lower lobe is particularly reduced.   *B.* Lateral view. The marked hyperradiolucency is associated with a flat diaphragm, a wide anteroposterior diameter of the chest, and an increase in the retrosternal space.

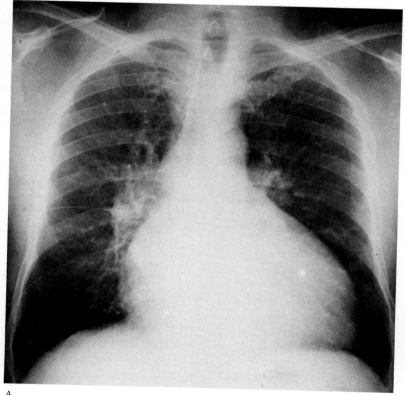

A

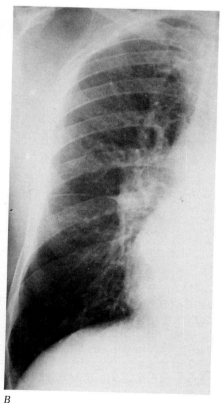

B

FIGURE 35-18   Pulmonary vasculature in mitral stenosis.   *A.* PA view. The enlarged left atrium is seen as a double density within the cardiac shadow. Cephalization of the pulmonary blood vessels is also present, the result of an increase in blood flow to the apexes in conjunction with a decrease to the lung bases.   *B.* Close-up view. The increase in vascular markings at the apexes is more striking.

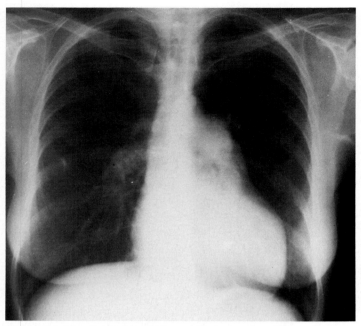

FIGURE 35-19 Primary pulmonary hypertension. The pulmonary trunk and its right and left main bronchi are markedly enlarged. In contrast, the peripheral vasculature is sparse.

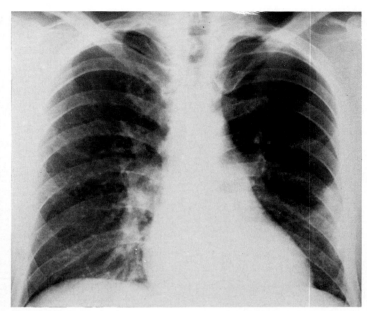

FIGURE 35-21 Massive pulmonary embolus. The PA view demonstrates marked diminution of the pulmonary vasculature to the left lung, secondary to a chronic massive pulmonary embolus in the left main pulmonary artery.

Zone		Behavior of capillary	Flow depends on
I $P_A > Ppa > Ppv$	P_A / Ppa □ Ppv	Collapsed	No flow*
II $Ppa > P_A > Ppv$	P_A / Ppa □ Ppv	Starling resistor	$Ppa - P_A$
III $Ppa > Ppv > P_A$	P_A / Ppa □ Ppv	Open or distended	$Ppa - Ppv$

*Except for flow through corner vessels.

FIGURE 35-20 Schematic representation of the behavior of small vessels in different parts of the lung. The lung is pictured as consisting of three vertical zones. In zone I, alveolar pressure is greater than arterial pressure so that collapsible vessels in the pulmonary microcirculation close; there is no flow. In zone II, arterial pressure exceeds alveolar pressure, which exceeds venous pressure. The pulmonary arterial-alveolar pressure difference determines the blood flow. Microvessels in this zone behave like the Starling resistors. The arterial-alveolar pressure difference increases linearly from top to bottom of the lung and produces corresponding changes in blood flow. In zone III, blood flow is determined by the difference between pulmonary arterial and venous pressures since venous pressure exceeds alveolar. The collapsible vessels are open, and the pressure difference is constant throughout the zone. (After West, 1977.)

pattern of the lungs distal to a large pulmonary embolus (Fig. 35-21). In primary pulmonary hypertension, the peripheral vessels are small and the central vessels are quite large, resulting in the "pruned tree" appearance of the central pulmonary vasculature (Fig. 35-19). In emphysema, local destruction of pulmonary vasculature results in bizarre and unpredictable patterns of pulmonary blood flow (Fig. 35-17A).

DISTRIBUTION OF AIR WITHIN THE LUNG

The distribution of ventilation, as of pulmonary blood flow, is affected by gravity. Normally, the ventilation of the base is greater than that of the apex because of distortion of the lung by gravity and the higher transpulmonary pressure at the apex than at the base (see Chapter 13). Changes in ventilation from top to bottom of the upright lung are much more modest than are changes in blood flow. When the lung is supine, ventilation, as well as blood flow, is much more uniform. If the lung is turned upside down, the normal pattern is reversed so that the apex is better ventilated than the base.

Radiographic techniques can be of considerable value in providing information about the distribution of air within the lungs. For example, fluoroscopy of the chest and comparison of chest radiographs taken during inspiration and expiration are useful in detecting and localizing air trapping; blebs and bullae appear as avascular and excessively radiolucent areas. Extensive pleural encasement of one lung often is associated with a disproportionately small thorax and diminished ventilation of the affected side. Marked reduction in pulmonary vascular shadows also occurs in unilateral hypoventilation or hypoplasia of the pulmonary artery (Swyer-James, or Macleod's syndrome); the hemithorax on the affected side is also usually small. Syndromes associated with unilateral hypoplasia often show air trapping on the affected side.

Obstructive Airways Disease

The radiologist generally has little to offer in the early diagnosis of obstructive disease of the airways. Chest radiographs are nearly always normal in patients in whom the obstructive disease of the airways is reversible. For example, in asthma, the chest radiograph is usually normal, except during an acute episode of status asthmaticus in which the lungs often appear to be hyperinflated.

Similarly, the diagnosis of chronic bronchitis is primarily a clinical one, based on the history of chronic expectoration supplemented by tests of pulmonary performance. The radiograph rarely provides substantive help. Vascular markings throughout the lung fields are sometimes prominent, but this finding is nonspecific.

Even the practice of using the radiograph to assess the coexistence of emphysema and chronic bronchitis is generally unrewarding unless emphysema is marked. The classic radiographic appearance of emphysema is one of overinflation and diminution of vascular markings (Fig. 35-17). Hyperinflation is manifested by increasing radiolucency of the lungs, low and flat diaphragm, exaggerated verticality of the heart, increase in the anteroposterior diameter of the chest, and widening of the retrosternal space. Of these criteria, diaphragmatic flattening is probably most reliable.

Hyperinflation can be simulated by a normal, *robust* person who exerts a maximal inspiratory effort. The lungs also appear hyperinflated in very slender individuals. Therefore, it is unwise to make the radiographic diagnosis of pulmonary emphysema based upon hyperinflation alone.

Supplementary evidence about the presence of emphysema is afforded by the state of the pulmonary vessels. Two distinctly different vascular patterns have been identified in patients with chronic bronchitis and emphysema: (1) arterial deficiency and (2) increased markings. Those who manifest the arterial deficiency pattern (Fig. 35-17) often prove to have panlobular emphysema and manifest the clinical syndrome of the "pink puffer"; those who have the increased markings pattern (Fig. 35-22) often prove to have centrilobular emphysema and are designated clinically as "blue bloaters." It must be emphasized that these radiographic findings are relatively late manifestations of pulmonary emphysema.

Patients with chronic bronchitis and emphysema who develop pulmonary hypertension usually show the

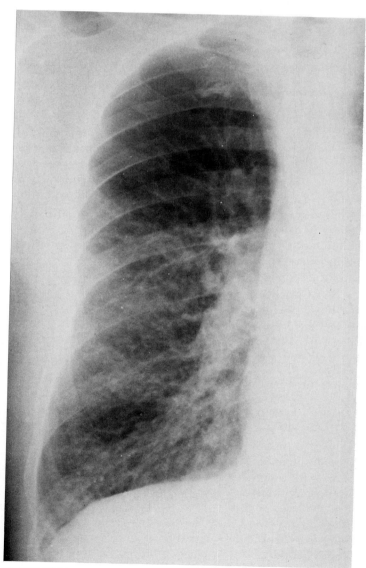

FIGURE 35-22 Increased markings pattern. The vascular markings are prominent throughout the lung fields. The patient has chronic bronchitis and emphysema. Hyperaeration is minimal.

characteristic features of hyperinflation and abnormal vascular pattern. In addition, they may show a distinctive enlargement of the hilar pulmonary arteries and oligemia of the peripheral lungs. These findings constitute important evidence for the existence of pulmonary hypertension and cor pulmonale.

Attempts have been made over the years to use radiographic techniques to determine lung volumes in chronic bronchitis and emphysema. Multiple measurements, using PA and lateral films, have been the basis for the calculations; the results have compared favorably with those obtained directly using spirometric or body plethysmographic techniques. Recently, the radiographic approach has been reinforced by the availability of sophisticated computer techniques. However, this approach has not been widely adopted because of the availability and accuracy of body plethysmography.

Heart Failure Complicating Chronic Bronchitis and Emphysema

Both right and left ventricular failure occur in the patient with chronic bronchitis and emphysema, but the mechanisms and the radiographic expressions are different. Right ventricular failure in chronic bronchitis and emphysema is generally a consequence of pulmonary hypertension secondary to severe hypoxia and respiratory acidosis. As a part of the right ventricular failure, the quantity of water in the lungs increases but rarely to the point of overt pulmonary edema. In contrast, left ventricular failure is generally caused by unrelated disease of the coronary circulation and the left ventricular myocardium: as a result, pulmonary venous pressure is abnormally high, favoring the formation of "hemodynamic" pulmonary edema.

Recognition of left ventricular failure in patients with chronic bronchitis and emphysema is difficult. The low diaphragm and the rarefied lungs obscure enlargement of the heart. The changes in pulmonary vasculature that are associated with left ventricular failure are difficult to recognize in the patient with an "increased markings" pattern. Moreover, pulmonary edema often assumes unusual appearances. Most helpful is the comparison of recent and old chest radiographs, looking for changes in cardiac size and vascular pattern. Frequently, the presence of left ventricular failure is recognized retrospectively, as the heart becomes smaller, and many of the vascular markings attenuate following a brisk diuresis and response to a cardiotonic program.

DISEASES AFFECTING THE PULMONARY PARENCHYMA

In determining the nature of a pulmonary disease, it is quite useful to know if the disease process involves primarily the alveoli of the lung or whether it involves primarily the interstitium; frequently this distinction can be made on the radiograph. It is worthwhile to attempt to distinguish alveolar from interstitial disease, even though, in some instances, distinction is difficult or impossible.

Alveolar involvement by a pulmonary process results in filling of the alveoli with some material—blood, pus, exudate. The radiograph should reflect this alveolar filling. The characteristic radiographic features of alveolar filling disease are shown in Figs. 35-23 to 35-25. They are: (1) coalescence of densities, thereby creating large homogeneous shadows; (2) the presence of an air bronchogram, i.e., visualization of peripheral bronchi due to consolidation of surrounding alveoli; (3) fluffy, irregular margins to localized areas of consolidation; and (4) rapid changes in the areas of consolidation.

Localized Alveolar Disease

Localized alveolar disease assumes two primary patterns: (1) patchy consolidation of airspaces *without* a decrease in the volume of the affected area, and (2) consolidation of airspaces associated *with* a decrease in the volume of the affected area (atelectasis). The differential diagnosis depends heavily on the extent to which volume is decreased.

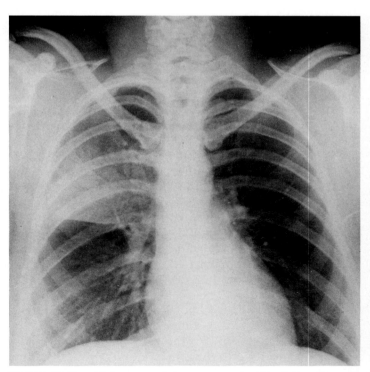

FIGURE 35-23   Right upper lobe pneumonia. The PA radiograph shows diffuse consolidation of the right upper lobe. The alveolar pattern is characteristic. The radiolucent streaks that run through the consolidation represent air in the bronchi (air bronchogram).

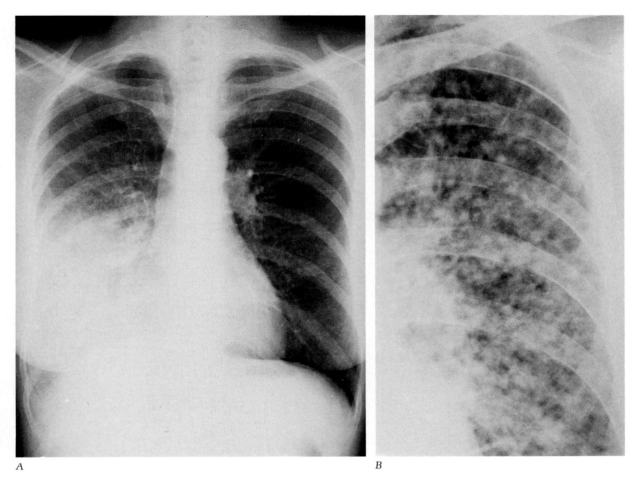

A   B

FIGURE 35-24   Patterns of alveolar cell carcinoma. *A.* A large area of consolidation in the right lower lobe in which the alveolar pattern suggests pneumonia. *B.* The more distinctive pattern for alveolar cell carcinoma consists of multiple alveolar nodules. These nodules have irregular or fuzzy margins that are characteristic of alveolar, rather than interstitial, nodulation.

Localized consolidation of alveolar airspaces without loss of volume, or with minimal loss, is generally a sign of pneumonia (Fig. 35-23). Consolidation may be localized to a lobe or a pulmonary subsegment, or it may be more diffuse. Consolidation of a pulmonary subsegment causes a characteristic radiographic pattern (Figs. 35-26 and 35-27). Among the other causes of consolidation without loss of volume is pulmonary edema, which occasionally occurs as a local consolidation even though more often it is diffuse. Pulmonary infarction is a common cause of localized consolidation.

In most instances, localized pulmonary consolidation without loss of volume indicates an acute inflammatory process. However, if consolidation persists without change for several weeks, then a less common pathologic process becomes likely. Among these are alveolar cell carcinoma (Fig. 35-24); lymphoma; metastatic carcinoma, particularly from the breast; fungus disease; eosinophilic lung disease (PIE syndrome); and granulomatous vasculitis, such as Wegener's disease.

A loss of volume (atelectasis) commonly accompanies localized consolidations of the lung. However, most instances of atelectasis detected radiographically are lobar, since collapse of pulmonary segments smaller than lobes seldom occurs because it is prevented by collateral airdrift. The patterns caused by atelectasis of the different lobes are illustrated in Figs. 35-28 to 35-32. It is extremely important to recognize the various patterns of lobar atelectasis since atelectasis is a very common manifestation of carcinoma of the lung and its presence immediately suggests an endobronchial neoplasm. Atelectasis is also common in the postoperative patient, presumably due to hypoventilation of dependent parts of the lungs and inadequate clearing of secretions. It also occurs as a consequence of inflammatory disease of the airways and of aspiration of a foreign body.

Diffuse Alveolar Disease

The prototype of a pathologic process that affects alveoli diffusely is pulmonary edema (Fig. 35-25). Most often,

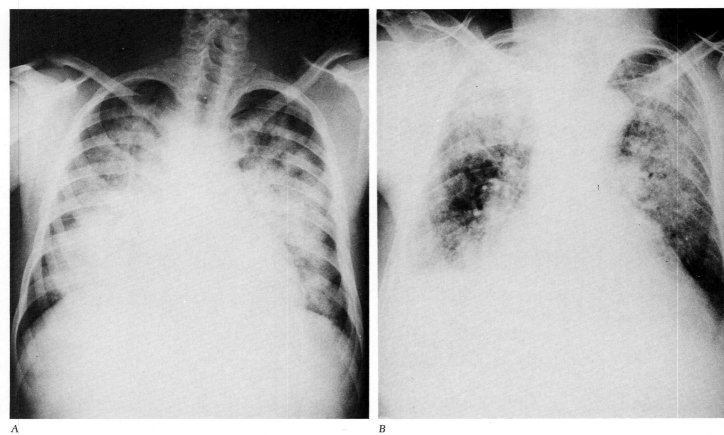

A   *B*

FIGURE 35-25   Pulmonary edema. Pulmonary edema may be either localized or diffuse. Most distinctive, but not most common, is a "bat wing" pattern of central alveolar consolidation *(A)*. More often, pulmonary edema affects one or more areas of the lung and appears as a patchy pattern of alveolar consolidation *(B)*.

pulmonary edema is secondary to left ventricular failure. But, noncardiac pulmonary edema is now also common. The etiologies of noncardiac pulmonary edema are diverse, e.g., hypersensitivity reactions to drugs or inhaled toxins, adult respiratory distress syndrome, uremia, drug overdose, O_2 toxicity, and near-drowning. Cardiac pulmonary edema characteristically clears rapidly following appropriate therapy, whereas noncardiac pulmonary edema often requires days or weeks to clear.

If diffuse alveolar consolidation persists for weeks or months, chronic disorders, such as pulmonary alveolar proteinosis (Fig. 35-33), alveolar-cell carcinoma (Fig. 35-24), sarcoidosis, metastastic carcinoma, desquamating interstitial pneumonitis, and lymphoma, are among the disorders that can also cause this rather unusual radiographic pattern.

Interstitial Lung Disease

The radiographic features of interstitial disorders differ from those of the alveolar disorders (Fig. 35-34): the pattern is discrete and sharp rather than fluffy and irregular; the lesions tend to be diffuse rather than localized; coales-

cence is not a feature; and the small densities are characteristically either nodular, reticular, or linear.

Pathologic processes of the pulmonary interstitial space tend to be chronic rather than acute. Of the acute processes, a pattern of interstitial disease that changes in hours to days usually represents interstitital pulmonary edema; occasionally it is pneumonia secondary to a virus or to *Mycoplasma*. These acute interstitial disorders typically cause a linear or reticular pattern which is characterized by prominent Kerley lines throughout the lung fields (Fig. 35-34*A*). In the original description of these lines in 1951, Kerley identified these lines with left ventricular failure and recognized three types: A, B, and C. At first, these lines were thought to represent swollen pulmonary lymphatics. Now it is recognized that they usually represent edematous septa within the pulmonary interstitium. Type B lines are the most familiar and are particularly prominent at the lung bases, where they appear as straight, thin lines approximately 1 cm in length that parallel the diaphragm. Type A lines represent septa deep within the substance of the lungs and radiate from the hili. Type C lines probably represent coalescence of A and B lines.

498

(Text continued on page 507.)

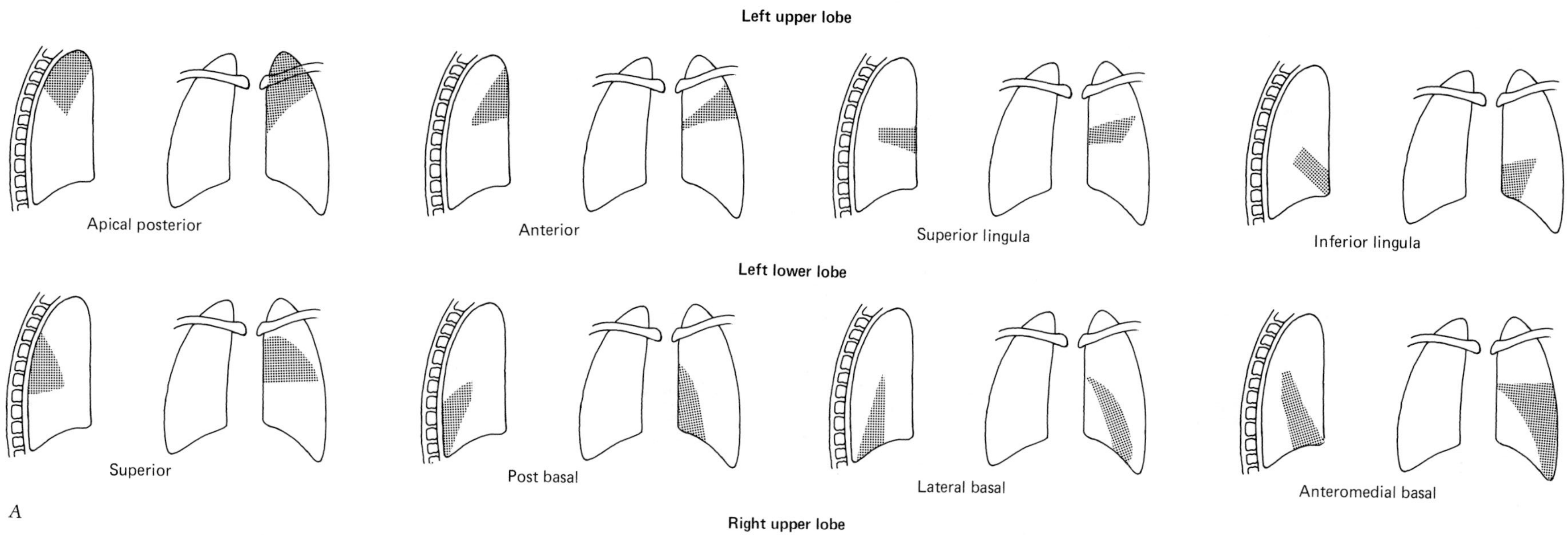

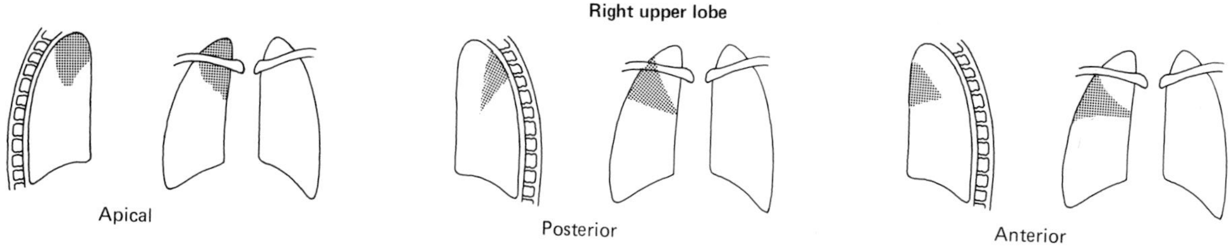

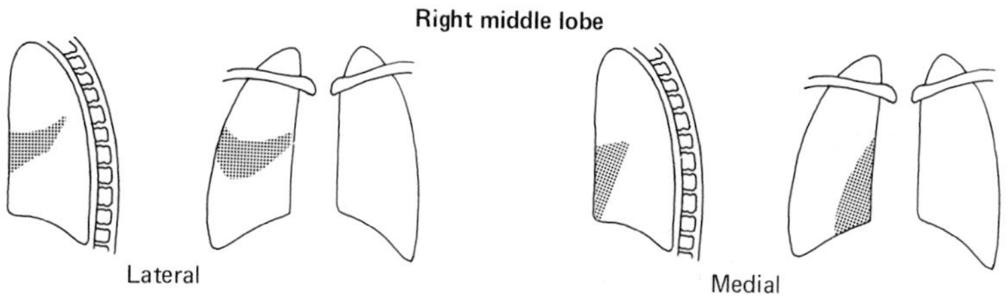

Left upper lobe

Apical posterior

Anterior

Superior lingula

Inferior lingula

Left lower lobe

Superior

Post basal

Lateral basal

Anteromedial basal

Right upper lobe

Apical

Posterior

Anterior

Right middle lobe

Lateral

Medial

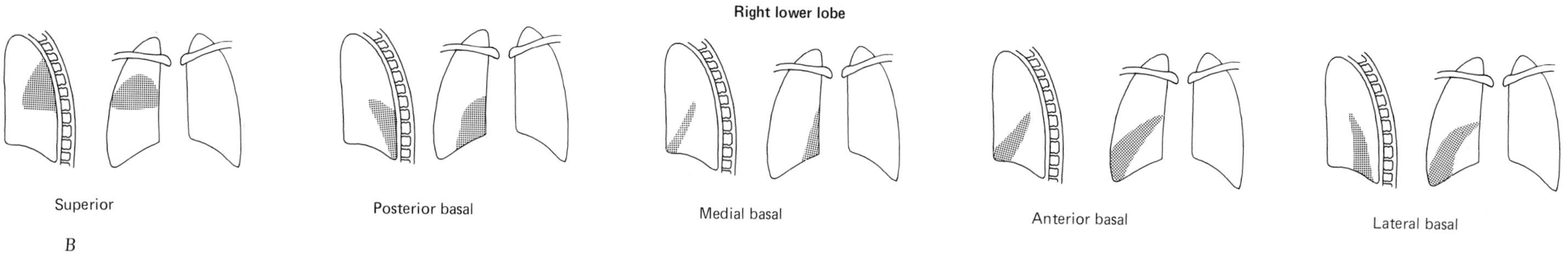

Right lower lobe

Superior

Posterior basal

Medial basal

Anterior basal

Lateral basal

A

B

FIGURE 35-26 Radiographic anatomy of the pulmonary subsegments. Schematic representations of the characteristic patterns of consolidation for each of the pulmonary subsegments. *A.* Left lung. *B.* Right lung.

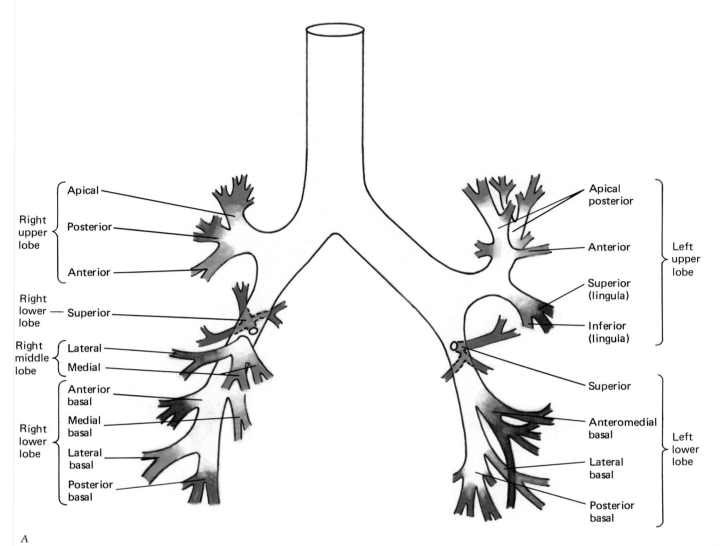

Right
upper
lobe
{ Apical
Posterior
Anterior

Right
lower
lobe — Superior

Right
middle
lobe
{ Lateral
Medial

Right
lower
lobe
{ Anterior
basal
Medial
basal
Lateral
basal
Posterior
basal

Apical
posterior
Anterior
Superior
(lingula)
Inferior
(lingula)
} Left
upper
lobe

Superior
Anteromedial
basal
Lateral
basal
Posterior
basal
} Left
lower
lobe

A

FIGURE 35-27 Topographic anatomy of the tracheobronchial tree ▶
and pulmonary subsegments. *A.* Tracheobronchial tree. *B.* Left
anterior. *C.* Left lateral. *D.* Left cutaway. *E.* Left posterior.
F. Right anterior. *G.* Right lateral. *H.* Right cutaway. *I.* Right posterior.

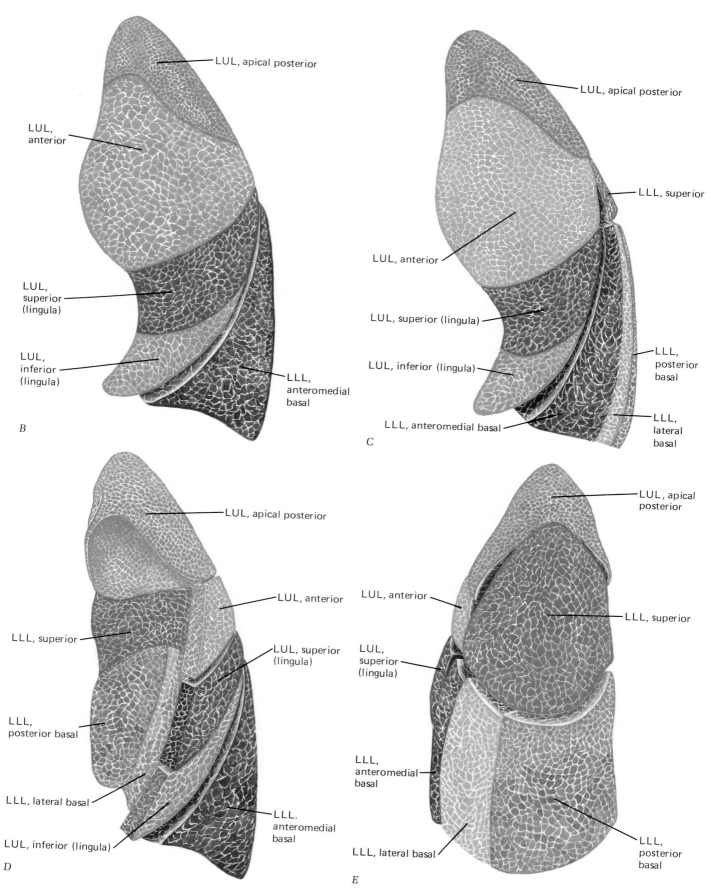

LUL, apical posterior

LUL,
anterior

LUL,
superior
(lingula)

LUL,
inferior
(lingula)

LLL,
anteromedial
basal

B

LUL, apical posterior

LLL, superior

LUL, anterior

LUL, superior (lingula)

LUL, inferior (lingula)

LLL, anteromedial basal

LLL,
posterior
basal

LLL,
lateral
basal

C

LUL, apical posterior

LLL, superior

LUL, anterior

LUL, superior
(lingula)

LLL,
posterior basal

LLL, lateral basal

LUL, inferior (lingula)

LLL.
anteromedial
basal

D

LUL, apical
posterior

LUL, anterior

LLL, superior

LUL,
superior
(lingula)

LLL,
anteromedial
basal

LLL, lateral basal

LLL,
posterior
basal

E

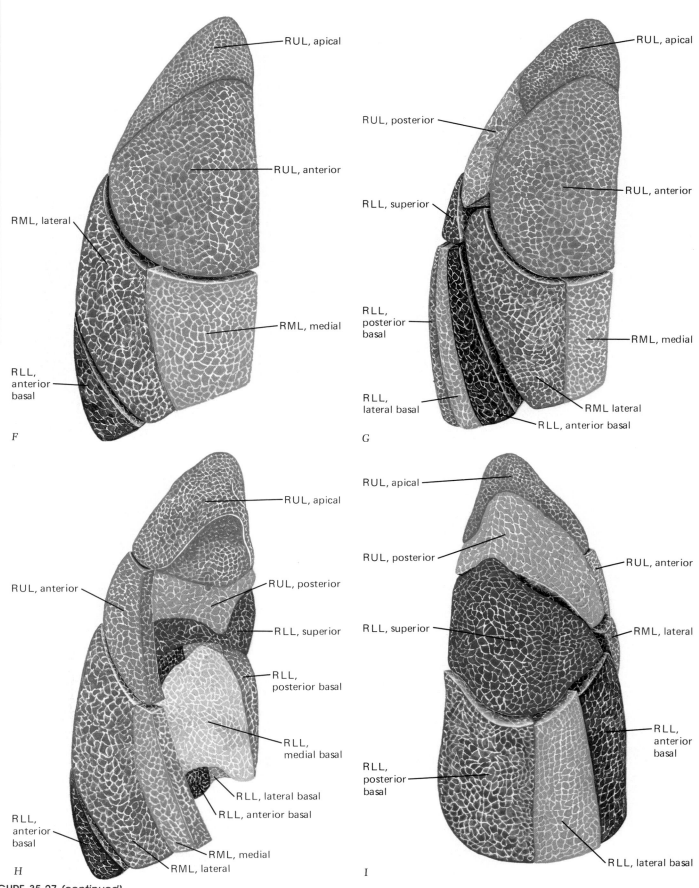

F

RUL, apical

RUL, anterior

RML, lateral

RML, medial

RLL,
anterior
basal

G

RUL, apical

RUL, posterior

RUL, anterior

RLL, superior

RLL,
posterior
basal

RML, medial

RLL,
lateral basal

RML lateral

RLL, anterior basal

H

RUL, apical

RUL, anterior

RUL, posterior

RLL, superior

RLL,
posterior basal

RLL,
medial basal

RLL, lateral basal

RLL, anterior basal

RLL,
anterior
basal

RML, medial

RML, lateral

I

RUL, apical

RUL, posterior

RUL, anterior

RLL, superior

RML, lateral

RLL,
anterior
basal

RLL,
posterior
basal

RLL, lateral basal

FIGURE 35-27 *(continued)*

502

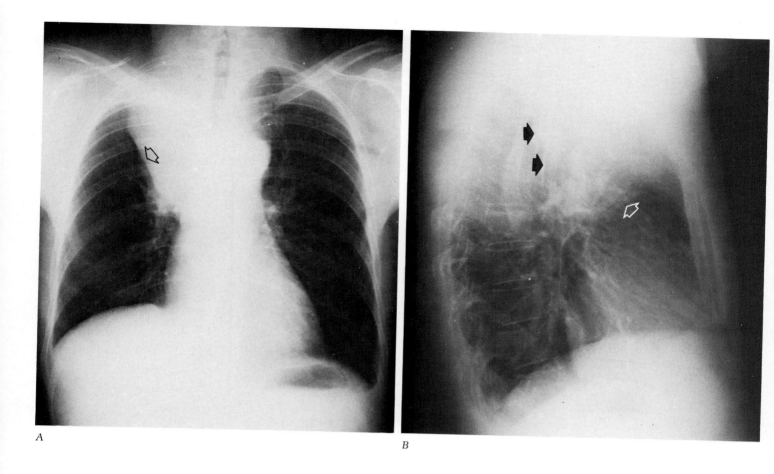

A

B

FIGURE 35-28 Right upper lobe atelectasis secondary to carcinoma of the lung. *A.* PA view. The minor fissure is elevated (arrow). *B.* Lateral view. The minor fissure is displaced upward (open arrow), and the major fissure is displaced anteriorly (closed arrows). *C.* Schematic representation of atelectasis of the right upper lobe.

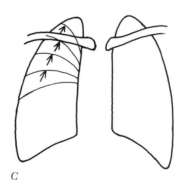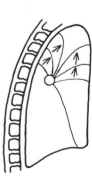

C

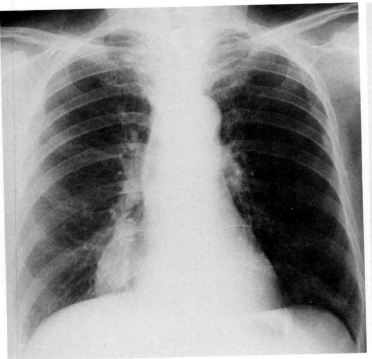

A

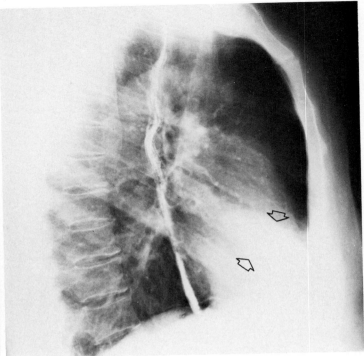

B

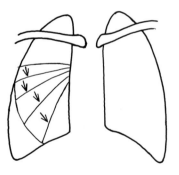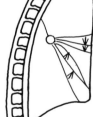

C

FIGURE 35-29 Right middle lobe atelectasis secondary to right middle lobe syndrome. *A.* PA view. The middle lobe is collapsed against the right side of the heart. *B.* Lateral view. The major and minor fissures are drawn together (arrows), creating a density that overlies the cardiac shadow. *C.* Schematic representation of right middle lobe atelectasis.

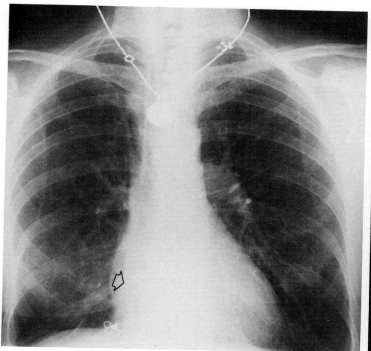

A

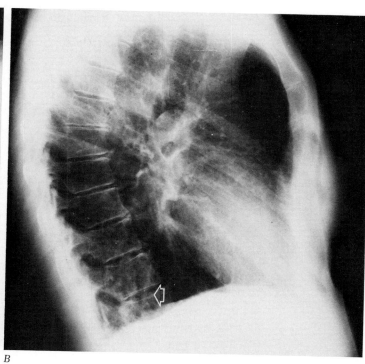

B

FIGURE 35-30 Atelectasis (severe) of the right lower lobe due to chronic inflammatory disease. *A.* PA view. Secondary signs of atelectasis are present in the right lung: small hemithorax, stretching of the pulmonary vessels, hyperlucent lung, small hilus. In addition, there is downward displacement of the right hilus, and the collapsed lower lobe can be seen through the right heart border (arrow). *B.* Lateral view. The entire right lower lobe appears only as a diffuse density overlying the spine (arrow). The posterior portion of the right hemidiaphragm cannot be identified (silhouette sign). *C.* Schematic representation of right lower lobe collapse.

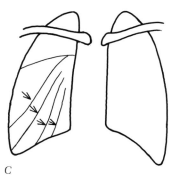

C

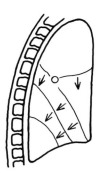

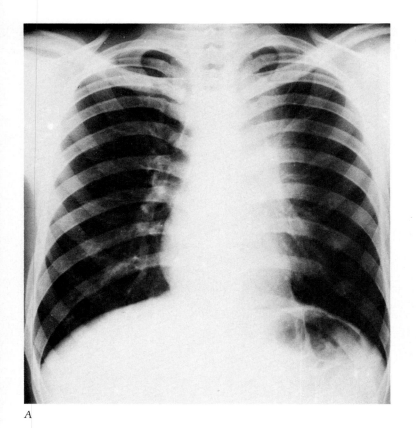

A

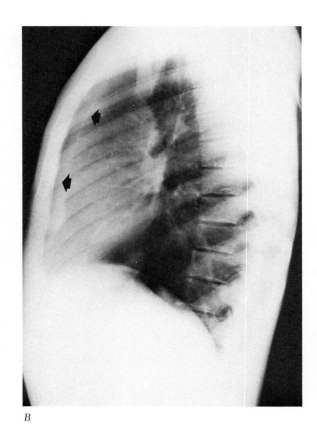

B

FIGURE 35-31   Left upper lobe atelectasis secondary to carcinoma of the lung.   *A.* PA view. The left superior mediastinum and the left side of the heart are indistinct owing to collapse of the left upper lobe medially.   *B.* Lateral view. The collapsed lung is seen as a density anterior to the major fissure (arrows) which is displaced far anteriorly.   *C.* Schematic representation of left upper lobe collapse.

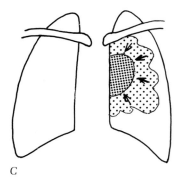
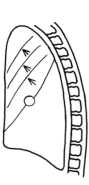

C

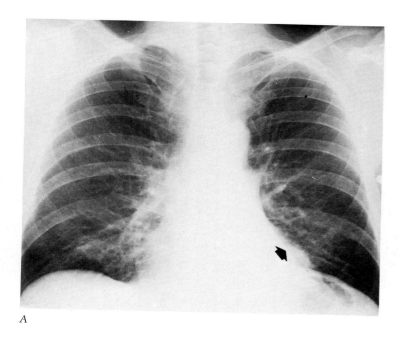

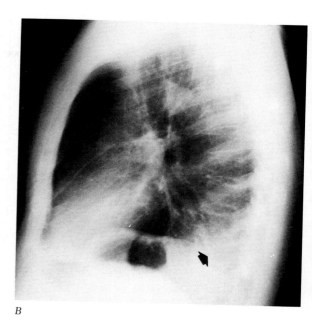

A

B

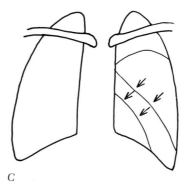

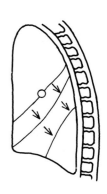

FIGURE 35-32   Left lower lobe atelectasis (postoperative). *A.* PA view. The collapsed left lower lobe is seen as a straight line (arrow) behind the left heart border. No vasculature can be seen through the heart shadow, and the medial border of the left hemidiaphragm is obscured by the collapsed left lower lobe (arrow). *B.* Lateral view. Density over spine and absence of left posterior diaphragm. *C.* Schematic representation of left lower lobe collapse.

C

Chronic interstitial lung disease is caused by a variety of disease processes (Figs. 35-34 and 35-35). A partial list includes: pneumoconioses; sarcoidosis; lymphangitic spread of tumors; infections, such as miliary tuberculosis, interstitial pneumonia, and fungus diseases; allergic lung disease; the collagen vascular diseases; eosinophilic granuloma; and idiopathic interstitial fibrosis. It is often helpful in differential diagnosis to characterize the type of interstitial lung disease as nodular, reticular, or linear, since many of the interstitial lung diseases adopt, almost exclusively, one of these three patterns.

Interstitial nodules range in size from minute to massive. Large nodules generally represent metastatic tumor. Smaller nodules are found in pneumoconioses, such as coal worker's pneumoconiosis or silicosis, miliary tuber-

culosis, sarcoidosis (Fig. 35-34*B*), and allergic lung disease.

Linear densities, as previously noted, are more characteristic of acute lung disease, e.g., interstitial pulmonary edema (Fig. 35-34*A*) or interstitial pneumonia. A similar but chronic pattern occurs in lymphangitic spread of metastatic malignancy (Fig. 35-34*C*).

Reticular patterns suggest collagen vascular disease when they are tiny and primarily confined to the lung bases (Fig. 35-34*D*). Asbestosis, desquamative interstitial pneumonitis, and usual interstitial pneumonitis also cause a basilar reticular pattern. Eosinophilic granuloma of the lung causes a similar reticular pattern at the lung apexes. A larger reticular pattern suggests idiopathic pulmonary fibrosis or the end-stage lung pattern that is often

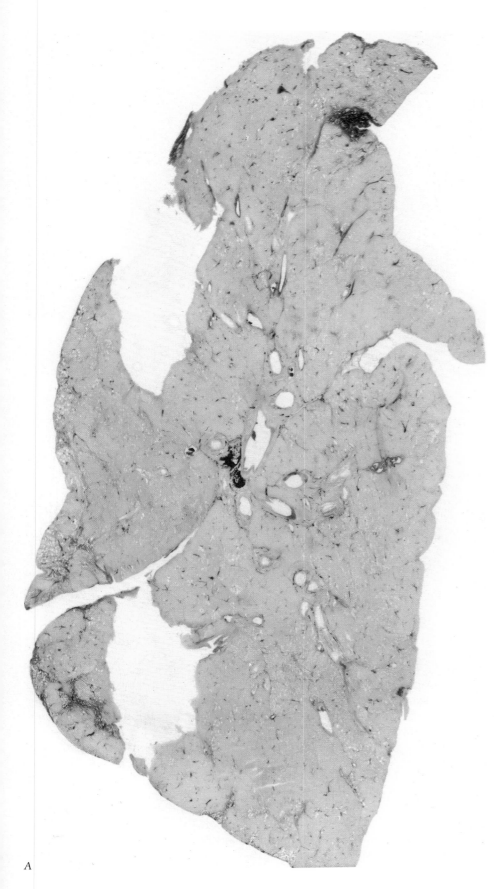

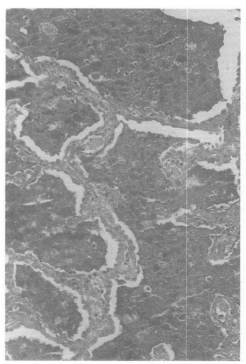

FIGURE 35-33 Anatomic changes in alveolar proteinosis. *A.* Sagittal section of the lung showing homogeneous filling of alveoli as though the lung had been embedded in the proteinaceous material. *B.* Alveolar spaces are filled with granular PAS-positive material. The alveolar septa are minimally thickened and are lined by hyperplastic type II pneumocytes. PAS, ×540. (*A, courtesy of Dr. S. Moolten; B, courtesy of Dr. G. G. Pietra.*)

A

B

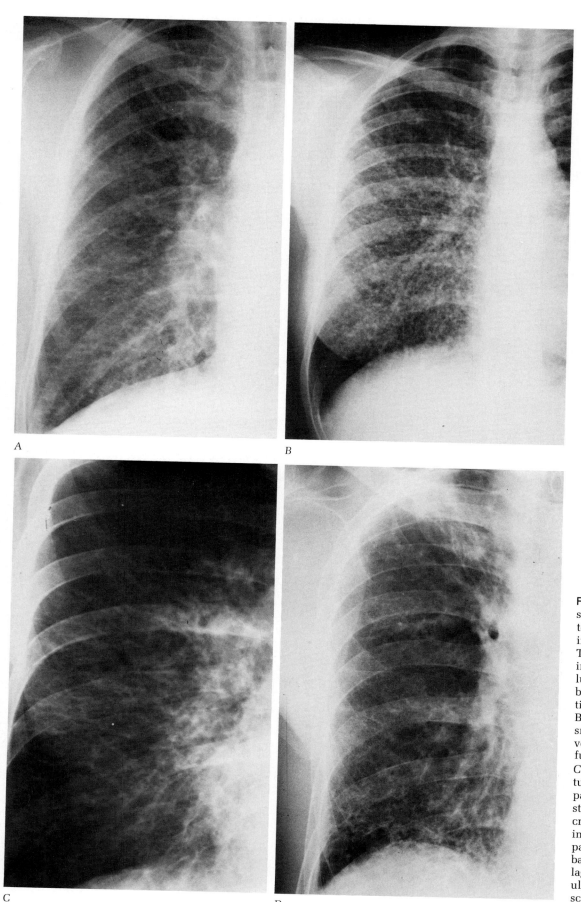

A

B

C

D

FIGURE 35-34 Diffuse interstitial disease. *A*. Linear interstitial pattern produced by interstitial pulmonary edema. The pattern is caused by fluid in the interstitial spaces of the lungs, particularly in interlobar septa. *B*. Nodular interstitial pattern produced by Boeck's sarcoid. Multiple small, discrete nodules involve both lung fields diffusely. Adenopathy is absent. *C*. Lymphangitic spread of tumor. The linear interstitial pattern was caused by metastatic carcinoma of the pancreas. *D*. Reticular or cystic interstitial lung pattern. The pattern is most marked at the bases, characteristic of the collagen vascular disease, particularly, as in this patient, of scleroderma.

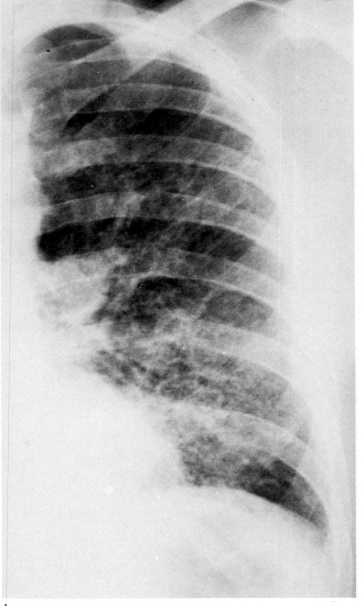

A

FIGURE 35-35 Different types of interstitial pneumonia. *A.* Chest radiograph of fibrosing alveolitis (usual interstitial pneumonia). *B.* Usual interstitial pneumonia (UIP). The alveolar septa are irregularly thickened by collagen (blue) and mononuclear cells. The airspaces contain desquamated epithelial cells, macrophages, and newly formed fibrous tissue. Masson trichrome, ×540. *C.* Bronchiolitis obliterans (BIP). The lumen of a small bronchus is obliterated by fibrin (bright red), collagenous tissue, and macrophages. H&E, ×540. *D.* Desquamative interstitial pneumonia (DIP). The airspaces are filled with desquamated epithelial cells and occasional eosinophils. The alveolar walls are lined by hyperplastic type II cells. Giant cells are also present. H&E, ×400. *E.* Lymphocytic interstitial pneumonia (LIP). The alveolar septa are infiltrated by mononuclear cells, primarily mature lymphocytes and plasma cells. H&E, ×405. *(B to E, courtesy of Dr. G. G. Pietra.)*

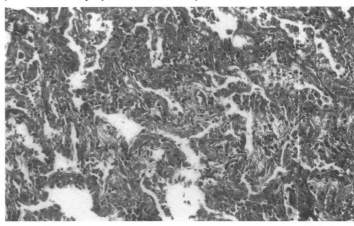

B

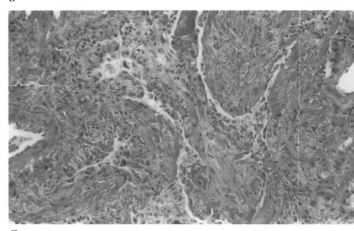

C

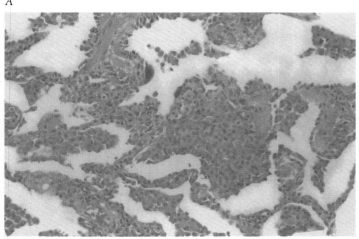

D

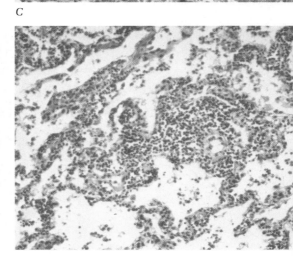

E

the final common denominator of a variety of chronic interstitial lung diseases (Fig. 35-35).

The Solitary Nodule

A wide variety of pathologic processes appear on the chest radiograph as a solitary nodule (see Chapter 124). Among the more common lesions that are first manifested as solitary nodules are primary carcinoma of the lung, granuloma due to tuberculosis or fungus disease, metastatic carcinoma, and organizing pneumonia. Less common are hamartoma, bronchogenic cyst, bronchial adenoma, arteriovenous malformation, pulmonary sequestration, necrobiotic nodule due to rheumatoid arthritis or Wegener's granulomatosis, lymphoma, inflammatory pseudotumor, and lipoid granuloma. Although the radiograph is invaluable for detection of a pulmonary nodule, it is usually of little help in deciding the pathologic nature of the nodule. Although certain radiographic aspects of a nodule may suggest its nature, in most instances, histologic or cytologic proof is required.

One radiologic clue to the etiologic nature of a pulmonary nodule may be the character of its border: ill-defined margins suggest an inflammatory lesion, e.g., tuberculosis, pneumonia; a very sharply circumscribed pulmonary nodule with a regular contour is more likely to be a granuloma or hamartoma—even though metastatic malignancy often presents with a sharply circumscribed contour, and a primary neoplasm of the lung may present either as a sharply circumscribed nodule or with ill-defined margins.

The age of the patient is useful in the differential diagnosis of a solitary nodule: primary carcinoma of the lung is extremely rare in patients less than 30 years old, whereas in patients older than 50 years, more than half of solitary nodules are primary carcinoma of the lung.

Occasionally, the radiograph may be sufficiently convincing about the benignity of a pulmonary nodule to avoid diagnostic thoracotomy. Extensive calcification within the nodule suggests that the process is benign; laminography may be helpful in displaying the calcification. Benignity is also suggested by calcification that is central, concentric, diffuse, or punctate (popcorn). On the other hand, eccentric calcification is of no diagnostic help since it also occurs in malignant disease, presumably as a consequence of envelopment of a preexisting calcified focus within an expanding neoplastic process. In some clinics, CT numbers have been definitive in identifying benign pulmonary nodules; unfortunately, this experience has not been universal.

Prominent vascular shadows (that prove to be veins) extending from a nodule suggest that the nodule is an arteriovenous malformation; arteriography confirms the vascular nature of the shadows (Fig. 35-5). A nodule at the lung base suggestive of pulmonary sequestration can be identified arteriographically by demonstrating an anomalous artery to the mass arising from the abdominal aorta.

The lung is uniquely suited for serial radiographic estimates of the size of a solitary pulmonary nodule. This feature has led to the practical concept of doubling time, i.e., the time required for tumor to double in volume. Most useful as a baseline for estimating the growth rate of a solitary nodule is a previous radiograph on which the nodule was present, even if unrecognized. If a nodule does not change in size for 2 years, it can be assumed that the process is benign. Conversely, any growth of the node within 1 year is evidence of malignancy. Usually, malignant tumors grow quickly, doubling in volume between 1 and 15 months (Fig. 35-36). Not uncommonly, however, a slowly growing nodule proves to be a primary carcinoma of the lung, usually in adenocarcinoma or alveolar cell carcinoma.

Cavitation within a pulmonary nodule rarely settles whether a nodule is benign or malignant. Other radiographic features, including stranding, satellite lesions, or associated pleural disease, are seen in both benign and malignant processes and do not constitute bases for distinction.

It should be emphasized that definite diagnosis is rarely possible by using radiographic techniques alone. To establish the diagnosis, sputum for cytology, bronchoscopy with transbronchial biopsy, percutaneous biopsy, or open lung biopsy are necessary.

Multiple Pulmonary Nodules

Although a solitary pulmonary nodule can be benign or malignant, multiple nodules strongly suggest metastatic malignancy. The occasional exception to this rule includes rheumatoid nodules (Fig. 35-37), fungus disease, alveolar sarcoid, and Wegener's granulomatosis.

Left Ventricular Failure

Failure of the left ventricle is generally easy to recognize on the chest radiograph: the heart is enlarged, and the pulmonary vasculature is unduly prominent. Changes in the size of the heart and vessels are most evident on consecutive radiographs.

In chronic left ventricular failure, due to chronic dependent edema and interstitial fibrosis at the lung bases, pulmonary blood flow is directed from the bases toward the apexes; the vessels of the upper lobes then become more prominent than those of the lower lobes ("cephalization"). Interstitial edema often accompanies pulmonary venous congestion and is manifested by a diffuse increase in interstitial markings, usually in a linear fashion (Fig. 35-34B); Kerley lines are characteristic features of interstitial edema. Alveolar edema succeeds interstitial edema and is characterized by diffuse bilateral consolidation (Fig. 35-25).

Pleural effusions often accompany *combined* ventricular heart failure. At first, the pleural effusions are accompanied by prominence of the pulmonary vascular

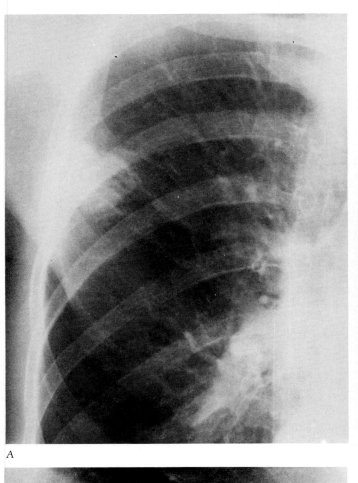

A

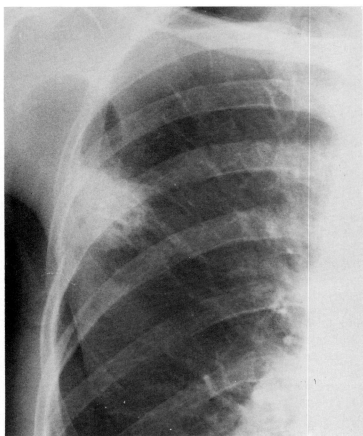

B

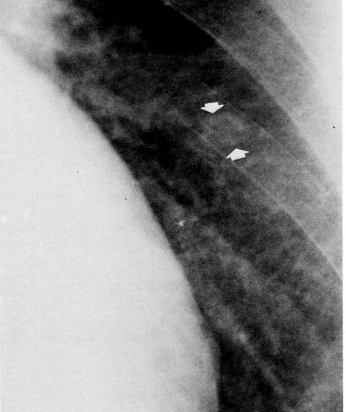

C

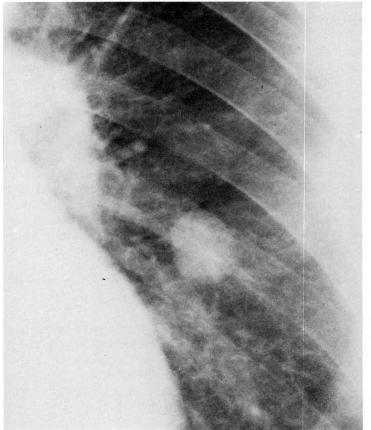

D

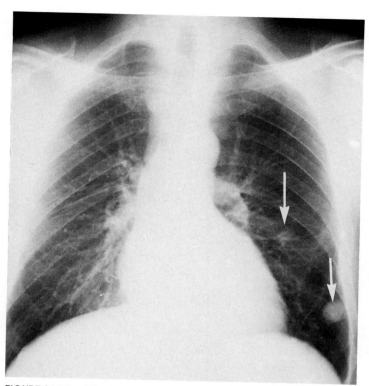

FIGURE 35-37   Rheumatoid nodules. The nodules in the left lung of this patient with rheumatoid arthritis regressed 4 months later.

markings and/or cephalization. But, even though the pulmonary congestion clears in response to therapy, a pleural effusion often remains after the pulmonary vessels have returned to normal size. Pleural effusion in congestive heart failure can affect one or both pleural cavities. If unilateral, the effusion almost invariably occurs on the right side. As indicated above, recognition of left ventricular failure is difficult in the patient with obstructive lung disease because the hyperinflated lungs and the elongated heart make it difficult to recognize cardiomegaly and pulmonary vascular engorgement. Comparison with previous films is paramount in recognizing subtle changes in cardiac size and in pulmonary vascular engorgement.

THE MEDIASTINUM

As pointed out in Chapter 133, different authors and specialties advocate different designations for the "compart-

◀ **FIGURE 35-36**   *Top,* carcinoma of the lung with a long doubling time. An interval of 18 months elapsed between *A* and *B*. The right upper lobe lesion, which only enlarged minimally during that time, proved to be a squamous cell carcinoma of the lung. *Bottom,* carcinoma of the lung with a short doubling time. An interval of 4 months elapsed between *C* and *D*. The nodule was not detected on the first radiograph *(C)*. It proved to be an oat cell carcinoma of the lung.

ments" of the mediastinum. For radiographic diagnosis, we have adopted a simple classification (Fig. 35-38): (1) The *anterior* compartment, which extends from the sternum anteriorly to the heart, aorta, and brachiocephalic vessels posteriorly, includes only the thymus and a few lymph nodes; surgeons use a more elaborate classification (see Table 133-1), generally preferring *anterosuperior mediastinum* that includes certain structures, such as trachea, esophagus, aortic arch, vena cava, and azygos vein, which the radiologist assigns to the middle (*visceral*) compartment. (2) The *middle* (visceral) compartment contains the heart, great vessels, trachea and its branches, esophagus, and descending aorta. It extends from the posterior border of the anterior compartment to the anterior border of the vertebral column. These boundaries differ from the anatomist's classification (Fig. 35-39), which relegates portions of the esophagus and the descending aorta to the posterior mediastinum. (3) The *posterior* compartment contains the vertebrae and the paravertebral sulci. Applying this approach to the lateral chest radiograph, mediastinal masses can readily be categorized according to their position within the mediastinum.

In the anterior compartment are characteristically to be found enlarged lymph nodes, substernal goiter, thymus and thymic tumors, and teratomas. Distinction among these can also be made on the basis of their position within the anterior mediastinum and their appearance: thyroid masses almost invariably lie high in the anterior mediastinum and displace the trachea and esophagus (Fig. 35-39*A* and *B*); thymomas and teratomas generally lie below the aortic arch and present as a single, well-demarcated mass (Fig. 35-39*C* and *D*). Lymph node enlargement is generally more diffuse and often nodular or lumpy in character (Fig. 35-40). Lymph node enlargement can be produced by metastatic tumor, particularly from a primary neoplasm of the lung, sarcoidosis, lymphoma, and primary tuberculosis. Less common causes of mediastinal lymphadenopathy are other inflammatory processes such as fungus disease or infectious mononucleosis. Malignant thymoma or malignant teratoma may be diffuse and, therefore, indistinguishable from diffuse lymphadenopathy.

The middle compartment of the mediastinum contains all the viscera as well as lymph nodes. Lymphadenopathy in the middle compartment is quite common and is generally seen as a diffuse mass, often associated with enlargement of one or both hili (Fig. 35-41). A localized mass can be caused by anomaly or aneurysm of the aorta or the great vessels; its vascular nature is suggested by proximity to the aortic shadow and is readily confirmed by aortography (Fig. 35-42*A*, *B*, and *C*). Computed tomography and nuclear magnetic resonance are also extremely well suited to demonstrate vascular lesions (Fig. 35-42*D* and *E*); nuclear magnetic resonance is somewhat safer since it does not require intravenous contrast material to

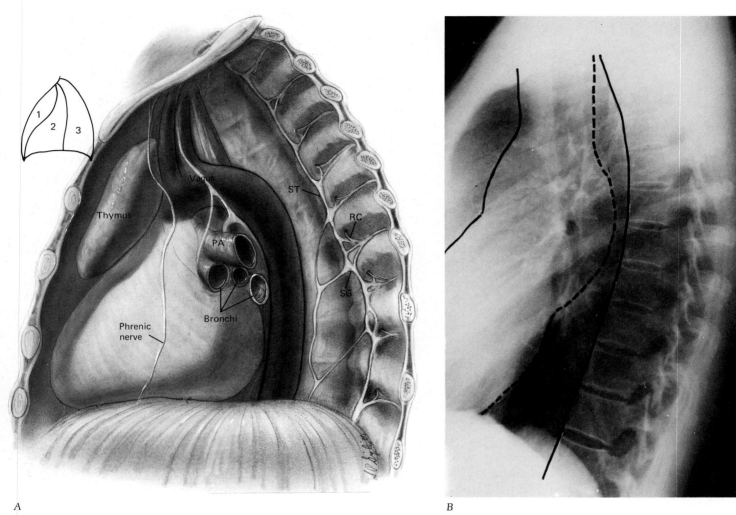

FIGURE 35-38 Compartments of the mediastinum. *A.* Anatomic view of the compartments of the mediastinum. The subdivisions in the small schematic *(top left)* correspond to the white boundary line in the larger figure. PA = pulmonary artery; ST = sympathetic trunk; SG = sympathetic ganglion; RC = ramus communicans. *(From Jones, Pietra, Sabiston, 1980.)* *B.* Radiographic division of the mediastinum. The closed lines delineate the anterior, middle, and posterior compartments. The dashed line represents the division of the middle and posterior mediastinum that is conventionally used by anatomists (cf. Fig. 133-5 and Table 133-1).

demonstrate the lesion. Duplication cysts of the esophagus and the tracheobronchial tree are also common in the visceral department. These localized masses are smooth and well circumscribed and generally do not contain air. Bronchogenic cysts commonly occur at the tracheal carina, whereas esophageal duplication cysts are characteristically located near the end of the esophagus (Fig. 35-43A and B). However, esophageal cysts or bronchogenic cysts may occur anywhere within the middle compartment.

A dilated esophagus is sometimes seen on the chest radiograph as a long tubular mass in the visceral compartment (Fig. 35-43C and D); tumors of the esophagus or trachea may also present as more localized mediastinal masses. Radiographs taken with barium in the esophagus

are particularly helpful in characterizing masses in the visceral (middle) mediastinal compartment.

In the posterior (paraspinal) compartment, the characteristic mass is the neurogenic tumor (Fig. 35-44). But tumors or infections of the vertebral column may also present as a mass in the posterior compartment (Fig. 35-45).

Various lines or stripes occur about the mediastinum on the PA radiograph. Very useful among these is the posterior paraspinal line which is a pleural reflection to the left of the thoracic spine (Figs. 35-5 and 35-45). This line is related to the descending aorta; it is seen on the right side if the descending aorta is on the right. Tumors or inflammatory diseases involving the vertebral bodies displace the posterior mediastinal line to the left and create a

514

(Text continued on page 519.)

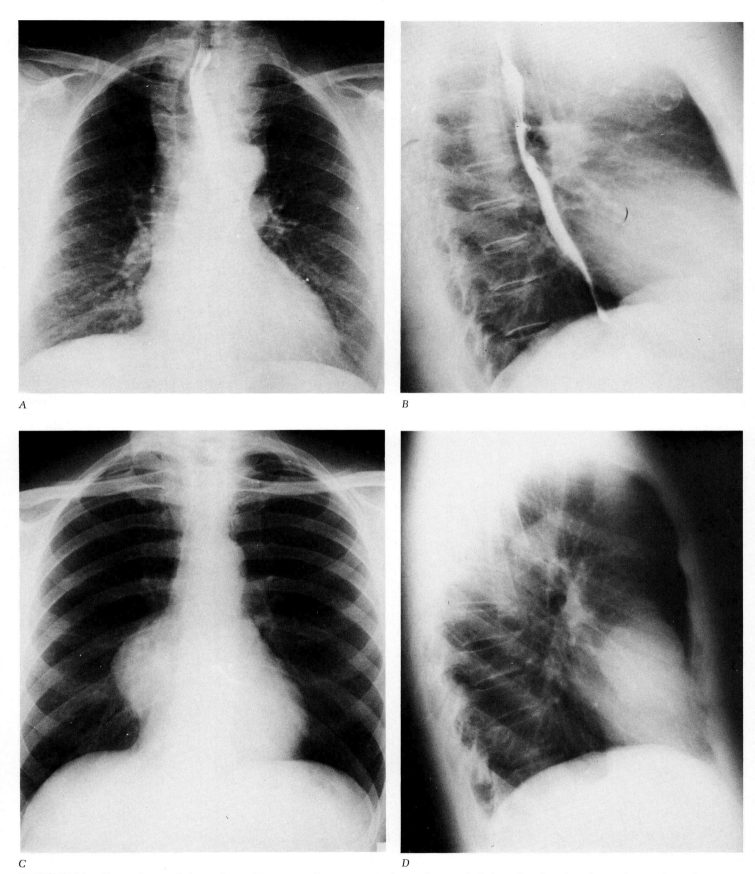

A

B

C

D

FIGURE 35-39 *Top*, substernal thyroid. *A*. PA view. A large mass in the neck extends below the clavicle. The trachea and esophagus are displaced to the right. *B*. Lateral view. The trachea and esophagus are also displaced posteriorly. Several calcifications are present within the mass. *Bottom*, thymoma. *C*. PA view. A discrete mass (thymoma) lies along the right heart border. *D*. Lateral view. The mass also overlies the anterior portion of the cardiac shadow.

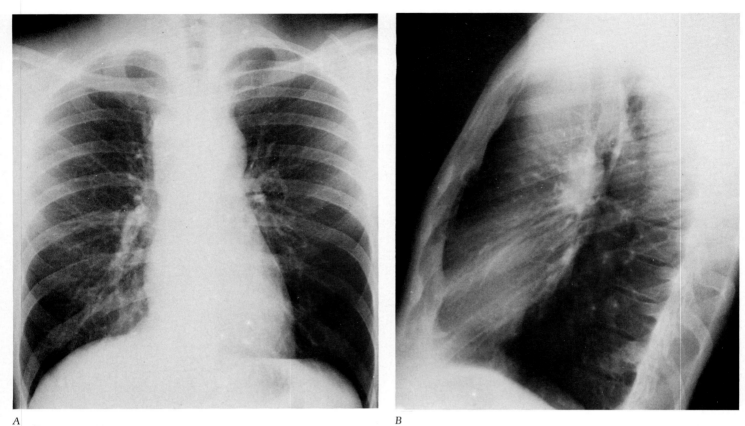

A　　　　　　　　　　　　　　　　　　　　　　B

FIGURE 35-40　Hodgkin's disease.　*A*. PA view. A lobulated mass widens the mediastinum on both sides of the trachea.　*B*. Lateral view. The mass lies anterior to the trachea.

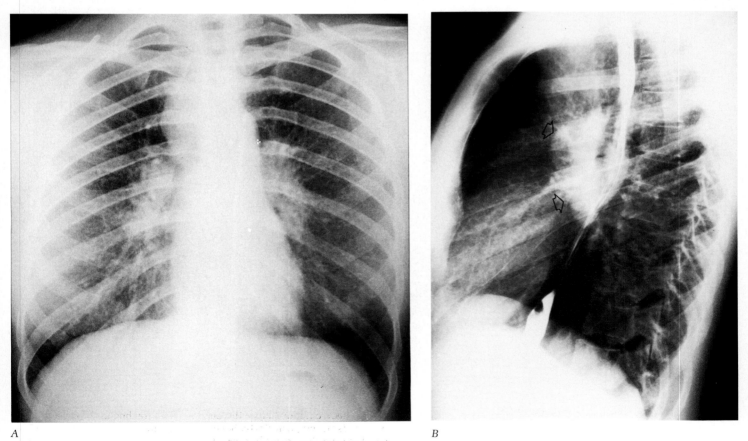

A　　　　　　　　　　　　　　　　　　　　　　B

FIGURE 35-41　Sarcoidosis.　*A*. PA view. A mass is present in the right paratracheal area, and both hili are enlarged.　*B*. Lateral view. The hilar enlargement (arrows) is striking. Enlargement in these three node-bearing areas is characteristic of sarcoidosis.

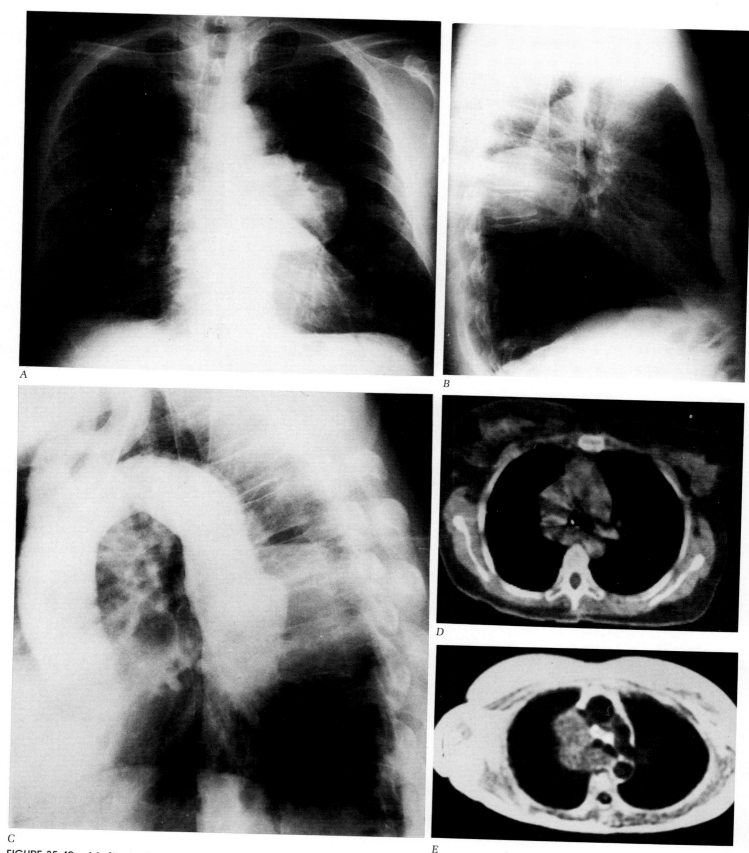

FIGURE 35-42 Mediastinal mass. *A.* Aortic aneurysm, PA view. A mass is seen on the left of the aorta. *B.* Aortic aneurysm, lateral view. The mass is also posterior to, and intimately associated with, the aorta. *C.* Aortic aneurysm, aortogram. An irregularity in the wall of the opacified aorta indicates the aneurysm. Most of the aneurysm is filled with clot. This type of mass is often mistaken for a neurogenic tumor in the posterior mediastinal compartment. *D.* Magnetic resonance imaging. An enhanced CT scan of the chest fails to clearly demonstrate a mediastinal mass seen by routine chest radiograph. This is in part due to a technically poor scan. *E.* Magnetic resonance imaging. A magnetic resonance scan clearly shows the mass as mediastinal adenopathy in the right paratracheal and subcarinal areas. The ascending aorta, descending aorta, and pulmonary artery are easily identified owing to lack of signal.

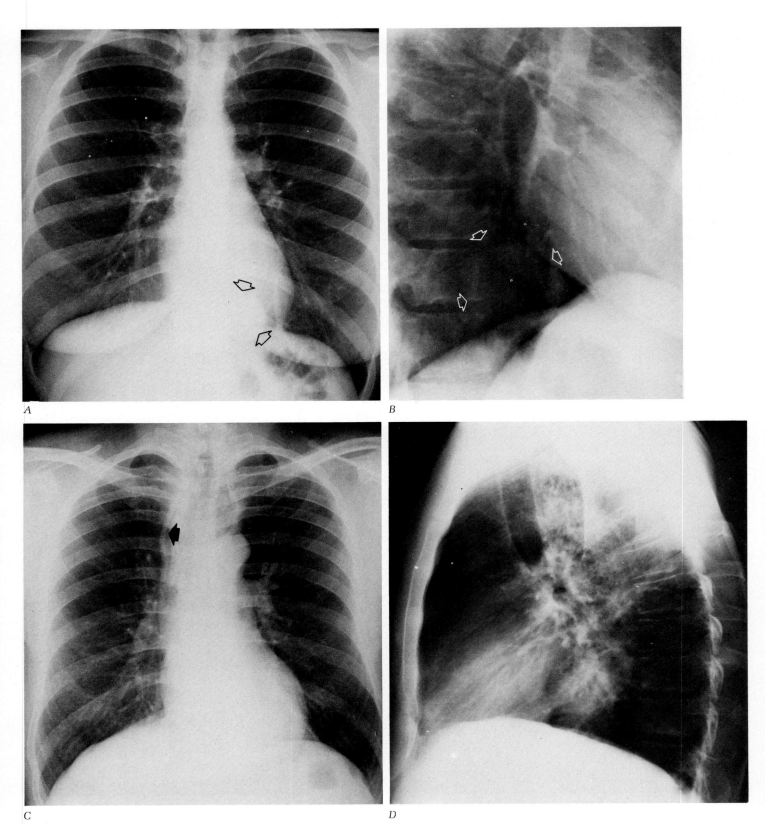

FIGURE 35-43 *Top,* esophageal duplication cyst. *A, B.* The small round mass behind the heart (arrows) has the characteristic location and appearance for an esophageal duplication cyst. *Bottom,* achalasia. *C.* PA view. The dilated esophagus is visible as a mass in the mediastinum. Air outlines the wall of the upper esophagus above the aortic arch (arrow). *D.* Lateral view. The mass appears to consist of an amorphous cluster of material lying posterior to the trachea and the heart.

518

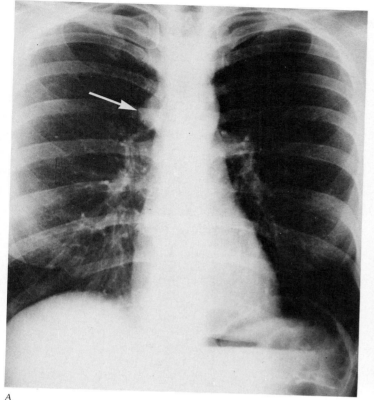 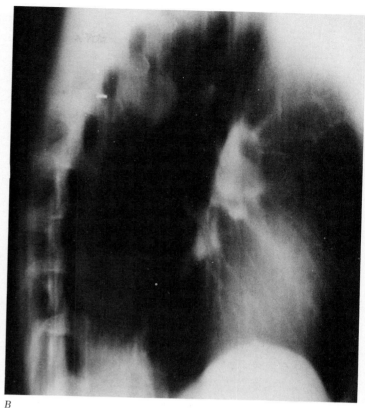

A

B

FIGURE 35-44 Neurogenic tumor (pheochromocytoma). *A.* PA view. A small mass (arrow) lies to the right side of the spine. *B.* Lateral view. The mass overlies the spine. The location is typical for a neurogenic tumor, usually a neurofibroma or neurolemmoma. This mass proved to be a thoracic pheochromocytoma.

posterior mediastinal line on the right where one is not ordinarily present. Large spurs arising from the vertebral body on the right also push out the pleura, creating a paraspinal line on the right that is clinically unimportant (Fig. 35-5A).

While the plain chest radiograph is quite good in detecting mediastinal lesions, it requires that a mass must get large enough to project into the lung before it can be detected. CT and MRI are specifically suited to study the mediastinum, since they can detect masses hidden deep in the mediastinum even if the masses are surrounded, or obscured, by other mediastinal structures that render the mass invisible on the plain chest radiograph (Fig. 35-46).

THE DIAPHRAGM AND CHEST WALL

The left hemidiaphragm is generally lower than the right; only in about 9 percent of patients is the left hemidiaphragm higher than the right. Variations in diaphragmatic contour are common. Most common is a localized eventration (Fig. 35-47) in which a segment of diaphragmatic muscle is replaced by a thin fibrous membrane. The use of fluoroscopy in identifying local eventration of the diaphragm has been described above.

Foramina traverse the normal diaphragm to connect the thorax and abdomen. Sometimes they enlarge sufficiently to allow herniation of abdominal viscera into the chest. The paired foramina of Morgagni lie anteriorly and medially; hernias through one of these foramina occur frequently on the right (Fig. 35-47A and B) but rarely on the left. Generally, these hernias contain only omentum or fat. Hernias through the centrally placed esophageal hiatus (Fig. 35-47C to E) are much more common than through the foramina of Morgagni. The stomach is the usual herniating viscus; less often the hernia contains colon or small bowel. Traversing the diaphragm posteriorly and slightly laterally are the paired foramina of Bochdalek. The massive congenital hernias occasionally seen in newborns generally occur through a large foramen of Bochdalek, usually on the left side. Hernias through the foramina of Bochdalek are unusual in adults and may contain a kidney.

Masses of the chest wall generally cause bone destruction or erosion, and usually protrude as a mass into the lung. Most lesions of the chest wall are metastatic tumors to the ribs, but primary tumors of the ribs or soft tissue sarcomas also occur. Their protrusion into the lung causes a characteristic shadow that has smooth margins and tapering edges and is generally seen well in only one

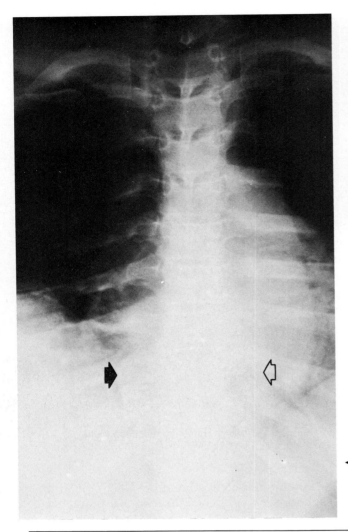

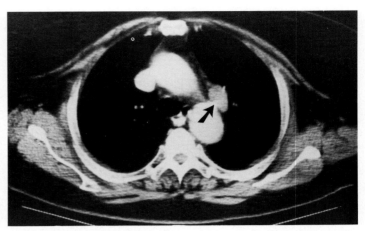

FIGURE 35-46 Mediastinal mass not seen on the routine chest radiograph. A large lymph node (arrow) is well seen on the CT scan lying just anterior to the descending aorta. This could not be seen on the routine chest radiograph. This node contained adenocarcinoma and was important in staging a primary carcinoma of the left lower lobe.

◀ **FIGURE 35-45** Tuberculosis. The normal left paraspinal line is displaced laterally (open arrow) by a paraspinal mass; the right paraspinal line, which is usually not seen, is present and displaced laterally (closed arrow). These findings are characteristic of infection about the spine, in this case, tuberculosis.

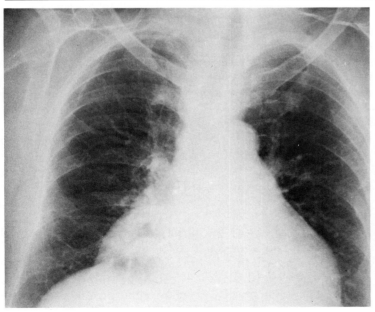

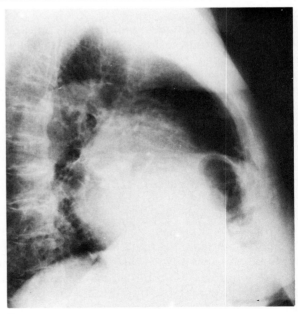

A

B

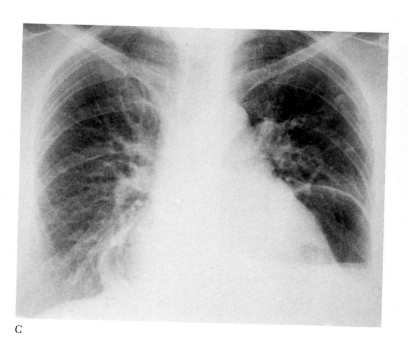

C

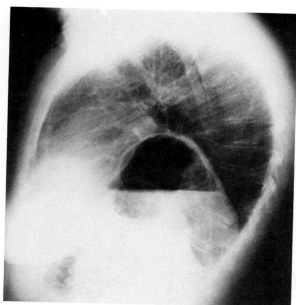

D

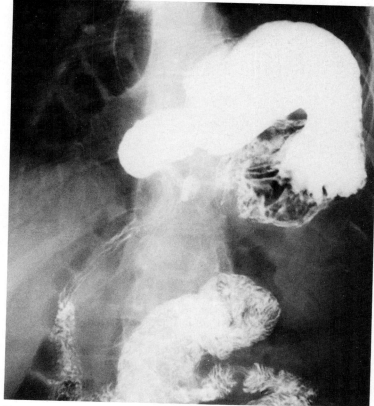

E

FIGURE 35-47 *Facing page*, foramen of Morgagni hernia. *A.* PA view. A mass containing a loop of bowel is just to the right of the cardiac silhouette. *B.* Lateral view. The mass is also anterior to the cardiac silhouette. The location of the mass is characteristic for a foramen of Morgagni hernia. The hernia usually contains only omentum but, in this instance, contained a loop of colon. *Above*, hiatus hernia. *C.* PA view. An air-fluid level is present on the left. *D.* Lateral view. The mass is also posterior to the heart. *E.* An upper gastrointestinal series demonstrates the air-fluid level to be within the stomach, which has herniated into the chest and lies in an upside-down position.

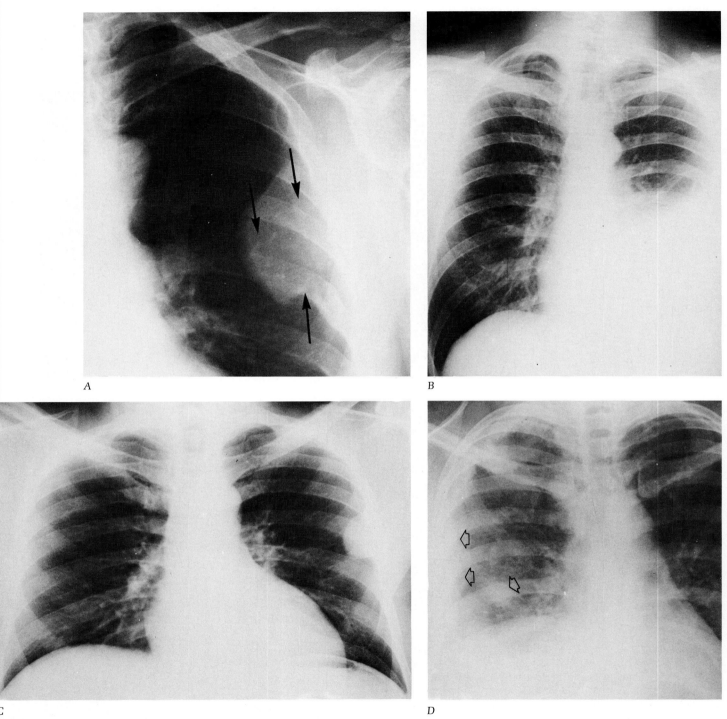

A

B

C

D

FIGURE 35-48   *A*. Rib metastases (extrapleural sign). A smooth mass protrudes into the lung. This mass has tapering edges, characteristic of an extrapleural lesion. The destroyed anterior rib (arrows) is secondary to a metastatic tumor that is invading the rib.   *B*. Rheumatoid effusion. The characteristic meniscus of a free pleural effusion is seen in the left hemithorax. This patient had rheumatoid arthritis.   *C*. Pleural lipoma. A smooth mass along the left lateral chest wall proved to be a lipoma.   *D*. Pleural metastases. A right pleural effusion, showing a meniscus, blunts the right costophrenic sulcus. The lobulation along the right lateral chest wall is characteristic of tumor nodulation (arrows).

of the two radiographs of the chest (PA or lateral) Fig. 35-48A); this characteristic configuration has been designated the *extrapleural sign* by Felson. Since many pleural lesions mimic the extrapleural sign, bone destruction is the key to accurate identification of an extrapleural mass.

In addition to hernias through the diaphragm, tumors of the diaphragm occasionally present as a mass on the chest radiograph.

THE PLEURA

The pleura and its disorders are considered in Chapters 135 and 136. Radiographic involvement of the pleura is generally manifested either by pleural fluid, localized or diffuse pleural thickening, or pleural nodules.

Pleural Effusions

Fluid in the pleural cavity appears radiographically as a homogeneous opacity that generally occupies a dependent position in the pleural cavity. A small pleural effusion that is barely perceptible or overlooked on the PA view is often readily apparent on the lateral radiograph as blunting of the posterior costophrenic sulcus (Fig. 35-2). The best radiographic technique for demonstrating small quantities of pleural fluid is the lateral decubitus film. (Fig. 35-3C). By this technique, as little as 25 ml of fluid can be detected. Larger pleural effusions usually blunt the lateral costophrenic sulcus on the PA radiograph as well (Fig. 35-48B). Occasionally, the fluid remains between the diaphragm and the lung (infrapulmonary), displacing the lung upward so that the lateral costophrenic angle remains sharp (Fig. 35-3). The presence of an infrapulmonary accumulation of fluid is suspected if the diaphragm appears elevated, if the costophrenic sulcus is blunted posteriorly, or if the stomach bubble is separated from the dome of the apparent hemidiaphragm by more than a few millimeters. Computed tomography is especially sensitive in identifying small pleural effusions (Fig. 35-49).

Pleural fluid sometimes is loculated and difficult to distinguish from localized pleural thickening. A pleural effusion generally has a convex border toward the hilus, whereas pleural thickening more often presents a concave border toward the hilus. Loculated pleural fluid in an interlobar fissure assumes a cigar-shaped configuration on the lateral radiograph and sometimes simulates a mass. This mass disappears as the fluid is eliminated ("phantom tumor").

Common causes of pleural effusion are tuberculosis, pneumonia, pulmonary infarction, metastatic tumor, primary pleural tumor, lymphoma, collagen vascular disease, chest trauma, and intra-abdominal inflammatory processes such as subphrenic abscess or pancreatitis. Tho-

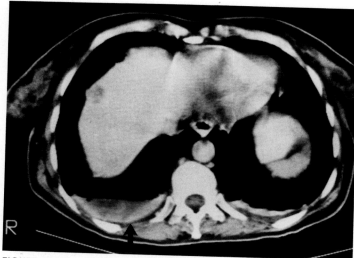

FIGURE 35-49 Right pleural effusion seen by CT. A right pleural effusion (arrow) is identified by CT. This was not seen on the routine chest radiograph. Pleural thickening is seen in a similar location on the left side.

racentesis and pleural biopsy are generally necessary to establish the nature of a pleural effusion that has been recognized radiographically.

Pleural Thickening

Fibrosis of the pleura is localized or generalized. Localized pleural thickening is common at the lung apexes and is suggestive of tuberculosis. But most often, apical scarring remains unexplained and is attributed to aging. Blunting of the costophrenic sulcus is an occasional residue of a previous pleural effusion. A costophrenic sulcus that appears to be blunted laterally on the PA radiograph but not posteriorly on the lateral radiograph usually represents pleural thickening rather than pleural fluid.

Generalized pleural thickening confined to one hemithorax is usually secondary to previous tuberculosis, empyema, or hemithorax. Bilateral pleural thickening that is either localized or generalized is strongly suggestive of asbestosis. Although this thickening is sometimes accompanied by pleural calcification or interstitial lung disease, it is important to recognize that pleural thickening may be the sole radiographic manifestation of asbestosis.

Pleural Nodules

A localized pleural nodule suggests a benign pleural tumor (Fig. 35-48C and D). This nodule may be difficult to distinguish from a localized area of pleural thickening but generally is larger and more symmetric in contour. Diffuse pleural nodulation (Fig. 35-48D) indicates diffuse mesothelioma or metastatic malignancy. These are impossible to distinguish radiographically and often difficult to distinguish histologically. Either is commonly associated with pleural effusion. As with pleural effusion, computed tomography is extremely useful in identifying localized or diffuse pleural abnormalities.

Pneumothorax

In the conventional upright radiograph, air within the pleural cavity is best seen at the tops of the pleural spaces. There, the thin line of visceral pleura surrounding the partially collapsed lung is easily identified. If doubt exists, a radiograph taken during expiration may make a pneumothorax more obvious. In supine patients or in patients with pleural adhesions, pneumothorax may be seen only at the bases medially or laterally.

Trauma, iatrogenic or other, is the most common cause of pneumothorax. Spontaneous pneumothorax is caused by a variety of conditions. Most often the etiology is unknown. On occasion, it may be clearly seen to be due to a ruptured apical bleb. Diffuse lung disease, such as eosinophilic granuloma, is sometimes the cause of spontaneous pneumothorax.

When a pneumothorax is chronic, it is invariably associated with fluid in the pleural space. When associated with air in the pleural space, the fluid assumes a very flat line (Fig. 35-50) rather than the usual curved line (menis-

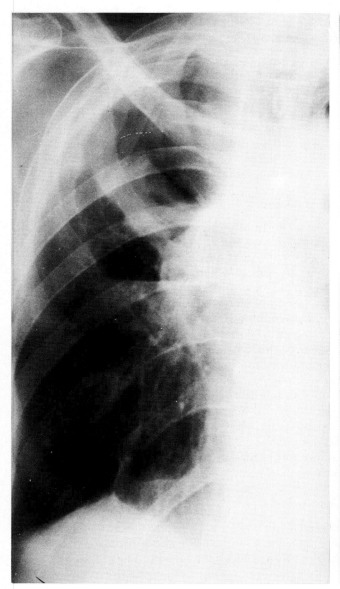

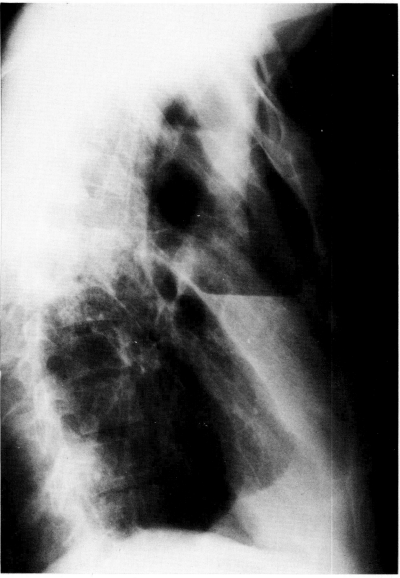

A   *B*

FIGURE 35-50   Hydropneumothorax.   *A.* Posteroanterior view. A distinct air-fluid level is seen overlying the left hilus.   *B.* Lateral view. The fluid and air are anterior to the hilus, indicating that they are in the pleural space. The hydropneumothorax was secondary to a postoperative bronchopleural fistula.

cus) seen when air is absent. A pneumothorax is ordinarily rapidly reabsorbed or replaced by fluid in the pleural space. A chronic pneumothorax is strongly suggestive of a bronchopleural fistula.

PORTABLE CHEST EXAMINATION

Portable radiographic examination of seriously ill patients has become routine in most large hospitals. Interpretation of the portable radiograph is oftentimes difficult because of poor technical quality. Despite its problems, the portable radiograph may provide useful information in the postoperative patient who may be difficult to examine clinically and in the very ill patient in the intensive-care unit who is undergoing assisted mechanical ventilation.

Localized pulmonary consolidation on the postoperative radiograph generally indicates one of three possibilities: pulmonary contusion, pneumonia, or atelectasis (segmental or lobar). Pulmonary contusion is common after thoracic surgery. It is generally noted immediately after the surgery and gradually improves. In contrast, pneumonia generally occurs after the second or third postoperative day; it is diffuse or localized. If localized, it is often difficult to distinguish from atelectasis; if diffuse, it is often difficult to distinguish from pulmonary edema.

Atelectasis is a frequent postoperative complication. It occurs most often in the lower lobes, more commonly on the left than on the right. An increased density behind the cardiac shadow or obliteration of the diaphragmatic shadow behind the cardiac silhouette constitutes presumptive evidence of left lower lobe atelectasis. It is frequently difficult to distinguish between atelectasis and pleural fluid on the portable radiograph.

Basilar atelectasis (platelike atelectasis, Fleischner lines, or discoid atelectasis) frequently occurs in the very ill, particularly after abdominal surgery. It is manifest by linear densities at the bases that tend to parallel the diaphragm; they do not follow the usual patterns of lobar collapse. It is generally considered to be an indication of poor diaphragmatic motion and is often a concomitant of abdominal pain. Basilar atelectasis can be seen in patients who are obese and have poor diaphragmatic motion or in patients with eventration of their diaphragms (Fig. 35-51).

Pleural effusion is often difficult to identify on a portable examination, since that patient is rarely upright in bed or optimally positioned, and a lateral radiograph is not available. On occasion, a large pleural effusion mimics lower lobe atelectasis. Although difficult to perform, portable decubitus radiographs can be useful in distinguishing a pleural effusion from atelectasis.

In the patient with recent thoracic surgery, fluid may accumulate in the extrapleural space in the area of the incision, where it simulates a loculated collection of pleural fluid. If a mediastinal incision has been made, fluid may accumulate in the mediastinum and be seen as a diffuse widening of the mediastinal shadow. Once again, comparison with earlier films is particularly useful in determining that a changing situation is present, i.e., further accumulation of fluid.

Left ventricular failure is another common complication that is often difficult to recognize on the portable radiograph because of distortions in heart size produced by inconsistent distances of the radiographic tube from the patient's chest. The size of the pulmonary vessels is probably the most reliable sign of left-sided heart failure. This evidence must also be interpreted with care, however, since the portable radiograph is often made while the patient is supine, thereby promoting redistribution of blood flow toward the apexes. Pulmonary interstitial edema and alveolar edema are additional signs that are generally recognizable on the portable radiograph.

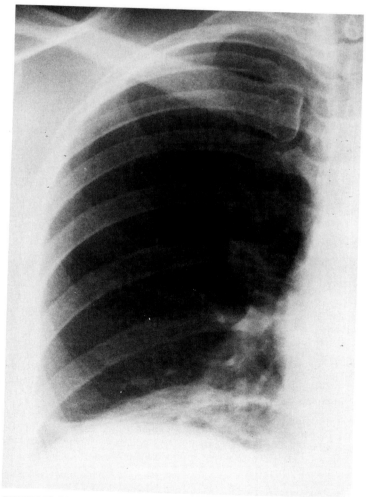

FIGURE 35-51 Platelike atelectasis. A linear density above the right hemidiaphragm in this postoperative patient represents platelike atelectasis. The configuration of this density does not correspond to that of any pulmonary subsegment, and it crosses segmental boundaries.

Diffuse alveolar consolidation on the portable radiograph generally signifies the presence of pulmonary edema, just as it does on the routine radiograph. However, in the critically ill patient, edema is often noncardiac in origin, caused by overtransfusion, O_2 toxicity, or the adult respiratory distress syndrome. Massive aspiration pneumonia or sepsis can also produce the radiographic picture of diffuse alveolar consolidation.

BIBLIOGRAPHY

Albelda SM, Epstein DM, Gefter WB, Miller WT: Pleural thickening: Its significance and relationship to asbestos dust exposure. Am Rev Respir Dis 126:621–624, 1982.
  Emphasizes pleural disease as an indicator of asbestos exposure.

Clinton JE, Yaron M, Tsai SH: Chest radiography in the emergency department. Ann Emerg Med 15:254–256, 1986.
  Guidelines for cost-effective and safe use of chest radiography in the emergency department.

Currie DC, Cooke JC, Morgan AD, Kerr IH, Delany D, Strickland B, Cole PJ: Interpretation of bronchograms and chest radiographs in patients with chronic sputum production. Thorax 42:278–284, 1987.
  Plain chest radiographs were insensitive in distinguishing between bronchiectasis and chronic bronchitis.

Favis EA: Planigraphy (body section radiography) in detecting tuberculous pulmonary cavitation. Dis Chest 27:668–673, 1955.
  Value of routine tomography in evaluating tuberculosis.

Feigin DS: Nocardiosis of the lung: chest radiographic findings in 21 cases. Radiology 159:9–14, 1986.
  The chest radiographic manifestations of nocardiosis are pleomorphic and not specific. Consolidations and large irregular nodules, often cavitary, are most common; nodules, masses, and interstitial patterns also occur. Pleural effusions are quite common, and lymph nodes may be enlarged.

Felson B: Chest Roentgenology. Philadelphia, Saunders, 1973.
  Basic textbook in chest radiology with emphasis on various signs for recognizing pathology.

Felson B: Lung torsion: radiographic findings in nine cases. Radiology 162:631–638, 1987.
  The radiographic findings in nine patients with pulmonary torsion are analyzed.

Fraser RG, Pare JAP: Diagnosis of Diseases of the Chest, 2d ed. Philadelphia, Saunders, 1978.
  Outstanding general text on chest disease with emphasis on radiology.

Gurney JW, Harrison WC, Sears K, Robbins RA, Dobry CA, Rennard SI: Bronchoalveolar lavage: radiographic manifestations. Radiology 163:71–74, 1987.
  Benign, self-limited radiographic changes are common after bronchoalveolar lavage and may simulate pulmonary edema, aspiration, or hemorrhage.

Hessén I: Roentgen examination of pleural fluid. A study of the localization of free effusions, the potentialities of diagnosing minimal quantities of fluid and its existence under physiological conditions. Acta Radiol 86(suppl):1–80, 1951.
  Classic article on detection of pleural fluid.

Jones KW, Pietra GG, Sabiston DC: Primary Neoplasms and Cysts of the Mediastinum, in Fishman AP (ed), Pulmonary Diseases and Disorders, 1st ed. New York, McGraw-Hill, 1980, pp 1490–1521.
  A comprehensive review focusing on the anatomic nature of the abnormalities of the mediastinum and their clinical implications.

Koval JC, Joseph SG, Schaefer PS, Tenholder MF: Fiberoptic bronchoscopy combined with selective bronchography. A simplified technique. Chest 91:776–778, 1987.
  A simplified method is presented for performing selective bronchography in conjunction with fiberoptic bronchoscopy.

Lavender JP, Doppman J, Shawdon HE, Steiner RE: Pulmonary veins in left ventricular failure and mitral stenosis. Br J Radiol 35:293–302, 1962.
  Early article recognizing the importance of vascular changes in left heart disease.

Lillington GA: The solitary pulmonary nodule—1974. Am Rev Respir Dis 110:699–707, 1974.
  Good review of the solitary pulmonary nodule.

Lloyd HM, String ST, DuBois AB: Radiographic plethysmographic determination of total lung capacity. Radiology 86:7–14, 1966.
  Pioneering article on the use of the chest radiograph in determining total lung capacity.

Milne EC: Correlation of physiologic findings with chest roentgenology. Radiol Clin North Am 11:17–44, 1973.
  Basic correlative study of the chest radiograph, especially pulmonary vasculature and pulmonary and cardiac physiology.

Nadel JA, Wolf WG, Graf PD: Powdered tantalum as a medium for bronchography in canine and human lungs. Invest Radiol 3:229–238, 1968.
  Interesting approach to bronchography.

Nadich D, Zerhouni E, Siegelman S: *Computerized Tomography of the Thorax.* New York, Raven, 1984.
  Good general textbook on chest CT.

Nathan MH, Collins VP, Adams RA: Differentiation of benign and malignant pulmonary nodules by growth rate. Radiology 79:221–232, 1962.
  Doubling time as a determinant of malignancy.

Ochsner SF: Pulmonary tuberculosis: Contributions of radiology in diagnosis and treatment. South Med J 79:1416–1424, 1986.
  This review records the important place that radiologic examinations have had in the diagnosis and treatment of pulmonary tuberculosis in the past nine decades.

Pratt PC: Role of conventional chest radiography in diagnosis and exclusion of emphysema. Am J Med 82:998–1006, 1987.
  Review of existing literature that deals solely with papers in which radiographic observations have been related to morphologic evidence of emphysema in inflation-fixed lungs at autopsy.

Rinker CT, Templeton AW, MacKenzie J, Ridings GR, Amond CH, Kiphart R: Combined superior vena cavography and azygography in patients with suspected lung carcinoma. Radiology 88:441–445, 1967.
  Early attempt to stage lung cancer.

Shackelford GD, Sacks EJ, Mullins JD, McAlister WH: Pulmonary veno-occlusive disease. Am J Roentgenol 128:643–648, 1977.
  Good discussion of an unusual entity.

Silverman PM, Godwin JD: CT/bronchographic correlations in bronchiectasis. J Comput Assist Tomogr 11:52–56, 1987.
  CT was compared with bronchography to assess the utility of CT in diagnosing and determining the extent of bronchiectasis. Twenty-six bronchograms were performed in 14 patients. In 77 percent (20/26) of the lungs examined, CT correctly detected or excluded bronchiectasis. But CT was less sensitive than bronchography and underestimated the number of diseased segments.

Simon G: *Principles of Chest X-Ray Diagnosis.* New York, Appleton-Century-Crofts, 1971.
  Basic textbook.

Spencer H: *Pathology of the Lung,* 3d ed. Oxford, Pergamon, 1977.
  Basic lung pathology text.

Swyer PE, James GOW: A case of unilateral pulmonary emphysema. Thorax 8:133–136, 1953.
  Original description of a classic radiologic syndrome.

Tape TG, Mushlin AI: The utility of routine chest radiographs. Ann Intern Med 104:663–670, 1986.
  The authors recommend that the practice of doing routine chest radiographs on admission and preoperatively be stopped and that the procedure be reserved for patients with clinical evidence of chest disease and patients having intrathoracic surgery.

Thurlbeck WM: *Chronic Airflow Obstruction in Lung Disease,* in Bennington JL (ed), *Major Problems in Pathology,* vol. 5. Philadelphia, Saunders, 1976.
  Excellent review of chronic obstructive lung disease.

Tuddenham WJ: Problems of perception in chest roentgenology, facts and fallacies. Radiol Clin North Am 1:277–289, 1963.
  Early work with a good review on the importance of visual perception in radiology.

Viamonte M Jr: Angiographic evaluation of lung neoplasms. Radiol Clin North Am 3:529–542, 1965.
  Review of the merits of angiography and lung cancer.

West JB: *Regional Differences in the Lung.* New York, Academic, 1977.
  Outstanding discussion of pulmonary physiology with major applications to the chest radiograph.

Chapter 36

Computed Tomography and Magnetic Resonance of the Chest

David M. Epstein / Warren B. Gefter
Alfred P. Fishman

Computed Tomography
  Concepts and Techniques
  Normal Anatomy
  Clinical Applications
  Radiographic Indications
  Clinical Applications

Magnetic Resonance
  Concepts and Techniques
  Clinical Applications

The past decade has witnessed a phenomenal growth in medical imaging technology. Computed tomography (CT) and more recently magnetic resonance (MR) are two such technologies which have been applied to disorders of the thorax. CT is now well established, although points of uncertainty in its application to chest disease are still being actively evaluated. MR has only recently moved from an investigational technique to the clinical armamentarium, although its availability is still quite limited. Although these two techniques differ significantly in their physical basis and the type of information they can offer, both CT and MR do provide highly similar and informative cross-sectional images of the chest.

This chapter reviews the concepts and techniques governing these two methods of imaging and discusses their applications to chest disorders. Clinicians who do have access to both modalities need to be familiar with the information that each technique can provide, the limitations of each technique, and the advantages of one over the other, particularly in a world that is increasingly concerned with obtaining the maximum diagnostic yield at the lowest cost.

COMPUTED TOMOGRAPHY

A decade of experience with computed tomography has established the technique as a powerful and sensitive diagnostic tool for evaluating the thorax. Its strength is in its ability to provide a cross-sectional image that affords far greater delineation of soft tissues than can be obtained by conventional radiography. With respect to evaluating intrathoracic structures, its major value is in the exploration of the mediastinal contents by providing extraordinary anatomic detail and enabling differentiation among solid, cystic, lipomatous, and vascular structures.

Computed tomography has also greatly expanded the boundaries of methods used to evaluate the pulmonary parenchyma. The traditional chest radiograph takes advantage of the air in the lung as natural contrast material in assessing lesions within the substance of the lungs. CT has added a new dimension to conventional chest radiography by enhancing the detection of occult metastases, the differentiation between pleural and parenchymal pulmonary disease, and the assessment of the solitary pulmonary nodule.

Concepts and Techniques

CT is based on the passage of multiple, highly collimated radiographic beams through the anatomic plane of interest from which the radiographic image is reconstructed. The density of tissue that the x-rays traverse en route to the detectors determines the degree to which the beams are attenuated. The projections of tissue density obtained from the detectors are mathematically reconstructed by a computer into a radiographic image.

Thoracic CT is not a screening procedure. Ideally, each CT examination should be tailored to address a particular clinical problem. This goal requires on-line participation by the radiologist at the time of scanning to set certain parameters that will determine the content and quality of the radiographic image. The following operator-dependent parameters warrant special attention.

SLICE THICKNESS

Most CT scanners deal with slice thicknesses of between 1 and 10 mm. The thicker the slice, the more will the densities of adjacent structures be included in the density averaging—the so-called partial volume averaging. In contrast, thin slices decrease the number of sampling photons and increase image noise unless the radiation dose to the patient and the workload on the x-ray tube are increased. Since the detection of a lesion depends on the density gradient between the lesion and the surrounding normal tissue, thick sections are appropriate for detecting most diseases of the pulmonary parenchyma. Because the lung is intrinsically low in density, the much greater density of most pathologic processes in the lungs suffices for them to be easily recognized even if only a sliver of the abnormality appears on a particular slice. For example, on a slice 10 mm in thickness, nodules as small as 1 mm can be identified. This thickness has the additional advantage over thin sections in that vessels that run obliquely through the scan are readily distinguished from lung nodules.

In contrast, thinner sections are more useful in examining the mediastinum where the density gradient between normal and pathologic structures is far less than within the pulmonary parenchyma. For example, thinner sections are useful in detecting small mediastinal lymph nodes, particularly if there is little mediastinal fat.

SLICE SPACING

The spacing of the slices depends on the size of the abnormality to be imaged. When the abnormality is expected to be larger than the slice thickness, contiguous slice spacing is unnecessary since it will only increase the radiation dose to the patient and prolong the examination. Oppositely, contiguous spacing is needed if the lesion is apt to be smaller than the slice (e.g., as an occult metastasis), or if areas of complex anatomy (e.g., the pulmonary hili) are to be closely scrutinized.

SCAN TIME

Respiratory motion severely degrades the quality of the CT image. Most scanners can acquire the data needed for an image during a single period of breath holding. This procedure requires instruction of the patient about proper breathing technique, and data are gathered either at end-inspiration or at end-expiration.

FIELD OF VIEW

Image quality is strongly influenced by the size of the picture elements (*pixels*) composing the image. Ideally, pixel size should be smaller than the minimal distance resolvable by the scanner, i.e., usually less than 0.6 to 1 mm. Larger pixel size results in loss of spatial resolution, whereas smaller pixel size is impractical owing to the inordinate number of computer calculations involved in creating the image. The selection of an appropriate field of view, based on the patient's thoracic diameter, will optimize pixel size and enhance image resolution and quality.

CONTRAST ENHANCEMENT

Contrast agents administered intravenously are useful in thoracic CT, particularly in evaluating the pulmonary hili and mediastinal vascular structures. However, not every thoracic CT requires intravenous contrast. When contrast agents are used, satisfactory opacification of hilar and mediastinal vessels can usually be achieved by scanning from just below the carina toward the apex after the intravenous injection of a 100-cm³ bolus of contrast material; the study is then completed by scanning from the carina to the diaphragm.

DYNAMIC SCANNING

Dynamic scanning enables several scans to be obtained in a brief period of time. It can be used to determine the vascularity of a lesion, e.g., arteriovenous malformation or pulmonary varix, or to examine an aortic aneurysm or dissection. By delivering multiple small boluses of contrast, a series of scans, with considerable vascular enhancement, can be obtained at different levels in a short period of time. The limitations of dynamic scanning are the heat capacity generated by the x-ray tube, the time required for the table to move, and the breath-holding capacity of the patient.

CT NUMBERS

Differences in tissue density are expressed in terms of CT numbers. Typical CT numbers range from approximately -1000 (air) to $+1000$ (dense cortical bone). Structures of the same density as water have a CT number of approximately 0; in contrast, fat is approximately -100. These numbers are not absolute. Many factors can affect a CT number and cause it to differ from examination to examination and/or from one CT scanner to another. The relative CT number between structures is usually far more informative than the absolute value.

INFORMATION DISPLAY

The full scale of CT numbers generated by the CT reconstruction process cannot be displayed in a single image because current electronic display systems use only a limited number of shades of gray. The operator has to select the portion of the CT number range to be displayed. This is done by manipulating electronic windows at the CT console to establish the width and level at which the window will be active. All CT images of the thorax should be viewed with at least two, and optimally three, window settings: one for the lungs, one for the mediastinum and chest wall, and one for the bony structures.

RADIATION DOSE

The radiation dose delivered by modern CT scanners is about 1.2 rads to lungs and 3.1 rads to the skin. These dosages are distinctly less than the 20 rads delivered to the lung and the 40 rads delivered to the skin during conventional whole lung tomography. With shielding, the dose reaching the gonads during chest CT is estimated at 2.8 mrad.

Normal Anatomy

Interpretation of mediastinal structures on thoracic CT requires familiarity with normal cross-sectional relationships in the mediastinum. These are illustrated in the figures that follow. In these figures, the CT images and corresponding schematic representations progress from cephalad to caudal. The symbols are listed alphabetically in Table 36-1.

Figure 36-1 is at the level of the sternal notch, through the lung apices. In this section, six mediastinal vessels

TABLE 36-1
Abbreviations Used in Figures

AA = aortic arch
AR = aortic root
AsA = ascending aorta
AzV = azygous vein
BCA = brachiocephalic artery
BCV = brachiocephalic vein
BI = bronchus intermedius
C = carotid artery
Ca = carina
Cl = clavicle
DA = descending aorta
DLPA = descending left pulmonary artery
E = esophagus
E(A) = air-filled esophagus
EF = epicardial fat
IA = innominate artery
IPV = inferior pulmonary vein
JV = jugular vein
LA = left atrium
LCCA = left common carotid artery
LIV = left innominate vein
LJV = left jugular vein
LLApex = apex of left lung
LLL-PA = pulmonary artery to left lower lobe
LN = lymph node
LPA = left pulmonary artery
LSA = left subclavian artery
LSV = left subclavian vein
LULBr = left upper lobe bronchus
LV = left ventricle
LVMyo = left ventricular myocardium
M = muscle
MF = mediastinal fat
MPA = main pulmonary artery
P = pericardium
PMF = periesophageal mediastinal fat
RA = right atrium
RCCA = right common carotid artery
RIV = right innominate vein
RLApex = apex of right lung
RPA = right pulmonary artery
RSA = right subclavian artery
RSPV = right superior pulmonary vein
RSV = right subclavian vein
RV = right ventricle
S = scapula
St = sternum
SC = subclavian arteries
SF = subcutaneous fat
SPV = superior pulmonary vein
SVC = superior vena cava
T = trachea
TA = truncus anterior
TVM = thoracic vertebral marrow

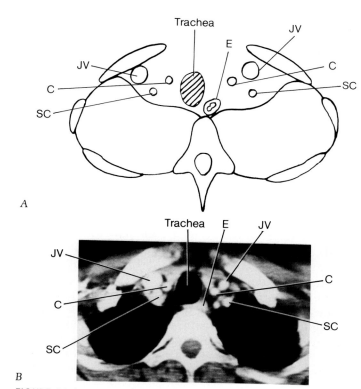

FIGURE 36-1 Normal anatomy at level of sternal notch. Six major mediastinal vessels are seen: the paired jugular veins (JV), carotid arteries (C), and subclavian arteries (SC), which may be tortuous. Other structures include the trachea and esophagus (E).

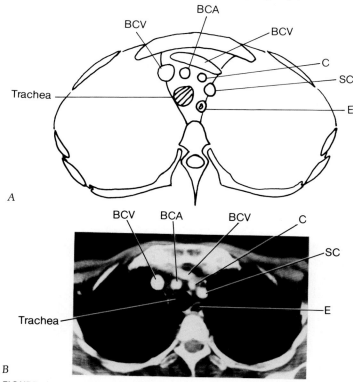

FIGURE 36-2 Normal anatomy at level of manubrium. The left brachiocephalic vein (BCV) courses anteriorly to join the right brachiocephalic vein (BCV), forming the superior vena cava (SVC) shown at the next lower level. The left subclavian (SC), left carotid (C), and right brachiocephalic artery (BCA) are seen.

can usually be identified. The paired jugular veins, variable in size, lie anteriorly. Medial to the jugular veins lie the paired carotid arteries; posteriorly lie the subclavian arteries. The thyroid gland is closely opposed to the anterior lateral aspects of the trachea. The thyroid often has a higher density than the muscle because of its high iodine content. The trachea and esophagus also appear on this section.

In Fig. 36-2, behind the manubrium, the left brachiocephalic vein courses anteriorly in a longitudinal direction as it crosses the midline to join the right brachiocephalic vein en route to form the superior vena cava at a slightly lower level. Also seen are the left subclavian, left carotid, and right innominate arteries.

In Fig. 36-3, at the level of the aortic arch, the superior vena cava is the only other vessel. The superior vena cava is ovoid or elliptical in configuration and oriented in the anterior posterior direction; it provides a slight convexity to the right superior mediastinum. The region between the posterior aspects of the superior vena cava and the anterior lateral aspect of the trachea is fat-filled; frequently lymph nodes less than 1 cm in diameter are also found in this region.

In Fig. 36-4, the left pulmonary artery is located posteriorly, just cephalad to the left main-stem bronchus where it forms the left lateral margin of the mediastinum. The right upper lobe bronchus is also seen at this level along with the ascending and descending thoracic aorta, superior vena cava, and truncus anterior branch of the right pulmonary artery.

In Fig. 36-5, the right pulmonary artery is seen extending posteriorly and to the right from the main pulmonary artery. It runs immediately behind the superior vena cava and anterior to the bronchus intermedius which appears as a circular lucency. The posterior wall of the right upper lobe bronchus and the posterior wall of the bronchus intermedius are contiguous with the aerated right lung. Any area of tissue density other than lung in this region is abnormal. The invagination of the right lung posterior to the bronchus intermedius into the mediastinum is referred to as the *azygoesophageal recess*. The pulmonary artery to the left lower lobe lies behind the left upper lobe bronchus at this level.

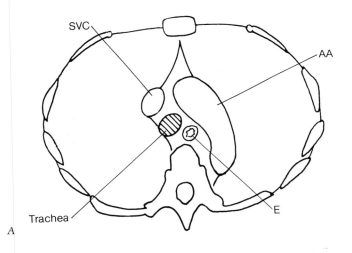

A

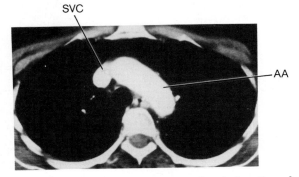

B

FIGURE 36-3   *A* and *B.* Normal anatomy at level of aortic arch (AA). The superior vena cava (SVC), trachea and esophagus (E) are seen.

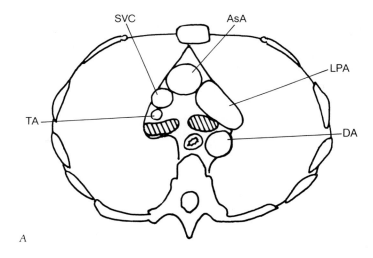

A

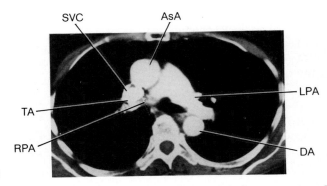

B

FIGURE 36-4   Normal anatomy at level of left pulmonary artery. The left pulmonary artery (LPA) courses posteriorly over the left upper lobe bronchus. Ascending aorta (AsA), descending aorta (DA), superior vena cava (SVC), and truncus anterior (TA) branch of the right pulmonary artery (RPA) are also seen. The uppermost part of the RPA is also partially visualized in this section.

Figure 36-6 shows the left atrium. Anteriorly lies the superior vena cava at the junction with the right atrium, ascending aorta, and main pulmonary artery. The main pulmonary artery is usually slightly anterior to the ascending aorta. At this level, subcarinal masses or adenopathy can be seen closely apposed to the left atrium.

The final section, Fig. 36-7, shows the cardiac chambers.

Clinical Applications

The mainstay for radiographic evaluation of the thorax is the chest radiograph, particularly comparison of radiographs taken sequentially in the evolution of a lesion. Chest CT scans afford a second level of radiologic examination. The remaining discussion of thoracic CT will divide the indications for thoracic CT into two main categories: (1) *radiographic indications*, to clarify an abnormality or suspected abnormality visualized on the conventional radiograph, and (2) *clinical indications*, to

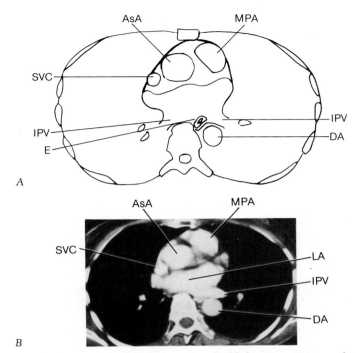

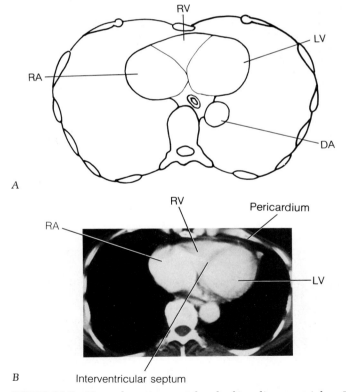

FIGURE 36-6 Normal anatomy at level of left atrium. Main pulmonary artery (MPA), AsA, left atrium (LA), and superior vena cava (SVC) are seen. The inferior pulmonary veins (IPV) on the left are seen entering the LA.

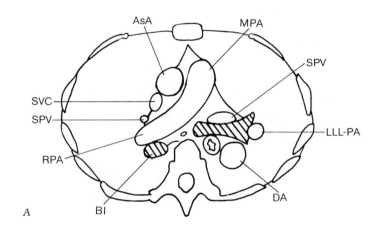

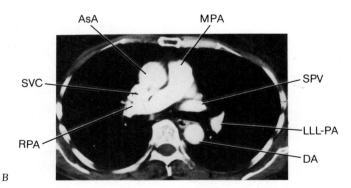

FIGURE 36-5 Normal anatomy at level of right pulmonary artery. Right pulmonary artery (RPA) extends posteriorly from the main pulmonary artery (MPA) to course anterior to the bronchus intermedius (BI). The left lower lobe pulmonary artery (LLL-PA) is posterior to the left main-stem bronchus. The ascending aorta (AsA), descending aorta (DA), superior vena cava (SVC), and superior pulmonary veins (SPV) are seen at this level.

FIGURE 36-7 Normal anatomy at level of cardiac ventricles. Left ventricle (LV), right ventricle (RV), interventricular septum, and right atrium (RA) are identified. The pericardium is seen as a thin line of soft tissue between the pericardial fat anteriorly and the epicardial fat posteriorly.

provide additional diagnostic information about a clinical problem.

Radiographic Indications

MEDIASTINAL MASSES

Interpretation of mediastinal masses seen on the conventional chest radiograph can be facilitated by CT because of its ability to distinguish between subtle differences in density. Uniformly solid lesions can be separated on CT from those that are cystic, and areas of necrosis or minute foci of calcification can be more sharply delineated than on conventional radiographs. Cross-sectional imaging can clarify relationships of a mass to other vital structures, and visualization of tissue planes is often helpful in planning surgery.

Thyroid

The diagnostic value of CT is limited for mediastinal masses that are similar in density and in certain other features, such as calcification and necrosis. The iodine content of a substernal thyroid on CT scans that are not contrast-enhanced is diagnostically helpful because of the greater density of the thyroid than of other solid mediastinal masses (Fig. 36-8). Other characteristics of a substernal thyroid gland on CT include extension of the mass from the mediastinum into the neck on contiguous CT sections, a well-defined border, punctate or ringlike calcifications, and nonhomogeneity that includes discrete, nonenhancing, low-density areas. Occasionally, a substernal thyroid may appear less dense than other mediastinal masses because of a relative lack of iodine in areas of cystic degeneration. CT cannot discriminate neoplastic dis-

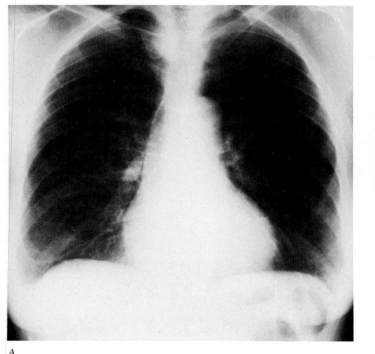

A

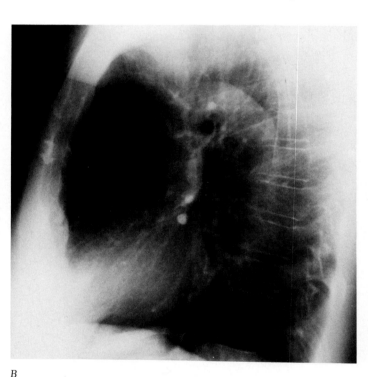

B

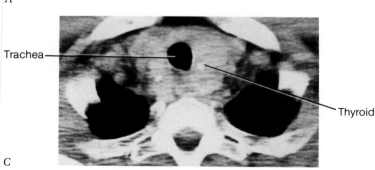

C   *D*

FIGURE 36-8   Intrathoracic goiter.   *A* and *B.* Chest radiograph demonstrates soft tissue fullness in the upper right paratracheal area suggesting a mediastinal mass.   *C* and *D.* Contiguous CT scans without contrast show a high-density mass with foci of calcification surrounding the trachea. The mass is more dense than muscle because of its intrinsic iodine content. Its density and continuity into the neck suggest a substernal thyroid gland.

ease of the thyroid gland unless adjacent structures are invaded.

Thymus

The thymus gland normally appears as a bilobed arrowhead shaped structure, often best visualized at the level of the aortic arch but frequently seen extending from the left brachiocephalic vein to the root of the aorta and pulmonary artery. Normal measurements vary with age; persons who are more than 30 years old tend to have decreased width, thickness, and density of the thymic gland because of fatty infiltration. But, normal thymic contours are usually preserved even in persons after the age of 40. In patients over 40 years of age, the presence of a spherical or ovoid mass in the expected location of the thymic gland or deformity of the adjacent pleura suggests a thymoma (Fig. 36-9). Diffuse enlargement of the thymic gland with preservation of its normal shape is more suggestive of hyperplasia.

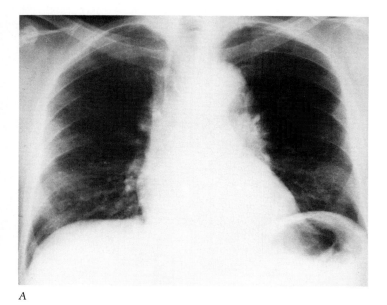

A

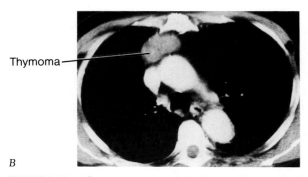

B

FIGURE 36-9 Thymoma. *A.* Subtle abnormality in the lateral contour of the ascending aorta in an elderly patient who previously had coronary bypass surgery. *B.* CT scans show a solid, ovoid nonenhancing mass anterior to the ascending aorta and superior vena cava. The mass is clearly separate from the aorta and represents a thymoma.

Thymic pathology is more difficult to exclude in the young who have not yet developed fatty infiltration. A diffusely and symmetrically enlarged thymus raises the possibility of infiltration of the gland by Hodgkin's disease. Radiation therapy often causes the thymus to appear cystic rather than solid.

Well-circumscribed thymic tumors are almost always benign, whereas tumors showing infiltration into adjacent fat are usually malignant. CT cannot consistently differentiate a benign from malignant thymoma unless there is evidence of metastatic disease to the mediastinum, pleura, or lungs. CT can also not consistently differentiate mediastinal lymph node enlargement from thymoma.

Teratomas

Teratomas are difficult to distinguish from lesions of the thymus by CT criteria alone: both are usually solid masses and may contain calcifications. Also, unlike pelvic dermoids, mediastinal teratomas rarely contain teeth. Either a teratoma or a thymic lesion can have areas of lower density mixed with the solid components. In a teratoma, a region of low density is due either to cystic areas or to fatty elements within the solid mass. A mediastinal mass that is predominantly low density in character suggests a cystic teratoma or a mediastinal germ cell tumor.

Lymphadenopathy

Lymphadenopathy in the mediastinum appears as a solid tissue mass. The lymphadenopathy may contain regions of lower density caused by necrosis or of calcification caused by granulomatous disease or radiation therapy. Lymph nodes sometimes undergo modest enhancement after the intravenous injection of contrast material, thereby complicating differentiation from mediastinal vessels. The histology of lymphadenopathy in the mediastinum cannot be predicted from CT evaluation.

Cystic Lesions

Most benign cystic lesions of the mediastinum are homogeneous, water-equivalent in density, and do not enhance following the intravenous administration of contrast material. Pericardial cysts occur in both the right and left cardiophrenic angle (Fig. 36-10). Bronchogenic cysts are typically round or ovoid, low-density structures (water equivalent) in the subcarinal region or the right paratracheal region (Fig. 36-11). The density of both pericardial and bronchogenic cysts occasionally exceeds that of water. Although most masses that have densities slightly greater than that of water represent cysts containing mucus or other debris, absolute confidence in diagnosing a pericardial or bronchogenic cyst using CT in these instances is not possible. Further evaluation, including biopsy and/or surgery, may be necessary.

Lipomatosis

Localized, benign mediastinal fat collections can be diagnosed by CT with almost complete assurance: the low

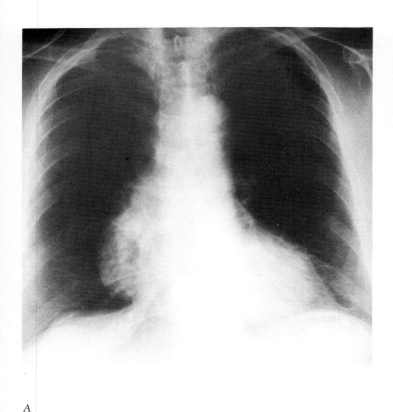

A

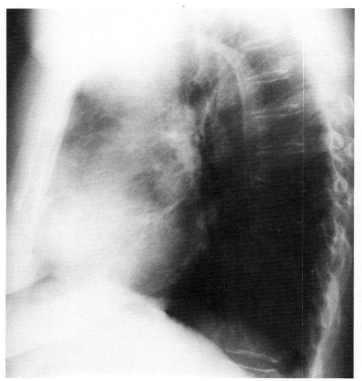

B

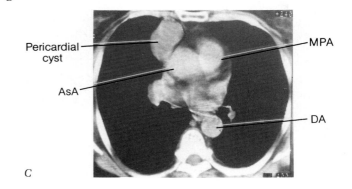

Pericardial cyst — MPA

AsA — DA

C

FIGURE 36-10 Pericardial cyst. *A* and *B*. Posteroanterior and lateral chest radiographs showing a mass obscuring the right heart border. Its density is indistinguishable from the heart. *C*. CT scan shows a well-marginated cardiophrenic angle mass. Its low density (water equivalent) confirms a pericardial cyst. Main pulmonary artery (MPA), ascending aorta (AsA), and descending aorta (DA) are identified.

density of fat enables distinction to be readily made between fat and lymphadenopathy (Fig. 36-12). Malignant liposarcomas, which are extremely rare, usually contain elements of higher tissue density than pure fat. Patients in whom CT discloses areas disposed like fat but having higher-density values than fat, need further evaluation by either biopsy or thoracotomy.

Neurogenic Tumors

Neurogenic tumors, the most common posterior mediastinal masses, are well evaluated by CT. CT allows precise localization, detection of destruction of vertebral bodies, and recognition of intraspinal extension (Fig. 36-13). In complicated cases, the use of CT, in conjunction with metrizamide administered intrathecally, provides an examination of the spinal canal that is comparable to myelography.

MEDIASTINAL WIDENING

When mediastinal widening is detected on the plain film, the cause may be normal variant (abundant fat or tortuous vessel), an aneurysm, or a soft tissue mass (primary neoplasm or enlarged lymph nodes). CT is ideally suited for analysis of the widened mediastinum. It can differentiate vascular from nonvascular lesions and often provides specific and conclusive diagnoses.

Abundant fat in the mediastinum is readily diagnosed because of its characteristic low CT density. It is common in patients taking corticosteroids or who have Cushing's syndrome. Vascular dilatation or aneurysm formation can be diagnosed in most cases after the administration of intravenous iodinated contrast material: the contrast agent causes enhancement and increased density of vascular structures well beyond the range of other solid

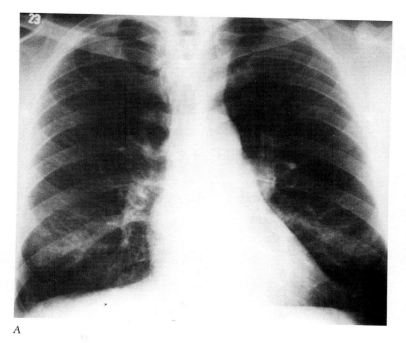

A

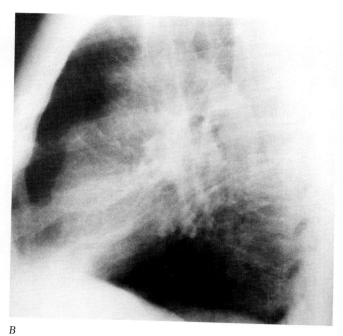

B

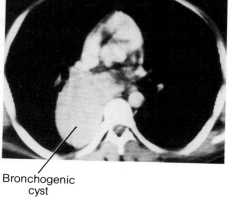

Bronchogenic
cyst

C

FIGURE 36-11 Bronchogenic cyst. *A* and *B*. Posteroanterior and lateral chest radiographs reveal increased density in the subcarinal location without a distinct mass. *C*. CT scan demonstrates a sharply circumscribed subcarinal mediastinal mass. This mass was more dense than water. A bronchogenic cyst may have higher density than water if it contains debris or blood or is infected.

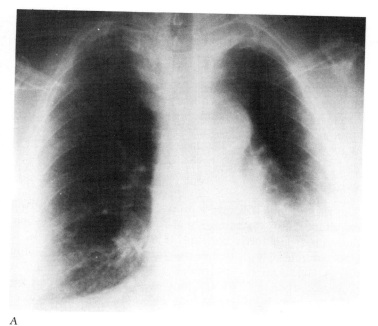

A

Lipomatosis

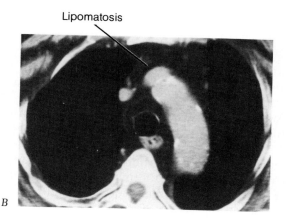

B

FIGURE 36-12 Lipomatosis. *A*. Chest radiograph reveals a widened superior mediastinal contour due to either lymph nodes, fat, or tortuous great vessels. *B*. CT scan demonstrates low-density tissue infiltrating the anterior mediastinum. This picture is characteristic of benign mediastinal lipomatosis.

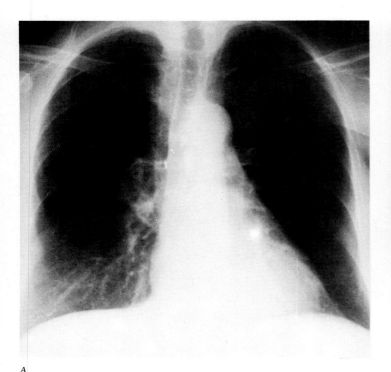

A

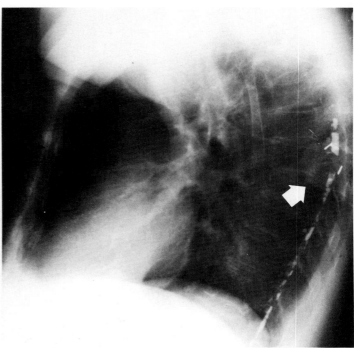

B

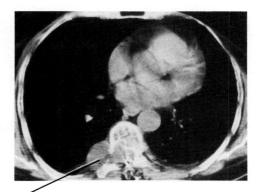

C Neurofibroma

FIGURE 36-13 Neurofibroma. *A* and *B*. Posteroanterior and lateral chest radiographs showing posterior mediastinal soft tissue mass overlying the spinal canal (arrowhead in *B*). Residual pantopaque is present in the subarachnoid space from prior myelography. *C*. CT scan confirms a paraspinal soft tissue mass and in addition shows direct invasion of the vertebral body and intraspinal extension of this neurofibroma. The detail of involvement is far greater with CT and is important in preoperative assessment.

mediastinal tissues. CT can also display an array of congenital vascular anomalies of the aortic arch and mediastinal vessels that cause abnormal contour of the mediastinum.

Aneurysms or dissection of the thoracic aorta can be identified by using dynamic CT scanning. The diagnosis of aortic dissection is confirmed by demonstrating medial displacement of intimal calcification on the precontrast CT scan, and then, after administering contrast material, a raised intimal flap with opacification of both the true and false lumens (Fig. 36-14). Not only can the origin of dissection be seen but also an associated hemothorax or hemopericardium. Occasionally an aortic aneurysm fails to enhance because it is filled with clot. In this instance, it will not be distinguishable from a solid mass.

Interpretation of posterior mediastinal paraspinal widening is often facilitated by CT: distinction can usu-

ally be made between enlarged lymph nodes and vessels; anatomic variants become evident. Although involvement of the vertebral body by extension of a paraspinal mass caused by either infection or metastatic tumor is readily seen, distinction between the two etiologies is rarely possible. CT-guided biopsy may then provide a definitive diagnosis.

PULMONARY HILI

The pulmonary hili are composed of airways, including segmental and subsegmental bronchi, pulmonary arteries, and veins. The fairly constant relationship between these structures is useful in the interpretation of the hili using CT. Analysis of the pulmonary hili based on bronchial anatomy displayed by CT may suffice without need for enhancement by contrast material. However, analysis of

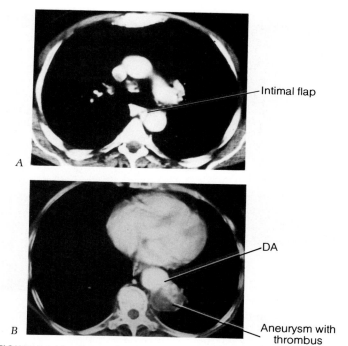

Intimal flap

DA

Aneurysm with thrombus

FIGURE 36-14 Aortic dissection and aortic aneurysm. *A.* CT scan with contrast reveals an intimal flap (lucency) with opacification of the true and false lumens in a dissection of the descending thoracic aorta. *B.* CT scan in which high-density intravenous contrast mixes with low-density thrombus in aortic aneurysm.

the hili is facilitated by contrast material, administered intravenously, which readily separates enhancing (vascular) from nonenhancing (nonvascular) structures. The demonstration of nonenhancement implies abnormality, i.e., either adenopathy or a mass. On rare occasions, lymph nodes undergo contrast enhancement that may obscure distinction from pulmonary vessels. This blurring in diagnosis has been noted in patients with angioimmunoblastic lymphadenopathy, small cell carcinoma, vascular metastases from renal and thyroid cancer, and viral infections.

Hilar adenopathy that is not apparent on a plain film may be detected by CT, especially posterior hilar adenopathy. CT compares favorably with oblique tomography in the evaluation of the pulmonary hili. The clarity of detail provided by cross-sectional CT imaging should make CT a preferable radiographic method for hilar evaluation.

SOLITARY PULMONARY NODULE

Using conventional radiography, distinction between a benign and a malignant solitary pulmonary nodule depends on its growth pattern and the presence of calcification. A nodule that fails to grow over a 2-year interval, or a nodule that has popcorn or concentric rings of calcification, is presumed to be benign. But, a dense nodule often poses a more perplexing problem. Indeed, it is difficult to

identify a solidly calcified nodule even if the conventional chest radiograph is supplemented by tomography. CT has been advocated as a method for distinguishing between benign and malignant lung nodules on the basis of density. The major problem in using CT this way is in getting thin sections through the lesions in order to eliminate artificially low density values from "volume averaging." As indicated previously, the artifact stems from the inclusion of surrounding, normal, low-density lung in the determination of the average density of the nodule.

Seigleman developed a technique based on density numbers that relied on thin-section (2 to 5 mm) computed tomography and a computerized printout of the data to distinguish benign from malignant lung nodules. Unfortunately, this technique has technical problems that have precluded its widespread use. An alternative approach relies on a commercially available phantom to mimic the environment of any given lung nodule. Although the CT number of a nodule does vary greatly with the scanner and technique; the size, position, and environment of the nodule; and the electronic drift, all scanners respond linearly to increasing density. This relationship indicates that two identical objects of different density can be compared on a given scanner providing the conditions under which the measurements are made are similar. Accordingly, the phantom technique permits the analysis of a lung nodule to be made by visual inspection without need for a printer; it also does away with the time-consuming process of first analyzing the numerical data for each section and then calculating a representative CT number.

Confidence in the diagnosis of a benign nodule is greatest when the entire lesion exhibits values in excess of the phantom. High-density values should be seen in several different sections. Some benign lesions are low in density and will give false positives that are suggestive of malignancy. CT yields false-negative results in patients with scar carcinoma or cancers that have dystrophic calcification. Although promising, the accuracy and reproducibility of the phantom approach requires further testing.

PULMONARY PARENCHYMA

The high natural contrast in the pulmonary parenchyma makes the chest radiograph difficult to surpass in formulating a differential diagnosis. CT has limited value in the evaluation of the pulmonary parenchyma and, as a rule, transbronchial or open lung biopsy is more rewarding in clinching the diagnosis. Assessment of pulmonary density using CT has been tried in patients with diffuse pulmonary disease. However, this approach is hindered by technical as well as physiological factors: since lung density represents an average of the densities of blood, air, lung tissue, and extravascular fluid, the individual component(s) responsible for an increase, or decrease, in global density are not distinguishable. Clearly, CT would be

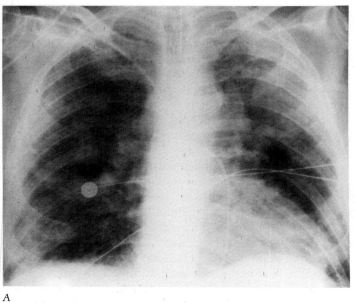

A

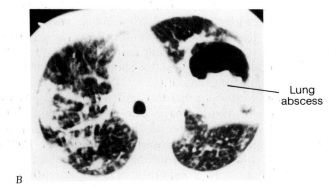

B

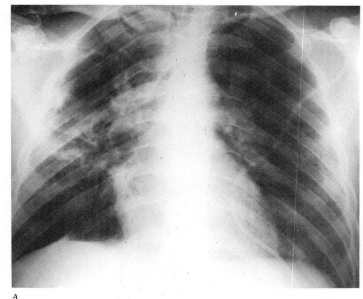

A

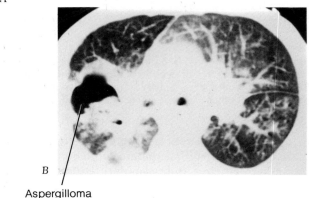

B

Aspergilloma

FIGURE 36-15 Lung abscess. *A.* Extensive bilateral infiltrates due to pneumonia with adult respiratory distress syndrome. *B.* CT scan shows a cavitary left upper lobe lung abscess which is not apparent on the chest radiograph.

— Lung abscess

FIGURE 36-16 Sarcoidosis. *A.* Bilateral interstitial lung disease due to sarcoidosis is present in a patient with hemoptysis. *B.* A well-defined thick-walled cavity in the right upper lobe with an intracavitary mass is typical of an aspergilloma.

more effective if it could visualize the abnormality directly rather than imply that it is there because of a change in the average density that it registers.

In the attempt to visualize abnormal pulmonary parenchyma directly, high resolution, thin-section, computed tomography has been coupled with magnification of the pulmonary parenchyma. As a result, morphologic analysis of the fine details of the pulmonary interstitium is now technically feasible, i.e., septal lines and their branching pattern can be visualized in various physiological states. Whether this technique will be clinically useful is still uncertain.

Computed tomography is helpful in localizing and characterizing cystic and cavitary parenchymal pulmonary disease. The size, wall thickness, and regularity of cystic lesions is better defined by the cross-sectional imaging afforded by CT than by conventional radiographs. In patients with bronchiectasis, CT reveals a greater extent of

disease than does the conventional chest radiograph, an observation that is useful with respect to guiding surgical resection. Also, transverse images that avoid the superimposition of vascular and osseous shadows can detect occult cavities in areas of dense parenchymal consolidation (Fig. 36-15). Intracavitary masses are far easier to define using CT than conventional radiography. One practical application of this advantage is in patients with underlying interstitial disease and hemoptysis who are suspected of having a mycetoma due to secondary noninvasive aspergillosis (Fig. 36-16).

Occasionally distinction between bronchopleural fistula and empyema on the one hand and a lung abscess on the other is difficult using conventional radiography. This distinction has considerable importance since tube thoracostomy is necessary for treating the empyema. CT can be of great help in clarifying matters: the typical CT appear-

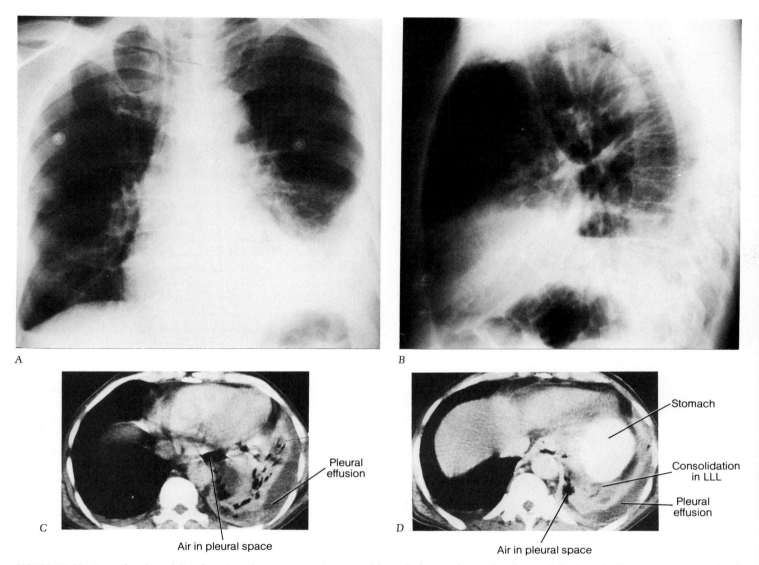

FIGURE 36-17 Bronchopleural fistula. *A* and *B*. Posteroanterior and lateral chest radiographs show a left pleural effusion with an air-fluid level behind the heart. The air-fluid level could be due to a hiatal hernia or lung abscess in the left lower lobe. *C* and *D*. CT scans at two different levels showing consolidation in the left lower lobe with a left pleural effusion. Multiple air lucencies are present in the left pleural space. The pleural air indicates the presence of a bronchopleural fistula.

ance of a lung abscess is a rounded mass with an irregular, thick wall and a nodular inner margin; in contrast, an empyema conforms to the shape of the pleural cavity and has a smooth, thin wall (Fig. 36-17).

The extent of bullous disease may also be assessed by thoracic CT: even though bullae can be seen or inferred on conventional radiographs in most patients with bullous emphysema, CT provides a more accurate assessment of the extent of disease.

ATELECTASIS

Lobar collapse is usually evident on conventional chest radiographs, and bronchoscopy generally identifies and

characterizes the underlying endobronchial obstructing lesion. CT can be a useful adjunct particularly in the patient with bronchogenic carcinoma, not only in localizing and visualizing the endobronchial lesions, but also in detecting abnormalities of the mediastinum, chest wall, hilus, and adjacent lung. In lobar atelectasis, the involved lobe loses its hemispheric contour on cross section and becomes pear-shaped (Fig. 36-18). The proximal portion of the lobe assumes a V shape, the apex of which is situated at the origin of the affected bronchus; the density of the lobe increases. A large tumor mass is sometimes manifest as a bulge in the contour of the collapsed lobe. If the entire lobe is replaced by tumor, the appearance of the lobe becomes lobular rather than wedge-shaped. Using

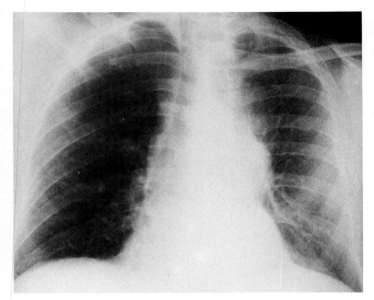

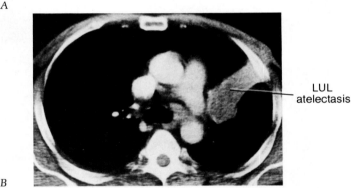

LUL
atelectasis

FIGURE 36-18 Atelectasis. *A.* Left upper lobe collapse secondary to an endobronchial carcinoma. *B.* Typical pear-shaped appearance of left upper lobe atelectasis when imaged cross sectionally on CT.

CT, fluid within the pleural space is often easily distinguished from underlying collapsed lung because of the difference in density between collapsed lung and the surrounding fluid.

PLEURA

The pleural fissures seen by CT serve as landmarks for the accurate localization of parenchymal disease. The CT appearance of the major fissure depends on its axis relative to the plane of cross section: most often it appears as a broad avascular band within the pulmonary parenchyma; less frequently, if the vertical axis of the major fissure is perpendicular to the plane of the CT section, the major fissure will be a thin, dense linear structure. Occasionally, the major fissure appears as a broad, dense band. The minor fissure appears as an area of decreased vascularity in the right mid-lung field at the level of the bronchus intermedius. Familiarity with the CT appearance of the pleural fissures is helpful in localizing lung infiltrates and

nodules and in distinguishing loculated fluid from parenchymal disease.

CT is of no help in differentiating transudative from exudative or chylous effusions. Likewise, it is difficult to distinguish pleural fluid from pleural thickening or fibrosis unless fluid can be shown to move with change in body position. CT suffers from similar difficulties as the conventional radiograph in distinguishing peripheral parenchymal masses from pleural or extrapleural densities. But CT can be helpful in identifying tumors of the pleura by enabling distinction between pleural nodularity and masses on the one hand and a surrounding pleural effusion on the other. Also, in individuals who have been exposed to asbestos, CT is useful in delineating subtle pleural plaques and in distinguishing the enface pleural plaque due to asbestos disease from a pulmonary nodule. With respect to the histologic nature of *pleural-based* masses seen on the conventional radiograph, a lipoma is the only one that can be identified with certainty because of its characteristic low density.

CT can be helpful in establishing the diagnosis of active tuberculosis in areas of fibrothorax: the active infection is suggested by medial displacement of calcification and by the identification of low-density fluid, not apparent on the conventional radiographs, within the fibrothorax.

Clinical Applications

PULMONARY NODULES IN EXTRAPULMONARY MALIGNANCY

In patients known to have an extrapulmonary malignancy, CT provides a sensitive, albeit nonspecific, means of identifying small pulmonary metastases (Fig. 36-19). Many pulmonary metastases are located subpleurally so that discrimination by conventional tomography is impractical because of the obscuring density of the overlying chest wall. The capability of visualizing the lung apex, the retrocardiac and retrosternal regions, and the posterior inferior lung recesses near the diaphragm make CT the most sensitive imaging modality in the detection of pulmonary nodules that are less than 6 mm in diameter.

Occasionally, parenchymal nodules may be indistinguishable from normal vascular structures on CT. But, as a rule, if a nodular density in the periphery is separate from, and larger than, adjacent vascular structures situated at a similar distance from the chest wall, then the density represents a lung nodule. However, if the visualized density is continuous with vascular structures, or if it changes in size and shape, then it is probably a blood vessel. A major problem in using CT imaging for the detection of occult metastases is its lack of specificity. For example, in endemic areas of histoplasmosis where granulomas or subpleural lymph nodes may constitute up to 25 percent of lung nodules, these benign lesions are generally indistinguishable from pulmonary metastases.

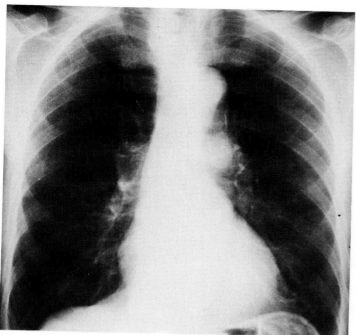

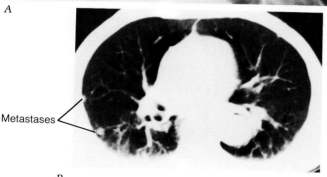

Metastases

FIGURE 36-19 Metastases. *A.* Normal chest radiograph in a patient with hypernephroma. *B.* CT shows two small subpleural nodules which are suspicious of occult metastases.

In patients with high-risk malignant melanoma, CT offers a chance of identifying a metastatic nodule that cannot be seen on the chest radiograph. In patients with extrathoracic malignancy in whom a single nodule is detected on the conventional chest radiograph, CT may help to distinguish a primary carcinoma of the lung from a pulmonary metastasis since the detection of additional nodules suggests metastatic disease.

THYMOMA

Ten to fifteen percent of patients with myasthenia gravis have a thymoma. CT is the imaging procedure of choice following chest radiography in patients with myasthenia gravis (Fig. 36-20).

Thymomas produce a focal soft tissue bulge that interrupts the normally smooth outer margin of the thymus. A thymoma may entirely replace the normal thymus by a round or ovoid mass. Thymoma is more easily recognized in patients over 30 years of age in whom fatty infiltration involves most of the thymus. Thymic hyperplasia, also associated with myasthenia gravis, is sometimes recognizable as diffuse glandular enlargement, especially by an increase in thickness. However, although CT can suggest hyperplasia and also exclude the presence of a thymoma, it cannot exclude hyperplasia. Finally, an invasive thymoma is suggested on CT by the appearance of widespread infiltration into the surrounding mediastinal fat and/or the appearance of localized masses along the pleural or pericardial surfaces.

THYMIC CARCINOID, PARATHYROID ADENOMA, OR HYPERPLASIA

CT may also be useful in localizing a thymic carcinoid tumor in patients suspected of having ectopic production of adrenocorticotropic hormone (ACTH). In patients with unexplained hypercalcemia, an aberrantly located parathyroid adenoma or a hyperplastic gland in the superior mediastinum is sometimes identifiable by CT.

BRONCHOGENIC CARCINOMA

The use of thoracic CT in determining operability of bronchogenic carcinoma varies from clinic to clinic. However, certain generalizations can be made. Patients with cancer of the lung and distinct mediastinal adenopathy on the plain film do not need CT; these patients only require tissue confirmation to prove mediastinal metastases. If involvement of the chest wall is considered to be a contraindication to surgery, then the detection of rib destruction on the conventional chest radiograph obviates the need for CT. Conversely, if chest wall involvement is not a contraindication to surgery, then CT provides a more accurate estimate than does conventional chest radiography of the extent of the tumor. In patients who have a small lung nodule in the periphery of the lung, the likelihood of mediastinal metastases is small, particularly if the carcinoma is squamous cell; in these individuals, a normal appearing mediastinum on the chest radiograph suggests that CT will not be rewarding. Finally, in those clinics that consider oat cell carcinoma to be a nonsurgical problem, histologic diagnosis of this neoplasm eliminates the need for CT.

Mediastinal invasion by a carcinoma of the lung is a contraindication to surgical intervention that is directed at cure. CT can demonstrate direct extension of tumor into the mediastinum that involves mediastinal fat and vessels (Fig. 36-21). However, it is worth emphasizing that contiguity of tumor with the mediastinal pleura, or the absence of a distinct plane between the tumor and the mediastinum, is insufficient evidence for tumor invasion.

Invasion of the chest wall by tumor is suggested by pleural thickening adjacent to the tumor, increased density in the extrapleural fat, rib destruction, and the pres-

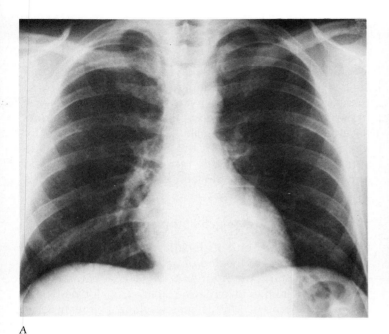

A

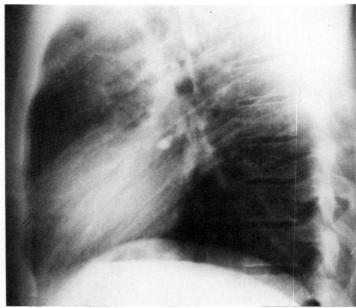

B

Thymoma

C

FIGURE 36-20 Thymoma. *A* and *B*. Posteroanterior and lateral chest radiographs in a middle-aged male with myasthenia gravis. The radiographs appear normal. *C*. CT scan reveals a discrete mediastinal mass representing a thymoma.

ence of soft tissue mass in the chest wall. However, these criteria are most useful when the CT scan indicates that the chest wall is normal and less reliable when abnormalities are seen. The most sensitive finding (pleural thickening) is least specific for chest wall invasion; although rib destruction is much more specific, it also occurs far less often (Figs. 36-22 and 36-23).

The importance of detecting chest wall invasion in the evaluation of lung cancer is unclear. In the absence of mediastinal metastases, a 35 percent survival for 5 years can be anticipated after en bloc resection of peripheral lung cancer and the adjacent chest wall. Therefore, in clinics that do not regard invasion of the chest wall by a peripheral tumor as a contraindication to surgery, the use of CT in preoperative detection may not be of much clinical significance, except to demonstrate mediastinal lymphadenopathy.

Currently under investigation is the reliability of CT in detecting metastases to mediastinal nodes and how CT compares with mediastinoscopy and mediastinotomy. One inherent difficulty posed for CT in this regard is that even though lymph nodes containing tumor are apt to be larger than normal, there is no absolute size beyond which

a lymph node must contain tumor; conversely microscopic metastases occur in lymph nodes that are normal in size (Fig. 36-24). Another inherent problem in CT imaging of lymphadenopathy is that some lymph nodes are vertically disposed and the technique does not provide reliable estimates of longitudinal dimension. The sensitivity and specificity of CT with respect to evaluating enlarged mediastinal nodes possibly due to metastatic disease depends on the criteria used for abnormal size and the method of lymph node sampling. To date, the criteria are not standardized. Moreover, enlarged mediastinal lymph nodes are common in normal individuals, and their size depends on their location in the mediastinum, i.e., they are larger in the precarinal, subcarinal, and aortopulmonary window areas than in the pretracheal and left innominate vein areas. Thus, choice of an arbitrary size as a criterion for judging whether mediastinal lymph nodes are enlarged with tumor obviously tinges the results with uncertainty.

The usefulness of CT in mediastinal nodal staging depends on the surgical criteria for operability in carcinoma of the lung. In clinics that accept mediastinal metastases as a contraindication to pulmonary resection, it is

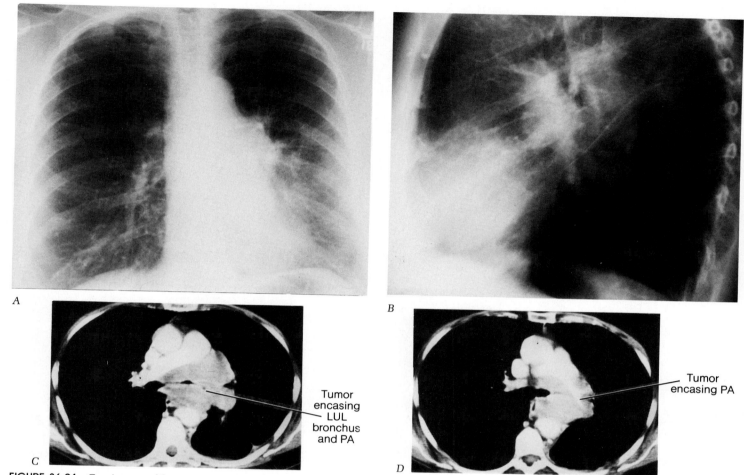

FIGURE 36-21 Carcinoma of lung. *A* and *B.* Posteroanterior and lateral chest radiographs showing a central mass in the left lung in the region of the left hilus and pulmonary artery. *C* and *D.* CT scans at different levels showing the extent of tumor mass directly invading the mediastinum with compression and severe narrowing of the left pulmonary artery and left main-stem bronchus. The mass is distinct from vascular structures which are enhanced by intravenous contrast. LUL = left upper lobe.

important to recall that lymph node size varies with location in the mediastinum, that enlarged lymph nodes need not harbor metastases, and that normal-sized lymph nodes may have metastases. Therefore, in the search for metastatic lymph nodes in the mediastinum, the advantage of CT over the chest radiograph is the ability to identify the precise mediastinal location of enlarged lymph nodes that should be evaluated for the presence of metastases at the time of surgical resection. Oppositely, a normal mediastinum on CT should, in principle, obviate the need for surgical staging, mediastinoscopy, or mediastinotomy. However, in practice, up to 10 percent of patients in whom the mediastinum appears normal on CT can be expected to provide histologic evidence of metastatic tumor in lymph nodes removed at thoracotomy.

To summarize, enlarged lymph nodes identified by CT require histologic confirmation. Since enlarged reactive nodes, secondary to proximal bronchial obstruction, particularly with collapse or pneumonia, are common,

enlarged nodes cannot be assumed to contain tumor without histologic assessment. CT should serve as a guide for selecting the appropriate surgical staging procedure in order to sample enlarged lymph nodes; no patient should be denied surgery on the basis of nodal size alone.

The relationship between tumor histology and the diagnostic information provided by CT is not known. In patients with alveolar cell carcinoma, who manifest lobar consolidation involving only one lobe on the conventional radiograph, CT often reveals occult disease either in other lobes or contralaterally, thereby confirming that the process is diffuse and that the prognosis is poor. After pneumonectomy, detection of tumor recurrence using conventional radiography is often difficult, whereas CT can single out discrete masses in a setting of organizing pleural fluid and soft tissue reaction in the post-pneumonectomy space. Most tumor recurrences occur at the site of the bronchial stump, and many can be seen on CT.

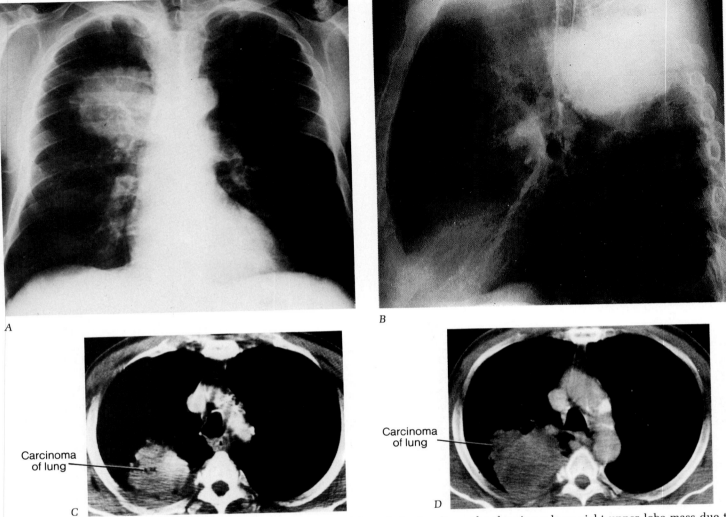

FIGURE 36-22 Carcinoma of lung.   A and B. Posteroanterior and lateral chest radiographs showing a large right upper lobe mass due to carcinoma.   C and D. CT scans at different levels showing that the mass is contiguous with the pleura and chest wall. At surgery there was no tumor invasion of the chest wall. Contiguity of a peripheral lung mass on CT with the pleura and chest wall does not necessarily indicate invasion and nonresectability.

Carcinoma of lung

Carcinoma of lung

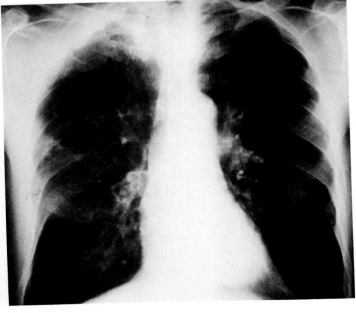

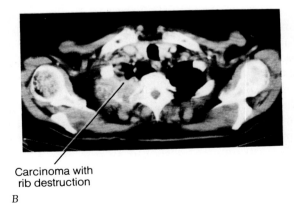

Carcinoma with rib destruction

FIGURE 36-23 Carcinoma of lung.   A. Peripheral mass in the right upper lobe due to squamous cell carcinoma.   B. CT scan demonstrates extension of the mass through the chest wall with rib destruction. Rib destruction is the most specific finding for chest wall invasion with CT.

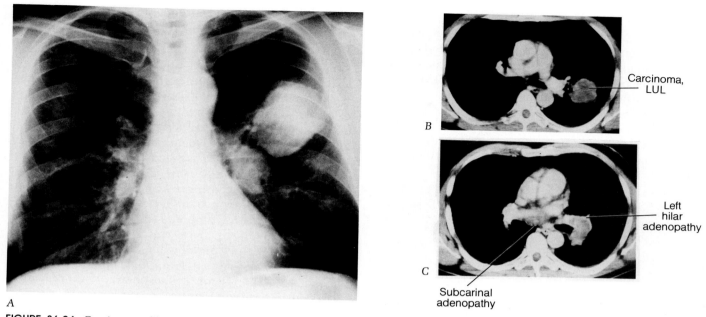

FIGURE 36-24 Carcinoma of lung. *A.* Posteroanterior chest radiograph showing left upper lobe carcinoma with left hilar adenopathy. *B.* CT scan showing left upper lobe mass separate from the left hilus. *C.* CT scan after contrasts showing nonenhancing areas in the left hilus and subcarinal regions that indicate hilar and mediastinal lymphadenopathy. Patient underwent a pneumonectomy. The hilar lymph nodes contained carcinoma. However, no carcinoma was found in the enlarged subcarinal nodes. Although in patients with carcinoma of the lung lymph node enlargement suggests metastases, not all enlarged lymph nodes contain metastatic carcinoma.

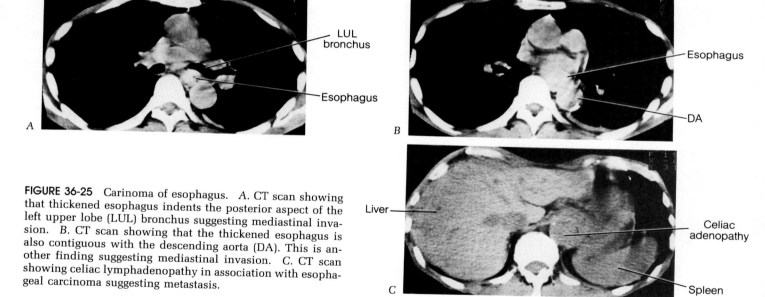

FIGURE 36-25 Carinoma of esophagus. *A.* CT scan showing that thickened esophagus indents the posterior aspect of the left upper lobe (LUL) bronchus suggesting mediastinal invasion. *B.* CT scan showing that the thickened esophagus is also contiguous with the descending aorta (DA). This is another finding suggesting mediastinal invasion. *C.* CT scan showing celiac lymphadenopathy in association with esophageal carcinoma suggesting metastasis.

ESOPHAGEAL CARCINOMA

Prompted by the fact that cancer of the esophagus is rarely diagnosed before it has invaded locally or spread to distant areas as metastases, CT has been advocated as a useful preoperative staging procedure. Its proponents suggest that if an esophageal mass displaces, or indents, the posterior wall of the trachea or bronchus, or envelops 50 percent of the circumference of the descending thoracic aorta, the tumor is locally invasive (Fig. 36-25). All agree that periesophageal lymph nodes, which are usually small and difficult to recognize or distinguish from the primary tumor, are difficult to use in staging. More useful is the detection of distant spread to celiac nodes, the liver, and the lung. Others have challenged the use of CT of the esophagus as a reliable guide to staging. They point out

547

that CT frequently overestimates the length of the esophageal tumor and is often falsely positive in identifying metastatic involvement of celiac lymph nodes. Nonetheless, CT does seem to offer the best nonsurgical estimate of the extent of esophageal carcinoma and of the details of anatomic relationships before surgical intervention.

After esophagectomy the mediastinal contour is widened in most patients because of the intrathoracic stomach. CT is helpful in detecting a postoperative mediastinal abscess or hematoma in these patients and in distinguish-

ing these lesions from the normal, postoperative, intrathoracic stomach (Fig. 36-26).

LYMPHOMA

CT has been helpful in planning treatment for lymphoma. It is more definitive than the chest radiograph in detecting areas and extent of nodal involvement. Using CT, it is possible to differentiate epicardial fat pads from pericardial effusion and pericardiac adenopathy. This is especially important in patients who have extensive mediastinal disease due to lymphoma because it enables the radiation therapist to exclude the heart from the radiation portal.

If the patient responds to therapy, serial CT examinations in patients with lymphoma may reveal a decrease in the extent of adenopathy. However, lymph nodes often do not regress completely, and the distinction between residual soft tissue masses due to lymphoma and fibrosis is not always possible by CT since fibrotic and lymphomatous lymph nodes may look identical on a CT scan. Nevertheless, the improved sensitivity of CT over conventional radiography in the delineation of lymph node size and location make CT the most useful modality in following the course of these patients.

MESOTHELIOMA

On CT, a malignant mesothelioma appears as a thick, pleural-based rind of soft tissue encasing the lung (Fig. 36-27). A variable quantity of fluid, usually loculated, is generally present. This fluid is usually less dense than the rind of soft tissue. Malignant mesothelioma spreads to involve the pericardium or contralateral lung or spreads directly into the mediastinum. It may also spread through the diaphragm to involve the abdominal and retroperitoneal viscera. CT is the most effective imaging modality available to identify the extent of involvement with malignant mesothelioma.

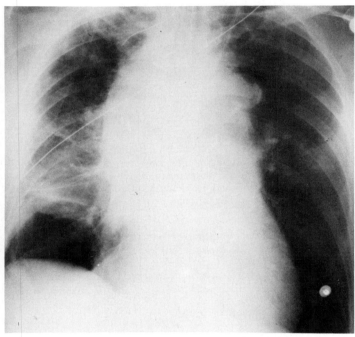

A

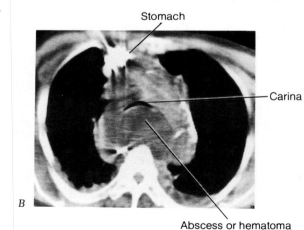

B

FIGURE 36-26 Postoperative mediastinal mass. *A.* Posteroanterior chest radiograph shows a widened mediastinal contour. This abnormal appearance is usually due to the intrathoracic location of the stomach after esophagectomy. *B.* CT scan shows contrast material taken by mouth in the anterior substernal stomach. A large soft tissue mass is present posteriorly compressing the airway. This mass represents a postoperative abscess/hematoma that could not be appreciated on the conventional radiographs.

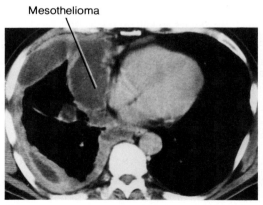

FIGURE 36-27 Malignant mesothelioma. A thick rind of low-density loculated pleural fluid encasing the right lung is typical of a malignant mesothelioma.

AORTIC DISSECTION

CT is useful in detecting aortic dissection in individuals who are hemodynamically stable. If the patient is hemodynamically unstable, or the risk of aortic dissection is high, it is advisable to resort directly to aortography rather than CT.

The CT findings of aortic dissection include a thickened aortic wall (greater than 1 cm), a septum between two opacifying lumens, differential time density between opacification of the two lumens, and compression of the true lumen. An aortic dissection is usually longer than a thoracic aneurysm. If the dissecting hematoma is acute, the false lumen usually appears denser than the true lumen; if it is chronic, the false lumen usually has a lower density. Occasionally only the true lumen enhances. In this instance, i.e., when the false lumen does not fill with contrast, it is difficult to distinguish aneurysm from dissection.

The reliable diagnosis of aortic dissection requires both the presence of an intimal flap and the filling of both the true and false lumens. Other findings that are more readily identified by CT than by aortography are hemothorax and hemopericardium.

CT also provides a noninvasive approach to following patients with chronic aortic dissection.

MISCELLANEOUS: TREATMENT AND DIAGNOSIS

The cross-sectional anatomy of the thorax visible on CT is useful in planning radiation therapy for thoracic malignancy. Indeed, many clinics have adopted CT as a routine guide to planning radiation therapy in patients with thoracic malignancy. CT-guided needle biopsy has also been tried but proved to be both cumbersome and time-consuming: the needle cannot be maneuvered under direct vision during the procedure, and the prolonged time for biopsy increases the risk of pneumothorax. However, CT is occasionally useful for biopsying a lesion that cannot be visualized on fluoroscopy, such as lesions at the lung apex or near the diaphragm. As indicated previously, CT has been successfully applied to the delineation of pleural plaques that may be due to asbestos and to the discrimination between pleural plaques and subpleural lipomatosis. In patients with tube thoracostomy for empyema, CT has helped in distinguishing between multiple pleural loculations and parenchymal consolidation, in determining if the tube has entered the lung or into a fissure, and in ensuring optimum position for drainage of a loculated empyema.

MAGNETIC RESONANCE

The revolution in diagnostic imaging resulting from the development of CT is rapidly being followed by the emergence of another highly technical modality which holds even greater potential for noninvasive diagnosis. Magnetic resonance (MR) offers fantastic possibilities for high-resolution anatomic imaging, analysis of tissue structure and metabolism by in vivo spectroscopy, and the noninvasive analysis of physiological processes such as blood flow. Owing to the abundance of hydrogen in biologic tissue, proton (^{1}H) imaging has had the widest clinical application. Unlike CT, MR can image the body directly in multiple planes, involves no ionizing radiation, and requires no intravenous contrast agents. The soft tissue contrast on MR is significantly greater than that of CT, and the spatial resolution is rapidly approaching that of fourth-generation CT scanners.

This portion of the chapter will review the basic principles of MR and discuss current clinical applications to disorders of the chest, emphasizing proton imaging. Although clinical experience with this modality is still in a very early stage, advantages and limitations of this technique and comparisons to CT will be reviewed.

Concepts and Techniques

The phenomenon of nuclear magnetic resonance (NMR) was discovered by Bloch and Purcell in 1946. NMR spectroscopy has been used since then in analytic chemistry, relying on powerful magnetic fields and small, homogeneous samples. In 1971, Damadian showed in vitro that NMR properties of benign and malignant tissues differed, suggesting exciting possibilities for the diagnosis of cancer. In 1973, Lauterbur's demonstration that magnetic field gradients could be used to encode spatial information in the NMR signal made it possible to obtain two-dimensional proton images of large, inhomogeneous objects.

MR is based on the fact that the nuclei of some elements that contain odd numbers of protons and/or neutrons (e.g., ^{1}H, ^{31}P, ^{13}C, and ^{23}Na) have magnetic moments produced by the spin of these charged subnuclear particles. Because of the magnetic moments, the nuclei behave like small bar magnets. When subjected to a strong, static magnetic field, these nuclei become polarized and align parallel to, or antiparallel to, the main magnetic field. Because of the different orientations of the nuclei, energy differentials develop that produce a net nuclear magnetization vector. The nuclei also wobble or "precess" around the axis of the main magnetic field. The frequency of this precession is directly related to the magnetic field strength, as expressed by the Larmor equation:

$$W\phi = \delta\, H\phi$$

where

$W\phi$ = the characteristic (Larmor) frequency
δ = the intrinsic characteristic property of the nucleus defined by its gyromagnetic ratio

Hϕ = the field strength of the magnet used to produce a homogeneous magnetic field and align the nuclei

The NMR signal is generated by exposure of the susceptible nuclei to a radio-frequency (rf) pulse. The nuclear spins absorb energy (resonate) when they are exposed to an rf pulse at the Larmor frequency. The rf pulse tips the net magnetization vector off its axis, the angle of displacement (e.g., 90°, 180°) being dependent on the duration of the rf pulse. Discontinuing the rf restores the stimulated nuclei to their equilibrium state, and rf energy at the same frequency is released. This emitted rf energy can be detected as small voltages induced in a nearby receiver coil which acts as an antenna.

It is because of the Larmor relationship that an MR image can be obtained from an inhomogeneous object such as the body. As indicated by the Larmor equation, the frequency of precession is dependent on the strength of the local magnetic field for a given nuclear species. If one varies the magnetic field strength as a function of distance by superimposing linear gradients on the main field, then the frequency of the spins will correlate directly with their position along the gradient. In this manner, appropriate rf's can be used to excite spins limited to a given plane or "slice" of the body. Likewise, spatial localization of the spins within each slice can be determined by the frequencies of the emitted signals. The resulting complex MR signal obtained after rf excitation is analyzed by means of a mathematical process known as 2-D Fourier transformation, performed by digital computers. The signal amplitude associated with each spatial location (defined by a unique frequency and phase) can be derived in this manner. The amplitude is then assigned according to a gray scale: the strongest signals usually appear white and the absence of signal as black.

After stimulation, a given nuclear species returns to its preexcitation state by two processes, each of which represents fluctuations in the local magnetic field surrounding the nuclei: (1) T1 (*spin-lattice relaxation* or *longitudinal relaxation*) is due to interaction between the nucleus and the molecules in its environs; and (2) T2 (*spin-spin relaxation* or *transverse relaxation*) is due to interaction between neighboring nuclei. T2 generally occurs more rapidly than T1.

The more free water in a tissue, the longer the relaxation times. Conversely, the more tightly organized the tissue structure (the less free water), the shorter the relaxation times. Because the state of water of various tissues varies more widely than their electron density or anatomic numbers, MR can achieve a greater degree of contrast between soft tissues than is possible with CT.

The signal intensity of MR images reflects several parameters, including the number of mobile protons (proton density), their T1 and T2 values, rate of motion (e.g., blood flow), and the chemical composition of the molecules containing the protons (largely lipid and water in human tissue). By varying the rf pulse sequences, images emphasizing each of these various contrast determinants can be obtained. In the commonly used *spin-echo* (SE) *sequence*, a 90° pulse is followed by a 180° pulse which results in a signal (spin echo). The time between the 90° pulse and the spin echo is the *echo time* (TE). This 90 to 180° sequence is then repeated. The interval between successive 90° pulses is the *repetition time* (TR). By varying the TR and TE, images emphasizing T1, T2, or proton density can be made. All the MR images illustrated below were made employing the SE sequence. The other commonly used pulse sequence, *inversion recovery*, consists of a 180° pulse followed by a 90° pulse. Inversion recovery images provide information about T1 and proton density.

The relationship of signal intensity to blood flow in large vessels is complex. In general, the more rapid the flow, the greater the loss of signal from blood. Modified pulse sequences have been developed that may permit measurement of blood flow.

MR IMAGER

The MR imager consists primarily of a large-bore magnet (50 to 100 cm), rf and gradient coils, a radio-frequency transmitter and receiver, and a computer. With the exception of the patient's couch, the system essentially has no mechanically moving parts. Scanners utilizing permanent, resistive, and cryogenic (superconducting) magnets are available. The permanent and resistive magnets are of low field strength, generally not exceeding 0.2 T (1 tesla equals 10,000 gauss; the earth's magnetic field is approximately 0.9 G). Resistive systems, although less expensive than superconducting units, have the disadvantages of unstable magnetic fields, lower signal-to-noise ratio, heat generation, and prolonged image acquisition times. The cryogenic magnets (up to 2.0 T) are more costly to install and operate, but have more homogeneous magnetic fields and significantly greater signal-to-noise ratios.

Current high field systems can obtain slices that are 3 to 5 mm thick. Greater resolution, i.e., to 0.5 by 0.5 mm, is possible by using a small field of view in combination with surface coils, i.e., small receiver coils placed directly on the patient. The average total examination time, which depends on the number of planes and number of pulse sequences used, is approximately 1 h. The current cost of an MR examination is nearly twice that of a contrast-enhanced CT scan.

The chest is routinely examined in the axial plane, using both T1- and T2-weighted pulsing sequences; coronal and sagittal scans can also be used for the lung apex or diaphragm, or to clarify craniocaudal relationships. Additional options, e.g., imaging in any desired plane, are being developed.

RESPIRATORY AND CARDIAC MOTION

Motion, both respiratory and cardiac, represents the major problem in MR imaging of the chest. This motion blurs the image and produces artifacts. Several approaches have been taken to try to minimize the influences of respiratory motion on the image. The principal approach has been that of respiratory gating, in which only signals obtained during the expiratory phase of the respiratory cycle are used. For example, nonferromagnetic devices have been used to monitor chest wall motion and provide a signal to trigger the rf excitation pulses only during the appropriate phase of respiration. Alternatively, the rf pulses can be allowed to proceed without interruption, but only the signals acquired during expiration are used to create the image. These approaches have reduced respiratory artifacts, but have approximately doubled the scan time, thereby seriously limiting the number of patients that can be tested. Alternative software modifications to circumvent this problem are currently under development.

The approach to cardiac motion is more straightforward. The electrocardiogram (ECG) is used to gate data acquisition to the cardiac cycle; the ECG signal is transmitted to the computer by means of a telemetry apparatus or fiberoptic systems. The rf pulses are then triggered by the R waves or delayed by any preset interval after the R wave, thereby obtaining images at different parts of the cardiac cycle. Cardiac gating serves not only to eliminate motion artifacts, but also to produce systolic and diastolic images. Cardiac gating does not appreciably prolong scanning time. For routine imaging of the mediastinum, hilus, or lung, cardiac gating may not be required. However, to image the heart and paracardiac masses properly, gating is generally mandatory.

HAZARDS

The only known hazards of MR imaging are the effect of strong magnetic fields on ferromagnetic material. Patients with cerebral aneurysm clips must be excluded from study, since the magnet may exert a considerable torque on these ferromagnetic clips. Since ferromagnetic objects in the vicinity of the magnet can be propelled like missiles, screening of personnel and patients to exclude such objects is strictly enforced. The reed switch of cardiac pacemakers may be activated, so that patients with such pacemakers as well as other implanted electronic devices cannot be examined. Likewise, it may not be possible to perform an MR study on patients requiring electronic monitoring equipment.

No harmful effects on human health have been demonstrated in experimental studies of static magnetic fields up to 2 T. RF pulses do cause tissue heating in the body. The amount of such heating depends on frequency (increasing with field strength), pulse sequences, number of images, body mass, etc. Although no harmful effects of this kind of heating have been reported, guidelines regarding rf power absorption are still being assessed. Another potential, but as yet clinically insignificant, hazard is the induction of current in the body by the rapidly changing field gradients.

Recent studies of long-term exposures of human lymphocytes and hamster ovary cells to MR conditions far in excess of those used in current clinical scanners have shown no evidence of cytogenetic damage in vitro. Although no adverse effects of MR imaging on pregnancy have been reported, and even though MR is an attractive alternative to imaging methods involving ionizing radiation, patients with normal pregnancies, particularly during the first trimester, are usually not examined.

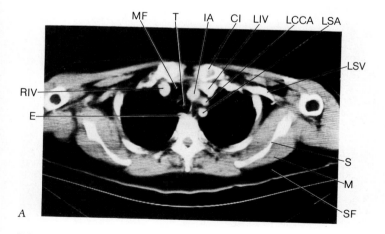

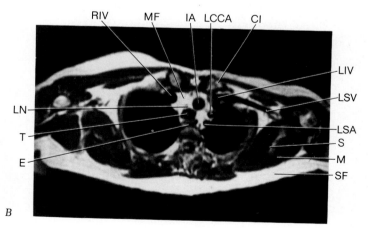

FIGURE 36-28 Normal chest. Axial sections at level above aortic arch. *A.* CT scan. Vessels are bright white following enhancement by intravenous contrast material. *B.* MR scan (T1-weighted; 1.5 T) at the same level. In contrast to CT, vessels appear black because of lack of signal from flowing blood. Fat in mediastinum and chest wall is bright white. Cortical bone is black, but there is relatively high signal from bone marrow due to fat.

Clinical Applications

MEDIASTINUM

The mediastinum is ideally suited for imaging by MR. The normal mediastinum is composed primarily of fat, vessels, airway, and a few small lymph nodes (Fig. 36-28).

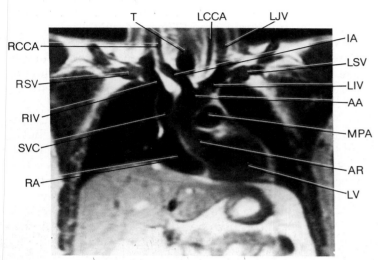

FIGURE 36-29   Normal cardiovascular anatomy. Coronal scan at level of aortic root. Absence of signal from flowing blood allows excellent depiction of great vessels and cardiac chambers.

Fat, having a relatively short T1 and long T2, has the highest signal intensity in the normal chest on both T1- and T2-weighted images. The tracheobronchial tree and most of the lung appear black, since air has little proton density. Since normally flowing blood generates little MR signal, mediastinal vessels appear relatively dark (Fig. 36-29). Most vessel walls can be imaged separately from the vascular lumens without the use of any intravenous contrast agents. Therefore, vascular anomalies (Fig. 36-30) and displacement or compression of vessels (Fig. 36-31) are easily demonstrated. Intravascular clot, tumor, or diminished flow can also be identified by increased signal intensity (Fig. 36-32). Aortic dissections can be demonstrated in a totally noninvasive fashion (Fig. 36-33).

Pathologic soft tissue masses have an intermediate T1 value, appearing gray on T1-weighted images, in great contrast to the white fat and dark bronchi and vessels. The contrast between masses and vessels is often better than with CT (Fig. 36-34). These masses, in which the water content is high so that T2 is prolonged, have a high signal intensity (brighter than fat) on heavily T2-weighted scans (Fig. 36-35). Direct mediastinal extension of adjacent lung tumors is sometimes better seen by MR (Fig. 36-36). Unlike CT, the craniocaudal extent of lesions of the aorta and esophagus can be directly imaged by MR using sagittal and coronal planes (Fig. 36-37). However, preliminary studies have shown that MR, like CT, has low accuracy in

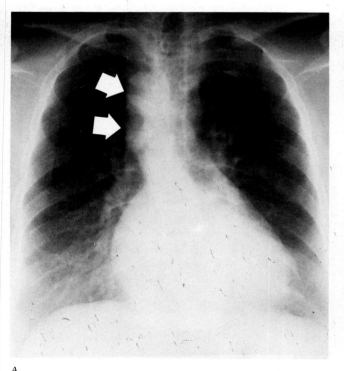

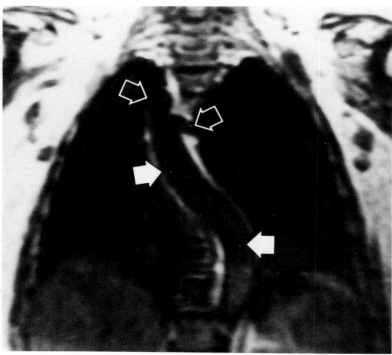

A   *B*

FIGURE 36-30   Congenital anomaly of the aorta.   *A.* PA radiograph shows paratracheal widening due to right aortic arch (arrows).   *B.* Posterior coronal MR image displays anatomy of anomalous aorta (solid arrows) without the need for intravenous contrast material. Aorta descends from right to left. A double aortic arch (open arrows) can be seen.

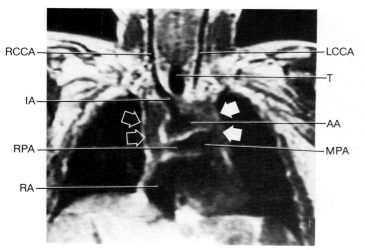

RCCA — LCCA
IA — T
RPA — AA
RA — MPA

FIGURE 36-31 Superior vena caval obstruction. Patient with Hodg-kin's disease presenting with superior vena caval obstruction. The normal superior vena cava (see Fig. 36-2) is not seen due to encasement by lymphoma (open arrows). Intermediate signal intensity mass due to adenopathy is also present in the left upper mediastinum (solid arrows). The areas of tumor are readily distinguished from vascular structure and high intensity fat.

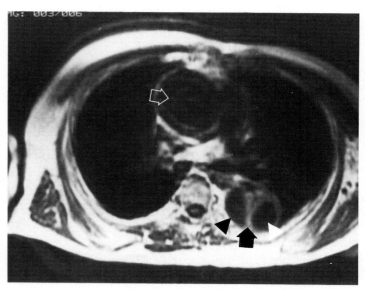

FIGURE 36-33 Aortic dissection. Axial MR image shows intimal flap (open arrow) in the descending thoracic aorta. Adjacent true and false lumens (arrowheads) are dark because of flowing blood. The ascending aorta (solid arrow) is markedly dilated, compressing the right pulmonary artery posteriorly.

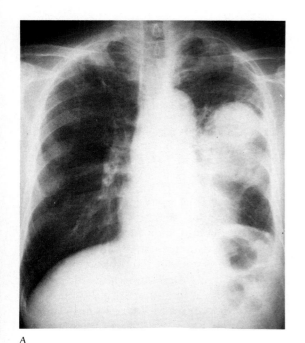

A

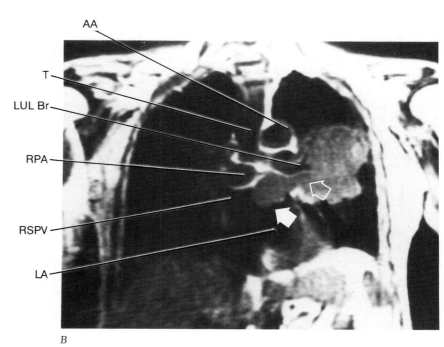

AA
T
LUL Br
RPA
RSPV
LA

B

FIGURE 36-32 Carcinoma of the lung. *A.* Posteroanterior radiograph shows large mass in the left mid-lung. *B.* MR scan demonstrates that mass extends through left superior pulmonary vein (open arrow) into superior aspect of the left atrium (closed arrow).

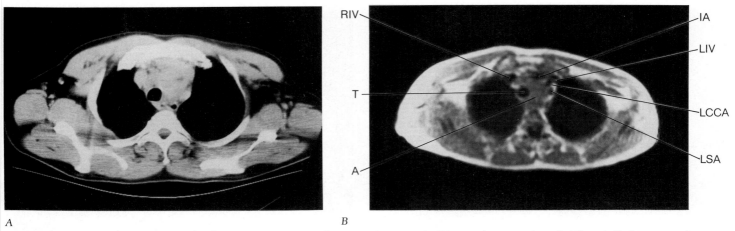

A

B

FIGURE 36-34 Mediastinal adenopathy due to metastatic anaplastic carcinoma. *A.* CT scan above aortic arch. There is little contrast between the adenopathy and normal vascular structures. *B.* MR scan (T1-weighted; 0.12 T) shows greater contrast between adenopathy (intermediate signal intensity = gray) (A), displaced mediastinal vessels (absent signal = black), and normal mediastinal fat (high signal = white).

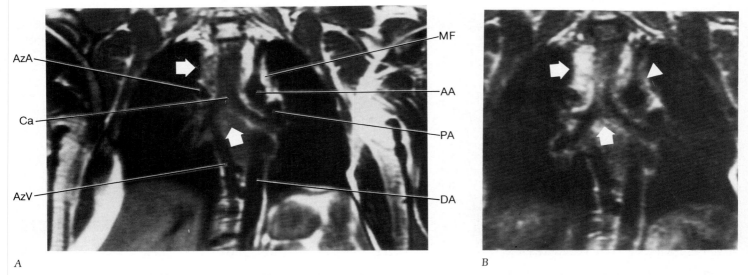

A

B

FIGURE 36-35 Mediastinal adenopathy due to Hodgkin's disease. *A.* Coronal MR image at level of tracheobronchial tree. Right paratracheal and subcarinal nodes (arrows) show intermediate signal intensity on this T1-weighted scan (TR 400 ms/TE 25 ms). *B.* The lymph nodes involved by lymphoma (arrows) show a relatively increased signal with T2-weighting (TR 2500 ms/TE 80 ms). (Fibrotic nodes should be expected to have a relatively shorter T2 and to remain low in signal intensity.) The signal from the mediastinal fat (arrowhead) is less intense than that of the T1-weighted image.

detecting esophageal tumor invasion through the muscle layer into periesophageal fat. Delineation of masses at the cervicothoracic junction, such as substernal thyroid, is excellent by MR (Fig. 36-38): soft tissue structures and vascular anatomy in this area are very well displayed. Unlike CT, MR images of this region do not require intravenous contrast and are not subject to streak artifacts from the shoulders.

The capability for detecting and quantifying adenopathy, particularly with respect to the staging of bronchogenic carcinoma, is similar to that of CT and relies on similar criteria of size. Subcarinal nodes are more easily

identified by MR owing to the marked contrast with the adjacent low-signal vascular structures. Unfortunately, metastatic adenopathy has not been found to have a distinctive appearance on MR images or to have specific T1 and T2 values. However, acute inflammatory nodes do have longer T1 and T2 relaxation times than do normal nodes or other types of lymphadenopathy. MR has also been able to differentiate fibrosis from tumor: on T2-weighted images fibrotic tissue, which has fewer mobile water protons than tumor, appears relatively dark (short T2) compared with tumor.

Disadvantages of MR as compared to CT in the medi-

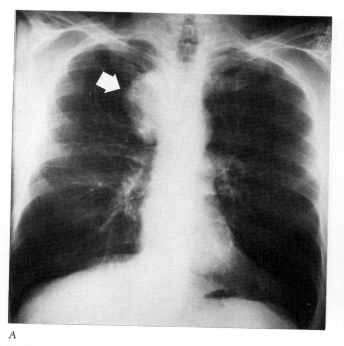

A

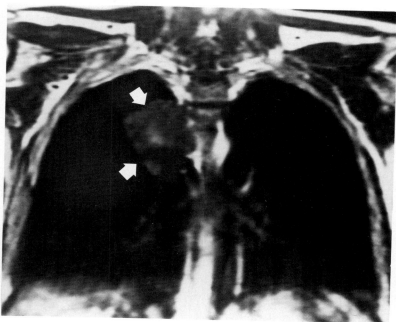

B

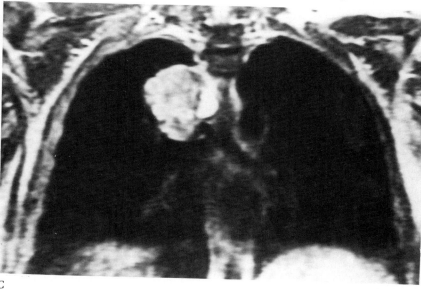

C

FIGURE 36-36 Carcinoma of the lung. *A.* Posteroanterior radiograph shows mass (arrow) abutting on right upper mediastinum. *B.* Coronal MR scan with T1-weighting (TR 400 ms/TE 25 ms) shows mass of intermediate intensity (arrows) invading the high signal mediastinal fat. *C.* With T2-weighting (TR 2500 ms/TE 80 ms) the tumor shows increased signal due to relatively long T2. The contrast between the tumor and normal mediastinal fat has decreased.

astinum include the lack of an intraluminal contrast agent for the esophagus and the difficulty in recognizing calcification. Macroscopic calcifications, like cortical bone, contain virtually no mobile proteins and, therefore, appear dark on both T1- and T2-weighted images.

Overall, diagnostic information obtained by MR in the mediastinum has been comparable to CT, despite the superior spatial resolution of the latter. MR is particularly useful for evaluating the mediastinum when the CT scan is nondiagnostic because of inadequate contrast enhancement or the presence of streak artifacts. MR, unlike CT, is not subject to artifacts from surgical clips (Fig. 36-39). MR

is an excellent alternative to CT in patients who are allergic to intravenous contrast agents.

HEART

Because flowing blood generates little signal, the blood within the cardiac chambers, in contrast to the cardiac structures, appears black (Fig. 36-29). Soft tissue contrast allows delineation of myocardium, pericardium, and the high-intensity pericardial fat (Fig. 36-40). The atrial and ventricular septa are usually well demonstrated. Sagittal images are advantageous in displaying the origins of the

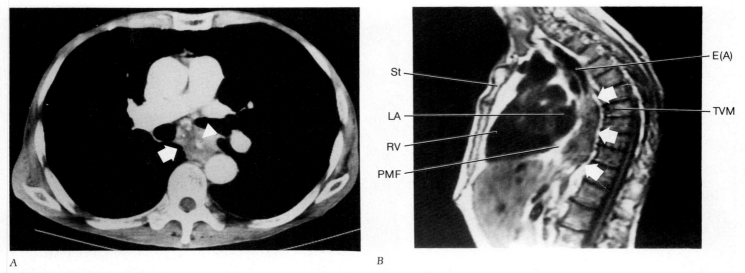

A   B

FIGURE 36-37 Carcinoma of the esophagus. *A.* CT scan at level of right pulmonary artery shows marked thickening of the esophageal wall (arrow) surrounding the narrowed contrast-filled lumen (arrowhead). *B.* Sagittal MR image shows cephalocaudal extent of the esophageal mass (arrows).

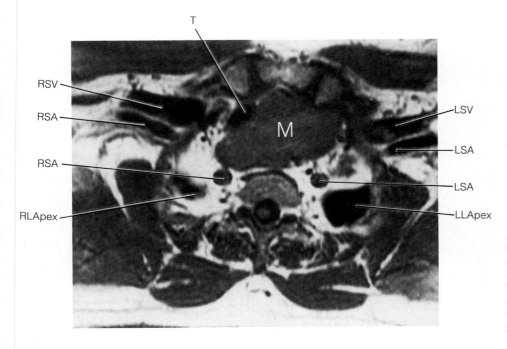

FIGURE 36-38 Substernal goiter. T1-weighted surface coil MR image (1.5 T) of superior mediastinum at level of sternoclavicular junction. Large mass (M) due to substernal extension of goiter. Displaced trachea (T) and adjacent vascular structures are displayed in great detail.

great vessels. Coronal imaging is useful in delineating the cardiac apex. Myocardial wall thickness and chamber size can be accurately measured. The extent of wall thickening in hypertrophic cardiomyopathy is more clearly delineated than with 2-D echocardiography. Areas of old infarction appear as regions of wall thinning or aneurysm (Fig. 36-40). Mural thrombus can be identified. Areas of acute myocardial infarction show regions of decreased intensity on T1-weighted images and increased intensity on T2-weighted scans, compatible with edema in the area

of infarction. The morphology of a large variety of congenital heart lesions has been identified, including ventricular septal defects (Fig. 36-41), transposition of the great vessels, coarctation, etc. MR has been quite useful in demonstrating pericardial abnormalities, including effusions and thickening. The extent of these pericardial abnormalities is better shown by MR than echocardiography. Chamber enlargement in congestive cardiomyopathy and valvular heart disease is easily demonstrated. The extent of intracardiac and paracardiac masses is well shown (Fig.

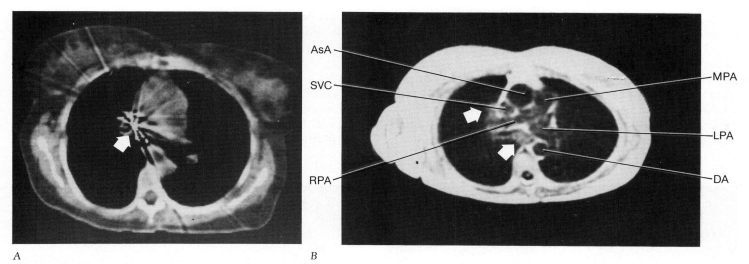

FIGURE 36-39 Advantages of MR in imaging the mediastinum. *A.* CT scan of mediastinum is degraded by streak artifacts from surgical clips (arrow). There is also poor contrast enhancement of the mediastinal vessels. *B.* MR scan (0.12 T) at same level. Absence of clip artifacts and improved visualization of vessels allow identification of intermediate signal tumor in the right hilus and subcarinal regions (arrows).

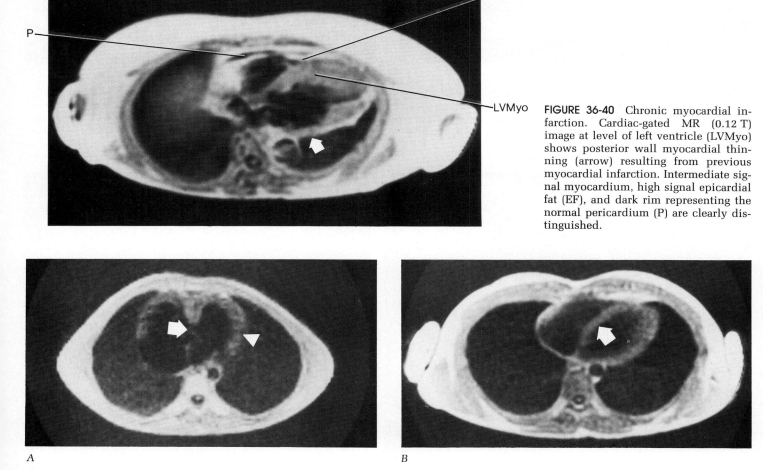

FIGURE 36-40 Chronic myocardial infarction. Cardiac-gated MR (0.12 T) image at level of left ventricle (LVMyo) shows posterior wall myocardial thinning (arrow) resulting from previous myocardial infarction. Intermediate signal myocardium, high signal epicardial fat (EF), and dark rim representing the normal pericardium (P) are clearly distinguished.

FIGURE 36-41 Ventricular septal defect. *A.* Large defect in interventricular septum (arrow). This patient also has corrected transposition resulting in myocardial hypertrophy (arrowhead) in transposed systemic right ventricle. *B.* Intact ventricular septum (arrow) in normal heart (0.12 T, nongated).

36-32), and MR is superior to echocardiography and contrast-enhanced CT in this regard.

To date, MR has been inferior to echocardiography for depicting cardiac valves and for evaluating ventricular function, since MR does not have the advantage of real-time imaging. However, methods for evaluation of myocardial function from images obtained at specified intervals throughout the cardiac cycle are currently being developed. Unlike radionuclide studies, MR does not

display blood flow in tissues, although the latter may become possible with the development of myocardial-specific paramagnetic contrast agents.

In vivo phosphorus spectroscopy of the heart has been achieved using surface receiver coils in small animals and very recently in humans. Such spectra permit noninvasive measurements of ATP and its metabolites and can be used to monitor myocardial ischemia. This technique has been shown in animal experiments to accu-

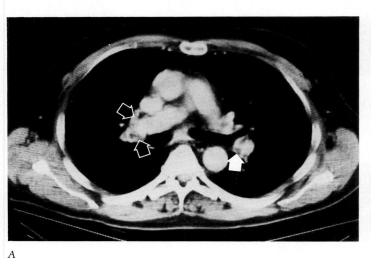

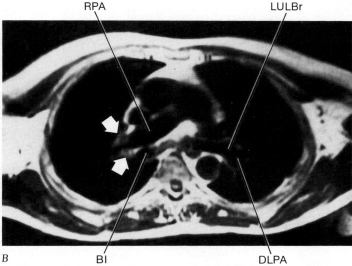

FIGURE 36-42   Unilateral hilar adenopathy in lymphoma.   *A.* Dynamic contrast-enhanced CT scan at level of hili shows probable adenopathy on the patient's right manifested by nonenhancing soft tissue (open arrows) and questionable abnormality in the left hilus (closed arrow). *B.* MR scan (1.5 T) at same level shows abnormal signal consistent with adenopathy (arrows) surrounding right pulmonary artery. In contrast, there is little signal seen in the normal left hilus, consisting of the signal-free descending pulmonary artery and left upper lobe bronchus.

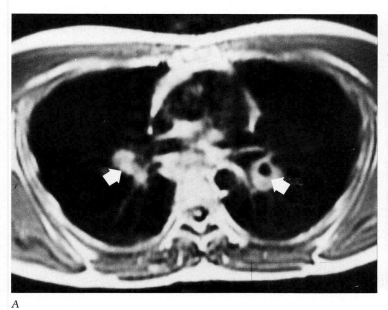

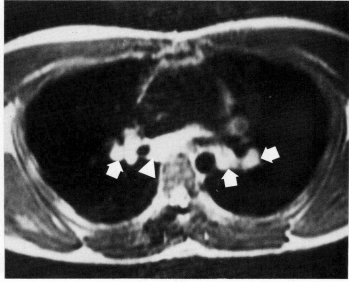

FIGURE 36-43   Bilateral hilar adenopathy due to lymphoma.   *A.* T1-weighted MR image (TR 600 ms/TE 25 ms; 1.5 T) shows soft tissue masses (arrows) in both hili. *B.* T2-weighted image (TR 2500 ms/TE 80 ms) at the same level shows bright signal from bilateral hilar adenopathy (arrows) as well as from subcarinal lymphadenopathy (arrowhead). The relatively long T2 of these tumor-bearing nodes makes them stand out from the normal mediastinum with a high degree of contrast.

rately detect early myocardial toxicity to doxorubicin hydrochloride (Adriamycin). The possibility of combining cardiac imaging with in vivo phosphorus spectroscopy, feasible at field strengths of 1.5 T or greater, offers the exciting potential to directly monitor the extent and severity of myocardial ischemia.

PULMONARY HILI

MR is an excellent technique for distinguishing the normal pulmonary hilus from that involved by tumor or lymphadenopathy. The normal hilus yields very little signal, since it comprises vessels and bronchi which have virtually no signal, along with a small amount of normal fat (Fig. 36-42). Hilar masses, therefore, are readily identified by their increased signal (Fig. 36-43). MR is comparable or superior to CT in identifying hilar masses; it does not require the carefully timed bolus of intravenous contrast which is often used for proper hilar evaluation by CT. The greater spatial resolution of CT, on the other hand, provides a more accurate display of endobronchial abnormalities. As in the mediastinum, although its sensitivity for detecting hilar lymph nodes is high, MR has not yet increased the capability for distinguishing between benign and malignant nodes.

PULMONARY VESSELS

The central pulmonary arteries and veins can be imaged directly by MR. The low-signal vascular lumens can be distinguished from the higher-signal wall. Therefore, vascular caliber and wall thickness can be determined. Involvement of proximal pulmonary arteries and veins by tumor or fibrosing mediastinitis can be assessed. Intraluminal masses, such as thrombi, emboli, or tumor, appear as areas of higher signal intensity within the lumen (Fig. 36-32). In addition, since signal intensity increases inversely in relation to velocity, diminished or absent flow in pulmonary arteries associated with emboli will also appear as increased signal. Cardiac gating may permit

the distinction between signal related to flow and that from clot, since flow-related signal may change in various portions of the cardiac cycle. Differentiation between clot and slow flow can also be obtained using a multiple spin-echo pulse sequence: thrombus shows diminishing intensity on successive spin echoes, whereas, in a multiecho sequence, flow-related signal increases with every other echo (the even-numbered echoes); the latter phenomenon is referred to as *even-echo rephasing*. Pulmonary emboli can be identified by MR. However, as yet, the application of MR to the diagnosis of pulmonary embolism remains investigational. Since it is possible to measure linear velocity and vessel diameter with MR, this modality has potential for measuring flow within the pulmonary vessels and for the noninvasive assessment of pulmonary arterial hypertension (Fig. 36-44).

PULMONARY PARENCHYMA

Except for the walls of central pulmonary vessels and bronchi, the low proton density of normal air-containing lung generates little MR signal. Any process which serves to replace the air (tumor, atelectasis, exudate, edema, etc.) will correspondingly increase the signal by increasing proton density. But, it is the T1 and T2 values of such processes that hold promise in allowing more specific characterization of these pathologic processes.

Although the spatial resolution of conventional radiography and CT is superior to that of MR, density measurements by these two radiographic methods cannot provide the same characterization as MR. For example, a direct relationship has been shown between extravascular lung water and T1 and T2 relaxation times in rats with alloxan-induced acute pulmonary edema. In atelectasis with superimposed bacterial pneumonia or superimposed chemical pneumonitis, T2 in rabbits is prolonged as compared to uncomplicated atelectasis. Also, in human studies, MR has been able to differentiate central tumor from associated distal obstructive atelectasis in 40 to 50 percent

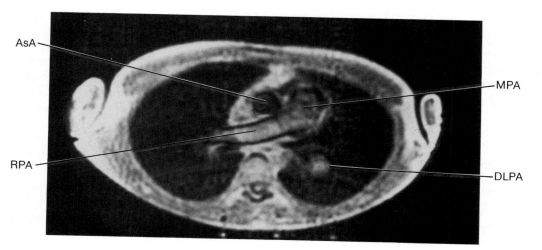

FIGURE 36-44 Pulmonary arterial hypertension. Increased intraluminal signal in dilated pulmonary arteries in a patient with severe primary pulmonary arterial hypertension. The increased vascular signal is felt to result from diminished velocity of blood flow.

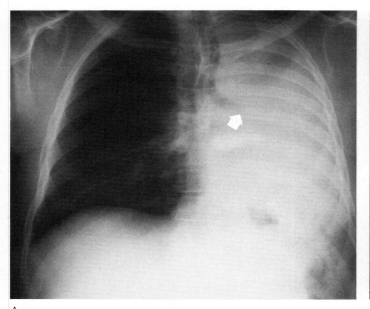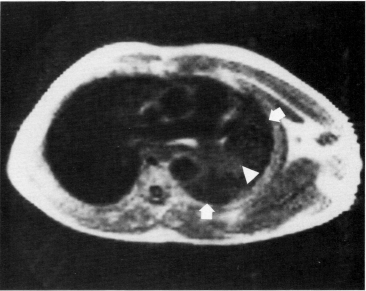

A   B

FIGURE 36-45   Atelectasis due to central obstructing carcinoma.   *A.* Posteroanterior radiograph shows complete opacification of the left hemithorax. Ipsilateral shift of the mediastinum and abrupt cutoff of left main-stem bronchus (arrow) indicate central obstruction although the size of the mass cannot be determined.   *B.* T1-weighted axial MR image (0.12 T) shows relatively little signal from left lung (arrows) due to the long T1 resulting from increased water content in the chronically obstructed lung. In contrast, the central tumor mass (arrowhead) can be identified by its higher signal.

of cases (Fig. 36-45): the peripheral obstructed lung shows a prolonged T1 and T2 relative to the tumor; this prolongation of relaxation times is probably due to edema and/or inflammatory exudate in the obstructed lung. Although this distinction between tumor and atelectasis can sometimes be made by CT after intravenous contrast enhancement, often it is not possible. In bleomycin-induced fibrosis in rats, T2 is relatively normal in the alveolitis phase, but significantly reduced with fibrosis. Although pulmonary hemorrhage has not been investigated, studies of hemorrhage and hematoma in the brain and elsewhere in the body by MR have shown a striking increase in signal from blood over time, probably related to conversion of hemoglobin to methemoglobin; the latter, being paramagnetic, causes a marked shortening of T1 relaxation. Therefore, pulmonary processes characterized by hemorrhage may be recognized by this T1 shortening.

It should be pointed out that accurate determination of T1 and T2 values is not a trivial matter. These determinations for the lung are further complicated by respiratory variation in lung volume and the effects of pulmonary blood flow. Moreover, although tissue characterization may be useful in differential diagnosis, it seems unlikely that the T1 and T2 values will be specific. Further pathophysiological information may be obtained by paramagnetic contrast materials which are selectively distributed in the vascular system or extracellular fluid. Such agents will likely become available in the near future.

Because of the relatively low signal-to-noise ratio in the lung, poorer spatial resolution, greater partial volume averaging, and motion blurring, the detection of pulmonary nodules is inferior to that of CT. The signal from such nodules can be maximized using a long TR/short TE (proton density) pulsing sequence. On the other hand, the distinction between a peripheral pulmonary nodule and a pulmonary vessel, which can be difficult using CT, is usually easily made with MR, since patent peripheral vessels generate little signal. The greater soft tissue contrast of MR enables necrosis within masses to be more easily identified than by CT. As indicated previously, difficulty in identifying calcification by MR is a significant limitation in the evaluation of pulmonary nodules.

PLEURA

Pure water has a very long T1 and T2 (on the order of 2 s). Because of this long T1, the TR must be sufficiently long to yield adequate signal from fluid, which would otherwise be invisible adjacent to the black air-containing lung. Increasing protein concentration is associated with shortening of relaxation times. Therefore, it would be theoretically possible to determine the protein concentration of a pleural effusion using MR imaging. Transudates would be expected to be relatively dark on T1-weighted images, compared to brighter exudative effusions (Fig. 36-46). However, calculations of this type are not straightforward

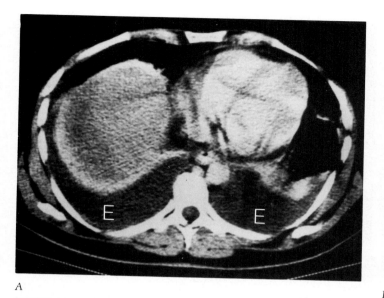
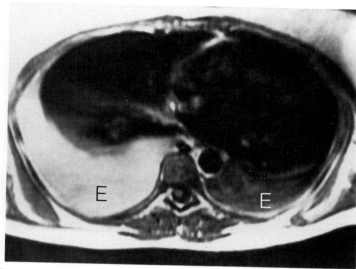

A

B

FIGURE 36-46 Hemorrhagic right pleural effusion. *A.* CT scan shows bilateral pleural effusions (E). There is very minimal increase in density of the fluid on the right compared with that on the left. *B.* T1-weighted (TR 400 ms/TE 25 ms) MR scan shows higher intensity (shorter T1) of the right effusion (white appearing) compared with the left effusion (gray-black appearing). The right effusion proved to be secondary to hemorrhage, the left a transudate related to ascites.

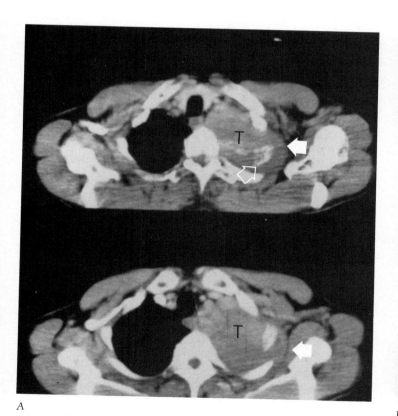
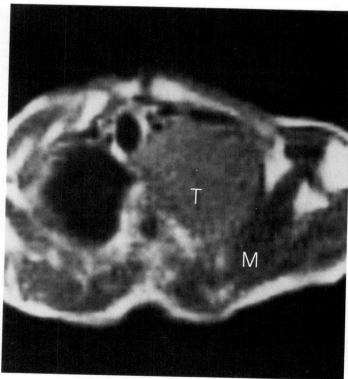

A

B

FIGURE 36-47 Carcinoma of the left apex with chest wall invasion. *A.* CT scans at the apices show tumor (T) with destruction of a rib (open arrow) and extension into adjacent chest wall fat (closed arrow). The mass has a density similar to the adjacent muscles. *B.* On MR scan (TR 286 ms/TE 20 ms; 0.12 T), the tumor (T) can be distinguished from adjacent muscle (M) by the higher signal intensity of the mass. The rib destruction evident on CT, however, was not clearly identified.

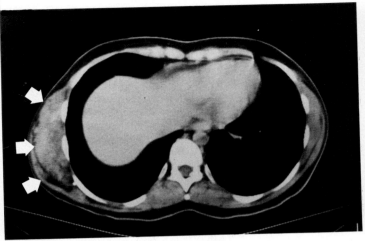

A

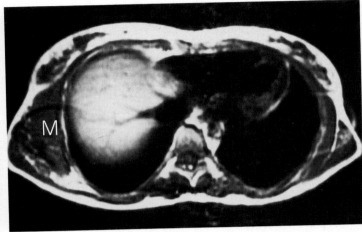

B

C

FIGURE 36-48 Hemangioma of the right chest wall. A. CT scan of lower chest shows soft tissue mass (arrows) in the right lateral chest wall. The density of the mass is similar to normal chest wall musculature. B. T1-weighted MR scan similarly shows mass (M) not separable from muscle. C. The mass (four open arrows) has markedly increased signal intensity relative to muscle on this T2-weighted (TR 2500 ms/TE 80 ms) image. The mass is seen to infiltrate the serratus anterior muscle. In contrast, the normal left serratus anterior muscle (two solid arrows) shows a relatively low signal.

since these exudates usually contain other constituents such as cells, hemoglobin, etc. Preliminary investigations have shown that some types of effusions may be distinguished by MR, a distinction which cannot be made by other imaging modalities. Loculated effusion can also be distinguished from thickened pleura by the longer T2 of fluid. Calcified pleural plaques are generally not detectable.

CHEST WALL

The exquisite soft tissue contrast of MR makes this a promising modality for evaluation of tumors involving the chest wall. Normal muscle groups are well displayed. The ribs, clavicles, and sternum show a very high intensity centrally from fat-containing marrow surrounded by a black rim representing cortical bone (Fig. 36-28). Although bone marrow involvement is more apparent on MR, CT is more useful in showing abnormalities in cortical bone (Fig. 36-47). Most tumors and inflammatory processes, having a significantly longer T2 than muscle,

stand out against the lower-intensity muscles of the chest wall (Fig. 36-48). This contrast is superior to CT. Coronal scans can also be used in showing the extent of chest wall abnormalities.

FUTURE PROSPECTS

Much of the clinical potential of MR is yet to be realized, and many significant advances are likely to take place in the near future since this technology is in a very rapid stage of development. Improvements in proton imaging will include faster scanning, higher resolution, and reduction in motion-induced artifacts. Tissue specificity, which to date has been somewhat disappointing, may improve with refinements in quantitative determinations of relaxation times as well as the use of more tissue-specific paramagnetic contrast agents. In vivo MR spectroscopy, currently in its infancy, promises to be a significant tool for noninvasive diagnosis and monitoring of therapy. Hydrogen, carbon, and phosphorus spectra have been obtained from a variety of intact human tissues including brain, liver, heart, and muscle. Considerable research being directed toward refinements in the spatial localization of these spectra will unify the imaging and tissue characterization capabilities of MR. The ability to obtain precisely localized phosphorus spectra, for example, would enable the monitoring of tissue pH, ischemia, and infarction. Imaging of nuclei other than hydrogen, e.g., sodium, has recently been shown to be feasible. Finally, MR offers the exciting potential for combining detailed imaging of vasculature with noninvasive quantitative determination of blood flow.

BIBLIOGRAPHY

Computed Tomography

Baron RL, Levitt RG, Sagel SS, Stanley RJ: Computed tomography in the evaluation of mediastinal widening. Radiology 138:107–113, 1981.
  CT correctly identified normal variants, soft tissue density masses, or vascular abnormalities as the cause of mediastinal widening in 92 percent of 71 patients.

Daly BD Jr, Faling LJ, Pugatch RD, Jung-Legg Y, Gale ME, Bite G, Snider GL: Computed tomography. An effective technique for mediastinal staging in lung cancer. J Thorac Cardiovasc Surg 88:486–494, 1984.
  The authors advocate CT for all patients with lung cancer in whom operation is contemplated. They believe CT directs the most appropriate surgical staging procedure for patients with positive findings and obviates invasive staging for patients with negative findings.

Fiastro JF, Newell JD: Quantitative computed tomography evaluation of benign solitary pulmonary nodules. J Comput Tomogr 11:103–106, 1987.
  The computed tomography chest phantom proved useful in identifying benign nodules in patients living in an area endemic for C. immitis pulmonary infections.

Genereux GP, Howie JL: Normal mediastinal lymph node size and number: CT and anatomic study. AJR 142:1095–1100, 1984.
  A study correlating mediastinal lymph nodes on CT with autopsy findings in normal patients. They assess lymph node frequency and size by location in the mediastinum.

Glazer HS, Aronberg DJ, Sagel SS: Pitfalls in CT recognition of mediastinal lymphadenopathy. AJR 144:267–274, 1985.
  Pictorial review of normal variants and artifacts that may be confused with mediastinal lymphadenopathy.

Heiberg E, Wolverson M, Sundaram M, Connors J, Susman N: CT findings in aortic dissection. AJR 136:13–17, 1981.
  CT findings in 11 patients with aortic dissection were correlated with aortographic, surgical, and postmortem findings. CT is a reliable noninvasive method for the diagnosis of aortic dissection.

Libshitz HI, McKenna RJ Jr, Haynie TP, McMurtrey MJ, Mountain CT: Mediastinal evaluation of lung cancer. Radiology 151:295–299, 1984.
  Provocative study on the utility of CT in the preoperative assessment of mediastinal lymph nodes in lung cancer using size as the basis for predicting metastases. They found a predictive value for tumor of only 35 percent if lymph nodes larger than 1 cm were considered abnormal. CT is not useful with T1N0 lesions, and its value in peripheral T2 and central cancers is questionable.

Moore AV, Korobkin MK, Olanow W, Heaston DK, Ram PC, Dunnick NR, Silverman PM: Age-related changes in the thymus gland: CT-pathologic correlation. AJR 141:241–246, 1983.
  Surgical correlation of the thymus gland in 64 patients. Thymoma could easily be distinguished from normal thymus if age-related fatty infiltration is appreciated.

Moss AA, Schnyder P, Thoeni RF, Margulis AR: Esophageal carcinoma: Pretherapy staging by computed tomography. AJR 136:1051–1056, 1981.
  Esophageal carcinoma was studied in 52 patients. CT correlated closely with surgical findings. Local extension, regional adenopathy, and tumor size were better evaluated by CT than by other methods.

Naidich DP, Zerhouni EA, Siegelman SS: Computed Tomography of the Thorax. New York, Raven Press, 1984.
  Comprehensive textbook on CT of the thorax which is extensively referenced and up to date.

Pennes DR, Glazer GM, Wimbish KJ, Gross BH, Long RW, Orringer MB: Chest wall invasion by lung cancer: Limitations of CT evaluation. AJR 144:507–511, 1985.
> *Study of 33 patients with peripheral lung cancer contiguous with a pleural surface. CT scanning had a low accuracy in assessing invasion of the chest wall.*

Pugatch RD, Faling LJ, Robbins AH, Spina R: CT diagnosis of benign mediastinal abnormalities. AJR 134:685–694, 1980.
> *CT was performed on 49 patients to evaluate a suspected mediastinal mass. Specific diagnoses were established in 14 cases including mediastinal lipomatosis, cysts, and anomalies or aneurysms of vessels. CT should be the initial procedure for evaluating most mediastinal abnormalities. If the patient is asymptomatic, and CT indicates a benign process, conservative management with careful follow-up is justified.*

Quint LE, Glazer GM, Orringer MB, Gross BH: Esophageal carcinoma: CT findings. Radiology 155:171–175, 1985.
> *Preoperative CT scans of 33 patients with esophageal cancer revealed poor correlations with surgical pathology. CT was not useful in assessing resectability.*

Schaner EG, Chang AE, Doppman JL, Conkle DM, Flye MW, Rosenberg SA: Comparison of computed and conventional whole lung tomography in detecting pulmonary nodules: Prospective radiologic-pathologic study. AJR 131:51–54, 1978.
> *In 25 patients with malignant tumors, the authors found that CT detected more nodules than conventional tomograms, particularly subpleural nodules. However, 60 percent of additional nodules detected by CT proved to be benign at thoracotomy.*

Silverman PM, Harell GS, Korobkin M: Computed tomography of the abnormal pericardium. AJR 140:1125–1129, 1983.
> *CT in 18 patients with pericardial disease detected effusions, thickening, calcifications, and cystic and solid masses. CT and echocardiography are complementary.*

Williford ME, Hidalgo H, Putman CE, Korobkin M, Ram PC: Computed tomography of pleural disease. AJR 140:909–914, 1983.
> *CT scans in 65 cases were studied to determine characteristics of pleural involvement. The CT feature most helpful in detecting pleural involvement was the angle formed by the interface of the lesion with the adjacent pleura.*

Zerhouni EA, Boukadoum M, Siddiky MA, Newbold JM, Stone DC, Shirey MP, Spivey J, Hesselman CW, Leo FP, Stitik FP, Siegelman SS: A standard phantom for quantitative CT analysis of pulmonary nodules. Radiology 149:767–773, 1983.
> *A promising new technique that may permit distinction between benign and malignant lung nodules using a commercially available phantom for comparison.*

Magnetic Resonance

Axel L: Blood flow effects in magnetic resonance imaging. AJR 143:1157–1166, 1984.
> *Review of the effects of blood flow on MR and of approaches to measurement of flow using MR.*

Bailes DR, Gilderdale DJ, Bydder GM, Collins AG, Firmin DN: Respiratory ordered phase encoding (ROPE): A method for reducing respiratory motion artifacts in MR imaging. J Comput Assist Tomogr 9:835–837, 1985.
> *An example of new approaches to the problem of artifacts due to respiratory motion in MR imaging.*

Bradley WG, Newton TH, Crooks LE: Physical principles of nuclear magnetic resonance, in Newton TH, Potts DG (eds), *Advanced Imaging Techniques, vol 2, Modern Neuroradiology Series.* San Anselmo, Calif., Clavadel Press, 1983, pp 15–61.
> *Clear, well-illustrated review of the fundamental principles of MR imaging including basic physics, relaxation times, pulse sequences, and instrumentation.*

Budinger TF, Lauterbur PC: Nuclear magnetic resonance technology for medical studies. Science 226:288–298, 1984.
> *State-of-the-art review of the clinical applications of MR including imaging, in vivo spectroscopy, and safety considerations.*

Cohen AM: Magnetic resonance imaging of the thorax. Radiol Clin North Am 22:829–846, 1984.
> *Well-illustrated review of MR imaging of the chest including normal anatomy and a variety of pathologic conditions.*

Cohen MD, Scales RL, Eigen H, Scott P, Tepper R, Cory DA, Smith JA: Evaluation of pulmonary parenchymal disease by magnetic resonance imaging. Br J Radiol 60:223–230, 1987.

Thirty-eight patients with a wide variety of different disorders of the lung were imaged using magnetic resonance. Magnetic resonance imaging identified all lesions seen on chest radiographs, but was not quite as sensitive as computed tomography for detection of very small abnormalities.

Dooms GC, Hricak H, Moseley ME, Bottles K, Fisher M, Higgins CB: Characterization of lymphadenopathy by magnetic resonance relaxation times: Preliminary results. Radiology 155:691–697, 1985.

Analysis of T1 and T2 values of benign and malignant lymph nodes in 93 patients, including 23 patients with metastatic bronchogenic carcinoma.

Elliott DO: Magnetic resonance imaging fundamentals and system performance. Radiol Clin North Am 25:409–417, 1987.

The underlying physical principles of magnetic resonance (MR) imaging are discussed.

Epstein DM, Kressel H, Gefter W, Axel L, Thickman D, Aronchick J, Miller WT: MR imaging of the mediastinum: A retrospective comparison with computed tomography. J Comput Assist Tomogr 8:670–676, 1984.

Comparison of MR at 0.12 T and CT in 30 patients with a variety of mediastinal abnormalities.

Fisher MR, Higgins CB: Central thrombi in pulmonary arterial hypertension detected by MR imaging. Radiolog 158:223–226, 1986.

MR may play an important role in excluding large central thrombi as the cause of pulmonary arterial hypertension.

Gamsu G, Webb WR, Sheldon P, Kaufman L, Crooks LE, Birnberg FA, Goodman P, Hinchcliffe WA, Hedgecock M: Nuclear magnetic resonance imaging of the thorax. Radiology 147:473–480, 1983.

Early report of MR imaging of the chest including normal anatomy, nine patients with advanced bronchogenic carcinoma and three with benign abnormalities.

Glazer GM, Gross BH, Aisen AM, Quint LE, Francis IR, Orringer MB: Imaging of the pulmonary hilum: A prospective comparative study in patients with lung cancer. AJR 145:245–248, 1985.

Prospective comparison of MR imaging, dynamic CT, and 55° posterior oblique tomography in evaluation of the pulmonary hilus in 19 patients with lung cancer.

Glazer HS, Lee JKT, Levitt RG, Heiken JP, Ling D, Totty WG, Balfe DM, Emani B, Wasserman TH, Murphy WA: Radiation fibrosis: Differentiation from recurrent tumor by MR imaging. Work in progress. Radiology 156:721–726, 1985.

Early results showing the potential of MR in differentiating radiation fibrosis from recurrent tumor based on T2 differences in 21 treated and 15 untreated tumors.

Higgins CB, Byrd BF, McNamara MT, Lanzer P, Lipton MJ, Botvinick E, Schiller NB, Crooks LE, Kaufman L: Magnetic resonance imaging of the heart: A review of the experience in 172 subjects. Radiology 155:671–679, 1985.

Large series reviewing the application of gated MR imaging to evaluate abnormalities of the heart and great vessels, including eight patients with pulmonary hypertension.

Kundel HL, Kressel HY, Epstein D: The potential role of NMR imaging in thoracic disease. Radiol Clin North Am 21:801–808, 1983.

Review of tissue properties that contribute to the MR image and of the prospects for tissue characterization of pulmonary processes using MR.

Levitt RG, Glazer HS, Roper CL, Lee JKT, Murphy WA: Magnetic resonance imaging of mediastinal and hilar masses: Comparison with CT. AJR 145:9–14, 1985.

Comparison of MR and CT of the mediastinum and/or hili in 37 patients with bronchogenic carcinoma.

Ross JS, O'Donovan PB, Paushter DM: Tracheobronchial tree and pulmonary arteries: MR imaging using electronic axial rotation. Radiology 160:839–841, 1986.

By the use of electronic axial rotation (EAR), however, MR is capable of imaging any plane.

Steinberg EP, Sisk JE, Locke KE: X-ray CT and magnetic resonance images. N Engl J Med 313:859–864, 1985.

MR imagers have as yet diffused more slowly than CT scanners. Tendency is noted to install imagers in outpatient rather than in hospital settings. The public policies relating to the different patterns of diffusion are considered.

Schmidt HC, Tsay DG, Higgins CB: Pulmonary edema: an MR study of permeability and hydrostatic types in animals. Radiology 158:297–302, 1986.
Magnetic resonance imaging can be used to estimate severity of hydrostatic and permeability pulmonary edemas.

von Schulthess GK, Fisher MR, Higgins CB: Pathologic blood flow in pulmonary vascular disease as shown by gated magnetic resonance imaging. Ann Intern Med 103:317–323, 1985.
Axial, dual spin-echo MR images taken at the level of the pulmonary arteries and gated to the cardiac cycle were assessed in a patient with primary pulmonary arterial hypertension. A correlation between pulmonary vascular resistance and the MR signal is interpreted as suggesting a potential of MR images for providing physiological information about blood flow in the large pulmonary arteries and the severity of pulmonary arterial disease in pulmonary hypertension.

Webb WR, Gamsu G, Stark DD, Moore EH: Magnetic resonance imaging of the normal and abnormal pulmonary hila. Radiology 152:89–94, 1984.
Review of MR images of the hilus in 25 normal subjects and 12 patients with hilar masses.

Webb WR, Jensen BG, Sollitto R, deGeer G, McCowin M, Gamsu G, Moore E: Bronchogenic carcinoma: Staging with MR compared with staging with CT and surgery. Radiology 156:117–124, 1985.
Prospective comparison of MR and CT in staging lung cancer in 30 patients.

Wehrli FW, MacFall JR, Newton TH: Parameters in determining the appearance of NMR images, in Newton TH, Potts DG (eds), *Advanced Imaging Techniques, vol 2, Modern Neuroradiology Series.* San Anselmo, Calif., Clavadel Press, 1983, pp 81–117.
Excellent discussion of the effects of various imaging methods and pulse sequences on MR images.

Chapter 37

Disability Evaluation

Gary R. Epler

The number of patients seen by internists and pulmonary physicians for determination of disability continues to increase. This is due in part to legislation entitling individuals to compensation whether work-related or not; it also reflects the changing attitudes within society so that, now more than formerly, impaired individuals are claiming disability. As a result, clinicians trained to diagnose and treat disease are often being asked to quantitate functional impairment.

Impairment is a medical term defined as an anatomic or functional abnormality; it designates an objective, measurable loss of function. Impairment may be either temporary or permanent; impairment that persists after appropriate therapy, without reasonable prospect of improvement, is permanent. The degree of impairment varies in severity from *mild* to *moderate*, which precludes some types of labor, to *severe*, which precludes any type of gainful employment.

Disability is a general term defined as an inability to work because of physical or mental impairment; it implies an inability to perform expected roles or tasks. Disability is affected by such diverse factors as age, education, and economic and social environment. *Disability* is categorized as *partial*, if the degree of impairment is such to allow some types of labor, to *total*, if the impairment is so severe to preclude any type of gainful employment.

Adjudication of disability by judicial panels and compensation boards entails the consideration of medical factors, as well as the educational level, society's physical and attitudinal barriers, and the availability of suitable work. In this process, the chest physician is expected to assess (rate) the impairment arising from pulmonary disease.

Individuals requiring pulmonary disability evaluation are referred from several sources. They may be seen as a "patient" for a pulmonary consultation, and subsequently they become a "claimant" requesting a disability review. More often, they are referred from public agencies, insurance companies, or attorneys. Generally, there are three distinct, but interrelated issues: (1) pulmonary diagnosis; (2) whether the condition is work-related or not; and (3) the degree of impairment/disability (Table 37-1). For example, the degree of impairment is the key question for social security disability evaluation, and although the diagnosis is important in some instances, whether the pulmonary disorder arose in the workplace or was aggravated there is not. The method of evaluating disability consists of several elements: obtaining a clinical data base of pulmonary symptoms, gathering information about occupational and environmental exposure, performing the physical examination, categorizing the chest radiograph, and quantifying the pulmonary function tests.

ESTABLISHING THE CLINICAL DATA BASE

Evaluating the patient for disability begins in the traditional manner with the gathering of clinical information. A respiratory questionnaire is used to record the history systematically. Categorizing the degree of dyspnea is an important first step because it is often the principal manifestation of impairment. Dyspnea can be coded from 0 (none) to grade 4 (very severe) (Table 37-2).

However, the use of dyspnea as a sole, or paramount, criterion for the determination of pulmonary disability has serious limitations. As indicated elsewhere (Chapter 165), not only are the mechanisms of dyspnea poorly understood, but individual responses to equivalent impairments of pulmonary function vary greatly. A complaint of shortness of breath requires first an awareness of a sensation and then an interpretation of whether the sensation is inappropriate or abnormal. These two steps are influenced by factors unrelated to the extent of pulmonary dis-

TABLE 37-1

Questions from Referral Sources

1. What is the diagnosis?
2. What is the degree of impairment/disability?
3. Is the pulmonary condition related to the workplace?

TABLE 37-2
Categorizing the Degree of Dyspnea

Grade	Degree	Description
0	None	Not troubled with breathlessness except with strenuous exercise
1	Slight	Troubled by shortness of breath when hurrying on the level or walking up a slight hill
2	Moderate	Walks more slowly on the level than people the same age because of breathlessness
3	Severe	Stops for breath after walking about 100 yards after a few minutes on the level
4	Very severe	Breathless when dressing or undressing; too breathless to leave the house

ease, such as difficulty of verbal expression, questions of comprehension, or preoccupation with health. Some persons being evaluated for disability emphasize or exaggerate their shortness of breath. In some instances, socioeconomic factors and educational attainments are more closely related to the work status than severity of dyspnea.

Insofar as possible, other pulmonary symptoms, such as cough, sputum production, and wheezing, should also be characterized and quantified, e.g., frequency and duration of cough, when sputum is produced and how much, the occurrence of symptoms at a particular time of day or throughout the day, on what days of the week the symptoms occur, and the persistence of cough and sputum, e.g., for more than three consecutive months. The timing and duration of wheezing could be explored in the same way. Finally, it should be ascertained if the cough, sputum, or wheezing are disabling by limiting the person's capacity to function in daily work activities.

Information concerning Occupations and Hazardous Exposures

Information concerning occupations and hazardous exposures is helpful to adjudicators in assessing the environment of the workplace and to physicians in determining causation. Data collection begins from the date and place of birth; it proceeds through summer employment and military service to a chronologic list of jobs beginning with the first and ending with the present. Job titles should be listed, but a brief description of duties is essential, because titles such as plasterer, fire fighter, or engineer may be of little value because titles tend to remain the same while job activities and hazardous exposures may change dramatically as the result of new technology. In some instances, such as asbestos or beryllium exposure, eliciting job or exposures of the spouse and family members is helpful. Exposures to pets, use of forced air

humidifiers, presence of neighborhood factories, and the nature of hobbies should be determined. The person should be questioned about specific hazardous dust or fume exposures. When such an exposure is found, it is important to document the following indices: (1) year first exposed to the agent; (2) total years exposed; (3) estimation of the exposure level: level 1 peripheral exposure (administrative personnel), level 2 indirect exposure (electricians), or level 3 direct exposure (insulation workers); and (4) years since last exposure.

Amount of cigarette smoking or tobacco use should be determined. Individuals can be classified as nonsmokers, ex-smokers (stopped for at least 1 year), or present smokers. Information concerning type of smoking (cigarette, pipe, or cigar), the depth of inhalations, and the use of filters may be of some help. The age first started and age stopped, and the average number of packs of cigarettes smoked daily should be recorded.

The Physical Examination

The physical examination should include careful attention to the patient's breathing, the presence of finger clubbing or cyanosis, the quality of the breath sounds, the presence of crackles or wheezes, and the cardiac findings. The description of the patient's breathing should include the use of accessory muscles, paradoxical movements of rib cage and abdomen, the use of pursed lips during exhalation, the presence of labored breathing at rest, and inability on the part of the patient to utter complete sentences. Signs of right ventricular failure secondary to pulmonary hypertension should be sought: neck vein distention, dependent edema, hepatomegaly, exaggerated intensity of the second heart sound, and a right ventricular gallop that occurs early in diastole and increases with inspiration. Although abnormal physical findings are sometimes helpful in establishing that pulmonary disease is disabling, more often, they do not help in quantifying disability, e.g., fine crackles are heard in 80 percent of patients with chronic interstitial pneumonia who are severely impaired, and yet they are heard almost as often in early disease and sometimes in asymptomatic patients.

THE CHEST RADIOGRAPH

Chest radiographs should be obtained for all persons being evaluated for disability, although radiographs, too, are of limited value. In disease of airflow obstruction, such as asthma and emphysema, the appearance of the chest radiograph often bears little relation to severity of disease and may be entirely normal despite severe obstructive airways disease. For this large group of diseases, no correlation between work status and radiographic findings has been noted. However, as part of an overall evaluation of disability, the chest radiograph should be described in terms of lung size, presence of bullae, flattened diaphragms, increased posteroanterior diameter, and findings consistent with cor pulmonale.

In contrast to obstructive airways disease, the abnormalities associated with diffuse interstitial disease have received considerable attention with respect to disability evaluation. Indeed, certain regulations, such as the Coal Mine Safety Act, have mandated disability payments based only on radiographic appearance. However, in coal worker's pneumoconiosis, and other pulmonary diseases that result in *diffuse rounded* opacities, poor correlation exists between physiological and radiographic abnormalities. Evidence of progressive massive fibrosis (PMF) is an exception: as PMF develops, physiological dysfunction generally progresses concurrently.

Diffuse reticular-nodular opacities, commonly seen in sarcoidosis, also tend to correlate poorly with physiological findings. There are two reasons for the poor correlation of the severity of diffuse rounded or reticular-nodular opacities with functional status: (1) rounded densities are detected early in the evolution of the disease since they are not seen on the normal chest radiograph, and (2) there are large volumes of normal lung between the nodular opacities.

Diffuse linear opacities, as seen in the chronic interstitial pneumonias, asbestosis, and other diseases, are associated with some correlation between severity of the radiographic abnormalities and pulmonary function. But the physiological impairment is sometimes underestimated because linear opacities become evident as abnormalities only late in the course of the disease and because linear opacities generally represent fibrosis. Thus, inconsistencies exist in correlating radiographic abnormalities and impairment. However, even though, as in diseases of airflow obstruction, the radiograph cannot be the sole basis for determining impairment/disability, in dealing with pneumoconiosis or interstitial lung disease, it is essential to categorize the chest radiographs according to a quantitative scheme, e.g., International Labor Office radiographic classification for pneumoconiosis, so that the information can be part of an overall evaluation for disability.

PULMONARY FUNCTION TESTING

Although the clinical data base is useful as part of the overall evaluation of impairment and disability, symptoms, physical findings, and radiographic abnormalities are often inconstant or nonspecific. The poor discriminatory value of such data explains the emphasis on physiological studies. The latter are useful in categorizing impairment from none to severe and for comparing the pulmonary performance of the claimant with that of a healthy reference population. Physiological testing can vary from minimal testing to elaborate, expensive, time-consuming, and sometimes invasive tests. The preferred approach to physiological testing as part of disability evaluation consists of three initial screening tests with provision for proceeding to more complex studies should discrepancies appear between clinical findings and screening values.

Pulmonary function should be tested in individuals after they have stabilized in response to optimal therapy. The tests should be performed by standardized techniques, and both the equipment used and the methods of calibration should meet published standard guidelines.

Recommended Pulmonary Function Tests for Screening

The *forced expired volume in 1 s* (FEV_1) is the single best test for determining impairment in patients with airflow obstruction. The FEV_1 has been accepted throughout the world for the past 25 years, is simple to perform, is not excessively fatiguing, does not place excessive demands upon instrumentation, and cooperation is generally such that there is little difference between first and subsequent trials. In a study of 147 patients with chronic obstructive airways disease who were in a rehabilitation program, the FEV_1 correlated well with the work status: among the 29 who were working after the program, the mean FEV_1 was 61 percent of predicted, whereas in the 67 who either did not return to work or stopped work, the mean FEV_1 was 45 percent of predicted. In another study of 30 patients, all those with an FEV_1 above 2 L were working. A value for FEV_1 40 percent or less of predicted, or $FEV_1/FVC\%$ 40 percent or less, indicates severe impairment.

The *forced vital capacity* (FVC) is the most valuable screening test for volume determination. It is easily performed routinely along with the FEV_1; it requires minimal time and effort; it is both valid and reliable; the variance is small; and adequate regression equations for predicted normal values are available.

The third screening test is the *single breath diffusing capacity* ($DL_{CO_{sb}}$). In a group of 821 patients with interstitial lung diseases, it was the single most important test for determination of severe impairment. In more than one-half of these patients, the $DL_{CO_{sb}}$ was the only test that indicated severe impairment. Furthermore, the $DL_{CO_{sb}}$ is noninvasive, is suitable for rapid screening, requires little cooperation or effort, and is a well-standardized test; adequate regression equations for prediction of normal values are available. In an analysis of 111 patients with chronic interstitial disease, sensitivity studies, using the response to exercise as an independent criterion, suggested that severe impairment was reflected in either a reduction of the FVC to 50 percent or less of predicted, or of the $DL_{CO_{sb}}$ to 40 percent or less of predicted.

Other Pulmonary Function Tests

The maximal voluntary ventilation (MVV) has become less important for disability determination. The test is fatiguing and often elicits cough, instrumental requirements are rigorous, and special technician training is necessary; most importantly, FEV_1 is simpler to perform, is highly reproducible, and correlates well with the MVV. The functional residual capacity (FRC) and residual volume (RV) are sometimes helpful because they are effort-dependent tests that may be useful in a poorly cooperative patient. The extra time and expense that they entail must be considered in comparison to the limited benefit. Certain tests such as the mid-expiratory flow ($FEF_{25-75\%}$), closing volumes, helium-oxygen flow-volume determinations, and compliance measurements have no place in assessing disabling impairment.

In principle, determination of arterial oxygenation would appear to be an ideal objective test. But, in practice, it is a poor initial screening tool because it is invasive, the results are difficult to standardize because of the effects of acute hyperventilation and altitude, and even more importantly, the results do not correlate with the work status. For example, in a rehabilitation study of patients with chronic obstructive airways disease, the mean resting value for arterial P_{O_2} of 72.3 mmHg was similar in the 29 patients who worked to the arterial P_{O_2} of 68.0 mmHg in the 67 who were not working; the FEV_1 was markedly reduced in the latter group. In the interstitial lung diseases, the value for arterial oxygenation at rest often underestimates the degree of impairment; determination of the level of arterial oxygenation during exercise has an important place in demonstrating pulmonary impairment in such patients. Unfortunately, exercise testing is both invasive and expensive.

Pulmonary Exercise Testing

The effects of exercise on cardiopulmonary function have been widely used in research on exercise physiology, control of breathing, and athletic training, but remarkably little has been written concerning their role in pulmonary disability evaluation. However, because of the increasing number of requests for exercise studies by referral sources and governmental agencies, knowledge of testing methods and interpretation of results are becoming increasingly important.

Tests designed for direct measurement of work capability seem desirable for evaluation of pulmonary disability. But, it is often impossible to reproduce in the laboratory the specific type of exertion involved in the various occupations. Nor is it possible to mimic the duration of effort entailed in regular work. Most occupations in our highly mechanized society are nearly sedentary so that work at levels requiring high to maximum levels of O_2 consumption are not required. Often, the main distress

associated with work experienced by patients with severe pulmonary impairment is related to a long duration of low-level activity and the exertion, frustration, and discomfort experienced in travel to and from the job. These experiences are not strongly related to the response to 3 to 10 min of treadmill exercise. Motivation is another consideration: those who desire rehabilitation tend to perform graded exercise tests to the best of their ability, whereas those claiming disability or seeking compensation may refuse to attempt to exercise. Although it is generally believed that claimants often behave in such a way that it may be impossible to distinguish unwillingness from genuine distress, in reality this type of behavior may be uncommon: in one study, fewer than 5 percent refused exercise testing, and no difference was found between the oxygen uptake of claimants as compared to patients referred for diagnostic evaluation.

The cycle ergometer and treadmill are both suitable for exercise testing. Each has advantages and disadvantages. A higher oxygen consumption and heart rate can be achieved on a treadmill because a larger muscle mass is used; the treadmill is preferred for disability evaluation. But arterial blood sampling and complex ventilatory studies are more easily performed while the patient is seated on a cycle ergometer. Cycling is not as universal as walking, and most elderly patients find it easy and more comfortable to walk on the treadmill.

The type of exercise used is determined by the purpose of the testing and population being studied. For example, elderly patients generally tolerate one of the levels of the six-stage treadmill protocol suggested by Naughton, whereas most younger and middle-aged patients can perform the more strenuous protocol of Bruce. Another choice is between steady-state testing that entails 5 to 6 min at each level and incremental studies in which the level of work during uninterrupted exercise is increased minute-by-minute. Incremental studies are becoming increasingly popular because of the ease and short duration of the test. However, the steady-state method is generally preferable for disability evaluation because it has been used in most laboratories for many years, most elderly patients do complete the study in 5 to 6 min, and it best reflects work-related activities.

The "estimated" $\dot{V}_{O_2}$ may be used in some situations such as evaluating the patient's progress in a rehabilitation program, but it is too variable for disability determination and should not be used. It is obtained indirectly by calculating power output (KPM per minute) of either the cycle ergometer or treadmill. A poor correlation has been found between the measured and estimated $\dot{V}_{O_2}$ at both low-level and high-level exercise.

For disability evaluation, it is especially important that patients attain an adequate level of exercise. Subjective findings noted by the patients as well as observations of testing personnel should be carefully recorded. However, this is insufficient documentation for defining an adequate, or maximal, test. Objective cardiac and pulmonary criteria are needed. The heart rate is used as the cardiac criterion because it is part of routine exercise monitoring, it is the easiest reflection of cardiac performance to quantify, and it correlates linearly with ventilation and $\dot{V}_{O_2}$. A value of 80 percent of predicted (210 − age × 0.65) can be used for the minimal limit. For subjects not attaining this requirement, an FEV_1 criterion can be used because it is also a routine measurement, it is subject to minimal mechanical error, and it correlates best with $\dot{V}_{O_2}$. A maximal expired minute volume (MEV) of 50 percent of predicted (actual FEV_1 × 35) can be used as a minimal limit. Therefore, for disability evaluation, an exercise study is considered adequate or maximal if the subject attains a heart rate of at least 80 percent of predicted or an MEV of at least 50 percent.

Exercise testing should be deferred in patients with any of the following conditions: acute illness, congestive heart failure, dissecting or ventricular aneurysms, limiting neuromuscular impairment, medications that may constitute significant risk, severe aortic stenosis, severe pulmonary hypertension, uncontrolled arrhythmias, uncontrolled severe hypertension, or unstable angina pectoris.

Among the reasons for terminating any exercise study are the following: (1) no further testing is necessary because adequate or maximal test criteria have been attained, (2) the patient stopped because of either dyspnea, muscle fatigue, or both, or (3) the physician stopped the test because of clinical concerns. Medical indications for stopping the test include: extreme fatigue; intolerable leg muscle pain; a decrease or lack of increase in systolic blood pressure with increasing workload; an increase in diastolic pressure of more than 20 mmHg or in systolic pressure of more than 260 mmHg; three or more successive premature ventricular contractions; recurring multifocal premature ventricular contractions; a major left ventricular conduction disturbance; symptomatic ST-T-segment depression or elevation greater than 2.0 mm; or signs of insufficient peripheral circulation or cardiac output, such as pallor, cyanosis, clammy skin, nausea, or dizziness.

The laboratory should be equipped to meet an emergency. Personnel should be capable of maintaining life until the patient can be managed by the resuscitation team. For purposes of safety, it is important to anticipate potentially low arterial oxygenation so that the appropriate monitoring and care can be provided. Ear oximetry is especially useful in this regard. The value for arterial oxygen saturation obtained by ear oximetry may be used to estimate the degree of impairment, but the direct P_{O_2}, P_{CO_2}, and pH measurements from an indwelling arterial cannula are preferable. Arterial studies during exercise often add new information in patients with interstitial lung disease, especially if the $DL_{CO_{sb}}$ is less than 70 percent of predicted.

Pulmonary Exercise Testing Interpretation

In healthy subjects, maximal exercise is limited by heart rate and cardiac output, and not by ventilation or pulmonary function. During maximal exercise, the minute ventilation approaches only about 70 percent of the maximum voluntary ventilation (MVV). With increasing age, the maximum heart rate decreases along with a decrease in maximal oxygen consumption. In healthy subjects, the magnitude of the increase in heart rate and ventilation elicited by a certain amount of exercise varies; it depends on body size, fitness, amount of training, and hemoglobin content. Because of these multiple factors, "work done" is best measured by quantifying oxygen consumption rather than determining the amount of external workload, another reason that estimated $\dot{V}_{O_2}$ is not recommended.

The maximal oxygen uptake gives an excellent estimate of an individual's aerobic fitness, i.e., the ability to perform a task for which aerobic demands are well-defined. A worker involved in manual labor who is more or less free to set the work pace, can work comfortably at approximately 40 percent of maximum aerobic power ($\dot{V}_{O_2}$max). During shorter periods of time, an individual can work without fatigue at about 50 percent of $\dot{V}_{O_2}$max. In a large group of volunteers and patients in whom screening pulmonary function tests were normal, virtually all could attain a $\dot{V}_{O_2}$ of 25 ml/kg/min without difficulty. Many patients who had borderline abnormal resting pulmonary function studies could also attain these $\dot{V}_{O_2}$ values. In contrast, virtually no patient with severe impairment according to resting measurement could attain these $\dot{V}_{O_2}$ values; most of these exhibited severe gas exchange abnormalities with an alveolar-arterial difference of greater than 50 mmHg. Only 30 percent of these patients with severe impairment could attain a $\dot{V}_{O_2}$ of 15 ml/kg/min.

It has been estimated that office work requires a $\dot{V}_{O_2}$ of 5 to 7 ml/kg/min, that moderate labor requires about 15 ml/kg/min, and that strenuous, heavy labor, such as lifting 100 lb or stevedore work, requires at $\dot{V}_{O_2}$ of 20 to 30 ml/kg/min. Personal and athletic activities, such as golf, require a $\dot{V}_{O_2}$ of 7 to 10 ml/kg/min, tennis a $\dot{V}_{O_2}$ of 12 to 15 ml/kg/min and marathon running or handball a $\dot{V}_{O_2}$ of 25 to 30 ml/kg/min.

Interpretation of pulmonary exercise testing can be based on the two concepts discussed above: (1) a worker can perform a job comfortably at 40 percent of $\dot{V}_{O_2}$max and (2) $\dot{V}_{O_2}$ values can be assigned to specific jobs. For example, if an individual can attain a $\dot{V}_{O_2}$ of 35 to 40 ml/kg/min, work requiring a $\dot{V}_{O_2}$ of 10 to 15 ml/kg/min could easily be performed. However, if an individual can attain a $\dot{V}_{O_2}$ of only 15 ml/kg/min, moderate to heavy labor jobs could not be performed because an individual could not expect to work at 100 percent of the $\dot{V}_{O_2}$max.

A SCHEME FOR DETERMINATION OF PULMONARY IMPAIRMENT

There are at least three approaches to the evaluation of pulmonary impairment. The first, which relies solely on history and clinical examination, is unsatisfactory except in situations of extreme illness. A second entails the use of a large number of tests of cardiopulmonary function from which a total functional profile is generated, analyzed, and graded by computer. This approach is rejected because in many instances traumatic, painful, and expensive tests could be performed unnecessarily; furthermore, such examinations can be performed only in exceedingly few, specialized centers. A third, more flexible, approach is preferred. It consists of recording a data base consisting of the degree of dyspnea and the amount of cough and sputum, the detection of crackles or wheezes, and a description of the chest radiograph. Most importantly, it consists of physiological noninvasive screening tests: the FVC to describe volume, the FEV_1 to characterize flow rate, and the $D_{L_{CO_{sb}}}$ to characterize the diffusion characteristics of the gas-exchanging surfaces of the lungs; depending on the outcome of these tests, more complex physiological testing can be done. Furthermore, a scheme can be based solely on the concept of "loss of function," detected by spirometry and diffusing capacity, or "remaining function," generally determined by exercise testing. The preferred flexible approach utilizes both concepts, the first as a screening process and the second for selected situations (Fig. 37-1).

Several schemes have been advocated to establish categories of impairment. Some are based on criteria for obstructive or restrictive disease; others are based on three classes of impairment; a few have only a category for the severely impaired; one scheme is based on 10 categories of 10 percentage points each. Most governmental agencies and medical societies now agree on the two ends of the impairment spectrum: in the nonimpaired individual, the screening values are greater than 80 percent predicted, whereas in the severely impaired, the vital capacity is either 50 percent or less of predicted, or the FEV_1 or $D_{L_{CO_{sb}}}$ is 40 percent or less of predicted. Thus, if the screening pulmonary function tests are entirely normal, the person is not disabled by physiological pulmonary impairment; if they indicate severe functional impairment, then pulmonary dysfunction is so severe as to preclude, per se, gainful employment, i.e., the individual is totally disabled.

Between these extremes of impairment there is less agreement because of the imprecise correlation that exists between the results of pulmonary function testing and whether the individual is working. For example, individ-

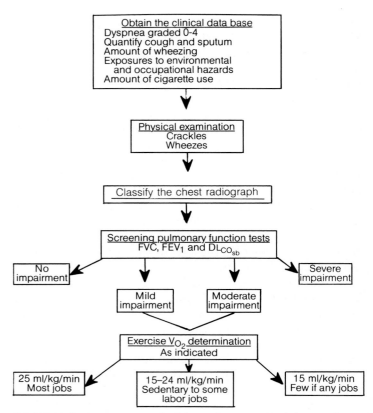

FIGURE 37-1 Summary method for pulmonary disability evaluation.

uals near the normal end of the spectrum can probably perform all types of jobs, despite slightly abnormal values, because of the large pulmonary functional reserve; if a work limitation does exist, it is more likely to be due to poor conditioning or to cardiac dysfunction. For individuals whose values range from 40 to 60 percent of predicted, the inability to perform certain types of work may be the result of pulmonary impairment, i.e. partial disability.

In accord with these considerations, the approach to pulmonary function testing consists of obtaining the vital capacity, the FEV_1, and the $D_{L_{CO_{sb}}}$ for each individual who is then categorized as normal, mildly impaired, moderately impaired, or severely impaired (Table 37-3). Mildly impaired individuals are usually not correlated with diminished ability to perform most jobs; moderately impaired individuals with progressively lower levels of lung function have diminishing ability to meet the physical demands of many jobs; and severely impaired individuals are unable to meet the physical demands of most jobs, including travel to work. Determination of exercise $\dot{V}_{O_2}$ should be limited in its use because of cost and time involved, but it may be useful in confirming the impairment category, in changing to a more severe category those individuals in whom a large discrepancy exists between perceived symptoms and screening tests, or in studying individuals who have very strenuous jobs. The

TABLE 37-3
Rating of Pulmonary Impairment

Pulmonary Function Tests	"Normal"	Mildly Impaired	Moderately Impaired	Severely Impaired
FVC, % predicted	≥ 80	60–79	51–59	≤ 50
FEV_1, % predicted	≥ 80	60–79	41–59	≤ 40
$FEV_1/FVC\%$	≥ 75	60–74	41–59	≤ 40
$DL_{CO_{sb}}$, % predicted	≥ 80	60–79	41–59	≤ 40

exercise $\dot{V}_{O_2}$ values that are useful in defining the work categories are as follows: (1) virtually all types of work if the individual can achieve a $\dot{V}_{O_2}$ of greater than 25 ml/kg/min, (2) desk work to light or moderate labor when the maximum $\dot{V}_{O_2}$ is between 15 and 25 ml/kg/min, and (3) no gainful employment when the maximum $\dot{V}_{O_2}$ is 15 ml/kg/min (Fig. 37-1). The 40 percent value of the individual's $\dot{V}_{O_2}$ can also be calculated and compared to the estimated $\dot{V}_{O_2}$ requirement for the particular job. If the job $\dot{V}_{O_2}$ requirement exceeds the worker's 40 percent $\dot{V}_{O_2max}$, then it would probably be difficult for this individual to work comfortably for a full workweek. This method can be applied only with caution because the job-specific $\dot{V}_{O_2}$ requirements are estimates and there is a large variability in $\dot{V}_{O_2}$ requirements among individuals and their work habits.

Although numerical limits to delineate degrees of impairment are necessary for use as guidelines by administrative personnel, such limits pose certain philosophical questions. For example, the Social Security Administration has published tables of lower limits for actual values of the FVC and FEV_1 based only on height, i.e., without regard to sex or age. Thus, the social security tables tend to favor women and elderly persons, while values expressed as percentages of predicted may not favor older workers because the respiratory cost of a given task remains unchanged with advancing age. The use of the 95 percent confidence interval for normal limits or the percentage of predicted values is preferable in most circumstances because physicians charged with rating impairment should compare organ function or function of the whole person to that of comparable, healthy persons.

SPECIAL CONSIDERATIONS AND OTHER IMPAIRMENTS

Cor pulmonale indicates severe impairment regardless of pulmonary function rating of impairment.

An asthmatic may be considered disabled if documented attacks of airflow obstruction require treatment in the emergency room or hospital at least once every 2 months, or an average of at least six times yearly despite optimal therapy. Exercise-induced bronchospasm requires special consideration of environmental conditions

and type of work; the degree of impairment should be assessed using postexercise values.

Persons with occupational asthma that has been documented, preferably by a 20 percent decrease in FEV_1 after exposure, have a specific impairment that will not allow them to work in an exposure-related job. Thus, they are totally and permanently "disabled" for those jobs even though they have neither measurable impairment nor manifestation of asthma after withdrawal from the inciting exposure. The same principle applies to individuals who have developed hypersensitivity pneumonia (extrinsic allergic alveolitis). In appropriate situations, this principle can also be applied to the pneumoconioses, e.g., a young worker with asbestos plaques should not work in any type of asbestos-related industry.

Upper airway obstruction can cause permanent respiratory impairment. The spirogram and flow-volume curve can be used for diagnosis. In such subjects, the increased work of breathing decreases exercise tolerance. If upper airway obstruction is documented, the individual should be considered impaired; moreover, if the individual retains CO_2, then the impairment is severe.

Some respiratory disorders lead to impairment because of their effect on overall body function rather than their respiratory effects, e.g., carcinoma of the lung, pulmonary hypertension, sleep apnea syndromes, and severe chronic respiratory infections. Impairment results from weight loss, muscle weakness, fatigue, loss of mental alertness, and general debility. Such impairments need to be documented as accurately as possible in each individual case.

There are individual circumstances leading to pulmonary impairments that are too numerous to mention and require case-by-case analysis. For example, an individual with bullous emphysema and mucous plugging should be disqualified from diving or aviation jobs because of risk of barotrauma.

Decisions concerning impairment should be made after appropriate therapy and when there appears to be no reasonable prospect of further improvement. If the participant is not being treated or has refused therapy, this should be recorded. When two diseases coexist, it is important to present a separate evaluation of each diagnostic entity and indicate the major impairing condition; the examination should be sufficiently detailed for this distinction to be made. Although each disease by itself may not be disabling, the sum of the disorders may be. If there is an unreasonable refusal or inability on the part of the claimant to cooperate in the performance of the requested studies, this should be recorded. A state of poor conditioning should be described when the level of impairment is primarily attributable to a deconditioned state resulting from illness, recent hospitalization, physical inactivity, obesity, or malnutrition. In case of death, it is important to obtain all medical evidence that may be helpful in assessing the impairment; the death certificate, per se, is not sufficient.

ESTABLISHING CAUSATION

Causation is a medical and legal term often used in requests for disability evaluation, i.e., is the pulmonary condition related to the workplace? The medical definition of cause and effect requires scientific proof, and the alleged positive element must be one recognized scientifically. Legal causation requires either a probability greater than 50 percent or that the event was "more likely than not" to be the cause. In a study of 128 medicolegal referrals, two-thirds did not fulfill the legal definition of cause. Among the reasons for failing to satisfy the legal definition were the following: (1) the alleged exposure often did not cause a known disease; (2) the temporal relationship between cause and effect was inappropriate; (3) objective clinical evidence of disease was lacking; or (4) another disease, such as cigarette-related obstructive airways disease, was the more likely cause of the symptoms. A thorough review of the clinical and epidemiologic literature, recording all available medical and occupational information, and objective determination of the nature of disease are essential elements to establish causation. Four principles of medical causation should be followed: (1) document the exposure and determine that it is a proven hazardous agent; (2) determine if there is an appropriate dose-response relationship and latency period of the exposure; (3) establish that the clinical, physiological, and radiographic findings are consistent with the known expected work-related lung disorder; and (4) determine that a more likely and established diagnostic explanation does not exist as the cause of the pulmonary condition.

BIBLIOGRAPHY

Astrand PO, Rodahl K: *Textbook of Work Physiology.* New York, McGraw-Hill, 1977.
    This textbook includes a review of the concept that a person can work comfortably at 40 percent of maximal $\dot{V}_{O_2}$.

Barnhart S: Evaluation of impairment and disability in occupational lung disease. State Art Rev Occup Med 2:227–241, 1987.
    An approach to whether a respiratory disease is caused or aggravated by a patient's occupation.

Becklake MR: Organic or functional impairment. Am Rev Respir Dis 129(Suppl):S96–S100, 1984.
    An overall prospective of disability evaluation is presented including a review of $\dot{V}_{O_2}$ requirements for specific jobs.

Chan Yeung M, Malo JL: Occupational asthma. Chest 91:130S–136S, 1987.
    A review of recent developments in the study of occupational asthma and implications for the overall understanding of asthma.

Disability Evaluation Under Social Security: A Handbook for Physicians. SSA Publication No. 05-10089:28–34, 1986.
    This government publication lists limit values for the forced vital capacity (FVC), forced expired volume in 1 s (FEV_1), maximal voluntary ventilation (MVV), and diffusing capacity ($DL_{CO_{sb}}$) that indicate respiratory impairment.

Epler GR, Saber FA, Gaensler EA: Determination of severe impairment (disability) in interstitial lung disease. Am Rev Respir Dis 121:647–659, 1980.
    A study of 821 patients with interstitial lung disease showed that a vital capacity less than 50 percent predicted or a diffusing capacity of less than 40 percent indicated severe impairment.

Evaluation of Impairment/Disability Secondary to Respiratory Disease. American Thoracic Society. Am Rev Respir Dis 133:1205–1209, 1986.
    This American Thoracic Society statement includes a scheme for determination of degrees of pulmonary impairment by using screening pulmonary function tests and exercise testing for selected cases.

Gaensler EA, Wright GW: Evaluation of respiratory impairment. Arch Environ Health 12:146–189, 1966.
    This classic publication describes a pulmonary function testing scheme for determination of mild, moderate, severe, and very severe impairment.

Gilbert R, Keighley J, Auchincloss JH: Disability in patients with destructive pulmonary disease. Am Rev Respir Dis 90:383–394, 1964.

The FEV_1 correlated best with work status at the extremes of the impairment scale, and exercise testing had some reliability for selecting patients unable to maintain full-time employment.

Guides to the Evaluation of Permanent Impairment. American Medical Association, 2d ed. AMA OP-254:85–101, 1984.

Revised AMA guidelines for classification of no impairment and mild, moderate, and severe impairment.

Harber P: Alternative partial respiratory disability rating schemes. Am Rev Respir Dis 134:481–487, 1986.

Twelve alternative schemes for using results of clinical physiologic testing to "rate" partial respiratory disability are compared with respect to "ratings" of 650 claimants with asbestos lung disease. The degree of disability indicated by different schemes varied considerably depending on the physiologic abnormality.

Harber P, Schnur R, Emery J, Brooks S, Ploy-Song-Sang Y: Statistical "biases" in respiratory disability determinations. Am Rev Respir Dis 128:413–418, 1983.

Selection of recording results of pulmonary function tests has minor to major implications that should be considered in the design and goals of a disability system.

Kass I, Dyksterhuis JE, Rubin H, Patil KD. Correlation of psychophysiological variables with vocational rehabilitation outcome in patients with chronic obstructive pulmonary disease. Chest 67:433–441, 1975.

Individuals with an FEV_1 of less than 50 percent of predicted had an unacceptably poor outcome for vocational rehabilitation.

Koskela RS, Klockars M, Jarvinen E, Kolari PJ, Rossi A: Mortality and disability among granite workers. Scand J Work Environ Health 13:18–25, 1987.

The study was designed to investigate the mortality, disability, and long-term morbidity of granite workers.

Marini JJ, Rodriguez RM, Lamb VJ: Involuntary breath-stacking. An alternative method for vital capacity estimation in poorly cooperative subjects. Am Rev Respir Dis 134:694–698, 1986.

A strategy for estimating the vital capacity in individuals incapable of cooperating properly because of impaired comprehension, altered mental status, or inability to sustain forceful effort.

Morgan WKC: Clinical significance of pulmonary function tests: Disability or disinclination. Chest 75:712–715, 1979.

A perspective of terminology and methods used for disability determination.

Oren A, Sue DY, Hansen JE, Torrance DJ, Wasserman K: The role of exercise testing in impairment evaluation. Am Rev Respir Dis 135:230–235, 1987.

A consideration of the usefulness of exercise testing in impairment evaluation of 348 asbestos-exposed shipyard workers. Exercise testing proved useful in the accurate assessment of work capacity and in the identification of the major limiting system in those with low work capacity.

Pineda H, Haas F, Axen K, Haas A: Accuracy of pulmonary function tests in predicting exercise tolerance in chronic obstructive pulmonary disease. Chest 86:564–567, 1984.

The FEV_1 can predict exercise tolerance with some accuracy. If a more accurate evaluation is required, exercise testing should be performed.

Ries AL: The role of exercise testing in pulmonary diagnosis. Clin Chest Med 8:81–89, 1987.

In the evaluation of pulmonary patients, exercise testing can be used to measure exercise tolerance, assess the limitation to exercise in patients with unexplained dyspnea, evaluate patients for respiratory disability, assess blood gas changes with exercise, and detect exercise-induced asthma.

Risk CG, Epler GR, Sicilian L: Exercise alveolar-arterial pressure differences in interstitial lung disease. Chest 85:69–74, 1984.

In patients with interstitial lung disease, the exercise test with arterial blood-gas measurement adds important information if the $D_{L_{CO_{sb}}}$ is less than 70 percent predicted. For disability evaluation, the invasive exercise study may be helpful when there is a wide discrepancy between clinical findings and resting physiological studies.

Sherman CB: Cardiopulmonary exercise testing to assess respiratory impairment in occupational lung disease. State Art Rev Occup Med 2:243–257, 1987.

A critical review of the role of cardiopulmonary exercise testing in occupational lung disease.

Sicilian L, Epler GR, Gaensler EA: Analysis of environmental causality in lung disease. Chest 78:540, 1980.
> *This study of 128 medicolegal referrals showed that one-third had sufficient data to meet the legal definition of causation.*

Soutar CA, Hurley JF: Relation between dust exposure and lung function in miners and ex-miners. Br J Ind Med 43:307–320, 1986.
> *A sample of men working in the British coal industry in the 1950s has been followed up and examined 22 years later to examine the relations between lung function and individual cumulative exposure to respirable dust.*

Standards for the diagnosis and care of patients with chronic obstructive pulmonary disease (COPD) and asthma. Am Rev Respir Dis 136:225–244, 1987.
> *This statement represents the combined efforts of a Task Group appointed by the Scientific Assembly of Clinical Problems of the American Thoracic Society.*

Woods BO'B, Epler GR, Risk CG, Gaensler EA: Determination of severe pulmonary impairment (disability) by exercise testing. Am Rev Respir Dis 125:155, 1982.
> *This study showed a poor correlation between the estimated $\dot{V}_{O_2}$ and actual $\dot{V}_{O_2}$ and compared resting screening pulmonary function tests to the exercise $\dot{V}_{O_2}$.*

Part 6

Immunologic Disorders (including Certain Interstitial Diseases)

Chapter 38

Cellular Communication in Respiratory Immunity

John Bienenstock / Ralph Scicchitano / Jack Gauldie

Immune Responses

Architecture
Antigen Processing
IgA Immune Responses
Tolerance

Other Influences on Respiratory Immunity
Diet
Adjuvants
T Lymphocytes and Natural Killer Cells
Mast Cells
Goblet Cells
Epithelium
Eosinophils
Cellular Communication
Neuropeptides

Conclusions

Immunologists, as other medical scientists schooled in a specific discipline, have a natural tendency to regard any other discipline through their own particular tinted glasses. While it is totally defensible and needs no apology or justification, this tendency often leaves the reader with unwanted and unneeded detail and a distinct feeling of helplessness when attempting to fit this new knowledge into a framework of understanding.

We have, therefore, written this chapter as an introduction to the immunology of the lung and have tried to indicate and stress, wherever possible, the network of communication that exists between central components of the immune system and their natural surroundings. Our hope is that the reader will begin to see immunity as part of the complex physiology of the lung. We have chosen to emphasize some things and have omitted others, solely to achieve this aim.

We begin with a short description of the structural basis for respiratory immunity, to provide a framework on which to hang some of the concepts and ideas that follow.

Before describing the architecture and the interplay of the immune system in the lung, we introduce two concepts. The first is that the immunologic apparatus of the respiratory tract differs from that of the blood and other tissues, both in respect of antibody and the cell types contained therein.

The most obvious example of this difference is the alveolar macrophage, which serves as a useful model to explore this concept. Although the alveolar macrophage derives from stem cells in the bone marrow, lodges in lung tissue after originating in the bone marrow, and is related to the circulating blood monocyte and to macrophages in other parts of the body, it has many distinctive characteristics when removed from the lungs by bronchoalveolar lavage. Thus, it seems likely that local environmental factors in the lung constitute an influence that has directed these cells into becoming characteristic alveolar macrophages. What these local factors are, where they come from in the lung, and from which cells they derive remains enigmatic. Nor is it clear how the synthesis and secretion of these factors is regulated, either in health or disease. Finally, no one really knows what is the end of the alveolar macrophage. Does it die, as many people think, in its own graveyard in the gastrointestinal tract, or does it find its way back from the lumen into the tissues? Could it even be that some alveolar macrophages, outside the lung environment and its local influences, change phenotypically and morphologically and are, therefore, not recognized in other sites as having passed some time in the lung?

These questions lead us to the second concept: "A cell is not a cell, is not always a cell." Many examples of this abound in immunology, and we will return to this issue later. For example, the lineage relationship between cytotoxic T cells and natural killer (NK) cells appears very close at this time. Exactly how they are related is not clear; however, it is thought by many immunologists now that despite the characteristically, clearly different, functional attributes of these two cell types, they may change one into the other. There are increasing examples of the close interrelationship between helper T cells and suppressor T cells, which under certain circumstances (in vitro) may apparently convert into the other cell type. The mast cell population gives us yet another example of these interrelationships, since even fully differentiated rat peritoneal mast cells may, when placed in the gastrointestinal tract in vivo, proliferate under local growth factor stimulation and convert into phenotypically and functionally different mast cells (see "Mast Cells," below). Therefore, local factors in the lung may be decisive in influencing cells to differentiate along a particular pathway.

While it is helpful to consider immune mechanisms as separate entities, the study of immunity in the rest of the body cannot substitute for its study in the lung, if we are interested in respiratory immunity. Its similarities and its differences must be compared with those seen in other tissues. Furthermore, it is obvious that the influence of the expression of immunity in the lung and on the lung and its functions must be studied. It is equally clear that the study of the effect of the normal physiological processes of the lung on immune mechanisms will provide us with a better understanding of the integrated physiology of the lung.

This chapter, then, deals with the extensive nature of the communication network between cells of the immune system and other cells, as well as the influence that neuroendocrine cells and nerves may have on immune function.

IMMUNE RESPONSES

Architecture

Beneath the ciliated mucosal lining of the tracheobronchial tree are found collections of lymphoid follicles (bronchus-associated lymphoid tissue, BALT). Despite some dissenting voices, it seems clear that BALT is a normal component of human respiratory tract.

These lymphoid follicles are covered by a specialized epithelium known either as *follicle-associated epithelium (FAE)*, by analogy with Peyer's patches in the intestine and the bursa of Fabricius in chickens, or as *M cells*. This apparently specialized epithelium seems to be capable of actively transporting into the interior of the follicle molecules that are potentially antigenic and particles that are as large as bacteria. As noted above, BALT in many ways resembles the gut-associated lymphoid tissue, including Peyer's patches. In certain infections, including tuberculosis, these lymphoid follicles may increase considerably in size and number. Indeed, they may expand so much in volume as to occlude the distal airways with an appearance similar to that seen in lymphoid nodular hyperplasia of the intestine.

The FAE overlying BALT is devoid of glandular and goblet cells, and of cilia. This arrangement possibly increases turbulence of airflow at these sites and may help to congregate soluble antigens and particulate matter. It has been suggested that macrophages and other cells may enter the lung tissues through the FAE from the lumen and enter the BALT. Lipscomb has suggested that alveolar macrophages transported by the cilia enter the BALT via this route. However, this issue is not yet settled.

Undoubtedly, the size of the inhaled particles and the way in which they pass down the respiratory tract will determine, in large measure, whether they will engage mucosal immune mechanisms or become deposited lower, in distal airways that contain the traditional elements for initiating immune responses, particularly those leading to an IgG-type of immunity.

Antigen Processing

Antigen is processed by specialized macrophages, usually found in lymphoid tissue, to initiate immune responses.

Such macrophages exist not only in the BALT but also elsewhere in the respiratory tract. It is established that alveolar macrophages, especially when activated, are capable of initiating immune responses by presenting antigen to T cells and also to B cells. Less well appreciated is the fact that normal epithelial cells activated by inflammatory processes may express Ia antigens on their apical surface, thereby acquiring the capability of processing and presenting antigen in traditional in vitro immune responses. Thus, the normal epithelium itself may be involved as an initiator of local immune responses since it has all the machinery necessary to do so.

IgA Immune Responses

Immune responses to specific antigens introduced into the respiratory tract occur locally. As far as immunoglobulin is concerned, the responses are primarily mediated by IgA antibody in the secretory form. As indicated above, evidence of local immunity is not necessarily reflected or accompanied by evidence of similar antibody specificity in the serum. As a rule, respiratory immunization is better achieved by local presentation of antigen than by parenteral immunization. Moreover, since most of the antigen introduced into the respiratory tract eventually finds its way into the gut via the ciliary escalator, the possible contribution of intestinal immunity to respiratory tract immunity must always be kept in mind.

Many of the immunologic responses of the upper respiratory tract resemble those of mucosal tissues elsewhere, especially the gut. In the upper respiratory tract, IgA predominates over other immunoglobulins. The IgA is in the secretory conformation, composed of two serum-type IgA molecules covalently linked to a secretory component that is added to the IgA dimer as it is transported through the respiratory epithelium. The secretory component functions as a transport protein for dimeric IgA and is expressed on both the basal and lateral epithelial cell surfaces. Receptor-mediated endocytosis transports IgA across the epithelium to the apical surface where it is secreted. In the process of secretion, proteolytic cleavage of secretory component occurs, leaving a short molecular structure in the epithelium and the full secretory IgA molecule in the respiratory secretions at the cell surface, now relatively resistant to proteolysis.

Some dimeric IgA synthesized elsewhere in the body may also be transported onto the respiratory epithelial surface. The extent to which this occurs is not known. However, this selective transport system for dimeric IgA without secretory component has been established for several glandular mucosal epithelia such as the breast and intestine, and includes the biliary epithelium in the human. Thus, the scope of local antigenic specificity can be broadened by local as well as distal synthesis of immunoglobulin.

Most of the local IgA is synthesized as dimeric IgA in B cells in the mucosal lamina propria. The number of IgA cells found in normal healthy respiratory mucosa is low with respect to other mucosal sites, such as the gut, presumably as a result of lower antigenic exposure.

If antigen is delivered to the gastrointestinal tract directly with due regard for amount, physicochemical nature, frequency of administration, and dosage, gastrointestinal immunity in the form of the local IgA is expressed and accompanied by dissemination of immunity, especially to other mucosal sites. This dissemination has been termed the *common mucosal immune system* in which cells that have been primed, either in gut-associated lymphoid tissue (Peyer's patches) or in the draining lymph nodes such as mesenteric lymph nodes, eventually seed distal mucosal sites via the bloodstream. These primed cells selectively localize in distal mucosal sites; in these sites, they seem to provide some protection because of their secreted products and their lifetime is normally short. However, if the seeded cells encounter antigen locally in these sites, they divide and amplify the specific immunity that they are geared to provide. The respiratory tract is no exception to this principle which has been shown to be operative in humans for adenovirus and influenza virus. More recently, oral immunization with *Hemophilus influenzae* has been shown to be effective in the reduction of the number of attacks of respiratory infection suffered by patients with chronic bronchitis.

The basis for selective localization of lymphocytes appears to depend, at least in part, on the expression of molecules on the surface of lymphocytes that are complementary to molecules on the endothelial surface of vessels within particular tissues. Additional factors in the tissues, outside the vascular compartment, may keep these cells in place after they have traversed the vascular endothelium.

The localization of lymphocytes in mucosal tissues is also influenced by many other factors, including the presence of antigen to which the lymphocytes are directed. Also, in tissues that are targets for the sex hormones, such as the mammary gland and cervix, IgA B-cell localization is influenced by the levels of estrogen, progesterone, and prolactin. Whether hormonal effects other than those due to sex hormones can influence lymphocyte localization in the respiratory tract is not known, but seems likely.

The influence of local inflammatory products on the expression of lymphocyte localization factors or on factors expressed by the endothelium is not known. However, it is known that inflammation causes postcapillary venules to change in structure and to become sites for the emigration of lymphocytes. Endothelial activation and expression of Ia antigens is also seen in inflammatory processes elicited by a variety of stimuli.

The propensity of mucosal-derived lymphocytes for localizing in mucosae is an important principle. Moreover, localization of mucosal-derived lymphocytes is also strongly influenced by the organ from which they derive. For example, intestine-derived lymphocytes are inclined to return primarily to the intestine and secondarily to other mucosal sites. The same is true for lung-derived lymphocytes. Since the majority of lung-derived lymphocytes are not derived from the mucosa, it is not surprising that many, if not most, of the lung-derived lymphocytes have a tendency to distribute elsewhere. However, the IgA-producing, lung-derived lymphocytes do tend to return to the lung. This is not exclusively the property of IgA-producing cells but may also be found in lung-derived, IgG-producing cells.

Tolerance

Tolerance is defined as immunologic unresponsiveness to challenge with specific antigen. It can be brought about by a variety of mechanisms, especially by active induction that is supported by T-suppressor cells, macrophages, and a variety of cell-cell interactions. Complete systemic tolerance can be induced via the intestinal tract if timing and dosage of antigen are appropriate. Similarly, tolerance can be induced by administering antigen to the respiratory tract. However, since most of the antigen in the respiratory lumen is eventually delivered into the gastrointestinal tract, it cannot be certain whether respiratory tolerance is totally separate from oral tolerance.

What is important to recognize, however, is that oral tolerance is a form of "split tolerance"; that is, no evidence of systemic immunity occurs, but mucosal expression of IgA is retained. Thus the presentation of antigen to the host via the lung can result in immunity which may be total or partial. This is a very complex area, and the many factors which control immune expression in the lung, or how best to harness this for respiratory protection are, at present, incompletely understood.

OTHER INFLUENCES ON RESPIRATORY IMMUNITY

Diet

Dietary factors and the state of nutrition can influence immune responses in a variety of ways. For example, malnutrition due to inadequate protein intake and/or vitamin A deficiency causes major effects on the expression of mucosal immunity, both as a result of direct effects on the epithelium and also as a result of interference in the localization of IgA B cells in mucosal tissues.

Adjuvants

The factors that ordinarily control antigen uptake by the respiratory tract are not known. But, it is likely that anything that promotes access of the antigen to the epithelium, and its subsequent binding, has adjuvant activity.

For example, antibiotics, such as streptomycin or lysozyme, increase intestinal mucosal immunity as does the extraneous administration of vitamin A. These may act by way of influence on the flora, as with the antibiotics, or through direct action on the epithelial membrane (vitamin A). Administration of cholera toxin also acts as an adjuvant. This is probably through its action via a surface membrane receptor for the β subunit, which in turn allows the γ subunit to increase cyclic AMP levels within the cell. Antigen coupled to the β subunit is increased in immunogenicity probably through increased binding to epithelium. Also, antigen delivered into the respiratory tract by aerosol containing a detergent improves the local specific immune response, possibly by increasing the permeability of the respiratory epithelium to antigen.

T Lymphocytes and Natural Killer Cells

B lymphocytes are not found in the epithelium of the respiratory tract. However, lymphocytes bearing T-cell markers are found in the intercellular spaces above the basement membrane. Many of these lymphocytes contain granules of an unknown nature that bear considerable resemblance to the intraepithelial leukocytes in the intestine. In this location, these cells resemble the "large granular lymphocytes" that are believed to be responsible for most of the natural killer activity in peripheral blood and lymphoid tissues. However, very little NK activity is associated with these cells. The functions of the intestinal epithelial leukocytes are several and include NK and cytotoxic T-cell activity, a natural killer type of activity capable of killing virus-infected cells, and precursors of T and mast cells. It is likely that these intestinal epithelial leukocytes are long-lived and migrate back into the tissues and not into the lumen after their stay in the epithelium. However, the fate and appearance of these cells after their sojourn in the epithelium is not known.

One of the questions about cellular protection of the lungs against invading pathogens is whether the cells can normally get from the bloodstream to the appropriate site of infection.

In experimental conditions, certain clones of influenza-specific, cytotoxic T lymphocytes, which are protective in vivo against lethal virus challenge in mice, tend to selectively localize in the respiratory epithelium after they are introduced into the circulation; this localization did not depend on the specific influenza virus antigens against which they were directed. Under appropriate conditions, then, protective T cells can migrate into and across the epithelium where they can be detected in bronchoalveolar lavage fluids.

Cytotoxic T cells are also found in the lamina propria of mucosal tissues. In these sites, however, under normal healthy conditions, the helper cell phenotype usually predominates. This predominance is reflected in bronchoalveolar lavage specimens from healthy volunteers. Thus, the cytotoxic T cells and NK cells, seen as a result of antigenic challenge of the lungs, may come either from the blood or lymphoid tissue, or have been locally influenced to divide in the lung tissue as a consequence to local inflammatory signals.

Mast Cells

Mast cells are heterogeneous in phenotype and function. Like the IgA B-cell system, the mast cell system in the mucosa appears to be different from that in other tissues.

In the rat, which has been best studied, the mucosal mast cell is differentiated from that found in connective tissue on the basis of its staining properties and its resistance or sensitivity to fixation with formalin (Table 38-1). The intestinal mucosal mast cell loses its ability to be stained after tissues have been fixed in formalin. This property is conferred on the cell by the proteoglycan content, which in the rat intestinal mast cell is chondroitin sulfate di-B and which in the connective tissue type cell is heparin. Mast cells contain many preformed mediators, as well as those which can be stimulated to be synthesized by an external stimulus, such as antigen. Histamine, the best known mediator, has a large number of well described and different effects on many separate biologic systems, as do many of the leukotrienes and prostaglandins. Indeed, apart from its effect on increase of permeability of capillary endothelium, histamine has profound immunosuppressive properties. However, here only the widespread effect of the proteoglycan, heparin, will be considered as an example of the multiplicity of effects and interactions found with a single secreted molecule.

Heparin is contained in the granules of the serosal (connective tissue) type of mast cell (Table 38-2). As indicated above, many differences exist between peritoneal

TABLE 38-1

Effect of Different Agents on Mast Cells

Agent	Mast Cell Source	
	Peritoneum	Intestine
Antigen, anti-IgE	++	++
Neutrophil cationic protein C3a, C5a, dextran, polylysine	++	?
48/80, bee venom peptide 401	++	0
Ionophores	++	+/++
Substance P	++	+
VIP, somatostatin, bradykinin, neurotensin	++	0
Dynorphin, β-endorphin, neoendorphin	++	0
Cortisone	0	++(depletion)
Cromoglycate	++	0
Quercetin, doxantrazole	++	+

and intestinal mast cells (Table 38-2). In the mucosa such as the intestine, growth of the mast cell is influenced by interleukin 3 (IL-3), a molecule synthesized by T lymphocytes. This molecule is not simply a mast cell growth factor. It also is capable of stimulating stem cells to differentiate into many different lineages and is also known as colony stimulating factor (multi-CSF). Similar factors have been found to be synthesized by epithelial cells, keratinocytes and some epithelial cell tumors, indicating again that local factors with specific immunologic properties may be synthesized and secreted by cells other than those ordinarily associated with immune responses.

Histochemically, the mast cells found in the pulmonary parenchyma of both humans and rats are of both types, whereas in the mucosa, the formalin-sensitive, or mucosal, type of mast cell predominates.

There is now good evidence that most cells in human bronchoalveolar lavage show significant functional differences when compared to their counterparts obtained from dispersed pulmonary parenchyma, in terms of responsiveness to secretagogues and antiallergic drugs. The mast cell growth factor (IL-3) may cause the precursor cell to grow and, in concert with other differentiation factors locally found in the mucosa, may direct the differentiation of this cell into the mucosal pathway. As mentioned previously, strong evidence exists to support the notion that the type of mast cell seen in a tissue site may be directed by factors locally secreted in the tissues. In humans, we have shown that mast cell precursors are present in the circulation and that these are increased in number in atopic patients. In addition, we have shown that these precursors can be found in the nasal mucosa of patients with nasal allergy and that growth factors for these cells are synthesized by local cells including the epithelium in atopic states. Thus, we can postulate that in allergic inflammation, the epithelium begins to secrete factors which attract and cause mast cell precursors to grow and proliferate. In the process, antigens more easily penetrate the epithelium and, if mast cells are sensitized with IgE antibody, cause these cells to release their mediators, and

so initiate and perpetuate an allergic inflammatory response which continues as long as the stimulus (antigen) presents itself (Fig. 38-1).

This is a useful model to contemplate since it invokes many of the principles of interaction to which we have earlier alluded.

Mast cell proliferation also follows immunization and occurs after administration of antigen by aerosol. Thus, injury and the associated repair processes may cause the synthesis and secretion of factors that promote mast cell growth. Depending on the site in which this occurs, i.e., mucosa or parenchyma, phenotypically different mast cells seem to emerge. A massive increase in the number of mast cells occurs in the lungs after the intratracheal administration of bleomycin into rats; in this case, the mast cell type appears to be a connective tissue type of cell. It is particularly interesting that fibroblasts secrete a mast cell growth factor which promotes the connective tissue mast cell growth and further that histamine may cause fibroblasts to proliferate depending on the stage of cell cycle reached. Here we see again the intimate association between cells of different types and their interdependence.

Goblet Cells

Goblet cells secrete mucus in response to a variety of local stimuli. Among these are the neuropeptides and neurotransmitters, and products of the arachidonic acid pathways, such as leukotrienes and prostaglandins. The number of goblet cells in a tissue appears to be influenced by the amount of immune stimulation that is occurring locally. This has been shown in the respiratory tract by aerosol administration of antigen. Furthermore, it has been shown that T cells from the thoracic duct may, on adoptive transfer to secondary recipients, influence the number of goblet cells present in the intestine of rats infected with the nematode *Nippostrongylus brasiliensis*. Since goblet cell proliferation and mucous secretion are characteristics of chronic inflammation, such as bronchitis and asthma, it is pertinent to consider these types of immunophysiological responses when exploring the pathophysiology of these disorders. Furthermore, the amount of mucus present on the epithelial surface can determine not only the efficiency of the ciliary beat as a clearance mechanism, but also the likelihood of antigen coming into contact with the epithelium and, therefore, immunogenicity.

Epithelium

As indicated above, the permeability and the capacity of the epithelium to handle antigen and particulate matter depends on the state of inflammation in the local microenvironment. Epithelial cell function, per se, is also likely to be altered as a result of local mucosal inflammatory events. For example, profound changes in ion flux, water

---

TABLE 38-2

Effects of Heparin

Blocks activated properdin

Blocks mitogen-induced blastogenesis

Inhibits phagocytosis by neutrophils

Enhances phagocytosis by Kupffer cells

Enhances pinocytosis by fibroblasts

Blocks some neutrophil enzymatic activity

Blocks tissue damage by eosinophil major basic protein

Inhibits smooth muscle growth

Causes osteoporosis

Stimulates angiogenesis

SOURCE: From Bienenstock et al., 1987.

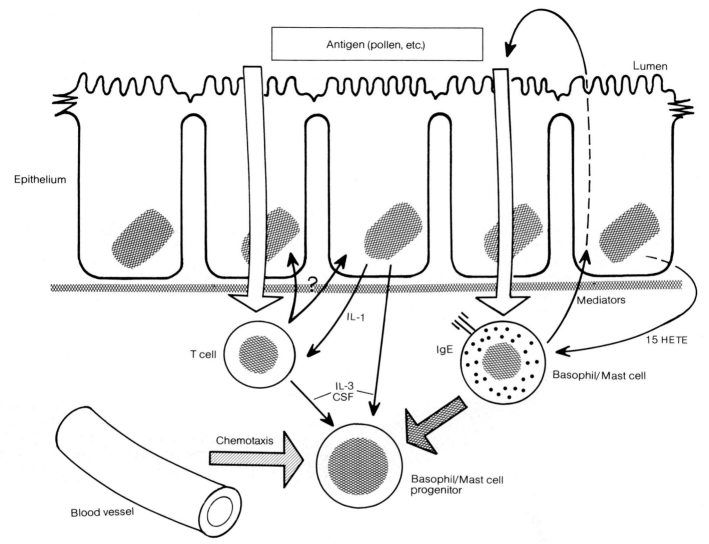

FIGURE 38-1 Schema showing how lymphocytes, mast cells, and the epithelium may interact to promote antigen ingress from the lumen and thus provide a vicious circle of inflammation which may be broken only by removal of the stimulus or a therapeutic intervention.

transport, and glucose uptake can be induced by antigen-specific challenge of the intestine that evokes local anaphylaxis in sensitized animals. This IgE-mediated response, apparently the result of mast cell degranulation, can be abrogated by the administration of doxantrazole, a compound that functionally inhibits secretion by the rat mucosal mast cells; in contrast, disodium cromoglycate has no effect on these cells or the physiological changes elicited. Similar types of effects have been elicited in the rat intestine by Castro and his colleagues long after infection with nematodes was removed, indicating that the intestine responded by epithelial physiological changes to specific antigenic challenge. Finally, short circuit current changes have been found to occur across the gut epithelium of guinea pigs sensitized to milk protein when challenged with specific antigens. Although these types of experiments have not yet been performed in relation to

the respiratory tract, they do illustrate common principles that are of major importance to the understanding of respiratory function and mucosal physiology.

Eosinophils

As do mast cells, eosinophils may depend on T-cell-derived growth factors for proliferation, and possibly also for maturation. T-cell-derived factors can activate eosinophils and cause them to secrete their products. Eosinophil products, such as major basic protein, have deleterious effects on respiratory epithelium. Therefore, the eosinophil may be considered to be directly involved in the pathogenesis of the different forms of respiratory disease in which they participate, and add yet another cellular player to the complex stage of local inflammatory responses on which they perform.

Cellular Communication

In the process of digesting antigen, be it in the airways or in the tissues, macrophages release interleukin 1 (IL-1); keratinocytes and epithelial cells also release IL-1 or IL-1-like molecules. The properties of interleukin 1 are summarized in Table 38-3, which illustrates the extraordinary and extensive nature of the paracrine secretion that also acts as a hormone on a number of tissues. For example, IL-1 appears to be responsible for the pyrexic effect of inflammation by acting directly, or indirectly, on the hypothalamus to alter the temperature set point. It can act on smooth muscle to cause muscle proteolysis and on fibroblasts—depending on the local circumstances—to cause either proliferation or inhibition of growth. Nevertheless, it clearly modulates the function of fibroblasts and their ability to secrete prostaglandins which, in turn, affect the growth and function of fibroblasts as well as other cells. IL-1 appears to be responsible for the production of acute phase reactants by way of a mechanism of communication that involves hepatocytes—which synthesize most of these glycoproteins. In this way, local production of IL-1 in one tissue causes a distal organ (the liver) to synthesize molecules that return via the bloodstream to modulate local tissue inflammation. IL-1 is chemotactic for T cells and leukocytes and increases the release of neutrophils from bone marrow stores. It also alters heavy-metal concentrations in the blood and, if delivered to the brain, appears capable of inducing γ-wave sleep and of acting as a somnogenic factor.

Cellular communication is also involved in the host of different signals that follow the initiation of each immune response; these signals to many tissues and organs have far-reaching biologic implications. Not all immune responses are triggered by specialized macrophages; moreover, immune responses may be modified by local factors including the physiological state of the epithelium, as discussed earlier in the section dealing with mast cells.

Against this background, it is germane to reconsider the association between mast cells and fibroblasts in pulmonary fibrosis. This association is involved in all forms of fibrotic reactions, ranging from keloids to scleroderma. It is known that fibroblasts avidly phagocytose mast cell granules, and this process influences fibroblast function. It is also known that alveolar macrophages contain products capable of degranulating mast cells and that various mast cell products, such as histamine, can modulate the growth of fibroblasts. Furthermore, fibroblasts may secrete "competence factors" that promote the differentiation of connective tissue types of mast cells. Therefore, it is clear that the network of communication between mast cells, alveolar macrophages, and fibroblasts is an important one. Since lymphocytes synthesize factors that can specifically sensitize mast cells, these cells may be extensively involved in delayed hypersensitivity reactions, in addition to those immediate reactions characteristic of allergy.

TABLE 38-3
Biologic Activities of Interleukin 1 (IL-1)

Lymphocytes	Increased T-cell proliferation and IL-2 production
	Chemotaxis of T cells
	Increased B-cell activation and antibody synthesis
Natural killer cells	Enhanced cytotoxicity
Hepatocytes	Increased uptake of amino acids and synthesis of acute phase reactants
	Decreased albumin synthesis
Bone marrow	Release of neutrophils into blood
	Chemotaxis of neutrophils and monocytes
Hypothalamus	Increased PGE_2 synthesis; pyrexia
Brain	Increased γ-wave sleep
Endothelial cells	Increased PGI_2 synthesis and neutrophil adhesiveness
Fibroblasts	Increased PGE_2 and collagenase synthesis
	Modulation of proliferation
Chondrocytes	Increased protease secretion and bone resorption
Muscle	Proteolysis
Systemic effects	Increased serum iron; decreased zinc and copper; decreased appetite

Neuropeptides

Immunity can be modulated by sensory neuropeptides. Somatostatin causes inhibition of growth of lymphocytes, and substance P enhances mitogen-induced proliferation. These opposing effects are somewhat similar to the bidirectional functional regulatory activities of these neuropeptides in the nervous system. Vasointestinal polypeptide causes connective tissue mast cells and basophils to degranulate. It also causes altered localization of T lymphocytes in the intestine, affects phagocytosis by polymorphonuclear leukocytes, and is probably contained in some mucosal mast cells. Substance P and somatostatin have organ-specific effects on immunoglobulin synthesis. Physiological concentrations of substance P increase IgA synthesis by Peyer's patch cells to 700 percent over controls. Somatostatin is generally without effect in these systems, except as a negative effect.

Interactions between mast cells and nerves have been displayed by diverse techniques ranging from electron microscopy to physiological interactions. For example, substance P is the only neuropeptide which causes both mucosal and nonmucosal mast cells to degranulate. Many other neuropeptides cause connective tissue mast cells and basophils, but not mucosal mast cells, to release their constituents. It has been known for some time that both substance P and mast cells are involved in the axon reflex, though the structural basis for this communication has only just been established. Nonmyelinated neurones appear to be intimately associated with mast cells in the intestine, skin, and diaphragm, indicating the existence of a communication network involving mast cells and nerves. Whether this is a two-way communication system or a one-way interaction is unknown. Because of this communication network, it is not surprising that the network of nerves containing neuropeptides may exert major effects on immunity in the respiratory tract and elsewhere when these substances are released.

nisms may be affected by and, in turn, affect local physiological processes in the lung. The intimate and nonrandom interaction of cells as diverse as fibroblasts, epithelial cells, macrophages, lymphocytes, mast cells, goblet cells, eosinophils, and nerves must be integrated into our understanding of normal physiological and altered (disease) states. In addition to improvement in our knowledge, as our horizons expand, we are slowly finding that as always with new knowledge, it may be possible to apply it to fundamental problems of disease and derive and introduce new and possibly more effective therapeutic approaches.

CONCLUSIONS

We have tried to provide a framework of understanding, by the use of selected examples, of how immune mecha-

BIBLIOGRAPHY

Ader R, Cohen N: CNS-Immune system interactions: Conditioning phenomena. Behav Brain Sci 8:379–394, 1985.
 A very good discussion of the whole area of psychological conditioning and immune responses.

Allardyce RA, Bienenstock J: The mucosal immune system in health and disease, with an emphasis on parasitic infection. Bull WHO 62:7–25, 1984.
 Review of the mucosal immune system.

Askenase PW, Loveren HV: Delayed-type hypersensitivity: Activation of mast cells by antigen-specific T-cell factors initiates the cascade of cellular interactions. Immunol Today 4:259–264, 1983.
 Review of involvement of mast cells in delayed hypersensitivity and mechanisms involved.

Barclay AN, Mason DR: Induction of Ia antigen in rat epidermal cells and gut epithelium by immunologic stimuli. J Exp Med 156:1665–1676, 1982.
 Immune responses induce capability of antigen presentation in epithelium.

Beer DJ, Rocklin RE: Histamine induced suppressor cell activity. J Allergy Clin Immunol 73:439–452, 1984.
 Review of role of histamine in immunity.

Befus AD, Bienenstock J, Denburg J: *Mast Cell Heterogeneity.* New York, Raven, 1986, pp 1–426.
 Many chapters of a review nature covering most aspects of mast cell heterogeneity.

Bienenstock J: *Immunology of the Lung and Upper Respiratory Tract.* New York, McGraw-Hill, 1984, pp 1–414.
 Up-to-date information on the lung as an immunologic organ. Includes basic and clinical information.

Bienenstock J: Bronchus-associated lymphoid tissue. Int Archs Allergy Appl Immun 76:62–69, 1985.
 Short review on the subject.

Bienenstock J, Befus AD: Mucosal immunology. Immunology 41:249–270, 1980.
 Fairly detailed review. Good source of references. A little outdated.

Bienenstock J, Befus AD: Regulation of lymphoblast traffic and localization in mucosal tissues, with emphasis on IgA. Fed Proc 42:3213–3217, 1983.
 Review of lymphocyte traffic as pertains to mucosal tissues.

Bienenstock J, Befus AD: Gut and bronchus-associated lymphoid tissue. Am J Anat 170:437–445, 1984.
 Comparative review.

Bienenstock J, Johnston N, Perey DYE: Bronchial lymphoid tissue. I. Morphological characteristics. Lab Invest 28:686–692, 1973.
Original paper outlining the BALT.

Bienenstock J, McDermott MR, Befus AD: The significance of bronchus-associated lymphoid tissue. Bull Europ Physiopath Resp 18:153–177, 1982.
Very complete review, includes extensive early references on the subject.

Bienenstock J, Tomioka M, Matsuda H, Stead RH, Quinonez G, Simon GT, Coughlin MD, Denburg JA: The role of mast cells in inflammatory processes: Evidence for nerve/mast cell interactions. Int Archs Allergy Appl Immun 82:238–243, 1987.
Short, up-to-date review of the subject.

Bitterman PB, Wewers MD, Rennard SI, Adelberg S, Crystal RG: Modulation of alveolar macrophage-driven fibroblast proliferation by alternative macrophage mediators. J Clin Invest 77:700–708, 1986.
In addition to the two primary growth promoting signals, fibronectin and alveolar macrophage-derived growth factor, alveolar macrophages are able to release other mediators that may have a potential role in modulating lung fibroblast replication in response to these primary signals, including interferon γ (IFNγ), prostaglandin E_2 (PGE$_2$), and interleukin 1 (IL-1).

Buck CA, Horwitz AF: Cell surface receptors for extracellular matrix molecules. Ann Rev Cell Biol 3:179–205, 1987.
An overview of the present state of understanding of cell-adhesion molecules that are involved in diverse biologic phenomena within the intercellular matrix.

Castro GA: Immunological regulation of epithelial function. Am J Physiol 243:G321–G329, 1982.
Review of interaction of immune mechanisms with physiological processes in the intestine.

Claman HN: Mast cells, T cells and abnormal fibrosis. Immunol Today 6:192–195, 1985.
Review of the role of mast and T cells in fibrosis.

Clancy R, Bienenstock J: A framework for immunization strategy, in Bienenstock J (ed), *Immunology of the Lung and Upper Respiratory Tract.* New York, McGraw-Hill, 1984, pp 216–231.
A review of immunization strategy to achieve the best lung responses.

Dinarello CA: Interleukin I. Rev Infect Dis 6:51–95, 1984.
Good review of this ubiquitous cytokine.

Dinarello CA: Interleukin-1 and the pathogenesis of the acute-phase response. N Engl J Med 311:1413–1418, 1984.
A concise review of the broad biologic significance of this inflammatory factor.

Ernst PB, Befus AD, Bienenstock J: Leukocytes in the intestinal epithelium: An unusual immunological compartment. Immunol Today 6:50–55, 1985.
Comprehensive review of function of epitheliae lymphocytes.

Gleich G, Frigas E, Filley W, Loegering DA: Eosinophils and bronchial inflammation, in Kay AB, Austen KF, Lichtenstein LM (eds), *Asthma: Physiology, Immunopharmacology and Treatment.* London, Academic, 1984, pp 195–207.
Review of role of eosinophils in pulmonary inflammation and asthma.

Herberman RB: Natural killer cells. Annu Rev Med 37:347–352, 1986.
Natural killer (NK) cells are a subpopulation of lymphocytes, that have spontaneous cytotoxicity against a variety of tumor cells, virus-infected cells, and some normal cells in the bone marrow and thymus. A central role in lysis by NK cells is played by a cytolytic protein contained within their cytoplasmic granules.

Ishizaka K: Mast cell activation and mediator release. Progr Allergy 34:1–336, 1984.
Contains detailed reviews. An excellent source of references and information on this subject.

Katzenstein AL: Pathogenesis of "fibrosis" in interstitial pneumonia: an electron microscopic study. Hum Pathol 16:1015–1024, 1985.
Seven cases in which interstitial fibrosis developed in patients who had acute interstitial pneumonia were studied ultrastructurally to explore the pathogenesis of the interstitial thickening seen by light microscopy.

Lanier LL, Le AM, Cwirla S, Federspiel N, Phillips JH: Antigenic, functional, and molecular genetic studies of human natural killer cells and cytotoxic T lymphocytes not restricted by the major histocompatibility complex. Fed Proc 45:2823–2828, 1986.
Cytotoxicity not restricted by the major histocompatibility complex (MHC) is mediated by two distinct types of lymphocytes: natural killer (NK) cells and non-MHC-restricted cytotoxic T lymphocytes (CTL). NK cells are distinct in lineage from T lymphocytes and do not use the T cell antigen receptor genes for target recognition.

Lee TDG, Swieter M, Bienenstock J, Befus AD: Heterogeneity in mast cell populations. Clin Immunol Rev 4:143–199, 1985.
  Careful and critical review of the evidence for, and significance of, mast cell heterogeneity.

Lipscomb MF, Toews GB, Lyons CR, Uhr JW: Antigen presentation by guinea pig alveolar macrophages. J Immunol 126:286–291, 1981.
  Investigation of the role of alveolar macrophages in the induction of immune responses within the lung.

McDermott MR, Befus AD, Bienenstock J: The structural basis for immunity in the respiratory tract. Int Rev Exp Pathol 23:47–112, 1982.
  Good review of respiratory immune mechanisms.

Meuwissen JH, Hussain M: Bronchus-associated lymphoid tissue in human lung: Correlation of hyperplasia with chronic pulmonary disease. Clin Immunol Immunopathol 23:548–561, 1982.
  Collection of patients with recurrent unexplained lung infections and a type of lymphoid nodular hyperplasia of the lung (BALT).

Payan DG, Levine JD, Goetzl EJ: Opinion: Modulation of immunity and hypersensitivity by sensory neuropeptides. J Immunol 132:1601–1604, 1984.
  Short review of the effect of neuropeptides on immune mechanisms.

Rankin JA, Hitchcock M, Merrill W, Bach MK, Brashler RJ, Askenase PW: IgE-dependent release of leukotriene C from alveolar macrophages. Nature 297:329–331, 1984.
  An original study that describes the IgE receptor on the alveolar macrophage. This is a new observation which has important implications for this cell type in mediating immune and nonimmune inflammatory responses.

Reynolds HY, Chretien J: Respiratory tract fluids: Analysis of content and contemporary use in understanding lung diseases. Dis Month 31:1–98, 1985.
  An overview of cells and mediators in bronchoalveolar lavage fluid.

Stanisz AM, Befus AD, Bienenstock J: Differential effects of vasoactive intestinal peptide, substance P, and somatostatin on immunoglobulin synthesis and proliferations by lymphocytes from Peyer's patches, mesenteric lymph nodes and spleen. J Immunol 136:152–156, 1986.
  Striking effects of some neuropeptides, especially substance P, on immunoglobulin synthesis, such as IgA.

Tomasi TB Jr: Oral tolerance. Transplantation 29:353–356, 1980.
  Review of phenomenon of oral tolerance.

Tomasi TB Jr: Mechanisms of immune regulation at mucosal surfaces. Rev Infect Dis 5:S784–S792, 1983.
  Current understanding of IgA by investigator who did pioneering work in the field.

Underdown B, Schiff JM: Immunoglobulin A: Strategic defense initiative at the mucosal surface. Ann Rev Immunol 4:389–417, 1986.
  Detailed review of role and function of IgA in mucosal defenses.

Young KR, Rankin JA, Naegel GP, Paul ES, Reynolds HY: Bronchoalveolar lavage cells and proteins with the acquired immunodeficiency syndrome: An immunologic analysis. Ann Intern Med 103:522–533, 1985.
  Immunology of AIDS lung disease presented.

Chapter 39

Immune Defenses of the Lung

Ronald P. Daniele

Macrophages and the Immune Response

Structure of the Lungs' Immune Defenses

Bronchoalveolar Airspaces

Lessons Learned from Lavage

The Secretory System

Lymph Nodes and Lymphatics

Fate of Inhaled Antigens in the Lung

The lung defends against respirable particles by two primary mechanisms: clearance by the mucociliary blanket in the proximal airways and phagocytosis by the alveolar macrophage in the distal airways (Fig. 39-1). Inhaled particles greater than 5 μm in diameter are generally trapped on the mucociliary blanket and are then redirected toward the mouth for elimination within hours by swallowing or expectoration. Most particles that are smaller than 5 μm in diameter reach the distal airways, where they are handled almost exclusively by alveolar macrophages which ingest them. The inhaled particles may then experience one of several fates: (1) complete degradation within the phagosome of the macrophage; (2) transport without degradation by alveolar macrophages, which migrate up the distal airways to reach the mucociliary escalator for elimination, usually within days; and (3) transport of engulfed particles by alveolar macrophages into interstitium and peribronchial lymphatics.

Particles that are conveyed to the interstitium by the latter route are often retained within the host for months to years and interact with collections of lymphoid cells beneath the bronchial mucosa and in the draining tracheobronchial lymph nodes. Also, there is evidence that bronchial epithelial cells may transport (e.g., by pinocytosis) antigenic particles directly across the mucosa. Nonetheless, by whatever route substances gain access to recognized pulmonary lymphoid tissue (e.g., secretory system), the full development of an immune response to substances recognized as antigens requires intimate collaboration between phagocytic cells and lymphocytes. Whether alveolar macrophages or tissue (or interstitial) phagocytes or both are involved in this interaction remains problematic. In any case, instead of being a solitary scavenger in the distal airways, the alveolar macrophage appears to be an active participant in the highly structured immune system of the lung.

MACROPHAGES AND THE IMMUNE RESPONSE

In other immune tissues (e.g., lymph node and spleen), the phagocyte assumes a crucial role in the recognition and disposal of antigen. The afferent or recognitive phase usually begins with antigen processing by the phagocyte. This processing not only includes degradation but also a poorly defined preparative step that allows optimal presentation of antigen to immunocompetent cells, thereby stimulating the production of antibody and/or sensitized cells.

Macrophages (including alveolar macrophages) are part of a group of cells, called *accessory cells*, that are capable of antigen presentation and include epidermal Langerhans cells, dendritic cells of lymphoid organs, and vascular endothelial cells. A common and essential feature of these cells is that they display class II major histocompatibility complex (MHC) antigens (HLA-DR, DP, DQ) which are recognized by T cells. For T cells to generate a cell-mediated or humoral response, they must recognize antigen in association with a genetically compatible expression of MHC surface determinants on macrophages (MHC restriction).

Depending on the type of antigen, presentation of antigens by the macrophage to lymphocytes within lymph nodes and spleen results in a predominantly cellular or humoral immune response. Whether a given antigen induces a cellular or humoral immunity depends on a number of ill-defined factors including the size, route of entry, and biologic properties of the antigen.

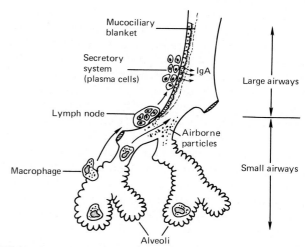

FIGURE 39-1 Components of lungs' defenses: Mucociliary escalator in proximal bronchi and alveolar macrophages in the distal airways. Arrows indicate possible routes alveolar macrophages may take in eliminating airborne particles.

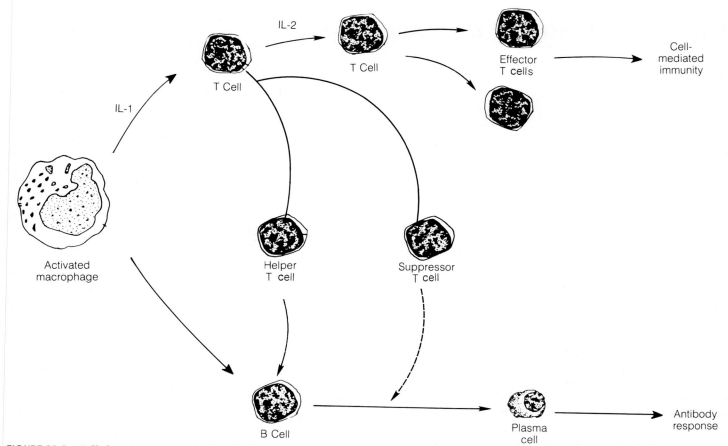

FIGURE 39-2 Cellular interactions involved in the generation of the immune response. Antigen presentation leads to stimulation of the T-cell or B-cell system. Factors involved in the T-cell system include interleukin 1 (IL-1), which stimulates T cells to acquire a receptor for a T-cell growth factor called interleukin 2 (IL-2); the same subpopulation of T cells may also secrete IL-2.

Cellular immune responses (delayed hypersensitivity) are mediated by thymus-derived lymphocytes or T cells. Antigen interaction with the T-cell system usually leads to cellular proliferation or activation. It is now recognized that T-cell proliferation and the generation of effector cells occur in at least two steps (Fig. 39-2). The first involves antigen interaction with macrophages and the release of a soluble factor, interleukin 1, which stimulates resting T cells so that they can respond to a second signal. The second product is derived from stimulated T cells and is mitogenic for T cells; this growth factor, called *interleukin 2,* signals responsive T cells to proliferate and differentiate into effector cells. Among the progeny of antigen-stimulated T cells are memory cells that respond more rapidly after challenge to the original antigen, killer cells which destroy alien cells, and effector cells that produce nonimmunoglobulin molecules called *lymphokines.*

Lymphokines are a diverse group of molecules secreted by T cells (and B cells) in response to certain antigenic stimuli. They can increase capillary permeability and influence the movement, activation, and function of phagocytic cells. Together, lymphokines probably play an important role in the generation of inflammatory responses, particularly those involving cell-mediated immunity.

Humoral responses are the end result of antigen interaction with bursal equivalent lymphocytes (B cells). B-cell function, however, is regulated by at least two subpopulations of T cells. One subset of cooperative T cells, called *helper* T cells, is required for optimal antibody production to most antigens (Fig. 39-2). Another distinct subpopulation of lymphocytes, called *suppressor* T cells, inhibits or modulates the humoral response once it is initiated.

Until recently, suppressor and helper T cells in humans were only functionally defined. Now, however, human T cell subsets have been shown to express distinct differentiation antigens, which can be identified with monoclonal antibodies (e.g., OK4 and OK8 antibodies to helper and suppressor T cells, respectively).

In the effector, or antigenic disposal, phase the macrophage again assumes a prominent role and interacts

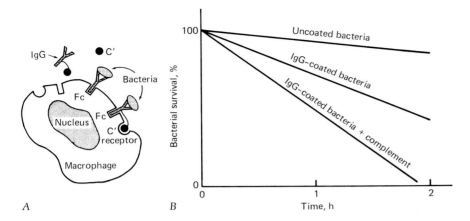

A *B*

FIGURE 39-3 *A.* Receptors on macrophages. Fc denotes macrophage receptors for C-terminal portions of immunoglobin molecules, predominantly IgG1 and IgG3. C' receptor represents receptor for complement components. *B.* An in vitro assay that demonstrates the importance of macrophage receptors. Macrophages are incubated with unsensitized bacteria, bacteria coated with specific antibody (IgG), and bacteria sensitized by IgG and complement (C'). The percent of surviving bacteria of the original inoculum are plotted as functions of time.

with the products of both T-cell and B-cell systems. The macrophage possesses a receptor for the Fc, or carboxy, portion of the IgG molecule (Fig. 39-3*A*). The Fc portion does not contain the antibody-combining site, but depending on the antibody class, it may fix complement and interact with a complementary receptor (Fc receptors) on certain cell types (e.g., macrophages, mast cells). When a specific antibody combines with a foreign substance (e.g., opsonizes) such as a bacteria, fixation via the macrophage membrane Fc receptor occurs, enhancing phagocytosis and promoting the killing of bacteria (Fig. 39-3*B*). Also, when antibody combines with specific antigen, certain classes of antibody, such as IgG and IgM, interact with and activate the complement system. One of the activated components, C'3b, binds to the Fc portion of antibody. Macrophages also possess a receptor for the activated components of complement, such as C'3b. Particles and organisms that are coated with both antibody and complement may interact with the C'3b receptor of the macrophage, resulting in optimal phagocytosis and killing (Fig. 39-3*B*). The human alveolar macrophage possesses both a C'3b and Fc receptor for IgG, suggesting that interaction with these protein systems may be important in respiratory defenses.

In promoting cellular immune responses, lymphokine production by T cells (or B cells) also has important effects on macrophages. Four examples of lymphokine molecules that are produced by T (or B) cells are macrophage inhibition factor, macrophage chemotactic factor, interferons, and macrophage-activating factor. These lymphokines serve to attract the monocytes or macrophages to the site of inflammation or antigenic stimulation, keep them there, and activate or arm them for enhanced phagocytosis and bacterial killing.

STRUCTURE OF THE LUNGS' IMMUNE DEFENSES

One operational model of the lungs' immune system is pictured as existing in three distinct compartments (Fig.

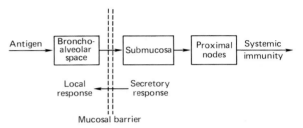

FIGURE 39-4 Three compartment model of the lungs' immune system.

39-4), each containing immunocompetent cells (lymphocytes and macrophages): (1) the bronchoalveolar airspaces, (2) the submucosal or secretory antibody system lying beneath the lamina propria of the tracheobronchial tree, and (3) a network of lymphatic vessels and lymph nodes lining the tracheobronchial tree. Within each of these compartments, the potential exists for lymphocyte-macrophage interaction for both antigen recognition and disposal.

Within the last 5 years, much of our knowledge about immune responses in the lung has come from studies involving cells recovered from bronchoalveolar airspaces by segmental pulmonary lavage in humans or total lung lavage in experimental animals.

BRONCHOALVEOLAR AIRSPACES

Until the advent of the flexible fiberoptic bronchoscope, little was known about the cells and secretions in the bronchoalveolar airspaces of the human lung. Since this technique was introduced, it has been observed that in nonsmoking adults cell yields equal 10 to 15 × 10⁶ cells per 100 ml of lavage fluid and alveolar macrophages are the predominant cell type (80 to 90 percent); lymphocytes constitute about 10 percent of the cells. Neutrophils, eosinophils, and basophils represent less than 1 percent of the cells (Table 39-1).

TABLE 39-1

Cellular and Soluble Constituents in Bronchoalveolar Lavage Fluid*

Cells	
Macrophages	84 ± 1
Lymphocytes	11 ± 1
T cells	62 ± 2
Helper T (T4)	46 ± 3
Suppressor (T8)	25 ± 2
B cells	5 ± 2
Neutrophils, eosinophils, basophils	<1
Soluble factors	
IgG, IgA	+
IgM	−
C4, C3, Factor B	+
C5	−

* All values are for normal nonsmokers; data expressed as mean ± standard deviation.

SOURCE: From Daniele, Elias, Epstein, Rossman, Ann Intern Med 102:93–108, 1985.

In smokers, the cell yield is up to four times greater; macrophages usually account for 90 percent or more of recovered cells and lymphocytes for 1 to 5 percent. There may also be a slightly higher proportion of neutrophils (1 to 4 percent).

The distribution of lymphocyte subpopulations in the lavage fluid is similar to that seen in blood, with T cells equaling 60 to 70 percent of the cells, and B cells equaling 5 to 10 percent. The ratio of helper cells to suppressor T cells is 1.6:1 and is comparable to what is found in blood.

The major soluble constituents in lavage fluid are IgG and IgA; their concentrations reflect the rate of active transport across the bronchial epithelium. Relatively little, or no, IgM is present. Components of both the classic and alternative pathways have also been identified in lavage fluid.

Much needs to be learned about the functional role of lymphocytes in the normal human lung, particularly with respect to their initiation and development of immune responses. The evidence, however, is more substantial in experimental animals. Lymphocytes recovered by total lung lavage in guinea pigs and rabbits respond to antigens introduced into the respiratory tract by producing antibody and lymphokines [e.g., macrophage migration inhibition factor (MIF)]. Furthermore, lung lymphocytes can demonstrate an anamnestic response to airborne antigens and, depending on the type and dose of antigen, exhibit a capacity to respond that is independent of systemic lymphoid tissue. Thus, animal experiments indicate that localized immune responses can occur within the bronchoalveolar airspaces.

Alternatively, it has been proposed that the cells and secretions in the bronchoalveolar airspaces are deployed there so as to prevent entry of antigenic particles beyond the mucosal barrier and to deter antigen interaction with organized lung lymphoid tissue. According to this notion of "immune exclusion," the primary function of the alveolar macrophage is to ingest and remove particles from the lung rather than to transport them to submucosal and tracheobronchial lymph nodes where interactions may occur between collections of lymphocytes and tissue macrophages. Which of these two hypotheses is correct remains to be settled.

The two hypotheses, however, may not be mutually exclusive. For certain inhaled inert substances, the nonspecific activities of the alveolar macrophage and mucociliary blanket in expelling these substances may be entirely adequate. For other antigens, such as microorganisms with capsular membranes that resist phagocytosis, nonspecific clearance mechanisms would not suffice and require the aid of specific antibody and cells in bronchial secretions to permit effective phagocytosis, killing, and clearance. The generation of a specific immune response consisting of either antibody or cells in bronchial secretions requires, however, that the inciting antigen in some way penetrates the mucosal barrier and stimulates submucosal lymphoid cells. This same condition applies to any inhaled particles (e.g., allergens, organic particles) that result in local humoral and cellular immune responses. It should also be emphasized that initially only a relatively small fraction of the inhaled antigenic load may actually be required to stimulate submucosal lymphoid tissue. Once initiated, the secretion of antibody or the appearance of sensitized cells in the airspaces would greatly enhance the exclusion of the same or similar inhaled antigens upon subsequent challenges.

The degree to which nonspecific defenses interact with specific immune responses in the lung remains ill-defined but probably depends on a number of factors: (1) the size of the particle, (2) the antigenic load, (3) the physicochemical characteristics of the particle which relate to its antigenicity, toxicity, and (4) perhaps most important, its biologic properties (e.g., type of virus, capsulated bacteria, etc.).

These are some of the variables which determine whether inhaled particles and microbes are contained or eliminated or result in lung injury and disease. Equally important is the unique genetic background of the host, especially the immune responses that are linked to the immune response genes. The latter consideration may be particularly relevant for two of the immunologic diseases, hypersensitivity pneumonitis and chronic berylliosis, which will be discussed elsewhere. In both of these disorders, only a minority of those exposed to specific airborne antigens develop disease.

LESSONS LEARNED FROM LAVAGE

The examination of cells and secretions in broncho-alveolar lavage fluid from patients with immunologic lung diseases has provided several important insights into pathogenesis. First, the lung may be the site of compartmentalized inflammatory response as in hypersensitivity pneumonitis, in which the disease is restricted to the lung. In other systemic disorders, the inflammatory response that evolves in the lung may not be reflected in the peripheral blood. Notably, in a systemic disease such as sarcoidosis, the immunologic abnormalities that occur within the airway and the pulmonary parenchyma are often opposite those in peripheral blood. The reason for this difference is unclear, but one hypothesis is that when the lung is involved, it appears to act as a selective target for acute (neutrophils) or chronic (lymphocytes and monocytes) inflammatory cells, which are increased in the pulmonary parenchyma as well as in the lavage fluid. Second, pulmonary lavage has established the existence of two predominant types of chronic inflammatory response in the lung, one involving neutrophils and macrophages (idiopathic pulmonary fibrosis), the other involving lymphocytes and macrophages (hypersensitivity pneumonitis and sarcoidosis). Finally, several laboratories have emphasized the heightened state of activation of these inflammatory cells. Lymphocyte activation probably reflects immune stimulation in cases of hypersensitivity pneumonitis, berylliosis, and possibly sarcoidosis (Chapters 42, 44, and 54).

THE SECRETORY SYSTEM

The secretory immune system consists of lymphocytes and plasma cells lining the tracheobronchial tree. These cells secrete antibody molecules, which are then transported by the epithelial cells into the bronchial lumen. During passage through the epithelial cell, the secretory immunoglobulin IgA acquires a glycoprotein molecule called the secretory piece. The function of the secretory piece is incompletely understood, but it seems to allow IgA dimers to resist proteolytic digestion by enzymes that are present in both the bronchial and gastrointestinal secretions. IgA antibody-secreting cells of the secretory system originate in subepithelial collections of lymphoid cells in the lung (bronchial-associated lymphoid tissue, BALT), which are similar in appearance and function to Peyer's patches in the gut (Figs. 39-5 and 39-6).

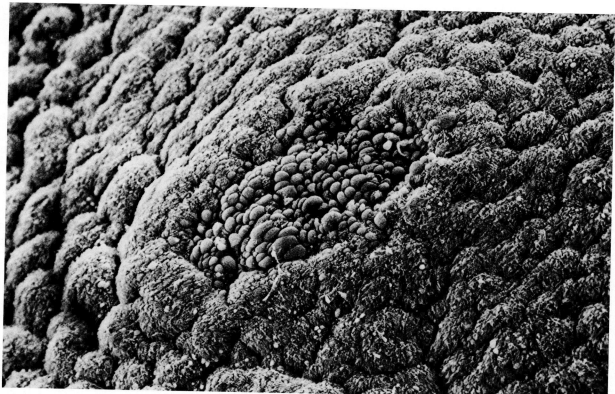

FIGURE 39-5 Scanning electron microscopic photograph of rabbit bronchial epithelium. The carpet of ciliated epithelial cells is interrupted by clusters of lymphoepithelial cells (BALT) which lack cilia but possess microvilli (×96). *(Courtesy of J. Bienenstock.)*

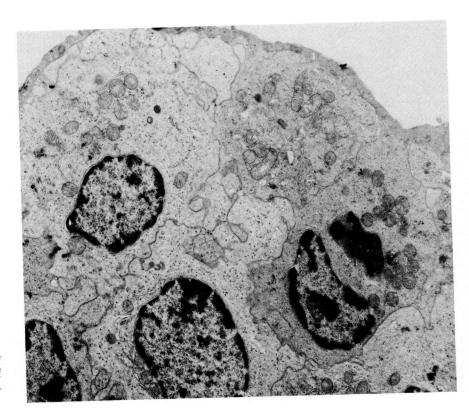

FIGURE 39-6 Transmission electron microscopy of BALT. Lymphocytes covered by thin extension of lymphoepithelium (×11,250). *(Courtesy of Q. N. Myrvik.)*

The IgA in bronchial secretions appears to protect the lung in several ways: (1) by inhibiting viruses from infecting epithelial cells; (2) by promoting clumping and decreasing adherence to mucosal surfaces of certain bacteria (streptococcus); and (3) in combination with lysozyme (and complement) present in bronchial secretions, by promoting phagocytosis of IgA-coated particles and bacteria.

Until recently, it was unclear how secretory IgA interacted with the alveolar macrophage. This uncertainty stemmed from two causes: (1) the alveolar macrophage lacks a receptor for IgA antibody and (2) IgA does not fix complement by the classic pathway. Thus, it first appeared that the enhanced phagocytosis (and killing) resulting from particles or bacteria that are coated (or opsonized) with antibody and complement might not be operative in the lung. A way out of this dilemma was suggested by two observations that allow macrophages to interact with secretory immunoglobulins in bronchial secretions. First, bronchial secretions have been shown to contain precursors for complement activation. This is of potential importance since, under certain conditions, IgA may fix complement via the alternative pathway and allow interaction of opsonized particles with the alveolar macrophage C′3b receptor. Second, regional differences in the class of actively secreted immunoglobulins have been found along the respiratory tract, and IgA has proved not to be the exclusive secretory immunoglobulin in bronchial secretions. Thus, IgA predominates in the nasal and upper respiratory secretions, whereas IgG is the major immunoglobulin in the lower respiratory tract. These distinctions are important since, as previously mentioned, the alveolar macrophage possesses an Fc receptor for IgG, but not for IgA. Moreover, alveolar macrophages express Fc receptors for IgG1 and IgG3 subclasses; both of these Ig subclasses actively bind complement. Bacteria have been shown to be more effectively phagocytized by the alveolar macrophages when coated or opsonized with IgG than with IgA molecules. Thus, immunoglobulins and precursors of complement in bronchial secretions interact in a specific manner with alveolar macrophages.

Secretory IgA also relates to the theory of immune exclusion. Because of its antiviral properties and capacity to agglutinate and impair the adherence of certain antigens to the mucosal surface, IgA is thought to prevent entry of antigens beyond the mucosal barrier by augmenting antigen elimination by phagocytosis and clearance mechanisms. This hypothesis is supported by the increased association of allergic disease and circulating antibodies to food proteins in patients with IgA deficiency.

IgE was once linked with IgA as a secretory immunoglobulin. This notion, however, needs revision in light of recent evidence indicating that IgE does not bind to secretory components and is not actively transported by epithelial cells. Moreover, earlier estimates of the distribution of IgE-bearing immunocytes in the lamina propria of the upper respiratory tract were inaccurate. Application of newer immunohistochemical techniques, which distinguish IgE B cells from mast cells, reveals fewer IgE B cells than previously thought.

The concentration of IgE in bronchoalveolar lavage fluid is barely detectable, but it may increase in certain allergic inflammatory states. Although the deleterious effects that follow mast cell and basophil sensitization by IgE molecules in the atopic individual have been well studied, the defensive role of IgE in bronchial secretions remains obscure. There is some evidence that IgE possesses antiviral properties and that IgE cooperates with IgA in defending against certain microorganisms. The latter is supported by the clinical observation that patients with combined deficiency of secretory IgE and IgA but not IgA alone have a greater incidence of sinopulmonary infections.

Recently, it was demonstrated that alveolar macrophages in humans and certain species possess Fc receptors for IgE. This finding provides an important and direct link between immune events in the airways and the secretory activities of the submucosal immune system. When alveolar macrophages are exposed to specific IgE-allergens or anti-IgE antibody, there is a rapid release of lysosomal enzymes, neutral proteases, and superoxide anion. Also, the binding and bridging of IgE receptors on alveolar macrophages causes the release of leukotriene C. Thus, in sensitized individuals, inhaled allergens may initiate an inflammatory response directly within the airways. The release of certain of these inflammatory mediators by allergen-IgE complexes may represent another mechanism by which bronchial epithelial permeability is altered, and allergens and particles gain access to the submucosal immune system.

LYMPH NODES AND LYMPHATICS

An extensive network of lymphatic channels drains the pulmonary parenchyma and communicates with submucosal lymphoid aggregates and tracheobronchial lymph nodes. Some of these lymphatic channels originate from respiratory bronchioles. Macklin considered these collections of lymphocytes and the specialized epithelial cells that cover them to be "sumps" for trapping and removing respirable particles. These lymphoepithelial aggregates, and the associated lymphatics, constitute another route for particles or particle-laden macrophages to reach organized lymphoid tissue.

FATE OF INHALED ANTIGENS IN THE LUNG

Having described the basic architecture of the lungs' immune system, it is important to consider an alternative to the "immune exclusion theory" and describe in some detail the ways by which antigenic particles may penetrate the bronchial submucosa and gain access to pulmonary lymphoid tissue. One pathway involves specialized sites along the tracheobronchial tree where antigen is transported across the bronchial epithelium to submucosal lymphoid tissue. As shown in Fig. 39-7, these include areas where specialized epithelium covers bronchial-associated lymphoid tissue (BALT) in the proximal airways and the less-defined lymphoid aggregates in the distal airways.

It was first thought that the major function of BALT was to provide the precursors of IgA plasma cells beneath the lamina propria. Newer evidence, however, indicates that the epithelium overlying BALT is capable of pinocytizing and transporting soluble as well as particulate antigens (Fig. 39-8). It is noteworthy that BALT is preferentially located at bifurcations in the tracheobronchial tree, increasing the probability for inertial impaction of inhaled particles at these sites.

In the more distal airways, particularly in the respiratory bronchioles, similar epithelial cells cover another collection of lymphoid aggregates, which Macklin originally called "pulmonary sumps." Again, it has been demonstrated that these specialized lymphoepithelial cells are capable of transporting antigens by a pinocytotic mechanism across the mucosal boundary. Morphologically, the epithelial cells covering BALT and lymphoid aggregates share several unique features: the cells are flattened and possess irregular microvilli and no cilia; the cytoplasm

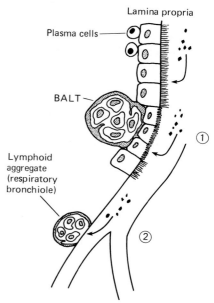

FIGURE 39-7 Locations in tracheobronchial tree where epithelial cells may transport antigenic particles across the mucosa: (1) BALT, (2) lymphoid aggregates that are close to respiratory bronchioles.

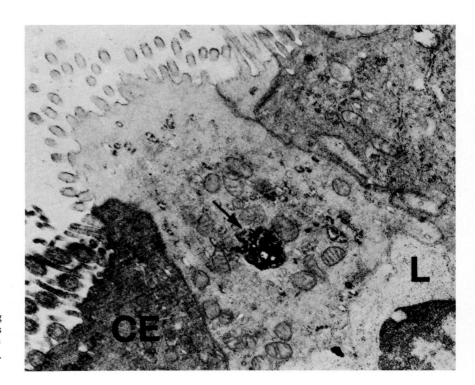

FIGURE 39-8 BALT. Lymphoepithelium containing pinocytosed horseradish peroxidase deposits (arrow) in vacuoles of a lymphoepithelial cell. L = lymphocyte; CE = ciliated epithelial cell. (×8,900). *(Courtesy of Q. N. Myrvik.)*

contains numerous vesicles and vacuoles (Fig. 39-8). Unlike BALT, the lymphoid aggregates in the distal airways are less organized and do not contain true germinal centers. Lymphatics originate from these lymphoid aggregates and probably connect extensively with lymphoid collections in the more proximal airways such as BALT and plasma cell collections beneath the lamina propria.

There is also some evidence that nonciliated epithelial cells scattered throughout the respiratory tree that are not associated with discrete lymphoid collections may also pinocytose and transport particles and antigens across the mucosal boundary. In fact, under certain circumstances, type I and type II cells have been shown to actively take up particulate antigens. Thus, a picture is emerging whereby discrete loci of respiratory epithelium act as ports of entry for inhaled antigens.

Until recently, it was unclear what role alveolar macrophages played in transporting antigen from the airways to organized lymphoid tissue. Recent experiments, however, using fluorescent-labeled microspheres that were instilled into canine lungs showed that alveolar macrophages can ingest inhaled particles and migrate directly to tracheobronchial lymph nodes. Thus, alveolar macrophages probably participate directly in the induction of immune responses in the lung.

In summary, the local immune system represents a component of the lungs' general defense mechanisms. Specific responses to inhaled antigens involve the transport of cells and antibodies into bronchial secretions and operate in concert with nonspecific mechanisms to eliminate antigens from the respiratory tract. Of particular importance are lymphocytes and antibody interactions with the alveolar macrophage in enhancing phagocytosis of particles and the killing of microbes. The degree to which the immune system cooperates with the nonspecific activities of the alveolar macrophage and the mucociliary blanket depends on a number of ill-defined factors which, for the most part, include the particle load and the biologic characteristics of the inhaled particle.

BIBLIOGRAPHY

Bienenstock J, McDermott MR, Befus AD: The significance of bronchus-associated lymphoid tissue. Bull Eur Physiopathol Respir 18:153–177, 1982.
  A review of the structure and function of bronchial-associated lymphoid tissue; it also describes the species variation for this immune stucture.

Brain JD, Sorokin SP, Godleski JJ: Quantification, origin and fate of pulmonary macrophages in Brain JD, Proctor DF, Reid LM (eds), *Lung Biology in Health and Disease, part II, vol 5, Respiratory Defense Mechanisms.* New York, Dekker, 1977, pp 849–892.
  An excellent and concise description of the development of pulmonary macrophages.

Daniele RP, Elias JA, Epstein PE, Rossman MD: Bronchoalveolar lavage: Role in the pathogenesis, diagnosis, and management of interstitial lung disease. Ann Intern Med 102:93–108, 1985.
  A current review on the methodologic approaches of bronchoalveolar lavage. It emphasizes the findings with respect to pathogenesis of immune diseases in humans.

Dinarello CA: Interleukin-1 and the pathogenesis of the acute-phase response. N Engl J Med 311:1413–1418, 1984.
  A concise review of the broad biologic significance of this inflammatory factor.

Fels AO, Cohn ZA: The alveolar macrophage. J Appl Physiol 60:353–369, 1986.
  In addition to its endocytic, phagocytic and microbicidal roles, the alveolar macrophage produces a wide variety of pro- and anti-inflammatory agents including arachidonic acid metabolites of the cyclooxygenase and lipoxygenase pathways, cytokines which modulate lymphocyte function and factors which promote fibroblast migration and replication.

Green GM, Jakob GJ, Low RB, Davis GS: Defense mechanisms of the respiratory membrane. Am Rev Respir Dis 115:479–514, 1977.
  A review on the nonimmune defenses of the respiratory tract; emphasizes the function of the alveolar macrophage.

Harmsen AG, Muggenburg BA, Snipes MB, Bice DE: The role of macrophages in particle translocation from lungs to lymph nodes. Science 230:1277–1280, 1985.
  An original study which describes an important pathway of the macrophage across the mucosal barrier to draining lymph nodes.

Racz P, Tenner-Racz K, Myrvik QN, Fainter LK: Functional architecture of bronchial associated lymphoid tissue and lymphoepithelium in pulmonary cell-mediated reactions in the rabbit. J Reticuloendothel Soc 22:59–83, 1977.
  A well illustrated study of the bronchial-associated lymphoid tissue in the rabbit; also describes its capacity to transport particles as well as microbes across the lymphoepithelium.

Rankin JA, Hitchcock M, Merrill W, Bach MK, Brashler RJ, Askenase PW: IgE-dependent release of leukotriene C from alveolar macrophages. Nature 297:329–331, 1984.
  An original study that describes the IgE receptor on the alveolar macrophage. This is a new observation which has important implications for this cell type in mediating immune and nonimmune inflammatory responses.

Reynolds HY: Lung inflammation: normal host defense or a complication of some diseases? Annu Rev Med 38:295–323, 1987.
  After a review of the normal interactions between alveolar macrophages, various opsonins, complement and chemotactic factors, and the responsiveness of PMNs, several examples of disease are presented.

Romain PL, Schlossman SF: Human T lymphocyte subsets: Functional heterogeneity and surface recognition structures. J Clin Invest 74:1559–1565, 1984.
  A clear and current review on the human T-cell lymphocyte subsets that are defined by monoclonal antibodies.

Unanue ER, Beller DI, Lu CY, Allen PM: Antigen presentation: Comments on its regulation and mechanism. J Immunol 132:1–4, 1984.
  A review of the molecular events involved in antigen presentation by accessory cells and monocytes. Although it is a general review, the descriptions of these mechanisms apply to alveolar macrophages.

Chapter 40

The Eosinophil

A. B. Kay

An increase in the number of eosinophils in the blood, tissues, or sputum is found in many pulmonary disorders. In fact, eosinophilia has been recognized in almost every type of lung pathology, although characteristically the cell is associated with bronchial asthma, allergic bronchopulmonary aspergillosis (ABPA), and "pulmonary eosinophilia" (Table 40-1). Traditionally, pulmonary eosinophilia has been used to describe those syndromes characterized by fleeting shadows visible on the chest radiograph, associated with a *blood* eosinophilia. Pulmonary eosinophilia can be conveniently divided into identifiable causes (fungi, helminths, and drugs), and unknown causes [cryptogenic pulmonary eosinophilia (chronic eosinophilic pneumonia) and the Churg-Strauss syndrome].

In adults the majority of eosinophils are produced in the bone marrow, probably under the influence of factors derived from T lymphocytes. Human *eosinophil colony stimulating factors* (EO-CSFs) have been identified from T cells challenged with specific antigen, monocytes (unstimulated), and T-cell clones challenged with specific antigen. These may all be identical with CSFα (obtained from human placental conditioned medium). The *eosinophil colony forming cell* (EO-CFC) is possibly a null cell. CSFα (colony stimulating factor) and other eosinophil colony stimulating factors also activate eosinophils directly.

Eosinophils are usually considered as "end-stage" cells although mitotic division is occasionally observed

within tissues. In vitro the cells can remain viable for several days. For every circulating eosinophil there are approximately 200 mature eosinophils in the bone marrow and 500 in loose submucosal connective tissue. Therefore, there is a dynamic turnover of eosinophils with production by the bone marrow and transport via the blood to certain tissue sites. The eventual fate of the cell is not fully understood, although intact or ruptured eosinophils may be engulfed by macrophages or pass through the intestinal and respiratory mucosae and be excreted.

STRUCTURE OF THE EOSINOPHIL

In all species the eosinophil is characterized by the presence of large intracytoplasmic granules (Fig. 40-1). Human eosinophils are approximately 10 to 15 μm in diameter and contain about 200 refractile granules which stain a yellow-pink color with acid aniline dyes such as eosin or chromotrope 2R. The granules are often spherical or ovoid and about 0.5 to 1.0 μm in diameter. Ultrastructural studies show that the granules contain a crystalline core (or *internum*) surrounded by a less-electron-dense matrix bounded by a double-layered membrane. The granules contain a number of unique proteins, although some of these enzymes are also present in neutrophils and basophils. The high content of a biochemically distinct peroxidase and the presence of at least three other basic proteins are the principal distinguishing features of the granules.

In addition to the large crystalloids, a smaller granule is present, but only in mature eosinophils. This does not contain a crystalline core but stains intensely for acid phosphatase and arylsulfatase. These smaller granules are thought to be derived from the Golgi apparatus.

TABLE 40-1
Diseases Associated with Pulmonary Eosinophilia

Bronchial eosinophilia
    Bronchial asthma
Pulmonary eosinophilia (PIE syndromes)
    Identifiable causes
    Allergic bronchopulmonary mycoses (particularly aspergillosis)
    Helminths (e.g., ascariasis, microfilariasis, schistosomiasis, *Toxocara canis*)
    Drugs (e.g., nitrofurantoin, sulfonamides, *p*-aminosalicylic acid, penicillin)
    Unknown causes
    Cryptogenic pulmonary eosinophilia (chronic eosinophilic pneumonia)
    Churg-Strauss syndrome
Other lung diseases
    Cryptogenic fibrosing alveolitis (interstitial pulmonary fibrosis)
    Carcinoma of the lung (uncommon)

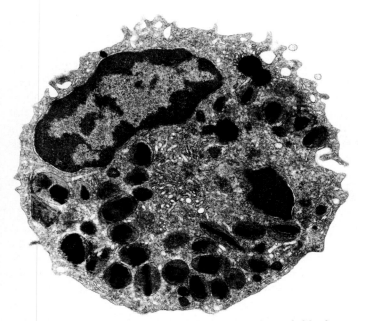

FIGURE 40-1 Electron micrograph of a human eosinophil leukocyte showing the typical crystalloid granules (×16,000). *(Courtesy of Anne Dewar, Cardiothoracic Institute, London.)*

The eosinophil nucleus is similar in appearance to those of other mature granulocytes and contains clumps of condensed chromatin distributed against the nuclear membrane with filamentary connections between nuclear lobes. Nucleoli, the site of ribosomal RNA production, are absent from the mature cell suggesting that major biosynthetic processes have ceased.

GRANULE CONSTITUENTS

The crystalloid core of the eosinophil is composed almost entirely of an arginine-rich *major basic protein* (MBP). Guinea pig and human MBP has been highly purified by isolating the granules and eluting the protein with dilute acids. Human MBP has a molecular weight of 10,000 and an isoelectric point of greater than 11. In vitro, MBP kills schistosomula of *Schistosoma mansoni* and other helminthic larvae. It is likely that this represents an important mechanism for larval killing in vivo, although this is yet to be proved conclusively. MBP may also act as a ligand to facilitate adherence of eosinophils to the surface of parasitic larvae. MBP has also been identified in human basophils suggesting that these two cell types may have common origins.

Another arginine-rich protein associated with human eosinophil granules is the *eosinophil cationic protein* (ECP) which has a molecular size of 21,000 and is immunochemically distinct from MBP. Associated with ECP, there are a number of properties which include alterations of the coagulation pathway and inhibition of T-cell blasto-genesis. ECP also damages schistosomula of *S. mansoni* in vitro in a similar fashion to that described for MBP, and on a molar basis ECP appears to be more potent. Monoclonal antibodies have been raised to both a storage and secreted form of ECP, thus enabling the ready identification of granule secretory products in tissues.

The matrix (or cortex) surrounding the core of the eosinophil granule is rich in a relatively cyanide-insensitive peroxidase which differs from myeloperoxidase of the neutrophil both antigenically and biochemically. Peroxidase has been shown to be discharged into phagosomes after phagocytosis and onto the surface of certain helminthic worms following adherence. Eosinophil peroxidase, in the presence of H_2O_2 and a halide, induced noncytotoxic mast cell degranulation. The precise in vivo significance of this observation is unknown, but it may be an important amplification mechanism in the release of pharmacologic mediators of hypersensitivity.

Genetic deficiency of eosinophil peroxidase has been reported, and it appears to be transmitted as an autosomal recessive mode of inheritance. The anomaly has been described in two families in the Middle East. The eosinophils had hypersegmented nuclei and gave negative histochemical staining for peroxidase but normal staining for basic proteins and acid phosphatases. These individuals appear to be clinically normal.

Eosinophils also possess a fourth cationic granule associated protein [*eosinophil-derived neurotoxin* (EDN)], which has a molecular weight of approximately 18,000. In experimental animals EDN was shown to damage Purkinje cells and myelinated neurons (the "Gordon phenomenon").

Charcot-Leyden crystals (CLC) are elongated, dipyramidal-shaped hexagonal crystals which have been recognized for more than 100 years and are associated with a number of conditions characterized by a tissue or peripheral blood eosinophilia in humans. For instance, the presence of CLC in sputa from asthmatic patients is indicative of an "eosinophilic response." It is now known that CLC is composed almost solely of a single, membrane-derived protein having a molecular size of approximately 13,000. The protein has been shown to be lysophospholipase ("phospholipase B") and may play a role in the inactivation of otherwise toxic lysophospholipids. More recently it was shown that basophils are also a source of CLC, indicating that the presence of these refractile crystals might be indicative of a broader spectrum of inflammatory cell infiltration than was originally supposed. In addition to the basic proteins, eosinophil granules contain several other hydrolytic and proteolytic enzymes. These include arylsulfatase B (type II), phospholipase D (previously associated only with tissues of plant origin), histaminase, acid phosphatase, β-glucuronidase, acid β-glycerophosphatase, ribonuclease, and cathepsin.

CELL SURFACE RECEPTORS

The eosinophil plasma membrane possesses a number of "recognition units" which include receptors for IgG (Fc) and IgE (Fc) (Fig. 40-2). The Fc-γ receptor on human eosinophils and neutrophils appears to be structurally distinct. Low-affinity Fc receptors for IgE on human and rat eosinophils have also been identified using both a rosette technique and radioligand binding studies using ^{125}I-labeled human IgE. Fc-ε receptor expression appears to be increased on light density ("hypodense") eosinophils obtained from patients with hypereosinophilia. These Fc-ε receptors on eosinophils were antigenically related to similar low-affinity receptors on lymphocytes and monocytes. A functional role for IgE receptors was suggested by their participation in eosinophil-mediated killing of schistosomula of *S. mansoni*, both in rats and humans. Direct evidence of the involvement of IgE in eosinophil-mediated killing of schistosomula has been obtained using an IgE-specific monoclonal antibody directed against haptenated schistosomula larvae.

After incubation with chemotactic factors, human eosinophils form increased numbers of rosettes with erythrocytes (E) coated with human myeloma IgG subclasses, i.e., E-IgG1, E-IgG2, E-IgG3, and E-IgG4. Whether this is the result of increased numbers of receptors or greater affinity of the eosinophil membrane for multivalent particles is unclear. However, this phenomenon of "receptor enhancement" might have pathologic significance and represents a feature of amplification of the inflammatory response.

It can be shown by the rosette technique that eosinophils bind E-C3b and E-C3bi, although complement receptor expression on eosinophils is weak when compared to neutrophils.

MEMBRANE-DERIVED MEDIATORS

Eosinophils preferentially generate the SRS-A sulfidopeptide leukotrienes (LTC$_4$, LTD$_4$, LTE$_4$) after stimulation with the calcium ionophore (Fig. 40-2). It was recently shown that a physiological stimulus (IgG-coated particles) also stimulated eosinophils to produce SRS-A leukotrienes and that greater amounts were generated by "activated" cells (i.e., eosinophils prestimulated in vitro by chemotactic factors) or by using light density cells. Eosinophils also generate substantial quantities of *platelet activating factor* (PAF) after ionophore stimulation. It has also been shown that ionophore-stimulated eosinophils produce predominantly 15-lipoxygenase pathway derivatives when incubated with radiolabeled exogenous arachidonic acid.

EOSINOPHIL CHEMOTAXIS

A large number of eosinophil chemotactic factors have been recognized, but the biologic significance of many of them is unclear (Table 40-1). PAF is the most potent eosinophilotactic agent so far described. Although mast cell-derived products might play a role in the recruitment of eosinophils during the early phases of allergic tissue reactions, T-cell and monocyte-derived agents are probably also involved in sustaining eosinophil infiltration. Mast cell-derived eosinophil chemotactic factors can be broadly divided into amines, acidic peptides, and lipid agents. The amines and peptides are of weak potency. Histamine and one of its major catabolites—imidazoleacetic acid—are both chemotactic and chemokinetic for human eosinophil over the dose range 10^4 to 10^6 M.

The *eosinophil chemotactic factor of anaphylaxis* (ECF-A) is a family of closely related acidic peptides, in the molecular weight range 360 to 1000, which reside preformed within mast cell granules. They possess a number of biologic activities for eosinophils and (to a lesser extent) neutrophils. These properties include chemotaxis, chemokinesis, eosinophil accumulation in vivo, chemotactic deactivation, and complement receptor enhancement. Currently only two of the peptides, valine-glycine-serine-glutamic acid and alanine-glycine-serine-glutamic acid have been identified. There are a number of higher molecular weight ECF-A mast cell peptides (i.e., 600 to 1000 daltons) that are more hydrophobic, appear to be more biologically active, but are not yet chemically characterized. Various lipid mediators, i.e., LTB$_4$ and some of the monohydroxy eicosatetraenoic acids, possess eosinophil, as well as neutrophil, chemotactic properties. None

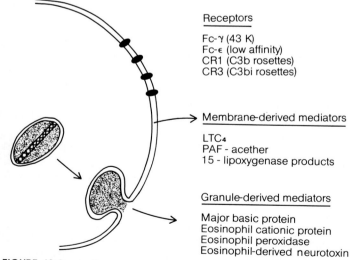

Receptors

Fc-γ (43 K)
Fc-ε (low affinity)
CR1 (C3b rosettes)
CR3 (C3bi rosettes)

Membrane-derived mediators

LTC₄
PAF - acether
15 - lipoxygenase products

Granule-derived mediators

Major basic protein
Eosinophil cationic protein
Eosinophil peroxidase
Eosinophil-derived neurotoxin

FIGURE 40-2 A diagrammatic representation of the human eosinophil. The mediators can be considered as membrane-derived (PAF-acether and lipoxygenase products) and preformed (the basic protein). The immunoglobulin and complement receptors have distinct features when compared to the neutrophil.

of these appear to be as potent as PAF. Bacterial products and material derived from metazoan parasites have eosinophil as well as neutrophil chemotactic properties. In experimental animals, several T-lymphocyte-derived eosinophil chemotactic factors have been described. These may be relevant to the eosinophilia which sometimes accompanies delayed-type hypersensitivity reactions and parasite-associated granulomata.

ACTIVATED EOSINOPHILS

Several investigators have shown that eosinophils are also heterogeneous in terms of their density after centrifugation on Percoll or metrizamide gradients. With discontinuous metrizamide gradients the cells can be separated into light ("hypodense") and normal ("normodense") density bands. Compared to normal density cells, light density cells from the same individual have increased expression of membrane receptors for Fc-γ and Fc-ϵ, are more cytotoxic for helminthic larvae in vitro, produce more LTC_4 than normodense cells after incubation with IgG-coated particles, are metabolically more active in terms of higher oxygen consumption, and have complete or partial loss of the crystalline granule core (which probably corresponds to the "vacuolated cells" previously observed in peripheral blood in the hypereosinophilic syndrome). On the other hand, normal density eosinophils from patients with raised blood eosinophil counts had markedly enhanced cytotoxicity for schistosomula compared to normal density eosinophils from normal subjects. Also, there is still some debate as to whether light density cells are indeed activated as a result of the disease process or merely represent a stage in maturation. Resident eosinophils, i.e., lung cells from patients with pulmonary eosinophilia, are of the light density type. Recent work using monoclonal antibodies to granulocyte membrane proteins indicates that the membranes of activated eosinophils possess altered amounts of antigenic determinants.

Several factors "activate" eosinophils for increased cytotoxicity and enhanced expression of membrane markers for C and IgG (Fc). These include T-cell-derived factors, monokines, CSFα, lipid mediators, mast cell-derived products, and products derived from helminths.

EOSINOPHILS AND HELMINTHIC PARASITIC DISEASE

There is a well-known association between eosinophils and helminthic infections. The precise nature of this association is difficult to define because of the extreme complexity of the life cycles of these organisms as well as the immune status of the host at the time observations are made (i.e., whether primary, secondary, or subsequent infections).

Despite the difficulties in studying the exact role of eosinophils in helminthic parasitic disease, it is possible to make several generalizations. In the sensitized, primed animal, an intense eosinophilia usually occurs when larvae are migrating in the tissues. Examples of helminthic infections having a lung phase associated with eosinophilia are shown in Table 40-2. As the infection becomes chronic, eosinophils usually tend to become less prominent, although not invariably so since, in schistosomiasis for example, they are often found in quite large numbers in association with granulomata around eggs.

Part of the immune response to worms involves the production of IgE as well as other immunoglobulin classes. Very raised levels of IgE are characteristic of tropical eosinophilia and indeed most helminth infections are accompanied by a sustained IgE response. It has been shown experimentally that, in the rat, there is a direct relationship between the IgE antibody response and resistance to infection since selective suppression of IgE production diminished both resistance and the eosinophil response to infection with *Trichinella spiralis*. In this sense the host has become sensitized, or allergic, to the parasite as is shown, for example, by the intense asthmatic reaction which often accompanies pulmonary ascariasis. The intense itching associated with the cutaneous phase of repeated exposure to hookworm infections, strongyloidiasis, and filariasis is another example. Thus migrating larvae may come into contact with mast cells sensitized with parasite-specific IgE. At the same time, the parasitic larvae may become *opsonized* by antibody (IgG) and complement. It has been shown, for instance, that schistosomula and other helminthic larvae activate complement by the alternative pathway and that mast cells adhere to complement coated larvae.

As outlined above, a number of mast cell products are chemotactic for eosinophils. The IgE-mediated release of these agents as a result of contact with stage-specific surface antigens of the migrating parasite would lead to recruitment and infiltration of inflammatory cells and direct contact of eosinophils and neutrophils with the larval surface (Fig. 40-3).

A topic of particular interest relates to the special role of eosinophils as cytotoxic cells in antibody and/or complement-dependent killing of parasitic larvae in vitro. It was originally shown that the human eosinophil was a principal effector cell in antibody (IgG)-dependent damage to schistosomula of *S. mansoni*, in vitro. Later, in the rat, it was found that schistosomula, coated with C3 through alternative pathway activation, were also highly susceptible to eosinophil-mediated damage. It was then reported that human eosinophils *and* neutrophils killed schistosomula coated with antibody and/or complement but that the eosinophil appeared to be a more effective

TABLE 40-2

Examples of Helminthic Infections Having a Lung Phase Associated with Eosinophilia

Class	Genus	Species	Disease Caused	Comments
Trematoda	Schistosoma	haematobium mansoni japonicum	Schistosomiasis (bilharzia)	(1) Acute lung inflammatory reaction associated with migration of larvae. (2) Chronic eosinophilia as part of the inflammatory response against eggs.
	Paragonimus	westermani kellacotti africanus uterobilateralis	Paragonimiasis	(1) Eosinophilic pneumonia in initial stages. (2) Eosinophils around "egg tubercules."
Cestodea	Echinococcus	granulosus multilocularis	Hydatid disease	Leakage of fluid from hydatid cyst causes anaphylaxis with eosinophilia.
Nematoda	Strongyloides	stercoralis	Strongyloidiasis	Symptoms resembling tropical pulmonary eosinophilia may occur, especially with autoinfection.
	Ancylostoma	duodenale	Hookworm disease	Passage of larvae through lungs sometimes associated with asthmatic symptoms. Eosinophilia intense.
	Necator	americanus brasiliense	Hookworm disease Dog hookworm disease	
	Ascaris	lumbricoides	Roundworm disease	Intense pulmonary eosinophilia with asthma common.
	Wuchereria	bancrofti	?Tropical eosinophilic lung	Tropical eosinophilia is the consequence of an amnestic immune response against migratory microfilaria. The disease shows a mixed clinical picture with eosinophilia, cough, wheezing, and adenopathy.
	Brugia	pahangi	?Tropical eosinophilic lung	

SOURCE: After Spencer H: *Pathology of Lung*, 3d ed. Philadelphia, Saunders, 1977.

cytotoxic cell when complement was present, either alone or in combination with antibody. Similar findings have been made with in vitro models of filariasis. At present there is still some debate as to the effectiveness of neutrophils in these in vitro systems. Some investigators believe that they have little or no activity, whereas others find that their cytotoxic potential equals that of the eosinophil. For instance, human eosinophils and neutrophils were found to be equally effective in killing newborn larvae of T. spiralis.

However, a number of in vivo studies also support the view that the eosinophil is a major cytotoxic cell for parasitic larvae. For example, adoptive transfer of peritoneal eosinophils from immune rats to normal recipient rats induced a high degree of resistance to a challenge infection with S. mansoni.

Activation of eosinophils by agents of diverse origin leads to enhanced, or accelerated, killing of parasite lar-

vae and eggs. Mast cells and mast cell-associated mediators (i.e., histamine ECF-A tetrapeptides and leukotriene B_4) enhance IgG-, IgE-, and complement-dependent killing of schistosomula. Enhancement of human eosinophil-mediated killing of schistosomula by reversed-type (IgE-mediated) anaphylaxis has also been observed using human blood basophils. Similarly, supernatants from cultured *mononuclear cell preparations* (MCS) enhanced eosinophil killing in an antibody-dependent system. Interestingly, the activity in MCS was detected in supernatants prepared from patients with eosinophilia only and not by mononuclear cells from normal subjects. Preliminary evidence suggests that the activity in MCS is derived from the macrophage. It has also been shown that antibody- and complement-mediated cytotoxicity was enhanced by colony stimulating factor(s). These experiments on eosinophil activation in vitro indicate that the cell might be primed for more effective killing, both at the precursor,

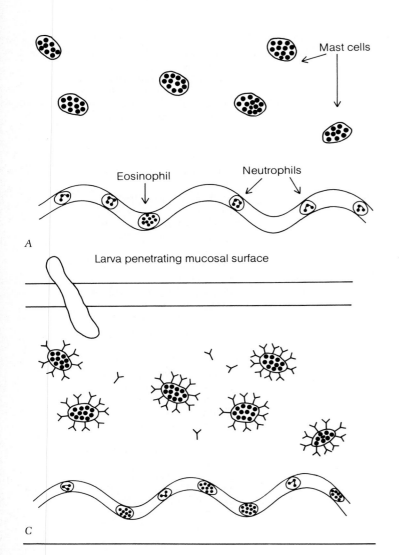

Mucosal surface

Mast cells

Eosinophil

Neutrophils

A

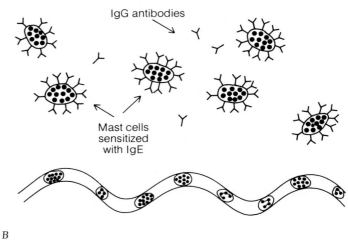

IgG antibodies

Mast cells
sensitized
with IgE

B

Larva penetrating mucosal surface

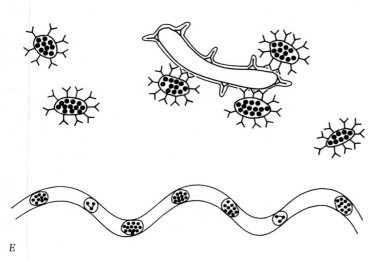

C

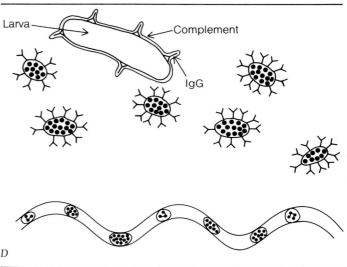

Larva

Complement

IgG

D

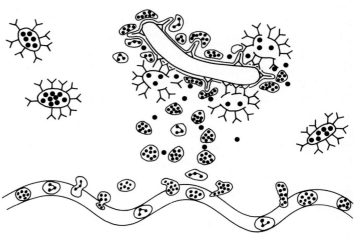

E

F

developmental stage in the bone marrow and by mast cell-derived products which regulate their migration in the tissues.

Thus many observations have led to the view that mediators of hypersensitivity might play a role in immunity to helminths by recruiting and activating cytotoxic effector cells, principally the eosinophil. Very recent studies have implicated leukotrienes in immune responses in the rat against secondary challenge with *Nippostrongylus brasiliensis* and *T. spiralis*. These experiments pointed to an association between high concentrations of enteral and parenteral leukotrienes (especially LTC_4/D_4) and increases in the numbers of tissue eosinophils and mucosal mast cells in the immune animals.

The precise mechanism of killing of larvae by eosinophils is still uncertain. As mentioned above, basic proteins such as MBP and ECP are active in in vitro systems. However, the role of oxidative processes such as those involving partially reduced products of oxygen and eosinophil peroxidase is controversial.

ALLERGY AND THE EOSINOPHIL

In general, the allergic diseases associated with eosinophilia are those in which an immediate-type hypersensitivity reaction is predominant, i.e., those reactions involving mast cells sensitized by IgE, triggered by specific allergen. Common examples are hay fever and other forms of allergic rhinitis, extrinsic bronchial asthma, and general anaphylactic reactions in subjects sensitive to, for example, certain drugs and stinging insects.

As discussed above, present evidence suggests that the interaction of sensitized mast cells (or other cells with Fc-ε receptors such as macrophages and T cells) with spe-

◄ FIGURE 40-3 Eosinophil and parasitic worms. The highly diagrammatic scheme depicts: A. Tissue mast cells and circulating eosinophils and neutrophils. B. Following an infection with parasitic worms, tissue mast cells become sensitized with IgE antibody directed against helminthic larvae. Larvae would also have ready access to IgG antibodies. The ratio of eosinophils to neutrophils in the blood increases, presumably as a result of initiation of T-cell-dependent eosinopoiesis. C. A helminthic larva penetrates the mucosal surface and undergoes transformation. An example is provided by the cercariae that develop into schistosomula following skin penetration in schistosomiasis. D. The transformed larvae are opsonized by antibody and complement. Complement coating will occur both by the alternative and classic pathways. E. Larvae migrate through the tissues and interact with sensitized mast cells. This initiates an immediate-type hypersensitivity reaction with a liberation of pharmacologic mediators. F. Mast cell mediators including eosinophil and neutrophil chemotactic agents (e.g., PAF-acether, histamine and ECF-A) lead to migration of granulocytes from the blood vessels. These mediators enhance eosinophils (and to a lesser extent, neutrophils) for more effective parasite killing. The combination of eosinophils, neutrophils, mast cells, IgE, and complement leads to parasite damage or destruction.

cific antigen leads to the release of factors which are chemotactic for eosinophils and that eosinophils migrate toward the site of degranulated mast cells as a result of chemotaxis and/or chemokinesis. The precise role of the eosinophil, once it has arrived at the site of an immediate-type reaction, is still the subject of some speculation. There is some evidence for believing that in these situations eosinophils may have an additional regulatory role in dampening mast cell activity. The eosinophil's content of histaminase might be relevant to its role in these reactions (although there are plenty of noneosinophil sources of this enzyme). It has also been shown that eosinophil peroxidase inactivated LTB_4, LTC_4, and LTD_4 in reactions dependent on H_2O_2 and a halide. The Charcot-Leyden crystal protein may also play a role in regulating mast cell events since lysophospholipases are known to inactivate potentially toxic lysophospholipids formed as a result of the action of phospholipase A_2. These observations are sometimes used to strengthen the argument that eosinophils down-regulate mast cell-dependent allergic reactions.

It has been suggested that immediate-type (IgE-mediated) hypersensitivity might have been retained in phylogeny because of the benefit this mechanism confers in adaptive immunity to metazoan parasites. Thus in evolutionary terms the *advantages* of mast cell/IgE/eosinophil interactions in limiting helminth infections greatly outweigh the *disadvantages*, i.e., the retention of relatively trivial diseases such as allergic rhinitis. This reasoning implied that helminths and common allergens stimulate comparable immunologic mechanisms, possibly as a result of shared antigens or perhaps because of similar modes of access to the same immunologically competent cells. Thus allergies and their attendant eosinophilia might simply be a case of mistaken identity, i.e., the host responds to allergens as if they were parasites. Since helminthic infections presumably exert some form of evolutionary selective pressure, eosinophils, mast cells, and IgE have been retained.

TISSUE DAMAGE CAUSED BY EOSINOPHILS AND THEIR PRODUCTS

It is apparent that the eosinophil, by virtue of its granule-associated and membrane-derived products, has considerable potential for tissue damage. MBP is cytotoxic for various mammalian cells, including ascites tumor cells, mononuclear phagocytes, and ciliated respiratory epithelial cells. LTC_4, the major 5-lipoxygenase product of pathophysiologically stimulated eosinophils, might substantially contribute to smooth-muscle contraction and mucous hypersecretion.

There is now considerable evidence to support the view that eosinophils may play a critical role in the pathogenesis of bronchial asthma. Durham and Kay (cited in Kay review) have shown an inverse correlation between blood eosinophils and the degree of nonspecific bronchial hyperreactivity. They also found a relationship between clinical improvement after treatment with the mast cell stabilizing agent disodium cromoglycate (DSCG) and the percentage of eosinophils in tracheobronchial secretions and lung lavage samples. Eosinophils and ECP are prominent in bronchial lavage fluid from patients who developed dual (early and late phase) reactions after antigen challenge, whereas this was not observed in the "single early responders." MBP is thought to play a special role in tissue damage since it was detected in mucous plugs, in damaged epithelial surfaces, and beneath the basement membrane from bronchi of autopsy material obtained from asthma deaths.

In less common pulmonary disorders, e.g., cryptogenic fibrosing alveolitis, the identification of eosinophils in bronchoalveolar lavage fluid is often predictive of a poor prognosis. Eosinophils purified from bronchoalveolar lavage of human interstitial lung disease also demonstrated spontaneous cytotoxicity for cat lung epithelial cells indicating a possible role for eosinophils in chronic inflammatory disorders of the lower respiratory tract.

There is increasing interest in the role of the eosinophil, especially eosinophil granule-derived enzymes, in eosinophilic endomyocardial disease, and in the cardiomyopathy often found in association with the hypereosinophilic syndrome.

PERSPECTIVE

Eosinophils share many biologic properties with neutrophils, but they also have very distinct features. These in-clude their content of large crystalloid granules, which contain a number of unique basic proteins, and their capacity to preferentially generate the SRS-A, sulfidopeptide leukotrienes, and 15-lipoxygenase products, as well as low-affinity receptors for IgE (Fc). Eosinophil-derived products probably play an important role in the destruction of helminthic larvae, whereas in some situations, e.g., chronic bronchial asthma and the hypereosinophilic syndrome, the cell might be responsible for considerable tissue damage. The role of eosinophils in IgE-mediated allergic disease is uncertain. There is some evidence to support the view that the cell dampens the allergic response by inactivating mast cell mediators. On the other hand, eosinophils might be inappropriately recruited in allergic disease due to a phylogenic failure in distinguishing between allergens and parasitic worms. At the present time there is growing interest in eosinophil heterogeneity, as exemplified by the fact that hypereosinophilia is associated with a population of light-density "activated" cells. In a variety of biologic systems these light density cells respond more vigorously than normal density eosinophils. A number of agents have been shown to selectively activate the eosinophil. The nature of these agents is diverse and involves factors associated with eosinophil maturation such as CSFα, various mast cell products, and other substances released during allergic tissue reactions and other inflammatory processes. Knowledge of eosinophils and eosinophil-associated events is growing rapidly, and there is a need to modify continuously our views on the precise role(s) of the eosinophil in the light of these new findings.

BIBLIOGRAPHY

Butterworth AE: Cell-mediated damage to helminths. Adv Parasitol 23:143–235, 1984.
  Concise review on eosinophil function in parasitic disease.

Colley DG: Lymphocyte products, in Mahmoud AAF, Austen KF (eds), *The Eosinophil in Health and Disease.* New York, Grune & Stratton, 1980, pp 293–309.
  Review with special reference to eosinophil activating factors derived from lymphocytes.

Gleich GJ, Adolphson CR: The eosinophilic leukocyte: Structure and function. Adv Immunol 39:177–253, 1986.
  A very comprehensive review, especially regarding the biochemistry of the basic proteins.

Kay AB: The cells causing airway inflammation. Eur J Respir Dis (suppl) 147:38–43, 1986.
  The eosinophil considered in the full context of cells causing airway inflammation.

Wardlaw AJ, Kay AB: The role of the eosinophil in the pathogenesis of asthma. Allergy 42:321–335, 1987.
  Well annotated review including a perspective of the eosinophil as an effector cell in immunity and hypersensitivity disorders.

Chapter *41*

Immune Mechanisms in Lung Injury

Peter A. Ward / Daniel G. Remick

Complement Activation Products Responsible for Acute Lung Injury

Lung Injury Produced by Immune Complexes

In Vitro Activities of IgG Immune Complexes

In Vivo Production of Acute Lung Injury by IgG Immune Complexes

In Vivo Production of Acute Lung Injury by IgA Immune Complexes

Cellular Immune Mechanisms in Lung Injury

Types of Granulomas

Immunopathogenesis of Granuloma Formation

Macrophage-Lymphocyte Interactions

Lymphocytes in Granulomas

Cytokines

The Fibrogenic Response

Clinical Relevance

There is abundant evidence that immune mechanisms are responsible for both acute and progressive lung injury. Animal models have established unequivocally the roles for both humoral and cellular immune mechanisms. Although these mechanisms have been incriminated in the pathogenesis of pulmonary parenchymal injury in human interstitial lung disease, the evidence is largely circumstantial and incomplete. This chapter focuses on the role of complement activation products, immune complexes, oxygen radicals, and T-cell-mediated events as determinants of lung injury in experimental models.

COMPLEMENT ACTIVATION PRODUCTS RESPONSIBLE FOR ACUTE LUNG INJURY

It has been known for some time that, when instilled into the airways of hamsters or rabbits, the complement-derived chemotactic peptide C5a and the formyl chemo-tactic peptides, such as N-formyl-methionyl-leucyl-phenylalanine (FMLP), produce acute mobilization of neutrophils into the distal airways. In the hamster, this procedure causes little evidence of injury. In the rabbit, parenchymal injury does occur after repeated exposure of the lung to chemotactic peptide. Although the peripheral intravenous infusion of C5a or FMLP, or the infusion of zymosan-activated plasma, causes neutrophil sequestration in the pulmonary interstitial capillaries, little evidence is found of vascular injury unless the animals have been first exposed to anoxia or to the infusion of prostaglandin E_2. In contrast, intravenous infusion in rats of the potent complement activator, cobra venom factor (CVF), causes acute injury of the pulmonary microvasculature. Cobra venom factor activates the complement system via the alternative complement pathway and causes the transient appearance in plasma of C5a. The acute damage to the lung microvasculature is associated with sequestration of neutrophils in the pulmonary interstitial capillaries. Where neutrophils are in contact with vascular endothelial cells, the lining cells seem to be necrotic. This process of endothelial cell injury seems to be diffuse and limited to a small area of the total endothelial surface of the lung microvasculature. Nevertheless, focal loss of endothelial cells does occur and is accompanied by fibrin deposition, interstitial edema, and intra-alveolar hemorrhage (Fig. 41-1).

In the pathogenesis of complement-induced injury of the type described above, the neutrophils and their toxic oxygen products play a critical role. The outline of events thought to be involved in the reaction sequence is depicted in Fig. 41-2. Flooding of the vascular compartment with C5a results in activation of neutrophils, this process being associated with adherence and aggregation of neutrophils and their entrapment within the pulmonary microvasculature, where intimate contact of these cellular aggregates with pulmonary capillary endothelial cells takes place. This process results in acute damage of the pulmonary microvascular endothelial cells due to the generation of toxic oxygen products from neutrophils.

The series of oxygen products generated by activated neutrophils is outlined in Fig. 41-3. C5a as well as a variety of other agonists can activate neutrophils via pathways that seem to be linked to activation of protein kinase C and nicotinamide-adenine dinucleotide phosphate hydrogenase (NADPH) oxidase, probably through prior activation of phospholipases in the cell membrane. NADPH oxidase initiates a series of steps featuring single-electron addition to molecular oxygen:

$$O_2 \xrightarrow{e^-} O_2^- \quad \text{(superoxide oxide anion)}$$

$$O_2^- \xrightarrow{e^-} H_2O_2$$

$$H_2O_2 \xrightarrow{e^-} HO^\cdot \quad \text{(hydroxyl radical)}$$

$$HO^\cdot \xrightarrow{e^-} H_2O$$

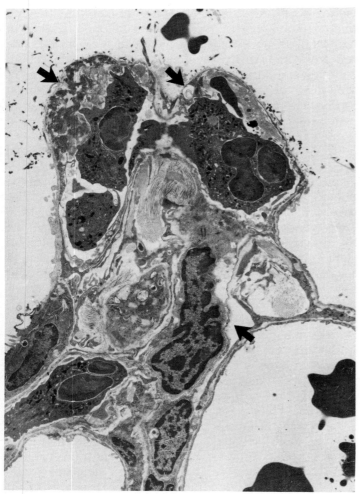

FIGURE 41-1 Transmission electron micrograph 30 min after the peripheral intravenous infusion of cobra venom factor into a rat. Shown is an area of interstitium of lung surrounded by alveolar spaces. The interstitial capillaries show intravascular neutrophils and areas where the lining endothelial cells have been replaced with a protein coagulum and fibrin, resulting in exposure of vascular basement membrane (arrows). Alveolar spaces contain red cells and fibrin deposits. (Uranyl acetate and lead citrate treated tissue, ×6100.)

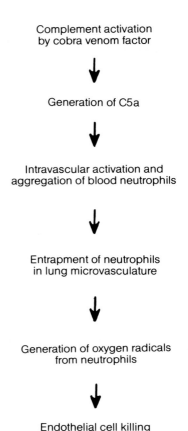

FIGURE 41-2 Pathogenic mechanisms leading to microvascular injury of lung after systemic activation of complement.

As shown in these steps that entail the net adduction of four electrons to a molecule of oxygen, three toxic products (O_2^-, H_2O_2, $HO^\bullet$) are generated. In Fig. 41-3, the central role of iron is shown in the conversion of H_2O_2 to $HO^\bullet$. Current evidence suggests that the source of iron in these reactions could be either the effector (neutrophil) or the target (endothelial) cell. Iron bound to ferritin is reduced by O_2^- to Fe^{2+}, which is the critical transition metal involved in the production of $HO^\bullet$ from H_2O_2. There is also a possibility that iron radicals such as the perferryl ion ($Fe^{3+}O_2^-$) may participate in tissue damage. H_2O_2 can be converted to toxic products, such as hypochlorous acid ($HOCl$), by neutrophil-associated myeloperoxidase in the

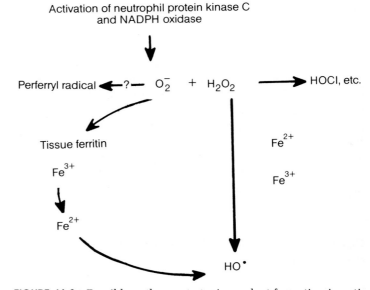

FIGURE 41-3 Possible pathways to toxic product formation in activated phagocytic cells.

presence of halide, although in vitro experiments that involve the killing of endothelial cells by activated neutrophils suggest that $HO^{\cdot}$ rather than HOCl is the critical oxygen derivative responsible for injury to endothelial cells.

On the grounds that oxygen-derived products play a key role in the microvascular injury following systemic (intravascular) activation of the complement system, several different therapeutic strategies have been tried and proved successful in protecting the vasculature from injury. These interventions are summarized in Table 41-1; they include the use of antioxidant enzymes, scavengers with high reactivity for $HO^{\cdot}$, nonspecific scavengers, and iron chelators.

As would be expected, catalase is a potent protective agent in the cobra venom factor (CVF) model of acute lung injury, since its use directly stops H_2O_2 from being converted, in the presence of a transition metal, to $HO^{\cdot}$. One possible drawback in the use of catalase is its relatively high molecular weight (400,000 s) which limits its ability to gain entry into extravascular locales. Superoxide dismutase has some protective effects in the complement-activation model of lung vascular injury, but the enzyme has proved to be much less effective than catalase. There is little evidence that O_2^- is itself toxic to either cells or tissues, and it seems likely that the main function of O_2^- may be to reduce Fe^{3+} to Fe^{2+}, which is necessary for iron to reduce H_2O_2 to $HO^{\cdot}$ (and in the process be reoxidized to Fe^{3+}, Fig. 41-3).

Other protective antioxidant enzymes are glutathione peroxidase and reductase, which maintain tissue levels of the antioxidant, glutathione. Oxygen radical scavengers with relative specificity for $HO^{\cdot}$ have been shown to be potent inhibitors of pulmonary microvascular injury following intravascular activation of complement. Dimethylsulfoxide and dimethylthiourea afford high degrees of protection against neutrophil-mediated injury to the lungs. Not surprisingly, nonspecific oxygen radical scavengers, such as vitamin E, will also protect against oxygen-radical-mediated injury of endothelial cells.

Finally, agents that chelate iron are also protective in the model of lung injury described above. Deferoxamine, which only chelates iron in its fully oxidized state (Fe^{3+}), and apolactoferrin, which can bind either Fe^{2+} or Fe^{3+}, are protective against both the lung injury that follows systemic activation of complement and the in vitro model of neutrophil-mediated injury to bovine pulmonary arterial endothelial cells. Prior saturation of either chelator with Fe^{3+} abolishes its protective effects.

LUNG INJURY PRODUCED BY IMMUNE COMPLEXES

Clinical studies in humans have demonstrated a correlation between the presence in serum of immune complex-like material (as measured by the RAJI cell assay) and the presence of interstitial inflammatory disease in the lungs. Subsequently, the finding of neutrophils and immune complex-like material in bronchoalveolar lavage fluids from patients with idiopathic pulmonary fibrosis increased interest in the possible role of immune complexes in causing pulmonary interstitial inflammatory diseases in humans. Abundant evidence now exists that immune complexes can acutely injure the lungs. But, because the pathways involved in producing the acute lung injury depend on the type of immune complexes, it is convenient to discuss separately the pathogenesis of IgG and IgA immune complex-induced injury of the lungs.

IN VITRO ACTIVITIES OF IgG IMMUNE COMPLEXES

The biologic properties of the complex formed in vitro by reacting rabbit polyclonal antibody of the IgG class with the antigen bovine serum albumin (BSA), vary considerably according to the ratio of antigen and antibody in the complex: human neutrophils, when exposed to IgG complexes preformed with the antigen-antibody ratio of 1:5 (wt:wt), are maximally active with respect to their ability to activate complement and to cause secretory release of lysosomal enzymes. In contrast, IgG complexes containing the same amount of antibody but with larger amounts of BSA (so that the immune complexes that are formed are more soluble and of lower molecular weight) are without complement-activating activity, and their ability to cause the release of lysosomal enzyme is greatly decreased; but the complexes containing a higher proportion of BSA now demonstrate maximal stimulatory activity with respect to generation of H_2O_2 and O_2^-. These observations suggest that in immune complex-induced injury two types of immune complexes (small and large) are probably involved in the events that ultimately lead to tissue damage.

TABLE 41-1

Protective Agents in Complement-Mediated Injury of the Pulmonary Microvasculature

Enzymes
    Catalase ($H_2O_2 \longrightarrow H_2O + O_2$)
    Superoxide dismutase ($O_2^- \longrightarrow H_2O_2$)
    Glutathione peroxidase and reductase
Scavengers of hydroxyl radical
    Dimethyl sulfoxide
    Dimethylthiourea
Nonspecific scavengers
    Vitamin E
Iron chelators
    Deferoxamine
    Apolactoferrin

IN VIVO PRODUCTION OF ACUTE LUNG INJURY BY IgG IMMUNE COMPLEXES

Formation of several types of immune complexes will cause acute lung injury. Aerosol exposure of sensitized guinea pigs to relevant antigen results in acute hemorrhagic pneumonia. So does the instillation by airway of preformed immune complexes (in conjunction with complement-fixing complexes) or the instillation by airway of IgG antibody while the antigen (BSA) is injected intravenously. In all models, acute injury of the interstitial microvasculature of the lung follows exposure to the IgG immune complexes and results in interstitial and intra-alveolar hemorrhage, edema, and large numbers of neutrophils. Also, in all models, prior depletion of neutrophils or of complement prevents the development of lung injury.

Mediator pathways have been most extensively explored in the previously described model of passive IgG immune complex–induced acute damage to the lungs. Current understanding of the pathogenesis of the pulmonary injury is shown in Fig. 41-4. The complexes deposited in the lungs are probably heterogeneous due to varying ratios of antigen to antibody; the heterogeneity is aggravated by the increasing vascular permeability that accompanies the evolving tissue damage and the resulting increase in the fraction of antigen. From the details presented above, it can be predicted that large, relatively insoluble, complement-fixing complexes would first be formed, followed by increasing amounts of soluble complexes that are more effective in activating phagocytic

cells for the production of oxygen radicals. Deposition of immune complexes in tissues ultimately leads to activation of complement and the influx of neutrophils. Although IgG complexes can stimulate neutrophils directly to produce oxygen radicals, the presence of C5a probably evokes maximal activation of neutrophils. The generation of O_2^- has been shown in vitro to convert arachidonic acid to chemotactic lipid. In the rat, lung injury produced by IgG immune complexes is attenuated for a while by treatment of the animals with superoxide dismutase (SOD). The protective effects of SOD are associated with the absence of infiltrates of neutrophils, findings that are consistent with the postulated role of O_2^- in promoting the influx of neutrophils. Because of the potent protective effects of catalase (which does not appear to interfere with the accumulation of neutrophils) in lung injury produced by immune complexes, H_2O_2 must play a key role in the events leading to damage of interstitial vascular endothelial and alveolar epithelial cells. Although H_2O_2 is toxic per se to cells (but only in relatively high concentrations), Fe^{2+}-catalyzed reduction of H_2O_2 to $HO^{\cdot}$ or to myeloperoxidase, and halide-dependent conversion of H_2O_2 to HOCl, are probably involved in immune complex-induced injury. That $HO^{\cdot}$ is the key toxic product is suggested by the observations that the killing of endothelial cells in vitro by activated neutrophils is highly sensitive to the presence of either catalase or iron chelator and to the presence of hydroxyl radical scavengers, whereas it is resistant to pretreatment of neutrophils with azide (which inactivates myeloperoxidase). In contrast to a wealth of knowledge about mechanisms that lead to in vitro damage or to the killing of endothelial cells by stimulated neutrophils, relatively few details are available concerning in vivo models except for immune complex-induced vasculitis; in this disorder, iron chelators (apolactoferrin or deferroxamine) or the $HO^{\cdot}$ scavenger dimethyl sulfoxide are protective; this, too, is consistent with a cardinal role for $HO^{\cdot}$.

Agonists that activate neutrophils to produce oxygen radicals also often cause secretory release of lysosomal enzymes that have many different substrates as targets, including connective tissue products (collagen, elastin, basement membranes). Hydrolysis of matrix material, to which the underlying surfaces of vascular endothelial cells are adherent, may occur as a result of secreted leukocytic proteases, causing endothelial cells to lift from the underlying basement membrane, possibly contributing thereby to increased vascular permeability. There is little doubt that IgG immune complex-induced injury is the result of the combined effects of proteases and oxygen radicals. Perhaps nowhere is this conclusion better underscored than in recent studies that suggest that hydrolysis of vascular basement membrane is greatly increased if the membrane is first exposed to nanomolar concentrations of H_2O_2.

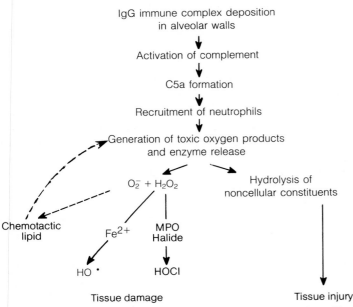

FIGURE 41-4 Pathogenic events leading to lung injury mediated by IgG immune complexes.

IN VIVO PRODUCTION OF ACUTE LUNG INJURY BY IgA IMMUNE COMPLEXES

Interest in the phlogistic potential of IgA-containing immune complexes has stemmed from the clinical observations that in IgA nephropathy and in Henoch-Schönlein purpura the glomerulitis and the vasculitis are associated with deposits of IgA and C3. The mechanisms by which these complexes injure the tissue are entirely unknown. The ineffectiveness of corticosteroids in improving the clinical state of these patients has caused considerable frustration.

It is known that the stimulating activity of IgA immune complexes via the alternative pathway is modest. Nonetheless, the experimental evidence that IgA immune complexes have potent lung-damaging activity is now unequivocal. Although the clinical relevance of this evidence to the human lung is unclear, the experimental studies have led to better understanding of the manner in which these complexes *can* inflict tissue injury.

Using myeloma protein, murine monoclonal antibody of the IgA class with reactivity to the hapten dinitrophenol (DNP) has been instilled into the airways of rats while the hapten (linked to a carrier protein) is injected intravenously. This procedure results in an acute lung-damaging reaction within 2 to 3 h. The mediator pathways that are presumably involved in the tissue damage are shown in Fig. 41-5, and in Table 41-2 the lung injury produced by IgG and IgA immune complexes are compared.

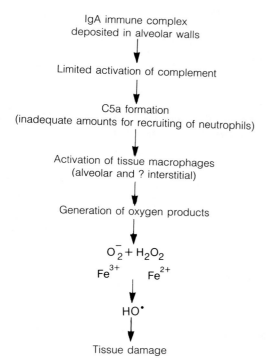

FIGURE 41-5 Pathogenic events leading to lung injury mediated by IgA immune complexes.

TABLE 41-2

Comparison of IgG and IgA Immune Complex-Induced Acute Lung Injury

Requirement or Mediator	Type of Immune Complex	
	IgG	IgA
Neutrophils	Required	Not required
Tissue macrophages	Not required	Required
Complement	Required	Required
Sensitivity to		
Superoxide dismutase	Yes, limited	Yes
Catalase	Yes	Yes
Dimethyl sulfoxide	??	Yes
Dimethylthiourea	??	Yes
Deferoxamine	??	Yes

The lung injury produced by IgA immune complexes is associated with increased vascular permeability, extensive blebing of capillary vascular endothelial cells, and intra-alveolar hemorrhage. Necrosis of type I and II alveolar epithelial cells also occurs. In marked contrast to the reaction involving IgG immune complex-induced lung injury, strikingly, neutrophils are absent in this type of reaction.

Preformed IgA immune complexes have measurable, albeit limited, complement-fixing activity that can be detected using electrophoresis to demonstrate conversion of C3. But, because complement activation via the alternative pathway is slight, the total hemolytic complement activity (CH_{50}) undergoes little, or no change. The latter observation underscores that conclusions based solely on CH_{50} assays are potentially misleading.

The response pattern disclosed by bronchoalveolar lavage fluid (BAL) obtained from animals in which saline was introduced into the airways differed strikingly from that elicited by the concomitant introduction of IgG or IgA antibody into the airways and the injection of antigen intravenously. As expected, the BAL from the saline-injected controls contained a preponderance of alveolar macrophages and very few neutrophils. The "basal" rate of O_2^- generation in nonstimulated neutrophils and in alveolar macrophages was very small (<2 nmol/h); the addition of phorbol myristate acetate (PMA) produced potent cellular responses.

In animals with ongoing IgG immune complex reactions in lung, as expected, large numbers ($\approx 33 \times 10^6$) of neutrophils were retrieved in BAL with no increase in the numbers of alveolar macrophages. When these cells were examined in vitro for basal and for PMA-stimulated production of O_2^-, increases were found in the basal amounts of O_2^- generation of both neutrophils and alveolar macrophages. In cells stimulated by PMA, the level of O_2^- production in neutrophils from animals with ongoing IgG immune complex reactions was virtually identical with that in the peritoneal neutrophils; in contrast, the O_2^- responses of alveolar macrophages from animals with ongoing IgG immune complex reactions were less than half of those for similar cells from control animals. The latter observation can be attributed to failure of the activated macrophages to be replenished by an influx of fully competent cells from the circulation, whereas the influx of neutrophils is apparently quite large. In animals with ongoing IgA immune complex-induced lung injury, the results differed considerably from those obtained in animals with IgG immune complex reactions. Neutrophils were not present within the BAL, whereas the number of alveolar macrophages increased threefold. The macrophages showed evidence of prior activation, as indicated by a doubling in the amounts of O_2^- generated in the absence of PMA. Also in contrast to the IgG immune complex model, in which alveolar macrophages showed a marked decrease in their ability to generate O_2^- after addition of PMA, the O_2^- response in macrophages from the IgA immune complex model was fully expressed.

As a result of the various manipulations using rats in vivo, the following generalizations can be made with respect to IgA immune complex-induced lung injury: neutrophil depletion does not affect the intensity of lung injury, whereas complement depletion is strongly protective; the in vivo administration of SOD or catalase is protective, whereas administration of heat-inactivated catalase is not protective; the iron chelator deferoxamine, but not iron-saturated deferoxamine, is protective against the development of lung injury. Although these data are still incomplete, they do support the proposed pathogenesis of acute lung reactions induced by IgA immune complexes (Fig. 41-5). It seems likely that the modest ability of IgA immune complexes to fix complement yields small amounts of C5a in the peripheral airways. These small amounts presumably suffice to "prime" or to enhance alveolar, and possibly interstitial, macrophages in mounting an oxygen radical burst in response to IgA immune complexes. The protective effect of SOD is probably due to O_2^- that is presumably generated in small amounts.

CELLULAR IMMUNE MECHANISMS IN LUNG INJURY

Cellular immune mechanisms are involved in a number of inflammatory reactions of the lungs in humans, perhaps best illustrated by pulmonary sarcoidosis, where granuloma formation is the predominant histopathologic feature. Large numbers of lymphocytes are found in the BAL fluid of these patients; the lymphocytes appear to be in a state of "activation" as defined by the elaboration of diverse soluble mediators. Cellular immune mechanisms are also involved in other granulomatous inflammatory diseases affecting the lungs and fibrogenic events can often also be closely linked to products of the cellular immune system. Granulomas may result from specific immune responses to antigens, such as those derived from infectious sources [e.g., Bacille bilié de Calmette-Guérin (BCG) or *Schistosoma mansoni*], or from the response to foreign body irritants, such as plastic or polysaccharide beads, and talc crystals. In many clinical instances, the etiologic agents responsible for granuloma formation have not been defined, e.g., sarcoidosis or Wegener's granulomatosis.

Granulomas play a protective mechanism against pathogenic organisms such as the tubercle bacilli by sequestering microorganisms, thereby limiting their spread from the lungs to the remainder of the body. Also, the close proximity of macrophages to T lymphocytes within the granuloma enhances cell-cell interactions and the local production of cytokines that facilitate the killing of the microorganisms.

TYPES OF GRANULOMAS

Based on experimental models, there are two functional classifications of granulomas: *delayed-hypersensitivity granulomas* that are characterized by antigen-specific immune responses to agents such as bacteria, bacterial wall products, viruses, fungi, and schistosome eggs; and *foreign body granulomas* that are independent of immune mechanisms and vary from minimally tissue-destructive reactions (as in the case of reactions to relatively inert particles) to the more destructive lesions that progress to fibrosis (e.g., those caused by silica crystals). The characteristics of both types of granulomas are summarized in Table 41-3.

Delayed hypersensitivity granulomas are characterized by several important features: the mixture of compo-

TABLE 41-3

Comparison of Foreign Body and Delayed-Type Hypersensitivity Granulomas

Characteristics	Foreign Body	Delayed-Type Hypersensitivity
Cellular composition	Macrophages, fibroblasts	Macrophages, T lymphocytes, eosinophils, mast cells, fibroblasts
Rate of cell turnover	Low	High
Antigen-specific responsiveness	Absent	Present
T-lymphocyte responsiveness	Absent	Present
IL-2 production by granuloma cells	Absent	Present
Modulation by arachidonic acid metabolites	Absent	Present

nents of the cellular immune system (T cells, their specific reactivity to antigens, the production of interleukin 2 by T cells isolated from the granulomas) and the modulation of granuloma formation by products of arachidonate metabolism. These features are absent in foreign body granulomas. It is not surprising that macrophage–T-cell interactions play an important role in the development of delayed hypersensitivity. An excellent animal model of pulmonary delayed hypersensitivity granuloma formation is produced by injecting S. mansoni eggs intravenously in mice: embolized eggs lodge in the microvasculature of the lung, resulting in granuloma formation with characteristic phases of growth, maintenance, and resolution that can be quantified morphometrically. Figure 41-6 shows the pattern of growth and resolution of pulmonary granulomas over a period from 4 to 32 days after egg embolization. The granulomas are synchronous morphologically, i.e., all the granulomas are at the same stage of development histologically and functionally. This model allows careful dissection of events responsible for the initiation and growth of the granulomas and the events responsible for resolution of the granulomas.

IMMUNOPATHOGENESIS OF GRANULOMA FORMULATION

Granulomas of the delayed hypersensitivity type evolve through a sequence of specific events, each step of which is critical for the fully expressed, granulomatous inflammatory response. This fact implies the ability to modulate the development of granulomas at any step in the series. The events are sequenced in a cascade that includes the release of soluble promoter and suppressor factors, the recruitment of blood cells, cell-cell interactions, and the local proliferation of inflammatory cells.

Delayed hypersensitivity granulomas in the lungs are initiated by antigens which reach the lungs via either the airways or the bloodstream. Macrophages are common features in granulomas, being among the first cells to interact with antigen. The macrophages of granulomas are derived from precursor cells in the bone marrow. Macrophages are recruited to the lungs as monocytes from the bloodstream by monocytic chemotactic factors that are produced locally in developing granulomas. The monocytes "mature" into tissue macrophages and take up antigen, sometimes partially degrading the antigen if it is large and complex.

The presentation of antigen by macrophages to T cells is a critical initial step in the series of immunologic events. Antigen "processing" by macrophages involves "activation" of the macrophages: in the mouse, activation is shown by expression of Ia antigen on the surface of the macrophage, by the presence of increased intracellular hydrolytic enzymes, and by the ability of the macrophage to release active oxygen species. Activation of the macrophage by interaction with antigen promotes the killing of ingested, intracellular organisms.

The kinetics of Ia expression have been carefully established in the synchronous schistosome granuloma where Ia expression is highest at day 16 when granulomas achieve their largest size. Arachidonic acid metabolism of the macrophages appears to be linked to the development of granulomas induced by schistosome eggs. The products of arachidonic acid metabolism probably reflect one way by which macrophages regulate the granulomatous response. The rate of arachidonic acid metabolism is inversely related to the state of activation (as defined by Ia content) of the macrophage; in "activated" macrophages the metabolism of arachidonic acid is greatly diminished. The arachidonic acid metabolism of macrophages from early schistosome granulomas increases when they are

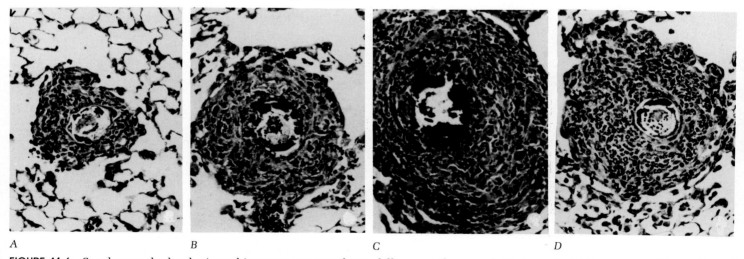

A   B   C   D

FIGURE 41-6 Synchronously developing schistosome egg granulomas following tail vein embolization of schistosome eggs. Time points of postembolization are: A. Day 4. B. Day 8. C. Day 16. D. Day 32. (All photos same magnification, ×400.)

incubated in vitro with zymosan particles, whereas later on arachidonate metabolism is relatively unaffected.

Arachidonic acids are metabolized via the lipoxygenase and cyclooxygenase pathways (Fig. 41-7). Products of the lipoxygenase pathway may be considered to be proinflammatory; they include the leukotrienes and the monohydroxyeicosatraenoic acids. Certain cyclooxygenase pathway products, including the prostaglandins PGE_2 and PGI_2, may be considered to be anti-inflammatory. The possible role of arachidonic acid metabolites has been explored by the exogenous administration of stable analogs of prostaglandins or by the treatment of mice with inhibitors of the lipoxygenase or cyclooxygenase pathways. Systemic administration of exogenous 15-methyl prostaglandin E_1 significantly inhibits both macrophage Ia expression and granuloma size in the schistosome egg granuloma model. In contrast, prostaglandin $F_2\alpha$ increases granuloma size. Neither of these arachidonic acid metabolites affects the size of foreign body granulomas, underscoring the importance of these compounds in the regulation of delayed-type hypersensitivity granulomas and the possible role of these lipid products from macrophages in the evolution of pulmonary granulomas.

Indomethacin, a cyclooxygenase inhibitor, augments both the size of granulomas and the expression of macrophage Ia. This is probably due to decreased production by macrophages of the E series of prostaglandins. Inhibition of the lipoxygenase pathway, using either nordihydroguaiaretic acid (NDGA) or BW755C, reduces the size of granulomas and the expression of Ia macrophages derived from the granuloma. Thus, products of the two pathways act in a counterregulatory manner to modulate the immune response.

MACROPHAGE-LYMPHOCYTE INTERACTIONS

As emphasized above, the granulomatous inflammatory response requires intimate interaction between macrophages and T lymphocytes. T lymphocytes do not respond to antigens in the absence of macrophages. This interaction is mediated by Ia antigens on the surface of the macrophage. Ia molecules vary structurally, are under strict genetic control, and represent one component of a group of membrane proteins that are coded for by the major histocompatibility complex (MHC); the MHC enables specific cell-cell interactions. For an effective immune response, the macrophage and T cell must exhibit the same Ia membrane glycoproteins. Thus, T cells will interact effectively with macrophages only if both the "processed" antigen and the appropriate Ia molecule are present on the surface of the macrophage. It is not known if the Ia molecule and antigen exist as a single complex on the cell surface or as two separate distinct entities. As indicated above, detection of Ia on the cell surface provides a measure of macrophage activation. The proximity of the macrophage and T cell in the granuloma facilitates the cell-cell communication necessary for an effective immune response.

LYMPHOCYTES IN GRANULOMAS

Lymphocytes are a requisite element in the formation of delayed hypersensitivity granulomas, especially T lymphocytes with the helper-inducer phenotype. The need for T cells is demonstrated by several lines of evidence. Nude mice, animals which are congenitally athymic and

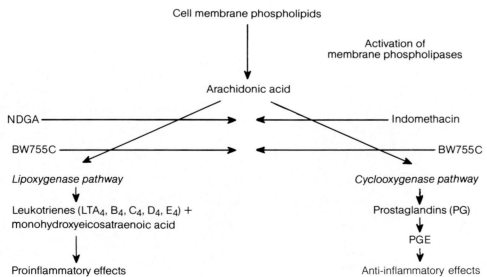

FIGURE 41-7 Arachidonic acid metabolism in granuloma macrophages. After stimulation, several metabolites are produced. Crossbars indicate enzyme inhibition by the compound shown; BW755C blocks both pathways.

lack T cells, develop poorly formed granulomas and do not develop delayed-type hypersensitivity reactions, such as footpad swelling, in response to antigen. A similar outcome is obtained in mice that are thymectomized, lethally irradiated, and then provided with lymphocyte preparations that are depleted of T cells. Antilymphocyte antisera also abrogate the granulomatous response.

The antigen specificity of the immune response is governed by the T lymphocytes and not by the macrophages. Certain clones of T cells replicate and secrete lymphokines after presentation of antigen. This is demonstrated by adoptive transfer studies in which sensitized T lymphocytes produce an enhanced immune response when transferred to nonimmunized animals. The response is antigen-specific since lymphocytes sensitized to one antigen do not produce an enhanced response if the recipient animal is challenged with a different antigen.

CYTOKINES

During macrophage–T-cell interaction, many soluble mediators are synthesized and released. Monokines are produced by macrophages and lymphokines by lymphocytes; collectively they are termed *cytokines*. A principal product of the activated macrophage is interleukin 1 (IL-1) which has a range of diverse effects, including lymphocyte activation. IL-1, formerly termed *lymphocyte activation factor*, appears to play a major role in granuloma formation. IL-1 is also chemotactic for T cells. The macrophage probably secretes IL-1 during the presentation of antigen. Thus, the T cell receives from the macro-phage both the antigen and the soluble mediator to promote T-cell activation.

In vitro, T cells in hypersensitivity granulomas produce a variety of lymphokines, the presence of which correlates with progression of the granuloma (Fig. 41-8). As noted above, the start of granulomas appears to be enhanced by the formation of monocyte chemotactic factor by T cells; this factor recruits peripheral blood monocytes to the site of inflammation. Migration inhibition factor prevents these recruited cells from departing. Macrophage activation factors from T cells enhance the ability of the macrophage to kill intracellular organisms. Lymphokines do not have specificity and induce their effects on macrophages irrespective of the type of Ia molecule on the surface of the macrophages. Eosinophil "stimulation promoter" is also a T-cell product that may explain the prominence of eosinophils in many types of granulomas.

Interleukin 2 (IL-2) acts as a lymphokine for T cells. The former term for IL-2, *T-cell growth factor*, describes the biologic antibody of this lymphokine which interacts with appropriately primed T cells, causing them to proliferate. IL-2 is produced by the helper subset of T cells. A soluble factor secreted by suppressor cells has also been described which down-regulates the granulomatous response and is found in the later stages of schistosomal infection. Lymphocytes also produce factors that are chemotactic for fibroblasts.

THE FIBROGENIC RESPONSE

Fibrosis often represents the final stage of granulomatous inflammation. In response to macrophage-generated me-

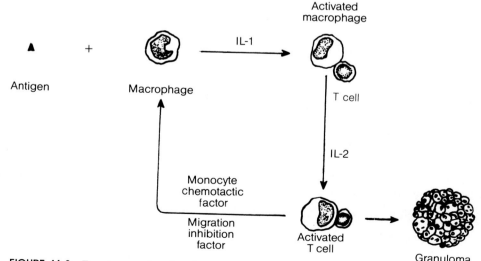

FIGURE 41-8 Events associated with macrophage- and T-cell-induced pulmonary granulomas. Interaction of antigen with macrophages leads to antigen presentation to specific T cells and interleukin 1 production. T cells then produce interleukin 2 which expands T-cell clones, resulting in granuloma formation. Activated macrophages produce other lymphokines which amplify the inflammatory response.

diators, fibroblasts are recruited by chemotactic signals to areas within the lung where they attach, proliferate, synthesize, and secrete collagen. Chemotactic recruitment of fibroblasts also occurs in response to fibronectin, collagenous peptides, or fragments derived from the fifth component of complement. Fibronectin from alveolar macrophages is not only a chemoattractant for fibroblasts but also mediates attachment and provides a signal for fibroblast replication. Alveolar macrophage-derived growth factor for fibroblasts stimulates these cells to produce their own fibroblast growth factor. Macrophages also produce fibroblast-activating factors. Lymphocytes produce chemotactic factors for fibroblasts and fibroblast-activating factors. The resulting fibrotic response in the lung is a combination of (1) increased numbers of pulmonary fibroblasts, due to chemotaxis, adherence to connective tissue, and local proliferation, and (2) increased collagen production by these fibroblasts.

The immune nature of the fibrotic response is suggested by experimental studies where immunosuppressive therapy effectively decreases the development of pulmonary fibrosis. At high concentrations, steroids inhibit pulmonary fibrosis, as does antilymphocyte globulin or thymectomy. Removal of macrophages by administering antimacrophage globulin also decreases fibrosis. The fibrotic response in delayed hypersensitivity reactions is governed by macrophages, lymphocytes, and mediators resulting from macrophage–T-cell interactions. In contrast, the fibrotic response in foreign body reactions is mediated almost exclusively by macrophages, as shown by their production of fibroblast-activating factors following exposure to silica or quartz crystals.

CLINICAL RELEVANCE

Immune responses that lead to progressive pulmonary injury, as described here, may also be operative in human pulmonary granulomatous diseases such as sarcoidosis. Many of the regulatory mechanisms described in experimental animals have been demonstrated in patients as well. Activation of alveolar macrophages also occurs as does an increase in the spontaneous release of IL-1. Human leukocyte antigen-DS (HLA-DS), the human counterpart of the mouse Ia antigen, is expressed on alveolar macrophages. Lung T cells from sarcoidosis patients also spontaneously release IL-2 and migration inhibition factor. Analysis of bronchoalveolar lavage fluid from patients with high intensity alveolitis shows a greater number of T cells, mostly with the helper phenotype, as compared to normal individuals or patients with idiopathic pulmonary fibrosis or sarcoidosis patients in whom alveolitis is of low intensity. The concentrations of fibronectin and alveolar macrophage-derived growth factor are also abnormally high in the lavage fluid of sarcoidosis patients. These observations suggest that cells mediating immune reactions probably represent an important mechanism in pulmonary inflammatory diseases.

BIBLIOGRAPHY

Bauman MD, Jetten AM, Brody AR: Biologic and biochemical characterization of a macrophage-derived growth factor for rat lung fibroblasts. Chest 91:15S–16S, 1987.
   In parenchymal lung disease that entails attraction of macrophages to sites of particle deposition or lung injury, local regulation of macrophage-derived growth factor, a PDGF-like growth molecule, may contribute importantly to the regulation of altered mesenchymal cell growth.

Bitterman PB, Wewers MD, Rennard SI, Adelberg S, Crystal RG: Modulation of alveolar macrophage-driven fibroblast proliferation by alternative macrophage mediators. J Clin Invest 77:700–708, 1986.
   In addition to the two primary growth promoting signals, fibronectin and alveolar macrophage-derived growth factor, alveolar macrophages are able to release other mediators that may have a potential role in modulating lung fibroblast replication in response to these primary signals, including interferon γ (IFNγ), prostaglandin E_2 (PGE_2), and interleukin 1 (IL–1).

Boros DL: Experimental granulomatous disease, in Fanburg BL (ed), Sarcoidosis and Other Granulomatous Disease of the Lung. New York, Dekker, 1983, pp 403–452.
   Provides a comprehensive review of experimental models of granulomatous diseases.

Buck CA, Horwitz AF: Cell surface receptors for extracellular matrix molecules. Ann Rev Cell Biol 3:179–205, 1987.
   An overview of the present state of understanding of cell-adhesion molecules that are involved in diverse biologic phenomena within the intercellular matrix.

Chensue SW, Kunkel SL, Ward PA, Higashi GI: Exogenously administered prostaglandins modulate pulmonary granulomas induced by Schistosoma mansoni eggs. Am J Pathol 111:78–87, 1983.
   Clearly shows the role of arachidonic acid metabolites in a well-defined model system of synchronous pulmonary granulomas.

Cross CE: Oxygen radicals and human disease. Ann Intern Med 107:526–545, 1987.
An edited and updated summary of a conference that focuses on the chemistry of oxygen radical production and the role of iron and of various oxidants.

Fantone JC, Ward PA: Review article: Role of oxygen-derived free radicals and metabolites in leukocyte-dependent inflammatory reactions. Am J Pathol 107:395–418, 1982.
A good general review of the phagocytic cell-induced tissue damage by oxygen radicals.

Fantone JC, Ward PA: Oxygen-derived radicals and their metabolites: Relationship to tissue injury, in Current Concepts, A Scope Publications. Kalamazoo, MI, Upjohn Company, 1985.
A good general review of the phagocytic cell-induced tissue damage by oxygen radicals.

Fels AOS, Cohn ZA: The alveolar macrophage. J Appl Physiol 60:353–369, 1986.
Recent investigations on the alveolar macrophage demonstrate an extensive synthetic and secretory repertoire including lysozyme, neutral proteases, acid hydrolases, and O_2 metabolites. In addition, these cells produce a wide variety of pro- and anti-inflammatory agents, including arachidonic acid metabolites of the cyclooxygenase and lipoxygenase pathways, cytokines which modulate lymphocyte function, and factors which promote fibroblast migration and replication.

Garrett KC, Richerson HG, Hunninghake GW: State of the art pathogenesis of granulomatous lung diseases. II. Mechanisms of granuloma formation. Am Rev Respir Dis 130:477–483, 1984.
This is an up-to-date, well-referenced review of pulmonary granulomatous inflammation and fibrosis.

Herberman RB: Natural killer cells. Annu Rev Med 37:347–352, 1986.
Natural killer (NK) cells are a subpopulation of lymphocytes, which have spontaneous cytotoxicity against a variety of tumor cells, virus-infected cells, and some normal cells in the bone marrow and thymus. A central role in lysis by NK cells is played by a cytolytic protein contained within their cytoplasmic granules.

Iozzo RV: Proteoglycans: Structure, function and role in neoplasia. Lab Invest 53:373–396, 1985.
A general review of current knowledge about structure, function, and localization of proteoglycans which feature prominently in connective tissue and influence a variety of biological processes, including cell recognition, cell proliferation, and cell differentiation.

Johnson KJ, Wilson BS, Till GO, Ward PA: Acute lung injury in rat caused by immunoglobulin A immune complexes. J Clin Invest 74:358–369, 1984.
Oxygen radical damage caused by oxygen products of tissue macrophages.

Karnovsky ML: Comparative aspects of the production of oxygen radicals by phagocytic cells, and aspects of other effector substances. Int J Tissue React 8:91–97, 1986.
The author reviews the information gleaned from a great variety of sources on the factors influencing the production of oxygen radicals by phagocytic cells, with reference to inflammation.

Katzenstein AL: Pathogenesis of "fibrosis" in interstitial pneumonia: an electron microscopic study. Hum Pathol 16:1015–1024, 1985.
Seven cases in which interstitial fibrosis developed in patients who had acute interstitial pneumonia were studied ultrastructurally to explore the pathogenesis of the interstitial thickening seen by light microscopy.

Lanier LL, Le AM, Cwirla S, Federspiel N, Phillips JH: Antigenic, functional, and molecular genetic studies of human natural killer cells and cytotoxic T lymphocytes not restricted by the major histocompatibility complex. Fed Proc 45:2823–2828, 1986.
Cytotoxicity not restricted by the major histocompatibility complex (MHC) is mediated by two distinct types of lymphocytes: natural killer (NK) cells and non-MHC-restricted cytotoxic T lymphocytes (CTL). NK cells are distinct in lineage from T lymphocytes and do not use the T cell antigen receptor genes for target recognition.

Martinet Y, Rom WN, Grotendorst GR, Martin GR, Crystal RG: Exaggerated spontaneous release of platelet-derived growth factor by alveolar macrophages from patients with idiopathic pulmonary fibrosis. N Engl J Med 317:202–209, 1987.
Observations suggesting that the accumulation of mesenchymal cells within the alveolar walls in patients with idiopathic pulmonary fibrosis may result partly from the exaggerated release of the potent mitogen platelet-derived growth factor by mononuclear phagocytes in the lower respiratory tract.

Phan SH: Fibrotic mechanisms in lung diseases, in Ward PA (ed), Immunology of Inflammation. New York, Elsevier, 1983, pp 121–162.
Provides a clear review of pulmonary fibrotic mechanisms.

Quinones F, Crouch E: Biosynthesis of interstitial and basement membrane collagens in pulmonary fibrosis. Am Rev Respir Dis 134:1163–1171, 1986.
An experimental study of the biosynthesis and matrix deposition of type IV procollagen and of interstitial collagens in rat lung explants in bleomycin-induced pulmonary fibrosis.

Rennard SI, Bitterman PB, Crystal RG: State of art pathogenesis of granulomatous lung diseases. IV. Mechanisms of fibrosis. Am Rev Respir Dis 130:492–496, 1984.
An up-to-date, well-referenced review of pulmonary granulomatous inflammation and fibrosis.

Salahuddin SZ, Rose RM, Groopman JE, Markham PD, Gallo RC: Human T lymphotropic virus type III infection of human alveolar macrophages. Blood 68:281–284, 1986.
The human T-cell lymphotropic virus type III (HTLV-III) not only preferentially infects T4 lymphocytes but also infects other cell types, notably B lymphocytes and other nonlymphoid cells. Macrophage infection with HTLV-III may be one mechanism for the establishment of viral persistence in infected hosts.

Schwarz MI, King TE Jr: Interstitial Lung Disease. Philadelphia, B.C. Dekker, 1988.
A multiauthored volume that covers the broad span of interstitial diseases and ranges from fundamental mechanisms to clinical applications.

Smedly LA, Tonnesen MG, Sandhaus RA, Haslett C, Guthrie LA, Johnston RB Jr, Henson PM, Worthen GS: Neutrophil-mediated injury to endothelial cells. Enhancement by endotoxin and essential role of neutrophil elastase. J Clin Invest 77:1233–1243, 1986.
The neutrophil has been implicated as an important mediator of vascular injury, especially after endotoxemia. This study examines neutrophil-mediated injury to human microvascular endothelial cells in vitro.

Till GO, Johnson KJ, Kunkel R, Ward PA: Intravascular activation of complement and acute lung injury. Dependency on neutrophils and toxic oxygen metabolites. J Clin Invest 69:1126–1135, 1982.
Sensitivity of the microvasculature to oxygen radical damage from neutrophils and a definition of the radicals involved.

Tomasi TB Jr: Mechanisms of immune regulation at mucosal surfaces. Rev Infect Dis 5:S784–S792, 1983.
Current understanding of IgA by investigator who did pioneering work in the field.

Unanue ER: Cooperation between mononuclear phagocytes and lymphocytes in immunity. N Engl J Med 303:977–985, 1980.
A succinct presentation of the cell interactions between macrophages and lymphocytes.

Ward PA, Till GO, Kunkel R, Beauchamp C: Evidence for role of hydroxyl radical in complement and neutrophil-dependent tissue injury. J Clin Invest 72:789–801, 1983.
Sensitivity of the microvasculature to oxygen radical damage from neutrophils and a definition of the radicals involved.

Warheit DB, Hill LH, George G, Brody AR: Time course of chemotactic factor generation and the corresponding macrophage response to asbestos inhalation. Am Rev Respir Dis 134:128–133, 1986.
Pulmonary macrophages have been implicated as significant mediators of the pathogenic process that follows inhalation of asbestos fibers. The present study demonstrates the time course of chemotactic factor generation and the corresponding macrophage response in vivo.

Warren JS, Kunkel RG, Johnson KJ, Ward PA: Comparative O_2^- responses of lung macrophages and blood phagocytic cells in the rat. Possible relevance to IgA immune complex induced lung injury. Lab Invest 57:311–320, 1987.
IgA immune complex-induced lung injury in the rat is oxygen radical mediated and partially complement-dependent but not neutrophil-dependent. Lung interstitial and alveolar macrophages produce O_2^- when stimulated by immune complexes in vitro suggesting that they contribute to the development of oxygen radical mediated lung injury.

Weissler JC, Nicod LP, Toews GB: Pulmonary natural killer cell activity is reduced in patients with bronchogenic carcinoma. Am Rev Respir Dis 135:1353–1357, 1987.
Natural killer (NK) cells are a subpopulation of lymphocytes capable of killing a variety of tumor targets. The NK activity of pulmonary lymphocytes obtained from the patients with lung cancer was significantly lower than the NK activity of normal lungs.

Young KR, Rankin JA, Naegel GP, Paul ES, Reynolds HY: Bronchoalveolar lavage cells and proteins with the acquired immunodeficiency syndrome: An immunologic analysis. Ann Intern Med 103:522–533, 1985.
Immunology of AIDS lung disease presented.

Chapter 42

*Sarcoidosis**

Carol Johnson Johns†

*This chapter contains excerpts from the chapter written by Louis E. Siltzbach in the previous edition of this book.

†Supported in part by The Hospital for the Consumptives of Maryland (Eudowood).

Sarcoidosis has been described as a multisystem granulomatous disorder of unknown etiology, most commonly affecting young adults and presenting most frequently with bilateral lymphadenopathy, pulmonary infiltrations, and skin or eye lesions. Other organs that are commonly affected include peripheral lymph nodes, liver, spleen, mucous membranes, parotid glands, phalangeal bones, muscles, heart, and nervous system. The diagnosis is established most securely when clinical radiographic findings are supported by histologic evidence of widespread noncaseating epithelioid-cell granulomas in more than one organ, or a positive Kveim-Siltzbach skin test. Immunologic features include depression of delayed-type hypersensitivity suggesting impaired cell-mediated immunity and raised or abnormal immunoglobulin levels. Hypercalciuria with or without hypercalcemia may be observed. The course and prognosis may correlate with the mode of onset: an acute onset with erythema nodosum usually heralds a self-limiting course and spontaneous resolution, while an insidious onset may be followed by relentless progressive disease with pulmonary fibrosis. Corticosteroids usually relieve symptoms, produce clinical remissions and suppress inflammation and granuloma formation. Long-term treatment is often required.

Recent studies made possible by bronchoalveolar lavage have indicated that these disorders are characterized by enhanced cellular immune processes at sites of involvement. Studies of thymus-derived T-cell subsets identified by means of monoclonal antibodies have revealed increased numbers of thymus-derived T-helper or -inducer lymphocytes, with a relative decrease in the T-suppressor or cytotoxic lymphocytes. An intense interaction with alveolar macrophages and T cells produces an alveolitis with resultant alveolar capillary dysfunction. Detailed studies of the cells and mediators and modulation of the inflammatory and immune processes continue to elucidate the control and progression from alveolitis to granuloma formation and possible fibrosis or healing. Sarcoidosis is currently viewed as a disorder of immune regulation. The agent or agents responsible have not been identified, but further studies may provide new understandings of the etiology and optimal treatment of this persistently puzzling disease.

HISTORICAL BACKGROUND

Knowledge concerning sarcoidosis has been accumulated during the last century in roughly four historical periods. In 1869, almost simultaneously, two dermatologists, Jonathan Hutchinson of London and Carl William Boeck of Christiana (now Oslo), independently encountered skin eruptions of an unfamiliar type which, in retrospect, may have represented examples of chronic cutaneous sarcoidosis. In 1889, Besnier of Paris designated a cutaneous manifestation involving the nose, ear lobules, and fingers as "lupus pernio" which, as later reported in 1892 by two other French observers, Tenneson and Quainquaud, exhibited a typical sarcoidal histologic pattern dominated by epithelioid cell infiltration with few giant cells.

From 1899 forward, Caesar Boeck, of Christiana, nephew of Carl William Boeck, clearly set forth some of the clinical and histopathologic features of sarcoidosis which led, for a time, to its eponymic designation as Boeck's sarcoid. In the following two decades, piecemeal descriptions appeared of lesions of sarcoidosis involving bones, eyes, salivary glands, subcutaneous tissues, and lungs; but during the first historical period, none of the authors recognized that the local area of their particular concern was only the palpable part of a "whole elephant."

The second historical era began in 1917 with Schaumann's important clinical observations, which for the first time firmly established the multisystemic nature of sarcoidosis. Thereafter, until the 1940s, more than 1000 individual cases of sarcoidosis affecting almost every organ system were reported in the world literature. But even then, the diagnosis was limited to patients in the later stages of sarcoidosis when symptoms were usually present while the far more numerous group in the clinically silent earliest stage went virtually undetected.

It was in the third historical period of the 1940s and 1950s, the era of mass chest radiography, when Löfgren's pioneering observations stimulated a general awareness that sarcoidosis most often began with asymptomatic symmetric bilateral hilar lymphadenopathy that was sometimes accompanied by an acute attack of erythema nodosum. The proper diagnostic interpretation of the widespread finding of asymptomatic bilateral hilar adenopathy in chest radiographs laid the groundwork for exploring for the first time the epidemiologic aspects of sarcoidosis in various countries around the world.

During that same period Longcope from Johns Hopkins and Freiman of the Massachusetts General Hospital published their classic monograph describing the broad spectrum of disease identified as *sarcoidosis*.

The fourth and current historical phase has been marked by an intense interest in the characteristics of the cellular and immune processes in sarcoidosis. The advent of modern cell biologic techniques and monoclonal antibodies has resulted in extensive study of the alveolar macrophage and T-cell and B-cell interactions as well as mediators and modulators of the immune and inflammatory responses.

EPIDEMIOLOGY

Sarcoidosis has been detected with varying frequency among populations of virtually every country in the world. The national prevalence and annual incidence rate remain vague approximations, being weighted, in part, by the frequency with which systematic mass radiography is carried out among the general population of each country and by the level of the medical community's awareness of the multifaceted manifestations of sarcoidosis. In countries where tuberculosis is prevalent, it is difficult to determine the frequency of sarcoidosis. This is especially true in Africa and India, where a few cases have been identified. It is clearly recognized that significant but unknown numbers of cases of sarcoidosis remain undetected. Figures clearly vary with the case finding method and the frequency of chest radiographs. The reported data have been extensively reviewed by James in his recent book. Prevalence rates per 100,000 vary from 64 in Sweden to 12 in Japan and 80 in blacks in New York City.

The disease is most frequent in the third and fourth decades of life. However, the age range begins in the preadolescent period and extends to the sixth and seventh decades in small numbers of patients. The prevalence of sarcoidosis in American blacks is 10 times higher than the prevalence in whites. The frequency of erythema nodosum varies between ethnic groups and between males and females. The highest incidence is in young, childbearing women, often following pregnancy and lactation as noted by Löfgren. This has been particularly noted in young Irish women in London and in Puerto Ricans in New York City. It is less common in black and Japanese women and uncommon in men in all countries. In Denmark and Sweden, where the rates for tuberculosis have sharply decreased, the rates for sarcoidosis have remained virtually unchanged.

ETIOLOGY

The cause of sarcoidosis is still not known. Suspicion that it was a special form of *Mycobacterium tuberculosis* has not been substantiated. The hypothesis that pine pollen is the cause was suggested by the geographic distribution in military recruits from the southeastern United States, but this thought has had to be abandoned. No organic or inorganic chemical has been consistently identified within sarcoidal tissue. It is unclear whether one or several infectious or other exogenous agents might be responsible and whether these are acquired through inhalation, ingestion, or dermal contact.

A genetic susceptibility has been suggested by studies of familial clusters of sarcoidosis. HLA studies have not demonstrated consistent patterns in whites, blacks, or other racial groups. It is likely that factors which determine and regulate the immunologic response may be as important as the inciting agent in causing the disease manifestations. International studies using the Kveim-Siltzbach material have demonstrated a common responsiveness to the same material and support the concept of a single cause.

PATHOLOGY

The characteristic noncaseating tuberculoid epithelioid cell granulomas are widely distributed in numerous organs and tissues even when bilateral hilar adenopathy may be the only clinical abnormality. Such granulomas are frequently present both in the lung and in the liver as well as other organs rich in lymphoreticular elements. Occasionally some central fibrinoid necrosis is identified. The typical epithelioid cell granulomas are not pathognomonic, as almost identical granulomas may occur in beryllium disease, tuberculosis, leprosy, hypersensitivity pneumonitis, Crohn's disease, primary biliary cirrhosis, fungal disease, and local "sarcoid reactions," which occur in lymph nodes that drain neoplastic or chronic inflammatory areas.

Most granulomas in sarcoidosis gradually undergo resolution, leaving behind few or no residual changes. On the other hand, even a decade or more after complete clinical recovery, a few scattered epithelioid granulomas are often discernible in lymph nodes, lung, liver, and spleen. At autopsy others who once had sarcoidosis, but died of other causes, often have only a few stellate scars or hyalinized foci as the only remnants of granulomatous involvement that years ago may have been florid.

The predominant cell within a sarcoidal granuloma is the epithelioid cell with elongated, waist-pinched, vesicular nucleus and its eosinophilic cytoplasm (Fig. 42-1). The epithelioid cells are arranged compactly in a whorled, tuberculoid conformation near the center of which may be a small area of fibrinoid necrosis. On electron microscopy, the epithelioid cell has a characteristic interdigitation of cell membranes, extensive rough endoplasmic reticulum, enlarged Golgi apparatus, and numerous cytoplasmic transport vesicles. Giant cells that result from fusion of macrophages are also present and sometimes contain cytoplasmic inclusions, particularly the calcium- and iron-containing lamellar concretions (Schaumann bodies), as well as asteroids and crystalline material, none of which is diagnostically specific.

Pulmonary granulomas tend to congregate in areas that are rich in lymphatic vessels such as subpleural, perivascular, and peribronchial regions. Adjacent and accom-panying nonspecific inflammatory changes are also frequently noted, and alveolitis with cellular infiltrates has been observed. Initially, most of the granulomas lie widely scattered within the alveolar septae, and, in most instances, they undergo resolution with little or no residual fibrosis. In progressive disease, the granulomas proliferate, become more densely packed, and fuse. Alveolar spaces may be obliterated with reduction in the area available for alveolocapillary gas exchange. Bronchioles and small bronchi are often involved and may narrow progressively because of granulomatous lesions on the surface as well as from peribronchial fibrosis. Healing of granulomas in the lung may be followed by fibrosis and hyalinization and may result in extensive lung fibrosis. Such scarring sometimes causes traction on adjacent lung tissue and may result in large cystic lesions. Granulomatous angiitis and perivascular granulomas and fibrosis may increase pulmonary vascular resistance and promote the gradual development of cor pulmonale and ultimately intractable right ventricular failure.

In patients who are in the chronic stage of disease, fresh granulomas exist side by side with granulomas that exhibit various stages of healing by fibrosis and hyalinization. Extensive lung fibrosis sometimes leads to severe pulmonary insufficiency; scarring in the uveal tracts may

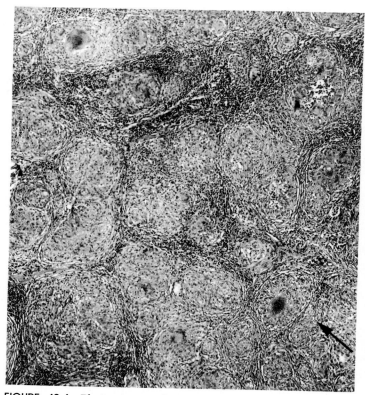

FIGURE 42-1 Photomicrograph showing lymph node substance almost entirely replaced by discrete and confluent epithelioid cell tuberculoid granulomas without necrosis. Several giant cells are visible. ×88.

result in secondary glaucoma and blindness. Persistent hypercalcemia and hypercalciuria with renal calculi are sometimes complicated by hydronephrosis, pyelonephritis, nephrocalcinosis, and, finally, renal failure.

Comparable extensive scarring may occur in the liver with resultant cirrhosis and portal hypertension. The extent and localization of the granulomas and possible scarring determine the clinical manifestations. Factors which determine the persistence, progression, or resolution of these lesions are poorly understood.

PHYSIOLOGY

The abnormalities in pulmonary performance correlate closely with the histopathologic changes at successive stages of sarcoidosis. Particularly the pulmonary parenchyma, but also the airways, become progressively affected by the granulomatous and fibrosing process. As a result, changes in lung volumes, diffusing capacity, and airflow become more manifest as the disease persists.

In type I, which is characterized by hilar node enlargement but radiographically clear lung fields, granulomas and nonspecific cellular infiltration are often present in the alveolar septa even though they are radiographically unrecognized. At this early stage, the only abnormality in lung function is apt to be an impairment in diffusing capacity. On the average, lung volumes are within the normal range even though they tend to fall at the lower limits.

In type II, in which distinct radiographic mottling of lung fields accompanies hilar node enlargement, changes in pulmonary function tests become characteristic of restrictive lung disease; lung volumes are abnormally low, and the diffusing capacity is more often abnormal. Occasionally, these are all within normal predicted values but may go above the normal range after treatment. The lungs become "stiff" as indicated by a decrease in pulmonary compliance and an increase in static transpulmonary pressure. If the airways are involved, conventional tests of airways resistance and of the distribution of inspired gas are sometimes abnormal. More often, however, obstruction of the airways in type II is confined to the small airways so that only "sensitive" tests are abnormal.

In type III, gross pulmonary fibrosis is often associated with cystic and bullous transformation and with severe obstruction of the airways. As a result, some of the features of chronic bronchitis and emphysema are superimposed upon the pattern of restrictive lung disease. However, in sarcoidosis, the residual volume generally does not become abnormally large, and total lung capacity is reduced. The decrease in the rate of airflow is disproportionally large for the decrease in lung volume; the discordance is readily demonstrated by the reduced FEV_1/FVC ratio. In the patient with progressive disease, respiratory failure may supervene, characterized by arterial hypoxemia, pulmonary hypertension, cor pulmonale, and right ventricular failure. Granulomatous angiitis and perivascular fibrosis contribute to the pulmonary hypertension.

IMMUNOLOGY AND PATHOGENESIS

Sarcoidosis is a disorder characterized by widespread granulomas which form in response to an unidentified stimulus. The granulomas may continue to appear, may eventually resolve completely, or may undergo fibrosis. While the lung is the predominant site of involvement, almost every organ system may be involved.

In the 1980 edition of this book Siltzbach emphasized "three features which epitomize the patterns of immune responsiveness in sarcoidosis: first, impaired cell mediated responses as exemplified by deficient delayed hypersensitivity cutaneous reactivity; second, intact humoral immune mechanisms enabling heightened immunoglobulin production; and third, a novel capacity, acquired early in the disease to respond specifically by forming granulomas at sites of intracutaneous injection of special sarcoidal tissue suspensions."

In recent years, modern techniques of cell biology coupled with bronchoalveolar lavage have expanded our understanding of this disorder. At this writing, the characteristic pathogenetic features of sarcoidosis are: (1) an *enhanced* cellular response at sites of disease involvement as exemplified by pulmonary alveolitis and granuloma formation, and (2) an altered regulation of humoral immunity as demonstrated by peripheral hyperglobulinemia. Still unexplained are the cutaneous anergy to common delayed-type hypersensitivity antigens, and the Kveim reactivity. It is hoped that further study will provide explanations for these phenomena as well as indicate the basic stimulus or defect which initiates these processes. The presence of activated lymphocytes and macrophages at sites of disease involvement is similar to the nonspecific, effector phase of models of a delayed-type hypersensitivity reaction such as the tuberculin skin test. However, the initiating stimulus for the inflammatory reaction in sarcoidosis is unknown. Delayed-type hypersensitivity reactions classically are initiated by interaction of an antigen with a preexisting clone of T cells which exhibit both specificity and memory for the antigen.

In sarcoidosis an antigen has been postulated but not identified. However, it is increasingly recognized that inflammatory reactions may also be initiated by nonspecific activation of T cells, bypassing the usual, immunologic, antigen-lymphocyte interaction. Host factors may also affect the response to a given stimulus.

In the following section, the specific pathogenetic features of sarcoidosis are reviewed in greater detail. Table 42-1 and Fig. 42-2 are intended to supplement the discussion.

TABLE 42-1
Inflammatory and Immune Factors in Sarcoidosis

Alveolar Macrophages

Derived chiefly from blood monocytes

Two types—resident tissue macrophages and inflammatory macrophages

Both may be activated and are indistinguishable by routine staining

May proliferate locally in the lung

Functions

Microbicidal function

Antigen presentation

Features of activated macrophages

Express immune-associated (Ia) surface molecules essential for antigen recognition by T cells

Release mediators

Secretory products

Alveolar macrophage-derived growth factor (AMDGF)

A progression factor for growth of fibroblasts

Interleukin 1 (IL-1)

Increases the interleukin 2 receptors on T cells and may stimulate T cells to release IL-2

Initiates lymphocyte activation and/or cell division

Chemotactic factor for T cells

Augments fibroblast replication in response to fibronectin and AMDGF

Increases immunoglobulin synthesis by B cells

May stimulate type II alveolar cell proliferation

Increases collagenase from fibroblasts, affects degradation

Affects protein degradation in muscle cells; causes weakness and weight loss

Increases protein synthesis, i.e., fibrinogen, haptoglobin, ceruloplasmin and C-reactive protein

Causes fever (the leukocyte pyrogen)

Fibronectin—adhesive and opsonic glycoprotein

Mediator of interactions between cells and extracellular matrix

Predominant *competence* factor for growth of fibroblasts

Gamma or immune interferons

Macrophage-activating factor

Affect antigen presenting capacity of alveolar macrophages

Inhibit fibroblast replication

Augment or inhibit lymphocyte activation and/or cell division

Gamma or Immune Interferons (cont.)

May augment effects of interleukin 1

Potent immunoregulatory factor in both humoral and cellular immune processes, depending on amount, timing, and interactions

Thymus-derived lymphocytes (T cells)—responsible for cellular immunity

Classified in subsets based on surface markers

Helper-inducer OKT4$^+$ (Leu-3$^+$) responsible for delayed-type hypersensitivity

Suppressor cytotoxic (OKT8$^+$)

Functions

Interact with antigen bound to antigen presenting cells

Initiate and amplify cellular inflammatory reactions

Features of activated T-helper cells

Express interleukin 2 (IL-2) cell surface receptor

Secrete mediators

Mediators released

Interleukin 2 (IL-2)

Proliferation and differentiation of activated T cells

Chemotactic factor for T cells

Monocyte chemotactic factor—(may be IL-2)

Attracts and activates monocytes

Immune interferons (see above)

Released by T-helper cells with DR antigen on the surface (Leu-3$^+$ DR$^+$)

Macrophage activating factors

Assist in formation of granulomas

Macrophage migration inhibitory factor (MIF)

B-cell growth factor (BCGF)

B-cell differentiation factor (BCDF)

Bone marrow derived (B-cell) lymphocytes

Responsible for humoral immunity

Secrete a variety of classes of immunoglobulins, produce polyclonal hypergammaglobulinemia

Fibroblasts

Produce collagen and cause scarring

Both competence and progression growth factors involved

Balance of stimulation and inhibition determines scarring

Type II alveolar cells

Responsible for re-epithelialization and tissue remodeling

More desirable than fibrosis

NOTE: Italic entries are demonstrated in sarcoidosis by in vitro study of cells from bronchoalveolar lavage.

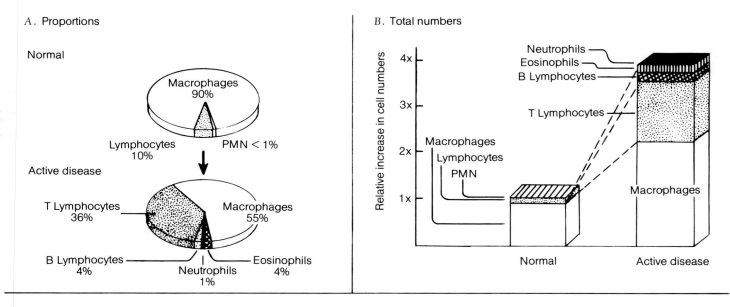

A. Proportions

Normal

Macrophages
90%

Lymphocytes
10%   PMN < 1%

Active disease

T Lymphocytes
36%

Macrophages
55%

B Lymphocytes
4%

Neutrophils
1%

Eosinophils
4%

B. Total numbers

Relative increase in cell numbers

Neutrophils
Eosinophils
B Lymphocytes

T Lymphocytes

Macrophages
Lymphocytes
PMN

Macrophages

Normal   Active disease

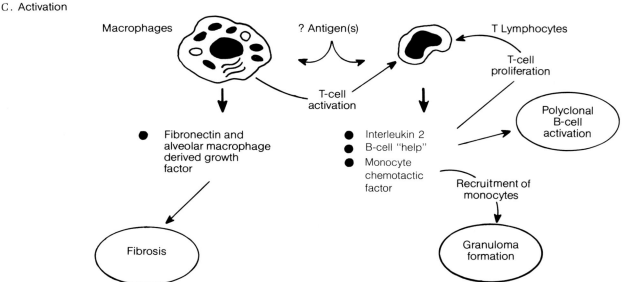

C. Activation

Macrophages   ? Antigen(s)   T Lymphocytes

T-cell
proliferation

T-cell
activation

● Fibronectin and
alveolar macrophage
derived growth
factor

● Interleukin 2
● B-cell "help"
● Monocyte
chemotactic
factor

Polyclonal
B-cell
activation

Recruitment of
monocytes

Fibrosis

Granuloma
formation

FIGURE 42-2   Current concepts of the pathogenesis of pulmonary sarcoidosis. Data from a typical patient are shown.   A. Proportions of effector cells are different from those normally observed. B. Total numbers of effector cells are increased, but to a different extent for each cell type.   C. Two cell types, alveolar macrophages and T lymphocytes, actively release mediators thought to be important in the pathogenesis of the disease. *(From Crystal, Bitterman, Rennard, Hance, Keogh: N Engl J Med 310:235–244, 1984.)*

Enhanced Cellular Response

The first, pathogenetic feature of sarcoidosis is an enhanced cellular response at sites of disease involvement. This has best been demonstrated in the lung. Using bronchoalveolar lavage, it has been appreciated that alveolitis is a major feature of the lung pathology, and it has been postulated that the alveolitis precedes and mediates granuloma and fibrosis formation. Both lavage and lung biopsy demonstrate an increase in lymphocytes and macrophages in sarcoidosis.

T-CELL LYMPHOCYTES

The lymphocytes include a higher proportion than normal of T-helper lymphocytes as demonstrated by fluorescent monoclonal antibody stains. The T cells are activated: they spontaneously secrete the protein called interleukin 2 (IL-2) or T-cell growth factor. IL-2 stimulates the growth of T-helper or cytolytic cells after an initial stimulus (which has not been identified in sarcoidosis). As a monocyte chemotactic factor, IL-2 attracts blood monocytes to sites of sarcoid involvement and may thus contribute to granuloma formation. Another T-cell mediator released is γ or immune interferon. γ-Interferon is a macrophage activator and induces an immune-associated (Ia) macrophage surface marker necessary for antigen recognition and delayed-type hypersensitivity.

ALVEOLAR MACROPHAGES

Alveolar macrophages are also present in increased numbers in sarcoidosis. They include both activated resident tissue macrophages and newly differentiated inflammatory macrophages recruited from the blood monocyte pool. Evidence for their activation in sarcoidosis includes the demonstration of class II mixed histocompatibility antigens (Ia surface molecules) on their surface and their elaboration of interleukin 1, a T-cell activator.

Mediators released by activated alveolar cells may also modulate fibrosis formation. Alveolar macrophages in sarcoidosis release fibronectin, a fibroblast chemotactic factor which mediates macrophage attachment to the extracellular matrix. Alveolar macrophage-derived growth factor and IL-1 may also promote fibrosis. By contrast, blood and lung mononuclear supernatant from some sarcoidosis patients will inhibit fibroblast growth. This suggests the presence of balancing cellular mechanisms which modulate the development of fibrosis.

Cutaneous Anergy

The cutaneous anergy in sarcoidosis remains an enigma. It is paradoxical that increased numbers of activated lymphocytes and macrophages are present at sites of disease involvement and yet are not recruited to a site of specific antigen stimulation. The common occurrence of cutaneous lesions in sarcoidosis argues against a nonspecific inhibition of migration of inflammatory cells to the skin. It is perhaps of note that similar though more severe cutaneous anergy occurs in lymphoma. Tuberculin anergy is common in sarcoidosis.

The Kveim Reaction

Kveim reactivity can be defined as a state of cutaneous sensitivity expressed by the formation of a slowly evolving, granulomatous papule at the site of injection of certain human sarcoidal tissue suspensions (Fig. 42-3). Little is known about the nature of the active principle in sarcoidal tissue responsible for a positive Kveim reaction. Kveim suspensions are thermostable, and the active fraction is relatively insoluble in water and in ether in the cold. All indications are that Kveim activity resides within the subcellular particles of the test suspension, in particular, in association with cytoplasmic particles of unknown origin. It has been suggested that these particles

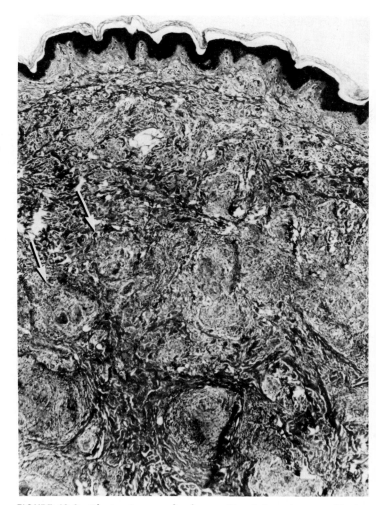

FIGURE 42-3 Photomicrograph of a positive intracutaneous Kveim reaction showing several discrete, noncaseating epithelioid cell granulomas in the midcorium. The granulomas show no necrosis and contain an occasional giant cell. ×120.

represent exogenous material that has been phagocytized and processed by the epithelioid cells of the sarcoid granulomas.

Efforts to devise an in vitro Kveim test have proved disappointing. The pathogenesis of the Kveim reaction remains unexplained. The value of Kveim reactivity persists as a research tool.

Abnormalities in Peripheral Lymphocytes

Abnormalities of peripheral lymphocytes also exist. Lymphopenia is common. Studies using circulating lymphocytes show a depressed proliferative response to mitogens and antigens but increased DNA synthesis. They also show increased spontaneous blast transformation and proliferation in culture and lymphokine release.

625

Immune Globulins

The increased immunoglobulin production may represent another example of altered T-cell regulation. T cells in sarcoidosis elaborate a B-cell growth factor. This factor could relate to the increased immunoglobulin response to viral infection seen in sarcoidosis or to the nonspecific hyperglobulinemia. The elevation of immune globulins is polyclonal. Increased IgG predominates, but elevations of IgA and IgM may also be present. Increased IgG is also observed in bronchoalveolar lavage fluid from sarcoidosis patients.

Circulating immune complexes may be seen in the early stages of the disease, particularly in association with erythema nodosum. Rheumatoid factor may occur in up to one-third of patients with active lesions. Antinuclear antibodies and cryoglobulins have been detected on occasion.

Angiotensin Converting Enzyme

Increased serum levels of angiotensin converting enzyme are thought to reflect the body's "granuloma load" in sarcoidosis. Epithelioid cells of the granuloma appear to be the source of this enzyme, and serum levels decrease with corticosteroid treatment. Increased levels of this enzyme also occur with diseases such as tuberculosis, biliary cirrhosis, leprosy, Gaucher's disease, and diabetes.

Cell Injury

In animal studies, oxygen radicals produced by inflammatory macrophages, as metabolic products from arachidonic acid, have been identified as important factors in lung injury. The lipoxygenase pathway seems essential for granuloma formation. Inhibitors of this, such as indomethacin, may diminish granuloma formation. The cyclooxygenase pathway seems to downregulate the lipoxygenase pathway by production of prostaglandins, prostacyclin, and thromboxane. Prostaglandins of the E class are thought to serve an immunoregulatory function, inhibiting T-helper cell aggregation and macrophage cytotoxicity. These and other substances are under study in the lavage fluid from the lungs of sarcoidosis patients. Studies of the schistosome lung granulomas in mice have demonstrated that inhibitors of the cyclooxygenase pathway can enhance granuloma formation. This animal model of granuloma formation has been useful in concepts potentially relevant to sarcoidosis.

SUMMARY

Sarcoidosis is now regarded as an inflammatory disorder of unknown etiology characterized by an intense interaction of activated lymphocytes and macrophages which result in disease expression and tissue injury. Alterations in immune regulation are suspected, with an exaggerated T-helper network. Recent studies have yet to alter the diagnosis, management, or treatment of sarcoidosis, except in the research setting.

CLINICAL FEATURES

Specific clinical manifestations depend on the extent and localization of organ involvement and the duration and progression of the disease. There is variation from a totally asymptomatic patient, with an incidental radiographic finding of bilateral hilar adenopathy, to a seriously breathless or blind patient. Many instances of this disease may be undetected, and it is likened to an iceberg, with only the tip identified. Spontaneous resolution is often observed. General constitutional symptoms of fatigue and weight loss may be noted in a quarter of the patients. Fever may be prominent in approximately 15 percent of the diagnosed patients.

The onset is generally insidious with gradual worsening. Exceptions to this are those with an acute *erythema nodosum* picture as described by Löfgren in 1952, with fever, red tender skin lesions, usually on the shins, arthralgias which may be seriously incapacitating, and bilateral hilar lymphadenopathy. This acute presentation occurs in only approximately 10 to 15 percent of the patients and is particularly common among young women of Swedish, Irish, and Puerto Rican backgrounds. Another abrupt onset may be noted with the appearance of an acute iritis with pain, photophobia, redness, and blurred vision. Again, a chest radiograph is likely to reveal bilateral hilar lymphadenopathy. It appears that the more acute the onset, the more favorable the prognosis.

Most frequently sarcoidosis is encountered either in a subacute or chronic form. The dividing point between the subacute and chronic phases empirically has been set at 2 years, although dating the onset of sarcoidosis is, at best, a rough approximation. Previous radiographs are of great assistance in dating the onset of the disease.

Abnormal Chest Radiograph

This is identified in about 90 percent of patients in most series. By international convention, the appearance is classified according to the presence of enlarged hilar lymph nodes, pulmonary infiltrates, and fibrosis.

The radiographic types may roughly parallel the evolution of the disease but there is no certainty that these occur as stages in all patients. The relative frequency of these types depends on the particular series reviewed and how it has been assembled. Data from Siltzbach indicate that about 10 percent will have a normal chest radiograph. Approximately 40 percent will have hilar lymphadenopathy. The presence of hilar lymphadenopathy and pulmonary infiltrates is the most frequent appearance in symptomatic patients and occurs in 30 to 50 percent. Infiltrates without lymphadenopathy, with or without fibrosis, will be observed in approximately 15 percent.

TYPE 0: NORMAL CHEST RADIOGRAPH

Although no abnormalities are obvious, adenopathy sometimes can be demonstrated by computed tomography when other clinical features suggest sarcoidosis.

TYPE I: BILATERAL HILAR ADENOPATHY

This is often accompanied by enlargement of the right paratracheal nodes (Fig. 42-4). Furthermore, computed tomography will frequently demonstrate anterior mediastinal and subcarinal adenopathy. About 50 percent of patients will exhibit this as their first radiographic manifestation of sarcoidosis. The nodes have been described as "potato nodes," and they typically stand away from the right border of the heart in contrast to nodes in lymphomatous and neoplastic disorders. The massive enlargement of nodes in the superior and anterior mediastinum

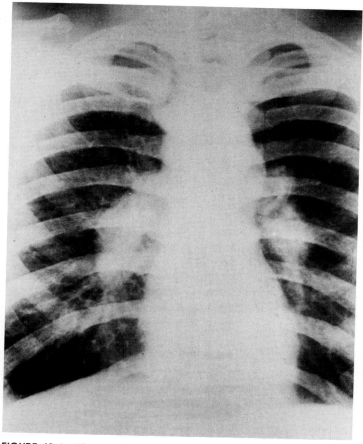

FIGURE 42-4 Chest radiograph showing bilateral hilar adenopathy as well as enlargement of nodes in both paratracheal regions. The enlarged hilar nodes characteristically stand away from the cardiac borders. The lung fields are virtually clear.

that is often seen in Hodgkin's disease is uncommon in sarcoidosis. The hilar and mediastinal adenopathy is only occasionally unilateral in sarcoidosis. This unusual form most often affects the left tracheal, bronchial, and periaortic areas and is thought to represent a residuum of resolving bilateral type I adenopathy. Asymmetric disease more often suggests primary tuberculosis, fungal infection, or metastases from a bronchogenic neoplasm. In three quarters of the patients with type I presentation, the enlarged hilar nodes regress within 1 to 3 years (Fig. 42-5). In about 10 percent hilar node enlargement becomes chronic and may persist for a decade or more. This is often seen in association with chronic skin sarcoid. Type I disease may progress to type II disease with obvious parenchymal changes.

TYPE II: BILATERAL HILAR ADENOPATHY WITH PULMONARY INFILTRATES

The infiltrates may be fine linear markings, coarse reticulonodules, or fluffy cotton wool confluent shadows. A ground glass appearance may cloud the lungs. Modern radiographic techniques demonstrate that the infiltrates are mostly peribronchial and subpleural in location. Pulmonary mottling appears most often within the first or second year of illness and occasionally occurs within weeks of the onset. Extensive micronodular densities sometimes resemble those of miliary tuberculosis, pneumoconiosis, beryllium disease, lymphangitic carcinoma, idiopathic hemosiderosis, and alveolar microlithiasis. The cotton wool fluffy infiltrations sometimes mimic those of exudative tuberculosis, eosinophilic pneumonia, Wegener's granulomatosis, and certain forms of extrinsic allergic alveolitis.

TYPE III: PULMONARY INFILTRATES WITHOUT LYMPHADENOPATHY

This is sometimes divided into subgroups A and B, according to the evidence for pulmonary fibrosis. It most frequently represents a later stage of the disease. Evidences of fibrosis and fibrocystic or bullous changes are often observed (Fig. 42-6). The radiographic patterns of this type are easily confused with the similar configurations of pulmonary tuberculosis involving the upper zones, fibrosing alveolitis, progressive systemic sclerosis, extrinsic allergic alveolitis, rheumatoid lung, congestive heart failure, and advanced bullous emphysema. These large cystic or bullous spaces are often found to contain fungus balls or mycetomas which most frequently are *Aspergillus fumigatus* (Fig. 42-7). Although the term *cavitary* disease is sometimes used, it is not clear that there has been necrosis and excavation of tissue, as in cavitary tuberculosis. The pattern is more likely the effect of fibrosis with traction or partial bronchial obstruction resulting in cystic lesions.

At the time of first diagnosis, about one of every seven patients exhibits the features of this fibrotic irreversible

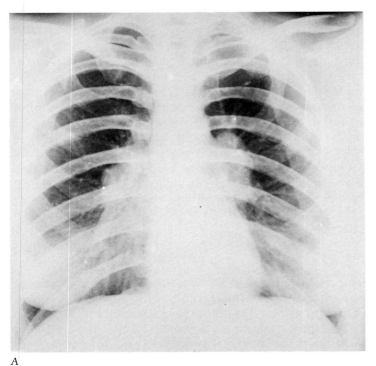 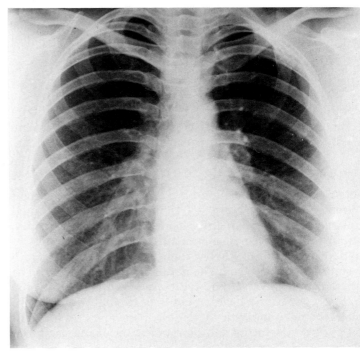

A   B

FIGURE 42-5   Especially rapid spontaneous resolution of hilar adenopathy.   A. Chest radiograph made in February 1977 after auto accident revealing unrelated characteristic bilateral hilar node enlargement.   B. Chest radiograph made in May 1977 shows virtually complete regression of node enlargement.

stage of pulmonary sarcoidosis. The degree of fibrosis ranges from clinically inconsequential linear streaks and nodular densities of limited extent, to widespread scarring and bullae that are totally disabling. Extensive scarring may shrink the lung fields, elevate the diaphragm, and cause upper retraction of one or both lung roots, sometimes leaving surprisingly clear lung fields. The hilar structures may become frozen masses of hyalinized scar tissue that distort major bronchi and narrow the pulmonary arteries and veins at the lung roots. Enlargement of the heart with cor pulmonale may ensue. Pneumothorax may follow rupture of the bullous lesions. Extensive pleural thickening is frequently noted over areas of cystic changes with mycetomas. Pleural effusion is infrequent and usually should raise the question of alternative diagnoses, although occasionally small effusions have been attributed to sarcoidosis when there is no other obvious explanation and pleural granulomas are identified. Occasionally, calcification is prominent in both nodes and pulmonary parenchyma (Fig. 42-8A and B).

Respiratory System

COUGH AND BREATHLESSNESS

These are the most common clinical complaints and occur in between one-third and two-thirds of the patients. The severity of symptoms may vary from mild to severe and incapacitating. Paroxysms of cough occasionally may even induce vomiting. Respiratory disease has been prominent in 85 percent of our patients with chronic persistent sarcoidosis of more than 5 years duration. The extent of radiographic change often far exceeds the findings of cough and breathlessness. In white patients it is common to find an absence or paucity of symptoms, in spite of extensive and progressive radiographic changes. However, the degree of breathlessness is extremely variable and may be marked even in the early stages. Prompt reversal with corticosteroid therapy is usual, except when irreversible fibrosis has ensued. In severe late stage disease, chronic hypoxia, cor pulmonale and right-sided congestive failure are frequent. Retention of carbon dioxide is unusual.

SPUTUM

The sputum is usually scanty or absent, except when chronic pulmonary changes have resulted in distortion and fibrocystic changes with persistent bacterial and/or fungal infections. The picture then resembles bronchiectasis. The sputum may be thick and yellowish green with 4 to 8 oz daily. Blood streaking is not uncommon. Temporary amelioration usually follows a course of broad spectrum antibiotics.

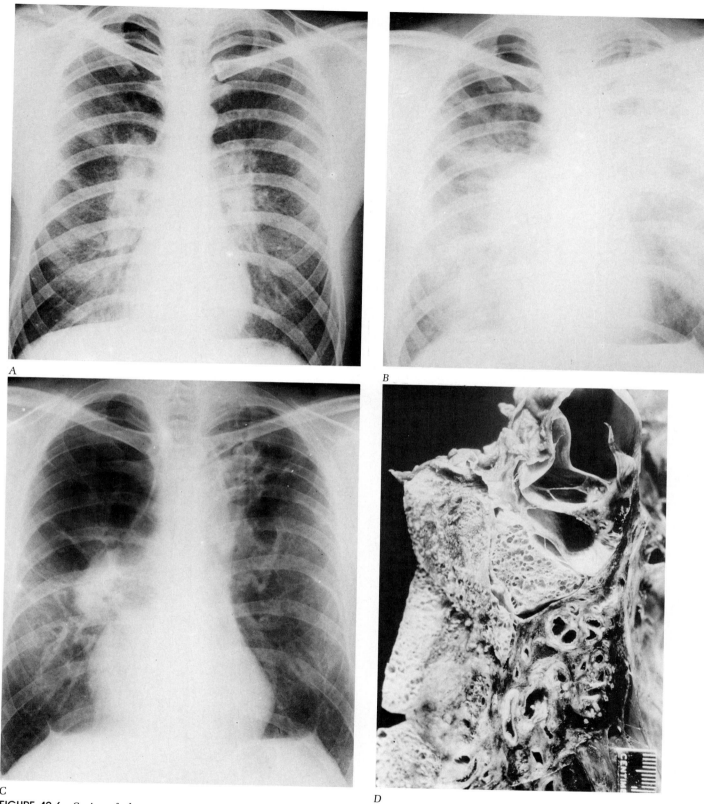

A

B

C

D

FIGURE 42-6 Series of chest radiographs covering a 15-year span illustrating progression through three stages of pulmonary sarcoidosis.
A. Chest radiograph taken November 1940 in an asymptomatic patient with hilar adenopathy discovered during U.S. Army induction examination (stage I). *B.* During the next 8 years, gradual opacification of the major portions of both lung fields by confluent mottling with persistence of hilar node enlargement bilaterally (stage II). *C.* Chest radiograph dated June 1955, 15 years after detection, shows progression to end stage (stage III) with giant bullae in right upper zone, an ill-defined density at the right lung root, and upward retraction of the left lung root with dense strands in the left upper zone. Corticosteroid therapy begun in 1952 had effected clearing of some lung densities and considerable relief of dyspnea which endured for 3 years before patient succumbed to right-sided heart failure in late 1955. *D.* Cut section of right lung at autopsy showing bullae and honeycombing with dense anthracotic scarring of right lung root that distorts and partially com-presses major blood vessels and bronchi.

629

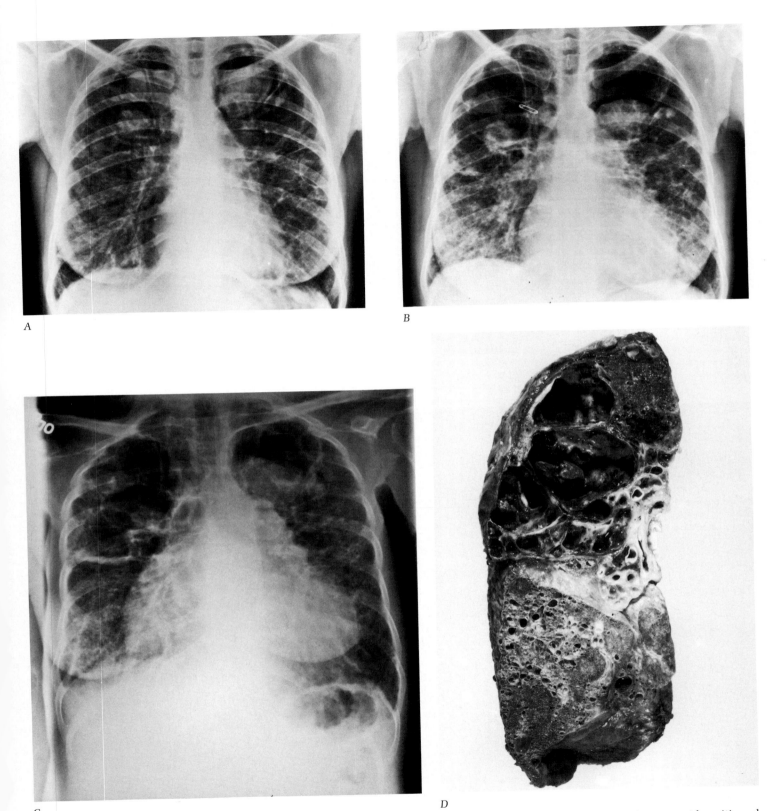

A

B

C

D

FIGURE 42-7 Chest radiographs of a black woman with sarcoidosis diagnosed at age 16. Patient developed blindness from sarcoid uveitis and extensive fibrocystic and bullous changes in the lungs. Course complicated by persistent and varying bilateral aspergillomas over a 17-year period. Occasional mild hemoptysis but persistent purulent sputum. *A*. Age 26 (1968). Bilateral mycetomas with crescentic overlying air shadows. *B*. Age 39 (1981). Persistent mycetomas and enlarging heart, on prednisone 10 mg daily, with no antifungal therapy. *C*. Age 41 (1984). Progressive cardiomegaly and congestive failure with cor pulmonale and pulmonary insufficiency. *D*. Age 42 (1985). Autopsy specimen of right lung after 26 years of sarcoidosis with multiple cysts containing necrotic material, with bronchiectasis.

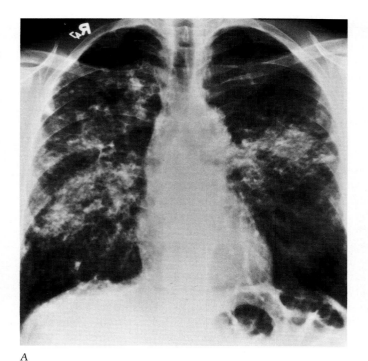

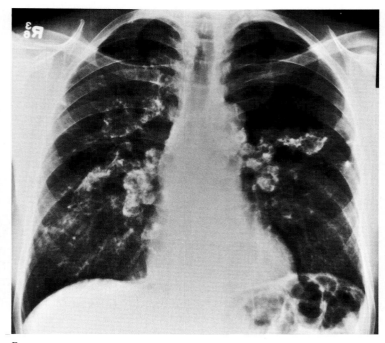

A   *B*

FIGURE 42-8   Chest radiographs of a white male with diffuse parenchymal infiltrates responding to corticosteroids. Biopsy proven sarcoidosis, renal calculi, hilar adenopathy, and lung infiltrates since 1964. Occasional hypercalcemia of 11.0 mg/dl.   *A.* Age 37 (1977). Corticosteroids begun because of gradual progression of infiltrates, with slight cough, but no dyspnea. Vital capacity and diffusing capacity always above normal.   *B.* Age 44 (1984). Still on 10 mg prednisone daily. Regression of infiltrates with egg-shell calcification of hilar nodes and calcified parenchymal lesions. No further renal calculi. Calcium normal. No respiratory symptoms.

HEMOPTYSIS

In early disease, the sputum is occasionally blood-streaked because of endobronchial granulomas. Later, recurrent hemoptysis of several hundred milliliters may occur in association with mycetomas in chronic fibrocystic disease with accompanying chronic bacterial infection. This is occasionally massive and may be fatal. Management of this is discussed subsequently.

ENDOBRONCHIAL DISEASE

The mucosal and submucosal layers of bronchi are frequent sites of involvement in sarcoidosis. The mural granulomas are usually nonulcerating and often silent but may present a pebbly appearance evident at bronchoscopy. There may be narrowing of segmental bronchi with focal and segmental atelectasis. In addition to cough, wheezing may occur. Middle lobe atelectasis has been observed. This is more likely the result of endobronchial disease than the effect of pressure from lymph nodes and usually improves promptly with corticosteroids.

MUCOSA OF THE UPPER RESPIRATORY TRACT

Mucosal lesions of the nose, sinuses, or larynx may be extensive, causing nasal obstruction, chronic sinusitis, and severe hoarseness. This occurs most frequently in chronic sarcoidosis with skin lesions. Surgical attempts to improve the airway usually result in destruction of the nasal septum, and a "saddle nose" may occur. Chloroquine can be very effective in alleviating the symptoms and reducing the granulomatous reaction in both skin and mucosa.

LARYNGEAL DISEASE

Chronic granulomatous laryngeal changes may result in hoarseness and narrowing of the airway with vocal cord thickening and stiffness and stridor. Such mucosal changes usually are accompanied by skin lesions. Indirect laryngoscopy is required to elucidate the status of the airway. Vocal cord paralysis and narrowed airway also may result from recurrent laryngeal nerve palsy in neurosarcoidosis. Direct laryngeal involvement can respond dramatically to corticosteroids, but tracheostomy is occasionally required.

Ocular Disease

About one quarter of the patients exhibit involvement of the eyes at some time in the course of sarcoidosis. In about 5 percent, ocular symptoms constitute the presenting manifestation usually accompanied by bilateral hilar lymphadenopathy. The sudden onset of redness, photophobia and blurred vision is dramatic and may be unilateral or bilateral. The prognosis for such a picture is generally good. A granular appearance of the conjunctiva is occasionally observed, and granulomas may be found on biopsy. When the conjunctiva appears normal, a blind biopsy is rarely productive. Keratoconjunctivitis and the sicca syndrome may be a late manifestation. Enlargement of the lacrimal glands may occur in about 3 percent, and biopsy may provide histologic support for the diagnosis. The triad of anterior uveitis, parotid enlargement, and facial palsy is known as *Heerfordt's syndrome*. A routine slit lamp examination will often demonstrate subtle anterior uveitis which may be otherwise overlooked. Chronic uveitis is observed in about one-fifth of the patients who have chronic persistent sarcoidosis and is probably more frequent in black patients. In a Hopkins series, 15 of 34 patients presenting with anterior uveitis continued with chronic smoldering uveitis. Some patients develop secondary glaucoma and severe vision loss. Cataracts may be secondary to chronic inflammation. Retinal periphlebitis and leakage demonstrated by fluorescein studies may require laser photocoagulation. The classic "candle wax dripping" appearance has been described for the retinal vessels with periphlebitis. Posterior uveitis was noted in 8 percent of 181 patients with chronic persistent sarcoidosis. Chorioretinitis and optic neuritis have also been noted. Retroorbital masses, usually with enlarged lacrimal glands, are occasionally observed and occur in late disease, and sometimes years after otherwise apparently quiescent disease.

Skin and Subcutaneous Tissues

ERYTHEMA NODOSUM

This is the most common skin manifestation in many groups of sarcoidosis patients. The red tender nodules, several centimeters in diameter, are most frequently observed on the legs. The presence of diffuse erythema, ecchymoses, and swelling around the ankle may be mistaken for thrombophlebitis. These skin changes are associated with severe joint pains, particularly in the feet, ankles, and knees and occasionally in the wrists and elbows. This is almost invariably accompanied by hilar lymphadenopathy, and the systemic reaction with fever may be striking. The onset is abrupt, but remission within a few weeks is the usual outcome. Bed rest and nonsteroidal anti-inflammatory agents often suffice to control symptoms. Salicylates are frequently helpful. Persistent incapacity can be abruptly terminated by the use of corticosteroid therapy. Tapering over a period of a few months usually is not followed by recrudescence. Biopsy usually shows only vasculitis, but occasionally granulomas are identified.

CUTANEOUS GRANULOMAS

These are of varying types. Maculopapular lesions may appear early and regress as the disease remits, with or without corticosteroid therapy. Small nodular lesions may develop in old traumatic or surgical scars, or even at the sites of venipuncture. Large raised, reddish, or pigmented plaques may be persistent and occur especially at the rear of the neck at the hairline, around the eyes, ears, nose, and mouth, on the eyelids, and even in the lips. *Lupus pernio* or "purple lupus" represents severely disfiguring chronic violaceous skin lesions covering the nose and cheeks and around the eyes. Lesions may be noted in the scalp, with alopecia. Large nodular lesions are most often distributed on the extensor surfaces of the arms and legs as well as the face. Areas of depigmentation may overlie firm subcutaneous granulomatous infiltrations. Skin changes are more frequent and extensive in black patients, although a few small isolated skin lesions may be noted in some white patients. Women are more often affected than men, and other sites of involvement frequently include bones, eyes, and upper respiratory tract. Hilar adenopathy is usually persistent in association with chronic skin lesions. Persistent disfiguring skin lesions of many years duration may occasionally spontaneously regress and flatten out, with only minimal residual scarring. In some mysterious way, the granulomatous process has turned itself off.

Superficial Lymph Nodes

Discrete, firm, painless enlargement of cervical, supraclavicular, pre- and postauricular, epitrochlear, axillary, inguinal, and femoral nodes are observed in about one of seven patients. Lymph node involvement is usually bilateral and relatively symmetric. Biopsy of any palpable lymph node is likely to reveal the characteristic granulomatous changes and provide readily available histologic support for the diagnosis. Lymph nodes often regress spontaneously, and although responsive to corticosteroids, they are not usually considered a sufficient justification for treatment. Hilar lymphadenopathy almost invariably accompanies peripheral lymphadenopathy. In the past, blind scalene fat pad biopsies were found to reveal the characteristic changes in about 75 percent of the patients, even in the absence of palpable nodes. This procedure is rarely utilized now since the advent of transbronchial lung biopsy.

Liver

Although the liver is clinically enlarged at some time during the course of illness in 20 percent of the patients, liver biopsy in patients with or without hepatomegaly reveals granulomas in 75 percent or more. It is recognized that these granulomas are never pathognomonic. However, in the setting of a picture highly compatible with sarcoidosis, hepatic granulomas can provide appropriate histologic support for the diagnosis. The concentration of alkaline phosphatase in serum is often elevated. Intense pruritis may be a major clinical problem, and the picture may resemble biliary cirrhosis. Antimitochondrial antibodies are absent. The level of transaminases and bilirubin are less often abnormal. Healing is often spontaneous or in response to corticosteroid therapy, and the granulomas will resorb, with inconsequential scarring of liver parenchyma or portal spaces. Fever may be a common feature when active inflammatory liver disease is present. Cirrhosis, jaundice, ascites, and esophageal varices may be the end result in a few cases in which granulomatous involvement pursues a progressive unremitting course. Corticosteroid treatment suppresses the active inflammatory process but is without effect when irreversible cirrhosis has resulted.

Spleen

Splenomegaly may occur in 20 to 30 percent of patients. Prompt regression usually follows corticosteroid treatment. Splenic enlargement may be persistent but is generally without complication. The author is not aware of any documented splenic rupture. Infrequently, the spleen may reach giant size with signs of hypersplenism, i.e., anemia, leukopenia, and moderate thrombocytopenia. This usually does not result in bleeding, although a few patients with thrombocytopenic purpura have been observed.

Bone

Osteal involvement by granuloma occurs in about 3 percent of patients and is confined to chronic sarcoidosis. There is a predilection for the small bones of the hands and feet usually with swelling and tenderness and overlying skin changes. Other bones such as skull, vertebrae, and long bones are much less frequently affected. Involvement takes the form of punched out lytic areas of cystlike structure or fine or coarse reticular changes. No correlation exists between osseous lesions and the concentration of calcium in serum.

Joints

The acute arthritis associated with erythema nodosum is severe and incapacitating but regresses over a period of weeks or months, either spontaneously or concomitant with therapy.

Chronic polyarthralgias with synovial thickening involving the hands and feet may be recurrent and painful and are often associated with chronic skin and bone lesions. Transient knee effusions sometimes are observed. Synovial granulomas may be demonstrated on biopsy.

Antinuclear antibody and rheumatoid factor are occasionally elevated. Chloroquine may be helpful.

Salivary and Lacrimal Glands

Bilateral, nontender, firm, enlarged parotid glands may be observed, usually early in the course of the disease. Spontaneous regression is frequent. Gallium scans may show increased uptake in both parotid and lacrimal glands. A syndrome known as *uveoparotid fever* includes bilateral lacrimal and parotid gland enlargement, fever, and anterior uveitis. Occasionally the sicca syndrome with dry eyes and dry mouth is observed, resembling Sjögren's syndrome. Facial nerve palsies are sometimes associated with parotid enlargement but are more frequently independent. Biopsy of minor salivary glands with a deep lip biopsy may provide histologic support in about one-fourth of the patients.

Heart

Chronic pulmonary hypertension and cor pulmonale are frequent complications of persistent severe pulmonary disease. Myocardial granulomatous involvement may result in conduction abnormalities, serious tachyarrhythmias, and myocardopathy. Sudden death is a frequent complication of such disease. Endomyocardial biopsy may demonstrate granulomas, but spotty distribution may cause sampling errors. Sarcoid myocardopathy may be a diagnosis of exclusion in a young adult without evidence of coronary artery disease. Other substantiating evidence for sarcoidosis is necessary to uphold this diagnosis and may be obtained from pulmonary function tests, transbronchial lung biopsy, or biopsy of suspicious skin lesions. Mitral valvular regurgitation may result from changes in the trabeculae and muscle wall. Corticosteroid treatment in modest dosages is generally felt to be indicated when sarcoid myocardopathy is suspected.

The management of cor pulmonale with right-sided congestive failure involves the usual measures of diuretics and attempts at afterload reduction. Nifedipine may be useful. The latter must be approached cautiously, as adequate filling pressures are required to maintain the circulation. Supplemental oxygen is often required to prevent worsening pulmonary hypertension.

Nervous System

Neurosarcoidosis has been observed in approximately 5 percent of patients. Cranial nerve palsies, especially the seventh nerve, are the most frequently observed abnormalities. The palsies may be asymmetric and recurrent and may remit. Patchy peripheral sensory changes may be observed. In order of frequency the cranial nerves affected are 7, 5, 8, 9, 10, and 11 with accompanying swallowing difficulties. Optic neuritis is also observed. Other manifestations include aseptic meningitis, hydrocephalus, and peripheral neuropathy. Spinal fluid changes may include increased numbers of cells and protein; spinal fluid sugars are occasionally reduced. Hypothalamic dysfunction with diabetes insipidus has been observed. Intraspinal lesions have been noted. CT scans may reveal intracranial mass lesions. Neurologic manifestations usually improve with corticosteroid therapy.

Muscles

Granulomatous myopathy is observed, and muscle biopsy may provide histologic support for the diagnosis, especially in association with arthralgias. Marked muscle weakness may be a presenting complaint and may respond dramatically to corticosteroid therapy. This has been observed in some elderly women and sometimes in association with hypercalcemia.

Hypercalcemia and Hypercalciuria

Abnormalities of calcium metabolism have been observed, and recent evidence suggests that granulomatous tissue and alveolar macrophages may produce 1,25-dihydroxyvitamin D_3. Increased calcium absorption results from the vitamin D effect, and this is readily reversed by corticosteroids. Hypercalcemia which fails to respond to corticosteroids suggests the possible concurrence of hyperparathyroidism. Persistent hypercalciuria may result in nephrocalcinosis, and renal insufficiency may occur even without hypercalcemia. Renal stones may be present. When renal disease is encountered, 24-h urine calcium determinations should be obtained.

Kidneys

Renal changes resulting from the hypercalcemia and hypercalciuria are as noted above. Improvement in function may result with corticosteroid treatment. Renal biopsy may occasionally demonstrate granulomas, but sampling errors may result in only nonspecific changes. The nephrotic syndrome or chronic glomerulonephritis have been noted.

Other Organs

Granulomatous changes may occur in the epididymis, but sarcoidosis of the testis, ovary, and uterus is very uncommon. Granulomatous changes have been noted in the pancreas, stomach, and even aorta. The significance of these always must be assessed in the light of the total clinical picture.

CLINICAL ASSESSMENT AND DIAGNOSIS

The diagnosis depends on a compatible clinical picture with appropriate histologic support, and clinical evidence of involvement of more than one organ system. Table 42-2 outlines the possible anatomic involvement to be noted. A thorough history and physical examination with review of all previous clinical information, especially previous chest radiographs, are of prime importance. Slit lamp examination of the eye is usually indicated to rule out a subtle anterior uveitis. Initial studies should include routine urinalysis, hematology, blood chemical tests including serum proteins, liver function tests and calcium, and posteroanterior and lateral chest radiograph. Sputum studies and simple pulmonary function tests are indicated. Tuberculin skin tests should be performed and are usually negative. Testing for cell-mediated immunity with *Monilia*, mumps, and trichophytin often will demonstrate generalized anergy. A previously positive tuberculin skin test may be shifted toward negative without becoming completely negative. An electrocardiogram should be obtained to determine the presence of conduction abnormalities, using a Holter monitor if arrhythmias are suspected.

Other Granulomatous Diseases

The differential diagnosis of sarcoidosis must include mycobacterial infections, leprosy, certain fungal infections, berylliosis, hypersensitivity pneumonitis, lymphoma, primary biliary cirrhosis, granulomatous arteritides, and lymphomatoid granulomatosis. All of these may reveal granulomatous reactions histopathologically identical to those found in sarcoidosis. A careful occupational history is essential to exclude berylliosis. Cultures and biopsies will assist in the exclusion of infectious agents. Bone marrow and other tissue biopsies are indicated when lymphoma is suspected. Open lung biopsy may be required for adequate study in some instances. Assessment of the total clinical picture usually will provide appropriate direction. Physicians must maintain an index of suspicion for other diagnoses when the clinical pattern or course is atypical.

Pulmonary Function Tests

Simple spirometry with forced vital capacity and 1-s forced expiratory volume and carbon monoxide diffusing capacity provide useful basic information for monitoring the course of lung disease and its response to treatment. These may be within normal limits even with definite radiographic changes. Helium lung volumes may be utilized to confirm restrictive disease, although small lung volumes are often obvious on physical examination and chest radiograph. Serial observations are important to document: (1) the initial response after 2 to 3 months, (2) the maximal improvement after 6 to 8 months, (3) the status just prior to tapering of corticosteroids, and (4) studies 1 to 3 months after cessation of corticosteroid treatment when relapse may occur. Restrictive changes on spirometry are characteristic, but obstructive airways disease is also noted. This latter seems more common in white pa-

TABLE 42-2
Possible Anatomic Features in Suspected Sarcoidosis

Head

Nervous system

Cranial nerve lesions: VII (Bell's palsy), V, I, VIII, IX, X, XI

Extraocular movements: III, IV, VI

Pituitary

Diabetes insipidus

Hypopituitarism

Chronic meningitis

Localized brain lesions, internal hydrocephalus

Eyes

Anterior uveitis, iridocyclitis, corneal opacities, photophobia, redness, vision loss

Posterior uveitis, chorioretinitis, retinal periphlebitis, candle wax dripping appearance

Periorbital nodules and plaques on lids

Conjunctival nodules

Keratoconjunctivitis, sicca syndrome

Sjögren's syndrome

Lacrimal gland enlargement

Optic neuritis

Glaucoma, cataracts

Retroorbital mass, may occur late

Face

Skin plaques—or nodules: forehead, periorbital, perinasal, perioral and at posterior hairline

Lupus pernio: large violaceous nodules on cheeks, nose, and forehead

Bell's palsy

Nose

Bilateral nasal obstruction

Nasal mucosal granulomatous lesions with crusting and bleeding

Chronic sinusitis

Perforated nasal septum, usually secondary to corrective surgery

Perinasal plaques, often involving the alae nasae

Salivary glands

Bilateral enlargement of parotids and submaxillary glands

Mouth

Lip nodules

Dryness, sicca syndrome

Mouth (cont.)

Minor salivary gland granulomas on biopsy

Hoarseness or stridor, laryngeal disease

Lymph node enlargement

Superficial

Cervical: anterior and posterior

Supraclavicular, axillary, epitrochlear

Femoral and inguinal

Thorax

Lungs

Abnormal radiograph

Restriction

Basal end-inspiratory crackles, common

Wheezes, occasionally significant

Often no adventitious sounds

Heart

Cor pulmonale

Heart block

Tachyarrhythmias

Mitral regurgitation

Congestive failure

Abdomen

Nodules in surgical scar

Hepatomegaly

Splenomegaly

Kidneys, renal calculi, or hypercalciuria

Genitalia

Occasional epididymal thickening or nodules

Extremities

Erythema nodosum, especially on shins

Diffuse swelling, pain, tenderness, and erythema, especially around ankles

Skin plaques

Traumatic scar nodules

Muscle weakness and occasional tenderness

Irregular sensory changes

Swollen distal phalanges with bone cysts and overlying skin changes

Painful joints, ankles, knees, feet, hands, with tendinitis

Occasional knee effusions with synovitis

tients than in blacks. Airway obstruction may result from endobronchial disease or peribronchial fibrosis. Bronchial hyperreactivity with asthmalike symptoms has been documented in a few patients. Arterial blood gases to assess hypoxia may be indicated with dyspnea at rest. Carbon dioxide retention is unusual.

Biopsy

Histologic support for the diagnosis is required to substantiate the compatible clinical picture. Treatment usually should not be initiated without obtaining biopsy tissue support. But biopsy may not be necessary for the incidental finding of bilateral hilar lymphadenopathy. Lymphoma would be most unlikely in a patient with no symptoms or other abnormalities on physical examination or laboratory study. The choice of biopsy site depends on the clinical manifestations. Search always should be made for superficial lesions of the skin or mucosa or palpable lymph nodes, as they are very likely to demonstrate the characteristic granulomatous changes.

BRONCHOSCOPY

The use of the flexible bronchoscope for transbronchial lung biopsy and/or transtracheal needle biopsy of paratracheal or subcarinal lymph nodes is the procedure of choice when superficial lesions are not available. Transbronchial lung biopsy is a safe and effective procedure. Noncaseating granulomas will be obtained in 60 to 90 percent of patients with pulmonary infiltrates, depending on the type and profusion of the lesions. At least four to five transbronchial lung biopsy specimens should be obtained at the time of bronchoscopy. Material can also be obtained for culture and cytologic studies.

Bronchoscopic biopsy of paratracheal or subcarinal nodes using a number 18 needle has been successfully employed with the finding of well-formed noncaseating granulomas. Early experience necessitated rigid bronchoscopy for this, but newer techniques and experience enable the use of the flexible bronchoscope.

MEDIASTINOSCOPY

Mediastinoscopy will provide good tissue specimens of mediastinal nodes and can readily confirm the diagnosis of sarcoidosis. This is a procedure requiring general anesthesia but is useful when lymphoma is a serious question.

OTHER BIOPSY SITES

Liver biopsy can be helpful in patients who have the classic features of sarcoidosis. It must be recalled that sarcoid liver granulomas are indistinguishable from those of many other liver disorders. Random muscle biopsies may show the characteristic changes, especially in association with significant arthritis. Biopsy of enlarged conjunctival follicles or irregular nasal and palatal mucosa may be revealing and are well tolerated. Minor salivary gland biopsies are occasionally useful. Priority is generally given to the site that is easily sampled with minimal inconvenience and expense to the patient.

THE KVEIM REACTION

The clinical diagnostic use of the Kveim reaction was pioneered and championed by the late Louis E. Siltzbach. He was a meticulous worker and observer who possessed some carefully standardized splenic material for intracutaneous injection to determine the potential for granuloma formation. With careful attention to avoidance of any foreign bodies, and experienced cautious interpretation, he provided a useful tool to support the diagnosis of sarcoidosis. The current lack of available safe adequately standardized material limits its future diagnostic use. However, it is of both historic and pathologic significance as a feature of sarcoidosis. Kveim reactivity occurs almost exclusively in patients with sarcoidosis, mainly during the active phase of the disease and most often associated with lymphadenopathy.

A positive reaction is indicated by a slowly enlarging papule, 3 to 8 mm in diameter, consisting of epithelioid follicles, occasionally showing some fibrinoid necrosis, an admixture of nonspecific inflammatory cells and few, if any, birefringent bodies. It usually reaches its largest diameter in 4 to 6 weeks. The papule is then biopsied and reveals epithelioid cell follicles which morphologically, histochemically, and ultramicroscopically mimic the epithelioid cell granulomas of the natural disease (Fig. 42-3).

False-positive reactions occur in 1 to 5 percent of nonsarcoid patients and are characterized by small papules and a feeble proliferation of epithelioid cells. Not all human sarcoidal tissue has proved to be useful for the Kveim test. Certain rigid criteria have to be met for sensitivity and specificity. Presently, safety precautions for potential transmissible agents, such as retroviruses, make it unlikely that preparations could be available and receive Federal Drug Administration (FDA) approval.

Bronchoalveolar Lavage

The technique of bronchoalveolar lavage (BAL) provides a remarkable research tool and insights into the cellular biology and pathogenesis of the lung disease of sarcoidosis. Increased numbers of activated T-helper lymphocytes have been found frequently in patients with pulmonary sarcoidosis, in contrast to increased numbers of neutrophils in patients with idiopathic pulmonary fibrosis and in smokers. Increased lymphocytosis is suggestive of sarcoidosis. The technical procedures of obtaining, handling, and analyzing the fluid and the cells are not yet standardized. The percent lymphocytosis has not proven to be a reliable guide to treatment. Uncertainty of interpretation and the expense and inconvenience to the patient do not justify its routine use.

Nonspecific Tests

ANGIOTENSIN CONVERTING ENZYME

This enzyme has been studied in both serum and lavage fluid, and its concentration is often found to be elevated in sarcoidosis. The epithelioid cells of the granulomas are felt to be the source of angiotensin converting enzyme. Continued studies have increased the awareness of the nonspecificity and variability of this finding. In general, elevated levels decrease as the disease appears to regress spontaneously or in response to corticosteroid treatment. Though relatively inexpensive and noninvasive, the results do not provide a reliable guide for treatment.

GALLIUM SCANS

Gallium scanning has been found to reveal avid uptake in tissues where there is any active inflammatory process. Again, the results are nonspecific. Patients with old pulmonary fibrosis do not demonstrate gallium accumulation in the lungs except where secondary bacterial infection is present. A lack of uptake does markedly diminish the likelihood of an active inflammatory process. Corticosteroids are known to suppress the gallium uptake. Gallium studies are not routinely recommended because of cost, radiation burden, nonspecificity, and clinical variation.

COURSE AND PROGNOSIS

In general, the outcome of sarcoidosis is favorable, particularly if account is taken of the 4:1 ratio of undiagnosed (asymptomatic) to diagnosed sarcoidosis in any community and the high incidence of complete spontaneous recovery in asymptomatic patients. Of the patients with manifest sarcoidosis (more than 90 percent of these with abnormal chest radiographs), two-thirds either clear completely within 2 to 3 years or improve to the point of minor residual pulmonary shadows but no active extrathoracic lesions. Of the remaining one-third, most have a smoldering course often with little change over a decade or more. Less than one-half of this group with persistent activity progress to a fatal outcome, generally from pulmonary insufficiency and cor pulmonale.

Serial observations of the severity of symptoms and extent of disease provide direct clues to the long-term outcome. Severely symptomatic patients are most likely to have persistent disease. Cough is the most important finding in suggesting the likelihood of progression of the lung disease. Racial factors are of importance. In a series of patients in Baltimore, black patients were more likely to continue with chronic persistent disease and more frequently demonstrated severe ocular, skin, mucosal, and joint involvement. The type of manifestations evident in the first year portend the nature of subsequent chronic manifestations, whether they be pulmonary, ocular, mucocutaneous, hepatic, neurologic, etc. Review of this series of 181 patients showed that very few patients had later major manifestations different from those at the onset. The pattern of disease usually seems to declare itself at the outset in the individual patient.

Extrathoracic disease is probably present very frequently and may not indicate a poor prognosis. Liver biopsies have demonstrated incidental granulomas in at least 75 percent of patients, even in the absence of enlargement or abnormal function tests of the liver. These have been observed in association with erythema nodosum, which is known to have a spontaneous remission in most instances. Overt symptomatic extrathoracic disease does tend to be persistent and often requires corticosteroids.

The death rate for patients with sarcoidosis who are followed for 5 years is about 4 percent, i.e., twice that for all causes in the general population of similar age and sex. Causes of death other than respiratory failure and cor pulmonale are azotemia from renal damage caused by chronic hypercalciuria, cardiac arrest resulting from myo-cardial involvement, and massive hemoptysis secondary to colonization of bullae by *Aspergillus fumigatus* in advanced pulmonary sarcoidosis.

Prognosis is strongly influenced by the type of pulmonary disease with which the patient is first seen and by the presence of clinically apparent extrathoracic lesions. Patients with asymptomatic hilar adenopathy (type I), with or without erythema nodosum, generally do best: the adenopathy usually subsides in 1 to 3 years without sequellae and rarely recurs. Less than 10 percent of patients presenting in stage 1 progress to pulmonary mottling (type II), and exceedingly few manifest extrathoracic lesions. For type I patients, a fatal outcome is rare.

For patients with type II disease with apparent pulmonary infiltrations and hilar lymphadenopathy, the prognosis is less favorable even though spontaneous remission of the pulmonary lesions, or clearing in the course of corticosteroid therapy is common.

The poorest outcome is experienced by patients with type III chest radiograph, without hilar node enlargement, with pulmonary fibrosis, with or without bullous transformation. This type frequently progresses to pulmonary insufficiency and cor pulmonale. The pulmonary lesions respond poorly to therapy, presumably because of the predominance of fibrosis. Moreover, in this chronic phase of the illness, chronic visual disturbances and nephrocalcinosis often add to the patient's burdens.

Extrathoracic lesions such as peripheral lymphadenopathy, salivary gland enlargement, and Bell's palsy generally subside spontaneously. Acute uveitis usually regresses in response to topical steroid therapy. Chronic ocular and cutaneous lesions tend to persist unchanged or to fluctuate in activity. Progression to glaucoma and blindness often follows persistent uveitis in spite of treatment.

TREATMENT

The Need for Treatment

Assessing the extent of the active inflammatory process and its potential reversibility is generally subsumed in the term *disease activity*. This has sometimes been confused to include an assessment of the likelihood of progression or need for treatment. There is no doubt that the acute erythema nodosum syndrome is a very active inflammatory process. Yet this is well recognized for a high potential of complete and permanent remission. Thus, a stage of active inflammation does not preclude spontaneous remission. This has sometimes been confused with a quite different situation in an infectious process such as tuberculosis, where the term "active" clearly implies a need for treatment.

Access to the lung by bronchoalveolar lavage (BAL) has revealed correlations with the inflammatory process identified on lung biopsy and the cellular content of the lavage fluid. Earlier enthusiasm for the arbitrary dividing line of 28 percent or more lymphocytes in the lavage fluid denoting "high intensity alveolitis" has waned. It was originally felt that this denoted a high likelihood of worsening of the disease and the need for treatment to deter the process, but individual aberrations on all sides have been observed. Studies show that a low BAL lymphocyte count does not exclude the possibility of deterioration or response to corticosteroid treatment. Conversely, a high lymphocyte count does not necessarily mean deterioration if the patient is untreated. Persistent lymphocytosis after 1 year does make a complete spontaneous remission unlikely. A panel chaired by Gordon Snider at the Tenth International Sarcoidosis Conference in 1984 concluded "that at the present time there is no evidence that bronchoalveolar lavage can be used to monitor the activity of sarcoidosis, to monitor the course of its therapy with corticosteroids, or to predict the outcome of the disease."

Other attempts to delineate markers of "activity" have included angiotensin converting enzyme (ACE) and gallium scans, as noted previously. The nonspecificity and patient variation of both of these remain a problem. Broad correlations do exist, and both tend to decrease in response to corticosteroids. Changes in lymphocytosis tend to lag behind.

Symptoms, serial radiographic alterations, and measurements of vital capacity generally change in parallel as the disease progresses or in response to corticosteroid treatment. These provide useful clinical parameters for guiding therapy. Studies of immunoglobulins both in serum and in lavage fluid tend to parallel the findings noted above. No single criterion has been identified to determine definitively the need for further treatment. Clinical, biochemical, metabolic, and immunologic markers of activity are not necessarily synonymous with extent or likelihood of progression of the disease, and none can define the prognosis.

Corticosteroid Treatment

In view of the frequency of spontaneous remission in asymptomatic sarcoidosis, it is understandable that only about one-third of all patients ever require treatment. Such spontaneous remissions are usually permanent, and patients need not fear relapse.

Considerable controversy persists about the need for and benefits of corticosteroid therapy in the individual patient. The extent and stage of the inflammatory process clearly influence the outcome. Earlier treatment is more likely to be beneficial for symptomatic disease. Extensive fibrosis and bullous disease are not likely to be reversible, although some improvement may be achieved. A therapeutic trial for at least several months is justified. Occasionally there is increasing infiltration in the chest radio-graph over 1 to 2 years, even though symptoms are minimal. A trial of corticosteroids is justified when the disease results in significant disruption of the normal pattern of life or shows definite progression. Documentation with objective parameters is essential to evaluate the course. Subjective euphoria can be misleading and result in prolonged steroid dependence. Similarly, documentation of the course during tapering of the dose is necessary to identify a relapse and the possible need for continued treatment.

Because of early enthusiasm for the apparent benefits of corticosteroids, no adequate controlled studies of the use of corticosteroids have ever been performed. Short courses of corticosteroids for approximately 6 months produce short-term benefits, but prompt relapse usually occurs when treatment is withdrawn. Longer-term treatment is usually necessary. Incapacitating erythema nodosum proves an exception to this in that it may respond promptly to low-dose corticosteroid (prednisone 30 mg daily), and tapering usually can be successfully achieved within a few months. The frequent impressive clinical response makes it unethical to withhold treatment from symptomatic incapacitated patients. At the other extreme, with mild asymptomatic disease there is no justification for any risk from corticosteroid treatment, unless there is evidence of progression of the disease. The degree of existing clinical bias and information precludes the optimal control study in symptomatic patients.

INDICATIONS FOR CORTICOSTEROIDS

Ocular disease with active anterior uveitis usually responds promptly to local corticosteroid drops and ointment, and systemic therapy usually is not necessary. Posterior uveitis, with retinitis and fluorescein evidence of leakage, requires systemic treatment. Laser treatment also may be needed.

Pulmonary disease is the most frequent indication for systemic treatment (88 percent). This is discussed in detail in other sections. *Liver disease*, often accompanied by fever, anorexia, weight loss, and elevated alkaline phosphatase, is the next most common problem requiring corticosteroids. The constitutional symptoms of *fever* and *weight loss* respond promptly to systemic corticosteroid therapy. Failure to respond suggests alternative diagnoses, especially lymphoma. Persistent significant *hepatosplenomegaly* usually regresses promptly unless cirrhosis and portal hypertension have intervened. *Nervous system disease*, especially cranial nerve palsies, meningitis, or mass lesions, justify treatment, usually with a favorable response.

Evidence of *myocardial disease* with conduction defects, tachyarrhythmias, and evidence of myocardopathy indicate need for prompt treatment, as the risks of sudden death and congestive failure are serious. The response is often difficult to assess, as prior irreversible damage often has occurred. In the face of devastating alternatives, moderate dose therapy as outlined for pulmonary disease with maintenance on 10 to 20 mg of prednisone daily seems reasonable. No advantages of high-dose treatment have been demonstrated. Antiarrhythmic agents, pacemakers, and automatic implantable defibrillators are often required.

Hypercalcemia and persistent *hypercalciuria* serve as further indications for corticosteroid treatment. Low dose treatment with maintenance on 10 to 15 mg daily usually produces prompt response. Calcium determinations guide therapy, which often can be discontinued as the disease remits over several years. Failure to respond will strongly suggest some other explanation, such as hyperparathyroidism.

Skeletal myopathy may respond slowly but dramatically to corticosteroid treatment. This has been observed in several older white women with associated hypercalcemia.

Thrombocytopenia usually responds promptly to corticosteroids and is a strong indication for treatment. *Hemolytic anemia* is very unusual and makes lymphoma a more likely diagnosis.

Pregnancy is not contraindicated in most sarcoidosis patients. Amenorrhea and reduced fertility may occur during debilitating disease, but many young women have delivered healthy infants while on treatment. With severe lung disease, bed rest may be necessary in the third trimester. Corticosteroid treatment should be continued with the usual doses during pregnancy. If treatment is withdrawn, relapse may occur a few weeks after the pregnancy. Patients must be monitored in the postpartum period.

DOSAGE OF CORTICOSTEROIDS

Prednisone and prednisolone are most widely used. The treatment schedule with prednisone is outlined in Table 42-3 and discussed below. Prednisolone is recommended when liver disease is significant. Initial doses of 40 mg daily, reduced at 2-week intervals to 30, 25, and 20 mg, usually bring the disease under prompt control. Doses higher than 40 mg are rarely necessary. Twice-daily split doses may be indicated for the first 2 to 4 weeks, especially to control fever. A maintenance dose of 10 to 15 mg daily usually is sufficient to maintain improvement. This is continued for at least 8 months until a plateau of improvement is achieved. A single 8 am daily dose facilitates compliance and is recommended after the first month. Alternate day treatment has been widely recommended, but the necessity and the advantages are not obvious at the lower maintenance doses of 10 to 15 mg, except in growing children. Compliance is facilitated by the use of a single daily dose, which can become a regular event in the daily routine. The initial use of alternate day

TABLE 42-3

*Recommended Prednisone Treatment Schedule**

Duration	Dose	Comment
2 weeks	40 mg daily	(Or 20 mg twice daily)
2 weeks	30 mg daily	(Or 15 mg twice daily)
2 weeks	25 mg daily	(Single 8 am dose)
2 weeks	20 mg daily	(Document response)
6 months	15 mg daily	(Document maximal response)
Every 2–4 weeks	Reduce by 2.5 mg to 12.5, 10.5, 7.5, 5.0, 2.5 mg level	[Monitor course monthly, observing for relapse; re-institute treatment at dosage known to control disease (i.e., 15–20 mg daily) if relapse persists]

* Use 5-mg tablets throughout to avoid dosage confusion. Alternate day maintenance therapy can be used, but advantages are poorly documented and compliance is more difficult.

therapy is unwise because of more erratic and slower responses, though its effectiveness has been clearly demonstrated in some patients.

MONITORING CORTICOSTEROID THERAPY

The efficacy of corticosteroids in relieving symptoms and producing a clinical remission is undisputed in many patients. The response may be dramatic. Respiratory symptoms improve within a few days, and radiographic clearing may be impressive within 2 weeks. Two-thirds of patients with fresh lesions show either clearing of pulmonary densities or substantial improvement. Soft patchy lesions and fine miliary lesions respond most dramatically. Enlarged hilar and mediastinal nodes regress at an uneven pace and may persist. Improvement in vital capacity is noted more frequently than changes in the diffusing capacity. Serial blood gases or exercise studies are not necessary. In a few patients with long-standing irreversible pulmonary fibrosis, no benefit will be achieved. If no objective improvement is observed in the first 2 to 3 months, therapy should be tapered and discontinued. Changes in symptoms tend to correlate directly with other objective abnormalities. It is not necessary to monitor patients with serial bronchoalveolar lavage studies, gallium scans, or angiotensin converting enzyme. The chest radiograph seems to be the single most valid criterion for response and stability. Serial observations should be made at least after 2, 6, and 8 months and at 1- to 2-month intervals during tapering. The patients usually can readily serve as their own control. Relapses generally occur within 1 to 2 months after stopping treatment but may begin at any dose of prednisone below 15 mg daily. When a relapse is documented and persistent, treatment should be reinstituted at a maintenance dose (10 to 15 mg) known to control the disease in that patient. The general effort is that of maintaining the patient at the minimal dose which will suffice. Relapses occur in one-half to two-thirds of the patients. Long-term treatment for 5 to 20 years, or even a lifetime, may be required.

DURATION OF CORTICOSTEROID THERAPY

The occurrence of relapse usually dictates the duration of treatment. One-quarter to one-third of patients will respond dramatically to the initial course of treatment with no subsequent relapses or problems. In chronic persistent disease, the need for prolonged treatment often has not been appreciated. Assessing symptoms and relevant clinical findings, it is not difficult to determine if the disease worsens as treatment is slowly tapered or terminated. Occasionally a relapse is temporary as a rebound when corticosteroids are withdrawn. It is justified to attempt tapering at the end of an initial course of 8 to 12 months of treatment and again at 1- to 3-year intervals. After repeated relapses over a 10-year period, it seems justified simply to continue the low-maintenance dose required to prevent the overt relapse. It is the conviction of this author that progressive fibrosis can be avoided or minimized with such an approach. Patients sometimes discontinue their own treatment or fail to return. In such intervals, relapse and significant progressive fibrosis are often observed. Johns and her colleagues reported on a series of 171 patients treated with corticosteroids for chronic disease of more than 5-years duration. Relapse occurred in 75 percent and tended to be recurrent in at least half of the patients. Continued low-dose corticosteroid was required to prevent relapse in 53 percent. The mean duration of treatment was 8 years. These recurrent relapses are noted most frequently in black patients.

COMPLICATIONS OF CORTICOSTEROID THERAPY

Excessive weight gain is the most frequently observed problem and was noted in 24 percent of a series of 171 patients with a mean treatment period of 8 years. It occurred more frequently in women. Diabetes mellitus was observed in 8 percent and seemed more frequent in patients with significant liver disease. Aseptic necrosis of bone was observed in only three patients. Peptic ulcer or minor gastrointestinal bleeding was observed in three patients, and cataracts unrelated to ocular sarcoidosis were noted in two patients. Tuberculosis has not been observed in recent series, as the disease has become less prevalent. Patients with a positive tuberculin skin test usually receive 300 mg of isoniazid for at least 9 months. When tuberculosis does intervene, the skin test, which had been previously negative, is found to be positive. Periodic monitoring of the tuberculin skin reactivity and sputum studies are indicated whenever a suspicion of tuberculosis arises.

Management of Hemoptysis

Blood streaking caused by endobronchial disease is usually readily controlled by corticosteroids. More significant bleeding is noted with advanced fibrocystic disease and the presence of saprophytic mycetomas in cysts. Conservative management with cough suppressants and broad spectrum antibiotics has frequently been effective in controlling the bleeding. Continued corticosteroid treatment is often necessary to control the underlying disease. A number of patients with multiple mycetomas have been successfully managed for many years with death unrelated to hemoptysis (Fig. 42-7). Bronchoscopy may be indicated to localize the bleeding, which is occasionally massive and may be fatal. Surgical resection usually is not feasible because of the diffuse underlying disease with limited pulmonary function and risk of fistula and empyema. Furthermore, mycetomas are often bilateral, and bleeding may originate from either side. With experienced personnel, interventional radiologic techniques with therapeutic embolization have been successfully utilized in several patients to control massive recurrent bleeding. Unfortunately, a fatal recurrence continues to be a real possibility.

Management of Chronic Skin Nodules

Small plaques presenting early in the disease usually clear promptly when systemic corticosteroids are necessitated by serious disease of other organs. When skin plaques are the major finding, systemic treatment usually is not justified. Local steroid creams with tape occlusion may be helpful when the lesions are localized and small. Steroid injections may be used, but results are usually disappointing and temporary at best. Skin plaques may be widespread, large, and disfiguring and are often associated with extensive mucosal changes; even systemic corticosteroids are often disappointing in their effect.

CHLOROQUINE

Severe chronic skin sarcoid usually responds dramatically to systemic chloroquine. An initial loading dose of 500 mg daily for 2 weeks is followed by 250 mg daily for 6 months. The response usually occurs within 2 to 3 months. Because of concerns about ocular toxicity, with potential reversible corneal opacities or irreversible retinal damage, ocular examination is performed before and after each treatment period. Treatment is usually for 6 months followed by 6 months without chloroquine. Occasionally longer periods of treatment have been used. Repeated 6-month courses often have been necessary because of gradual relapse with no ocular toxicity observed with this regimen. The benefits usually exceed those achieved with corticosteroids. Hydroxychloroquine (PLAQUENIL) 200 mg daily has also been utilized but seems less effective. Chloroquine and hydroxychloroquine have also occasionally been helpful with chronic joint pains. Occasionally, for no obvious reason, severe disfiguring cutaneous lesions will spontaneously remit and remain inactive.

Other Immunosuppressive Agents

Although corticosteroids may not be the perfect answer, the general success with their use has deterred aggressive attempts to find better drugs. A study is currently underway at the National Institutes of Health with *cyclosporin* in a few patients with progressive ocular disease. To date, results are limited and concern for renal toxicity is significant.

James has described success in managing severe skin sarcoid with lupus pernio with small weekly doses of 5 mg of *methotrexate* for 3 months. Repeated courses at 6-month intervals are usually necessary.

Other Treatment

The appropriate use of oxygen for hypoxia and antibiotics for complicating bacterial infection make significant contributions to the well-being of the patient. Antifungal agents are of no value for mycetomas, as they fail to penetrate the fungal mass and invasive disease is almost never seen. Antituberculous treatment is of no value unless there is evidence of complicating tuberculous infection.

BIBLIOGRAPHY

Bascom R, Johns CJ: The natural history and management of sarcoidosis. Adv Intern Med 31:213–241, 1986.
 A comprehensive review with extensive bibliography.

Bell NH, Stern PH, Pantzer E, Sinha TK, DeLuca HF: Evidence that increased circulating 1 alpha, 25-dihydroxyvitamin D is the probable cause for abnormal calcium metabolism in sarcoidosis. J Clin Invest 64:218–225, 1979.
 Original work, substantiated by others, identifying the defect as impaired regulation of 1α, 25-dihydroxyvitamin D, with resultant excessive absorption of calcium, with the level of 1α, 25-dihydroxyvitamin D reduced by prednisone.

Buck AA, Sartwell PE, McKusick VA: Epidemiological investigations of sarcoidosis. Am J Hyg 74:137–201, 1961.
 A family study of 62 index cases with 363 individuals reviewed. Multiple cases were found in five families, with a total of 14 cases in first-degree relatives and none in controls or spouses.

Crystal RG, Herman PB, Rennard SI, Hance AJ, Keogh BA: Interstitial lung diseases of unknown cause. Disorders characterized by chronic inflammation of the lower respiratory tract. N Engl J Med 310:154–166, 235–244, 1984.
 Excellent review of current concepts, well referenced, with good diagrammatic representations of alveolitis, cellular recruitment and activation, tissue injury, repair, and fibrosis in sarcoidosis.

Crystal RG, Roberts WC, Hunninghake GW, Gadek JE, Fulmer JD, Line BR: Pulmonary sarcoidosis: A disease characterized and perpetuated by activated lung T-lymphocytes. NIH Conference. Ann Intern Med 94:73–94, 1981.
 This reports the early studies of lung lavage and T cells of 45 patients with clinically active biopsy proven disease, reviewing the alveolitis, cellular studies, gallium scanning, and therapy.

Cullen MR, Kominsky JR, Rossman MD, Cherniack MG, Rankin JA, Balmes JR, Kern JA, Daniele RP, Palmer L, Naegel GP et al: Chronic beryllium disease in a precious metal refinery. Clinical epidemiologic and immunologic evidence for continuing risk from exposure to low level beryllium fume. Am Rev Respir Dis 135:201–208, 1987.
 In five workers at a precious metal refinery who developed granulomatous lung disease, the original diagnosis was sarcoidosis. Four of the workers subsequently proved to have hypersensitivity to beryllium by in vitro proliferative responses of lymphocytes obtained by bronchoalveolar lavage.

DeRemee RA: The present status of treatment of pulmonary sarcoidosis: A house divided. Chest 71:388–392, 1977.
 A concise review of the debate about the efficacy of corticosteroids.

Edmondstone WM, Wilson AG: Temporal clustering of familial sarcoidosis in non-consanguineous relatives. Br J Dis Chest 78:184–186, 1984.
A report of sarcoidosis developing within a short time in non-consanguineous members of two families, suggesting environmental factors.

Eighth International Conference on Sarcoidosis and Other Granulomatous Diseases. Jones Williams W, Davies BH (eds). Cardiff, Wales, Alpha Omega, 1980.
Proceedings of the conference held in 1979, with many studies of angiotensin converting enzyme.

Fanburg BL: *Sarcoidosis and Other Granulomatous Diseases of the Lung,* in Fanburg BL (ed), *Lung Biology in Health and Disease,* vol 20. New York, Dekker, 1983.
A multi-authored book with good general review.

Gumpel JM, Johns CJ, Shulman LK: The joint disease of sarcoidosis. Ann Rheum Dis 26:194–205, 1967.
Review of the joint manifestations found in 45 of 118 unselected patients attending a sarcoid clinic. Early transient polyarthritis, erythema nodosum, and later chronic arthritis were observed.

Hillerdal G, Nou E, Osterman K, Schmekel B: Sarcoidosis: Epidemiology and prognosis, a 15-year European study. Am Rev Respir Dis 130:29–32, 1984.
A study of serial chest radiographs in Uppsala, Sweden, with 50 percent of patients with bilateral hilar adenopathy showing a normal radiographic picture 15 months after discovery of the disease.

Hirsch JG, Cohen ZA, Morse SI, Schaedler RW, Siltzbach LE, Ellis JT, Chase MW: Evaluation of the Kveim reaction as a diagnostic test for sarcoidosis. N Engl J Med 265:827–830, 1961.
Good controlled objective evaluation of the Kveim reaction with 75 percent positive in subacute active sarcoidosis, 64 percent in chronic sarcoidosis for more than 2 years, and false positives of 5 percent of persons with other diseases.

Hunninghake GW, Kawanami O, Ferrans VJ, Young RC Jr, Roberts WC, Crystal RG: Characterization of the inflammatory and immune effector cells in the lung parenchyma of patients with interstitial lung disease. Am Rev Respir Dis 123:407–417, 1981.
Early report of comparisons of open lung biopsy and lavage and the lymphocytosis identified in sarcoidosis.

Israel HL, Lenchner GS, Atkinson GW: Sarcoidosis and aspergilloma. The role of surgery. Chest 82:430–432, 1982.
Review of 38 patients, with surgical resection for hemoptysis in 14, rarely followed by uncomplicated convalescence, and outcome usually related to the severity of the diffuse underlying lung disease.

James DG, Jones Williams W: *Sarcoidosis and Other Granulomatous Disorders,* in Smith LH (ed), *Major Problems in Internal Medicine,* vol 24. Philadelphia, Saunders, 1985.
Excellent, easily read, well referenced, clinical review, with data from 818 patients seen and followed in London.

Johns CJ: Management of hemoptysis with pulmonary fungus balls in sarcoidosis. Editorial. Chest 82:400–401, 1982.
Successful use of conservative management is reviewed with interventional radiologic techniques with therapeutic embolization recommended in preference to surgery for life-threatening massive bleeding.

Johns CJ, Zachary JB, Ball WC Jr: A 10-year study of corticosteroid treatment of pulmonary sarcoidosis. Johns Hopkins Med J 134:271–283, 1974.
Serial pulmonary function studies of 152 patients, predominantly black, demonstrated significant increase in vital capacity in 72 percent. Prolonged treatment was often necessary.

Kaplan J, Johns CJ: Mycetomas in pulmonary sarcoidosis: Nonsurgical management. Johns Hopkins Med J 145:157–161, 1979.
Review of the long-term course of 12 patients with minor and major hemoptyses, with nine successfully managed for many years with supportive therapy only.

Koerner SK: Transbronchial lung biopsy for the diagnosis of sarcoidosis. N Engl J Med 293:268–270, 1975.
Early report of the safe successful use with low risk and positive results in 21 of 23 patients.

Lawrence EC, Teague RB, Gottlieb MS, Shingran SG, Lieberman J: Serial changes in markers of disease activity with corticosteroid treatment in sarcoidosis. Am J Med 74:747–756, 1983.
Twelve patients with "active" sarcoidosis were studied. Significant improvement was noted in many clinical parameters, but changes in lavage lymphocytes were less impressive.

Lieberman J: Elevation of serum angiotensin-converting enzyme level in sarcoidosis. Am J Med 59:365–372, 1975.
Early studies showed increased levels in active sarcoidosis compared to controls, and patients receiving corticosteroids, or patients with resolved disease.

Longcope WT, Freiman DG: A study of sarcoidosis: Based on a combined investigation of 160 cases including 30 autopsies from The Johns Hopkins Hospital and Massachusetts General Hospital. Medicine 31:1–132, 1952.
The classic monograph reviewing the history and observations in this disease, with well illustrated descriptions of the varied manifestations.

Maddrey WC, Johns CJ, Boitnott JK, Iber FL: Sarcoidosis and chronic hepatic disease. A clinical and pathological study of 20 cases. Medicine 49:375–395, 1970.
A review of the spectrum of hepatic disease in sarcoidosis ranging from incidental granulomas to cirrhosis.

Mayock RL, Bertrand P, Morrison CE, Scott JH: Manifestations of sarcoidosis: Analysis of 145 patients with a review of nine series selected from the literature. Am J Med 35:67–89, 1963.
The most detailed and careful analysis of observed and reported clinical manifestations in 1254 patients.

Mitchell DN, Scadding JG: Sarcoidosis. Am Rev Respir Dis 110:774–802, 1974.
State-of-the-art review of the disease, with expanded discussion of pathology, the Kveim reaction, and possible etiology. Studies in mice suggested a transmissible agent causing granulomas in the mouse footpad, but these were not substantiated by others.

Morse SI, Cohn ZA, Hirsch JG, Schaedler RW: The treatment of sarcoidosis with chloroquine. Am J Med 30:779–784, 1961.
Original report of studies in seven patients with documented disease for more than 2 years, with considerable improvement in skin and mucosa, but other lesions were variable in their response.

Nessan VJ, Jacoway JR: Biopsy of minor salivary glands in the diagnosis of sarcoidosis. N Engl J Med 301:922–924, 1979.
Positive in 58 percent of 75 patients.

Neville E, Walker AN, James DG: Prognostic factors predicting the outcome of sarcoidosis: An analysis of 818 patients. Quart J Med 208:525–533, 1983.
A computerized retrospective study analyzing the clinical details and outcome. A favorable prognosis was associated with erythema nodosum, acute arthritis, and bilateral hilar lymphadenopathy. Chronicity was noted with mucosal, skin, and bone sarcoidosis.

Reisner D: Observation on the course and prognosis of sarcoidosis. Am Rev Respir Dis 96:361–380, 1967.
A review of 86 consecutive patients observed from 1937 to 1952 in New York City, with 69 followed for a mean of 8 years, revealed an extremely variable natural course.

Reynolds HY: Bronchoalveolar lavage, State of the art. Am Rev Respir Dis 135:250–263, 1987.
Review of the practicalities and usefulness of the procedure.

Reynolds HY, Newball HH: Analysis of proteins and respiratory cells obtained from human lungs by bronchial lavage. J Lab Clin Med 84:559–573, 1974.
The original study of bronchial lavage in 42 subjects, using transnasal fiberoptic bronchoscopy, in smokers and nonsmokers.

Roberts WC, McAllister HA Jr, Ferrans VJ: Sarcoidosis of the heart. A clinicopathologic study of 35 necropsy patients (Group I) and review of 78 previously described necropsy patients (Group II). Am J Med 63:86–108, 1977.
Autopsy series with retrospective review of the clinical features revealed sudden death in 60 percent.

Rohatgi PK, Goldstein RA: Immunopathogenesis, immunology and assessment of activity of sarcoidosis. Ann Allergy 52:316–325, 1984.
Good current review with practical suggestions for the clinician.

Sarcoidosis and Other Granulomatous Disorders. Ninth International Conference, Chretien J, Marsac J, Saltiel JC (eds). Paris, Pergamon, 1981.
Publication of proceedings with many bronchoalveolar lavage studies.

Sequeria W, Stinar D: Serum angiotensin-converting enzyme levels in sarcoid arthritis. Arch Intern Med 146:125–127, 1986.
The level of serum angiotensin-converting enzyme (SACE) is abnormally high in 75 percent of patients with sarcoidosis, often in association with activity of the disease. Levels of SACE may be helpful in the differential diagnosis of patients with "seronegative polyarthritis."

Seventh International Conference on Sarcoidosis and Other Granulomatous Disorders, Siltzbach LE (ed). New York, Ann NY Acad Sci 278:1–751, 1976.
  Full conference proceedings include discussions.

Sharma OP: *Sarcoidosis—clinical management.* Kent, England, Butterworths, 1984.
  A clinically oriented book which antedates the intense interest in the cellular immune processes in the lung.

Siltzbach LE: Sarcoidosis: Clinical features and management. Med Clin N Am 51:483–502, 1967.
  A clinical review of 311 patients observed from 1946 to 1961.

Siltzbach LE: Sarcoidosis, in Fishman AP (ed), *Pulmonary Diseases and Disorders,* 1st ed. New York, McGraw-Hill, 1980, pp 889–908.
  Review chapter in earlier edition. Source of many illustrations used in present edition.

Siltzbach LE, James DG, Neville E, Turiaf J, Battesti JP, Sharma OP, Hosoda Y, Mikami R, Odaka M: Course and prognosis of sarcoidosis around the world. Am J Med 57:847–852, 1974.
  Retrospective analysis of 1609 patients in five cities, London, New York, Paris, Los Angeles and Tokyo, with impressive parallelism of findings.

Silverman KJ, Hutchins GM, Bulkley BH: Cardiac sarcoid: A clinicopathologic study of 84 unselected patients with systemic sarcoidosis. Circulation 58:1204–1211, 1978.
  Complete autopsy survey at Johns Hopkins revealed 23 with myocardial granulomas.

Smellie H, Hoyle C: The natural history of pulmonary sarcoidosis. Quart J Med 20:539–558, 1960.
  Review of the clinical and radiographic features and natural course of 125 patients observed in London for more than 2 years.

Tenth International Conference on Sarcoidosis and Other Granulomatous Disorders, Sept 17–22, 1984, Baltimore, Maryland. Johns CJ (ed). Ann NY Acad Sci 465:1–749, 1986.
  Proceedings of the conference with papers on both basic mechanisms and clinical aspects with discussions of pathogenesis, clinical course, and bronchoalveolar lavage.

Thomas PD, Hunninghake GW: Current concepts of the pathogenesis of sarcoidosis. Am Rev Respir Dis 135:747–760, 1987.
  An up-to-date review of the inflammatory response in sarcoidosis.

Thrasher DR, Briggs DD Jr: Pulmonary sarcoidosis. Clin Chest Med 3:537–563, 1982.
  A general review, including 227 patients from Alabama, and the authors' approach to patients with suspected sarcoidosis.

Winterbauer RH, Belec N, Moores KK: A clinical interpretation of bilateral hilar adenopathy. Ann Intern Med 78:65–71, 1973.
  Bilateral hilar adenopathy in asymptomatic patients with negative physical examination or with erythema nodosum or uveitis should be considered a priori evidence of sarcoidosis, and biopsy is not necessary.

Chapter 43

Pulmonary Manifestations of Collagen-Vascular Diseases

Burton F. Dickey / Allen R. Myers

Rheumatoid Arthritis
  Pleurisy
  Intrapulmonary Nodules
  Caplan's Syndrome (Rheumatoid Pneumoconiosis)
  Interstitial Lung Disease
  Bronchiolitis Obliterans
  Miscellaneous

Ankylosing Spondylitis

Systemic Sclerosis (Scleroderma)

Polymyositis and Dermatomyositis

Systemic Lupus Erythematosus
  Pleurisy
  Alveolar Hemorrhage
  Pneumonitis
  Interstitial Lung Disease
  Diaphragmatic Weakness
  Miscellaneous

Sjögren's Syndrome

The collagen-vascular diseases are a diverse group of systemic illnesses of unknown etiology that share many clinical and pathologic features. Generally, however, each can be distinguished by a clinical constellation of signs, symptoms, and laboratory abnormalities. Although multisystem involvement is the hallmark of these diseases, each tends to affect certain organ systems more than others, thereby enabling the clinician to identify the specific disease by distinctive major features (Table 43-1).

Traditionally, rheumatoid arthritis (RA), systemic lupus erythematosus (SLE), and polymyositis-dermatomyositis (PM-DM) were the collagen-vascular diseases. This categorization, which was based on pathologic and clinical similarities, is now outmoded because of recent immunopathologic information and the clinical descriptions of large groups of patients. However, no satisfactory substitute term, including connective tissue disorders, vasculitides, etc., has proved more satisfactory. Hence, the term collagen-vascular disease has been retained even

though it is used in a somewhat different context from the original. The subsequent discussion is predicated on the awareness that collagen-vascular diseases are not primarily collagen disorders per se; instead, they are pathologic manifestations of processes that affect the connective tissues of the body, which include collagen as a constituent.

For several reasons, pulmonary involvement in collagen-vascular disorders is being recognized with increased frequency (Table 43-2). In addition to increasing precision in diagnosis, the incidence of pulmonary involvement has increased as a result of longer survival in response to treatment. Moreover, the possibility exists that new environmental stimuli are pathogenetically responsible for the pulmonary abnormalities. Because of this increased incidence, pulmonary involvement is now an important feature of the collagen-vascular diseases and significantly contributes to morbidity and mortality.

The lung responds to injury in only a few ways. Therefore, the pleural, vascular and parenchymal abnormalities caused by collagen-vascular diseases are generally indistinguishable clinically and pathologically from other causes. The identification of the pulmonary disorder as a manifestation of a collagen-vascular disease depends on demonstrating the existence of an associated, generalized extrapulmonary disorder of connective tissue.

RHEUMATOID ARTHRITIS

Rheumatoid arthritis is a chronic inflammatory disease that is primarily manifested by articular involvement, often in association with abnormalities in many other organ systems. Genetic and immunologic factors play important roles in the pathophysiological process. Its prevalence in the population is approximately 2 percent; the female-to-male ratio is 3:1. The onset is gradual with complaints of joint pain and swelling (arthritis not arthralgias), and morning stiffness. Characteristically, a symmetric polyarthritis affects the small joints in the hands and feet, as well as large peripheral joints, i.e., wrists, knees, elbows, shoulders, hips, and ankles. However, the disease can involve any joint of the body. Systemic features of the disease include low grade fever, malaise, weight loss, and easy fatigability.

The diagnosis of rheumatoid arthritis is based on the clinical picture of joint involvement and typical laboratory studies. The hematologic abnormalities are those of a nonspecific, chronic inflammatory or infectious disease, i.e., normocytic hypochromic anemia, diffuse hypergammaglobulinemia, hypoalbuminemia, and increased erythrocyte sedimentation rate. Synovial fluid is characteristically inflammatory in nature and demonstrates a polymorphonuclear leukocytosis, low viscosity, and poor mucin precipitate; the concentrations of complement and glucose are generally subnormal.

TABLE 43-1
Clinical Features of the Major Collagen-Vascular Diseases

Clinical Features	Rheumatoid Arthritis	Systemic Sclerosis	Polymyositis and Dermatomyositis	Systemic Lupus Erythematosus
Arthritis	100	30	35	90
Raynaud's phenomenon	15	90	30	20
Skin lesions	0	95	40	70
Renal	0	10	0	50
Gastrointestinal	0	90	50	0
Central nervous system	0	0	0	50
Myositis	0	10	100	2
Laboratory Tests				
Rheumatoid factor	70–80	25	40	20
Antinuclear antibodies	25	40	0	>95
ds DNA	3	0	0	60
Lupus erythematosus cells	5	0	0	70–80
Serum C3 or CH50	4	0	0	60
Sm antibody	0	0	0	25
Jo-1 antibody	0	0	30	0
Anticentromere antibody	0	50	0	0
Scl-70 antibody	0	25	0	0

TABLE 43-2
Pulmonary Manifestations of the Major Collagen-Vascular Diseases

Pulmonary Manifestations	Rheumatoid Arthritis	Systemic Sclerosis	Polymyositis and Dermatomyositis	Systemic Lupus Erythematosus
Pleural				
Thickening	++	+	0	++
Effusion	++	0	0	+++
Parenchymal				
Acute pneumonia	0	0	0	+
Diffuse intersititial fibrosis	++*	+++	++*	+
Nodules	++	0	0	0
Primary pulmonary vasculopathy	0	++	0	+
Aspiration	0	++	+++	0
Ventilatory insufficiency	0	+	++	+

*A rapidly progressing variant may occur.

NOTE: 0 = Absent or rare; +=uncommon; ++=recognized manifestation; +++=important feature of disease.

Rheumatoid factor (autoantibodies reactive with IgG) as manifested by a positive latex fixation test (titer of 1:160 or higher) is present in 70 to 80 percent of patients with rheumatoid arthritis. If rheumatoid factor (RF) does appear, it is usually detectable when the patient first presents with arthritic complaints, and it persists despite waning of disease activity or even complete remission. Titers vary little with the state of activity. Unfortunately, rheumatoid factor is not specific and occurs in a variety of chronic disorders: infectious (tuberculosis, subacute bacterial endocarditis, syphilis, and leprosy), inflammatory [systemic lupus erythematosus, idiopathic pulmonary fibrosis (IPF), sarcoidosis, and hepatitis], or immunologic (posttransplantation and repeated transfusion). Therefore, interpretation of the presence of rheumatoid factor depends on the clinical setting.

Other immunologic laboratory abnormalities may occur in rheumatoid arthritis: positive lupus erythematosus preparations, positive antinuclear antibodies, and decreased concentration of complement in serum. The first two of these are nonspecific; the last occurs only with severe necrotizing or "malignant" vasculitis. The presence of cryoglobulins as a measure of immune complexes appears to correlate with an increased prevalence of extra-articular disease, including pulmonary.

Extra-articular manifestations of the disease occur in patients with erosive arthritis with deformities and high titers of rheumatoid factor ("highly expressed" rheumatoid arthritis). Among these extra-articular features are subcutaneous nodules; vasculitic lesions, such as digital infarcts, gangrene, and visceral necrotizing arteritis; skin ulcerations; lymphadenopathy; ocular changes, such as episcleritis, scleritis, or scleromalacia; pericarditis and cardiomegaly; peripheral neuropathy; Felty's syndrome; Sjögren's syndrome; and pulmonary disease. Interestingly, the kidney is usually spared by the pathologic process underlying rheumatoid arthritis.

Although rheumatoid arthritis is a disease of antiquity, involvement of the lungs has been recognized only within the past 40 years. Curiously, although rheumatoid arthritis is more common in women, pulmonary manifestations are more common in men. Currently, several types of pulmonary disorders are recognized to be part of the syndrome of rheumatoid arthritis: (1) pleurisy, with or without effusion, (2) intrapulmonary rheumatoid nodules, (3) rheumatoid pneumoconiosis, (4) diffuse interstitial fibrosis, and (5) bronchiolitis.

Pleurisy

Evidence of rheumatoid pleural disease with effusions or fibrosis is found in about one-half of rheumatoid patients at autopsy, but it is expressed clinically only in about 5 percent of patients. The lifetime incidence of rheumatoid pleurisy among males is about 12 percent compared with 1 to 2 percent among females. It is rarely seen in patients younger than 40 years old. Effusions most often develop in the first decade after the diagnosis of rheumatoid arthritis, but they can precede the onset of articular disease by more than a decade, or can first appear several decades after the initial arthritic manifestations. Pleurisy usually appears in patients with more severe arthritis, often accompanied by subcutaneous nodules and a high titer of rheumatoid factor. Effusions may be asymptomatic, or may present with pleuritic chest pain or dyspnea. Fever is infrequent, in contrast to lupus pleuritis. A small to moderately sized unilateral effusion is the most common radiographic finding, but large or bilateral effusions occur (Fig. 43-1). A pleural rub may be the only manifestation of pleurisy.

Uniformly, the effusions are exudates, and lymphocytes are usually the predominant white cell present. The most useful diagnostic finding at thoracentesis is a low pleural fluid glucose, which is almost universally accompanied by a pleural fluid pH less than 7.3. Eighty percent of patients at presentation have a glucose level below 50 mg/dl, and in most of the remaining 20 percent, the glu-

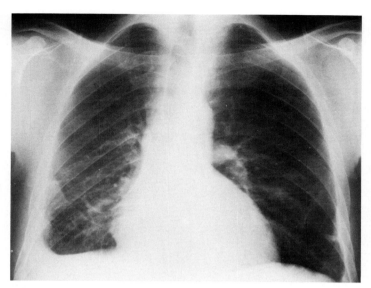

FIGURE 43-1 Rheumatoid arthritis. Right pleural effusion.

cose concentration will fall if the effusion persists for several weeks. Strikingly low or even absent glucose may be seen. Experimental studies have indicated that there is a relatively selective block of glucose transport into the pleural space, probably accompanied by increased metabolism by the inflamed pleurae. Pleural fluid total hemolytic complement levels and complement components tend to be low, while the rheumatoid factor is usually at least as high as serum titers. The gross appearance occasionally may be pseudochylous because of cholesterol accumulation in chronic effusions. A cytologic picture consisting of large, elongated histiocytes, multinucleated giant cells, and a granular, necrotic background is thought to be diagnostic. Pleural biopsy is generally not helpful, since most rheumatoid nodules are found on the visceral pleural surface.

Rheumatoid effusions generally resolve over several months, although they may persist for years or may recur. Residual pleural thickening is common, and marked thickening requiring decortication may rarely occur. The role of anti-inflammatory therapy is unclear, although both nonsteroidal drugs and corticosteroids have been used in an effort to prevent lung entrapment. Thoracentesis, and even pleural space obliteration may be needed in the management of the occasional case of recurrent or persistent symptomatic effusion. Empyema, generally due to staphylococci and resulting from a bronchopleural fistula secondary to subpleural nodule disruption, rarely supervenes.

Intrapulmonary Nodules

Discrete intrapulmonary nodules are a relatively rare (less than 1 percent) but dramatic finding in patients with

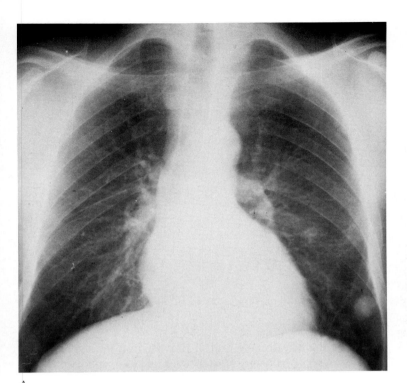

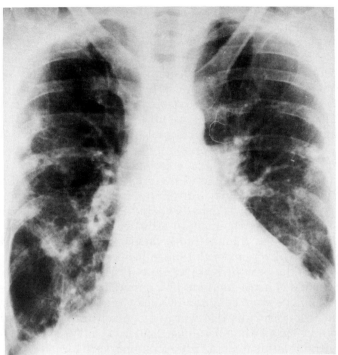

FIGURE 43-2 Rheumatoid arthritis. *A.* Single rheumatoid nodule in left lower lobe. *B.* Multiple rheumatoid nodules, left pleural reaction, and interstitial lung disease. *C.* Rheumatoid lung disease. The interstitial lung disease is both cellular and fibrotic.

C

rheumatoid arthritis. As with rheumatoid pleurisy, necrobiotic lung nodules occur predominantly in men. They may appear at any time during the course of rheumatoid arthritis and, rarely, even precede the clinical manifestations of arthritis by years. The rheumatoid factor is virtually always positive, especially when arthritis precedes the appearance of nodules. Often, pulmonary nodules are associated with other evidence of pulmonary and extraarticular disease.

Necrobiotic pulmonary nodules are usually multiple and pleural based, but may occur as solitary pulmonary nodules (Fig. 43-2A and B). The average diameter is 1 to 2 cm, but they range in size from a few millimeters to 7 cm. Cavitation is not uncommon and may leave only a thin-walled cystic shadow on the chest radiograph; more commonly a thick-walled cavity results. Nodules are generally asymptomatic, but they may cause cough and hemoptysis if they cavitate, bronchial obstruction when they occur endobronchially, and troublesome pneumothoraxes when they cavitate in a subpleural location. Even when asymptomatic, necrobiotic pulmonary nodules may present an obvious clinical diagnostic problem in differentiating malignancy and infection as alternative etiologies, especially if a nodule is solitary.

The histologic appearance of the pulmonary nodule is identical to that of the subcutaneous nodule. There is a three-layered structure that includes an irregular central area of fibrinoid necrosis that is surrounded by a well-defined margin of palisaded, large mononuclear cells and enveloped by a zone of granulation tissue. As in the case of the subcutaneous nodule, histologic identification of a necrobiotic nodule in the lung is strongly suggestive although not pathognomonic of rheumatoid arthritis.

The course of pulmonary nodules varies; they may undergo spontaneous resolution, cavitate, recur, or simply persist for years. They appear to wax and wane to some degree along with subcutaneous nodules and the activity of the arthritis. Corticosteroids do not have an established role in treatment, and therapeutic surgical intervention is indicated only for serious complications, such as persistent localized infection or bronchopleural fistula.

Caplan's Syndrome (Rheumatoid Pneumoconiosis)

Caplan's syndrome is the association of clinical rheumatoid arthritis, pulmonary necrobiotic nodules, and coal worker's pneumoconiosis (silicosis). Since Caplan's original description in 1953, the same radiographic picture has been observed in rheumatoid arthritis with other pneumoconioses, particularly asbestosis.

The nodules usually are multiple, occur at the periphery of the lung fields, are well circumscribed, and range in size from 0.5 to 5 cm (Figs. 43-3 and 43-4). They are seen most commonly on a background of mild

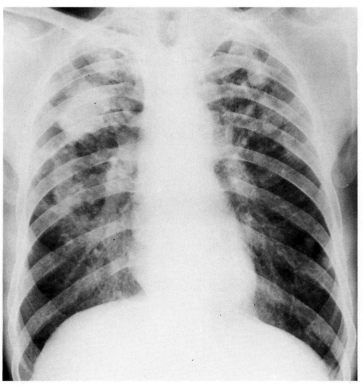 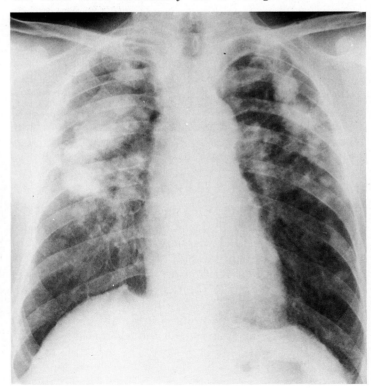

A   *B*

FIGURE 43-3 Chest radiographs in Caplan's syndrome. *A.* Coal miner with deforming rheumatoid arthritis of the hands complaining of mild shortness of breath on exertion. *B.* Two years later. The discrete nodules on the right have become conglomerate.

is frequently seen in addition. It is thought that mineral dust exposure may initiate inflammation leading to the formation of nodules. In miners with rheumatoid arthritis, the incidence of these nodules is 40 times greater than in miners with silicosis alone. Functional impairment due to Caplan nodules appears to be minimal and is related more to the underlying pneumoconiosis and to smoking. No specific treatment for this condition is indicated.

Interstitial Lung Disease

Evidence of interstitial lung disease (ILD) can be found radiographically in 2 to 5 percent of patients with rheumatoid arthritis. In another subset of rheumatoid arthritis, the chest radiographs are unremarkable, but the lung volumes show concentric reduction, the diffusing capacity is low, and interstitial lung disease is found on lung biopsy. In about half of the patients in whom pulmonary function tests are suggestive of interstitial disease, the chest radiograph is also abnormal.

As with pleurisy and nodules, interstitial lung disease in rheumatoid arthritis affects men predominantly; the ratio of men to women is 2:1. Clinical manifestations include dyspnea, nonproductive cough, and occasionally chest pain or fever. Dyspnea may be masked by immobility from arthritis. Late inspiratory crackles and clubbing occur when the pulmonary disease is severe. Although interstitial lung disease may precede overt joint symptoms in highly expressed disease, it usually follows arthritis in conjunction with high titers of rheumatoid factor and subcutaneous nodules.

The chest radiograph typically reveals bilateral, sometimes asymmetric, reticular or reticulonodular infiltration, which may progress to honeycombing (Fig. 43-5).

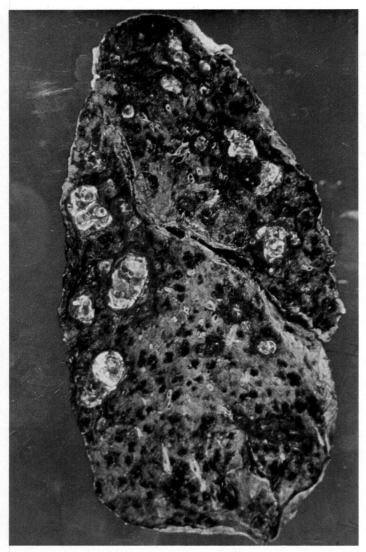

FIGURE 43-4 Whole lung section from a coal miner with Caplan's syndrome. *(Courtesy of R. M. E. Seal, Llandough Hospital, Wales.)*

pneumoconiosis and develop rapidly in crops over weeks to months. Arthritic manifestations of rheumatoid disease precede or occur simultaneously with the appearance of nodules in more than one-half of patients, but they may not develop until several years after the appearance of nodules. Rheumatoid factor is present in almost all patients with classic Caplan's syndrome.

Nodules of this syndrome are readily distinguished from nodules or masses seen in the progressive massive fibrosis (PMF) of pneumoconiosis. The opacities in PMF develop slowly on a background of severe pneumoconiosis, tend to be irregular in outline, and rarely cavitate or calcify.

Pathologically, nodules in Caplan's syndrome resemble typical rheumatoid nodules, except that mineral dust

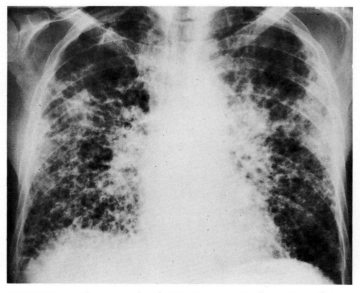

FIGURE 43-5 Rheumatoid arthritis. Coarse reticular pattern (honeycombing) of interstitial lung disease.

Progression is generally much slower and the course more benign than that of idiopathic pulmonary fibrosis. However, some patients present with a diffuse ground-glass appearance and severe respiratory impairment that may be rapidly fatal.

The pathogenesis of interstitial lung disease in rheumatoid arthritis remains obscure. Insoluble rheumatoid factor complexes are believed to be involved. Immunofluorescent staining of rheumatoid lung tissue has demonstrated large quantities of immunoglobulin in association with circulating immune complexes.

There is no apparent difference between the histology of interstitial lung disease that accompanies rheumatoid arthritis and that associated with other collagen-vascular diseases or idiopathic pulmonary fibrosis. A spectrum of abnormalities from predominantly cellular infiltration to highly fibrotic changes may be seen; often they coexist within the same patient and even within different areas of a single biopsy. Although corticosteroid therapy has generally not been given to patients with rheumatoid arthritis and interstitial pulmonary disease, occasionally it is helpful in patients in whom biopsy reveals that the interstitial process is cellular or to those in whom the pulmonary disease appears to be active according to clinical criteria.

Bronchiolitis Obliterans

Case reports beginning in the late 1970s have now established a rare association between rheumatoid arthritis and rapidly progressive obliterative bronchiolitis that is not attributable to drugs. (For drug-induced bronchiolitis, see below.) Patients typically present with the complaint of dyspnea progressing over several weeks, and examination usually reveals coarse, early inspiratory crackles and a characteristic high-pitched, midinspiratory squeak. The chest radiograph is normal. Pulmonary function testing demonstrates air trapping and irreversible obstruction to airflow which is most marked at low lung volumes, but normal total lung and diffusing capacities are present. Airways obstruction is generally progressive and usually fatal within several months, despite treatment with corticosteroids. Pathologically, bronchioles and small bronchi are obliterated by submucosal inflammation and fibrosis, without the polypoid intralumenal granulation tissue noted in bronchiolitis obliterans of other etiologies.

Some uncertainty exists as to whether chronic mild airways obstruction is more prevalent in patients with rheumatoid arthritis than in the population at large. However, in patients with rheumatoid arthritis who smoke cigarettes, airways obstruction is quite prevalent, suggesting that the healing process in response to inflammatory stimuli is abnormal. This observation may also relate to the etiology of Caplan's syndrome.

Miscellaneous

Among the pulmonary disorders that have been reported to be associated with rheumatoid arthritis is an unexplained ("primary") pulmonary vasculopathy. In most reported cases, some uncertainty exists about the diagnosis, since the manifestations have included Raynaud's phenomenon or other features of the collagen-vascular diseases that are known to be associated with a pulmonary vasculopathy. By default, in the few remaining cases the pulmonary hypertension that coexists with rheumatoid arthritis is relegated to the category of "primary" (unexplained) pulmonary hypertension.

Upper airway involvement may result from cricoarytenoid arthritis that produces sore throat, hoarseness, and inspiratory airflow obstruction. Symptoms are present in one-third of patients with cricoarytenoid arthritis; asymptomatic abnormalities are noted by laryngeal computed tomography or indirect laryngoscopy in others.

Upper lobe fibrocavitary disease, not due to tuberculosis or to necrobiotic nodules, has been described. The appearance is similar to infiltrates seen in ankylosing spondylitis. Amyloidosis may occur in long-standing rheumatoid arthritis, but pulmonary involvement is more often seen in primary amyloidosis. The incidence of pulmonary infections, particularly bronchitis and bronchiectasis, is reportedly increased in rheumatoid patients.

Pulmonary disease due to therapeutic drugs is an important cause of morbidity among patients with rheumatoid arthritis. Treatment with gold salts sometimes causes a type of interstitial lung disease which may be confused with the interstitial lung disease that is associated with rheumatoid arthritis. Distinguishing features are the clinical features of a hypersensitivity drug reaction, e.g., rash, fever, eosinophilia, thrombocytopenia, and increased concentrations of IgE in the serum. These manifestations appear soon after the initiation of gold therapy. The radiographic infiltrates generally resolve after the drug is discontinued; sometimes corticosteroid therapy is necessary. Among the patients with rheumatoid arthritis who are treated with gold but without obvious manifestations of "gold lung," pulmonary function testing shows no evidence of subclinical lung disease.

On rare occasions, penicillamine causes interstitial lung disease, generally only after prolonged treatment at high doses. A pulmonary hemorrhage syndrome has also been attributed to penicillamine. But, more often, penicillamine administered to patients with rheumatoid arthritis is associated with a severe, rapidly progressive bronchiolitis. Concentric bronchiolar constriction, rather than the more typical intraluminal polypoid obstruction of bronchiolitis obliterans, is seen histologically.

Pulmonary involvement in juvenile rheumatoid arthritis differs from that of adult rheumatoid arthritis in that necrobiotic nodules and adult-type interstitial lung disease occur rarely if at all. Lymphocytic interstitial pneumonitis has been reported in juvenile rheumatoid arthritis.

ANKYLOSING SPONDYLITIS

Ankylosing spondylitis is a chronic inflammatory disease, especially of males (male-to-female ratio 5:1). The spine and sacroiliac joints are primarily affected, but occasionally peripheral large joints are involved. Because of the pattern of joint involvement, this disease is generally easily distinguishable from rheumatoid arthritis. Moreover, it lacks the serologic abnormalities seen in rheumatoid arthritis. Genetic predisposition is marked as indicated by the existence of the HLA antigen B27 in more than 90 percent of patients with ankylosing spondylitis.

Extraskeletal manifestations of the disease include iritis, cardiac conduction defects, aortitis, and fibrocavitary (fibrobullous) disease of the apices of the lungs; this pulmonary complication occurred in 1.3 percent of 2080 patients with ankylosing spondylitis. Males with fibrocavitary lung disease outnumber females approximately 25 to 1. The average interval from the onset of ankylosing spondylitis to the radiographic appearance of fibrobullous disease is 15 to 20 years, and the skeletal disease is generally inactive by then. The pulmonary lesion begins with apical pleural thickening and patchy consolidation of one or both apices and usually progresses to dense bilateral fibrosis and airspace enlargement. The lesions may progress steadily, or they may remain stable with only mild radiographic disease (Fig. 43-6). The appearance is often indistinguishable from pulmonary tuberculosis. Histologic examination reveals nonspecific changes of chronic inflammation and fibrosis.

Hemoptysis from upper lobe traction bronchiectasis or spontaneous pneumothorax from rupture of a bulla occasionally complicates the course, but usually fibrobullous disease remains asymptomatic unless secondarily infected. *Aspergillus* infection is most common, and it frequently results in hemoptysis. Surgical treatment should be approached cautiously, since the postoperative course among these patients is frequently complicated by empyema or a bronchopleural fistula.

Pulmonary dysfunction may also occur in ankylosing spondylitis as a consequence of skeletal disease. Most patients with significant spinal ankylosis experience some restriction of motion of the thoracic cage due to fusion of costovertebral joints. The bucket handle motion of the thorax is impaired, as indicated by a marked decrease in thoracic excursion during ventilation. However, unlike the case with kyphoscoliotic restrictive disease, lung function is well-preserved because the thorax becomes fixed at higher lung volumes. Increased diaphragmatic function appears to compensate well for decreased thoracic motion, and total lung capacity and vital capacity are only mildly decreased, while residual volume and functional residual capacity are normal or slightly increased. Airflow parameters remain normal. Care must be taken after abdominal surgery, however, that ventilatory failure does not ensue when diaphragmatic function is compromised.

Cricoarytenoid involvement may lead to upper airway obstruction and respiratory dysfunction, although involvement of the cricoarytenoid joints in ankylosing spondylitis is much less common than in rheumatoid arthritis.

SYSTEMIC SCLEROSIS (SCLERODERMA)

Scleroderma or systemic sclerosis (SSc) is a generalized disorder of connective tissue; its cause is unknown. Scleroderma was the original designation because the skin was the most obvious manifestation. Currently, *systemic sclerosis* is preferred because of the associated visceral involvement. The disease is not only systemic but often progressive, although at times the rate of progression is almost imperceptible. The onset is usually in the third to fifth decades of life; women are affected almost three times as often as men. The incidence has been estimated to be at least 4.5 to 12 cases per million population per year.

The presenting manifestations of systemic sclerosis are quite variable but usually include either Raynaud's phenomenon, insidious swelling and/or thickening of the skin of the fingers, or musculoskeletal symptoms. Raynaud's phenomenon (cold-induced vasospasm manifested by a three-color sequence of skin reactions consisting of blanching, cyanosis, and then erythema) occurs in approximately 90 percent of patients. Although often associated with changes in the skin of the fingers, Raynaud's phenomenon frequently antedates specific evidence of the disease by many years.

Skin abnormalities, the hallmark of the disease, occur in 95 percent of patients (see Chapter 27). They are generally divided into two major categories on the basis of distribution: sclerodactyly, or acrosclerosis, which involves primarily distal upper extremities, and diffuse scleroderma, which involves the face, trunk, and extremities. In contrast, localized scleroderma or morphea is rarely associated with systemic disease. Skin changes frequently begin with an edematous phase, and the diagnosis of scleroderma is usually not considered until the indurative or "hide-bound" stage is evident. Skin thickening is invariably associated with either depigmentation or hyperpigmentation. Further diagnostic clues are telangiectasis, especially of face, tongue, lips, and hands and draining calcific deposits of the fingertips. CREST syndrome (calcinosis, Raynaud's, esophageal hypomotility, sclerodactyly,

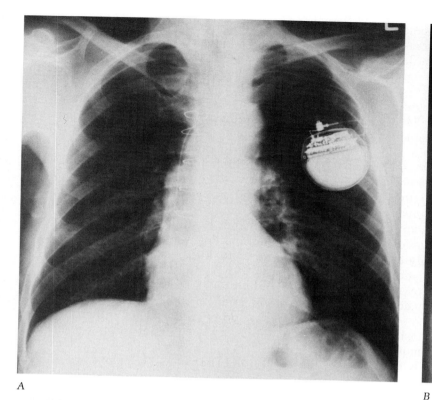

A

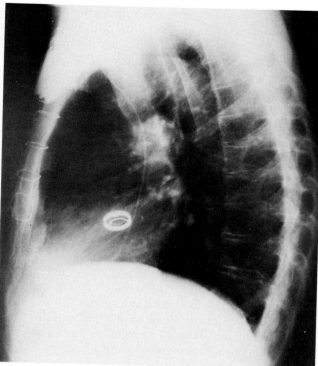

B

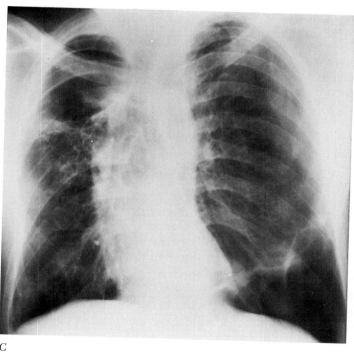

C

FIGURE 43-6 Ankylosing spondylitis. *A* and *B*. 60-year-old male with bilateral apical bullae. Aortic valvular insufficiency has been dealt with by replacing the aortic valve. A pacemaker was required for the conduction defect. *C*. Ankylosing spondylitis resembling old tuberculosis. A bulla is seen at the right apex and left base. The intervening lung is densely scarred.

and telangiectasis) is generally considered to be a special subset of scleroderma that has a better prognosis; but late visceral manifestations do occur and may be severe.

In about one-third of patients, the onset of systemic sclerosis is indistinguishable from that of early rheumatoid arthritis, i.e., articular symptoms that range from ar-

thralgias to frank polyarthritis. Late in the disease, inflammatory joint symptoms are uncommon because manifestations then predominate of either fibrosis in tendons or of contractures of the joints of the fingers caused by overlying skin pathology. A proximal myopathy that is indistinguishable from polymyositis sometimes occurs as part of the disease rather than as a concurrent, separate illness. Radiographs of the joints of the hands are sometimes unremarkable but often show resorption of terminal finger tufts, atrophy of soft tissue, or calcinosis circumscripta.

The visceral organs affected by the disease include the gastrointestinal tract, kidneys, heart, and lungs. The gastrointestinal tract is commonly involved and characteristically manifests diminished, or absent, peristalsis of the lower portion of the esophagus and evidence of esophageal reflux. Small intestinal and colonic involvement sometimes cause malabsorption or constipation to the point of obstipation. Cardiomyopathy secondary to myocardial fibrosis may produce chronic congestive heart failure. Renal disease that results from obliterative changes of interlobular renal arteries generally progresses rapidly to the stage of severe hypertension, renal insufficiency, and death unless very aggressive antihypertensive therapy is introduced. Renal and pulmonary disease are the major causes of death in systemic sclerosis.

Laboratory studies are rarely helpful in diagnosis. Mild anemia and hypergammaglobulinemia are common. A microangiopathic anemia sometimes occurs, usually in association with renal disease, and indicates a grim prognosis. Immunologic abnormalities include a positive rheumatoid factor test in approximately 25 percent of patients and a positive test for antinuclear antibodies in up to 75 percent of patients. The immunofluorescent pattern of the antinuclear antibodies is generally of the "speckled" or nucleolar variety and differs from the types that usually occur in systemic lupus erythematosus. Anticentromere antibodies occur in 90 percent of patients with the CREST variant but only in occasional patients with diffuse scleroderma.

The etiology of systemic sclerosis is not known. However, the evidence favors a generalized vascular process. Vessels of various sizes, including small arteries and capillaries, demonstrate abnormalities even in the absence of sclerosis. Pharmacologic studies of lower esophageal motility are consistent with a neurovascular disorder. Just how the vascular abnormality relates to the biochemical disorder of connective tissue is unclear.

Pathologic changes in the lungs of patients with systemic sclerosis were first recognized at the end of the nineteenth century. Subsequent reports have emphasized that it is common. Although respiratory symptoms occur in only one-half of patients, physiological dysfunction or abnormalities on the chest radiograph occur in most patients. The extent of interstitial disease seen radiographically and determined physiologically does not always correlate. The typical radiographic picture, seen in about one-half of patients, is one of bibasilar reticulonodular infiltrates (Fig. 43-7), often associated with honeycombing. The clinical manifestations are those of interstitial lung disease; however, clubbing is usually absent.

In between two-thirds and 95 percent of patients with systemic sclerosis, pulmonary function tests are abnormal. The diffusing capacity of the lungs for carbon monoxide becomes abnormally low early in the course of the disease, often before the chest radiograph becomes abnormal and while other manifestations of systemic disease are minimal. Later in the disease, lung volumes decrease. In most instances conventional tests reveal no evidence of obstructive disease of the airways unless the patient is a heavy smoker, or peribronchial fibrosis is present. Despite obvious and extensive involvement of the chest wall in this disorder, compliance of the chest wall is usually within normal limits and is not a cause of the pulmonary dysfunction. In general, despite the high prevalence of physiological abnormalities, the mean rates of change in lung volumes and diffusing capacity do not differ from those that occur with aging in a normal reference population. However, individuals vary widely in this regard, i.e., some improve, some remain stable, and some deteriorate. The rate of progression is not predicted either by the severity at presentation or by regression of proximal scleroderma.

Histologically, the characteristic lesions are interstitial fibrosis and thickening of the alveolar septa (Fig. 43-7). In advanced disease, extensive fibrosis replaces alveolar spaces. For mysterious reasons, the fibrotic changes are most marked at the lung bases. Honeycombing (enlargement of respiratory airspaces) occurs within areas of fibrosis, presumably the result of mechanical stresses originating with the fibrotic lesions. Interstitial lung disease is such a characteristic feature of systemic sclerosis that there is no reason for routine lung biopsy.

Pulmonary vascular disease occurs in systemic sclerosis independently of pulmonary fibrosis. Indeed, it may elicit pulmonary hypertension even though interstitial changes are minimal or absent. In this circumstance, unless there are other manifestations of systemic sclerosis, the pulmonary hypertension is apt to be categorized as *primary* (*unexplained* or *idiopathic*). The possibility has been raised that pulmonary vasospasm contributes to the pulmonary hypertension of systemic sclerosis. However, this idea has had no support from conventional pressor tests, which have failed to evoke a pulmonary pressor response in patients with systemic sclerosis even though systemic blood pressure and systemic vascular resistance have increased briskly in response to immersion of the hands in cold water.

Histologically, the vascular lesions involve arterioles and muscular arteries and show concentric intimal proliferation (Fig. 43-7), fibrosis, and medial hypertrophy. The major consequence of the pulmonary arterial disease in systemic sclerosis is cor pulmonale with right ventricular failure (Fig. 43-7). Once right ventricular failure has set in, thromboembolism sometimes contributes to the pulmonary hypertension.

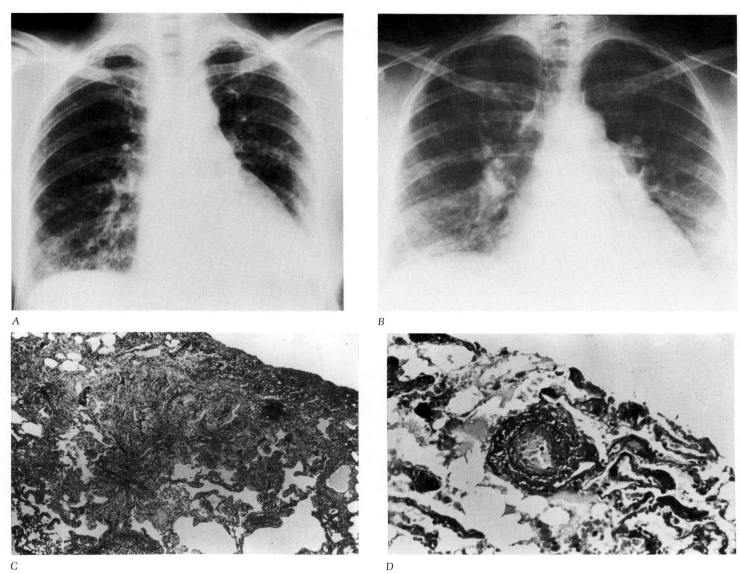

A

B

C

D

FIGURE 43-7 Scleroderma. *A.* Reticulonodular pattern of interstitial disease in the lower lobes. *B.* Cor pulmonale and right ventricular failure. *C.* Marked pulmonary fibrosis. *D.* Arteriolar intimal proliferation.

The prevalence of interstitial lung disease is less in patients with CREST syndrome than in systemic sclerosis. The presence of anticentromere antibody correlates with the reduced prevalence of interstitial lung disease. However, the occurrence of primary pulmonary vasculopathy appears to be equally high in CREST patients.

Respiratory failure is a rare but important consequence of pulmonary disease in systemic sclerosis. The compromise in ventilatory function stems from respiratory muscle weakness due to a noninflammatory myopathy. The ventilatory insufficiency may range from mild impairment to hypercapnic respiratory failure. The muscle weakness sometimes responds to corticosteroids.

Pleural effusions in systemic sclerosis are quite rare unless there is infection or congestive heart failure.

Pulmonary complications of scleroderma include spontaneous pneumothorax, aspiration pneumonitis, and pulmonary neoplasms. "Scar carcinoma," most often a bronchioloalveolar cell carcinoma histologically, is associated with long-standing interstitial lung disease in systemic sclerosis. This neoplasm appears to arise in areas of severely disordered architecture with epithelial metaplasia. Carcinoma should be suspected when a change occurs in a patient's respiratory symptoms, or when a new nodule or infiltrate appears on the chest radiograph, particularly when associated with an air bronchogram. Pneumothorax is rare and results from the rupture of subpleural or peribronchial cysts in an end-stage fibrotic lung. Aspiration pneumonitis occurs with an increased incidence in systemic sclerosis secondary to esophageal dilatation and aperistalsis.

There is no effective treatment for scleroderma or its visceral manifestations, including pulmonary fibrosis and pulmonary vascular disease. Corticosteroids have been uniformly disappointing so that most clinicians no longer even attempt therapeutic trials with these agents. Clinical trials evaluating bronchoalveolar lavage as a means of identifying a subgroup of patients with active inflammation which may respond to corticosteroid therapy are in progress. Currently, interest has been rekindled in the use of D-penicillamine. This chelating agent interferes with intermolecular cross-linking of collagen. The results have been more successful in treating the integumentary changes of progressive systemic sclerosis than the visceral disease. The prognosis of systemic sclerosis generally depends on the type and extent of visceral involvement. Patients with overt pulmonary, renal, or cardiac involvement have a worse prognosis than those in whom the lungs, kidney, and heart do not appear to be affected. A reduced $D_{L_{CO}}$ appears to be a strong predictor of early mortality.

Several syndromes which share clinical features with systemic sclerosis are also associated with similar pulmonary disorders. Both primary pulmonary hypertension and interstitial lung disease have been described in association with isolated Raynaud's disease. Mixed connective tissue disease has overlapping clinical features with progressive systemic sclerosis (as well as with systemic lupus erythematosus and polymyositis-dermatomyositis). It is associated with high titers of antibody to nuclear ribonucleoprotein. Originally thought to be a relatively benign disorder, mixed connective tissue disease has more recently been found to sometimes pursue a severe or fatal course, primarily because of pulmonary complications. Proliferative pulmonary vasculopathy and interstitial lung disease have been reported in up to 80 percent of patients in recent series. The lesions often respond to corticosteroids or a combination of corticosteroids and cytotoxic agents.

POLYMYOSITIS AND DERMATOMYOSITIS

Polymyositis and dermatomyositis (PM-DM) are inflammatory diseases of striated muscle that produce a characteristic clinical picture of proximal-muscle weakness. Their causes are unknown. They affect females twice as often as males, usually in the fifth and sixth decades; the incidence is approximately 1 per 200,000 to 300,000 population per year.

Myopathy is the distinctive clinical feature; the other clinical and serologic features overlap those of the other collagen-vascular diseases. When the myopathy is associated with skin disease (dermatomyositis), the diagnosis is usually obvious. Skin manifestations occur in approximately 40 percent of patients: the characteristic dermatitis is a bright erythematous, scaling eruption that affects the face, neck, shoulders, and chest, as well as the elbows, hand joints, knees, and ankles. Periorbital edema and purplish discoloration of the upper eyelids ("heliotrope rash") often occurs; the latter is considered to be pathognomonic of dermatomyositis.

The weakness begins insidiously. In most patients, it gradually involves the proximal aspects of both upper and lower extremities; distal weakness occurs in about one-quarter of patients. Weakness of the posterior pharyngeal muscles is responsible for the characteristic nasal voice and the dysphagia. Raynaud's phenomenon occurs in approximately 30 percent, and rheumatic symptoms, in the form of polyarthritis or arthralgias, are seen in one-quarter of patients. Subcutaneous calcifications often occur in areas of previous inflammation.

Laboratory studies are useful in confirming the inflammatory myopathy. They include determinations of the concentration of muscle enzymes in serum (aldolase, transaminase, and creatine phosphokinase) and electromyographic evidence of myositis. Muscle biopsy is mandatory. Positive serologic studies are less conspicuous in PM-DM than in other collagen diseases, although antinuclear factors and rheumatoid factor may be present. A more specific abnormality is the Jo-1 precipitating antibody found in 30 percent of idiopathic polymyositis and 10 percent of dermatomyositis patients.

Pulmonary disease is an important cause of morbidity and mortality among patients with PM-DM. Almost 50 percent of patients develop some form of clinically apparent lung disease during the early years after the diagnosis of muscle disease, and lung disease still contributes directly to death in about 10 percent of all PM-DM patients.

Aspiration pneumonitis is the most common pulmonary disorder encountered in PM-DM. Severe diffuse muscle weakness is generally at the root of this problem. Weakness of the expiratory muscles leads to impairment of the protective cough; weakness of the extremities interferes with protective body movements, such as turning and bending in response to vomiting; and most importantly, weakness of the striated muscles of the soft palate, pharynx, and upper esophagus impairs deglutition. Dysphagia is a presenting symptom in 25 to 50 percent of patients, and most patients with clinically apparent episodes of aspiration will have complained of dysphagia. Pharyngeal and upper esophageal dysfunction can be objectively demonstrated manometrically or radiographically.

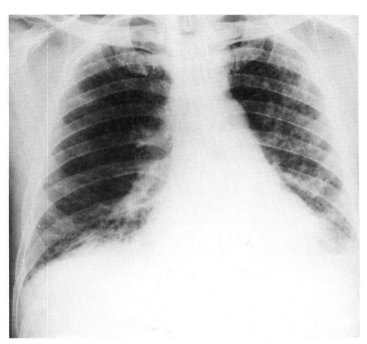

FIGURE 43-8 Polymyositis. Reticular pattern of interstitial lung disease most marked at the lung bases.

Radiographically evident interstitial lung disease is seen in 5 to 10 percent of PM-DM patients. It presents either as diffuse reticulonodular infiltration which is predominantly bibasilar (Fig. 43-8) or as diffuse ground-glass shadowing. Although reduced lung volumes and a decrease in diffusing capacity due to muscle weakness can complicate the interpretation of pulmonary function tests in PM-DM, physiological evidence of interstitial lung disease can be obtained in about one-third of all patients.

The spectrum of clinical presentations is broad, ranging from asymptomatic nonprogressive disease, through slowly progressive fibrosis, to an aggressive, often rapidly fatal Hamman-Rich type of presentation. Most of the typical signs and symptoms of interstitial lung disease, such as dyspnea on exertion, nonproductive cough, and bibasilar rales, are regular features, but clubbing is unusual. A strong association exists between interstitial lung disease and the presence of arthritis in PM-DM; however, the basis for this relationship is unclear. The onset of the interstitial lung disease is usually at the same time as or soon after the presentation of muscle disease. However, sometimes it precedes the muscle disease by months; in this circumstance, it may mask the clinical appearance of myopathy by limiting activity because of dyspnea. Serologic studies, with the exception of the Jo-1 antibody, have not been helpful. The presence of Jo-1 antibody seems to correlate strongly with the presence of interstitial disease in PM-DM. No histologic features distinguish the interstitial disease of PM-DM from that of other col-

lagen-vascular diseases or from idiopathic pulmonary fibrosis. However, in PM-DM, the response to the early use of corticosteroids in the more acute types of interstitial lung disease is often dramatic, thereby distinguishing it from the responses in other collagen-vascular diseases; in PM-DM, about 50 percent of patients respond with clearing of the chest radiograph, improvement in pulmonary function tests, and lessening of dyspnea; the response appears to correlate with the cellularity found on biopsy and a younger age of the patient. In patients with rapidly progressive disease, failure to respond promptly to corticosteroids portends that the prognosis is grim even if cytotoxic agents are added.

Ventilatory insufficiency is a serious manifestation of diffuse muscle weakness in patients with PM-DM. The weakness is evenly distributed between the inspiratory and expiratory muscles. Most patients develop some degree of respiratory muscle weakness as determined by measurement of maximal inspiratory and expiratory pressures, and 4 to 8 percent of patients go on to develop overt ventilatory failure. Marked respiratory muscle weakness generally becomes apparent in patients with the most severe generalized weakness and is frequently associated with pharyngeal dysfunction such as dysphagia and dysphonia. Aspiration, atelectasis, and pneumonia often dominate the clinical course of these patients before the onset of clinically apparent ventilatory insufficiency. Vital capacity and static pressures should be followed closely to avoid unanticipated, precipitous ventilatory failure: a decrease in vital capacity to less than 55 percent of predicted or in static inspiratory and expiratory pressures to less than 50 percent of predicted heralds the development of hypercapnia. Although the duration of profound muscle weakness may be prolonged, sometimes lasting for several months, the prognosis for eventual recovery of ventilatory function appears to be good.

Pleural disease independent of interstitial lung disease has not been reported in PM-DM. Nor has an association been established between PM-DM and a primary pulmonary vasculopathy. While no specific immune defects predisposing to infection have been described in PM-DM, the use of anti-inflammatory and immunosuppressive drugs in this disorder has become widespread leading to opportunistic lung infections caused by a wide range of pathogens. The therapeutic use of cytotoxic agents (especially methotrexate) for the myopathy may lead to interstitial lung disease; the resulting clinical picture can be confusing.

SYSTEMIC LUPUS ERYTHEMATOSUS

Systemic lupus erythematosus (SLE) is a chronic inflammatory disorder of unknown etiology that may affect virtually every organ system of the body. It is about four to five times more common in women than in men; its onset is usually between the ages of 15 and 45. It seems to be more common in black than in white women. The clinical manifestations of SLE vary greatly and range from asymptomatic disease that is limited to serologic abnormalities and involvement of few organs to lethal multisystem disease. In most patients, the cause is unknown, but some pharmacologic agents, e.g., procainamide, diphenylhydantoin, and hydralazine, can evoke a clinical syndrome that is often indistinguishable from the spontaneous disease.

Although SLE is protean in its clinical expressions, certain features are more apt to be present than others. For example, the skin is commonly involved, but the butterfly rash, one of its most distinctive features, is less common than originally described. Other skin manifestations include facial erythema, discoid lesions, and periungual erythema.

Photosensitivity, a rare phenomenon in other collagen diseases, occurs in approximately one-third of patients with SLE. Raynaud's phenomenon occurs in 15 to 20 percent of patients. Alopecia, patchy or diffuse, especially in the frontal area, is quite common in patients with active disease. Oral or nasal septal ulcerations are common, the latter often resulting in septal perforation.

Arthralgias and/or polyarthritis occur in more than 90 percent of patients with SLE and may be indistinguishable from early rheumatoid arthritis. However, the joint effusions are most often noninflammatory or mildly inflammatory, and erosive joint changes and deformity are quite rare. Nephritis occurs in over one-half of patients and is the major cause of mortality in SLE. It is the renal disease that frequently determines the major therapeutic interventions and eventual prognosis of the disease. Neurologic disorders occur in approximately one-half of patients and include seizures, cranial nerve disorders, focal neurologic changes, and psychosis. Cardiovascular abnormalities consist of pericarditis and atypical verrucous endocarditis (Libman-Sacks endocarditis). The endocarditis rarely elicits any clinical manifestations. Conversely, pericarditis occurs in 10 to 20 percent of patients with SLE and in some produces tamponade. Lymphadenopathy is common while the disease is active. Splenomegaly occurs in 10 percent of patients with SLE.

In contrast to other collagen diseases, laboratory tests in SLE are helpful in establishing the diagnosis. Some of the tests are characteristic, although nonspecific. Among these are the evidences of anemia which are common during active disease but not distinctive unless there is associated evidence of an autoimmune hemolytic process. The sedimentation rate is generally increased, and the concentration of albumin in serum is often decreased—as in any chronic inflammatory disease. Hypergammaglobulinemia is common. Leukopenia and thrombocytopenia are cardinal features of the disease. Proteinuria, microscopic he-

maturia, and cellular casts are seen in patients with nephritis, the nephrotic syndrome, or renal insufficiency.

In addition to these nonspecific indices of chronic disease or of organ involvement, there are certain serologic hallmarks of SLE: positive LE cell preparation occurs in 70 to 80 percent of patients and positive antinuclear antibodies (ANA) in greater than 95 percent. The ANA pattern using an immunofluorescent technique is usually homogeneous or shows peripheral staining. If the ANA test is negative, the diagnosis of SLE is in serious question. The presence of antibodies to native (double-stranded) DNA is currently being used for diagnosis and prognosis of SLE; these antibodies correlate well with active disease, particularly glomerulonephritis. Antibodies to small nuclear ribonucleoproteins, such as Sm antigen, appear to be specific for SLE but are present in less than one-half of the patients; antibodies to SS-A (Ro) or SS-B (La) may be present in SLE but are less specific. Low serum complement levels also correlate with active disease. Other serologic abnormalities include a chronic biologic false-positive test for syphilis (15 percent of patients) and positive rheumatoid factor test (20 percent of patients). Circulating anticoagulants occur in 10 percent of patients.

Serologic tests are often central to the diagnosis of SLE. However, positive serologic studies also occur in patients with interstitial pulmonary disease who have no evidence of SLE or rheumatoid arthritis. For example, the incidence of positive antinuclear antibodies and/or rheumatoid factor tests is high in unexplained pulmonary fibrosis and pneumoconiosis. In neither of these instances is there clinical evidence for collagen-vascular disease. Instead, the serologic findings appear to be nonspecific responses to stimuli that are not understood.

Pleuropulmonary disorders are frequently encountered in SLE, and they occur at some time during the disease course in many patients. However, extrapulmonary disorders such as uremia may also be manifested in the chest and must be considered in differential diagnosis. In addition, infection is common in SLE. Thus, pulmonary or pleural abnormalities are often infectious in origin rather than a consequence of the collagen-vascular disease per se.

Pleurisy

The most common pleuropulmonary abnormality in SLE is pleurisy. At least one-third of patients have pleurisy with or without effusion at sometime during the course of their disease, and it is the presenting manifestation in approximately 5 percent. The most common symptom is chest pain, which is present in almost all patients with lupus pleurisy. Other common symptoms are cough and dyspnea. A pleural friction rub and fever are found in most patients. In contrast, chest pain and fever in rheumatoid effusions are unusual. Effusions are most often small and bilateral, but unilateral or massive effusions are not uncommon. Characteristically, pleural fluid is a clear yellow exudate, but it may be turbid or frankly hemorrhagic. Cell counts are typically low, and either polymorphonuclear neutrophilic leukocytes (PMNs) or mononuclear cells can predominate, depending on the timing in relation to the onset of pleurisy. The concentration of glucose in pleural fluid and the pH are usually not depressed, and the lactic dehydrogenase (LDH) is generally below 500 UL; these chemistries can be useful in distinguishing the effusions of SLE from rheumatoid effusions. The components of complement are characteristically decreased. A pleural fluid ANA titer either higher than the serum titer or greater than 1:160 is helpful diagnostically, as is the presence of LE cells. LE cells are more commonly seen when the fluid is allowed to stand for several hours before examination. Pleural biopsy is not usually helpful unless the specimen is examined for immunofluorescence.

Before considering treatment of the pleural effusion, it is important to rule out infection or causes of effusion other than SLE. Small or asymptomatic effusions generally do not need treatment. But, if deemed necessary, effusions usually respond promptly to large doses of corticosteroids; after they clear, the corticosteroids are tapered rapidly.

Drug-induced SLE characteristically presents with arthritis and serositis; pleurisy is a common feature.

Alveolar Hemorrhage

Alveolar hemorrage is a rare but often fatal form of lung disease in SLE. Occasionally it is the initial manifestation of SLE. Patients present with the sudden onset of cough, dyspnea, rales, and fever. Hemoptysis generally occurs soon afterward, although it may not despite massive intra-alveolar hemorrhage. The diagnosis may then be supported by finding hemosiderin-laden macrophages in the sputum or lavage fluid. Also, the diffusing capacity in alveolar hemorrhage is sometimes markedly increased, since the intra-alveolar red blood cells act as a sump for carbon monoxide. However, an open lung biopsy is sometimes required to establish the diagnosis. The chest radiograph typically shows bilateral fluffy or reticulonodular infiltrates, and the hematocrit may fall because of the sequestration of blood in the lungs. Other features of active SLE are usually present, such as arthritis, fever, hypocomplementemia, and glomerulonephritis. Most patients are treated with corticosteroids, and some with cytotoxic agents or plasmapheresis as well. Despite treatment, mortality is high, i.e., about 70 percent.

The pathogenesis of this disorder is not clear. Massive intra-alveolar hemorrhage is the principal histologic feature; vasculitis and septal necrosis are generally not seen. Factors that might predispose to hemorrhage, such as uremia, thrombocytopenia, or infection, have been present in only few patients. Immunofluorescent microscopy often reveals granular deposits of IgG and complement components in the alveolar septa. Although this pattern does indicate that immune complexes have been deposited, it does not prove that the immune complexes play a pathogenetic role.

Pneumonitis

Acute lupus pneumonitis is a serious disorder characterized by tachypnea, dyspnea, cyanosis, high fever, and tachycardia without evidence of sepsis. The chest radiograph shows patterns of diffuse alveolar consolidation (Fig. 43-9), with a predilection for the lung bases. Effusions may be present. Because the presentation is nonspecific, other entities such as chest infections and cardiogenic or noncardiogenic pulmonary edema must be ruled out.

The acute pneumonitis usually responds to high dose corticosteroids or to a combination of a cytotoxic drug with steroids. However, some patients succumb from respiratory failure despite treatment; other deaths are due to infections or other complications. Histopathology reveals acute alveolar damage with hyaline membranes and interstitial edema with a mononuclear cell infiltration. Granular deposits of IgG, C3, and DNA have been demonstrated by immunofluorescence, and anti-DNA antibody has been eluted from pathologic specimens. The case for immune complexes playing a pathogenetic role in lupus pneumonitis is much stronger than that for alveolar hemorrhage.

It is unclear whether acute pneumonitis represents an intermediate form of lung injury between acute massive hemorrhage and chronic interstitial lung disease. Hemoptysis of small amounts of blood has been reported in patients with the typical histopathology of acute pneumonitis. Conversely, survivors of acute pneumonitis may be left with residual infiltration on chest radiograph and a restrictive defect on pulmonary function testing.

Interstitial Lung Disease

Chronic diffuse interstitial lung disease is an uncommon finding in SLE, from 0 to 4 percent. Clinical features such as dyspnea on exertion, basilar rales, and a basilar reticulonodular radiographic pattern (Fig. 43-9) are typical of interstitial lung disease in general. The pathologic findings are also nonspecific (see Chapter 49). Occasionally, the interstitial lung disease progresses rapidly.

In contrast to the rarity of radiographic evidence of interstitial lung disease, approximately 50 percent of patients upon physiological testing show a low diffusing capacity and a pattern of restrictive lung disease. However, these physiological findings are probably related to extrapulmonary dysfunction, such as respiratory muscle weakness, rather than to interstitial lung disease per se.

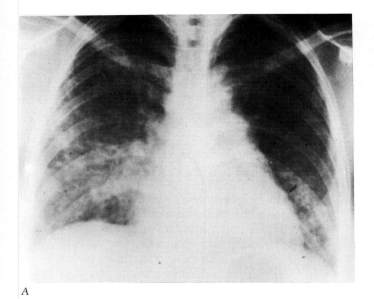

A

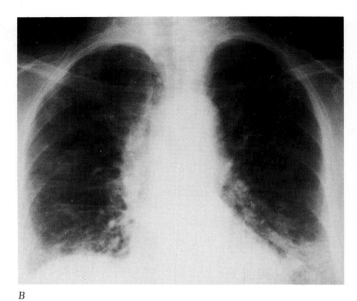

B

C

FIGURE 43-9 Lupus erythematosus. *A.* Acute bilateral pneumonitis. *B.* Chronic diffuse interstitial lung disease. *C.* Elevation of diaphragm and atelectasis ("shrinking lung").

Diaphragmatic Weakness

Impairment of ventilation due to ventilatory muscle weakness is well-described in PM-DM. It also occurs occasionally in other collagen-vascular diseases. However, until recently it was not appreciated that diaphragmatic weakness in SLE is relatively common. In retrospect, the common findings of "shrinking lungs," a radiographically elevated diaphragm, and unexplained basilar atelectasis noted in earlier reports can be largely attributed to diaphragmatic weakness (Fig. 43-9).

Muscle involvement in SLE appears to have a predilection for the ventilatory muscles because significant ventilatory impairment occurs without overt weakness of the extremities. Almost half of unselected outpatients with SLE have a restrictive defect on routine pulmonary function testing. More extensive evaluation reveals reduced inspiratory and expiratory pressures with reduced transdiaphragmatic pressure. Patients are typically more dyspneic when recumbent. Histopathology of the diaphragm reveals muscle atrophy and fibrosis with scant inflammation. The response to corticosteroids is often favorable.

Miscellaneous

Several other disorders rarely reported in SLE are also common to other collagen-vascular diseases. Pulmonary hypertension which is clinically and histopathologically indistinguishable from primary pulmonary hypertension occurs in a small number of patients with SLE (Fig. 43-10). The symptoms of pulmonary hypertension generally occur within a few years after the clinical presentation of SLE, but occasionally precede it. Raynaud's phenomenon

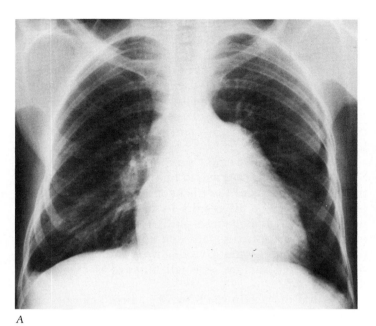

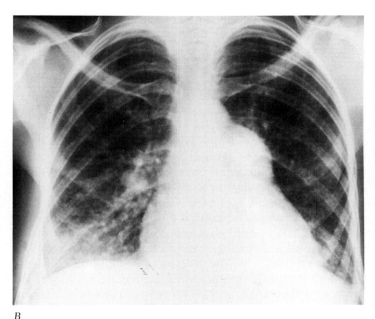

A   B

FIGURE 43-10 Pulmonary hypertension in lupus erythematosus. A 33-year-old woman with the clinical diagnosis of primary pulmonary hypertension and positive serologies for SLE. At autopsy the findings were those of collagen-vascular disease, consistent with SLE. *A.* 1975. Cardiomegaly, prominent central pulmonary arteries and diminished peripheral pulmonary vascular markings. Blunting of right costophrenic angle. *B.* 1978. In the interim, developed bilateral pleural effusions, persistent hyperproteinemia, and positive antinuclear antibodies. Cardiomegaly is increased, and bibasilar infiltrates are present in conjunction with right pleural effusion.

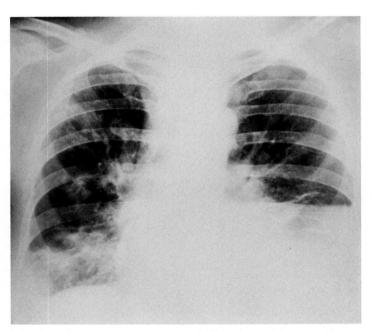

FIGURE 43-11 Sjögren's syndrome. Diffuse interstitial lung disease and pleural involvement. There was no underlying collagen disease.

is usually present, and immune complexes have been found in the walls of pulmonary arteries. Occasionally the pulmonary hypertension responds to corticosteroids.

Lymphocytic interstitial pneumonia, which is most commonly associated with Sjögren's syndrome, is occasionally seen in SLE. Some evidence of obliterative bron-

chiolitis can be found in almost any collagen-vascular disease, and there are occasional reports in SLE. Laryngeal involvement which occurs primarily in rheumatoid arthritis can be seen in SLE, and the lesions include mucosal edema and ulceration, laryngitis, cricoarytenoid arthritis, and vocal cord paresis. These patients present clinically with hoarseness or pain and may progress to upper airways obstruction.

SJÖGREN'S SYNDROME

Sjögren's syndrome is a chronic inflammatory disorder of lacrimal and salivary glands characterized by keratoconjunctivitis sicca (dry eyes) and xerostomia (dry mouth). In over one-half of the cases, a collagen-vascular disease, particularly rheumatoid arthritis, systemic lupus erythematosus, progressive systemic sclerosis, or polymyositis is associated. The disorder is a systemic disease with important renal, hematologic, and immunologic features. Also, patients can develop pseudolymphoma or true lymphoma. Rheumatoid factor is present in 95 to 100 percent of patients even when there is no clinical evidence of rheumatoid arthritis; antinuclear antibodies occur in 70 percent. Antibodies to the nuclear antigens SS-A (Ro) and SS-B (La) occur much more commonly in patients with the sicca complex alone than in Sjögren's syndrome associated with rheumatoid arthritis.

Interstitial lung disease may be detected radiographically (Fig. 43-11) in approximately 4 percent of patients

661

with Sjögren's syndrome, including both primary Sjögren's syndrome and Sjögren's syndrome associated with collagen-vascular diseases. Physiological studies of small patient populations have revealed a restrictive pattern with a reduced diffusing capacity in a large proportion of patients. Clinically and pathologically, this disorder resembles idiopathic pulmonary fibrosis.

A more distinctive type of interstitial infiltration occurs in Sjögren's syndrome with the spectrum of infiltrative lymphocytic disorders. Lymphocytic interstitial pneumonia, pseudolymphoma, and malignant lymphoma are all rare disorders that have an increased incidence in Sjögren's syndrome. *Lymphocytic interstitial pneumonia* resembles typical interstitial lung disease clinically, radiographically, and physiologically. However, the lesion is found histologically to be composed almost exclusively of lymphocytes and plasma cells; amyloid may also be found. Pseudolymphoma presents a more nodular radiographic appearance, and air bronchograms are characteristic; the lesions are composed of mature lymphocytes with true germinal centers, but the lymph nodes are free of lymphoma. Both of these nonmalignant disorders have been treated with corticosteroids and immunosuppressive drugs but their efficacy is uncertain since the natural history of the untreated diseases is not well known. Malignant lymphomas in the course of Sjögren's syndrome are usually poorly differentiated. Malignancy should be suspected when nodules are not associated with diffuse infiltration. The involvement of lymph nodes by malignant cells is helpful in distinguishing malignant lymphoma from pseudolymphoma.

Other characteristic pulmonary complaints of Sjögren's syndrome are due to lymphocytic infiltration of the mucous glands of the tracheobronchial tree. Atrophy of the mucous glands results in inspissated secretions, persistent cough, atelectasis, and an increased incidence of infection. Approximately one-third of patients complain of a troublesome dry cough; physiological studies reveal that obstruction of small airways is common in these patients.

Pleural disease in the form of pleuritic chest pain or pleural effusion occurs rarely; the pleural effusions have not been well characterized.

BIBLIOGRAPHY

General

Hunninghake GW, Fauci AS: Pulmonary involvement in collagen-vascular diseases. Am Rev Respir Dis 119:471–503, 1979.
  Comprehensive general review.

Light RW: Pleural disease in collagen-vascular disease, in Light RW (ed), *Pleural Diseases.* Philadelphia, Lea and Febiger, 1983, pp 163–171.
  An excellent source for pleural involvement in collagen-vascular diseases.

Wallaert B, Hatron PY, Grosbois JM, Tonnel AB, Devulder B, Voisin C: Subclinical pulmonary involvement in collagen-vascular diseases assessed by bronchoalveolar lavage. Relationship between alveolitis and subsequent changes in lung function. Am Rev Respir Dis 133:574–580, 1986.
  Subclinical pulmonary involvement in collagen vascular disease was assessed by bronchoalveolar lavage (BAL) in 61 patients free of clinical pulmonary symptoms and who had normal chest radiographs. Abnormal differential count of BAL cells was noted in 29 of 61 patients (48%).

Rheumatoid Arthritis

Benedek TG: Rheumatoid pneumoconiosis: Documentation of onset and pathologic considerations. Am J Med 55:515–524, 1973.
  Review of three cases with good longitudinal data, as well as literature review.

Caplan A: Certain unusual radiologic appearances in the chest of coal miners suffering from rheumatoid arthritis. Thorax 8:29–37, 1953.
  Original description of rheumatoid pneumoconiosis.

De Horatius RJ, Abruzzo JL, Williams RC: Immunofluorescent and immunologic studies of rheumatoid lung. Arch Intern Med 129:441–446, 1972.
  Immunopathologic study with some clinical data.

Frank ST, Weg JG, Harkleroad LE, Fitch RF: Pulmonary dysfunction in rheumatoid disease. Chest 63:27–34, 1973.
  Clinical, physiological, and radiographic series, including histopathology. Although the unusually high prevalence of abnormalities suggests patient selection, correlations can be made among these parameters.

Geddes DM, Corrin B, Brewerton DA, Davies RJ, Turner-Warwick M: Progressive airway obliteration in adults and its association with rheumatoid disease. Quart J Med 46:427–444, 1977.
   *Pioneering and detailed report of a series of rheumatoid arthritis patients with obliterative bron-
   chiolitis.*

Jurik AG, Davidsen D, Grandal H: Prevalence of pulmonary involvement in rheumatoid arthritis
and its relationship to some characteristics of the patients. Scand J Rheumatol 11:217–224, 1982.
   Large series which includes relationship between radiographic findings and clinical features.

Payne CR: Pulmonary manifestations of rheumatoid arthritis. Br J Hosp Med 32:192–197, 1984.
   Well-referenced and comprehensive review.

Pratt DS, Schwartz MI, May JJ, Dreisen RB: Rapidly fatal pulmonary fibrosis: The accelerated variant of interstitial pneumonitis. Thorax 34:587–593, 1979.
   *Useful recent look at the Hamman-Rich syndrome, with relevance to SLE and rheumatoid arthri-
   tis.*

Roschmann RA, Rothenberg RJ: Pulmonary fibrosis in rheumatoid arthritis: A review of clinical
features and therapy. Semin Arthritis Rheum 16:174–185, 1987.
   *Review of subject with discussion of therapy and selected cases that emphasize some complexi-
   ties of this manifestation.*

Sahn SA: Immunologic diseases of the pleura. Clin Chest Med 6:83–102, 1985.
   An excellent review of pleural involvement in collagen-vascular diseases.

Sassoon CS, McAlpine SW, Tashkin, DP, Baydur A, Quismorio FP, Mongan ES: Small airways
function in nonsmokers with rheumatoid arthritis. Arthritis Rheum 27:1218–1226, 1984.
   *Physiological study of a nonsmoking population of rheumatoid arthritis patients showing no
   increase in indices of small airways obstruction.*

Scott DL, Brady GVH, Aitman TJ, Zaphiropoulos GC, Hawkins CF: Relationship of gold and penicillamine therapy to diffuse interstitial lung disease. Ann Rheum Dis 40:136–141, 1981.
   *Good description of the clinical features of drug-induced pulmonary disease caused by specific
   rheumatoid arthritis disease-modifying agents.*

Scott TE, Wise RA, Hochberg MC, Wigley FM: HLA-DR4 and pulmonary dysfunction in rheumatoid arthritis. Am J Med 82:765–771, 1987.
   *An association between HLA-DR4 and obstructive lung disease in patients with rheumatoid
   arthritis.*

Walker WC, Wright V: Diffuse interstitial pulmonary fibrosis and rheumatoid arthritis. Ann Rheum
Dis 28:252–259, 1969.
   Early but large and useful clinical series.

Ankylosing Spondylitis

Grimby G, Fugl-Meyer AR, Blomstrand A: Partitioning of the contribution of rib cage and abdomen
to ventilation in ankylosing spondylitis. Thorax 29:179–184, 1974.
   *Pulmonary physiology in ankylosing spondylitis including analysis of individual muscle
   groups.*

Rosenow EC III, Strimlan CV, Muhm JR, Ferguson RH: Pleuropulmonary manifestations of ankylosing spondylitis. Mayo Clin Proc 52:641–649, 1977.
   Most comprehensive clinical series available with a useful literature review as well.

Systemic Sclerosis

Chausow AM, Kane T, Levinson D, Szidon JP: Reversible hypercapnic respiratory insufficiency in
scleroderma caused by respiratory muscle weakness. Am Rev Respir Dis 130:142–144, 1984.
   Initial report of reversible ventilatory failure in scleroderma.

Greenwald GI, Tashkin DP, Gong H, Simmons M, Duann S, Furst DE, Clements P: Longitudinal
changes in lung function and respiratory symptoms in progressive systemic sclerosis. Prospective
study. Am J Med 83:83–92, 1987.
   *In 61 patients with PSS, the progression of PSS-related lung disease was slow, with substantial
   individual variability.*

Owens GR, Fino GJ, Herbert DL, Steen VD, Medsger TA, Pennock BE, Cottrell JJ, Rodnan GP, Rogers
RM: Pulmonary function in progressive systemic sclerosis. Comparison of CREST syndrome vari-
ant with diffuse scleroderma. Chest 84:546–550, 1983.
   Good study of pulmonary function in the major subgroups of systemic sclerosis.

Owens GR, Paradis IL, Gryzan S, Medsger TA, Follenbee WP, Klein HA, Dauber JH: Role of inflammation in the lung disease of systemic sclerosis: Comparison with idiopathic pulmonary fibrosis. J Lab Clin Med 107:253–260, 1986.
  Interesting study that finds pulmonary inflammation in patients with systemic sclerosis and lung involvement that differs from idiopathic pulmonary fibrosis.

Peters-Golden M, Wise RA, Hochberg MC, Stevens MB, Wigley FM: Carbon monoxide diffusing capacity as predictor of outcome in systemic sclerosis. Am J Med 77:1027–1034, 1984.
  Interesting study of a single laboratory parameter of lung disease used as a predictor of outcome in systemic sclerosis.

Peters-Golden M, Wise RA, Schneider P, Hochberg M, Stevens MB, Wigley F: Clinical and demographic predictors of loss of pulmonary function in systemic sclerosis. Medicine 63:221–231, 1984.
  Fine longitudinal study of pulmonary functional tests (PFTs) in systemic sclerosis patients.

Shuck JW, Oetgen WJ, Tasar JT: Pulmonary vascular response during Raynaud's phenomenon in progressive systemic sclerosis. Am J Med 78:221–227, 1985.
  Interesting study which examines the relationship between peripheral Raynaud's phenomenon and pulmonary vascular responses in systemic sclerosis.

Steen VD, Owens GR, Redmond C, Rodnan GP, Medsger TA: The effect of D-pencillamine on pulmonary findings in systemic sclerosis. Arthritis Rheum 28:882–888, 1985.
  The use of D-penicillamine in a large group of scleroderma patients resulted in improvement in diffusing capacity and stabilization of symptoms compared with an untreated group.

Steen VD, Siegler GL, Rodnan GP, Medsger TA: Clinical and laboratory associations of anticentromere antibody in patients with progressive systemic sclerosis. Arthritis Rheum 27:125–131, 1984.
  Study confirming the decreased prevalence of interstitial lung disease in CREST compared to diffuse scleroderma and the correlation with anticentromere antibody.

Stupi AM, Steen VD, Owens GR, Barnes EL, Rodnan GP, Medsger TA Jr: Pulmonary hypertension in the CREST syndrome variant of systemic sclerosis. Arthritis Rheum 29:515–524, 1986.
  Pulmonary hypertension (PHT) occurred in 59 (9%) of 673 systemic sclerosis patients with the CREST syndrome (calcinosis, Raynaud's phenomenon, esophageal dysmotility, sclerodactyly, telangiectasias).

Sullivan WD, Hurst DJ, Harmon CE, Esther JH, Agia GA, Maltby JD, Lillard SB, Held CN, Wolfe JF, Sunderrajan EV, Maricq HR, Sharp GC: A prospective evaluation emphasizing pulmonary involvement in patients with mixed connective tissue disease. Medicine 63:92–107, 1984.
  Study focusing on pulmonary involvement in mixed connective tissue disease.

Taormina VJ, Miller WT, Gefter WB, Epstein DM: Progessive systemic sclerosis subgroups: Variable pulmonary features. Am J Roentgen 137:277–285, 1981.
  Radiologic study of pulmonary disease in systemic sclerosis based on clinical subgroups.

Ungerer RG, Tashkin DP, Furst D, Clements PJ, Gong H, Bein M, Roberts N, Cabeen W: Prevalance and clinical correlates of pulmonary arterial hypertension in progressive systemic sclerosis. Am J Med 75:65–73, 1983.
  Good study which explores the correlation between catheterization-documented pulmonary hypertension in systemic sclerosis and various noninvasive studies.

Young RH, Mark GJ: Pulmonary vascular changes in scleroderma. Am J Med 64:998–1004, 1978.
  Good pathologic study of pulmonary vasculopathy in systemic sclerosis.

Polymyositis and Dermatomyositis

Braun NM, Aurora NS, Rochester DF: Respiratory muscle and pulmonary function in polymyositis and other proximal myopathies. Thorax 38:616–623, 1983.
  Fine study of ventilatory function in a large group of patients with PM-DM.

Dickey BF, Myers AR: Pulmonary disease in polymyositis/dermatomyositis. Semin Arthritis Rheum 14:60–76, 1984.
  Retrospective analysis of a large series examining all types of lung disease in PM-DM with review of the literature.

Duncan PE, Griffin JP, Garcia A: Fibrosis alveolitis in polymyositis: A review of histologically confirmed cases. Am J Med 57:621–626, 1974.
  Good pathologic and clinical study of interstitial lung disease in PM-DM.

Frazier AR, Miller RE: Interstitial pneumonitis in association with polymyositis and dermatomyositis. Chest 65:403–407, 1974.
  Large clinical series with much useful data.

Lakhanpal S, Lie JT, Conn DL, Martin WJ II: Pulmonary disease in polymyositis/dermatomyositis: a clinicopathological analysis of 65 autopsy cases. Ann Rheum Dis 46:23–29, 1987.
  A review of the clinical and autopsy records of 65 patients with either polymyositis (24) or dermatomyositis (41) and pulmonary disease.

Schumacher HR, Schimmer B, Gordon GV: Articular manifestations of polymyositis and dermatomyositis. Am J Med 67:287–292, 1979.
  Study establishing association between arthritis and interstitial lung disease in PM-DM.

Schwartz MI, Matthay RA, Sahn SA: Interstitial lung disease in polymyositis and dermatomyositis: Analysis of six cases and review of the literature. Medicine 55:89–104, 1976.
  Good study of interstitial lung disease in PM-DM.

Yoshida S, Akizuki M, Mimori T: The precipitating antibody to an acidic nuclear protein antigen, the Jo-1, in connective tissue disease: A marker for a subset of polymyositis with interstitial pulmonary fibrosis. Arthritis Rheum 26:604–611, 1983.
  Explores association between Jo-1 antibody and interstitial lung disease in PM-DM.

Systemic Lupus Erythematosus

Asherson RA, Hackett D, Gharavi AE, Harris EN, Kennedy HG, Hughes GR: Pulmonary hypertension in systemic lupus erythematosus: a report of three cases. J Rheumatol 13:416–420, 1986.
  Three women with systemic lupus erythematosus (SLE) developed pulmonary hypertension as a terminal feature of their illness.

Carette S, Macher AM, Nussbaum A, Plotz PH: Severe, acute pulmonary disease in patients with systemic lupus erythematosus: Ten years experience at the National Institutes of Health. Semin Arthritis Rheum 14:52–59, 1984.
  Illustrates the importance of considering diagnoses other than acute lupus pneumonitis in patients with that clinical picture.

Eagan JW, Memoli VA, Roberts JL, Mathew GR, Schwartz MM, Lewis EJ: Pulmonary hemorrhage in systemic lupus erythematosus. Medicine 57:545–560, 1978.
  Report of four cases with an excellent review of the literature.

Eisenberg H, Dubois EL, Sherwin RP, Balchum OJ: Diffuse interstitial lung disease in systemic lupus erythematosus. Ann Intern Med 79:37–45, 1973.
  The most comprehensive study of chronic interstitial lung disease in SLE.

Gibson GJ, Edmonds JP, Hughes GR: Diaphragm function and lung involvement in systemic lupus erythematosus. Am J Med 63:926–932, 1977.
  Excellent study which establishes the link between commonly noted pulmonary dysfunction in SLE and diaphragmatic dysfunction.

Halla JT, Schrohenloher RE, Volankis JE: Immune complexes and other laboratory features of pleural effusions: A comparison of rheumatoid arthritis, systemic lupus erythematosus, and other diseases. Ann Intern Med 92:745–752, 1980.
  Some clinical as well as laboratory features of pleurisy in SLE and rheumatoid arthritis.

Inoue T, Kanayama T, Ohe A, Kato N, Horiguchi T, Ishii M, Shiota K: Immunopathologic studies of pneumonitis in systemic lupus erythematosus. Ann Intern Med 91:30–34, 1979.
  Pathologic study of pulmonary immune complex deposition.

Matthay RA, Schwarz MI, Petty TL, Stanford RE, Gupta RC, Sahn SA, Steigerwald JC: Pulmonary manifestations of systemic lupus erythematosus: Review of twelve cases of acute lupus pneumonitis. Medicine 54:397–409, 1974.
  Series of acute lupus pneumonitis describing clinical features, response to treatment, and prognosis.

Nadorra RL, Landing BH: Pulmonary lesions in childhood onset systemic lupus erythematosus: analysis of 26 cases, and summary of literature. Pediatr Pathol 7:1–18, 1987.
  In 26 patients (21 female, 5 male) with systemic lupus erythematosus, autopsy revealed systemic lupus erythematosus. Chronic interstitial pneumonitis in all, acute pneumonia in 20, and alveolar hemorrhage in 18.

Quismorio FP, Sharma O, Kors M, Boylen T, Edmiston AW, Thornton PJ, Tatter D: Immunopathologic and clinical studies in pulmonary hypertension associated with systemic lupus erythematosus. Semin Arthritis Rheum 13:349–359, 1984.
  Demonstration of immune complexes in the pulmonary arteries of two patients with lethal pulmonary hypertension and SLE. Extensive literature review emphasizes clinical features, treatment, and prognosis.

Rubin LA, Urowitz MB: Shrinking lung syndrome in SLE—A clinical pathologic study. J Rheumatol 10:973–976, 1983.

Case study with correlations between clinical, radiographic, functional, and pathologic findings.

Segal AM, Calabrese LH, Ahmed M, Tubbs RR, White CS: The pulmonary manifestations of systemic lupus erythematosus. Semin Arthritis Rheum 14:202–224, 1985.

Review of subject with selected case reports exemplifying the major manifestations.

Turner-Stokes L, Turner-Warwick M: Intrathoracic manifestations of systemic lupus erythematosus. Clin Rheum Dis 8:229–241, 1983.

Useful basic information on this topic.

Wallaert B, Aerts C, Bart F, Hatron PY, Dracon M, Tonnel AB, Voisin C: Alveolar macrophage dysfunction in systemic lupus erythematosus. Am Rev Respir Dis 136:293–297, 1987.

Alteration of antibacterial activity of alveolar macrophages may contribute to the increased susceptibility to lung infections observed in SLE.

Sjögren's Syndrome

Constantopoulos SH, Drosos AA, Maddison PJ, Moutsopoulos HM: Xerotrachea and interstitial lung disease in primary Sjögren's syndrome. Respiration 46:310–314, 1984.

Useful study of respiratory tract dryness and pulmonary function in Sjögren's patients.

Constantopoulos SH, Moutsopoulos HM: Respiratory involvement in patients with Sjögren's syndrome: is it a problem? Scand J Rheumatol (Suppl) 61:146–150, 1986.

A comprehensive study of the pulmonary involvement in 40 patients with primary Sjögren's syndrome and 26 patients with secondary SS.

Kamholz S, Sher A, Barland P, Rosen N, Rakoff S, Becker N: Sjögren's syndrome: severe upper airways obstruction due to primary malignant tracheal lymphoma developing during successful treatment of lymphocytic interstitial pneumonitis. J Rheumatol 14:588–594, 1987.

After dramatic radiographic improvement of the lymphocytic interstitial pneumonitis occurred during 14 months of corticosteroid therapy, a rare primary malignant lymphoma of the trachea developed.

Segal I, Fink G, Machtey I, Gura V, Spitzer SA: Pulmonary function abnormalities in Sjögren's syndrome and the sicca complex. Thorax 36:286–289, 1981.

Good study of pulmonary function in patients with Sjögren's syndrome.

Strimlan CV, Rosenow EC III, Divertie MB, Harrison EG: Pulmonary manifestations of Sjögren's syndrome. Chest 70:354–361, 1976.

Large clinical series with much useful information.

Chapter 44

Hypersensitivity Pneumonitis (Extrinsic Allergic Alveolitis)

Hal B. Richerson

Etiology

Pathology

Pathogenesis

Clinical Features
    Environmental History
    Clinical Presentation

Diagnosis

Differential Diagnosis

Prevention and Management
    Prevention
    Management

Hypersensitivity pneumonitis is an immunologically mediated inflammation of the pulmonary parenchyma, involving alveolar walls and terminal airways, secondary to the repeated inhalation of sensitizing agents including organic dusts and simple chemicals. Histopathology typically reveals a granulomatous interstitial pneumonitis with occasional bronchiolitis obliterans. In early stages granulomata are prominent and fibrosis is mild. The clinical picture is that of an interstitial pneumonitis; the presentation may be acute, subacute, or chronic.

Farmer's lung is the prototype of this group of allergic interstitial lung diseases, and in the United States it afflicts primarily dairy farmers. An initial series of exposures to a causative agent produces sensitization in susceptible subjects who then develop clinical disease with continuing exposure. Inhalation of agricultural dusts has caused various respiratory symptoms recognized by physicians for centuries. Campbell in 1922 reported a group of five English farmers with progressive symptoms following work with moldy hay. His farmers were afflicted with a subacute form of the disease which progressed over several days or weeks to severe respiratory distress and cyanosis. Following removal from the environment the symptoms cleared over several weeks. Chest radiographs showed a fine generalized stippling "reminiscent of silicosis."

In 1962, Pepys, Riddell, Citron, and Clayton showed that precipitating antibodies against moldy hay extracts could be demonstrated in the sera of patients with farmer's lung and the next year attributed farmer's lung hay antigens to thermophilic actinomycetes. These findings were followed by descriptions of other examples of hypersensitivity pneumonitis developing in a variety of occupational and domestic environments and associated with serum precipitins to incriminated environmental antigens.

ETIOLOGY

Inhalational exposure to appropriate antigens is a necessary but insufficient condition for the development of hypersensitivity pneumonitis. The majority of individuals so exposed remain well, suggesting host factors that are as yet poorly understood.

Etiologic agents implicated in hypersensitivity pneumonitis are listed in part in Table 44-1. The most important of these are thermophilic actinomycetes, fungal antigens, and bird proteins. The usual sources of antigen, other than exotic environmental and occupational exposures, are "moldy" hay, silage, or grain; bird droppings; and heating, cooling, and humidification systems. Recent reports, however, indicate that etiologic agents are not limited to organic dusts; chemicals such as the isocyanates have also been implicated.

Farmer's lung, pigeon breeder's lung and bird fancier's lung are well documented, classic examples of hypersensitivity pneumonitis. Hypersensitivity pneumonitis secondary to forced-air humidification and air-conditioning systems is well established, but the etiologic agents responsible have often been elusive. Heating of the unit in such systems and delivery of aerosols or fog, rather than simple evaporation, appear to be important for dispersal of responsible agents.

Actinomycetes are gram-positive organisms whose filamentous, hyphalike appearance was responsible for their earlier, erroneous classification as fungi; they are in fact bacteria. Thermophilic actinomycetes are ubiquitous, saprophytic organisms which grow best in warm, moist, decaying organic matter. They are abundant in compost, soils, foods, and freshwater and have been isolated from the atmosphere. The most important species implicated in hypersensitivity pneumonitis include *Micropolyspora faeni*, *Thermoactinomyces vulgaris*, *T. viridis*, and *T. candidus*. The antigenic composition of the thermoactinomycetes is complex and includes polysaccharides and glycoproteins with various enzymatic activities. The immunologic and clinical significance of these constituents is not understood.

The special properties of antigens capable of causing hypersensitivity pneumonitis have not been elucidated.

TABLE 44-1
Hypersensitivity Pneumonitis (Extrinsic Allergic Alveolitis)

Disease	Antigen	Source of Particles	Reference
Farmer's lung	Thermophilic actinomycetes	Moldy hay, grain, silage	Rankin et al, Ann Intern Med 57:606, 1962
Bird fancier's, breeder's, or handler's lung	Parakeet, budgerigar, pigeon, chicken, turkey proteins	Avian droppings or feathers	Reed et al, JAMA 193:261, 1965
Humidifier or air-conditioner lung	Thermophilic actinomycetes, *Aureobasidium pullulans,* or other	Contaminated water in humidification and air-conditioning systems	Fink et al, Ann Intern Med 84:406, 1976
Bagassosis	Thermophilic actinomycetes	Moldy bagasse (sugar cane)	Salvaggio et al, Ann Intern Med 64:748, 1966
Malt worker's lung	*Aspergillus fumigatus* or *A. clavatus*	Moldy barley	Channel et al, QJ Med 38:351, 1969
Mushroom worker's lung	Thermophilic actinomycetes	Mushroom compost	Stewart, Thorax 29:252, 1974
Sequoiosis	*Pullularia, Graphium* species	Redwood sawdust	Cohen et al, Am J Med 43:785, 1967
Maple bark disease	Cryptostroma corticale	Maple bark	Emanuel et al, N Engl J Med 274:1413, 1966
Woodworker's lung	Wood dust; *Alternaria*	Oak, cedar, and mahogany dusts; pine and spruce pulp	Sosman et al, N Engl J Med 281:977, 1969
Cheese washer's lung	*Penicillium casei*	Moldy cheese	Schlueter, Ann Intern Med 78:606, 1973
Suberosis	Cork dust mold	Cork dust	Avila, Villar, Lancet 1:620, 1968
Sauna taker's lung	Unknown	Contaminated sauna water	Metzger et al, JAMA 236:2209, 1976
Pituitary snuff taker's lung	Animal proteins	Heterologous pituitary snuff	Harper et al, Ann Intern Med 73:581, 1970
Coffee worker's lung	Coffee bean dust	Coffee beans	Van Toorn, Thorax 25:399, 1970
Miller's lung	Infested wheat flour	*Sitophilus granarius* (wheat weevil)	Lunn, Hughes, Br J Industr Med 24:158, 1967
Fish meal worker's lung	Fish meal dust	Fish meal	Avila, Clin Allergy 1:343, 1971
Furrier's lung	Animal fur dust	Animal pelts	Pimental, Thorax 25:387, 1970
Lycoperdonosis	Puffball spores	*Lycoperdon* puffballs	Strand et al, N Engl J Med 277:89, 1967
Chemical worker's lung	Isocyanates	Polyurethane foam, varnishes, lacquer, foundry casting	Charles et al, Thorax 31:127, 1976

Immunogenicity and adjuvanticity are of undoubted importance, as is the dose delivered to the lung. A farmer working with moldy hay can inhale and retain in the lungs as many as 750,000 organic particles per minute of which 98 percent are actinomycetes.

PATHOLOGY

The pathology of farmer's lung is typically a granulomatous interstitial pneumonitis consisting of lymphocytes, macrophages, epithelioid cells, and a few giant cells and variable degrees of interstitial fibrosis (Figs. 44-1 and 44-2). The alveolar septa are swollen with numerous lymphocytes and some plasma cells together with a variety of mononuclear and histiocytic forms. Large histiocytes, in which the cytoplasm is foamy or finely vacuolated with lipid, are interspersed with chronic inflammatory cells or occur as compact clusters in alveolar spaces. Although the inflammatory infiltrate is predominantly confined to alveolar walls, similar cells are seen within alveolar spaces. Granulomas are characteristic of the acute stage, appearing within 3 weeks and slowly resolving over 12 months. They are less likely to be seen in the chronic form.

Obstructive lesions of the bronchi (bronchiolitis obliterans) are common (Fig. 44-3). These lesions are usually found in areas with confluent disease and are characterized by nodular fibroblastic masses with an admixture of

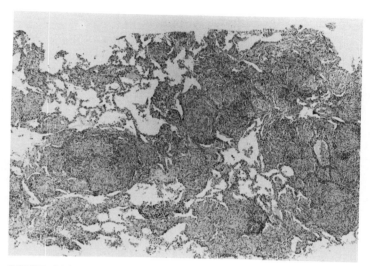

FIGURE 44-1 Granulomatous interstitial pneumonitis. Histologic section from a patient with farmer's lung. ×22.

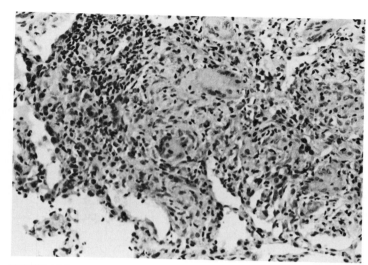

FIGURE 44-2 Hypersensitivity pneumonitis. Typical lesion containing histiocytes, giant cells, and lymphocytes that have formed small granulomas within alveolar septa. ×85.

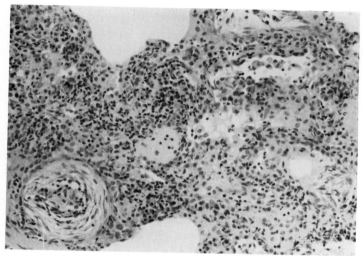

FIGURE 44-3 Bronchiolitis obliterans and interstitial pneumonitis in a patient with humidifier lung. ×85.

chronic inflammatory and histiocytic cells that project into, and sometimes occlude, the lumina of the bronchioles. Immunofluorescent studies of biopsy specimens have shown localized antigens in the walls of bronchioles; IgG, IgA, and IgM in plasma cells; lymphocytes widely scattered throughout the diseased lung; and great numbers of histiocytelike cells containing C3. Blood vessels were not involved. No convincing pathologic evidence has been presented for immune complexes in hypersensitivity pneumonitis.

Histopathology in 60 patients with farmer's lung biopsied during the active phase of their disease included an interstitial alveolar infiltrate consisting of plasma cells, lymphocytes, and occasional eosinophils in 100 percent and granulomata in 70 percent of the patients. Interstitial fibrosis was seen in 65 percent of the biopsy specimens but was unexpectedly mild; bronchiolitis was seen to some degree in 50 percent and foreign body material was demonstrable by polarized light in 60 percent of the patients. No vasculitis was observed in any case. Differentiation of the histopathology of farmer's lung from infectious fungus disease requires careful search for fungal elements. Certain histopathologic features typically differentiate sarcoidosis and farmer's lung. In sarcoidosis, granulomas are found not only in the submucosa of larger bronchi and in interstitial tissues, but also in perivascular and intramural areas of blood vessels. A variable infiltration of lymphocytes and plasma cells involving the pulmonary parenchyma at sites distant from granulomas is present in farmer's lung, whereas such infiltrates are found only in and around granulomata in sarcoidosis.

In other forms of hypersensitivity pneumonitis, the pathologic changes resemble those of farmer's lung. They, too, are characterized by a diffuse lymphohistiocytic interstitial infiltrate consisting of occasional small, often poorly formed granulomas and prominent collections of foamy histiocytes. Accordingly, the various entities cannot be distinguished on a morphologic basis alone.

PATHOGENESIS

Early reports of hypersensitivity pneumonitis postulated that the disease was infectious or resulted from the toxic properties of the inhaled organic dusts. The finding of precipitating antibodies to moldy hay in farmers afflicted with farmer's lung suggested a role for antibody in pathogenesis, and a type III (antigen-antibody complex-mediated or Arthus') hypersensitivity reaction based on the classification of allergic reactions by Gell and Coombs was postulated. Subsequent studies have indicated the importance of cell-mediated (delayed) hypersensitivity (type IV). It must be recognized that hypersensitivity mechanisms are quite complicated and that the classification of Gell and Coombs is an oversimplification; interreacting humoral and cellular responses are typical of most hypersensitivity reactions of whatever classic type as originally defined. The prime importance of T-cell and macrophage-mediated inflammation in hypersensitivity pneumonitis, however, is indicated by histopathology, animal models, and in vitro correlates in humans. There is no direct evidence to support contributions by precipitins, complement, or genetic host factors in the pathogenesis of hypersensitivity pneumonitis, nor are there studies as yet of cellular cytotoxicity contributions. Cellular and antibody interactions may lead to immunosuppressive processes modulating inflammatory responses and preventing disease despite immunogenesis.

CLINICAL FEATURES

Environmental History

Occupational exposure is unique and specific for many of the forms of hypersensitivity pneumonitis, and it is reflected in picturesque names. At times, however, the exposure is subtle and difficult to elicit and requires particular alertness and environmental investigation on the part of the physician. The diagnosis should be suspected in all cases of recurrent pneumonia or unexplained interstitial lung disease.

Farmer's lung is most apt to occur in farming operations requiring heavy exposure to warm, moist, stored hay within a confined area. Dairy farming is particularly well suited to the growing of thermophilic actinomycetes in hay and silage used to feed cows inside warm barns. Many other farming operations are more open, the hay is drier, and the farmer is less exposed. Thus, geographic location and specialized farming operations are of great importance in determining the incidence of this disease.

Many types of hypersensitivity pneumonitis potentially affect only very small occupational groups (malt workers, maple bark strippers, mushroom workers, cheese washers, coffee workers, redwood sawyers, bagasse workers, pigeon breeders) and can often be minimized by awareness of the problem and occupational hygiene. The more subtle forms include bird breeder's lung and humidifier's lung, where routine history taking often fails to provide key information.

Clinical Presentation

The clinical presentation may be acute, subacute, or chronic, depending on frequency, intensity, and duration of inhalational exposure and perhaps on host or other factors determining immunopathogenesis. Both systemic and respiratory symptoms may occur. In the *acute form*, influenzalike symptoms often predominate, consisting of chills, fever, sweating, myalgias, lassitude, headache, and nausea which come on 2 to 3 h after exposure, peak typically between 6 and 24 h, and last from hours to days. Respiratory symptoms such as cough and dyspnea are common but not universal. The *subacute form* may appear gradually over several days to weeks, is marked by cough and dyspnea, and may progress to severe dyspnea with cyanosis leading to urgent hospitalization. The *chronic form* has an insidious onset over a period of months with increasing cough and exertional dyspnea. Fatigue and weight loss may be prominent complaints.

Physical examination may be within normal limits or may disclose bibasilar or more generalized crepitant inspiratory rales in any of the forms of presentation. Fever is common after acute exposure. Cyanosis may be seen in severe disease. Clubbing is not expected.

Laboratory studies are nonspecific except for certain precipitins described below. A mild leukocytosis without eosinophilia is often present in acute cases. The erythrocyte sedimentation rate is either normal or slightly increased. Sometimes the rheumatoid factor is transiently positive, and immunoglobulins are mildly increased. Antinuclear antibodies are uncommon.

The *chest radiograph* may be normal, even in symptomatic patients. The acute phase is associated with small nodulation that is poorly defined, uniform, and rather discrete and symmetrically spares the apexes or the bases (Fig. 44-4*A* and *B*). Sometimes a diffuse, soft, stringy, or patchy interstitial infiltrate occurs, with or without nodulation (Fig. 44-5). In the chronic, fibrotic phase the linear element becomes more distinct, and the periphery is more prominently involved. As the disease progresses, a decrease in the air volume of the lungs accentuates the above changes. Certain abnormalities are rarely, if ever, seen in hypersensitivity pneumonitis. Among these are pleural effusion or thickening, hilar adenopathy, calcification, cavitation, atelectasis, and coin lesions.

DIAGNOSIS

A history of exposure to moldy hay, birds, or other occupational or environmental antigen in a patient with clinical and radiologic features suggestive of hypersensitivity pneumonitis should prompt an examination for serum precipitins to the suspected antigen in order to help establish the diagnosis. Exposure history is more difficult to

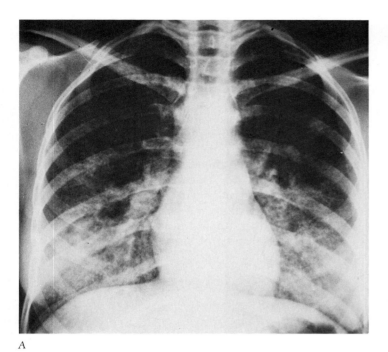
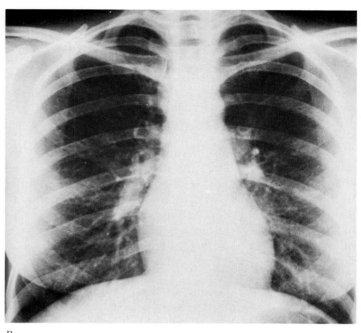

A   *B*

FIGURE 44-4 Chest radiographs taken during and following recovery from recurrent acute episodes of hypersensitivity pneumonitis. The patient is an 18-year-old female tourist guide. Her brother kept pet doves; precipitins to dove plasma were found in the patient's serum, and no further bouts occurred after the doves were removed from the home. *A.* On admission. Cough and shortness of breath. *B.* Five weeks later, when symptoms were absent. A predominantly alveolar pattern is present, symmetrically involving the lower lung fields and sparing the apexes.

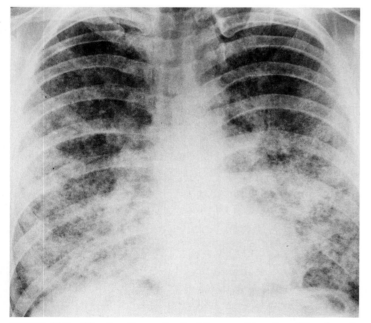

FIGURE 44-5 Chest radiograph of a 37-year-old male with subacute farmer's lung, who developed a nonproductive cough and progressive exertional dyspnea 2 weeks prior to hospitalization. Diffuse alveolar and interstitial infiltrates are present bilaterally. There are no pleural effusions or hilar adenopathy.

elicit in domestic situations including humidification and air-conditioning systems. A careful environmental history is essential. Indeed, at times, the physician must inspect the patient's environment personally.

The attempted demonstration of *precipitating antibodies* (precipitins) against suspected antigens is an important part of the diagnostic work-up. If found, precipitins indicate sufficient exposure to the causative agent to generate an immunologic response. Although at one time considered important in disease pathogenesis, precipitins are currently considered to be markers of exposure to an antigen source. Precipitins are not demonstrable in all patients, and available antigens are not standardized. False-negative results may occur because of poor antigens or the wrong choice of antigens. Extraction of antigens from the patient's environment may at times be helpful. False-positive precipitin reactions are quite common and must be interpreted with careful clinical correlations.

Many centers are using fiberoptic bronchoscopy and *bronchoalveolar lavage* to aid in diagnostic evaluation of interstitial lung diseases. Hypersensitivity pneumonitis and sarcoidosis are typically associated with an increase of lymphocytes, particularly T cells, whereas idiopathic pulmonary fibrosis is characterized by the presence of neutrophils in lavage fluids. Insufficient information is now available to know to what extent this procedure is useful in the routine diagnostic workup of interstitial lung diseases.

In patients without sufficient clinical criteria to make a definitive diagnosis, *lung biopsy* may be indicated, especially to rule out other diseases requiring different treatment. Open lung biopsy will usually provide adequate material, whereas transbronchial biopsy may not. Although the histopathology is distinctive, it is not pathognomonic.

Inhalation challenge using aerosolized material suspected as causative in individual patients has produced acute changes and substantiated the clinical impression in many reports. Few of these reports have included appropriate controls. No standardized antigens or techniques are available. In one recent study, positive findings most helpful included fever, neutrophilia, lymphopenia, decreased forced vital capacity, and decreased exercise minute ventilation.

In many patients, purposeful exposure to the suspected natural environment may be practical, useful, and preferable to laboratory challenge. Interpretation of results may be difficult, however, and routine use of either method of inhalational challenge is not recommended, especially in patients with forms of the disease other than simple, acute, recurrent, transient attacks.

Skin test antigens prepared and used experimentally in patients with hypersensitivity pneumonitis and appropriate controls have been irritating and nondiscriminatory. Skin testing is therefore not practical at this time.

DIFFERENTIAL DIAGNOSIS

Viral and other *infective pneumonias* (e.g., tuberculosis, histoplasmosis, psittacosis) can be distinguished by appropriate serologic studies, cultures, or histopathology. *Idiopathic pulmonary fibrosis* (fibrosing or intrinsic alveolitis) clinically resembles chronic hypersensitivity pneumonitis, and the pathology may also be similar in the chronic stages, but autoimmune phenomena are more common in fibrosing alveolitis. *Eosinophilic pneumonias* are usually accompanied by peripheral eosinophilia and associated with bronchial asthma; pathophysiology and histopathology are usually distinctive. *Allergic bronchopulmonary aspergillosis* is distinguished from hypersensitivity pneumonitis by the presence of eosinophilia and the predominance of obstructive airways, rather than restrictive lung disease. *Sarcoidosis* often causes hilar adenopathy and involves other organ systems. *Collagen-vascular diseases* and the *granuloma-angiitis syndromes* are also multisystem diseases. *Silo-filler's disease* is a chemical pneumonia produced by oxides of nitrogen produced in newly filled silos. A more chronic presentation may occur associated with bronchiolitis obliterans.

A condition termed *pulmonary mycotoxicosis* or *atypical farmer's lung* has been described in which acute massive exposure to moldy silage was followed in a few hours by fever, chills, and cough. The illness lasted from a few days to a week. The chest radiograph revealed diffuse infiltrates; lung biopsy showed an exudative bronchiolitis and alveolitis and a large number of fungal organisms. At least five different fungi, including *Fusarium* and *Penicillium*, were cultured from the specimen. No precipitins could be demonstrated in patients' sera. A similar but less severe condition is *grain fever*, which presents as a flu-like syndrome occurring several hours after exposure to stored corn, oats, or other grains. Chest symptoms may be absent, chest radiograph and pulmonary function testing are normal, and no precipitins are found.

PREVENTION AND MANAGEMENT

Prevention

Hypersensitivity pneumonitis can be prevented by avoidance of antigen inhalation. Masks, filters, industrial hygiene, and awareness of disease potential are all of importance in various occupational environments. Education of the public concerning the hazards of pet birds is essential. The same is true about the importance of proper cleaning and maintenance of humidification and air-conditioning systems, especially those involving aerosolization. Such educational measures and awareness have greatly reduced the incidence of hypersensitivity pneumonitis in groups at risk including dairy farmers, maple bark strippers, and bagasse workers.

Management

Management of hypersensitivity pneumonitis involves primarily antigen avoidance and the occasional use of adrenocorticosteroid therapy.

ANTIGEN AVOIDANCE

The most effective way to avoid an incriminated agent is to separate the patient from the source. In many instances the source is an area or place of employment, and avoidance may require a job change, a recommendation which cannot be lightly given and requires thoughtful consideration of alternatives. The dairy farmer with acute recurrent episodes may be able to avoid areas and activities associated with heavy burdens of respirable thermophilic organisms and may be persuaded to wear protective equipment (masks, respirators, ventilated helmets, filtration devices). The prognosis appears to be good in such patients if acute febrile episodes do not recur. Bird fanciers should avoid exposure completely but may demand compromise, and the use of protective equipment may prove useful. Contaminated humidification, air-conditioning, and ventilation systems can be removed, replaced, or thoroughly cleaned at intervals. Other occupational and environmental hazards may be avoidable. Of recent recognition is the potential for various chemicals, many known to cause occupational asthma, to result in hypersensitivity pneumonitis. These chemicals are ordinarily encountered in industry, but they have been reported in bathtub finishers and insulation installers. Protective equipment must be much more elaborate in such situations, since masks and filters do not remove low-molecular-weight substances.

Recurrence of symptoms demands more drastic measures for complete environmental control. In such cases, compromise measures are not recommended except in patients with acute, recurrent, self-limited episodes of hypersensitivity pneumonitis for which clinical monitoring is practical.

DRUG THERAPY

Acute, recurrent episodes of hypersensitivity pneumonitis are typically self-limited and do not require drug therapy. Severe symptoms or progressive impairment may, however, warrant corticosteroid therapy, provided the diagnosis has been established.

Progressive, *subacute* hypersensitivity pneumonitis often requires corticosteroid therapy. Prednisone 60 mg daily in divided doses is initiated, continued for 7 to 14 days, depending upon the response, tapered over 1 week to 20 mg daily in a single dose, and gradually reduced unless a relapse occurs.

Patients with *chronic* disease should gradually improve following avoidance of the antigen source; recovery may take 6 to 12 months. Corticosteroids may be indicated in some cases to expedite recovery if symptoms or impairment warrant. A regimen similar to that used for subacute disease is appropriate while monitoring the response. In general, corticosteroids are not necessary or recommended in patients with improving mild to moderate disease unless recovery has plateaued despite appropriate environmental control.

BIBLIOGRAPHY

Barrios R, Selman M, Franco R, Chapela R, Lopez JS, Fortoul TI: Subpopulations of T cells in lung biopsies from patients with pigeon breeder's disease. Lung 165:181–187, 1987.
  Monoclonal antibodies were used to determine surface phenotypes of T cells in tissue obtained by open lung biopsies from patients with chronic hypersensitivity pneumonitis (pigeon breeder's disease).

Burrell R, Rylander R: A critical review of the role of precipitins in hypersensitivity pneumonitis. Eur J Respir Dis 62:332–343, 1981.
  This extensive review maintains that precipitins have no role in disease but may be used to identify agents in the environments to which the patient has been exposed.

Coombs RRA, Gell PGH: Classification of allergic reactions underlying disease, in Gell PGH, Coombs RRA (eds): *Clinical Aspects of Immunology.* Oxford, Blackwell, 1962, pp 317–337.
  Classic classification of allergic reactions.

Daniele RP, Elias JA, Epstein PE, Rossman MD: Bronchoalveolar lavage: Role in the pathogenesis, diagnosis and management of interstitial lung disease. Ann Intern Med 102:93–108, 1985.
  Review of the types of information provided by evaluation of lavage fluid and cells with the conclusion that lavage is still an investigative procedure for most lung disorders.

Dewair M, Baur X, Fruhmann G: Lung-reactive antibodies in sera of patients with farmer's lung disease. Respiration 51:146–154, 1987.
  The titers of anti-lung antibodies in sera from patients with farmer's lung were 2 to 5 times greater than those of healthy persons.

Emanuel DA, Kryda MJ: Farmer's lung disease. Clin Rev Allergy 1:509–532, 1983.
  A definitive review of the subject from a group with extensive experience with dairy farmer's lung.

Feigin DS: Allergic diseases in the lungs. CRC Crit Rev Diagn Imaging 25:159–176, 1986.
  An understanding of the four basic reactions responsible for the common allergic disease of the lungs [hypersensitivity pneumonitis, asthma, allergic bronchopulmonary fungal disease, chronic eosinophilic pneumonia, hypereosinophilic syndrome, Goodpasture's syndrome and idiopathic pulmonary hemosiderosis (IPH), Wegener's granulomatosis, and allergic granulomatosis (Churg-Strauss disease)] is critical for interpreting the clinical, pathologic, and radiographic manifestations of these disorders.

Fink JN: Pigeon breeder's disease. Clin Rev Allergy 1:497–508, 1983.
  A comprehensive review of the subject by an active investigator.

Grammer LC, Patterson R: Occupational immunologic lung disease. Ann Allergy 58:151–159, 1987.
  Occupational immunologic lung diseases, either asthma or hypersensitivity pneumonitis, occur in a wide variety of occupations from numerous antigens. These disorders are considered here from the point of view of prevention.

Hendrick DJ, Marshall R, Faux JA, Krall JM: Positive "alveolar" responses to antigen inhalation provocation tests: Their validity and recognition. Thorax 35:415–427, 1980.
  Results of 144 antigen and control tests in 31 subjects with suspected hypersensitivity pneumonitis.

Hodgson MJ, Morey PR, Simon JS, Waters TD, Fink JN: An outbreak of recurrent acute and chronic hypersensitivity pneumonitis in office workers. Am J Epidemiol 125:631–638, 1987.
  Three episodes of an acute, flulike illness were associated with manipulations on the central air handling system of an office building.

Karol MH: Respiratory effects of inhaled isocyanates. CRC Crit Rev Toxicol 16:349–379, 1986.
  The industrial chemicals that cause allergic reactions in the lungs are isocyanates, the starting material in the production of polyurethanes. Syndromes of immediate respiratory reactivity, delayed-onset sensitivity, and hypersensitivity pneumonitis have all been associated with isocyanate exposure.

Kawanami O, Basset F, Barrios R, Lacronique JG, Ferrans VJ, Crystal RG: Hypersensitivity pneumonitis in man: Light and electron microscopic studies of 18 lung biopsies. Am J Pathol 110:275–289, 1983.
  Distinctive morphologic features of hypersensitivity pneumonitis.

Leatherman JW, Michael AF, Schwartz BA, Hoidal JR: Lung T cells in hypersensitivity pneumonitis. Ann Intern Med 100:390–392, 1984.
  Intensive study of T-cell subsets in blood and lavage of patients with chronic hypersensitivity pneumonitis, asymptomatic pigeon breeders, patients with sarcoidosis, and nonsmoking controls.

Merchant JA: Agricultural exposures to organic dusts. State Art Rev Occup Med 2:409–425, 1987.
  Occupational respiratory hazards in agriculture are varied and widespread, and farm workers have been found to have high rates of respiratory disability compared with other industrial sectors. The common denominator in most agricultural exposures is organic dust.

Murphy DMF, Fishman AP: Mushrooms and mushroom worker's lung, in Fishman AP (ed), Update: Pulmonary Diseases and Disorders. New York, McGraw Hill, 1982, pp 230–242.
  A comprehensive review of mushroom-associated hypersensitivity pneumonitis.

Pepys J: Hypersensitivity Diseases of the Lungs Due to Fungi and Organic Dusts. Basel, Karger, 1969.
  A review monograph by the investigator most responsible for early progress in the immunologic aspects of hypersensitivity pneumonitis.

Reyes CN, Wenzel FJ, Lawton BR, Emanuel DA: The pulmonary pathology of farmer's lung disease. Chest 81:142–146, 1982.
  Biopsies from 60 patients with farmer's lung are reviewed and compared for pathologic changes.

Reynolds HY: Louis E. Siltzbach Memorial Lecture. Concepts of pathogenesis and lung reactivity in hypersensitivity pneumonitis. Ann NY Acad Sci 465:287–303, 1986.
  A reflective overview of the mechanisms responsible for hypersensitivity pneumonitis, including a discussion of experimental models of both the acute and chronic disorders.

Reynolds HY: Lung inflammation: Normal host defense or a complication of some diseases? Annu Rev Med 38:295–323, 1987.
  Several examples of diseases that feature inflammation as part of their pathophysiology have been selected for this review: asthma (especially the late-phase reaction that involves PMNs), chronic bronchitis (in which irritants and bacterial products may stimulate mucus secretion and inflammatory cells), interstitial lung diseases, and acute lung injury leading to adult respiratory distress syndrome.

Richerson HB: Hypersensitivity pneumonitis—pathology and pathogenesis. Clin Rev Allergy 1:469–486, 1983.
  An extensive review of putative pathogenetic mechanisms in animal models and human disease.

Chapter 45

Immunologic Diseases of the Lung and Kidney (Goodpasture's Syndrome)

Curtis B. Wilson

Anti-Basement Membrane Antibody Mechanisms

Immunopathology

Diagnosis

Clinical Features

Management

Possible Immune Complex Mechanisms

Immunopathology

Diagnosis

Clinical Features

Treatment

Goodpasture's syndrome denotes simultaneous or sequential pulmonary hemorrhage and evidence of glomerulonephritis. This clinical presentation is most frequently caused by antibodies that react with the vascular basement membranes of the alveolus and the glomerulus. Some investigators include the presence of anti-basement membrane antibodies as an element of this syndrome. This usage, unfortunately, excludes consideration of other immunologic and unknown causes of a similar clinical picture, such as immune complex disease (Table 45-1).

The clinical picture of Goodpasture's syndrome is occasionally mimicked acutely by renal disease that is complicated by pulmonary edema, infection, or pulmonary embolism. However, Goodpasture's syndrome is generally an immunopathologic disorder whose etiologic mechanisms, i.e., anti-basement membrane antibody disease, immune complex disease, can be used to classify this fascinating, but fortunately rare, condition.

Two major immunopathologic mechanisms have been identified in renal disease; these mechanisms can cause pulmonary damage as well. The first involves the production of antibodies that react with an antigen that is present at the site of injury, such as the glomerular basement membrane (GBM), or potentially other structural glomerular antigens including those on glomerular cell membranes. In the second, antibodies form against antigens that are unrelated to the site of injury. These antigens and antibodies form immune complexes, generally in the circulation; the immune complexes are subsequently trapped in the renal or pulmonary vascular beds where they remain in dynamic equilibrium with their counterparts in the circulation. The continuing dynamic interchange is responsible for continuing modification of the immune complex composition of the deposit in situ. In addition, damaging immune complexes may form in situ in the glomerular capillary wall because of the combination of antibodies with antigens that become trapped in the capillary wall or mesangium for a variety of physiological and physicochemical reasons. The current view is that as much as 80 percent of the glomerulonephritis is caused by glomerular accumulation of immune complexes. Anti-basement membrane antibodies, specifically anti-GBM antibodies, probably account for less than 5 percent of glomerulonephritis; the pathogenesis, immune or nonimmune, of the remaining 15 percent is unclear. The tissue injury that either of the major immunopathologic mechanisms induces is produced by mediator systems including complement, polymorphonuclear leukocytes, monocytes/macrophages, and perhaps platelets, reactive oxygen species, arachidonic acid metabolites, vasoactive materials, and interplays related to the coagulation system. The presence of small numbers of T cells in glomeruli as well as peripheral cells sensitized to GBM antigens in some models or patients suggests that the cellular limb of the immune system also may be involved in some way. However, the extent of involvement remains to be defined.

TABLE 45-1

Pulmonary Hemorrhage and Glomerulonephritis (Goodpasture's Syndrome)

Anti-basement membrane antibody-induced

Presumed immune complex-induced (including vasculitic disorders)

    Systemic lupus erythematosus

    Mixed essential cryoglobulinemia

    Other exogenous and endogenous antigen-antibody systems

    ?? Other collagen vascular diseases, including progressive systemic sclerosis

    Polyarteritis nodosa

    Wegener's granulomatosis

    Lymphoid granulomatosis

    Allergic angiitis and granulomatosis (Churg-Strauss syndrome)

    Hypersensitivity angiitis

    Henoch-Schönlein purpura

    ?? D-penicillamine toxicity, trimellitic anhydride toxicity

Etiology undetermined

ANTI-BASEMENT MEMBRANE ANTIBODY MECHANISMS

About one-half of the patients with anti-GBM antibody-induced glomerulonephritis have clinical pulmonary involvement, generally manifested by hemorrhage. They are designated as having Goodpasture's syndrome. Anti-GBM antibody-induced Goodpasture's syndrome is generally severe, and can result in death either from renal failure and the complications of its management, or from pulmonary hemorrhage with respiratory failure. Milder and occasionally self-remitting forms of the disease have been identified, including a few that are confined largely or solely to the lung. How often anti-basement membrane antibodies may be responsible for the clinical presentation of "idiopathic pulmonary hemosiderosis" is unknown.

IMMUNOPATHOLOGY

That anti-basement membrane antibodies can cause renal injury in model systems is beyond doubt. Early experiments showed that heterologous antikidney antisera, and later that anti-GBM antisera, were nephrotoxic when administered to normal recipients. It was also possible experimentally to induce autologous production of anti-GBM antibodies by immunization with GBM or urinary basement membrane antigens in adjuvant. In humans, anti-GBM antibodies have been identified in the circulation, or bound in the kidney, in patients with anti-GBM nephritis; these antibodies have been used to transfer the disease to subhuman primates, thereby demonstrating their nephrotoxicity. The most compelling evidence for the nephritogenic importance of anti-GBM antibodies in humans is the recurrence of nephritis when a kidney is transplanted into an individual who has sufficient residual, circulating anti-GBM antibody.

Anti-basement membrane antibodies are also almost certainly involved in the accompanying pulmonary injury. However, the evidence, although less direct, is convincing: first, anti-basement membrane antibodies can be demonstrated in the alveolar basement membrane by immunofluorescence, and antibodies reactive with both the alveolar basement membrane and the GBM can be found in the circulation or can be recovered in acid eluates from lung tissue of affected individuals; also, immunization of animals with lung basement membrane, and to a lesser extent with GBM, induces anti-basement membrane antibodies that cause acute lung injury and hemorrhage. But, it has been much more difficult to induce lung injury than renal injury by these manipulations. Unlike the renal disease, it has not been possible to transfer the pulmonary component of anti-basement membrane disease to subhuman primates using antibody recovered from individuals with anti-basement mem-

brane antibody-associated Goodpasture's syndrome. This inability may be due to quantitative and qualitative differences in antibody, mediator system, and/or accessibility of the alveolar basement membrane antigens to the circulating antibody. Recent experimental observations have shown that toxic pulmonary injury induced by O_2 or hydrocarbon can cause fixation of anti-basement membrane antibodies in the lungs; this is not possible in unmanipulated controls, raising the possibility that, in humans, various types of injury, such as fluid overload, smoking, and infection, may contribute to the pulmonary toxicity of anti-basement membrane antibodies.

The events responsible for the induction of anti-basement membrane antibodies are poorly understood. Loose clinical associations have been observed between anti-basement membrane antibody diseases and diverse insults, such as influenza A2 infection, hydrocarbon solvent inhalation, renal ischemia, and neoplasia. The fact that the anti-basement membrane antibody response is generally self-limited, lasting only weeks to months, suggests that the stimulus for its formation is also brief and potentially identifiable. Whether infectious or toxic environmental stimuli alter basement membrane antigens, possibly in the lung, rendering them immunogenic, is unknown. Alternatively, such stimuli could denude antigen that is normally covered, thereby exposing it to anti-basement membrane antibodies that were formed for other reasons. Basement membrane antigens recovered from the urine can induce anti-GBM nephritis in animals; conceivably, such antigens could stimulate antibody production in humans.

DIAGNOSIS

Anti-GBM disease is diagnosed by: (1) a combination of immunofluorescence (Fig. 45-1) and elution studies of tissue, (2) demonstration of circulating anti-basement membrane antibodies using indirect immunofluorescence, or (3) radioimmunoassay. It should be stressed that detection using immunofluorescence of typical linear deposits of immunoglobulin (IgG, rarely IgA or IgM) along the glomerular or alveolar basement membrane is not sufficient to establish a diagnosis of anti-basement membrane antibody disease. Nonimmunologic linear deposits of immunoglobulin (usually accompanied by albumin) are sometimes seen in kidneys from patients with diabetes mellitus, in kidneys taken at autopsy, and occasionally in normal kidneys. Therefore, the results of studies using immunofluorescence must always be confirmed by demonstrating the specificity of eluted antibody in subsequent in vivo or in vitro assays, or by detecting antibody in the circulation. Generally, C3 is deposited along with immunoglobulin, suggesting that it participates in mediating the injury. About one-third of patients with anti-GBM dis-

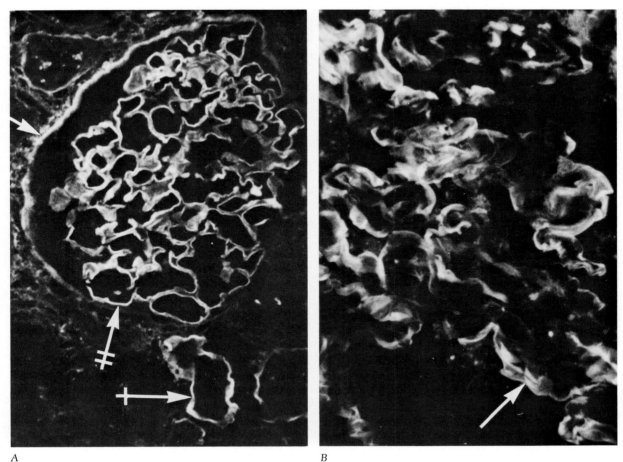

FIGURE 45-1 Typical linear deposits of IgG in Goodpasture's syndrome. A. Kidney. Anti-basement membrane antibodies react with Bowman's capsule (arrow) and the tubular basement membrane (barred arrow) in addition to the typical linear GBM localization (double-barred arrow). B. Lungs. Deposits are present along the alveolar basement membrane (arrow).

ease lack detectable C3 deposits, indicating that non-C3 mediator pathways may also be involved.

Circulating anti-GBM antibodies are best detected by radioimmunoassay or enzyme-linked assays that use solubilized GBM antigens remaining after collagenase digestion of the GBM. The physicians should be aware of the laboratory where the anti-GBM antibody measurements are being done, since the sensitivities, and perhaps specificities, of the assays vary. Because the salvage of the kidneys and of the patient depend so much on early diagnosis and aggressive therapy, accurate detection is critical. The major noncollagenous reactants immunopurified from the collagenase extract used in our radioimmunoassay are about 27 and 54 kD. Studies suggest that at least a portion of the reactivity in these digests is with the noncollagenous carboxyl-terminal regions of the type IV basement membrane collagen molecule. Just how many antigenic sites will be identified as the biochemical makeup of the basement membranes of the kidney and lung un-

folds is not yet known. It is hoped that better definition of the antigen systems will allow additional subdivision of patients with anti-basement membrane diseases, leading to corresponding refinements in clinical diagnosis, management, and prognosis.

To date, our radioimmunoassay has been positive in almost all patients early in the course of anti-GBM antibody-induced Goodpasture's syndrome. The assay is also useful in assessing the rate of disappearance of anti-GBM antibodies and the effects of therapy. Circulating antibody usually disappears within several months (varying from 1 month to 3 or 4 years). Nephrectomy does not have an immediate effect on antibody levels, although the rate of disappearance may be somewhat more rapid thereafter. No strict relationship exists between the level of circulating antibody detected by this assay and the episodes of severity of pulmonary involvement. Even though samples are generally not available at the onset of disease, a relationship does exist between the absolute amount of antibody detected and the overall severity of renal involvement. Roughly 10 percent of patients with pulmonary manifestations (frequently severe) and moderate levels of circulating antibody that persist for several months have only mild, and often nonprogressive, renal problems. In our laboratory a dozen or so patients have been identified whose clinical involvement was confined entirely to the lungs and whose diagnosis was idiopathic pulmonary hemosiderosis; antibody was bound in the kidney and/or lung on immunofluorescence study. It is unknown why the antibody failed to induce sufficient renal injury to be detected clinically; qualitative, quantitative, and temporal aspects of binding may be responsible.

CLINICAL FEATURES

In general, patients with Goodpasture's syndrome have severe renal lesions, and the clinical course is that of a rapidly progressive glomerulonephritis. A nephrotic syndrome is unusual. A prodromal period of flulike illness frequently occurs. Arthralgia and arthritis are prominent in about 5 percent of patients. The disease may begin with either renal manifestations or pulmonary problems (generally hemoptysis). Usually both organs are involved more or less simultaneously; but the interval between may be prolonged up to 1 year. Both sexes are affected, the ages ranging from less than 10 years to more than 70 years; the

age distribution is bimodal, peaking at about 30 and 60 years. Goodpasture's syndrome most often affects young men; kidney involvement alone occurs most often in older women. Hemoptysis is generally episodic; occasionally it is so extreme that it floods the lungs to produce asphyxia and death (Fig. 45-2). Anemia, a general feature of Goodpasture's syndrome, is microcytic and hypochromic; it is often severe. Macrophages in the sputum contain red blood cell fragments and stain for hemosiderin with Prussian blue. The chest radiograph is usually normal between episodes of hemorrhage; the hemorrhage, if large, produces clear-cut alveolar infiltrates (Fig. 45-3). Carbon monoxide uptake has been advocated as a test for sequestered blood within the lungs. As noted earlier, the severity of hemorrhage does not relate directly to the amount of circulating antibody, and episodes of hemorrhages can recur repeatedly at any time during the course of antibody production. The larger the hemorrhage, the more likely is a drop in hematocrit, the appearance of hemosiderin-laden macrophages in the sputum, and the appearance of fluffy infiltrates on the chest radiograph.

MANAGEMENT

In general, the course seems to be dictated by the severity of the initial immunologic insult. Dialysis is often required for the management of renal failure. Plasmapheresis combined with immunosuppression, most often using prednisone and cyclophosphamide/azathioprine, is used to lower rapidly the levels of circulating antibody. The response of the renal disease is related to the severity of damage at the time of therapy; the severity is assessed by the serum creatinine level and by the degree of crescent formation on renal biopsy. For a successful outcome, therapy has to be started before irreversible renal damage has occurred. The combined approach is reasonable in theory and the clinical results to date are promising, albeit largely uncontrolled. Careful evaluation is difficult in the crisis setting in which these infrequent patients are usually seen. It should be kept in mind that mild, self-remitting forms of the disease sometimes occur, and controlled clinical trials are needed. Study of the mechanisms responsible for long-term deterioration of renal function seen in some patients with initial favorable responses to treatment are also needed.

The occurrence of pulmonary involvement in antibasement membrane antibody-induced Goodpasture's syndrome is episodic and, as indicated above, seems to be precipitated in many instances by nonimmunologic factors, such as fluid overload, smoking, toxic exposure, or infection. Management should include a search for and correction of any such factors. Pulse doses of methylprednisolone appear to be helpful in treating episodes of pulmonary hemorrhage, even though controlled studies have

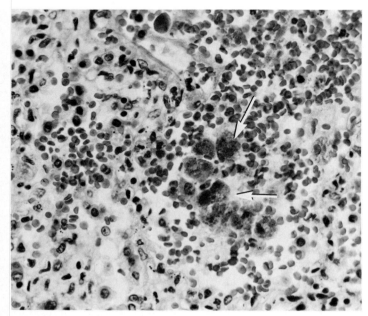

FIGURE 45-2 Histologic changes in the lung from a patient with Goodpasture's syndrome induced by anti-GBM antibody. Severe pulmonary hemorrhage has led to extravasation of red blood cells and to the presence of hemosiderin-laden macrophages (arrows) within an alveolar lumen.

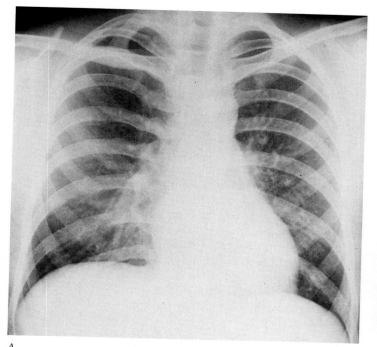

A

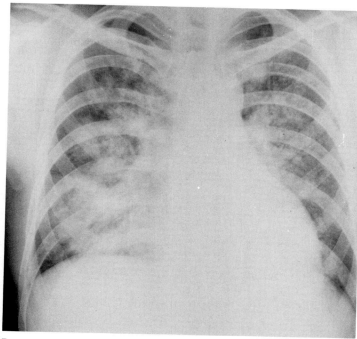

B

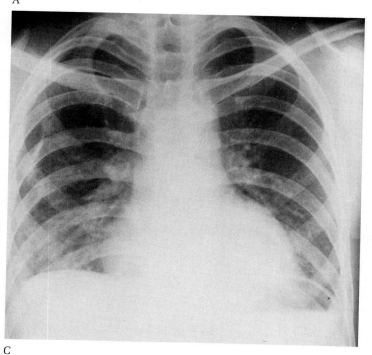

C

FIGURE 45-3 Goodpasture's syndrome. A. First admission. Two-year history of uremia. Left ventricular hypertrophy on electrocardiogram. No respiratory symptoms. B. Six months later. Acute shortness of breath of hemoptysis. Diffuse alveolar changes throughout both lung fields attributed to aspirated blood and edema. C. Seventeen days later. One week after bilateral nephrectomy for Goodpasture's syndrome and intensive respiratory therapy, including assisted ventilation. Small right pneumothorax. Left lung clear. Right lung clearing.

not yet been done to prove their value. The immunosuppression and plasma exchange regimens lower the levels of circulating antibody, and the risk of pulmonary hemorrhage subsides with the disappearance of circulating antibody. Nephrectomy, once suggested as beneficial for the pulmonary hemorrhage, is now seldom, if ever, used. Once antibody has disappeared, exacerbations of anti-basement membrane antibody production are infrequent.

POSSIBLE IMMUNE COMPLEX MECHANISMS

A third or more of patients with pulmonary hemorrhage and glomerulonephritis have etiologies other than anti-basement membrane antibodies (Table 45-1). Although the causes are often not well defined, they include typical immune complex disease, such as systemic lupus erythematosus, in which the lung and kidney are generally only two of many organs involved. Lung and kidney manifestations are also common in patients with other vasculitic conditions, including Wegener's granulomatosis, in which evidence for an immune complex etiology is less clear. In some patients with pulmonary hemorrhage and glomerulonephritis no specific immunopathologic etiology can be identified; this group probably represents a number of different pathogenetic mechanisms.

IMMUNOPATHOLOGY

The concept of immune complex disease arose from observations made on animals with serum sickness: in these animals, the administration of an antigen (generally a foreign serum protein) that persisted in the circulation until antibodies were formed was followed by complexing of the antigen and antibody, leading to vascular deposition and initiation of inflammation. Immune complex disease also occurs in situ if antigen (or antibody) first localizes in the tissue and later reacts with antibody (or antigen), as in Arthus' reaction. The lung is also subject to this in situ type of immune complex disease when it is exposed to inhaled antigens.

Serum sickness models of immune complex disease have been extensively studied in the rabbit. In these models, radiolabeled antigens (bovine serum albumin) allow quantification of the deposits of immune-complexed antigen. Almost all the immune-complexed antigen is removed rapidly from the circulation by the reticuloendothelial system; less than 1 percent of the immune complexed antigen deposits in the kidney. In the lungs, the deposition of immune complexes as reflected in the quantity of radiolabeled antigen that persists after 24 h is second only to that in the kidneys. Indeed, a pulmonary lesion has been induced in rabbits by producing experimental chronic serum sickness.

The factors that influence the particular tissue site of immune complex deposition are poorly understood but seem to include the immune complex size, determined in part by the relative antigen-antibody ratio, predilection for tissue binding because of physicochemical reasons such as charge of the immune complex components, changes in vascular permeability caused by immune release of vasoactive materials, function of the reticuloendothelial system, and dynamics of blood flow. As noted above, once deposited, the immune complex remains in equilibrium with antigen and antibody in the circulation, so that its composition is subject to continuous modification. For example, it is possible to use the known ability of antigen excess to solubilize immune complexes to treat experimental serum sickness in rabbits: by creating a huge antigen excess, the glomerular immune complex deposits can be removed.

In humans, an increasing number of endogenous and exogenous antigens are being identified in the glomerular deposits that presumably consist of immune complexes. Best known as potential contributors of exogenous antigens for nephritogenic immune complex formation are infectious agents—bacterial, parasitic, and viral. Other sources of exogenous antigens are medications and immunizations.

Endogenous antigens include the nuclear materials present in systemic lupus erythematosus, tumor antigens in neoplasia-associated immune complex formation, and immunoglobulins in cryoglobulinemia. The majority of

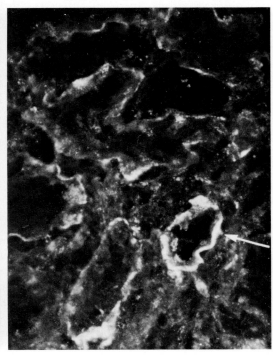

FIGURE 45-4 Granular deposits of IgG (arrows), typical of immune complexes, are seen within the glomerular capillary walls and mesangium (A) and within the tubular basement membrane and renal interstitium (B) in a renal biopsy from a patient with systemic lupus erythematosus.

A   *B*

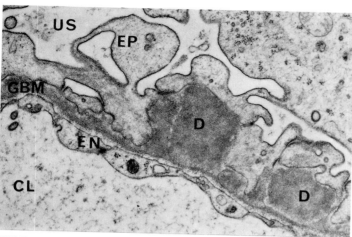

FIGURE 45-5 Electron-dense deposits (D) are seen along the subepithelial aspect of a GBM in immune complex-induced glomerulonephritis. EP = epithelial cell; EN = endothelial cell; CL = capillary lumen; US = urinary space.

antigens in presumed nephritogenic immune complex formation, particularly in primary forms of immune complex glomerulonephritis, remain to be identified. Parallel studies of the deposition of presumed pulmonary immune complexes have only just begun.

DIAGNOSIS

Tentative diagnosis of immune complex disease is based on the immunofluorescent detection of granular deposits of immunoglobulin and complement in tissue, generally in close association with vessels (Fig. 45-4). The deposits sometimes can be visualized also as dense accumulations by electron microscopy (Fig. 45-5). Confirmation that they are immune complexes depends on identifying specific antigen-antibody systems contributing to the immune complex deposit. This is done by identifying the antigen with immunohistochemical techniques or by eluting the immune complex in buffers that are known to dissociate antigen-antibody complexes, subsequently identifying the specificity of the antibody.

A lowering of serum complement levels and the appearance of cryoglobulins suggest the presence of immune complexes in the circulation. Methods to detect immune complexes themselves can facilitate diagnosis and be helpful in monitoring therapy. In Wegener's granulomatosis, autoantibodies that are reactive with extranuclear components of polymorphonuclear granulocytes have been reported to be of value in the diagnosis and in the estimation of disease activity. Evidence of vasculitis and granuloma formation can be sought by biopsy of lung, kidney, or more accessible tissues. Immunofluorescence studies should be included in the evaluation of tissues obtained by biopsy.

CLINICAL FEATURES

Clinical features of renal and pulmonary "immune complex and vasculitic disorders" are diverse and are also considered elsewhere in this book. Here it is worth noting that the disorders can generally be sorted into two major categories: in one, the kidney and lungs are involved as part of a systemic immune complex disorder, such as systemic lupus erythematosus or, less often, Wegener's granulomatosis, polyarteritis, Henoch-Schönlein purpura, or cryoglobulinemia; in the other, glomerulonephritis is secondary to pulmonary infection, neoplasia, or sarcoidosis, disorders that can supply antigens for the formation of nephritogenic immune complexes.

TREATMENT

Treatment of the various systemic, presumed immune complex disorders discussed in this section is broadly based on the use of steroids, immunosuppression, and often plasma exchange. As a group, the non-anti-basement membrane antibody forms of pulmonary hemorrhage and glomerulonephritis tend to respond more readily to treatment than do their anti-basement membrane antibody-positive counterparts. Cyclophosphamide therapy of Wegener's granulomatosis and vasculitis is often successful but, in contrast to patients with anti-basement membrane-induced Goodpasture's syndrome, a relapsing course is to be expected. One prospect for the future is the identification of the antigenic makeup of the immune complexes and either elimination of the source or manipulation of the specific immune response. For those patients in which no immunopathologic etiology can be identified, treatment is similar to that noted above; however, the outcome is variable, probably related to the particular etiology responsible for the disorder in the individual patient.

BIBLIOGRAPHY

Donaghy M, Rees AJ: Cigarette smoking and lung hemorrhage in glomerulonephritis caused by autoantibodies to glomerular basement membrane. Lancet 2:1390–1393, 1983.
  Describes the irritant effect of smoking on hemoptysis in anti-basement membrane antibody-induced Goodpasture's syndrome.

Fishman AP: Pulmonary hemorrhage in Goodpasture's syndrome. N Engl J Med 295:1430–1432, 1976.
  Describes the use of carbon monoxide uptake for detection of pulmonary hemorrhage.

Jennings L, Roholt OA, Pressman D, Blau M, Andres GA, Brentjens Jr: Experimental anti-alveolar basement membrane antibody-mediated pneumonitis. I. The role of increased permeability of the alveolar capillary wall induced by oxygen. J Immunol 127:129–134, 1981.
  Presents data suggesting that O_2 toxicity can alter the lung binding of anti-basement membrane antibodies.

Johnson JP, Moore J Jr, Austin HA, Balow JE, Antonovych TT, Wilson CB: Therapy of anti-glomerular basement membrane antibody disease: Analysis of prognostic significance of clinical, pathologic, and treatment factors. Medicine 64:219–227, 1985.
  Describes the results of immunosuppression with or without plasma exchange in the treatment of anti-basement membrane antibody diseases.

Johnson JP, Whitman W, Briggs WA, Wilson CB: Plasmapheresis and immunosuppressive agents in antibasement membrane antibody-induced Goodpasture's syndrome. Am J Med 64:354–359, 1978.
  Describes the induction, treatment, and outcome of patients with anti-basement membrane antibody disease.

Kefalides NA: The Goodpasture antigen and basement membranes: The search must go on. Lab Invest 56:1–3, 1987.
  A current review of the Goodpasture antigen.

Kleppel MM, Kashtan CE, Butkowski RJ, Fish AJ, Michael AF: Absence of 28 kilodalton non-collagenous monomers of type IV collagen in glomerular basement membrane. J Clin Invest 80:263–266, 1987.
  Recent evidence that the Goodpasture antigen is absent from kidneys in some patients with hereditary nephritis.

Peters DK, Rees AJ, Lockwood CM, Pusey CD: Treatment and prognosis in antibasement membrane antibody-mediated nephritis. Transplant Proc 14:513–521, 1982.
  Gives the results of therapy in a series of patients treated with an aggressive immunosuppression and plasma exchange protocol.

Pusey CD, Dash A, Kershaw MJ, Morgan A, Reilly A, Rees AJ, Lockwood CM: A single autoantigen in Goodpasture's syndrome identified by a monoclonal antibody to human glomerular basement membrane. Lab Invest 56:23–31, 1987.
  Development of a monoclonal antibody to the Goodpasture antigen.

Rees AJ, Lockwood CM, Peters DK: Enhanced allergic tissue injury in Goodpasture's syndrome by intercurrent bacterial infection. Br Med J 2:723–726, 1977.
  Describes the possible role of infection in triggering pulmonary hemorrhage in patients with anti-basement membrane antibody-induced Goodpasture's syndrome.

van der Woude FJ, Rasmussen N, Lobatto S, Wiik A, Permin H, van Es LA, van der Giessen M, van der Hem GK, The TH: Autoantibodies against neutrophils and monocytes: Tool for diagnosis and marker of disease activity in Wegener's granulomatosis. Lancet 1:425–429, 1985.

Wieslander J, Bygren P, Heinegard D: Isolation of the specific glomerular basement membrane antigen involved in Goodpasture's syndrome. Proc Natl Acad Sci USA 81:1544–1548, 1984.
  Provides some biochemical identification of at least one antigen reactive with human anti-basement membrane antibodies.

Wilson CB: Anti-GBM glomerulonephritis, in Rosen S (ed), Roth LM (series ed), *Pathology of Glomerular Disease*, vol 1, *Contemporary Issues in Surgical Pathology*. New York, Churchill-Livingstone, 1983, pp 171–194.
  Reviews the immunopathologic and clinical features of anti-basement membrane antibody-induced glomerulonephritis and Goodpasture's syndrome.

Wilson CB, Dixon FJ: Anti-glomerular basement membrane antibody-induced glomerulonephritis. Kidney Int 3:74–89, 1973.
  Presents the immunopathologic and clinical features of the first large group of patients with anti-basement membrane antibody disease prior to the current era of aggressive therapeutic management.

Wilson CB, Dixon FJ: The renal response to immunological injury, in Brenner BM, Rector FC Jr (eds), *The Kidney*, 3d ed. Philadelphia, Saunders, 1986, pp 800–889.
  Offers an extensive review of the basic immunopathologic processes responsible for both anti-basement membrane antibody and immune complex-initiated disease.

Chapter 46

The Eosinophilic Pneumonias

Robert L. Mayock / Renato V. Iozzo

Since the recognition of the eosinophil as a distinct cell type in 1879 by Ehrlich, pathologists have found that this cell is commonly seen in many forms of lung disease and can occur in the bronchial secretions, in the alveoli, or in the interstitium.

The term *eosinophilic pneumonia* refers to disease processes in which the parenchyma of the lung is involved with an inflammatory process that consists largely of eosinophils and histiocytes but also may contain other inflammatory elements: lymphocytes, neutrophilic granulocytes, plasma cells, and mast cells. Frequently, eosinophilia of blood and sputum accompanies the lung infiltrate; constitutional symptoms are often minimal or absent.

Occurrence of eosinophils in the bronchial and the nasal secretions has been a hallmark of allergic reactivity, of both the intrinsic and extrinsic types. The presence of eosinophils in the interstitium and in the alveoli is presumed to be the result of a similar hypersensitivity process, although in some syndromes the nature of the inciting compound or compounds has not been discovered.

The pathologic findings of eosinophilic pneumonia, either on biopsy or at postmortem examination, are not specific since a variety of etiologic factors may produce the same pathologic picture. Only by the finding of specific agents or of a typical picture can one give the syndrome a name. However, in one usage, the designation of eosinophilic pneumonia refers to a distinct entity, chronic eosinophilic pneumonia, to be discussed later. It is often loosely applied to eosinophilic pulmonary infiltrates (pulmonary eosinophilia) that accompany asthma, periarteritis nodosa, and other diseases of hypersensitivity.

HISTORY

Loeffler originally described a syndrome in which radiographic evidence of fleeting and migratory pneumonia was associated with blood eosinophilia; there was no evidence of systemic disease; symptoms were absent or minimal; no pathology was available.

It was von Meyenburg who provided the first pathologic description of eosinophilic pneumonia, reporting necropsy observations in four patients with Loeffler's syndrome who died an accidental death. The lesions consisted of intra-alveolar as well as interstitial infiltrations with eosinophils and both serous and fibrinous organizing exudates. Proliferating alveolar cells were present, including the formation of giant cells. The bronchi, bronchioles, and some veins were infiltrated by eosinophils; the liver also showed focal collections of eosinophils. Two of von Meyenburg's four patients had *Ascaris* worms in the intestines, but larvae were not seen in the lungs. Parasites, such as *A. lumbricoides* and *A. suum*, are a major cause of eosinophilic pneumonia. Their larvae pass through the lungs. Because in many instances, like those reported by von Meyenburg, the parasites are not present in the lung tissue, it has been suggested that the accumulation of eosinophils may result from the filtering of these cells by the lung capillaries while the actual cause resides elsewhere, i.e., intestinal parasites. In 1949, Sprent sensitized mice to various *Ascaris* extracts and induced pulmonary changes including an infiltrate with eosinophils. This observation also suggests that a sensitivity reaction, rather than larval migration per se, plays an important role in the production of the pathologic changes in the lungs. Crofton et al. extended Loeffler's description to include patients with tropical eosinophilia, pneumonia associated with asthma, and eosinophilic pneumonia associated with periarteritis nodosa. Later, Reeder and Goodrich introduced the term *pulmonary infiltration with eosinophilia (PIE) syndrome*, thereby enlarging further the restrictive term *Loeffler's syndrome*. Chronic eosinophilic pneumonia was first described by Christoforidis and Molnar in 1960 and later expanded on by Liebow, Carrington, and their associates.

CLASSIFICATION

Over the years a satisfactory classification of these conditions has been elusive. The earliest classifications (and even more recent attempts) have been a combination of radiographic, clinical, and etiologic bases. Since therapy depends on etiology, we believe that the classification developed in the earlier edition is more satisfactory to the practicing clinician (Table 46-1). This permits a review of possible etiologic or predisposing factors in patient evaluation.

It should be noted that, although many agents may produce characteristic clinical and pathologic changes, the changes in themselves are not diagnostic and there are many exceptions to classic presentations. Once the pathologic picture has been found, a careful search for an etiology should be undertaken.

TABLE 46-1
Etiologic Classification of Eosinophilic Pneumonia

Eosinophilic pneumonia due to parasitic infestation (Loeffler's syndrome)

Eosinophilic pneumonia induced by chemicals

Eosinophilic pneumonia associated with the asthmatic syndrome
    Bronchial asthma
    Mucoid impaction of bronchi
    Bronchopulmonary aspergillosis

Eosinophilic pneumonia seen with infections

Eosinophilic pneumonia in association with hypersensitivity disorders and systemic angiitis
    Periarteritis nodosa
    Allergic angiitis and granulomatosis (Churg-Strauss disease)

Eosinophilic pneumonia of unknown etiology

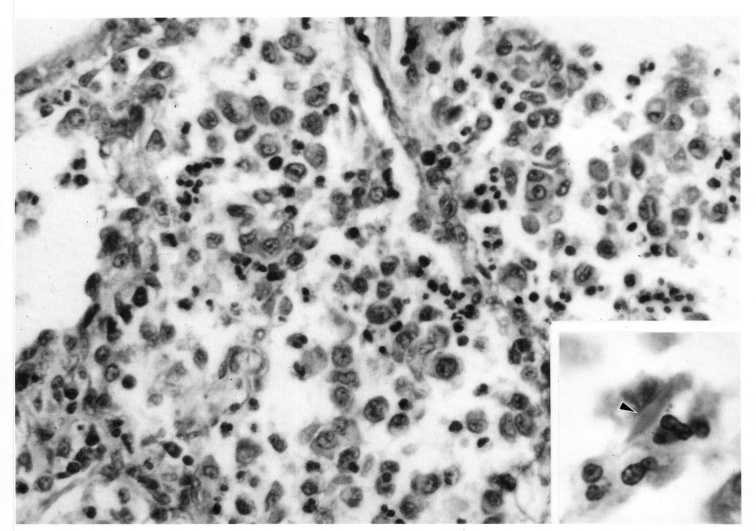

FIGURE 46-1   Light micrograph of eosinophilic pneumonia showing the filling of alveolar spaces with eosinophils and macrophages. The inset shows a Charcot-Leyden crystal (arrowhead) within the cytoplasm of a macrophage. Luna stain ×485; inset ×650.

PATHOLOGY

The Eosinophil

With recent advances in cellular biology, the knowledge of the eosinophil's structure and function has dramatically expanded. Chapter 40 presents the current status of our information concerning the eosinophil. As Kay points out, there are many gaps between structure and function. The precise role of the eosinophil in disease production is still to be elucidated.

Pathologic Findings

The predominant feature of eosinophilic pneumonia is the filling of alveolar spaces by eosinophils together with mononuclear and giant cells. Interestingly, the histopathologic changes are identical regardless of their causative agent, suggesting that the eosinophilic response is not specific for any particular type of etiology. The chronic form of eosinophilic pneumonia is likely to require lung biopsy for diagnosis. The consolidated areas observed grossly are due to extensive leukocyte infiltration of the interstitium and alveolar spaces. Eosinophilic leukocytes are generally seen within the alveoli and the edematous interstitium (Fig. 46-1). The Luna stain can help in identifying eosinophils, especially when they are not numerous, since their cytoplasm is stained bright red (Fig. 46-1). The proportion of eosinophils and macrophages varies widely; although eosinophils are generally predominant, the macrophages can constitute the major cellular component (Fig. 46-2A). Almost invariably, the alveolar spaces contain a number of multinucleated giant cells (Fig. 46-2A). Often the histiocytes and giant cells contain eosinophilic granules and minute, brightly eosinophilic crystals (Fig. 46-1, inset), the so-called Charcot-Leyden crystals. Necrosis of intra-alveolar exudate with formation of small eosinophilic abscesses (Fig. 46-2B) can cause focal de-

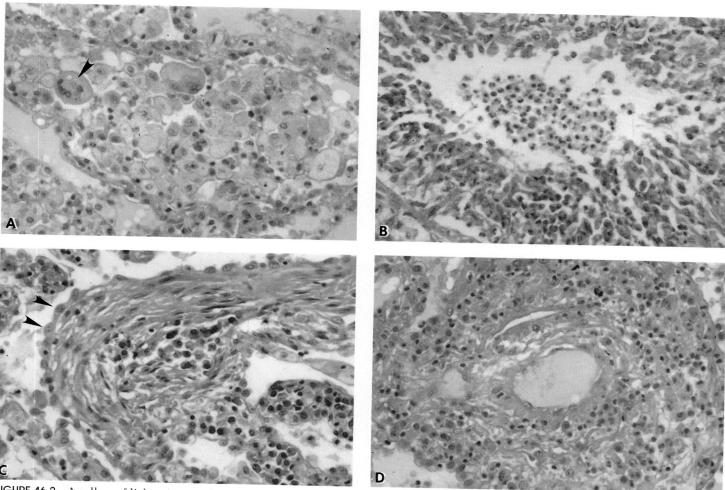

FIGURE 46-2 A gallery of light micrographs showing various histologic aspects of eosinophilic pneumonia. *A.* Alveolar infiltrate composed of foamy macrophages, multinucleated giant cells (arrowhead), and eosinophils. *B.* A small intra-alveolar eosinophilic abscess surrounded by a palisade of histiocytes and few lymphocytes. *C.* Interstitial chronic inflammation and hyperplasia of type II pneumocytes (arrowheads) *D.* Perivascular inflammation composed of eosinophils and lymphocytes. Note the lack of necrosis. H&E, *A* to *C* ×250.

struction of the alveolar wall and can lead to subsequent fibrosis. As expected from a lesion which damages the alveolar wall, there is often desquamation and hyperplasia of type II pneumocytes (Fig. 46-2C). An interstitial infiltrate is often associated with the intra-alveolar changes. The alveolar septa are often widened by edema and a mixed inflammatory cell infiltrate composed of lymphocytes and plasma cells with or without eosinophils. A mild, nonnecrotizing vasculitis involving a few small vessels, mostly venules, is often noted. This lesion is characterized by a perivascular infiltrate of lymphocytes and eosinophils without disruption of the normal vascular architecture (Fig. 46-2D). Occasionally, there is organization of the intra-alveolar and interstitial cell infiltrate with deposition of collagen and granulation tissue similar to that observed in bronchiolitis obliterans. However, a common cause of small airway obstruction is mucous plugging.

Since at least some cases of eosinophilic pneumonia can be associated with identifiable organisms, a series of special stains should be performed routinely. Silver stain for fungi and acid-fast stain for mycobacteria should be performed. These two stains are particularly important since in some conditions, such as in the acquired immunodeficiency syndrome (AIDS), macrophages can be the predominant cell in the intra-alveolar exudate admixed with a rare eosinophil.

Morphologically, however, only two pulmonary conditions pose a real challenge in differential diagnosis. They are desquamative interstitial pneumonia (DIP) and eosinophilic granuloma. The characteristic feature of DIP is the massive proliferation and accumulation of type II pneumocytes within the alveolar spaces. Generally, the interstitial infiltrate is quite sparse, and the eosinophils and plasma cells are present only in relatively small numbers, primarily in the interstitium. Finally, neither necrosis of the intra-alveolar exudate nor angiitis is a significant feature of DIP.

In eosinophilic granuloma the infiltrate is also composed of a mixture of eosinophils and histiocytes. However, there are several important differences: (1) The infiltrate differs topographically since it is confined primarily to the interstitium rather than being located in the alveolar spaces. (2) In the eosinophilic granuloma the histiocytes are often atypical with abnormal nuclei. (3) The lesions of eosinophilic granuloma are well defined and patchy, separated by intervening zones of normal-appearing pulmonary parenchyma, in contrast with the eosinophilic pneumonia that tends to be a more diffuse process. These pathologic changes are reflected in the radiographic appearances of these two conditions. Eosinophilic granuloma usually shows a finely reticulonodular pattern in contrast to the more homogeneous areas of consolidation in eosinophilic pneumonia.

ETIOLOGY

Pulmonary infiltrates with eosinophilia appear to result from the introduction of foreign material into the system by a variety of routes: ingestion, injection, inhalation, skin contact, vaginal absorption.

Two etiologic categories that have been specifically related to eosinophilic pneumonia are parasitic infestation and drug reaction. In tropical areas of the world, parasites have been identified with this disease since the earliest descriptions. Control of human parasites and vectors has resulted in a marked decrease in the simpler, more benign forms of the disease (Loeffler's syndrome, simple pulmonary eosinophilia), but the eosinophilic pneumonias continue to pose a major problem in parts of the world where the human population is still heavily parasitized. A partial list of parasites that cause this syndrome is found in Table 46-2. Tropical eosinophilia is discussed in detail below.

In contrast to the decreasing role of parasitism as the cause of eosinophilic pneumonia, drugs and elements in the environment have become more important etiologically (Table 46-3). The conclusion is unavoidable that this list will continue to grow as new drugs and synthetic substances are created.

In temperate climates, bronchial asthma is the most common disease state associated with eosinophilia and pulmonary infiltrations. Although eosinophilia is a common feature of asthma, a pulmonary infiltrate in these patients may represent multiple possibilities: fungal, bacterial, viral, or mycoplasmal infection; atelectasis; or eosinophilic pneumonia. However, diagnosis is generally possible on clinical grounds without recourse to pathologic confirmation. Moreover, the administration of steroid therapy for the asthma generally clears the eosinophilic pneumonia.

Interest is high in the role of the *Aspergillus* species as a cause of bronchopulmonary disease and eosinophilic

TABLE 46-2

Parasites Most Commonly Associated with Eosinophilic Pneumonia

Ascaris lumbricoides
Necator americanus
*Ancylostoma duodenale**
Trichinella spiralis
Fasciola hepatica
*Strongyloides stercoralis**
*Dirofilaria immitis**
*Wuchereria malayi**
*Toxocara canis**

* A cause of tropical eosinophilia.

TABLE 46-3

Partial List of Compounds and Elements Reported to Be Associated with Eosinophilic Pneumonia

Acetylsalicylic acid
Aminosalicylic acid (PAS)
Amiodarone
Azathioprine
Beclomethasone diproprionate inhaler
Beryllium
Bleomycin
Carbamazepine
Chlorpropamide
Chromoglycate
Clofibrate
Desipramine
Gold salts
Isoniazid
Mecamylamine
Mephenesin
Methotrexate
Methylphenidate
Nickel carbonyl
Nitrofurantoin (Furandantin)
Penicillins
Poison ivy desensitization
Pollen inhalation
Salazopyrin
Smoke inhalation
Streptomycin
Sulfonamides
Sulfonylureas
Talazamide
Tetracyclines
Thiazides
Thiopramine
Tolbutamide
Tricyclic antidepressants

pneumonia in patients with extrinsic bronchial asthma (Fig. 46-3). This coincidence has been reported more often in the United Kingdom than in the United States. The reason for this disparity is either better recognition or a greater prevalence of this mold in the United Kingdom. Because patches of eosinophilic pneumonia occur in so many diseases of hypersensitivity, they must be interpreted according to the clinical context in which they are encountered. For example, eosinophilic infiltrates in the lung are seen in the syndrome of allergic angiitis with granulomatosis (Churg-Strauss syndrome). The hallmark of this disorder is the coexistence of systemic manifestations of the syndrome.

Although it is usually possible to implicate one of the etiologic agents discussed above, in some instances of eosinophilic pneumonia no cause can be identified. Whether the idiopathic types represent a response to an as yet unrecognized sensitizing agent or develop endogenously in preconditioned individuals is unknown.

CLINICAL DISORDERS

Loeffler's Syndrome

Eosinophilic pneumonia varies from transient to chronic, from mild to severe; at times it is life-threatening. The mildest form is Loeffler's syndrome. Since the diagnosis is usually made radiographically, the disorder is usually uncovered in the course of chest radiography for other purposes. Respiratory symptoms are either minimal or absent; when present, they consist of a cough that is either dry and hacking or productive of mucoid sputum, wheezing, or mild shortness of breath. Systemic symptoms consist of a low-grade fever, grippelike sensations, and myalgias. Serial chest radiographs (Fig. 46-4) generally suggest the diagnosis. They are characterized by fleeting densities in any part of the lung fields; the densities are usually homogeneous, located peripherally, and nonsegmental; they can come and go over a 1- to 2-day period. Characteristically, one lesion disappears while another appears elsewhere. Cavitation, pleural effusion, and lymph node enlargement are ordinarily not part of this disorder.

Eosinophilia in blood and/or sputum is a major diagnostic feature. As indicated above, the initial inquiry concerning etiology focuses on parasitism, either intestinal (*Ascaris*) or systemic (filariasis), exposure to exogenous compounds, and the ingestion of medications or drugs. In looking for evidence of parasitism it should be noted that, in newly infected individuals, larval migration and sensitization occur before eggs or parasites appear in the stool. Therefore, the radiographic abnormalities sometimes have cleared and the patient has been discharged before the detection of ova and parasites in the stool becomes possible.

By definition, prognosis in Loeffler's syndrome is excellent. The disease generally remits spontaneously where the inciting agent is controlled; if corticosteroid therapy is required, the response is generally gratifying.

Tropical Eosinophilia

The term *tropical eosinophilia* was coined by Weingarten in 1943 for what he considered to be a new disease entity occurring in certain regions of India. It is now recognized that, in the tropics, the condition described by Weingarten and others usually represents filarial infestation. The geographic distribution of tropical eosinophilia corresponds

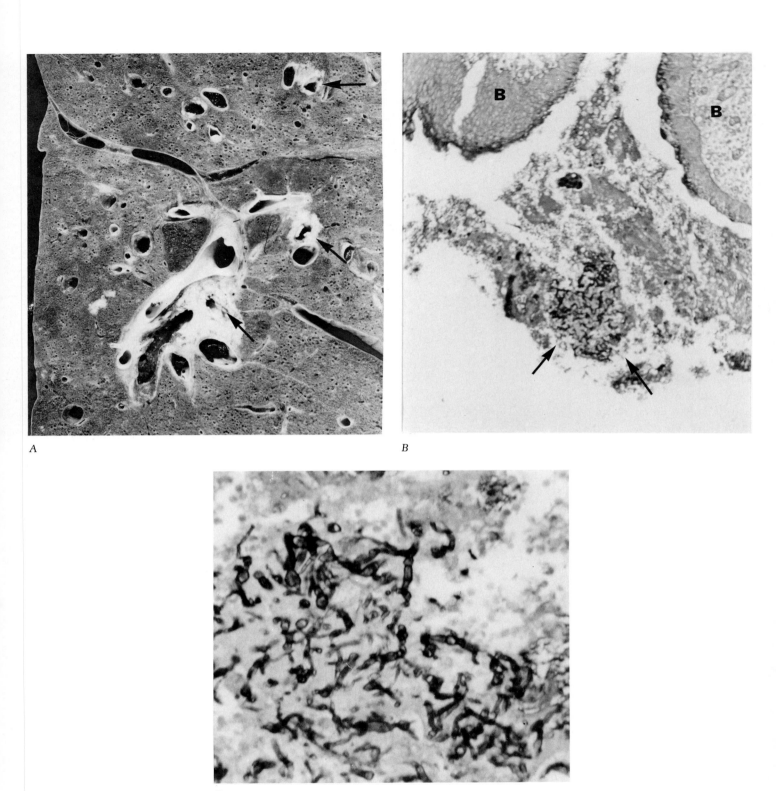

A

B

C

FIGURE 46-3 Bronchopulmonary aspergillosis in a 48-year-old man with severe asthmatic symptoms for 2 years. *A.* A sagittal section of the formaldehyde-perfused right lung shows destruction and plugging of bronchi by inspissated mucous secretions (arrows), ×2.1. *B.* Microscopic view of the bronchial wall (B) shows squamous metaplasia of the epithelium. The bronchial lumen is occupied by mucoid exudate containing *Aspergillus* hyphae (arrows). Methenamine silver, ×42. *C.* High-power view of the intrabronchial exudate reveals a large collection of hyphae with features of aspergillus. Methenamine silver, ×336.

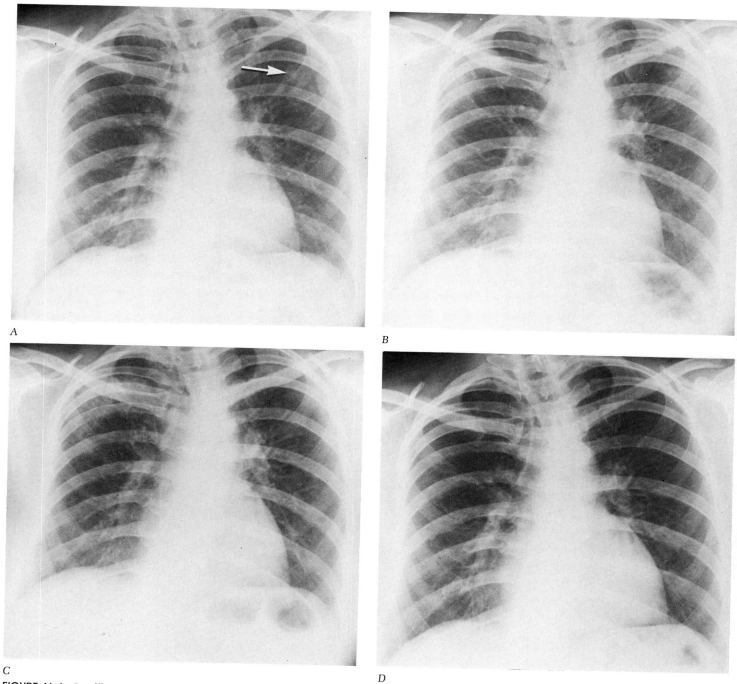

FIGURE 46-4 Loeffler's syndrome (simple eosinophilia). Patient with onset of fever and malaise 1 week before admission. No allergic history. Physical examination negative. Eosinophilia of 10 percent. *A.* Radiograph on admission. A soft infiltrate is present in left upper lobe (arrow). Scoliosis. *B.* One week later. Left upper lobe infiltrate persists, and new lesion has appeared in the right upper lobe. *C.* Two weeks later (4 weeks after onset). Spontaneous clearing of left upper lobe lesion; the infiltrate on the right is more marked. *D.* One month after C (8 weeks after onset). Complete spontaneous subsidence of symptoms and radiographic clearance. No cause found for infiltrates. No pathologic specimen was obtained.

to that of Bancroft's filariasis and filariasis malayi (Brug's filariasis). The disease is most common in southern Asia although it also occurs in Africa and South America. It is probably transmitted to humans by mosquitoes. An analogous condition exists in the United States where *Dirofilaria* infections occur in dogs, which serve as primary hosts.

The typical onset of tropical eosinophilia is insidious, generally beginning with a paroxysmal, dry cough that is worse at night and is frequently associated with dyspnea, wheezing, and hemoptysis. Scattered rales and rhonchi are sometimes heard all over the chest; enlargement of the liver and lymph nodes is common. The lymphadenopathy of tropical eosinophilia is sometimes difficult to distinguish from Hodgkin's disease, not only on clinical grounds but also histologically.

Eosinophilia is a regular feature and is often quite marked, occasionally constituting 90 percent of the total white count; leukocytosis is common, ranging from 15,000 to 50,000 cells per cubic millimeter. In about one-half of the patients, the radiograph shows diffuse mottling of both lung fields (Fig. 46-5), although at times the lesions are more localized. Hilar glandular enlargement sometimes occurs, particularly in children. The demonstration of the causative organism in circulating blood is difficult, and complement-fixing antibodies to filariae, although commonly present, are nonspecific. However, the causative parasite is often found in a biopsy of involved lymph nodes.

The treatment of tropical eosinophilia is diethylcarbamazine given orally, 5 to 6 mg/kg per day for 2 to 3 weeks. Aggravation of the clinical manifestations sometimes occurs early in the course of treatment. Over several weeks, however, the eosinophil count drops, and the radiographic changes disappear.

Pulmonary infiltrates with eosinophilia accompany both cutaneous and visceral infestation with larva migrans. *Creeping eruption* is the designation for the skin involvement in this disease. It is usually caused by the burrowing in the skin of the filariform larva of *Ancylostoma braziliense*, a hookworm that naturally infects dogs and cats. Since the sputum of these patients does not contain larvae, the lung manifestations are generally considered to be immunologic in origin.

Visceral larva migrans is a disease of patients who are in contact with soil that has been contaminated by dogs and cats. Wheezing, pulmonary infiltrates, urticaria, joint pains, and hyperglobulinemia are common. When *Toxocara canis* larvae are the cause, hepatomegaly is a major sign. Histologically, the parasite evokes a granulomatous response that is rich in giant cells and eosinophils.

It should be emphasized that eosinophilic lung disease in the tropics also accompanies parasitic infection with organisms other than filariae. During World War II a large number of American troops who were stationed in the Pacific area acquired helminthic infections and eosinophilia; *Ancylostoma duodenale* and *Strongyloides stercoralis* were the common offenders.

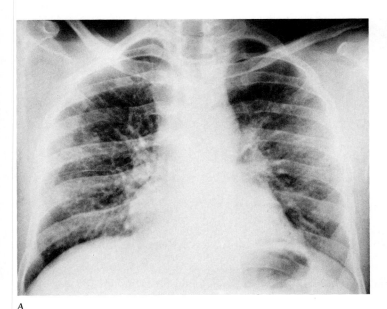 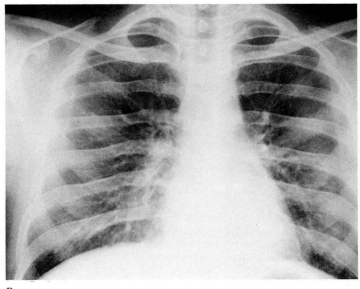

A   *B*

FIGURE 46-5 Tropical eosinophilia. A 24-year-old graduate student from India admitted with a 2-week history of cough with clear mucus. One year ago, he had identical cough with eosinophilia that responded in 20 days to diethylcarbamazine. On physical examination, inspiratory and expiratory wheezes and rhonchi were present over both lung fields. Eosinophilia 54 percent.   *A*. On admission. Disseminated linear and nodular interstitial changes with hilar and mediastinal prominence, possible nodes.   *B*. Radiograph, 3 weeks later. Complete clearing after a 12-day course of diethylcarbamazine 200 mg tid. At 12 h after onset of therapy, he had an acute onset of severe bronchospasm and dyspnea. This *Herxheimer* type of reaction, attributed to parasite death and release of antigen, is often seen in filariasis.

Drug-Induced Pulmonary Eosinophilia

A partial list of drugs and compounds that have been associated with eosinophilic pneumonia is given in Table 46-3. Nitrofurantoin (Furadantin) lung is the prototype. The prevalence of pulmonary disease due to nitrofurantoin reflects, in part, its widespread use as a prophylactic agent for urinary tract infections. Its reactions can be separated into two types, acute and chronic. The acute phase manifests with the clinical picture of eosinophilic pneumonia; the chronic phase begins insidiously and runs a more prolonged course, resembling chronic interstitial pneumonitis.

The acute phase usually begins 2 h to 10 days after the onset of a course of nitrofurantoin therapy. Clinical manifestations include dry cough, fever, chills, and dyspnea. Radiographically, the lung involvement is usually diffuse but is sometimes manifested by patchy infiltrates that neither migrate nor wax and wane as readily as those of Loeffler's syndrome. In addition to the blood eosinophilia, an important sign is the development of an eosinophilic pleural effusion: this finding has not been reported with drugs other than nitrofurantoin. Disappearance of the clinical, radiologic, and pathologic manifestations of the drug reaction along with the eosinophilia usually occurs when nitrofurantoin is discontinued. However, sometimes remission is slow, and steroid therapy is required to accelerate resolution. In some patients, residual fibrosis also occurs. Histologic confirmation of the diagnosis has been reported for the chronic variety but not for the acute. A feature of some diagnostic importance in drug-induced eosinophilic pneumonia is the development of systemic angiitis. It is quite likely that many instances of polyarteritis, periarteritis nodosa, and hypersensitivity angiitis that were associated with the use of sulfonamides in the late 1930s and 1940s fall within the spectrum of drug-related eosinophilic pneumonia.

Chronic Eosinophilic Pneumonia

At the other end of the spectrum from the benign Loeffler's syndrome is the uncommon, but distressing syndrome of chronic eosinophilic pneumonia described by Liebow, Carrington, and their associates. We have confirmed their descriptions in patients at the Hospital of the University of Pennsylvania. The clinical picture is that of an infection characterized by high fever, night sweats, loss of weight, and severe dyspnea. Most of the patients we have seen, like those in Carrington's series, have been white women. Most of Carrington's patients had previous clinical evidence of allergy; six developed asthma either a few months before the onset of the pulmonary lesions or coincident with them. Not all had peripheral eosinophilia; sputum eosinophilia was not mentioned. A major radiographic feature of the illness is the presence of dense pneumonic infiltrates that are distributed along the periphery of the lung in a pattern that has been likened to a photographic negative of the shadows seen in "butterfly" pulmonary edema (Fig. 46-6). Pathologic examination reveals an alveolar exudate consisting predominantly of a mixture of eosinophils and mononuclear cells.

Isolated case reports have added details to the clinical, radiographic, and pathologic picture described by Carrington et al. For example, instead of being a disorder exclusively of white women, the disorder has been reported in white men. The radiographic lesions may be less typical in distribution and occur in a more random pattern. Also, the inclusion of Charcot-Leyden crystals within alveolar macrophages has been emphasized. However, except for underscoring the probable immunologic bases for this disorder, few fresh insights have been provided into pathogenesis.

Corticosteroid therapy results in dramatic clinical, radiographic, and functional improvement generally within a few days. However, relapses are common after corticosteroids are discontinued, and the pulmonary lesions reappear in the original areas and pattern. Few long-term studies are available. But in a 5½- to 8-year follow-up of eight patients, two patients still required corticosteroids, four had been able to stop after an average of 4 years, and one patient had not required corticosteroids. Usually this entity is not associated with other diseases of hypersensitivity, but in one of our patients periarteritis nodosa developed 5 years later without any lung involvement.

Eosinophilic Pneumonia Associated with Bronchial Asthma

Eosinophilic pneumonia is associated with three forms of asthma: (1) uncomplicated bronchial asthma, (2) asthma with "mucoid impaction" of the bronchi, and (3) bronchopulmonary aspergillosis.

UNCOMPLICATED ASTHMA

Pulmonary eosinophilia appears to be uncommon in uncomplicated asthma. In a study of 5702 consecutive asthmatic individuals seen over a 5-year period, Ford (1966) identified only 20 patients with pulmonary eosinophilia. Some proved to have mucoid impaction (see below); whether a few others had aspergillosis is not clear. A wide variety of transient patterns were seen on the chest radiograph: 13 were patchy and confined predominantly to the upper zones, 3 were segmental, 2 hilar, and 2 miliary. In 14 of the 20 patients, the lesions disappeared in less than 3 weeks in response to antihistamines and sympathomimetic agents. Six required corticosteroid therapy to clear the infiltrate. Not all had uncomplicated asthma since some of the infiltrates cleared after aspiration of impacted mucus.

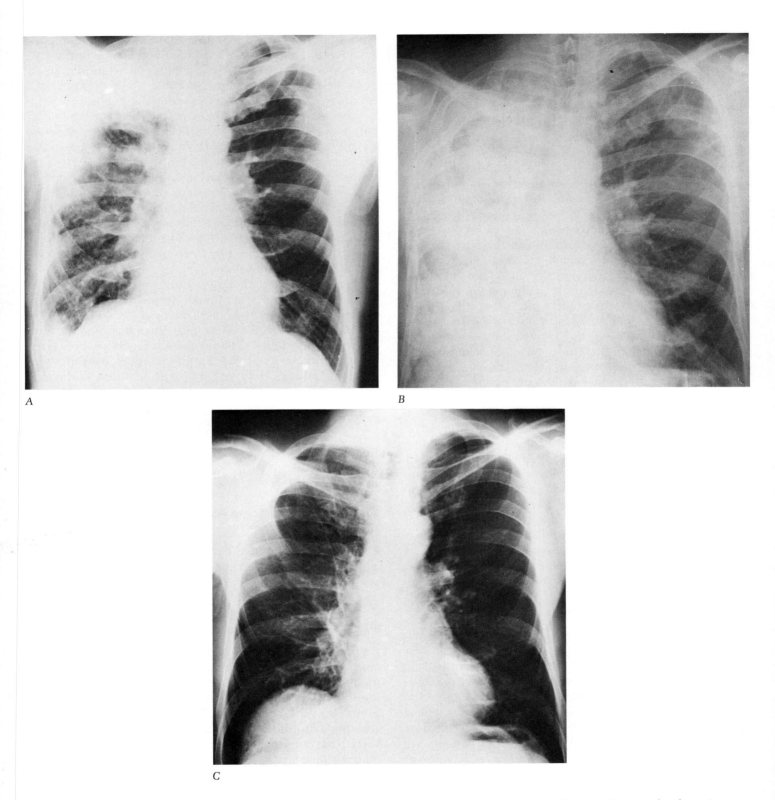

A

B

C

FIGURE 46-6 Eosinophilic pneumonia with bronchial asthma. A 43-year-old male with a history of childhood and seasonal asthma. Dyspnea for 3 months; fever and wheezing for 2 weeks. On admission, coarse rhonchi and fine rales over the right lung. White blood cell count; 39 percent eosinophils. *A.* Radiograph on admission. Bilateral, soft, peripheral, nonsegmental infiltrates. Lung biopsy showed classic pattern of eosinophilic pneumonia. *B.* Radiograph 3 weeks later. Progressive changes with almost complete consolidation of the right lung and additional peripheral infiltrates in the left lung. *C.* Radiograph, 7 weeks after *B*, after completing a course of prednisone 60 mg per day for 2 weeks, followed by gradual reduction of dose. Complete clearing of infiltrates.

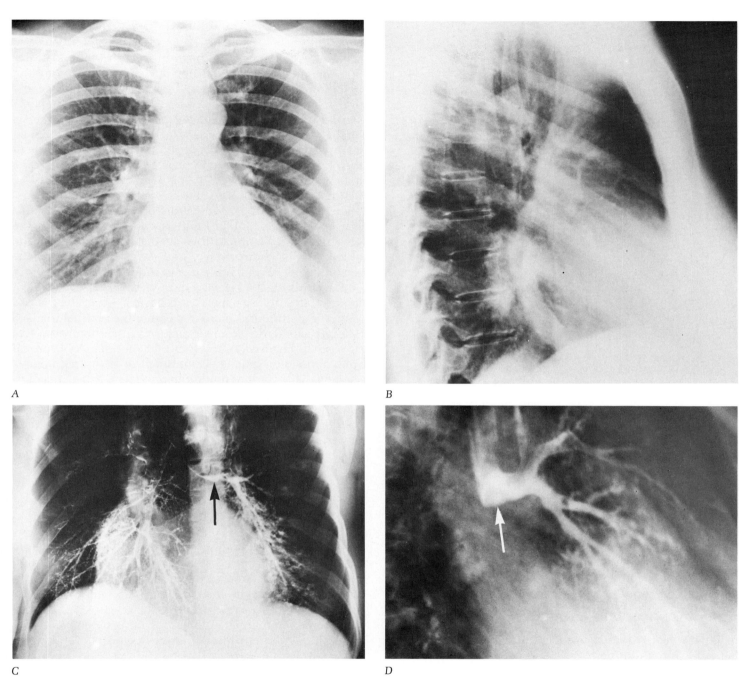

A *B*

C *D*

FIGURE 46-7 Mucoid impaction of bronchus. A 42-year-old white female with a 1-year history of cough. Physical examination normal. *A* and *B*. Radiographs on admission. Density is visible behind the heart on the lateral projection. *C* and *D*. Bronchograms showed cutoff of left lower lobe bronchus with a filling defect in the main bronchus (arrow). Bronchoscopy showed occlusion of left lower lobe bronchus; bronchoscopic biopsy showed "necrotic tissue." Lesions represent dilated impacted bronchi with associated pneumonitis. On resection, the patient proved to have mucoid impaction of right lower lobe bronchus with eosinophilic pneumonitis (see Fig. 46-8). No *Aspergillus* organisms were seen on silver methenamine stain.

MUCOID IMPACTION OF BRONCHI

Mucoid impaction of bronchi (Figs. 46-7 and 46-8) due to inspissated and trapped secretions is a vague and ill-defined entity and may occur without known allergy. It is seen most often in desert areas or areas of low humidity and may be due to desiccation of mucus under these con-ditions. It is essentially a bronchoscopic finding, as seen in postoperative patients who develop atelectasis from chest restriction due to pain. Mucoid impaction also oc-curs in patients with chronic bronchitis. Mucoid plugging may be present in asthma and in allergic bronchopulmon-ary aspergillosis. When mucoid impaction is associated

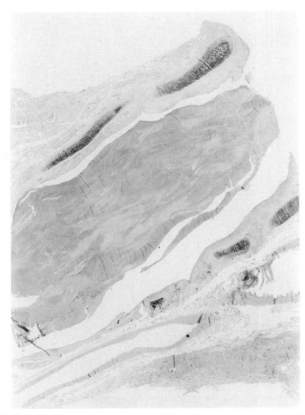

FIGURE 46-8 Mucoid impaction of bronchi in a 42-year-old female in Fig. 46-7. A large mucous plug fills the lumen of a major bronchus. Fibrosis of the bronchial wall and atrophy of cartilage. No fungi were seen on methenamine silver stain. H&E, ×10.

with a pulmonary infiltrate, it is reasonable to assume that the plug is producing an obstructive pneumonia or atelectasis, particularly if the pattern of the infiltrate is segmental. On the other hand, the infiltrate may represent an additional manifestation of hypersensitivity.

ALLERGIC BRONCHOPULMONARY ASPERGILLOSIS

In recent years allergic bronchopulmonary aspergillosis has come into prominence as a clinical entity. The disease was originally identified in the United Kingdom but is now recognized internationally. In Great Britain most instances of eosinophilic pulmonary infiltrations in extrinsic atopic asthmatics are attributed to *Aspergillus*. This association with aspergillosis does not seem to apply to intrinsic asthmatics who develop eosinophilic pneumonia. In the patient with bronchopulmonary aspergillosis, mucous plugging with expectoration of the plug occurs frequently, but infiltrates also appear without atelectasis. Allergic bronchopulmonary aspergillosis is suspected on the basis of five major criteria: (1) transitory pulmonary shadows, (2) eosinophilia of blood and sputum, (3) immunologic reactivity (IgE and IgG) to *Aspergillus fumigatus*

and rarely to other *Aspergillus* species, (4) asthma, and (5) isolation of the organism. The scattered patchy densities (Fig. 46-9) on the chest radiograph are attributed to eosinophilic pneumonia. In addition to changes of eosinophilic pneumonia, the central bronchi and bronchioles become dilated and bronchiectatic due to damage from the inspissated mucus in which hyphae can be identified. Diagnosis of allergic bronchopulmonary aspergillosis is established by repeated isolation of the organism, by demonstration of the characteristic septate hyphae by silver staining of the mucous plugs (Fig. 46-3*B*), or by immunologic testing. Characteristically, the patients have (1) a positive immediate skin test for *A. fumigatus*, (2) a delayed (type III) skin reaction (6 to 12 h) that is consistent with (3) the presence of IgG precipitins against *Aspergillus* in the blood, and (4) an extremely high level of total IgE in the serum. The level of IgE is a useful index of clinical activity and a guide to the effectiveness of therapy: the level of total IgE usually returns toward normal when the disease is under control and increases before the clinical relapse. Allergic aspergillosis sometimes progresses to obstructive disease of the airways and to bronchiectasis. As a general rule, permanent damage is more apt to follow asthma associated with bronchopulmonary aspergillosis than uncomplicated asthma. Therefore, continuing therapy with low levels of corticosteroids is commonly used in order to prevent repeated episodes and to decrease the likelihood of permanent damage.

DIFFERENTIAL DIAGNOSIS

Differential diagnosis of the eosinophilic pneumonias involves the consideration of a wide variety of pulmonary diseases; among these are bacterial pneumonia, pulmonary tuberculosis, and sarcoidosis. When blood and sputum eosinophilia are marked and associated with the distinctive radiographic changes, the diagnosis of eosinophilic pneumonia generally poses no problem. The emphasis then shifts to the etiologic diagnosis (Tables 46-2 and 46-3).

The conventional search for the etiology of eosinophilic pneumonia includes a detailed appraisal of clinical expressions of allergy, medications, environmental antigens, and parasites, followed by examination of blood and sputum for eosinophilia, and serial chest radiographs. Special attention is warranted for allergic bronchopulmonary aspergillosis. The essential diagnostic features have been itemized above. A few additional techniques are sometimes helpful. For example, mucous plugs require staining with a silver fungal stain, because *Aspergillus* organisms do not take the conventional stains that are used for histologic studies. Sometimes sputum cultures for tuberculosis, fungi, and other pathogens are in order.

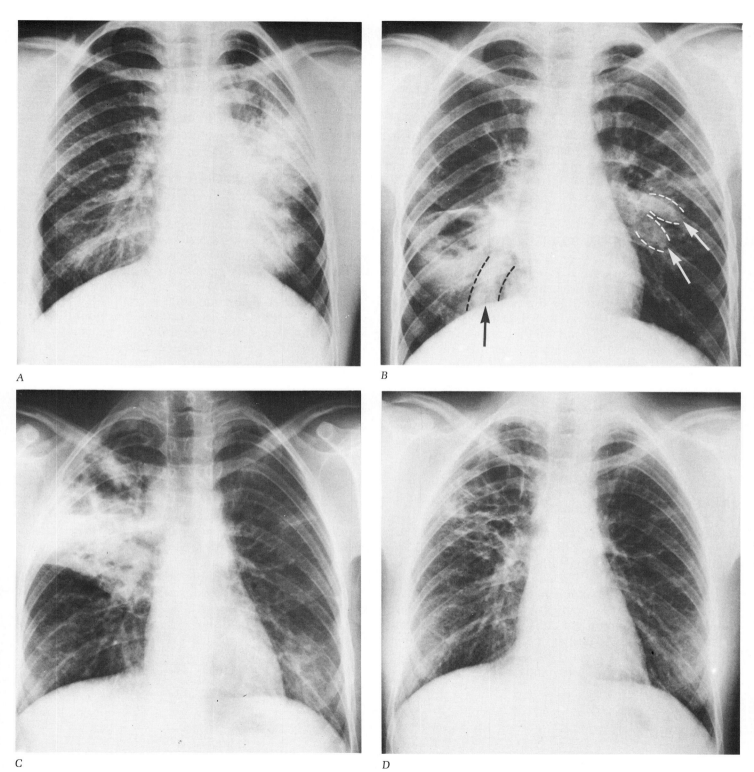

A

B

C

D

FIGURE 46-9 Bronchopulmonary aspergillosis. A 14-year-old girl with bronchial asthma and multiple episodes of pneumonitis, lung abscesses, and chronic bronchial infections. *A*. Radiograph on admission. Diffuse infiltrates, bilaterally, predominantly in right upper lobe. *B*. Six weeks later. A healed abscess is seen in the right lower lobe; bronchi are packed with mucous plugs (arrows). Dramatic resolution in response to antibiotic and steroid therapy. *C*. Ten years later. A right upper lobe cavitary, pyogenic pneumonia. At this time, eosinophilia of 20 percent, positive intermediate skin tests to *A. fumigatus*, precipitins to *Aspergillus*, and an IgE of 5000. She again responded to antibiotics plus prednisone. *D*. Ten weeks after *C*. Cystic residuals of the right upper lobe cavitary pneumonia with clear lung fields.

Since the eosinophilic pneumonia is generally self-limited, pathologic material usually is not sought. However, bronchoscopy is occasionally useful in collecting sputum or plugs for pathologic study, culture, or staining for eosinophils. In patients in whom the diagnosis of eosinophilic pneumonia is suspected but cannot be proved on clinical grounds, transbronchial lung biopsy sometimes settles the issue. Only on rare occasions is open lung biopsy undertaken: this procedure is generally reserved for those instances in which a specific diagnosis is needed to direct treatment and transbronchial biopsy has failed to provide the answer.

PULMONARY FUNCTION STUDIES

Pulmonary function studies in eosinophilic pneumonia are helpful in defining the type and extent of physiological impairment. Abnormalities are of three major types: (1) those of a restrictive variety when the parenchymal involvement is extensive and limits lung expansion; (2) an obstructive component that is usually reversible, which occurs in those patients with an underlying or associated bronchial asthma; (3) an increased intrapulmonic shunting with an increased alveolar-arterial gradient, reflecting ventilation-perfusion abnormalities in areas of consolidation and atelectasis. A mixed picture often results due to the presence of several or all of these components.

THERAPY

Therapy of eosinophilic pneumonia is prophylactic or therapeutic. Known atopic individuals are instructed to avoid exposure to potential allergens and to avoid indiscriminate use of drugs. Parasites are uncommon in the temperate climates, but exposure to dogs and cats is part of contemporary culture, and their parasites are a hazard to human beings. Careful search is undertaken for potential causative agents: parasites, drugs, allergens. If none are found, and if the process persists after a reasonable period of observation despite removal of potential causa-

tive agents, corticosteroid therapy is administered. A course of 40 to 60 mg of prednisone, or its equivalent, for 2 to 4 weeks is usually effective for control of the eosinophilic pneumonia. Relapses may occur after corticosteroids are discontinued and require resumption and more gradual withdrawal. The treatment of tropical eosinophilia due to filariasis with diethylcarbamazine was discussed earlier in this chapter.

EOSINOPHILIC PNEUMONIA IN COLLAGEN-VASCULAR DISEASE AND SYSTEMIC ANGIITIS

Eosinophilic pneumonia occurs as a part of the more serious hypersensitivity diseases. Periarteritis nodosa (PAN) was once considered to be the classic example of the association of eosinophilic pneumonia, systemic angiitis, and granulomatous disease. However, in 1951 Churg and Strauss distinguished from PAN a group of 14 patients with disseminated angiitis, asthma, eosinophilia, and fever. In this group, illness was fulminating, usually fatal, and was associated with a microscopic pattern of necrotizing angiitis, extravascular granuloma, and eosinophilic infiltration of tissues.

Differentiation between the conventional periarteritis nodosa (PAN) and the Churg-Strauss syndrome is based on several features of the two disorders: (1) neutrophilic leukocytes, rather than eosinophils, predominate in PAN; (2) the incidence of asthma is less in PAN, and extravascular granulomas are not found in PAN; (3) PAN affects small- and medium-sized arteries whereas the Churg-Strauss syndrome [allergic granulomatosis and angiitis (AGA)] affects small arteries and veins; and (4) elevated concentrations of IgE have been found in the serum of several patients with AGA, implicating the immediate hypersensitivity system in its pathogenesis.

Whether the separation of the Churg-Strauss syndrome from periarteritis nodosa will prove to be valid and of clinical value remains to be assessed. The prognosis of the Churg-Strauss syndrome, like that of periarteritis nodosa, is grave despite intensive corticosteroid therapy and immunosuppression.

BIBLIOGRAPHY

Archer GT, Blackwood A: Formation of Charcot-Leyden crystals in human eosinophils and basophils and study of the composition of isolated crystals. J Exp Med 122:173–176, 1965.
  Basic article on biochemistry of Charcot-Leyden crystals.

Carrington CB, Addington WW, Goff AM, Madoff IM, Marks A, Schwaber Jr, Gaensler EA: Chronic eosinophilic pneumonia. N Engl J Med 280:787–798, 1969.
  Additional cases and more detailed analysis of this syndrome (originally described by Christoforidis AJ and Molnar W, JAMA 173:157–161, 1960).

Chumbley LC, Harrison EG Jr, DeRemee RA: Allergic granulomatosis and angiitis (Churg-Strauss syndrome): Report and analysis of 30 cases. Mayo Clin Proc 52:477–484, 1977.
Relatively large number of cases with analysis of a relatively rare syndrome.

Cogen FC, Mayock RL, Zweiman B: Chronic eosinophilic pneumonia followed by polyarteritis nodosa complicating the course of bronchial asthma: Report of a case. J Allergy Clin Immunol 60:377–382, 1977.
Case showing interaction of these three diseases of altered immunity.

Cohen S: The eosinophil and eosinophilia. N Engl J Med 290:457–459, 1974.
Good summary of the literature to that period of time.

Cotran RS, Litt M: The entry of granule-associated peroxidase into the phagocytic vacuoles of eosinophils. J Exp Med 129:1291–1306, 1969.
Cellular biology of eosinophils and their granules.

Crofton JW, Livingstone JL, Oswald NC, Roberts ATM: Pulmonary eosinophilia. Thorax 7:1–35, 1952.
Early classification of the eosinophilia-associated syndromes.

Ehrlich P: Ueber die specifischen Granulationen des Blutes. Archiv fur Physiologie 1879:571–579 (abstract).
Ehrlich's discovery and description of the eosinophil.

Ford RM: Transient pulmonary eosinophilia and asthma: Review of 20 cases occurring in 5,702 asthma sufferers. Am Rev Respir Dis 93:797–803, 1966.
Most extensive study found in the literature.

Gonzalez EB, Swedo JL, Rajaraman S, Daniels JC, Grant JA: Ultrastructural and immunohistochemical evidence for release of eosinophilic granules in vivo: cytotoxic potential in chronic eosinophilic pneumonia. J Allergy Clin Immunol 79:755–762, 1987.
In a patient with relapsing idiopathic chronic eosinophilic pneumonia, evidence is provided for a cytotoxic potential of the eosinophil at the level of the pulmonary parenchyma.

Katzenstein A-L, Liebow AA, Friedman PJ: Bronchocentric granulomatosis, mucoid impaction, and hypersensitivity reaction to fungi. Am Rev Respir Dis 111:497–537, 1975.
Makes case for Aspergillus causing these syndromes.

Liebow AA, Carrington CB: The eosinophilic pneumonias. Medicine 48:251–257, 1969.
State of the art summary.

Liebow AA, Hannum CA: Eosinophilia, ancylostomiasis and strongyloidosis in the South Pacific area. Yale J Biol Med 18:381–392, 1946.
Description of these findings during World War II.

Loeffler W: Zur Differential-diagnoses der Lungeninfiltrierungen: Über flüchtige Succedaninfiltraten (mit Eosinophilie). Beitr Klin Tuberk 79:368–382, 1932.
Loeffler's original article bringing attention to the association of lung infiltrates, eosinophils, and parasites.

Lombard CM, Tazelaar HD, Krasne DL: Pulmonary eosinophilia in coccidioidal infections. Chest 91:734–736, 1987.
Two cases are reported of pulmonary eosinophilia associated with coccidioidal infections.

MacFadyen R, Tron V, Keshmiri M, Road JD: Allergic angiitis of Churg and Strauss syndrome. Response to pulse methylprednisolone. Chest 91:629–631, 1987.
In a steroid-dependent asthmatic patient with biopsy-proven Churg-Strauss syndrome, pulses of intravenous methylprednisolone resulted in dramatic clearing of widespread pneumonic process.

Ogushi F, Ozaki T, Kawano T, Yasuoka S: PGE2 and PGF2 alpha content in bronchoalveolar lavage fluid obtained from patients with eosinophilic pneumonia. Chest 91:204–206, 1987.
In two patients with eosinophilic pneumonia, the number of eosinophils and of prostaglandin (PG) E2 in BALF was greatly increased; treatment with corticosteroids restored the BALF to normal.

Pearson DJ, Rosenow EC III: Chronic eosinophilic pneumonia (Carrington's): A follow-up study. Mayo Clin Proc 53:73–78, 1978.
Gives prognosis of the cases of chronic eosinophilic pneumonia followed at the Mayo Clinic. Adds chronic eosinophilic pneumonia to Crofton's original classification of pulmonary eosinophilia.

Phills JA, Harrold AJ, Whiteman GV, Perelmutter L: Pulmonary infiltrates, asthma and eosinophilia due to *Ascaris suum* infestation in man. N Engl J Med 286:965–970, 1972.
    Review of Loeffler's syndrome.

Pinkston P, Vijayan VK, Nutman TB, Rom WN, O'Donnell KM, Cornelius MJ, Kumaraswami V, Ferrans VJ, Takemura T, Yenokida G, et al: Acute tropical pulmonary eosinophilia. Characterization of the lower respiratory tract inflammation and its response to therapy. J Clin Invest 80:216–225, 1987.
    Some of the abnormalities found in the lung in acute TPE are mediated by an eosinophil-dominated inflammatory process in the lower respiratory tract.

Reeder WH, Goodrich BE: Pulmonary infiltration with eosinophilia (PIE syndrome). Ann Intern Med 36:1217–1240, 1952.
    Description of the bases for their classification.

Rosenow EC III: The spectrum of drug-induced pulmonary disease. Ann Intern Med 77:977–991, 1972.
    Classic article of drug effects on lung (including those associated with eosinophilia).

Scadding JG: Eosinophilic infiltrations of the lungs in asthmatics. Proc R Soc Med 64:381–392, 1971.
    Early description of problem.

Sprent JFA: On the toxic and allergic manifestations produced by the tissue and fluids of *Ascaris*. Effect of different tissues. J Infect Dis 84:221–229, 1949.
    Demonstrates that metabolic products without parasites can cause pathologic picture of eosinophilic pneumonia.

Spry CJF: New properties and roles for eosinophils in disease. J Roy Soc Med 78:844–848, 1985.
    A succinct overview of the eosinophil as a primary mediator of the inflammatory response and of its relationship to the hypereosinophilic syndromes.

Urschel HC Jr, Paulson DL, Shaw RR: Mucoid impaction of the bronchi. Ann Thorac Surg 2:1–16, 1966.
    Surgical demonstration of this syndrome in southeastern United States.

von Meyenberg H: Das eosinophilie Lungeninfiltrat: Pathologische Anatomie und Pathogenese. Schweiz Med Wochenschr 23:809–811, 1942.
    First pathologic demonstration of parasites in lung tissue in cases of Loeffler's syndrome.

Wang JLF, Patterson R, Roberts M, Ghory AC: The management of allergic bronchopulmonary aspergillosis. Am Rev Respir Dis 120:87–92, 1979.
    Good summary of management.

Weingarten RJ: Tropical eosinophilia. Lancet 1:103–114, 1943.
    Excellent review of this disorder and parasites causing it.

Part 7

Interstitial Diseases

Chapter *47*

Nonimmunologic Defense Mechanisms

Joseph D. Brain

Inspired air contains considerable quantities of urban and occupational dusts, infectious particles, and cigarette smoke. Most of the pulmonary diseases discussed in the other chapters of this book are either initiated, or at least aggravated, by the inhalation of these particles and gases. Not only are the airways being reached by these pollutants, but also pharmacologic aerosols are being administered increasingly for therapeutic purposes, e.g., to relieve bronchospasm, for research in experimental pharmacology, and as probes of pulmonary function. After first considering how inhaled particles deposit in the respiratory tract, this chapter describes the clearance mechanisms of the lungs.

AEROSOL DEPOSITION

Depending on where aerosol particles land in the respiratory tract, deposition can be considered either as a defense mechanism or as a toxic threat. For example, nasal deposition prevents penetration of particles to airways and alveoli, whereas materials that settle in the respiratory tract pose a threat to vulnerable pulmonary structures. All particles that touch a surface are almost certain to deposit; the site of contact is the site of initial deposition. Physical forces operating on particles suspended in the inspired air cause them to move toward the surface of the respiratory tract; involved are inertial forces, sedimentation, Brownian diffusion, interception, and electrostatic forces.

Inertia is the tendency of moving particles to resist changes in direction and speed. Abrupt changes in the direction of airflow are caused by the repeated branching of the airways; because of inertia, particles tend to continue in their original direction, consequently impacting on airway walls. Gravity accelerates falling bodies downward, and terminal settling velocity is reached when viscous resistive forces are equal and opposite in direction to gravitational forces. Particles deposit when their settling causes them to strike airway walls or alveolar surfaces. Another mechanism of contact that leads to deposition of aerosol particles on respiratory surfaces is Brownian diffusion, a motion caused by collisions of gas molecules with particles suspended in the air.

The effectiveness of these deposition mechanisms depends on (1) the anatomy of the respiratory tract, (2) the aerodynamic diameters of the particles, and (3) the pattern of breathing. These factors determine the fraction of the inhaled particles that are deposited, as well as the site of deposition.

Effect of Anatomy

Deposition depends on the diameters of the airways, the angles of branching, and the average distances to alveolar walls. Along with the inspiratory flow rate, airway anatomy specifies the local linear velocity of the airstream. There are interindividual differences in the morphometry of the lungs; even within the same individual, the dimensions of the respiratory tract vary with changing lung volume, aging, and pathologic processes. Obstruction of airways or fibrotic parenchyma favors diversion of flow to healthy regions. Thus, in severe pulmonary disease, the remaining healthy airways and alveoli may be exposed to an increasing fraction of inspired irritant gases and particles. Narrowing of airways by mucus, inflammation, or bronchial constriction can increase linear velocities of airflow, enhance inertial deposition, and produce central patterns of deposition.

A highly significant change in the effective anatomy of the respiratory tract occurs when breathing switches from nose to mouth breathing, as during exercise or speech, or when the nose is bypassed by a tracheostomy or an endotracheal tube. In the nose, the combination of a small cross section for airflow, sharp curves, and interior nasal hairs all help to maximize linear velocity, turbulence, and impaction of particles. Large particles and water-soluble gases are removed efficiently. Bypass of the nose greatly increases the access of these inhaled materials to airways and alveoli.

Effect of Particle Size

The second major factor governing the effectiveness of deposition mechanisms is the size of the inspired particles. The effective aerodynamic diameter is a function of the size, shape, and density of the particles and affects the magnitude of forces acting on them. For example, while inertial and gravitational effects increase with increasing particle size, diffusion produces larger displacements as particle size decreases. Evaporation of particles or their hygroscopic growth may also alter size of particles, both inside and outside the respiratory tract.

Effect of Breathing Pattern

The remaining factor affecting deposition is the breathing pattern. Minute volume defines the average flow velocity of the air in the lung and the total number of particles entering the lungs. Respiratory frequency, tidal volume, and lung volume affect the time that aerosols reside in the lungs and, thereby, the probability of deposition of gravitational and diffusional forces. Changing lung volume also alters the dimensions of the airways and parenchyma.

Estimates of Deposition

The relationships among these parameters have been demonstrated by experiments and supported by theoretical treatments. Predictions indicate that changing the particle size not only affects the fraction deposited but alters the regional distribution of the retained particles as well.

Aerosol Retention

Deposition and clearance must be considered together when assessing risk of damage to the respiratory tract. It is the mass of the toxic substance in the lung not the amount in the air that is important. The actual amount of a substance present in the respiratory tract at any time is called the *retention*. When exposure to inhaled particles is continuous, the equilibrium concentration (achieved when the clearance rate matches the deposition rate) is also the retention. Thus, the relative rate constants of deposition and clearance determine the equilibrium levels; it is this equilibrium level, or retention integrated over time, and especially the properties of the particle that determine the probability, intensity, and duration of pathologic responses.

The distribution of particle size helps to determine the site of deposition and, hence, the clearance rates since some parts of the respiratory tract can clear much faster than others. Differences in particle size cause markedly different retentions even when the inhaled mass is the same. Figure 47-1 shows estimates of equilibrium retention levels in four compartments of the respiratory tract that followed inhalation of the same quantity of deposited particles; however, the particle size differed by factors of 10. It demonstrates that even when deposited mass is constant, changing particle size can dramatically affect the exposure of different parts of the respiratory tract. Solubility of the particles also has a great influence on clearance rates and, therefore, on retention.

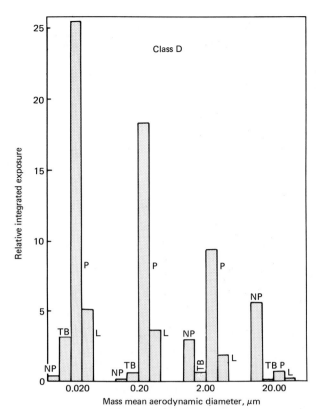

FIGURE 47-1 Equilibrium retention patterns in the respiratory tract as function of particle size. The respiratory tract is divided into four compartments: the nasopharynx (NP), the trachea and bronchi down to and including terminal bronchioles (TB), pulmonary (respiratory bronchioles to alveoli) (P), and pulmonary lymph vessels and nodes (L). *(From Brain and Valberg, 1974.)*

The clearance mechanisms of the lung are impressively effective. For example, in coal worker's pneumoconiosis, the diseased and blackened lungs of miners still contain less than 10 percent of the dust originally deposited there. Thus, even in the lungs seriously compromised by disease, the respiratory system remains surprisingly efficient at cleaning itself. The younger, healthy lung exhibits even greater potency in the pursuit of cleanliness.

CLEARANCE OF PARTICLES FROM THE RESPIRATORY TRACT

Different mechanisms are responsible for removal of deposited particles from the lungs. Highly soluble particles dissolve rapidly and are absorbed into the blood from the respiratory tract. Their metabolism and excretion resemble those of an intravenously injected dose of the same material. The role of high velocity airflow in removing deposited particles may become important when normal clearance mechanisms are either depressed or absent and when excess secretions are present. Irritation of the nose induces powerful physiological reflexes, such as sneezing, that help to remove unwanted particles from the nose. Similarly, the laryngeal epithelium and the airways contain cough and irritant receptors. Coughing creates airway narrowing as well as maximal expiratory flows. The very high linear velocities that are created in this way move mucus and debris along the airways. Momentum is transferred from gas moving at high velocity to the initially stationary, and much denser, mucus adhering to airway walls. Cough is effective in large airways but becomes less effective deeper in the lungs where total cross section for flow is greater and linear velocities are slower.

Mucociliary Transport and Airway Clearance

Although coughing can be important in dealing with excess secretions in central airways, in normal humans the major way of cleaning airways is by mucociliary transport. Particles that are deposited on the mucous blanket covering pulmonary airways are moved toward the pharynx by the cilia. Also present in this moving carpet of mucus are cells and particles which have been transported from the nonciliated alveoli to the ciliated airways. Similarly, particles deposited on the ciliated mucous membranes of the nose are propelled toward the pharynx. There, mucus, cells, and debris coming from the nasal cavities and the lungs meet, mix with salivary secretions, and after being swallowed, enter the gastrointestinal tract. Since the halftimes for removal of particles from the airways entail minutes to hours, there is little time for solubilization of slowly dissolving materials. In contrast, particles deposited in the nonciliated compartments have much longer residence times, and hence small differences to in vivo solubility can be of great importance there.

ANATOMIC BASIS

Most of the surface of the respiratory tract from the nose to the terminal bronchioles is covered with a mucous membrane composed of a pseudostratified ciliated columnar

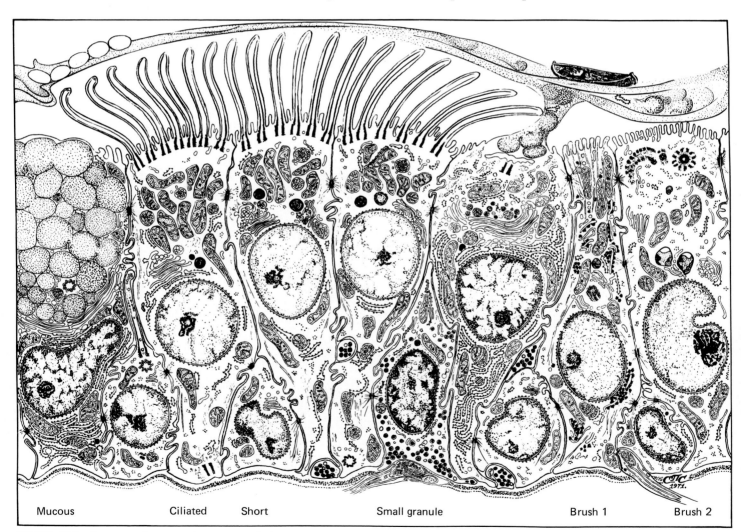

Mucous   **Ciliated**   **Short**   **Small granule**   **Brush 1**   **Brush 2**

FIGURE 47-2   Diagram showing ultrastructural characteristics of cells in the airway. (*Courtesy of Dr. S. P. Sorokin.*)

epithelium (Fig. 47-2). Although the term *pseudostratified* is used even though the nuclei found at different levels suggest that there are several layers of epithelial cells, serial sections show that each cell touches the basement membrane at some point. The primary cell type is the ciliated columnar cell which has numerous cilia extending from its free surface into the tracheal lumen (Fig. 47-3). There are approximately 270 cilia on each ciliated columnar cell or 1800 million cilia per square centimeter of mucosal surface. Also shown in Fig. 47-2 are the characteristic mucus-secreting cells called goblet cells. Chronic irritation of the tracheal or bronchial mucosa can lead to an increasing number of goblet cells.

Even more important in terms of the mass of secretions present are the submucosal glands which, in contrast to the goblet cells, are more influenced by the parasympathetic nervous system. The combined secretions of the goblet cells, submucosal glands, and other cells form a fluid layer which is located around, as well as above, the cilia and is moved mouthward by the cilia. This airway also contains cells, debris, alveolar lining fluid from the pulmonary parenchyma, secretions of airway cells, and transudates that reach the airways by passing through the bronchial epithelium.

PHYSIOLOGICAL BASIS

Particles that are deposited on the mucous blanket covering pulmonary airways are moved toward the pharynx by the cilia which beat at about 1000 times per minute. A number of factors affect the speed of mucous flow. They may be divided into two categories: those affecting the cilia themselves and those affecting the properties of the mucus. Certain aspects of ciliary action may affect mucous flow: the number of strokes per minute, the amplitude of each stroke, and time course and form of each stroke, the coordination of cilia, the length of the cilia, and the ratio of ciliated to nonciliated area. Intrinsic and extrinsic agents may also modify the rate and quality of ciliary motion.

The characteristics of the mucus are also of critical importance. The thickness of the mucous layer and its rheologic properties may undergo wide variations. Beginning with the classic work of Lucus and Douglas, others have shown that the mucous carpet is divided into two distinct layers: an outer, relatively viscous mucous layer that comes in contact with the cilia only during their active stroke; underneath the viscous layer is a more fluid layer (periciliary fluid) that surrounds the cilia and pro-

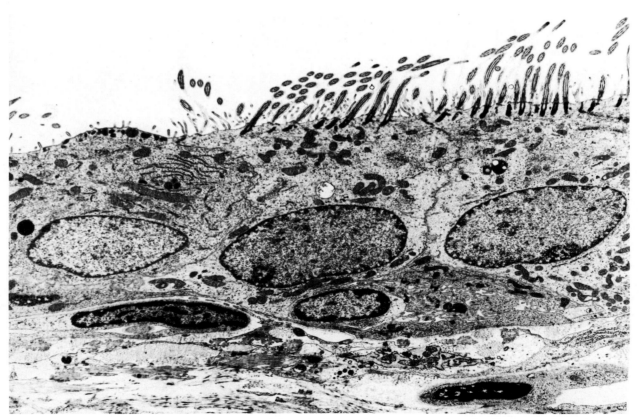

FIGURE 47-3 Electron micrograph of rat terminal bronchiolar epithelium. Two ciliated cells are on the right and a nonciliated bronchiolar epithelial (Clara) cell is on the left. ×6650. *(Courtesy of Dr. B. E. Barry.)*

vides a relatively frictionless medium in which the cilia move.

The quantity and quality of these two layers can profoundly affect the effectiveness of ciliary action. For example, slight drying could increase the viscosity of the mucous layer without affecting the underlying cilia; yet ciliary action might be less effective in moving the upper mucous layer. Or the fluid layer may become too deep, thereby elevating the viscous mucous sheet so that the cilia would no longer make effective contact with the fluid and would be unable to propel it along. Functional changes in mucociliary transport can be attributable primarily to alterations in the character of the secretions and not to direct injury to the ciliary mechanism. Unfortunately, distributions are not always made in published reports between ciliary motility on the one hand and the quantity and rheologic quality of the mucus on the other. As a result, they deal with interactions between the two processes, i.e., mucous transport rather than either one separately. Mucous secretion seems usually to be a more vulnerable process than is ciliary activity: in many instances, the quantity and rheologic characteristics of the polymeric gel that constitutes mucus can be affected independently of any change in the cilia.

Pulmonary Macrophages and Alveolar Clearance

ALVEOLAR MACROPHAGES

Pulmonary macrophages are credited with keeping the alveolar surfaces clean and sterile (Fig. 47-4). Alveolar macrophages are large, mononuclear, phagocytic cells found on the alveolar surface. The alveolar macrophages rest on the alveolar lining composed of pulmonary surface epithelial cells (type I pneumonocytes) and great alveolar cells (type II pneumonocytes). It is the phagocytic and lytic potential of the alveolar macrophages that provides most of the known bactericidal properties of the lungs. Like other phagocytes, alveolar macrophages are rich in lysosomes. The lysosomes attach themselves to the phagosomal membrane surrounding the ingested pathogen. Then the lysosomal membranes become continuous with the phagosomal membrane, and the lytic enzymes enter to kill and digest the bacteria. Among the hydrolases they are known to contain are proteases, deoxyribonuclease, ribonuclease, β-glucuronidase, and acid phosphatase. Generation of oxygen radicals is also important. Although these enzymes constitute an important aspect of the lung's defensive posture, the digestive capability of macrophages kept in a chronically activated state may damage

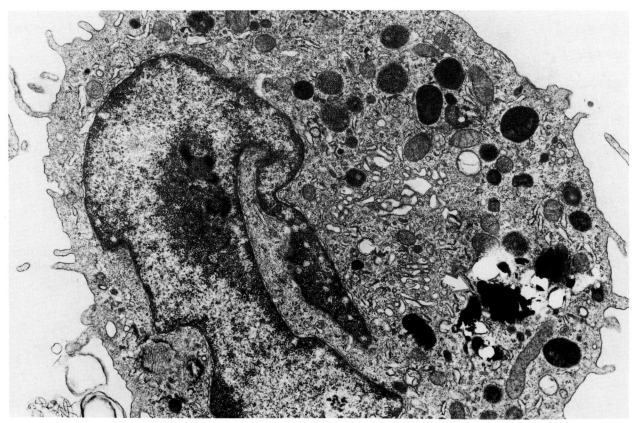

FIGURE 47-4 Alveolar macrophage recovered from a hamster by lung lavage. The cell contains ingested electron dense iron oxide particles (see arrow). About 1 month earlier the animal breathed an aerosol of Fe_2O_3. On the lower left, near the nucleus, another phagosome can be seen. This one contains tubular myelin probably derived from the alveolar lining layer. $\times 11,000$ *(Courtesy of Ms. R. C. Stearns.)*

pulmonary tissues. Release of lysosomal enzymes, particularly proteases, from macrophages and neutrophils may be involved in the development of emphysema; release may occur as a consequence of cell death, cell injury, or exocytosis. Increased deposition of inert or infectious particles acts to recruit additional macrophages and, thus, to reinforce the effect.

Another concern is the ability of macrophages to ingest nonliving, insoluble dust and debris. Figure 47-4 shows a hamster alveolar macrophage that has ingested considerable iron oxide. Rapid endocytosis of insoluble particles prevents penetration of particles through the alveolar epithelia and facilitates alveolar-bronchiolar transport. Macrophages laden with dust do not seem to be able to reenter the alveolar wall; free particles appear to have a greater likelihood of penetrating the alveolar epithelium. Thus, phagocytosis plays an important role in preventing the entry of particles into the fixed tissues of the lung. Once particles such as silica or asbestos leave the alveolar surface and penetrate the tissues subjacent to the air-liquid interface, their removal is slowed. Particles remaining on the surface are cleared with biologic half-lives estimated to be days to months, whereas the half-lives of particles that have penetrated into "fixed" tissues are much longer. The limiting factor is probably their in situ solubility. Therefore, the probability that particles will penetrate into fixed tissues is critical in determining their clearance from the lungs.

AIRWAY MACROPHAGES

During the last few years, it has become increasingly obvious that not all pulmonary macrophages are alveolar macrophages. Another important kind of pulmonary macrophage is the airway macrophage. These mononuclear cells are present in both large and small conducting airways. They may be present as passengers on the mucous escalator, or they may be found beneath the mucous lining, apparently adhering to the bronchial epithelium. These airway macrophages are probably alveolar macrophages transported to the airways from alveoli and bronchioles, although it is also possible that they are the product of direct migration of cells through the bronchial epithelium. The number, appearance, and distribution of airway macrophages is markedly influenced by the method of fixation; intravascular perfusion is preferred. Their ability to ingest particles and kill pathogens may be important to the airways.

INTERSTITIAL MACROPHAGES

The third kind of pulmonary macrophage is the interstitial macrophage found in the various connective tissue compartments in the lung. These include alveolar walls, sinuses of the lymph nodes and nodules, and peribronchial and perivascular spaces. Since interstitial macrophages may be in direct contact with elastin and collagen as well as with fibroblasts, their secretions are probably very important in the pathogenesis of interstitial lung disease.

OTHER PULMONARY MACROPHAGES

In addition to these three primary types, there are also other minor compartments of macrophages. For example, macrophages in the pleural space not only play a defensive role but may also act as miniature "roller bearings" that facilitate movements between the parietal and visceral pleura. A few macrophages may be found within the lumens of pulmonary capillaries (Fig. 47-5). These resemble the Kupffer cells within hepatic sinusoids; in ruminants and pigs, these macrophages are plentiful, prominent, and functionally important. They are capable of removing inert particles and bacteria from the circulation (Fig. 47-5C).

Macrophages from a single compartment need not be homogeneous. Heterogeneity is common both in structure and function. Considerable variability has been found among macrophages recovered by bronchoalveolar lavage. Using continuous-density gradients of colloidal silica, different fractions of macrophages recovered from normal rats by bronchoalveolar lavage were found to differ in their morphologic, cytochemical, and functional properties. Monoclonal antibodies have also been used to characterize heterogeneity. For example, Harbison et al., using an antibody against a specific antigen on the surface of hamster alveolar macrophages, showed that it is not present on macrophages from other organs or on other lung cells; this antigen develops after macrophages emerge onto the alveolar surface. They also separated pulmonary macrophages into four subpopulations that differed in both their length of time on the alveolar surface (as shown by [³H]-thymidine labeling) and the density of antigen on their plasma membrane.

FATE OF MACROPHAGES

Differences exist between the fates of the various classes of pulmonary macrophages: macrophages may be subject to alveolobronchiolar transport mechanisms; they may enter the lymphatics or connective tissue, or they may enter the circulation. Finally, it is also possible that some never leave the alveolar surface but persist for weeks or months, die there, and are then ingested and digested by younger, more vigorous siblings.

Despite much speculation, little is known about the mechanisms responsible for alveolar-bronchiolar transport. It is clear that most particles deposited in alveoli are ingested by alveolar macrophages. Some of these cells find their way to the bronchioles and are then carried to the pharynx by ciliary action. Although it is not possible to discount migration through alveolar pores, or other col-

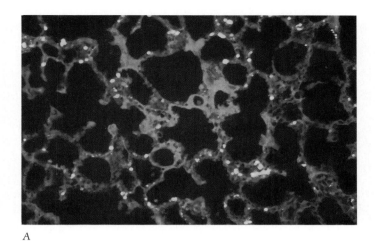

A

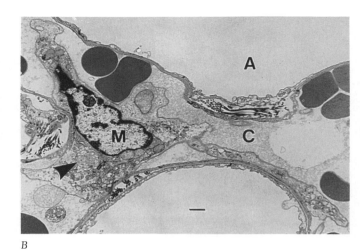

B

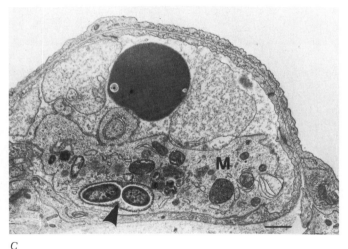

C

FIGURE 47-5 Intravascular macrophages in the sheep lung. A. Intravenous injection of fluorescent latex microspheres (1 μm in diameter) reveals a population of large phagocytic cells within alveolar walls (capillaries) containing the particles. ×225 (From Wheeldon and Hansen-Flaschen, 1986.) B. Electron micrograph showing a large pulmonary intravascular macrophage (M) in sheep lung. The macrophage is closely apposed to the capillary endothelial cell at some points. It is irregular in shape and has a large phagocytic vacuole (arrow). A = alveolar space; C = capillary lumen. ×4200. Bar = 1 μm. (Courtesy Dr. A. Warner.) C. Electron micrograph of a sheep lung capillary after intravenous injection of Pseudomonas aeruginosa. Two bacterial cells can be seen within a phagosome (arrow) of an intravascular macrophage (M). ×6600. Bar = 1 μm. (Courtesy Dr. A. Warner.)

lateral pathways between adjacent bronchial paths, almost all the macrophages that have been seen appear to be on the surfaces of alveoli and bronchi.

Since some macrophages find their way to airways, one important question is how these cells find the mucous escalator. One possibility is that macrophages exhibit directed locomotion by virtue of a concentration gradient of a chemotactic factor. The phenomenon of chemotaxis has been well studied in vitro, particularly for neutrophils, but far less for macrophages. Little is known about the chemotactic behavior of alveolar macrophages, and no observations have been made of alveolar macrophage movement in situ.

It has often been suggested that alveolar macrophages enter directly into lymphatic pathways and connective tissue; most of the available evidence is unconvincing. The mere presence of particle-containing macrophages in these compartments is not compelling evidence since it is not easy to distinguish between the entry of alveolar macrophages and the entry of bare particles that are subse-

quently ingested by preexisting connective tissue macrophages. It seems reasonable that, during alveolar clearance, some particles may travel via lymphatic or vascular channels from alveoli into the peribronchial, perivascular, or subpleural adventitiae, thereby entering the connective tissue of the lung; there, they are stored by resident macrophages. This route may be more accessible in permeability pulmonary edema when a greater number of particles might pass into lymphatic vessels via clefts between endothelial cells, to be carried along lymphatic drainage paths until filtered out by macrophages situated farther along in lymphoid foci.

However, recently convincing evidence was provided for the migration of surface macrophages into connective tissue compartments. Using red fluorescent and green fluorescent microspheres instilled into separate adjacent areas of dog lung lobes, Harmsen et al. showed that some particle-containing alveolar macrophages had indeed migrated to the tracheobronchial lymph nodes (Fig. 47-6). Although an uncommon event, macrophage migration

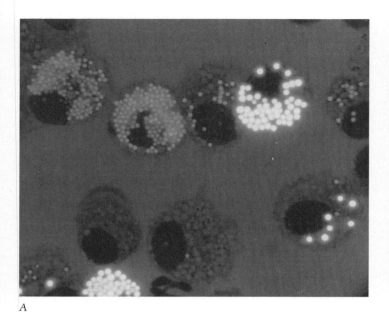
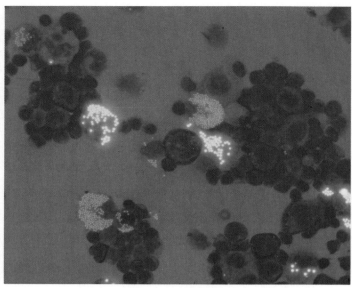

A   B

FIGURE 47-6 Migration of particle-laden macrophages from alveoli to regional tracheobronchial lymph nodes. Centrifugated preparations made 7 days after installation of red (orange) and green (yellow) fluorescent particles (1 to 3 μm in diameter) into adjacent lobes of a dog lung via a fiberoptic bronchoscope. *A.* Recovered by pulmonary lavage. ×1000. *B.* Recovered from cell suspension of regional transbronchial lymph nodes. As in *A,* the macrophages contain either the red (orange) or green (yellow) particles but rarely both, suggesting that alveolar macrophages had migrated to the regional nodes carrying particles with them. ×400. (*From Harmsen, Muggenburg, Snipes, and Bice, 1985.*)

may be important since it does provide a pathway for antigens, either in or on alveolar macrophages, to meet reactive lymphocytes in the connective tissue.

With respect to insoluble dusts, although estimates indicate that the percentage of particles cleared via the lymphatics is small, the importance of particles entering the lymphatics is great because particles in lymphatics are slowly cleared. Months and years after exposure to particles, these connective tissue burdens may constitute the major reservoir of retained particles.

SECRETION AND REGULATION

Macrophages have many functions in addition to phagocytosis. They secrete a variety of substances that interact with multienzyme cascades and with other cells such as lymphocytes, fibroblasts, and other macrophages. Thus, the macrophage both responds to, and regulates, its external environment. Interactions between alveolar macrophages and lymphocytes may be involved in the suppression or induction of immunologic pulmonary disease. Macrophages are also involved in the presentation of antigens and interact with the helper-inducer set of T lymphocytes.

Some macrophage secretions, e.g., collagenase, elastase, and lysosomal enzymes, are involved in the turnover of connective tissue. Other secretions affect lymphoid cells by helping to regulate mitogenesis and differentia-

tion. Macrophages release additional products such as interferon, fibronectin, lysozyme, and certain components of complement. Other biologically active materials secreted by macrophages include an angiogenesis factor, plasminogen activator, prostaglandins, nucleosides, cyclic nucleotides, pyrogens, granulopoietins, and factors influencing fibroblast proliferation and tumor growth. Still other agents may interact with humoral enzyme systems such as the clotting, complement, fibrinolytic, and kinin-generating systems.

PATHOPHYSIOLOGY OF PULMONARY MACROPHAGES

Although pulmonary macrophages are essential to host defense, the activity and movement of pulmonary macrophages may also cause harm. Because macrophages are professional phagocytes, inhaled toxic, radioactive, or carcinogenic particles become concentrated with them. What begins as a diffuse and uniform exposure becomes highly localized and nonuniform. "Hot spots" can be formed and be injurious.

Similarly, adherence of some airway macrophages to the airway epithelium may increase airway exposure to inhaled toxic materials. More important, perhaps, this close association with the bronchial epithelium can lead to transbronchial transport of inhaled particles and subsequent reingestion by subepithelial connective tissue macrophages. These cells, like their relatives in the alveolar and airway compartments, also segregate, retain, and perhaps metabolize carcinogenic and other toxic particles.

Another way in which macrophages may be involved is through diminution or failure of their defensive role. Studies using in vivo and in vitro bactericidal and phagocytic assays have shown that macrophage function can be compromised by environmental insults and pathologic changes. Such diverse agents as silica, immunosuppressives, surgical trauma, ethanol intoxication, cigarette smoke, air pollution, and oxygen toxicity can depress the ability of pulmonary macrophages to protect their host.

There are situations in which pulmonary macrophages not only fail but also contribute directly to the pathogenesis of pulmonary diseases. For example, macrophages play a pivotal role in the pathogenesis of two groups of pulmonary diseases involving aberrations of normal collagen and elastin balance, i.e., emphysematous and fibrotic disorders.

RELATED SYSTEMS

Although this book separates immunologic from nonimmunologic defense mechanisms, nature is far less compartmentalized. Specific recognition works in concert with more general defenses such as phagocytosis. All components of the immune system such as lymphocytes and immunoglobulins work with phagocytic cells. Both systemic and local respiratory immune mechanisms are involved in protection of the host and in the pathogenesis of some respiratory diseases, e.g., bronchial asthma or allergic alveolitis. Many other features of the airway and alveolar microenvironment are also involved. For example, factors regulating the production and degradation of surfactant, as well as other influences on alveolar stability, affect not only pulmonary mechanics, but also the ability of macrophages to function on alveolar surfaces. Pulmonary defenses must be appreciated as an integrated, overlapping system of considerable power.

BIBLIOGRAPHY

Brain JD: Macrophages in the respiratory tract, in Fishman AP, Fisher AB (eds), *Handbook of Physiology, sec 3: The Respiratory System, vol I: Circulation and Nonrespiratory Functions.* Bethesda, American Physiological Society, 1985, pp 447–471.
   A review of macrophages in the respiratory tract, emphasizing their origin, fate, physiological role, and methods of measuring the phagocytic property of pulmonary properties.

Brain JD, Proctor DF, Reid LM (eds), *Respiratory Defense Mechanisms, vol 5, parts I and II, Lung Biology in Health and Disease.* New York, Dekker, 1977.
   A two-volume, multiauthored book describing the diverse physiological mechanisms which prevent the accumulation and deleterious action of inhaled particles and gases.

Brain JD, Valberg PA: Models of lung retention based on the report of the ICRP Task Group. Arch Environ Health 28:1–11, 1974.
   Mathematical models of deposition and clearance of particles in the lungs.

Brain JD, Valberg PA, Sneddon SL: Mechanisms of aerosol deposition and clearance, in More F, Newhouse MT, Dolovich MB (eds), *Aerosols in Medicine—Principles, Diagnosis, and Therapy.* Amsterdam, Elsevier, 1985, pp 123–147.
   A review of mechanisms of particle deposition and clearance.

Chandler DB, Fuller WC, Jackson RM, Fulmer JD: Fractionation of rat alveolar macrophages by isopycnic centrifugation: Morphological, cytochemical, biochemical and functional properties. J Leukocyte Biol 39:371–383, 1986.
   Different populations of pulmonary macrophages are produced by differential centrifugation and then characterized in terms of their morphology, biochemistry, and function.

Fels AOS, Cohn ZA: The alveolar macrophage. J Appl Physiol 60:353–369, 1986.
   A recent comprehensive discussion of alveolar macrophages stressing their secretory and regulatory role.

Harbison ML, Godleski JJ, Mortara AM, Brain JD: Correlation of lung macrophage age and surface antigen in the hamster. Lab Invest 50:653–658, 1984.
   A monoclonal antibody and autoradiography are used to describe lung macrophage heterogeneity.

Harmsen AG, Muggenburg BA, Snipes MB, Bice DE: The role of macrophages in particle transloca-tion from lungs to lymph nodes. Science 230:1277–1280, 1985.
Fluorescent particles are used to trace the movement of lung macrophages into connective tissue.

Herscowitz HB: In defense of the lung: Paradoxical role of the pulmonary alveolar macrophage. Ann Allergy 55:634–648, 1985.
This review emphasizes the troublesome aspects of alveolar macrophages.

Leith DE, Butler JP, Sneddon SL, Brain JD: Cough, in Macklem PT, Mead J (eds), *Handbook of Physiology, sect 3: The Respiratory System, vol III: Mechanics of Breathing.* Bethesda, American Physiological Society, 1986, pp 315–336.
The physiology and pathophysiology of cough is described.

Lopez-Vidriero MT, Das I, Reid LM: Airway secretion: Source, biochemical and rheological proper-ties, in Brain JD, Proctor DF, Reid LM (eds), *Respiratory Defense Mechanisms, vol 5, part I, Lung Biology in Health and Disease.* New York, Dekker, 1977, pp 289–346.
The rheologic properties, biochemical constituents, and functional significance of airway secre-tions is discussed.

Satir P, Dirksen ER: Function-structure correlations in cilia from mammalian respiratory tract, in Fishman AP, Fisher AB (eds), *Handbook of Physiology, sect 3: The Respiratory System, vol I: Circulation and Nonrespiratory Function.* Bethesda, American Physiological Society, 1985, pp 473–494.
The structure and function of cilia are described as are general features of the mucociliary transport system.

Sorokin SP, Brain JD: Pathways of clearance in mouse lungs exposed to iron oxide aerosols. Anat Rec 181:581–626, 1975.
The fate of inhaled iron oxide in the murine lung is illustrated by extensive micrographs.

Valberg PA: Determination of retained lung dose, in Witschi HP, Brain JD (eds), *Toxicology of Inhaled Materials.* Berlin, Springer-Verlag, 1985, pp 57–85.
Methods for measuring retained particles in the respiratory tract, as well as principles influenc-ing their deposition, are described.

Warner AE, Barry BE, Brain JD: Pulmonary intravascular macrophages in sheep. Morphology and function of a novel constituent of the mononuclear phagocyte system. Lab Invest 55:276–288, 1986.
Through functional and anatomic studies, the presence of macrophages within pulmonary cap-illaries of ruminants is documented.

Warner AE, Molina RM, Brain JD: Uptake of bloodborne bacteria by pulmonary intravascular mac-rophages and consequent inflammatory responses in sheep. Am Rev Respir Dis 136:683–690, 1987.
Lung injury is caused by uptake of bacteria by macrophages within the alveolar capillaries of the sheep lung.

Werb Z: How the macrophage regulates its extracellular environment. Am J Anat 166:237–256, 1983.
A review of how macrophages influence their neighbors by secreting mediators.

Wheeldon EB, Hansen-Flaschen JH: Intravascular macrophages in the sheep lung. J Leukocyte Biol 40:657–661, 1986.
Fluorescent particles are used to demonstrate resident macrophages within the alveolar capil-laries of the sheep lung.

Winkler GC, Cheville NF: Postnatal colonization of porcine lung capillaries by intravascular mac-rophages: an ultrastructural, morphometric analysis. Microvasc Res 33:224–232, 1987.
In lungs of newborn pigs and 7- and 30-day-old pigs perinatal colonization of the porcine lungs by monocytes that replicate and differentiate into large, highly phagocytic, resident, intravascu-lar macrophages.

Chapter *48*

Reactions of the Interstitial Space to Injury

Ronald G. Crystal / Victor J. Ferrans

Anatomy of the Alveolar Interstitium
  Basement Membranes
  Connective Tissue Matrix
  Mesenchymal Cells
  Inflammatory Cells
  Other Molecules

Functions of the Alveolar Interstitium
  Defining the Alveolar Architecture
  Contribution to Mechanical Behavior
  Modulation of Alveolar-Capillary Exchange
    of Plasma Constituents
  Lower Respiratory Tract Defense

Maintenance of the Interstitium
  Production of Connective Tissue
  Degradation of Connective Tissue
  Turnover of Mesenchymal Cells
  Inflammatory Cell Traffic
  Fluid and Solute Movements through the Interstitium

Processes Mediating the Patterns of Injury to the Interstitium
  Inflammation
  Mesenchymal Cell Chemotaxis, Proliferation, and Deposition
    of Connective Tissue
  Locally Produced Injurious Products
  Xenobiotics
  Accumulation of Extracellular Molecules
  Ischemia

Consequences of Interstitial Injury to Lung Structure
  Distortion-Type Injury
  Fibrosis-Type Injury
  Destruction-Type Injury

Functional Consequences of Interstitial Injury
  Mechanical Consequences of Interstitial Injury
  Sensation of Dyspnea
  Alterations in Gas Exchange
  Reversibility of Lung Dysfunction

Familiar Examples of Interstitial Injury

The alveolar interstitium is a thin sheet of tissue in the alveolar wall that is bounded by the basal surfaces of the alveolar epithelial and endothelial cells. It is part of a continuum that includes the sheaths around the bronchial and pulmonary vascular trees, extends distally to all alveoli, and is connected to the perilobular and subpleural tissues. The alveolar interstitium plays a critical role in defining both the architecture and mechanical properties of the alveolar walls, providing the structural support for the epithelial and endothelial cells and modulating the behavior of the alveolar wall during respiration.

Although the alveolar interstitium may be the seat of infection and invasion by neoplastic cells, this chapter deals only with the nonmalignant, noninfectious, chronic disorders affecting the interstitium of the lower respiratory tract. The alveolar interstitium plays a central role in the major chronic diseases of the lower respiratory tract that are traditionally categorized into three groups: (1) the interstitial lung disorders of known etiology, (2) the interstitial lung disorders of unknown etiology, and (3) emphysema. However, from a pathogenetic point of view, they can be categorized differently, on the basis of the dominant pattern of injury to the alveolar interstitium (Figs. 48-1 to 48-4), including: (1) *distortion*, a process in which the interstitium is widened by the accumulation of cells and/or extracellular materials; (2) *fibrosis*, a process in which the normal interstitium is damaged and replaced by an increased number of mesenchymal cells and their connective tissue products; and (3) *destruction*, a process in which the integrity of the interstitium is lost.

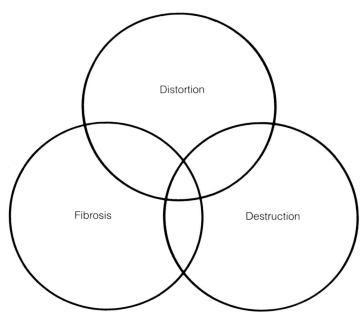

FIGURE 48-1   The three dominant patterns of injury to the alveolar interstitium in the chronic nonmalignant disorders of the lower respiratory tract. Although each defined disorder is almost always dominated by one form of injury over the others, many diseases include some mixture of two or all three types of injury.

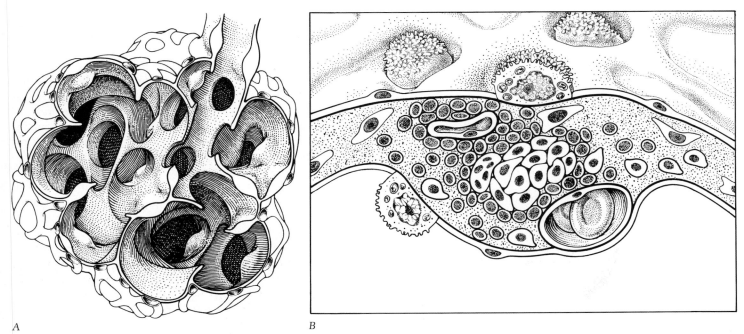

FIGURE 48-2 Schematic of the changes typical of distortion-type injury to the lower respiratory tract. *A.* Overview of many alveoli. *B.* Close-up view of a cutaway surface of an alveolar wall. Note that the alveolar wall is distorted, yet the individual cellular components are generally intact.

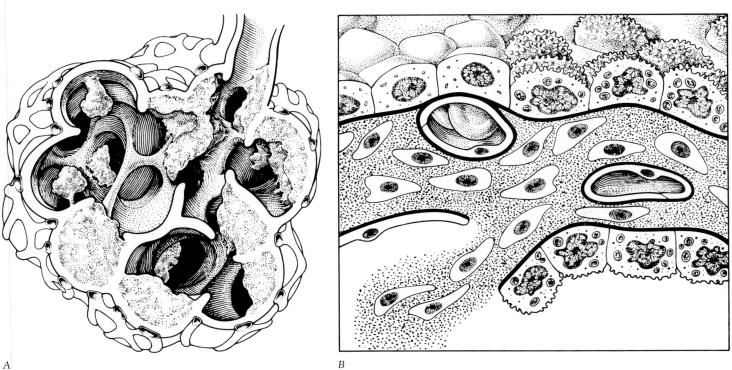

FIGURE 48-3 Schematic of the changes of fibrosis-type injury to the lower respiratory tract. *A.* Overview of many alveoli. *B.* Close-up view of a cutaway surface of one alveolar wall. The type I epithelial cells are damaged and replaced by cuboidal cells, including type II cells and epithelial cells migrating from the bronchioles. The endothelial cells are damaged and the pulmonary capillaries compressed. The interstitium is thickened by fibrous tissue. Intra-alveolar fibrosis is developing in some areas, mural incorporation in others (see text).

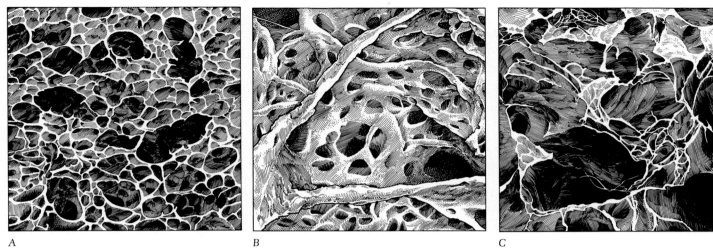

FIGURE 48-4 Schematic of the changes typical of destruction-type injury to the lower respiratory tract. *A.* Normal alveoli. *B.* Destruction-type injury in an area similar to that in panel *A.* *C.* Close-up view of an area of destruction. The alveolar walls are partially or completely destroyed, leaving large airspaces, i.e., emphysema.

In approaching diseases of the alveolar interstitium from the pathogenetic point of view, three caveats are necessary. First, although modifications of the interstitium cause alterations in lung function, the interstitium is not an isolated structure: the distortion, fibrosis, and destructive types of injury almost invariably involve the whole of the alveolar walls to some degree.

Second, the term *injury* refers to a change in the alveolar walls from their normal state, rather than only to overt damage. This concept is particularly relevant to the use of the term *fibrosis-type injury* to refer collectively to the processes of damage to the alveolar walls and the scarring which follows.

Third, although distortion, fibrosis, and destruction will be discussed as if they were distinct, independent processes, in practice they overlap considerably (Fig. 48-2, Table 48-1). Also, even though diseases affecting the interstitium are dominated by one form of injury, the other patterns of injury are often present, albeit usually to a lesser extent.

ANATOMY OF THE ALVEOLAR INTERSTITIUM

In the normal adult, the alveolar interstitium occupies approximately 50 percent of the volume of the alveolar walls. The interstitium itself is bounded by the epithelial and endothelial basement membranes, is made up of connective tissue (*stroma*), and includes the *interstitial (extracellular) matrix* and mesenchymal cells. The interstitium also contains alveolar machrophages and lymphocytes—inflammatory cells that, depending on the injury, play a vital role in defending the lungs on the one hand

and in injuring the interstitium on the other (Figs. 48-5 and 48-6). Also dispersed throughout the interstitium are proteins, lipids, carbohydrates, and small solutes derived from the plasma and the cells.

Basement Membranes

As indicated above, the alveolar epithelial and endothelial basement membranes are discrete, thin sheets of connective tissue located beneath the epithelial and endothelial cells, respectively (Figs. 48-5 to 48-7). At multiple places in the alveolar interstitium the two basement membranes fuse; at these sites, the distances between air and blood are the shortest and are likely the paths through which most gas exchange takes place. Transmission electron micrographs of both the alveolar epithelial and endothelial basement membranes demonstrate a lamina lucida subjacent to the basal surfaces of the epithelial and endothelial cells and a darker band, the lamina densa, beneath the lamina lucida.

Considered in toto, the basement membranes are composed of at least 50 proteins. The major components are type IV collagen, laminin, heparan sulfate proteoglycan, and nidogen (also called *entactin*). *Type IV collagen* [molecular weight (MW) 550,000 to 600,000] is composed of one α_1(IV) and two α_2(IV) chains; it has both a globular and triple helical structure that together form a long flexible rod that self-assembles through interactions at its ends. Type IV collagen is abundant in basement membranes and provides its structural backbone. *Laminin* (MW 850,000) is made up of light and heavy chains and has the overall shape of an asymmetric cross. It also is abundant and provides a major site for cell binding to the

TABLE 48–1

Classification of the Chronic, Nonmalignant Disorders of the Lower Respiratory Tract Based on the Type of Injury to the Alveolar Interstitium

Clinical Group	Disorder	Dominant Form of Injury*		
		Distortion	Fibrosis	Destruction
Interstitial lung disorders of known etiology	Inhalation of environmental agents†			
	Inorganic dusts	○	●	
	Organic dusts	●	○	
	Gases	○	●	
	Fumes	○	●	
	Vapors	○	●	
	Aerosols	○	●	
	Drugs†	○	●	
	Secondary to inflammation associated with lung infection†	○	●	
	Radiation	○	●	
	Poisons†	○	●	
	Recovery Phase of ARDS‡	○	●	
Interstitial lung disorders of unknown etiology	Sarcoidosis	●	○	
	Idiopathic pulmonary fibrosis	○	●	
	ILD§ associated with the collagen-vascular disorders	○	●	
	Histiocytosis X	○	○	○
	Chronic eosinophilic pneumonia	○	●	
	Idiopathic pulmonary hemosiderosis	○	●	
	Goodpasture's syndrome	○	●	
	Hypereosinophilic syndrome	○	●	
	Immunoblastic lymphadenopathy	●	○	
	Undefined lymphocytic infiltrative disorders			
	Lymphocytic interstitial pneumonitis	●	○	
	Pseudolymphoma	●	○	
	Lymphangiomyomatosis	●	○	
	Amyloidosis	●	○	
	Alveolar proteinosis	○	○	
	Bronchocentric granulomatosis	●	○	
	Inherited disorders			
	Familial idiopathic pulmonary fibrosis	○	●	
	Tuberous sclerosis	○	○	
	Neurofibromatosis	○	●	○
	Hermansky-Pudlak syndrome	○	●	
	Niemann-Pick disease	●	○	
	Gaucher's disease	●	○	
	ILD associated with liver disease			
	Chronic active hepatitis	●	○	
	Primary biliary cirrhosis	●	○	
	ILD associated with bowel disease			
	Whipple's disease	○	●	
	Ulcerative colitis	●	○	
	Crohn's disease	●	○	
	Weber-Christian disease	○	○	
	ILD associated with pulmonary vasculitis			
	Wegener's granulomatosis	○	●	
	Lymphomatoid granulomatosis	●	○	

TABLE 48-1 (continued)

Clinical Group	Disorder	Dominant Form of Injury*		
		Distortion	Fibrosis	Destruction
	ILD associated with pulmonary vasculitis (cont.)			
	Churg-Strauss syndrome	○	●	
	Systemic necrotizing vasculitis (overlap vasculitides)	○	●	
	Hypersensitivity vasculitis	○	●	
	ILD associated with chronic cardiac disease			
	Left ventricular failure	○	●	
	Left to right shunt	○	●	
	ILD associated with chronic renal disease with uremia	○	●	
	ILD associated with graft versus host reaction	○	●	
Destructive lung disorders	α_1-Antitrypsin deficiency			●
	Acquired emphysema			●

*Indicated are the types of injury that dominate typical examples of each disorder;
● = most dominant; ○ = present, but to a much lesser extent.

†See Davis and Crystal, 1984, for a complete list of all agents that can cause these disorders.

‡ARDS = adult respiratory distress syndrome.

§ILD = interstitial lung disease.

basement membranes. The *heparan sulfate proteoglycan* (MW 650,000) is composed of four heparan sulfate glycosaminoglycans bound to a small protein core that comprises 10 percent of the structure. The heparan sulfate proteoglycan serves diverse functions since it can bind to type IV collagen and laminin. *Nidogen* (MW at least 150,000) consists of a single chain that self-assembles with similar molecules; it binds to laminin and may serve to aggregate basement membrane components into nest-like structures.

These and other proteins are densely packed in a supramolecular complex that forms the 50- to 80-nm-wide basement membranes. It is generally believed that the overall biochemical composition of the alveolar epithelial and endothelial basement membranes is similar. Although the precise structural arrangement of the component proteins is not known, it is thought to be a continuous interlocking network of type IV collagen that serves as a backbone for the other components. All the differences between the lamina densa and lamina lucida are not known. However, type IV collagen seems to be localized to the lamina densa whereas laminin is more abundant in the lamina lucida; the other components are more diffusely distributed. The outer edges of the lamina densa include heparan sulfate that has been proposed to constitute an anionic barrier that retards the movement of proteins.

Connective Tissue Matrix

The connective tissue matrix, bounded by the epithelial and endothelial basement membranes, comprises fibrous, elastic, and amorphous components (Fig 48-5A). The fibrous components are the collagens, mostly type I and type III, but with small amounts of type V and, possibly, of other types. Type I collagen, a rigid molecule (MW 300,000) composed of two α_1(I) and one α_2(I) chains, is the most abundant, making up approximately 65 percent of the total collagen mass. In histologic sections, type I collagen stains positively with Masson's trichrome, and in transmission electron micrographs it appears as cross-banded fibrils that are disposed in parallel. Scanning electron micrographs of the interstitium show these fibers as thick bundles of ropelike structures that form interlocking, random weave. Type III collagen (MW 300,000) is composed of three α_1(III) chains and represents approximately 35 percent of the interstitial collagens. Type III collagen is poorly visualized by light microscopy, although it is detected, at least in part, by reticulin stains. Unlike type I collagen, type III does not condense into large fibers but tends to form loose, randomly dispersed fibrils, sometimes in association with type I collagen. The remaining fibrous components, such as type V collagen, are poorly characterized for the lungs, and their roles, if any, are unknown.

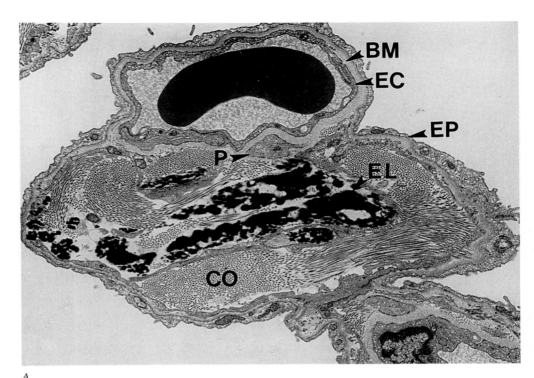

A

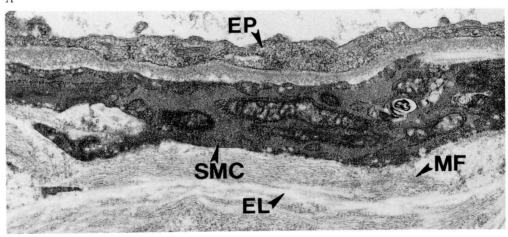

FIGURE 48-5   A. Electron micrograph of normal alveolar septum showing a capillary, collagen (CO), and elastic fibers (EL). Note the endothelial cells (EC), a pericyte (P) located within the capillary basement membrane (BM), and the type I alveolar epithelial cells (EP). Kajikawa stain. ×11,100.   B. Electron micrograph showing a type I alveolar epithelial cell (EP), a smooth-muscle cell (SMC) and elastic fibers, which are composed of an electron-lucent amorphous component (elastin, EL) surrounded by microfibrils (MF). Note the two components, lamina lucida and lamina densa, of the epithelial basement membrane. Lead citrate and uranyl acetate stain. ×18,500.

B

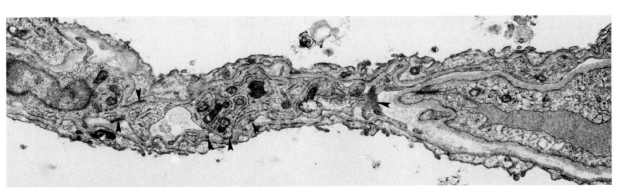

FIGURE 48-6   Myofibroblast with elongated cytoplasmic processes extends through alveolar septum, coming into close approximation with type I alveolar epithelial cells lining both septal surfaces. This cell has moderate numbers of cisterns of rough-surfaced endoplasmic reticulum and peripherally located dense areas (filament insertion sites) (arrowheads), which are similar to those in smooth-muscle cells. A basement membrane is not present in this myofibroblast. ×8820.

716

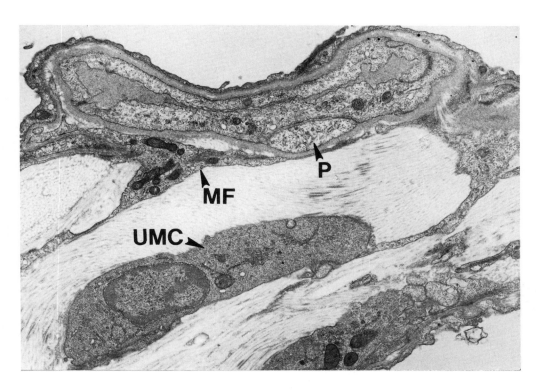

FIGURE 48-7 Undifferentiated mesenchymal cell (UMC), which has few cytoplasmic organelles and lacks a basement membrane, is subjacent to a capillary and is surrounded by collagen fibrils. A pericyte (P) and a myofibroblast (MF) are subjacent to the capillary. ×11,250.

The elastic components of the interstitium are the elastic fibers that represent 20 to 30 percent of the interstitial connnective tissue. The elastic fibers are actually made up of two components, elastin and microfibrils. The elastin gives the fibers their elastic properties, whereas the microfibrils provide a supporting structure. The elastin is composed of tropoelastin (MW 70,000) molecules that are tightly cross-linked, whereas the microfibrils are composed of poorly defined glycoproteins. In electron microscopic preparations stained with lead citrate and uranyl acetate, the elastin appears amorphous, whereas the microfibrils appear as 10- to 12-nm tubular structures (Fig. 48-5). In the adult alveolar interstitium, the amorphous component occupies the center of the elastic fiber; the microfibrils are on the periphery.

The amorphous component of the matrix, i.e., the "ground substance," includes proteoglycans and fibronectin. The proteoglycans are proteins linked to polysaccharides known as *glycosaminoglycans*. The normal alveolar interstitium contains several types of glycosaminoglycans. Among these are hyaluronic acid, chondroitin-4-sulfate, chondroitin-6-sulfate, dermatan sulfate, and heparin. Together, these components represent about 5 percent of the interstitial connective tissue. The proteoglycans stain with ruthenium red on electron microscopic preparations and are associated with both collagen and elastic fibers. Fibronectin (MW 440,000) is a glycoprotein composed of two identical chains joined by disulfide cross-links. Through its ability to interact with cells, collagen (particularly type I), and proteoglycans, fibronectin

plays a central role in cell-matrix interactions. Fibronectin is found diffusely through the interstitial matrix and represents less than 5 percent of the total connective tissue matrix.

Mesenchymal Cells

The mesenchymal cells represent 30 to 40 percent of the parenchymal cells present in the alveolar walls. There are several subtypes of mesenchymal cells, including fibroblasts, myofibroblasts, smooth-muscle cells, pericytes, so-called interstitial cells (myofibroblast-like cells, which often contain cytoplasmic lipid droplets), and undifferentiated mesenchymal cells (Figs. 48-6 to 48-9). It is assumed, but not proven, that the undifferentiated cells are the precursors of the others. By number, the fibroblasts and myofibroblasts dominate the mesenchymal cell populations of the normal lung.

The major functions of the mesenchymal cells are twofold: (1) to produce the interstitial connective tissue matrix and (2) to modulate the mechanical properties of the interstitium. The major connective tissue products of the mesenchymal cells are collagens (type I > type III at a ratio of 5:1 to 10:1), fibronectin, and proteoglycans. It is unclear which mesenchymal cells produce the elastic fibers found in the interstitium, although smooth-muscle cells may contribute, as may the capillary endothelial cells. Because they are abundant and contain contractile elements, the myofibroblasts mediate most of the mechanical effects of the mesenchymal cells. The disposition of

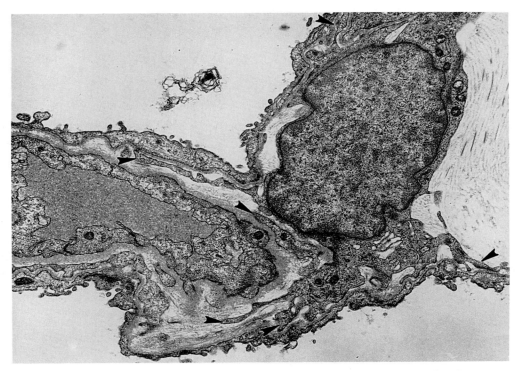

FIGURE 48-8 Myofibroblast has cytoplasmic processes which extend through alveolar septum and around a capillary (arrowheads). ×5920.

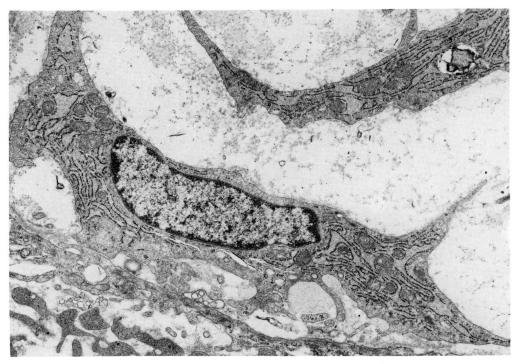

FIGURE 48-9 Fibroblasts have elongated shapes and contain typical cisterns of rough-surfaced endoplasmic reticulum. ×11,250.

the myofibroblasts—which normally have cytoplasmic processes that extend toward both sides of the interstitium (Figs. 48-6 and 48-8)—may have an important influence on both blood flow and airflow.

Inflammatory Cells

On the alveolar epithelial surface and within the interstitium there are about 65 alveolar macrophages and 15 lymphocytes per alveolus. The alveolar macrophages are derived from blood monocytes. They also proliferate slowly within the interstitium. Overall, the alveolar macrophage population turns over approximately every 3 months. The lymphocyte populations include T lymphocytes (T cells) and B lymphocytes (B cells). The T cells include helper-inducer and suppressor-cytotoxic cells, usually in the same proportions as in blood, i.e., 2 to 1. The interstitium contains proportionally fewer B lymphocytes than T lymphocytes than does the blood. The B cells in the lower respiratory tract synthesize and secrete immunoglobulins.

Other Molecules

The contents of the interstitium include a filtrate of plasma and, hence, the whole spectrum of molecules present in plasma. The relative amount of each macromolecule present in the interstitium depends largely on its molecular weight; the concentration of albumin (MW 69,000) in the interstitium is approximately 60 to 70 percent of that in plasma. Although few of the molecules in the interstitium have any direct bearing on lung function, the presence of others, such as α_1-antitrypsin, is critical in the defense of the lung (see below).

In addition to its connective tissue components, the interstitium also contains molecules secreted by the epithelial, endothelial, and mesenchymal cells. For example, the alveolar interstitium is thought to contain large amounts of prostaglandins of the E series, molecules that suppress inflammatory and immune processes. Furthermore, the interstitium contains, at least transiently, the constituents of parenchymal cells that are released when these cells die as a part of normal cell turnover. Certain of these molecules, such as catalase, play an important role in defending the interstitium against oxidants.

FUNCTIONS OF THE ALVEOLAR INTERSTITIUM

The alveolar interstitium serves four functions. First, it provides the structural support for the cells of the alveolar walls and, as such, helps to define the architecture of the alveolar airspaces. Second, the basement membranes, connective tissue matrix, and mesenchymal cells have a major influence on the mechanical behavior of the lower respiratory tract during respiration. Third, as part of the tissue barrier interposed between blood and air, the interstitium modulates the passage of fluid and solutes between the endothelial and epithelial surfaces. Finally, the interstitium poses a mechanical barrier that, together with the population of inflammatory cells normally present within the interstitium, contributes to the defense of the lower respiratory tract.

Defining the Alveolar Architecture

The concept that the alveolar interstitium provides the supporting framework that defines the alveolar architecture is fundamental to understanding the consequences of injury to the interstitium. Although the connective tissue components that form the matrix between the epithelial and endothelial basement membranes provide the bulk of the structural support, the basement membranes play an important role in delineating alveolar architecture.

The epithelial basement membrane is a critical component of the interstitium. If alveolar epithelial cells are damaged, they can be replaced by the surviving epithelial type II cells, which use the denuded epithelial basement membrane as a scaffold to form a new continuous lining. However, if the alveolar epithelial basement membrane is not largely intact, either the replacement epithelial cells must produce their own basement membrane or the epithelial surface of that alveolus cannot be restored.

In contrast to the distinct role of the epithelial cell basement membrane in organizing the alveolar lining, the role of the endothelial basement membrane in the disposition of endothelial cells (and hence capillaries) in the alveolar wall is unknown. Endothelial cells can produce basement membrane components; probably they produce basement membranes subjacent to the alveolar capillaries. However, it is not known if loss of pulmonary capillary endothelial cells is followed by migration and proliferation of the remaining endothelial cells to cover the capillary basement membrane, or if the outgrowth of new capillaries begins with endothelial cells that produce their own basement membranes.

Inflammatory cells move across the endothelial and epithelial basement membranes drilling holes for their passage, probably using proteases that are specific for the connective tissue components of the basement membranes. How these holes in the basement membrane are then sealed is not known, but since both endothelial and epithelial cells are capable of secreting basement membrane components, they presumably fill in the gaps.

Contribution to Mechanical Behavior

In normal inspiration, as the alveolar airspace diameter increases, the interstitium is subjected to tremendous mechanical forces. The basement membrane network of type IV collagen and laminin is expandable, somewhat less than the rubberlike elastic fibers, but more than the relatively rigid type I collagen fibers. Within the matrix, the type I and type III collagen fibers maintain the shape of the interstitium and help limit alveolar distention, whereas the more continuous elastic fibers provide elastic recoil. In addition, studies of the mechanical behavior of the lung parenchyma in vitro suggest that the mesenchymal cells in the interstitium, particularly the myofibroblasts and smooth-muscle cells, contribute to regulating local alveolar size and blood flow by contracting or relaxing in response to various stimuli.

Modulation of Alveolar-Capillary Exchange of Plasma Constituents

Fluid and macromolecular exchange between plasma and air are considered elsewhere in this book (Chapter 60). Here it will suffice to underscore that, in general, the exit of macromolecules from plasma into the interstitium and the passage from interstitium into alveolar spaces are largely a matter of the relative "tightness" of the endothelial and epithelial cell barriers: the endothelial cell junctions are relatively "loose" and the epithelial cell junctions far "tighter." The interstitium per se forms an additional barrier to passage of macromolecules: since the basement membranes are negatively charged, they can presumably retard the movement of the negatively charged plasma proteins. In addition, the proteoglycans of the interstitial matrix can absorb water molecules. The structural arrangement of the interstitial matrix constitutes another potential barrier to the movement of fluids and macromolecules from endothelium to epithelium. Finally, lymphatic capillaries in the interstitium of the alveolar ducts direct the interstitial fluid back toward the circulating blood.

Lower Respiratory Tract Defense

Because the lungs are exposed to both the outside environment and the entire cardiac output, alveolar structures are continuously burdened with a variety of potentially injurious agents, including infectious organisms, particles, and xenobiotics. The brunt of this burden is borne by the linings of the alveoli and capillaries. The continuity of both the epithelial and endothelial basement membranes contributes a mechanical barrier to the passage of these agents; so does, to a lesser extent, the interstitial connective tissue matrix. Alveolar macrophages and lymphocytes in the interstitial connective tissue matrix are also involved in lung defense. The defense mechanisms of the lungs are considered in detail elsewhere in this book (Chapters 39 and 47).

MAINTENANCE OF THE INTERSTITIUM

The components of the interstitium, including the connective tissue and the different cell populations, are con-

tinuously undergoing death and replacement, albeit at different rates. This dynamic character of the interstitium has important consequences for the maintenance of normal alveolar structure and for the pathogenesis of the diseases of the lower respiratory tract.

Production of Connective Tissue

As indicated above, the epithelial and endothelial cells can produce the components of basement membranes and provide, thereby, for the normal turnover of their respective basement membranes. The epithelial and endothelial cells also contribute to the maintenance of the interstitial matrix by producing collagen types I and III, fibronectin, and proteoglycans.

The mesenchymal cells produce collagen types I and III, fibronectin, and proteoglycans. However, their major secreted product is type I collagen; in culture, mesenchymal cells produce types I and III collagen in a ratio of 5:1 to 10:1. Interestingly, the ratio of type I to type III collagen in the normal interstitium is only 2:1, probably because the epithelial and endothelial cells contribute relatively more type III collagen to the interstitial matrix than do the mesenchymal cells. These facts are relevant to understanding the shift in collagen types observed in the interstitium in association with fibrosis-type injury. In these disorders, the number of mesenchymal cells in the interstitium is markedly increased and the number of endothelial cells is decreased, resulting in a relative increase in the number of cells that produce predominantly type I collagen. This realignment is consistent with the increase in the ratio of type I to type III collagen in the interstitium in these disorders.

Fibronectin produced by the mesenchymal cells mediates the attachment of mesenchymal cells to the matrix. Fibronectin is also involved in the pathogenesis of the intra-alveolar fibrosis that occurs in many of the interstitial lung disorders. Thus, if the interstitium sustains an injury sufficient to cause large holes in the epithelial basement membrane and localized capillary leaks, components of plasma, such as fibrin, move into the alveolar airspaces along with interstitial fibroblasts, thereby forming a nidus for the development of intra-alveolar fibrosis (Figs 48-10 and 48-11). Fibronectin is involved in this process by binding, with high affinity, to fibrin as well as to fibroblasts, providing a link for the attachment of fibroblasts to the "matrix" developing within the airspaces. This process is an example of how a mechanism that is operative during normal wound healing can also play an important pathogenetic role under suitable circumstances. In this example, injury to the endothelial and epithelial layers and their associated basement membranes permits fibronectin-mediated binding of fibroblasts to fibrin to initiate the development of an intra-alveolar scar.

The connective tissue products of the other subpopulations of mesenchymal cells are unknown. However, it is

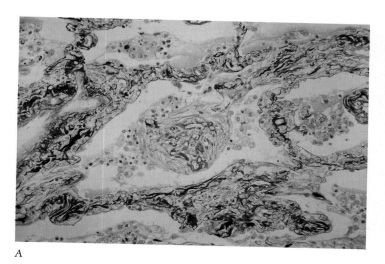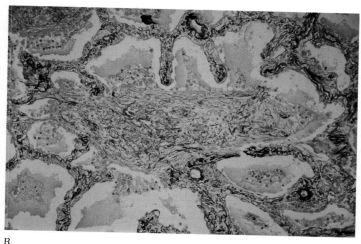

A   B

FIGURE 48-10   *A.* Area of intra-alveolar fibrosis is beginning to develop in lung of patient with hypersensitivity pneumonitis. This area is composed of collagen (stained black) and associated inflammatory cells. A narrow stalk connects the area of intra-alveolar fibrosis to the alveolar wall from which it originated. Periodic acid-methenamine silver stain. ×110. *B.* Large area of intraluminal fibrosis involves an alveolar duct and extends into the openings of several adjacent alveoli. Periodic acid-methenamine silver stain. ×110.

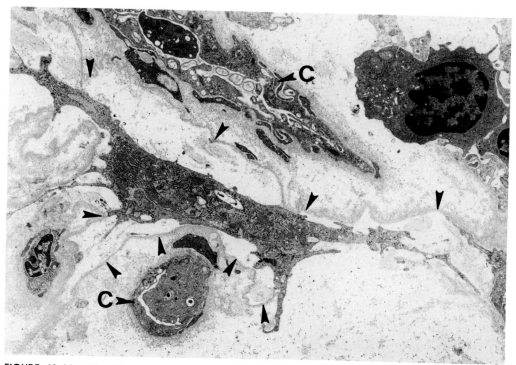

FIGURE 48-11   Fibroblast with elongated cytoplasmic processes appears to be passing through defect in the denuded alveolar epithelial basement membrane from a patient with hypersensitivity pneumonitis. The fibroblast is adjacent to the luminal sides of the two basement membranes (arrowheads), and a capillary (C) is found on the septal side of each basement membrane. ×9000.

likely that pericytes, which are found only within the confines of the endothelial basement membranes, secrete basement membrane components. Similarly, it is probable that smooth-muscle cells produce the components of the basement membrane that surrounds them.

Degradation of Connective Tissue

Since the alveolar interstitial connective tissue is being produced continuously, and yet its quantity in the normal lung remains unchanged, connective tissue must be continuously degraded in the interstitium. Although connective tissue proteins are generally difficult to degrade, a variety of connective tissue-specific proteases, including collagenases, elastases, and cathepsin G, carry out this task.

Collagenases, as the name suggests, attack and cleave collagens; cleavage is usually at a specific site, approximately two-thirds from the N terminus of the molecule. In the normal lung, fibroblasts and alveolar macrophages release a collagenase capable of cleaving collagen types I and III, although the amount produced by the macrophages is small. In addition, in inflammatory states that involve neutrophils, the connective tissue is exposed to a neutrophil collagenase that is specific for type I collagen. Should the inflammation entail eosinophils, an eosinophil collagenase is added; like the fibroblast and macrophage enzymes, the eosinophil collagenase attacks both collagen types I and III.

Elastases are enzymes capable of cleaving elastin, a molecule that is resistant to most proteolytic enzymes. The only known source of elastase in the normal lung is the alveolar macrophage. However, the human alveolar macrophage can release only modest amounts of this enzyme, consistent with the concept that elastin turnover in the normal alveolar interstitium proceeds at a very low rate. The most potent elastase known is produced by the neutrophil. This enzyme is stored in the neutrophil's azurophilic granules and is released when the neutrophil is activated or when it disintegrates in tissues at the end of its short life span. Although it readily cleaves elastin, neutrophil elastase is actually an omnivorous protease that cleaves most, if not all, connective tissue proteins making up the basement membranes and the interstitial matrix. If the interstitium is exposed to neutrophil elastase that is uninhibited, the consequences are profound and usually culminate in a destruction-type injury of the alveolar wall.

Cathepsin G is another neutrophil proteolytic enzyme. Although not normally present in large amounts, the alveolar wall must contend with it whenever there is an inflammation involving neutrophils. Cathepsin G has a proteolytic spectrum similar to that of neutrophil elastase but is less potent.

In addition to proteases, oxygen radicals (i.e., electron acceptors) can degrade connective tissue. Whether this actually occurs within the normal lung is unknown. But, it may play a role in inflammatory states in which the alveolar walls are exposed to heavy concentrations of oxidants.

Turnover of Mesenchymal Cells

Normal alveolar interstitial mesenchymal cells are continuously turning over, but at a slow rate. This process is accelerated in diseases characterized by fibrosis-type injury, in which enhanced mesenchymal cell proliferation

is followed by the accumulation of connective tissue components in the interstitium (Fig. 48-12). This process is central to understanding the mechanisms leading to fibrosis of the interstitium. For example, one consequence of an increase in the number of mesenchymal cells in the alveolar walls is an increase in the total amount of connective tissue—particularly type I collagen, the major secreted product of the fibroblast and myofibroblast—that is deposited in the interstitial matrix (Fig. 48-13); even though the mesenchymal cells produce the same amounts and types of collagen as they do in the normal lung, because there are more mesenchymal cells, there is more collagen secreted, hence fibrosis.

Like mesenchymal cells elsewhere, the alveolar interstitial mesenchymal cells are normally quiescent and require exogenous growth factors to stimulate them to enter the cell cycle and replicate. For convenience, these growth factors are grouped as *competence factors* (mediators that stimulate the cells to enter the cell cycle) and *progression factors* (mediators that stimulate competence factor-stimulated cells to proceed through the cell cycle and proliferate). Of all the known mesenchymal cell growth factors, at least four are possibly relevant to stimulation of the alveolar interstitial mesenchymal cells: (1) fibronectin, the glycoprotein component of the interstitial matrix, can act as a competence factor; it is continuously produced by alveolar macrophages and fibroblasts; (2) platelet-derived growth factor (PDGF, MW 32,000), the product of c-sis proto-oncogene, is a potent competence factor produced continuously by alveolar macrophages; (3) alveolar macrophage-derived growth factor (AMDGF, MW 18,000) is released by activated, but not quiescent, alveolar macrophages and acts as a progression factor; together, fibronectin and AMDGF, or PDGF and AMDGF, are sufficient to stimulate nonproliferating lung fibroblasts to enter the cell cycle, proceed through it, and proliferate; and (4) interleukin 1 (IL-1, MW 16,000) is released only by activated alveolar macrophages; although IL-1 can augment the proliferation of fibroblasts stimulated by fibronectin and AMDGF, IL-1 per se does not stimulate quiescent lung fibroblasts to proliferate.

In contrast to the growth stimulating potential of these growth factors, mesenchymal cell proliferation is suppressed by prostaglandins of the E series (PGE). This is relevant to the alveolar interstitium, because the lower respiratory tract has PGE levels 50 times that of serum, levels sufficient to suppress fibronectin-AMDGF-stimulated lung fibroblast proliferation in vitro. In this context, control of the rate of proliferation of mesenchymal cells within the interstitium can be seen as involving a balance between growth regulatory signals (e.g., fibronectin, PDGF, AMDGF, and IL-1) and growth inhibitory signals (e.g., PGE).

In addition to the rate of mesenchymal cell growth, the existence of several subtypes of mesenchymal cells in

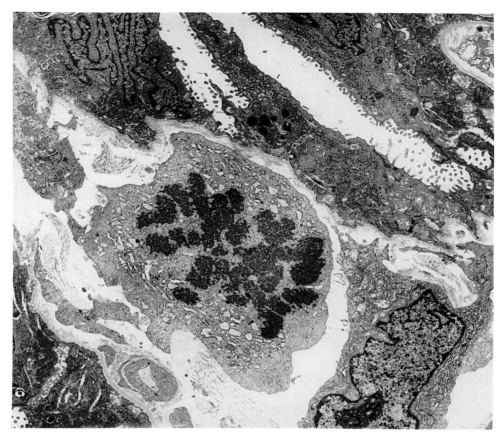

FIGURE 48-12   Fibroblastlike cell undergoing mitosis is subjacent to alveolar epithelial cells in lung of patient with IPF. ×10,000. *(Courtesy of Dr. F. Basset and Dr. P. Soler, INSERM U82, Hôpital Bichat, Paris.)*

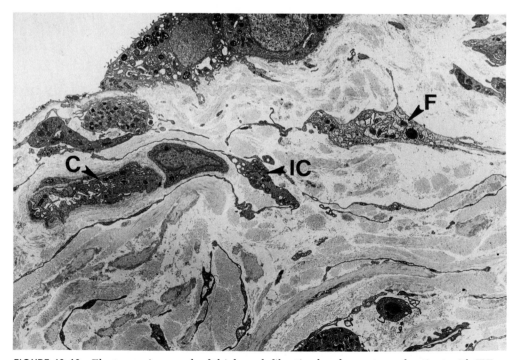

FIGURE 48-13   Electron micrograph of thickened, fibrotic alveolar septum of patient with IPF, showing type I and type II alveolar epithelial cells, overlying area of marked accumulation of collagen. Note capillary (C), fibroblasts (F), and thin, elongated interstitial cells (IC). ×4100.

the interstitium adds another layer of complexity to the concepts of mesenchymal cell turnover. For example, mesenchymal cells can differentiate from a fibroblast to a myofibroblast, to a smooth-muscle cell. Also, the accumulation of mesenchymal cells in a local region of the interstitium can result not only from enhanced proliferation but also from *chemotaxis*, i.e., the directed migration of cells toward a chemical stimulus. Thus, fibronectin is chemotactic for fibroblasts, as are elastin and collagen fragments. Finally, certain chemotactic signals may be more specific for one mesenchymal cell subtype than for another: PDGF is more highly chemotactic for smooth-muscle cells than for other mesenchymal cells.

Inflammatory Cell Traffic

In the normal lung, macrophages and lymphocytes in the interstitium undergo a slow but continuous turnover. In inflammatory disorders of the lower respiratory tract, the numbers and types of inflammatory cells in the interstitium change dramatically (Fig. 48-14). Moreover, the increased rate and type of inflammatory cell traffic to the interstitium are modulated by the amount and type of chemotactic signals that are released by cells residing in the alveoli. For example, alveolar macrophages can release leukotriene B$_4$, a chemotactic signal for neutrophils, as well as PDGF, a chemotactic factor for both monocytes and neutrophils. In contrast, activated T lymphocytes can release not only monocyte chemotactic factor, and thereby recruit monocytes, but also interleukin 2 (IL-2, the T-cell growth factor) that can also attract T cells.

In addition to chemotactic signals, the number of inflammatory cells in the interstitium can be markedly augmented by proliferation in situ. In this regard, most inflammatory states affecting the lower respiratory tract are associated with an enhanced rate of alveolar macrophage replication (Fig. 48-15); in sarcoidosis, the accumulation of T lymphocytes in the interstitium results from the enhanced rate of T-cell proliferation locally.

Fluid and Solute Movements through the Interstitium

There is constant movement of fluid and solutes from blood across the capillary endothelium to the alveolar interstitium. It is estimated that in the entire lung, 5 to 15 ml of interstitial fluid move through the alveolar interstitium each hour. This is likely an underestimate, as some of the fluid moving from plasma to the interstitium moves across to the alveolar epithelial surface, where at least a portion is removed by the cephalad movement of epithelial fluid from the alveolus to the trachea.

Along with the fluid moving from blood to the interstitium comes a variety of molecules, representing the whole spectrum of protein, lipids, carbohydrates, and other molecules present in plasma. The combination of endothelial junctions and endothelial basement membrane sieving retards the movement of the larger molecules more than those of the smaller ones, so that molecules like urea diffuse freely while IgM (MW 1,000,000) moves across in only small amounts. When there is injury to the endothelial cells or basement membrane, the amounts of fluid and amounts and types of plasma molecules present in the interstitium can change significantly. Likewise, if there are changes in the epithelial basement membrane, epithelial cell junctions, lymphatic function, or the rate of clearance of epithelial fluid, the rate of clearance of interstitial fluid and solutes is also affected.

PROCESSES MEDIATING THE PATTERNS OF INJURY TO THE INTERSTITIUM

The general classes of processes that are injurious to the alveolar walls are inflammation, locally produced toxic products, xenobiotics, accumulation of extracellular products, and ischemia.

Inflammation

Either directly or indirectly, whether it be the distortion, fibrosis, or destruction patterns of injury, most interstitial injuries that characterize the chronic noninfectious, nonmalignant disorders of the lower respiratory tract are mediated by inflammatory cells present in the alveolar structures. Even in the disorders in which the initiating stimulus is known, such as those caused by inorganic dusts, drugs, or cigarette smoke, it is inflammation that is responsible for most of the injury to the interstitium. The specific pattern of injury depends on the intensity, character, and state of activation of the cells in the inflamma-

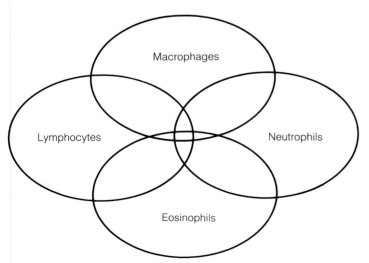

FIGURE 48-14 Inflammatory cells participating in the injury to the interstitium. To some extent, for most of the chronic disorders of the lower respiratory tract, the inflammation includes all four cell types. However, for each disorder, one cell type usually dominates, thus dictating the form of the injury to the interstitium.

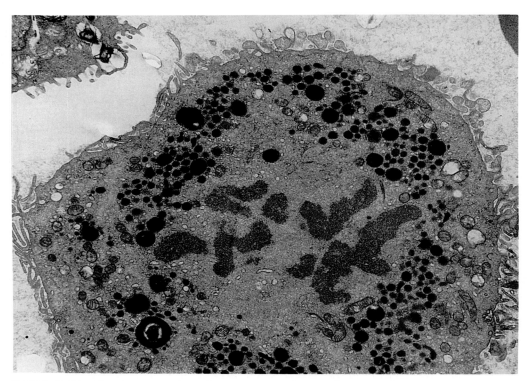

FIGURE 48-15 Alveolar macrophage from patient with sarcoidosis is undergoing mitosis. ×9840.

tion as well as the state of the defenses of the alveolar walls against these processes.

Inflammatory cells alter the interstitium in three ways: (1) their presence takes up space, thereby distorting the normal architecture; (2) the inflammatory cells can damage the cells and connective tissue components that form the interstitium itself; and (3) the inflammatory cells can damage the epithelium and endothelium, thus indirectly altering interstitial structure and function.

In the normal interstitium, about 82 percent of the inflammatory cells are alveolar macrophages and 17 percent are lymphocytes; neutrophils, eosinophils, basophils, and mast cells contribute, at most, only 1 percent of the population. Chronic disorders of the lower respiratory tract generally change these numbers and proportions appreciably, often dramatically; the total numbers of inflammatory cells often increase two- to tenfold, and the relative proportion of the individual cell types varies from disorder to disorder (Fig. 48-14): some disorders are characterized by a lymphocytic inflammatory process; others by a predominance of macrophages, neutrophils, or eosinophils. Since the different inflammatory cells can release different mediators, they can cause different types of damage. Furthermore, not only do the different inflammatory cells have a different armamentarium of mediators, but for each cell, certain classes of stimuli evoke some mediators while other stimuli evoke others. Finally, the alveolar walls contain a variety of defensive mechanisms

that work well against some mediators but are relatively ineffective against others.

Despite this complexity, certain general relationships can be drawn. Most importantly, the types of activated inflammatory cells in the interstitium play a major role in determining the type of injury that results. Thus, inflammation dominated by T lymphocytes commonly results in distortion-type injury, whereas inflammation dominated by alveolar macrophages, neutrophils, and eosinophils usually results in fibrosis-type injury. Neutrophils add the prospect of destruction-type injury because they carry an armamentarium that is capable of severely damaging all connective tissue components of the interstitium and, as a consequence, of completely destroying the architecture of the interstitium.

In general, the major categories of mediators involved in the pathogenesis of inflammatory diseases of the lower respiratory tract include: proteases; oxidants; chemotactic factors that recruit additional inflammatory cells, thereby amplifying the inflammation; the "immune" mediators; and the chemotactic and growth factors that mediate the accumulation of mesenchymal cells. Pitted against these processes are clearance mechanisms that prevent the inflammation from being initiated, antiproteases, antioxidants, immunosuppressants, inhibitors of chemotaxis, "antiproliferation" factors, and the ability of the interstitium to remove, or to wall off, stimuli that may initiate inflammatory processes.

PROTEASES

Neutrophils, alveolar macrophages, and eosinophils can release proteases. On a per cell basis, the neutrophil exceeds the others by far. Each of these cells also releases a different spectrum of proteases: activated neutrophils release a collagenase, elastase, and cathepsin G; eosinophils release a collagenase; activated alveolar macrophages release plasminogen activator, a protease that can activate complement, generate kinins, initiate fibrinolysis, and degrade connective tissue components. Although the alveolar macrophage can also release a collagenase and elastase, it does so in such small amounts that the role of these mediators in the pathogenesis of interstitial damage is unknown.

The lower respiratory tract is well protected against neutrophil elastase but has little or no protection against the other enzymes. Approximately 95 percent of the barrier to neutrophil elastase is provided by α_1-antitrypsin (MW 52,000), an antiprotease produced by hepatocytes and mononuclear phagocytes, including alveolar macrophages. Additional protection against neutrophil elastase is provided by α_2-macroglobulin, a very large molecule (MW 720,000) produced by mesenchymal cells, and by the bronchial proteinase inhibitor, a small antiprotease (MW 12,000) produced by airway cells. In contrast to this protection against neutrophil elastase, except for α_2-macroglobulin, which is present in very small amounts, the lower respiratory tract has little protection against neutrophil, macrophage, or eosinophil collagenases; macrophage elastase; or plasminogen activator. α_1-Antichymotrypsin serves as the major protection against cathepsin G, with α_1-antitrypsin serving as a backup.

Faced with a surfeit of connective tissue specific proteases, the antiproteases serve a critical role in protecting the connective tissue of the interstitium; should a protease-antiprotease balance tip in favor of the protease, the connective tissue components are apt to be destroyed. Although these proteases probably play some role in the normal turnover of interstitial connective tissue, they certainly play a major role in damaging the interstitium in chronic inflammatory states. The proteases attack not only the basement membrane and the components of the interstitial matrix, but also the proteins by which cells attach to the matrix, such as laminin for epithelial cells and fibronectin for mesenchymal cells. As indicated above, unopposed neutrophil elastase is the most dangerous protease, capable of destroying alveolar walls. The consequences of unopposed collagenases, cathepsin G, or plasminogen activator are less clear, but all are capable of inflicting at least some damage to the interstitial connective tissue, the kind of damage that is most relevant to the development of the fibrosis type of injury.

OXIDANTS

Stimulated neutrophils, alveolar macrophages, and eosinophils can release toxic oxidants, including superoxide anion ($O_2^{\dot{-}}$), hydrogen peroxide (H_2O_2), and hydroxyl radical (OH·). In addition, in the presence of a halide such as Cl^- and myeloperoxidase, an enzyme contained in neutrophils and young macrophages, H_2O_2 is converted to the very toxic hypohalide radical ($OHCl^-$). Of the various inflammatory cells that can release these oxidants, the neutrophil is the most potent. These oxidants can directly damage the epithelial, endothelial, and mesenchymal cells that make up the alveolar walls, although it is thought that type I epithelial cells and endothelial cells are the most sensitive. In addition, the connective tissue components of the interstitium can be modified by these oxidants, causing disruption of their interactions and integrity and rendering them more susceptible to proteases. These combined processes of damage to the parenchymal cells and connective tissue constitute the type of lesion that is fundamental to the development of fibrosis-type injury to the interstitium.

Oxidants can also profoundly affect the interstitium by interfering with the antiprotease protection of the interstitial connective tissue matrix. In this regard, α_1-antitrypsin, the molecule that provides the major antineutrophil elastase protection to the lower respiratory tract, is rendered impotent by oxidants by virtue of their ability to modify the active site of the antiprotease. When this occurs, the α_1-antitrypsin functions poorly and can no longer inhibit neutrophil elastase and prevent it from degrading the interstitium; the result is destruction-type injury.

The alveolar walls are protected from oxidants by several mechanisms: (1) intracellular antioxidants, i.e., superoxide dismutase, catalase, and the glutathione system; (2) extracellular antioxidants, such as vitamins E, C, and A; (3) small molecules, such as glutathione, methionine, and bilirubin; and (4) intracellular antioxidants, particularly catalase, released by parenchymal cells during their normal turnover. Thus, the ability of inflammatory cells to injure the alveolar walls by releasing oxidants can be depicted in terms of a balance between the intensity of the burden of oxidants on the one hand, and the ability of the antioxidant defenses to contend with this burden on the other.

CHEMOTACTIC FACTORS FOR INFLAMMATORY CELLS

Inflammatory responses are amplified by chemotactic factors, chemical signals that modulate the directed migration of inflammatory cells. Although how this process occurs is not entirely clear, it does take place along a concentration gradient of the chemotactic factor, which interacts with specific receptors on the target cell surface. Four chemotactic factors are known to be related to the pathogenesis of diseases of the interstitium: (1) leukotriene B$_4$, a low molecular lipid product of activated alveolar macrophages that attracts neutrophils and, to a lesser extent, monocytes and eosinophils; (2) monocyte chemotactic factor, a protein that is released by activated T lymphocytes and attracts monocytes; (3) platelet-derived growth factor (see above), a mediator that attracts monocytes and neutrophils; and (4) interleukin 2, a product of activated T cells that, in addition to serving as a T-cell growth factor, is chemotactic for T-helper cells. Although eosinophils are found in very small numbers in the normal lower respiratory tract and probably accumulate there only in response to specific chemotactic factors, the mediators responsible for eosinophil accumulation in those diseases that are dominated by eosinophil inflammation in the interstitium are not known.

Like antiproteases and antioxidants, antichemotactic factors, i.e., chemotactic factor inhibitors, have also been described. The role played by such defensive molecules is enigmatic. The possibility exists that they serve to dampen the amplifying effects of inflammatory cells on inflammatory processes in the lower respiratory tract.

"IMMUNE" MEDIATORS

All cells involved in immune processes, including mononuclear phagocytes, T-helper-inducer lymphocytes, T-suppressor-cytotoxic lymphocytes, and B lymphocytes, are present in the normal interstitium, and their numbers increase, albeit to different degrees, in almost all chronic diseases of the interstitium. Immune mediators, including immunoglobulins and complement, are also present in the lower respiratory tract. But, a role for these mediators has been identified in only three disorders: (1) idiopathic pulmonary fibrosis, in which locally synthesized immunoglobulins in the alveolar walls form immune complexes that interact with alveolar macrophages through the macrophage immunoglobulin Fc receptors; (2) hypersensitivity pneumonitis, in which antigen-specific immunoglobulins in the lower respiratory tract presumably are involved in the pathogenesis of the disease, probably via alveolar macrophages as in idiopathic pulmonary fibrosis; and (3) Goodpasture's syndrome, in which antibodies specific for basement membrane components shared by the basement membranes of the lungs and kidneys, probably by way of cryptic antigenic sites on type IV collagen, are found in blood and lungs.

Although both the classic and the alternative complement pathways are present in the lower respiratory tract, the normal lung contains little of the C5 component of complement, C5 levels do not increase in chronic inflammatory disorders of interstitium, and C5a, a cleavage product of C5 and a potent chemotactic factor for neutrophils, does not play an appreciable role in any of the chronic diseases of the interstitium.

Interleukin 1 (IL-1), a mediator produced by activated mononuclear phagocytes, including human alveolar macrophages, is considered to be an important mediator that augments T-cell responses. Its role as an immune mediator in the pathogenesis of diseases involving the interstitium is unclear.

The T-lymphocyte mediators, IL-2, monocyte chemotactic factor, and interferon-γ play a central role in sarcoidosis: IL-2 increases the number of T-cells in the lung; monocyte chemotactic factor recruits monocytes to the lungs; and interferon-γ activates alveolar macrophages. As a result, T lymphocytes and mononuclear phagocytes accumulate in the interstitium, and granulomas form. Although T lymphocytes with the suppressor-cytotoxic phenotype are present in the normal lung and are present in exaggerated numbers in diseases such as hypersensitivity pneumonitis, there is no evidence that cytotoxic T cells play a role in the pathogenesis of these, or any other, noninfectious, nonmalignant diseases of the lower respiratory tract.

T-suppressor cells present in the alveoli presumably dampen immune processes to prevent inordinate reactions. Prostaglandin E, which is present in the lower respiratory tract in greater concentration than in blood, also may play a suppressive role. It has recently been proposed that in some instances a relative deficiency in PGE in the alveolar walls is responsible for inordinate immune responses.

Mesenchymal Cell Chemotaxis, Proliferation, and Deposition of Connective Tissue

Mesenchymal cells in the interstitium are mobile and can respond to certain chemotactic factors. The most relevant are fibronectin and platelet-derived growth factor (see above), mediators produced by activated alveolar macrophages. Chemotaxis for mesenchymal cells is responsible for the accumulation of mesenchymal cells in the region where the chemotactic factor was released (Fig. 48-16). For example, although smooth-muscle cells are rare in the normal interstitium, the continuity of the interstitium with bronchiolar walls and alveolar ducts provides a source for these cells and a path along which they can migrate into the interstitium.

It has been noted above that even though mesenchymal cells are normally quiescent, they respond to exogenous growth signals by proceeding through the cell cycle and replicating. As in the normal lung, the growth signals in interstitial disease appear to originate with

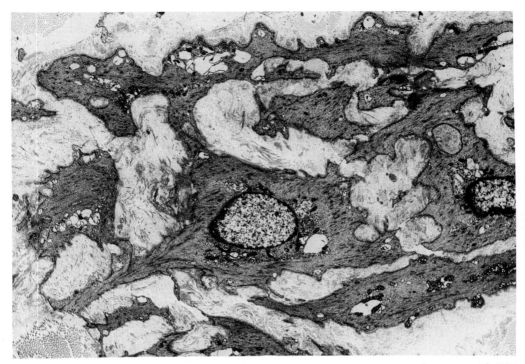

FIGURE 48-16 Cluster of smooth muscle cells in thickened alveolar septum of patient with IPF. ×6000.

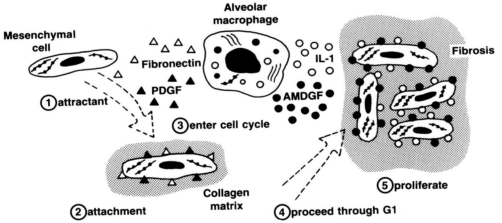

FIGURE 48-17 The central role of the alveolar macrophage in the development of fibrosis. By virtue of its ability to release mediators such as fibronectin, platelet-derived growth factor (PDGF), alveolar macrophage-derived growth factor (AMDGF), and interleukin 1 (IL-1), the macrophage can: (1) recruit mesenchymal cells, (2) modulate their attachment to the matrix, (3) stimulate the mesenchymal cells to enter the cell cycle, (4) direct them to proceed through the G1 phase of the cycle, and (5) proliferate. The result is an accumulation of mesenchymal cells and their products, i.e., connective tissue proteins, in the local milieu, resulting in fibrosis. See text for details.

greater intensity from alveolar macrophages (Fig. 48-17). In accord with this pathogenetic mechanism, activated alveolar macrophages recovered from the lungs of individuals with interstitial disease evoked by fibrosis-type injury of the interstitium release increased amounts of fibronectin, platelet-derived growth factor, and alveolar macrophage-derived growth factor. The role of T lymphocytes as a source of mesenchymal growth factors is unsettled.

Although it is reasonable to expect that suppressive signals are evoked in the attempt to modulate these growth signals, the only such mediator that has been clearly defined is PGE, the same mediator that suppresses exaggerated immune processes.

CLEARANCE PROCESSES

In addition to mechanisms that directly suppress inflammatory processes, the interstitium also has mechanisms to remove some of the initiating stimuli of inflammation. For example, if inhaled inorganic dusts, such as asbestos, silica, or coal, bypass the defenses of the upper respiratory tract and the alveolar epithelial surface and reach the interstitium, they can be removed by the combination of alveolar macrophages and movements of the interstitial fluid. The continuous movement of fluid from plasma through the endothelial layer and from the interstitium to the lymphatics constitutes a cleansing mechanism for the interstitium. Furthermore, after ingesting the dust, alveolar macrophages move out of the interstitium along with interstitial fluid flow en route to the lymphatics.

"WALLING OFF" POTENTIAL INJURIOUS SUBSTANCES

As an alternative to clearance, the interstitium is capable of "walling off" inorganic dusts, thereby rendering them innocuous. A classic example of this process is formation of ferruginous bodies (Fig. 48-18), a process by which inorganic dusts, such as asbestos fibers, are covered with iron and proteins. These bodies are presumably inert and do not stimulate inflammatory processes.

Locally Produced Injurious Products

The concept of local *toxins* as a source of injury to the interstitium is best exemplified by *oxygen toxicity*, in which the hyperoxia promotes the generation of excess oxygen radicals by the parenchymal cells of the lungs. As

with exogenous oxidants, probably the most vulnerable cells are the type I epithelial cells and endothelial cells. The result is a fibrosis-type injury. Oxygen toxicity is considered in detail in Chapter 151.

Xenobiotics

Among the xenobiotics that cause interstitial injury are paraquat, ionizing radiation, nitrofurantoin, bleomycin, and amiodarone. The result, as in oxygen toxicity, is injury of the alveolar epithelial and endothelial cells and a fibrosis-type injury of the interstitium.

Accumulation of Extracellular Molecules

In some relatively rare diseases, the primary mechanism of injury to the alveolar wall is the accumulation of extracellular material in the connective tissue matrix of the interstitium. The best example is amyloid deposition (Fig. 48-19). The result is primarily a distortion-type injury. Much more common is the distortion-type injury produced by a mild leak of fluid into the interstitium (Fig. 48-20). Distortion-type injury, caused by the predominant extracellular deposition of connective tissue, often is superimposed on fibrosis-type injury in certain interstitial lung disorders (Fig. 48-13).

Ischemia

Vasculitides, such as Wegener's granulomatosis, often produce ischemia distal to the involved segments of the vessels. Inflammation in the interstitium is sometimes followed by necrosis. In general, the injury is of the fibrosis type but patchy, reflecting the distribution of the vessels involved in the primary disease process.

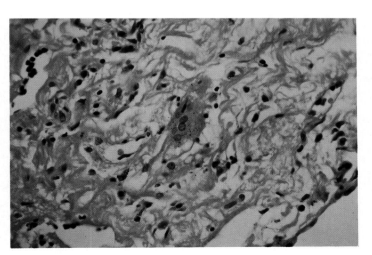

FIGURE 48-18 Asbestos bodies have been ingested by multinucleated giant cell in alveolar interstitium of patient with asbestosis. H&E stain, ×150.

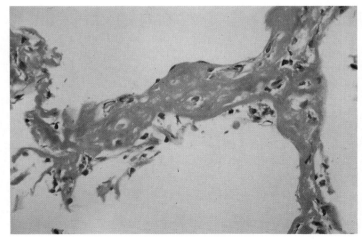

FIGURE 48-19 Alveolar septum of patient with pulmonary amyloidosis is thickened and distorted by deposits of amyloid material in the interstitium. H&E stain, ×150.

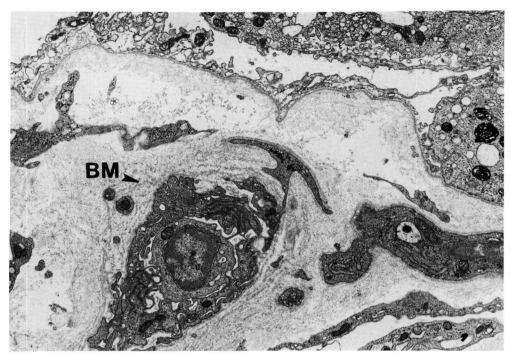

FIGURE 48-20 Damaged type I epithelial cell and type II cell with lamellar bodies line the surface of a fibrotic, edematous alveolus from a patient with IPF. Several myofibroblasts are present in the interstitium, close to a capillary which is distant from the surface and has a reduplicated basement membrane (BM). ×6660.

CONSEQUENCES OF INTERSTITIAL INJURY TO LUNG STRUCTURE

The type of injury is critical with respect to reversibility of the process and restoration of the architecture of the alveolar walls.

Distortion-Type Injury

This type of injury may be caused by the accumulation of cells (Fig. 48-21), water, or other materials (Fig. 48-19). Often, distortion-type injury coexists with fibrosis-type injury. But, since fibrosis-type injury is more disruptive of alveolar capillary function, the role of the distortion is often overridden (Fig. 48-22). As a rule, distortion-type injury is the most reversible of the forms of injury to the interstitium. However, if the distortion is extensive and long-lasting, permanent "mechanical injury" may result. Typical disorders in which distortion-type injury dominates are sarcoidosis, berylliosis, the early stages of hypersensitivity pneumonitis, and amyloidosis.

Fibrosis-Type Injury

Among the prototypes of injurious processes that result in fibrosis-type injury are inflammation, locally produced injurious products, xenobiotics, and ischemia. The disorders in which fibrosis-type injury dominates are the interstitial lung disorders ("fibrotic lung disorders") such as idiopathic pulmonary fibrosis, asbestosis, silicosis, the chronic drug-induced interstitial lung disorders, and paraquat poisoning. As indicated previously, a more circumscribed, patchy fibrosis-type injury also dominates in the pulmonary vasculitides, such as Wegener's granulomatosis.

In contrast to distortion-type injury, fibrosis-type injury is largely irreversible for two reasons: (1) the damage that precedes the fibrosis is generally sufficient to prevent reestablishment of the normal architecture of the interstitium, and (2) mesenchymal cells and the collagen that they deposit in the matrix are long-lived and not readily removable.

DAMAGE TO THE NORMAL INTERSTITIAL STRUCTURES

Inflammation, secondary to an injurious process, is responsible for most of the damage to the alveolar architecture (Figs. 48-23 to 48-25). The typical damage caused by these processes includes loss of type I epithelial cells, loss of capillary endothelial cells, breaks in the basement membranes, loss of intercellular junctions, interstitial edema, and disorganization of the interstitial connective tissue matrix (Figs. 48-10, 48-11, 48-13, 48-20, 48-22, 48-26, 48-27).

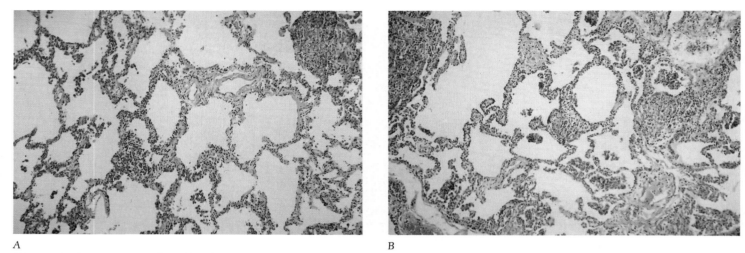

A   B

FIGURE 48-21   A. Macrophage-lymphocyte alveolitis distorts the alveolar septa of patient with sarcoidosis. H&E stain, ×110.   B. Small granuloma, lymphocytes, and macrophages are present within alveolar walls of patient with sarcoidosis. H&E stain, ×110.

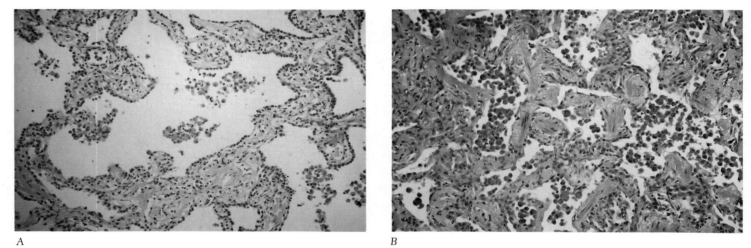

A   B

FIGURE 48-22   A. Alveolar septa of patient with early IPF are thickened by deposition of collagen and are lined by proliferating cuboidal epithelial cells. Inflammatory cells are present in the septal walls and in the interstitium. H&E stain, ×1100.   B. Lung of patient with IPF in midcourse, showing marked thickening of alveolar walls, inflammatory reaction and proliferation of smooth-muscle cells in septal walls, and numerous macrophages in alveolar lumina. H&E stain, ×110.

As a rule, the extent of the damage is related to the intensity and extent of the inflammation and the cell types that are involved: activated neutrophils are far more damaging than activated alveolar macrophages; in turn, the latter cause more damage than do activated eosinophils. In idiopathic pulmonary fibrosis, an aggressive disorder, an alveolar macrophage-neutrophil inflammation predominates. In asbestosis, which is generally slower and less severe than IPF, an alveolar macrophage inflammation predominates in association with very few neutrophils. In tropical pulmonary eosinophilia, a mild disease, the inflammatory process is dominated by eosinophils.

EXPANSION IN MESENCHYMAL CELL NUMBERS AND DEPOSITION OF CONNECTIVE TISSUE

A frequent sequel to interstitial damage is an increase in the number of mesenchymal cells; this process is driven by the alveolar macrophages. Once the number of mesenchymal cells has increased, fibrosis is the invariable consequence, since the mesenchymal cells continue to produce and secrete their connective tissue products. The increase in mesenchymal cells and the deposition of collagen need not be confined to the interstitium. As a result, two categories of disease can be identified: interstitial fibrosis (Fig. 48-22) and intra-alveolar fibrosis (Fig. 48-10).

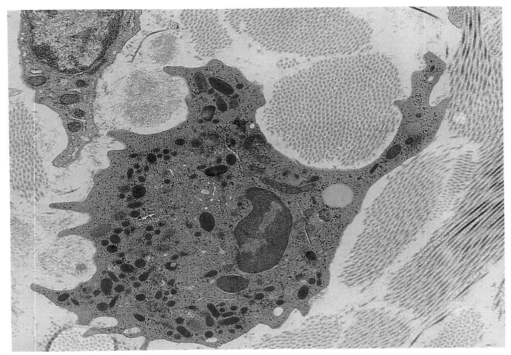

FIGURE 48-23 Electron micrograph showing neutrophil adjacent to collagen fibrils in fibrotic interstitium of patient with IPF. ×13,300.

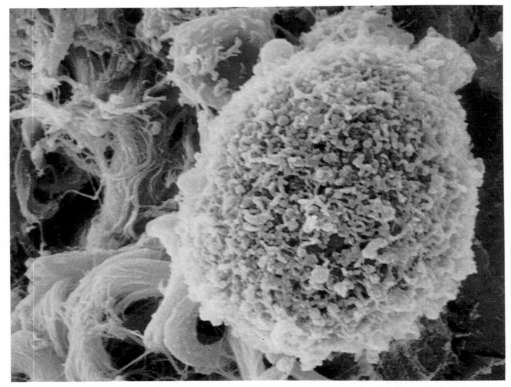

FIGURE 48-24 Macrophage in alveolar interstitium shows typical ruffled surface and is surrounded by collagen fibrils. Scanning electron micrograph. ×9700.

Interstitial fibrosis occurs entirely within the boundaries of the interstitium. The process is dominated by type I collagen, which is deposited by the mesenchymal cells as thick bundles arranged in a haphazard fashion (Fig. 48-27).

Not only does the deposition of connective tissue widen the interstitium between the epithelial and endothelial basement membranes, but the alveolar and endothelial basement membranes also thicken (Figs. 48-11 and 48-26). Indeed, in some instances, reduplication of the basement membranes is observed (Fig. 48-20).

Intra-alveolar fibrosis, in contrast to interstitial fibrosis, is characterized by the presence of mesenchymal cells and their products in the alveolar airspaces (Figs. 48-10 and 48-11). For intra-alveolar fibrosis to occur, the epithelial basement membranes must be damaged so that mesenchymal cells can migrate from the interstitium. For example, in hypersensitivity pneumonitis, the release of proteases into the interstitium by the neutrophils punches large holes in the epithelial basement membrane. When damage to the alveolar epithelial cells is extensive, a combination of intra-alveolar and interstitial fibrosis occurs to produce "mural incorporation" (Fig. 48-28), characterized by loss of the normal epithelium, fusion of the intra-alveolar mass with the underlying interstitium, and migration and overgrowth of epithelial cells to cause marked focal thickening of the alveolar wall.

Should the pathogenetic process continue unchecked, the end result of fibrosis-type injury is the "remodeling" or "end-stage lung" (Fig. 48-29). At this juncture, the anatomy of the alveolar walls is no longer recognizable: groups of fibrotic alveoli have collapsed into a mass of fibrous tissue, with the remaining airspaces represented by cystic spaces lined by cuboidal epithelium.

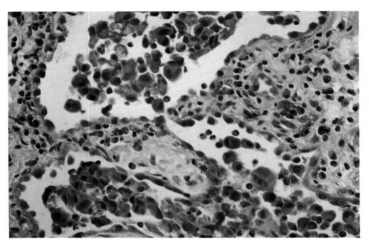

FIGURE 48-25 Numerous eosinophils and macrophages are present in alveolar walls and lumina of patient with chronic eosinophilic pneumonia. H&E stain, ×150.

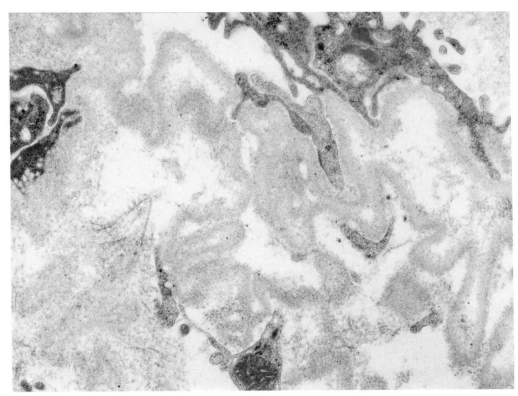

FIGURE 48-26 Multilayered, thickened basement membranes follow irregular courses just beneath an alveolar epithelial cell from a patient with IPF. ×18,750.

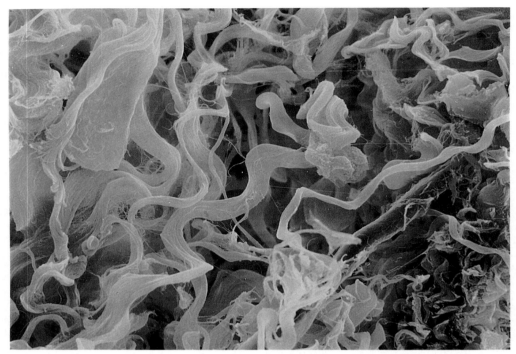

FIGURE 48-27 Scanning electron micrograph of fibrotic alveolar interstitium of patient with IPF, showing large bundles of collagen coursing in various directions. ×6000.

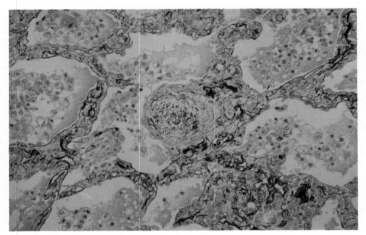

FIGURE 48-28 Area of intraalveolar fibrosis, similar to that shown in Fig. 48-10A, is being incorporated into septal wall, which is becoming focally thickened. Periodic acid-methenamine silver stain, ×150.

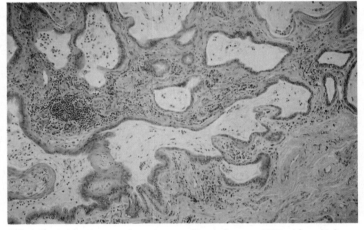

FIGURE 48-29 Lung of patient with end-stage IPF. Alveoli have been remodeled into cystic spaces that are lined by bronchiolar epithelium and are filled with mucus and inflammatory cells. The walls of these spaces are greatly thickened by fibrous tissue. H&E stain, ×110.

Destruction-Type Injury

In this type of injury, the interstitium is destroyed or dissolved (Figs. 48-4 and 48-30); the basement membranes and the interstitial connective tissue matrix have lost their identity. Although all connective tissue components are affected to some degree, the elastic fibers in the interstitial matrix are a primary target. Apparently, chronic inflam-

mation with a large number of neutrophils is necessary to destroy the interstitium, since (1) neutrophil elastase is the only protease that could conceivably destroy completely the interstitial connective tissue and (2) enough elastase must be present to overwhelm the natural defenses of the interstitium, which include α_1-antitrypsin.

The loss of alveolar walls consequent to the destructive-type injury causes irreversible enlargement of the dis-

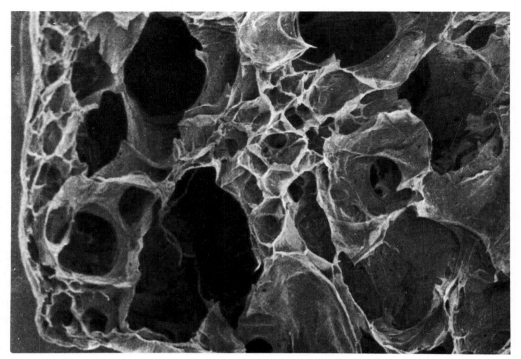

FIGURE 48-30 Scanning electron micrograph of lung from patient with emphysema, showing marked dilatation of airspaces. ×30.

tal airspaces. Typical examples of destructive-type injury are α_1-antitrypsin deficiency and the emphysema associated with cigarette smoking.

FUNCTIONAL CONSEQUENCES OF INTERSTITIAL INJURY

For interstitial disease to affect pulmonary function, the disease must be widespread. Moreover, although the mechanical consequences of distortion- and fibrosis-type injury differ from those of destructive-type injury, their overall effects on symptoms and gas exchange are quite similar.

Mechanical Consequences of Interstitial Injury

In both distortion- and fibrosis-type injury, the space available for air decreases, and the mechanical resistance to stretching the interstitium increases. In addition, fibrosis-type injury is associated with an increase in the number of myofibroblasts and smooth-muscle cells in the alveolar walls; this adds the capability for contractility to the mechanical forces that resist alveolar expansion. Consequently, the lung volumes—including vital capacity, residual volume and total lung capacity—are reduced, and the peak inspiratory intrathoracic pressures are inordinately negative. As a result, the static deflation volume-pressure curves are shifted downward and to the right, reflecting the high negative intrathoracic pressures that are required to expand the lungs to the limited extent permitted by the interstitial abnormalities.

Gross measures of airway function, such as FEV_1/FVC, are normal or supranormal. However, more sensitive tests, such as flow-volume curves, frequency dependency of compliance, and maximum flow-static recoil curves, may be abnormal, reflecting involvement of the small airways by the peribronchiolar interstitial process. Because of the loss of functional alveolar capillary bed, the diffusing capacity (carbon monoxide, corrected for volume) is abnormally low.

In contrast to distortion and fibrosis, destruction enlarges the space available for air and decreases the mechanical resistance to stretching of the interstitium. Consequently, the total lung capacity is increased, usually modestly. The destruction in the parenchyma also leads to obstruction of airflow, to an increase in the residual volume, and to a decrease in vital capacity.

The effect of the destruction is dramatically illustrated by changes in the static deflation volume-pressure characteristics of the lung: the decrease in parenchymal resistance to expansion and the less-than normal negative intrathoracic pressure required to expand the lungs cause the volume-pressure curve to be shifted up and to the left. In addition, the loss of interstitium, particularly the loss of the elastic continuum of the lung parenchyma, de-

735

creases elastic recoil. The decrease in the forces available to push air out causes a decrease in the rate of airflow during forced exhalation. The decrease in the forces of expiration together with the decrease in the tethering of small airways by the rarefied lungs promotes dynamic collapse of the small airways during expiration. Overall, the result of these structural abnormalities is a limitation of airflow during all phases of expiration. Also, like distortion and fibrosis, destruction-type injury is accompanied by a reduced diffusing capacity, reflecting the abnormalities and reduction in the gas-exchanging surfaces of the lungs.

Sensation of Dyspnea

Characteristically, interstitial injury evokes breathlessness, first at rest but later during exercise. Two major reasons are generally invoked to account for dyspnea in interstitial disease: (1) stimulation of breathing by intrapulmonary receptors, and (2) an increase in the work of breathing.

Alterations in Gas Exchange

Widespread, severe interstitial injury usually causes mild arterial hypoxemia at rest, which worsens during exercise. The arterial hypoxemia results from two processes: (1) mismatching of alveolar ventilation and of alveolar blood flow, and (2) an excessively rapid flow of red blood cells through the restricted pulmonary capillary bed, creating the equivalent of an alveolar-capillary diffusion limitation. Both processes worsen with exercise: the mismatching of alveolar ventilation and blood flow because of amplification of the mechanical derangements manifested at rest; the brief time red cells spend in the pulmonary capillaries because of the increase in the rate of blood flow during exercise through the curtailed capillary bed and past abnormal alveolar-capillary units.

Widespread interstitial injury, by restricting the pulmonary vascular bed through loss of pulmonary capillaries, generates pulmonary hypertension that strains the right heart. In time, the cardiac output falls, thereby compromising oxygen delivery from the pulmonary capillaries to the rest of the body.

Reversibility of Lung Dysfunction

The type of interstitial injury determines the reversibility of the damage: by definition, destruction-type injury is not reversible; at the opposite extreme is distortion-type injury, in which reversibility is the rule. In between the two is fibrosis-type injury, which is reversible only when the insult is sufficiently mild and short-lived for the normal architecture of affected alveoli to be restored. The effect of reversibility and nonreversibility on overall pulmonary function clearly depends on the number of affected alveoli and the constellation of injuries.

FAMILIAR EXAMPLES OF INTERSTITIAL INJURY

To illustrate the categories of interstitial injury—distortion-type, fibrosis-type and destruction-type—it may be useful to categorize five familiar entities. In this light, sarcoidosis is an example of distortion-type injury (Fig. 48-21 and 48-31); tropical pulmonary eosinophilia is an example of a mild form of fibrosis-type injury; asbestosis is a moderate form of fibrosis-type injury (Fig. 48-18); idiopathic pulmonary fibrosis is a severe form of fibrosis-type injury (Fig. 48-22); and α_1-antitrypsin deficiency is the classic example of destructive-type injury (Fig. 48-30). Each of these diseases is described in detail elsewhere in this volume.

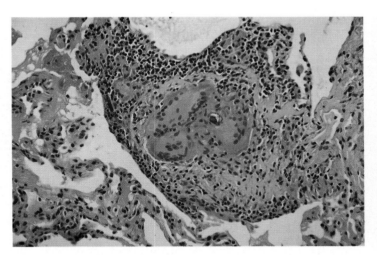

FIGURE 48-31 Granuloma distorting alveolar septum of patient with sarcoidosis is composed of multinucleated giant cells, epithelioid cells, macrophages, and lymphocytes. H&E stain, ×150.

BIBLIOGRAPHY

Basset F, Ferrans VJ, Soler P, Takemura T, Fukuda Y, Crystal RG: Intraluminal fibrosis in interstitial lung disorders. Am J Pathol 122:443–461, 1986.
Morphologic study of the patterns of fibrosis characterizing fibrosis-type injury.

Bitterman PB, Wewers MD, Rennard SI, Adelberg S, Crystal RG: Modulation of alveolar macrophage driven fibroblast proliferation by alternative macrophage mediators. J Clin Invest 77(3):700–708, 1986.

Recent study of the major alveolar macrophage mediators relevant to mesenchymal cell accumulation in fibrotic-type injury.

Brutinel WM, Martin WJ II: Chronic nitrofurantoin reaction associated with T-lymphocyte alveolitis. Chest 89:150–152, 1986.

Nitrofurantoin use was associated with the development of severe interstitial lung disease and a marked lymphocytosis, mostly of the T-helper subset, in bronchoalveolar lavage fluid.

Chapman HA, Allen CL, Stone OL: Abnormalities in pathways of alveolar fibrin turnover among patients with interstitial lung disease. Am Rev Respir Dis 133:437–443, 1986.

This study examined the cell-associated procoagulant activity of macrophages lavaged from patients with sarcoidosis (n = 14) or idiopathic pulmonary fibrosis (n = 13). Enhanced activity was demonstrated in the bronchoalveolar lavage fluid and correlated well with radiographic evidence of disease activity.

Crystal RG, Bitterman PB, Rennard SI, Hance A, Keogh BA: Interstitial lung disease of unknown cause: Disorders characterized by chronic inflammation of the lower respiratory tract. N Engl J Med 310:154–166, 235–244, 1984.

Comprehensive review of the current concepts of the pathogenesis, staging, and therapy of the interstitial lung disorders of unknown etiology.

Crystal RG, Gadek JE, Ferrans VJ, Fulmer JD, Line BR, Hunninghake GW: Interstitial lung diseases: Current concepts of pathogenesis, staging, and therapy. Am J Med 70:542–568, 1981.

Overview of the pathogenesis of the interstitial lung disorders.

Davis WB, Crystal RG: Chronic interstitial lung disease, in Simmons D (ed), *Current Pulmonology*, vol V. New York, Wiley, 1984, pp 347–473.

Detailed review of developments during the last few years of all the interstitial lung diseases; contains 668 references.

De Vuyst P, Dumortier P, Schandene L, Estenne M, Verhest A, Yernault JC: Sarcoidlike lung granulomatosis induced by aluminum dusts. Am Rev Respir Dis 135:493–497, 1987.

Aluminum can cause granulomatous lung disease accompanied by a helper T-lymphocyte alveolitis, similar to that of berylliosis and sarcoidosis.

Gadek JE, Crystal RD: α_1-Antitrypsin deficiency, in Stanbury JB, Wyngaarden JB, Fredrickson DS, Goldstein JL, Brown MS (eds), *The Metabolic Basis of Inherited Disease.* New York, McGraw-Hill, 1982, pp 1450–1467.

Detailed review of α_1-antitrypsin deficiency, the classic example of destruction-type injury.

Garcia JG, Munim A, Nugent KM, Bishop M, Hoie-Garcia P, Parhami N, Keogh BA: Alveolar macrophage gold retention in rheumatoid arthritis. J Rheumatol 14:435–438, 1987.

Although gold is retained for prolonged periods in pulmonary tissue macrophages, there is no relationship between gold and chronic rheumatoid lung disease.

Hance A, Crystal RG: Idiopathic pulmonary fibrosis, in Flenley DC, Petty TL (eds), *Recent Advances in Respiratory Medicine*, vol 3. Edinburgh, Churchill-Livingstone, 1983, pp 249–287.

Detailed review of the pathogenetic processes associated with idiopathic pulmonary fibrosis, the classic disease associated with fibrosis-type injury.

Haslam, PL, Dewar A, Butchers P, Primett ZS, Newman-Taylor A, Turner-Warwick M: Mast cells, atypical lymphocytes, and neutrophils in bronchoalveolar lavage in extrinsic allergic alveolitis. Comparison with other interstitial lung diseases. Am Rev Respir Dis 135:35–47, 1987.

Extrinsic allergic alveolitis (idiopathic pulmonary fibrosis) may be an example of a human disease in which a delayed hypersensitivity disorder involves mast cells as well as lymphocytes.

Kallenberg CG, Schilizzi BM, Beaumont F, De-Leij L, Poppema S, The TH: Expression of class II major histocompatibility complex antigens on alveolar epithelium in interstitial lung disease: relevance to pathogenesis of idiopathic pulmonary fibrosis. J Clin Pathol 40:725–733, 1987.

Class II major histocompatibility complex antigens are expressed on alveolar epithelium in patients with idiopathic pulmonary fibrosis, sarcoidosis, and microbial infections. However, their role in the pathogenesis of IPF is speculative.

Katzenstein A-LA, Askin FB: *Surgical Pathology of Non-Neoplastic Lung Disease.* Philadelphia, Saunders, 1982.

Most recent comprehensive description of the pathology of the nonmalignant lung disorders.

Kawanami O, Ferrans VJ, Crystal RD: Structure of alveolar epithelial cells in patients with fibrotic lung disorders. Lab Invest 46:39–53, 1982.
Changes to the epithelium characterizing fibrosis-type injury.

Myers JL, Veal CF, Jr, Shin MS, Katzenstein AL: Respiratory bronchiolitis causing interstitial lung disease. A clinicopathologic study of six cases. Am Rev Respir Dis 135:880–884, 1987.
Respiratory bronchiolitis is an uncommon cause of chronic interstitial lung disease.

O'Donnell K, Keogh B, Cantin A, Crystal RG: Pharmacologic suppression of the neutrophil component of the alveolitis in idiopathic pulmonary fibrosis. Am Rev Respir Dis 136:288–292, 1987.
Cyclophosphamide, alone or in combination with corticosteroids, is much more effective than corticosteroids alone in suppressing the neutrophil component of the inflammation of IPF.

Reynolds HY: Lung inflammation: normal host defense or a complication of some diseases? Annu Rev Med 38:295–323, 1987.
A review of inflammatory processes in the lungs as a prelude to considering particular disease entities.

Saltini C, Spurzem JR, Lee JL, Pinkston P, Crystal RG: Spontaneous release of interleukin-2 by lung T-lymphocytes in active pulmonary sarcoidosis is primarily from the Leu3$^+$ DR$^+$ T-cell subset. J Clin Invest 77:1962–1970, 1986.
Recent study of the mechanisms of T-lymphocyte accumulation in the lung in the distortion-type injury associated with sarcoidosis.

Takizawa H, Shiga J, Moroi Y, Miyachi S, Nishiwaki M, Miyamoto T: Interstitial lung disease in dermatomyositis: clinicopathological study. J Rheumatol 14:102–107, 1987.
In 14 cases of polymyositis-dermatomyositis (PM-DM), radiographic and histologic evidence of interstitial lung disease was found in 9 patients with DM.

Wewers MD, Casolaro MA, Sellers SE, Swayze SC, McPhaul KM, Wittes JT, Crystal RG: Replacement therapy for alpha$_1$-antitrypsin deficiency associated with emphysema. N Engl J Med 316:1055–1062, 1987.
Infusions of alpha$_1$-antitrypsin derived from plasma are safe and can reverse the biochemical abnormalities in serum and lung fluid that characterize this disorder.

Chapter 49

Structural-Functional Features of the Interstitial Lung Diseases

Larry K. Jackson / Jack D. Fulmer

Classification and Pathogenesis of the Interstitial Diseases

Pathophysiology of the Interstitial Diseases
   Volume-Pressure Relationships
   Work of Breathing and Control of Breathing
   Airway Mechanics
   Resting and Exercise Gas Exchange
   Pulmonary Hemodynamics

Structure-Function Alterations in Specific Interstitial Lung Diseases
   Sarcoidosis
   Idiopathic Pulmonary Fibrosis
   Organic Dust Disease
   Primary Pulmonary Histiocytosis X

Other Interstitial Lung Diseases
   Inorganic Dust Diseases
   Wegener's Granulomatosis

Clinical and Functional Assessment in the Management of the Interstitial Diseases

Future

The interstitial lung diseases are a diverse group of disorders classified together because of common clinical, radiographic, physiological, and pathologic features. Most patients present with the insidious onset of exertional breathlessness and a diffuse nodular, reticular, or reticulonodular pattern on the chest radiograph (Fig. 49-1). Physiological alterations are typically those of a restrictive defect: reduced lung volumes and compliance, reduced diffusing capacity, and arterial hypoxemia that worsens with exercise. The pathology of the interstitial diseases mainly involves parenchyma; in most, there is an inflammatory cellular infiltration and varying severity of fibrosis of alveolar septae (Fig. 49-1). Some of the interstitial diseases are also accompanied by airways disease, pulmonary vascular disease, and pleural disease.

Physiological assessment is important in the interstitial diseases. In patients who are at risk of interstitial disease, physiological testing is a useful means of detecting early disease. Also, although specific diagnosis depends on histopathology or identification of an etiologic agent, physiological testing can provide adjunctive data useful in establishing the diagnosis, in localizing and quantifying the component of the lungs, e.g., the alveolar-capillary membrane, which is predominantly affected, and in managing patients with interstitial diseases.

CLASSIFICATION AND PATHOGENESIS OF THE INTERSTITIAL DISEASES

More than 130 disorders have been associated with interstitial lung disease. Of these, only one-third have known etiologies. The interstitial diseases of unknown etiology can be separated into specific syndromes based on clinical, radiographic, physiological, and pathologic features (Table 49-1).

Despite the heterogeneous nature of the interstitial diseases, all share a common pathogenesis. As a result of an initial injury, inflammatory and immune effector cells accumulate in the pulmonary parenchyma. This accumulation of cells within alveoli is termed an *alveolitis*. In many of the interstitial diseases (e.g., idiopathic pulmonary fibrosis or asbestosis), the inflammatory cells are activated alveolar macrophages and polymorphonuclear leukocytes; in others (e.g., sarcoidosis or hypersensitivity pneumonitis), activated T lymphocytes and macrophages are the predominant inflammatory cells. Thus, although the character of the alveolitis varies from interstitial disease to interstitial disease, all have in common an accumulation of effector cells capable of altering the normal cellular and connective tissue elements of the alveolus. As the alveolitis becomes chronic, alveolar structures are damaged and areas of pulmonary parenchyma are replaced by fibrous tissue. Before the stage of fibrosis, the alveolitis is believed to be reversible; thereafter, it is irreversible. Histopathologically, advanced (end-stage) interstitial lung disease typically shows fibrotic replacement of alveoli, cystic lesions in the parenchyma, and distortion and dilatation of small airways.

Several pathologic terms are used to describe specific histologic patterns of interstitial diseases.

Desquamative interstitial pneumonitis (DIP) is characterized by a marked increase in intra-alveolar mononuclear cells with minimal interstitial fibrosis. DIP is generally viewed as the histologic expression of alveolitis caused by a variety of initiating mechanisms. It may also represent an early stage of idiopathic pulmonary fibrosis.

Usual interstitial pneumonitis (UIP) refers to a histologic pattern of interstitial and intra-alveolar cellular infiltrates, which ranges considerably in severity. Considerable fibrosis and destruction of alveolar septae accompanies the inflammatory reaction. It is likely that

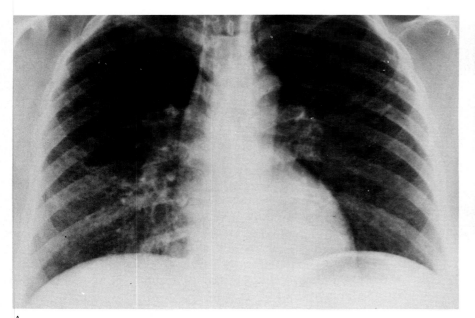
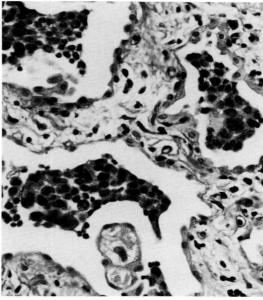

A   B

FIGURE 49-1   Diffuse interstitial lung disease in a 33-year-old female.   A. Chest radiograph shows a diffuse reticulonodular infiltrate. B. Lung biopsy shows thickened alveolar septae with interstitial and intra-alveolar inflammatory cells.

TABLE 49-1
Classification of the Interstitial Lung Diseases

Known Etiology	Unknown Etiology
Occupational and environmental inhalants	Sarcoidosis
Inorganic dusts	Interstitial lung diseases associated with collagen-vascular disorders
Organic dusts (hypersensitivity) pneumonitis)	Idiopathic pulmonary fibrosis
Gases	Inherited diseases
Fumes	Histiocytosis X
Aerosols	Lymphocytic infiltrative disorders
Drugs	Pulmonary hemorrhage syndromes
Poisons	
Radiation	Lymphangioleiomyomatosis
Infectious agents	Ankylosing spondylitis
Cardiac disease	Chronic eosinophilic pneumonias
Metabolic abnormalities	
	Veno-occlusive disease
	Pulmonary vasculitis

UIP represents late-stage interstitial disease of many causes.

Bronchiolitis obliterans and interstitial pneumonitis (BOP) is characterized by fibrous plugs that occlude small airways in association with the histologic appearance of usual interstitial pneumonitis.

These categories based on histologic patterns are useful to the extent that they provide prognostic information and limit diagnostic possibilities. However, they do not suffice for specific diagnosis.

PATHOPHYSIOLOGY OF THE INTERSTITIAL DISEASES

Structural changes in the lungs elicit changes in pulmonary function. Cellular infiltration and increased connective tissue elements within the pulmonary parenchyma cause an increase in the elastic recoil of the lungs, reducing lung volumes and increasing the work of breathing. Alterations in cellular and connective tissue elements of alveoli also interfere with the normal balance of ventilation and blood flow so that gas exchange becomes abnormal. In some interstitial diseases, airways and pulmonary blood vessels, as well as alveolar walls, are involved, thereby impairing airflow and blood flow.

Volume-Pressure Relationships

The increase in lung elastic recoil in the interstitial lung diseases generally has three consequences: reduced lung volumes, reduced pulmonary compliance, and increased work of breathing (see Chapter 163).

The increase in lung elastic recoil is responsible for a reduction in vital capacity (VC) and in total lung capacity (TLC) to less than the predicted normal values. Often, the residual volume (RV) and the functional residual capacity (FRC) do not decrease to the same extent as the VC so that RV/TLC (normally about 0.3) exceeds this value. The mechanism by which these lung volumes are preserved is unclear but may entail either premature closure of small airways and gas trapping, or revision of pulmonary parenchyma by cystic disease (and its attendant loss of recoil pressures at lung volumes below FRC), or both. The ratio RV/TLC is often markedly increased in certain interstitial

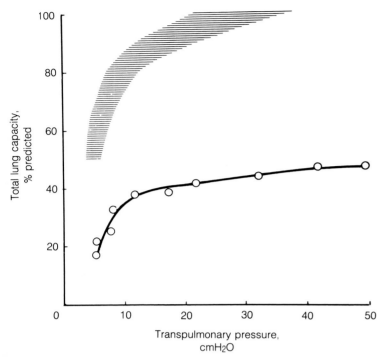

FIGURE 49-2 Volume-pressure curve in a 50-year-old male with chronic interstitial lung disease. The curve is shifted downward and to the right. Maximal transpulmonary pressure at TLC is increased. The shaded curve presents the normal relationship.

diseases, notably in primary pulmonary histiocytosis X, advanced sarcoidosis with cystic changes, some collagen vascular diseases, inorganic dust diseases, and lymphangioleiomyomatosis.

Characteristically, the compliance of the lungs measured at FRC is reduced and volume-pressure relationships are shifted downward and to the right (Fig. 49-2). In advanced fibrotic disease, when volume data are expressed as percent of *observed* rather than as percent of *predicted*, the volume-pressure data often fall within the normal range. This has raised the possibility that alterations in the volume-pressure relationship are due entirely to loss of functional alveolar units while the normal elasticity of remaining lung units is preserved. However, in less advanced disease, and in certain experimental models, the volume-pressure curve is shifted to the right when the data are expressed as a percent of *observed*. These results indicate that reduced compliance in the interstitial diseases is due to a combination of increased recoil of functional lung units as well as loss of other lung units.

Another common alteration of the volume-pressure relationship in the interstitial diseases is the abnormally high transpulmonary pressure at TLC (Fig. 49-2). However, pressure at maximal lung volume correlates inversely with TLC; therefore, the smaller the lungs, the greater the transpulmonary pressure that can be developed. Also, since the function of the inspiratory muscles in interstitial diseases is normal, the inspiratory muscles must work at a greater mechanical advantage at low lung volumes.

Work of Breathing and Control of Breathing

Because of the increased elastic recoil in the interstitial diseases, the elastic work of breathing is abnormally high. However, the increased work of breathing usually does not limit the minute ventilation ($\dot{V}E$). On the contrary, $\dot{V}E$ is usually increased above normal. However, the work of breathing does influence breathing pattern.

In patients with interstitial disease, the typical breathing pattern is one of reduced tidal volume VT and increased respiratory frequency f; the reduction in the VT is proportional to the reduction in VC. Measurement of respiratory times indicates that inspiratory time TI is decreased in proportion to the total respiratory cycle time TT; therefore, TI/TT remains normal. Mean inspiratory flow rate ($\dot{V}I$) is also increased, suggesting an increased respiratory drive. The result of these alterations in breathing pattern is a decrease in the peak force developed by contraction of the inspiratory muscles and minimization of the duration of development of peak force with respect to the duration of relaxation of the inspiratory muscles. These changes minimize both the perception of breathlessness and failure of the respiratory muscles.

The respiratory drive is increased in interstitial disease, as indicated by the fact that the slopes of the lines relating $\dot{V}E$ and $PaCO_2$ on the one hand and $Pm_{0.1}$ (the mouth pressure at 0.1 s of expiration) and $PaCO_2$ on the other are nearly normal, but the intercepts are not: for any value of $PaCO_2$, the $\dot{V}E$ or $Pm_{0.1}$ is higher than normal. Since the slopes are not significantly modified by either O_2 inhalation or administration of alkali, the increased respiratory drive is due to nonchemical (probably mechanical), receptor-mediated stimulation of the midbrain respiratory centers. The location of the receptors in the periphery remains speculative: because similar breathing patterns and CO_2 sensitivity studies can be produced in normal individuals who are subjected to external elastic loads, one possibility is that the receptors are in the chest wall; alternatively, the inverse correlation between CO_2 partial pressure and degree of alveolitis suggests that the receptors are situated within the pulmonary parenchyma.

Airway Mechanics

Although the interstitial diseases are considered to affect primarily the alveoli, many interstitial diseases are associated with morphologic and functional evidence of airways disease: in patients with idiopathic pulmonary fibrosis, sarcoidosis, collagen vascular disease, asbestosis, hypersensitivity pneumonitis, and histiocytosis X, small airways may be narrowed by fibrosis or inflammatory infiltrates (Fig. 49-3). Bronchiolitis obliterans also occurs in several of the collagen-vascular diseases. Obstruction of bronchi due to granulomatous lesions sometimes occurs in sarcoidosis and Wegener's granulomatosis.

Despite the histologic changes in the airways, functional obstruction to airflow using conventional tests is

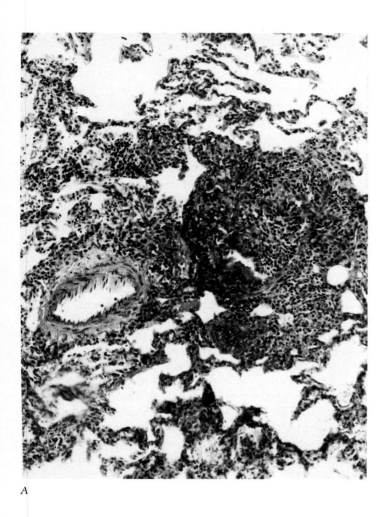

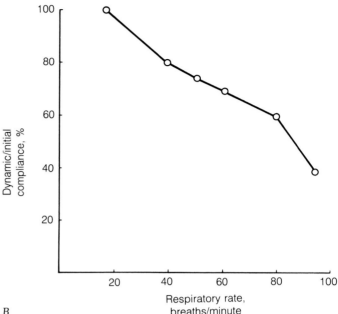

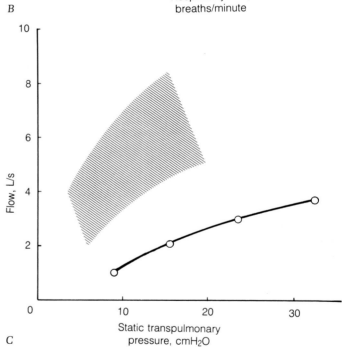

FIGURE 49-3 Small airways disease in idiopathic pulmonary fibrosis. *A.* Open lung biopsy showing a narrowed small airway from bronchiolitis and peribronchiolar inflammation and fibrosis. *B.* Dynamic compliance showing marked frequency dependence consistent with altered resistance of small airways. *C.* Maximum flow-static recoil curve showing reduced airflow for a given transpulmonary pressure. The normal flow-recoil pressure relationship is presented by the shaded curve.

uncommon in most of the interstitial diseases; e.g., the ratio of forced expiratory volume in 1 s to the forced vital capacity (FEV$_1$/FVC) is generally normal. Maximal midexpiratory flow rate (MMFR) is sometimes reduced in interstitial lung diseases, but usually in proportion to the decrease in lung volume. In some instances of interstitial disease, MMFR/FVC is increased, suggesting that an increase in the retractive forces of the lungs is keeping the airways more open than is normal at small lung volumes. However, there are notable exceptions to these generalizations. For example, FEV$_1$/FVC is abnormally low in some

interstitial diseases (Table 49-2): reversible airflow obstruction is encountered in allergic angiitis and granulomatosis (Churg-Strauss syndrome), in acute exacerbations of organic dust disease in the atopic patient, and in chronic eosinophilic pneumonitis. In addition, increased airways reactivity to a methacholine challenge occurs in sarcoidosis and in organic dust disease.

Routine spirometric measurements are relatively insensitive in detecting increased resistance in small airways. However, two physiological studies, i.e., the maximum expiratory flow-volume (MEFV) curves and the

TABLE 49-2
Interstitial Diseases That May Have an Abnormal FEV₁/FVC

$$\text{TABLE 49-2: Interstitial Diseases That May Have an Abnormal } FEV_1/FVC$$

Advanced sarcoidosis
Allergic angiitis and granulomatosis
Primary pulmonary histiocytosis X
Chronic eosinophilic pneumonia
Wegener's granulomatosis
Acute organic dust disease (in atopic patients)
Chronic organic dust disease
Lymphangioleiomyomatosis

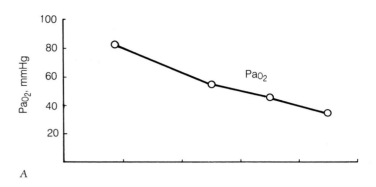

A

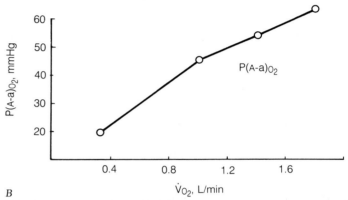

B

FIGURE 49-4 Resting and exercise oxygen tensions in a 50-year-old male with chronic interstitial disease. *A.* Mild resting hypoxemia is present and, during moderate exercise, severe hypoxemia develops. *B.* Alveolar-arterial oxygen gradient is mildly widened at rest and widens further with exercise.

dynamic compliance (Cdyn), do correlate well with involvement of the small airways in the interstitial diseases. A third test, the maximum flow-static recoil (MF-SR) curve, although occasionally useful for determining upstream airflow resistance (Fig. 49-3), is less sensitive than the MEFV and Cdyn curves in detecting small airways disease.

The clinical implications of involvement of the small airways in the interstitial diseases are uncertain. In sarcoidosis, the possibility has been raised that airways disease is a major determinant of dyspnea. However, probably the greatest significance of such involvement is a maldistribution of ventilation that causes abnormalities in gas exchange.

Resting and Exercise Gas Exchange

Arterial hypoxemia that worsens with exercise is a classic finding in the interstitial diseases. The oxygen tension gradient between alveoli and arterial blood [$P(A-a)_{O_2}$] is wide at rest and widens further during exercise (Fig. 49-4). Also, tests of gas transfer across the alveolar-capillary membranes, e.g., the single-breath diffusion capacity for carbon monoxide ($D_{L_{CO}}$), are reduced.

Although diffusion impairment was once thought to be the major mechanism for hypoxemia in these diseases (hence the term *alveolar-capillary block syndrome*), it now seems that diffusion impairment plays an insignificant role in the etiology of the arterial hypoxemia, except during vigorous exercise when capillary transit times decrease and diffusion limitation does occur. Instead of diffusion limitation, the major mechanism responsible for the arterial hypoxemia is mismatching of alveolar ventilation and pulmonary capillary blood flow; a lesser contribution is made by venous admixture, i.e., perfusion of nonventilated areas of the lungs. The transition from ventilation-mismatching ("physiological shunting" that is correctable by O_2 breathing) in interstitial disease to "true shunting" ("anatomic venous admixture") is a consequence of progressive fibrosis. In advanced interstitial disease, the anatomic venous admixture may increase to the point that restoration of arterial oxygen to tolerable

levels by administering supplemental O_2 may not be possible.

Minute ventilation is increased at rest and during exercise in patients with interstitial disease (Fig. 49-5), and the Pa_{CO_2} is generally below normal. However, hypercapnia does occur in severe, end-stage disease. Because tidal volumes are low and some of the ventilation is wasted on nonperfused lung units, the ratio of dead-space ventilation to tidal ventilation (V_D/V_T) is often increased. During exercise, (V_D/V_T) may increase as a result of further impairment in ventilation-perfusion matching (Fig. 49-5).

The high ventilatory requirements for a given workload and the associated high elastic work of breathing are the most common causes of exercise limitation in patients with interstitial lung disease (Fig. 49-4). Peak oxygen consumption ($\dot{V}_{O_2max}$) generally does not correlate with the degree of arterial hypoxemia during exercise, suggesting that most patients with these diseases can continue exercising despite arterial hypoxemia. A subgroup of patients with interstitial diseases is limited during exercise by pulmonary vascular disease (see "Structure-Function Alterations in Specific Interstitial Lung Diseases").

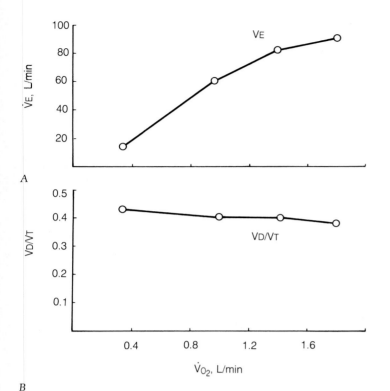

A

B

FIGURE 49-5 Resting and exercise minute ventilation and dead space ventilation in a 50-year-old male with chronic interstitial lung disease. *A.* Minute ventilation at rest is mildly elevated, but increases disproportionately to oxygen consumption; the average male has a $\dot{V}_E$ of 40 to 45 L/min at a $\dot{V}_{O_2}$ of 1.0 L/min. *B.* Ratio of dead space to tidal volume is elevated at rest and does not fall appropriately during exercise. Normal V_D/V_T at rest is 0.3, and usually falls below 0.2 at moderate workloads.

Pulmonary Hemodynamics

Pulmonary hypertension, which also worsens during exercise, is common in patients with advanced interstitial disease. In certain diseases that are categorized as interstitial diseases, e.g., scleroderma and rheumatoid lung disease, pulmonary vascular disease can occur independently of interstitial fibrosis; but, in most others, e.g., idiopathic pulmonary fibrosis and histiocytosis X, the pulmonary vascular disease is part of the interstitial process. The mechanisms responsible for pulmonary hypertension include destruction of blood vessels by the interstitial process, reduced distensibility of the pulmonary vascular bed, pulmonary vascular obstructive lesions (medial hypertrophy or intimal proliferation), and vasoconstriction elicited primarily by alveolar hypoxia.

The sustained and progressive pulmonary hypertension gradually overburdens the right ventricle: about two-thirds of patients with advanced pulmonary fibrosis have clinical evidence of cor pulmonale. In some patients with interstitial disease, transient failure of the right heart due to pulmonary hypertension is a cause of exercise limitation; in these patients, the $\dot{V}_{O_2max}$ and the anaerobic

threshold are very low, and the heart rate increases markedly during exercise.

STRUCTURE-FUNCTION ALTERATIONS IN SPECIFIC INTERSTITIAL LUNG DISEASES

Whereas early interstitial lung disease is mainly characterized by an alveolitis, advanced disease is characterized by extensive fibrosis, a reduction in air volume, and a loss of gas-exchange units. Presumably, the alveolitis is reversible; in contrast, the fibrosis and loss of alveoli are not. Tissue for histopathology is generally sampled only once in the attempt to establish a specific etiology and to assess the stage of the disease and the likelihood of response to therapy. With this exception, physiological testing and radiography are the mainstays for diagnosing, staging, and monitoring the disease process as well as for evaluating therapeutic regimens and evaluating disability. Underlying this usage of physiological testing and radiography is the assumption that they reflect structural changes in the lungs.

Sarcoidosis

Early pulmonary sarcoidosis is characterized by a mononuclear cellular alveolitis that is followed by the formation of noncaseating granulomas. The alveolitis in sarcoidosis is largely confined to the alveolar interstitium, although some cells may be found in the alveolar airspaces. The granulomata may resolve or undergo progressive fibrosis. In a small number of patients, sarcoidosis progresses to end-stage pulmonary disease. Granulomata can also involve bronchi, bronchioles, and pulmonary vessels and evoke clinical manifestations.

A number of radiographic classifications have been developed to group patients with sarcoidosis. These are considered in detail in Chapter 42. In essence, by international convention, the chest radiographs of patients are grouped according to the following scheme: *stage 0*, normal; *stage I*, bilateral hilar adenopathy; *stage II*, bilateral hilar adenopathy with diffuse parenchymal changes; and *stage III*, diffuse pulmonary infiltrates without hilar adenopathy. Patients with advanced fibrotic changes accompanied by cysts and bullae are usually assigned to stage III; however, some clinics add another stage, stage IV, for these patients. Few patients progress through the radiographic stages in a sequential fashion.

STRUCTURE-FUNCTION ALTERATIONS

Correlations have been made between histologic and radiographic appearance and physiological testing in sarcoidosis. Although stage I sarcoidosis has no radiographic evidence of parenchymal disease, lung biopsies have clearly established that virtually all patients have an alveolitis in which there are varying numbers of granulomata;

some have fibrosis of alveolar septae. Individual pulmonary function tests are insensitive in detecting parenchymal disease in stage I sarcoidosis: only one-fifth of patients have a reduction in VC and only 30 percent have a reduction in $D_{L_{CO}}$. In contrast, exercise hypoxemia seems to be more sensitive in detecting disease in stage I sarcoidosis: approximately 40 percent develop hypoxemia during exercise and up to 80 percent have widening of the $P(A-a)_{O_2}$ during exercise.

In contrast to the patients with stage I sarcoidosis, nearly two-thirds of those with stage II sarcoidosis have abnormalities in VC, $D_{L_{CO}}$, or pulmonary compliance. As a corollary, in at least one-third of patients with stage II sarcoidosis, any single routine test may be normal despite radiographically detectable disease. In approximately one-half of the stage II patients, the resting Pa_{O_2} is abnormal, nearly 60 percent develop arterial hypoxemia during exercise, and in nearly 90 percent the $P(A-a)_{O_2}$ is widened.

Comparisons of the severity of the physiological derangement and the histologic severity of disease in patients with sarcoidosis indicate that the $D_{L_{CO}}$ and exercise Pa_{O_2} generally correlate well with the overall histologic severity of disease. The diffusing capacity correlates best with the extent of granulomatous involvement and the overall severity of the fibrotic process: in individuals with few granulomata, the $D_{L_{CO}}$ is apt to be normal, whereas in those in whom granulomata are widespread, the $D_{L_{CO}}$ is often 65 percent or less of the predicted normal; in patients in whom the number of granulomata is moderate, the reduction in $D_{L_{CO}}$ is mild. In general, values of VC and resting Pa_{O_2} can distinguish mild from severe pathology, but cannot distinguish moderate from severe pathology. For the individual patient, the values are so variable that the pathologic severity of disease cannot be predicted reliably from the functional values. Radiographic-pathologic correlative studies suggest that the radiographic changes generally parallel the pathologic changes. The combination of normal pulmonary function studies and a stage I radiograph is associated with minimal pathology of the lungs and no fibrosis. But a stage I radiograph does not, per se, preclude extensive lesions or the presence of fibrosis.

Advanced radiographic abnormalities generally correlate with extensive lung pathology. Alveolar filling opacities on the chest radiograph generally signify an active alveolitis. In contrast, in radiographic stages III or IV, fibrotic disease is generally severe even though alveolitis and granulomata, in varying severities, may coexist. In general, reticular and linear densities accompanied by cysts and contraction are evidence of advanced fibrosis.

STRUCTURE-FUNCTION CORRELATES IN THE NATURAL HISTORY AND TREATED COURSE

The correlation between sequential chest radiographs and certain pulmonary function tests is reasonably good.

Among *untreated* patients with either stage II or stage III sarcoidosis who show radiographic improvement, the VC improves in 70 percent and the $D_{L_{CO}}$ in 30 percent; in most patients, neither VC nor $D_{L_{CO}}$ worsen in the face of radiographic improvement. Also, in patients in whom the radiograph remains unchanged or worsens, the VC decreases in one-fourth and the $D_{L_{CO}}$ in 43 percent. In contrast, the VC improves in 9 percent, but in none does the $D_{L_{CO}}$ improve. In essence, changes in VC generally reflect gross morphologic improvement as assessed by the chest radiograph.

The VC is also sensitive in detecting improvement in response to *treatment*. In 60 percent of nearly 300 patients with parenchymal sarcoidosis who improved, the VC improved by 10 percent or more; in 50 percent of these, the $D_{L_{CO}}$ also improved; and in 47 percent, pulmonary compliance increased. Rarely do VC and $D_{L_{CO}}$ deteriorate in face of radiographic improvement. Curiously, in nearly one-half of treated patients in whom the manifestations of parenchymal disease on chest radiography either remained unchanged or worsened, the VC improved, and in nearly 40 percent, the $D_{L_{CO}}$ improved; the reasons for the discrepancy between improved physiological performance and radiographic evidence of stability or deterioration are unclear.

Idiopathic Pulmonary Fibrosis

The pathology of idiopathic pulmonary fibrosis (IPF) consists primarily of a mononuclear and polymorphonuclear cellular infiltrate in the alveolar septae in association with varying degrees of interstitial fibrosis and no granulomata (Fig. 49-6). The acute stage of the disease is characterized by intra-alveolar exudates and hyaline membranes; the chronic stage is characterized by extensive fibrosis of alveoli and the development of cystic lesions. Varying degrees of peribronchiolar fibrosis and bronchiolitis are often present (Fig. 49-2); in some patients, there is a bronchiolitis obliterans.

STRUCTURE-FUNCTION ALTERATIONS

The chest radiograph is often normal in patients with symptomatic IPF: in a large but heterogeneous group of patients, most of whom seemed to have IPF, the chest radiograph was normal in nearly 23 percent in whom the pulmonary pathology was classified as DIP and in nearly 8 percent classified as UIP. In patients with interstitial lung disease in whom the chest radiographs were normal, the VC was low in nearly 60 percent, whereas the $D_{L_{CO}}$ was low in 70 percent; the TLC was significantly reduced in only 16 percent. Thus, reduction in $D_{L_{CO}}$ may be the earliest abnormality disclosed by routine pulmonary function tests in IPF. More limited experience suggests that arterial hypoxemia or widening of $P(A-a)_{O_2}$ is another early and sensitive functional aberration in IPF.

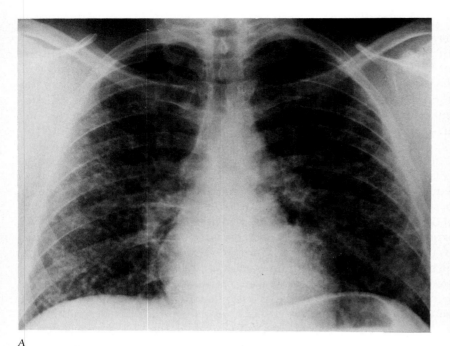
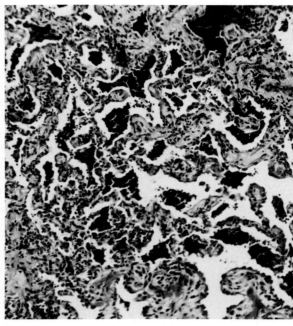

A   B

FIGURE 49-6 Early idiopathic pulmonary fibrosis.   A. Chest radiograph of a 28-year-old female showing a diffuse nodular and reticulonodular pattern.   B. Open lung biopsy showing interstitial and intra-alveolar cells with mildly thickened alveolar septae. This patient was early to midcourse in her disease.

Acute IPF is characterized by moderate reductions in both VC and TLC. In contrast, in the more typical pattern of the disease that is characterized by the insidious onset of breathlessness during exertion, the lung volumes are normal or near normal. Correspondingly, the acute phase of the disease is often characterized by reduced lung compliance at FRC and a shift in the volume-pressure relationship downward and rightward (Fig. 49-7), whereas the advanced stage of IPF is characterized by marked shifts in the volume-pressure relationship with dramatic increases in transpulmonary pressures at TLC; often, recoil pressure at FRC is decreased (Figs. 49-7 and 49-8), reflecting the replacement of large areas of pulmonary parenchyma by cystic lesions and fibrous tissue.

Although expiratory flow rates determined by spirometry are usually normal, up to two-thirds of patients with IPF have morphologic and physiological evidence of small airways disease. Published reports of the incidence of obstructive airways disease in DIP and UIP are difficult to interpret because of inclusion of cigarette smokers in the series.

In early IPF, arterial P_{O_2} is usually normal at rest in association with mild hypocapnia, whereas in both early and advanced disease arterial hypoxemia and widening of the $P(A\text{-}a)_{O_2}$ characteristically occur during exercise. Some patients with IPF exhibit resting hypoxemia but improve the level of oxygenation during exercise. This occurs primarily in patients with coexisting chronic obstructive airways disease in whom it has been attributed

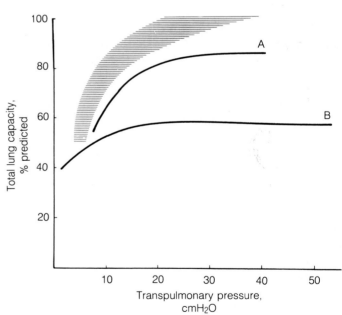

FIGURE 49-7 Volume-pressure curves in early and advanced idiopathic pulmonary fibrosis. Curve A presents the volume-pressure relationship of the case illustrated in Fig. 49-6 and is shifted downward and rightward. Curve B presents the volume-pressure relationship of the case illustrated in Fig. 49-8 and is shifted downward with marked increases in maximal transpulmonary pressure at TLC. In contrast, recoil pressures are decreased at and below FRC.

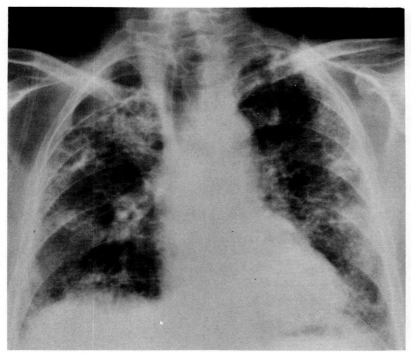
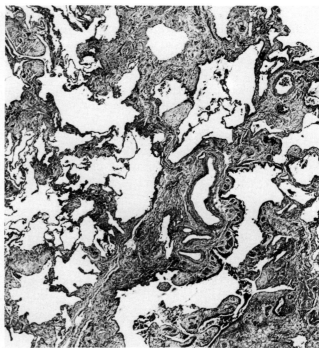

A   B

FIGURE 49-8   Advanced idiopathic pulmonary fibrosis in a 56-year-old male.   A. Chest radiograph shows marked volume loss with a coarsely reticular pattern with cystic lesions.   B. Open lung biopsy shows massive fibrosis with loss of alveoli and few inflammatory cells.

to improved ventilation-perfusion balance during exercise by either mobilizing secretions or by recruiting additional gas-exchange units with more nearly normal ventilation-perfusion ratios.

The severity of interstitial pulmonary fibrosis as judged from the chest radiograph correlates only weakly with the severity of disease as reflected in the lung biopsy. Nor is there a close relationship between the severity of the alveolitis (degree of cellularity and of fibrosis) and conventional pulmonary function tests. In contrast, virtually all indices derived from static deflation volume-pressure curve do correlate well with the morphologic assessment of the degree of fibrosis; of these, the best correlate is the pulmonary compliance at FRC. However, none of the indices of distensibility correlate with degree of cellularity.

Although neither the resting Pa_{O_2} nor $P(A-a)_{O_2}$ appears to bear much of a relationship to the morphologic evidence of the severity of disease, the $P(A-a)_{O_2}$ during exercise generally does parallel the pathologic severity of disease: virtually all patients with IPF who develop a $P(A-a)_{O_2}$ greater than 45 mmHg during exercise have severe disease.

In essence, of the various physiological tests used in assessing the morphologic severity of IPF, the volume-pressure relationship has proved valuable in estimating the degree of fibrosis (but not of cellularity), a feature

which may have prognostic significance. In contrast, although gas exchange during exercise correlates well with structural changes, they do not differentiate between the degree of cellularity and the severity of fibrosis.

STRUCTURE-FUNCTION CORRELATES IN THE NATURAL HISTORY AND COURSE, WITH AND WITHOUT TREATMENT

The natural history and course of IPF are variable. Although the original report by Hamman and Rich described an acute fulminant disease, more typical is a chronic progressive course in which death ensues after 4 to 5 years from pulmonary disease or its complications. However, in some instances, patients with IPF have survived for up to 20 years after the onset of symptoms.

In patients with IPF who were subdivided after lung biopsy on histologic grounds into DIP and UIP, about one quarter of 32 *untreated* patients with DIP improved, about two-thirds worsened, and the others remained unchanged. In contrast, in 48 *untreated* patients with UIP, none improved, only 15 percent were unchanged, and the remainder worsened. Treatment significantly affected the course of the disease: of 26 *treated* patients with DIP, nearly two-thirds improved, whereas only about one quarter worsened; of 26 *treated* with UIP, about 12 percent improved, more than two-thirds worsened, and the remainder were unchanged.

Cellularity and the absence of fibrosis on biopsy are useful in predicting a favorable response to therapy. Physiological measurements also have predictive value: those with a VC less than 60 percent of predicted and with a resting Pa_{O_2} less than 60 mmHg can be expected to die within 2 years; about a quarter of those with a resting Pa_{O_2} greater than 60 mmHg can be expected to be alive after 4 years.

Certain characteristics help to signal those patients with IPF apt to respond to corticosteroids: young age, little dyspnea, modest radiographic changes, and cellular histology. Among the factors that have no influence on survival are the degree of reduction in VC and TLC, the presence of an associated connective tissue disease, or any serologic or physical findings. Although the level of the VC had no prognostic significance, survival was significantly longer in patients in whom the $D_{L_{CO}}$ was greater than 45 percent of predicted.

In the patients who do respond favorably to corticosteroid therapy, pulmonary function usually improves within the first 8 weeks (Fig. 49-9); in some instances, improvement is more gradual, i.e., in 4 to 6 months. In general, VC and $D_{L_{CO}}$ show the most dramatic improvement; gas exchange during exercise may also improve dra-

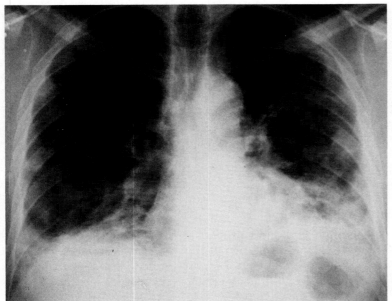

A

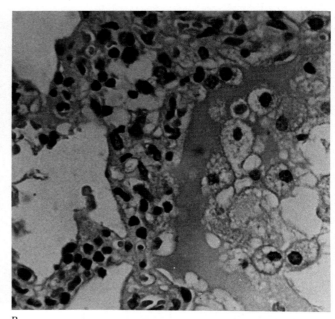

B

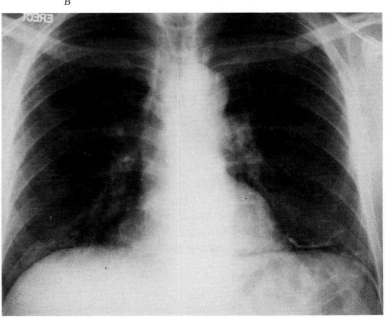

C

FIGURE 49-9 Chest radiograph and lung biopsy in a 40-year-old male with acute idiopathic pulmonary fibrosis. *A*. Chest radiograph before therapy showing a lower lobe, ground glass pattern. *B*. Lung biopsy showing intra-alveolar exudation with marked alveolar septal edema. *C*. Chest radiograph after 6 weeks on corticosteroids. There is marked clearing of the infiltrates.

matically. In the IPF patients in whom small airways are involved, corticosteroids may improve airflow. About 20 percent of the patients who do not respond to corticosteroid therapy survive for 4 to 5 years.

Organic Dust Disease

Sensitization to a variety of inhaled organic dusts can cause "the organic dust diseases," which are also known as *the hypersensitivity pneumonitides* and *the extrinsic allergic alveolitides*. In these diseases, the particles are sufficiently small as to bypass upper airway defenses and to be deposited in respiratory bronchioles and along alveolar walls producing a bronchioloalveolitis and, often, a bronchiolitis obliterans. The prototype of this disease is farmer's lung, which is caused by inhalation of spores from thermophylic bacteria present in moldy hay. However, there are nearly 30 well-described diseases which have been named according to either the occupational or environmental exposure to the antigen or the antigenic source.

The acute form of the disease is characterized by a mononuclear and often neutrophilic alveolitis accompanied by varying degrees of alveolar and interstitial edema and bronchiolitis; interstitial pneumonitis is an invariant finding. Interstitial granulomata may not be evident in very early or acute disease but are seen in up to 70 percent of biopsies of patients with repeated acute disease or subacute disease. Continued exposure to the offending antigen results in chronic interstitial pneumonitis and fibrosis. These diseases are considered elsewhere in this book (Chapter 44). Small airways may be totally obliterated with fibrous tissue. Often the mucous glands of large bronchi show marked hyperplasia.

STRUCTURE-FUNCTION CORRELATES

Acute organic dust disease is characterized radiographically by a fine nodular pattern or by patchy pneumonitis; uncommonly, there is a ground glass pattern. Less than 5 percent of patients have a normal chest radiograph. The physiological alterations in the acute form of the disease include a reduction in VC and in pulmonary compliance. Although asthma is not a feature of acute organic dust disease, unless there is atopy, obstructive disease of small airways is common, probably because of bronchiolitis. Air trapping, manifested by an enlarged RV and FRC, is also a common feature of acute organic dust disease.

Patients in the chronic stage of organic dust disease are often indistinguishable from those with IPF clinically, radiographically, and physiologically. The chest radiograph often shows coarse linear densities, retraction of the hili, and honeycombing. One-third of patients with chronic farmer's lung have a restrictive ventilatory defect with reduced D_{LCO} and hypoxemia that worsens with exercise. Major obstructive defects, e.g., reduction in

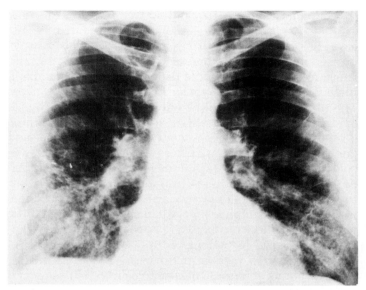

FIGURE 49-10 Chest radiograph of a 69-year-old male with chronic farmer's lung. There is maintenance of lung volumes with lower lobe coarse reticulation. Functional studies showed an abnormal FEV_1/FVC with a markedly increased RV/TLC.

FEV_1/FVC, occur in 25 to 75 percent of these patients. The chest radiograph indicates hyperinflation of the lungs (Fig. 49-10), the FRC is markedly increased, the D_{LCO} is low, and pulmonary recoil is decreased as in emphysema. The outcome of chronic organic dust disease is variable.

STRUCTURE-FUNCTION CORRELATES IN THE NATURAL HISTORY AND TREATED COURSE

The standard clinical response to acute exposure to the antigen is the onset of symptoms of pneumonitis 4 to 10 h after exposure; arterial hypoxemia and reduced lung volumes develop 8 to 12 h after exposure. In atopic patients, an acute asthmatic response with wheezing and reduction in FEV_1/FVC may follow immediately on inhalation of the antigen. If there is no further exposure, pulmonary function returns to normal within a few weeks to a month. Even after repeated acute attacks, pulmonary function often remains normal between exposures.

Radiographically, the acute organic dust disease manifests either a nodular pattern or a patchy pneumonitis. The more extensive the radiographic findings, the more apt is D_{LCO} to be severely compromised. However, the acute pattern does not predict the extent to which pulmonary function will return. Corticosteroid therapy does not appear to affect either the return of pulmonary function or the appearance of chronic fibrotic changes, but corticosteroids do appear to promote the disappearance of diffuse opacities. In the chronic stage of the disease, radiographic changes are severe; either diffuse or patchy opacities emerge, which are consistent with fibrosis.

Long-term changes in pulmonary function are now available for certain etiologies of chronic organic lung disease. In bird breeder's disease, in which small airways obstruction featured prominently during the acute and subacute stages, four of nine patients had recovered completely 30 months after exposure to the provoking antigen. The others were left with radiographic or physiological evidence of diffuse interstitial disease; in addition, three developed progressive obstructive airways disease, and one underwent progressive loss of lung recoil that was consistent with the development of emphysema. Although neither the clinical presentation, the nature, nor the degree of functional impairment predicted if there would be residual lung damage, elderly patients and those with intense antigenic exposure appeared to develop progressive disease. In patients with farmer's lung, most of whom average 15 years of the disease, about one quarter had symptoms of chronic obstructive airways disease and about one-third had radiographic evidence of interstitial lung disease. Symptomatic flare-ups of the pulmonary disease are probably the cardinal factor in determining if the disease will become progressive. The mainstay of treatment for chronic organic dust disease continues to be avoidance of exposure; corticosteroids do not appear to afford overall significant improvement.

Primary Pulmonary Histiocytosis X

Histiocytosis X can affect bone, skin, mucous membranes, lung, lymph nodes, or liver, either alone or in varying combinations. When only the lungs are involved, the condition is termed *primary pulmonary histiocytosis X*, or *eosinophilic granuloma of lung* (see Chapter 53). The histologic hallmark of this disease is the presence of discrete parenchymal nodules that range in size from several millimeters to more than 1 cm (Fig. 49-11). The nodules consist of characteristic histiocytosis X cells, monocytes, eosinophils, and fibrous tissue. Often, some lymphocytes and plasma cells are present; centering of the nodules around small airways causes obstruction. Involvement of bronchioles by granulomas can lead to their destruction. The lesions characteristically heal with a stellate scar that produces distortion and destruction of adjacent airspaces ("retraction emphysema") (Fig. 49-11). Advanced disease is characterized by fibrosis and destruction of alveoli and the formation of numerous thin- and thick-walled cysts or cavities.

STRUCTURE-FUNCTION ALTERATIONS

Early primary pulmonary histiocytosis X is characterized radiographically by nodular or reticulonodular infiltrates in the middle or lower lung fields; frequently, the costophrenic angles are spared (Fig. 49-12). The nodules range in size from 0.5 cm to more than 1 cm. Frequently, upper lobe cystic disease coexists with histiocytosis (Fig. 49-12), even when the disease is apparently early in its course. Rarely are the chest radiographs normal. On occasion, the radiograph shows a diffuse, ground glass pattern that reflects an active alveolitis and intra-alveolar exudation. Early in the disease, TLC is maintained, whereas VC is generally decreased; as a result, the RV/TLC is increased.

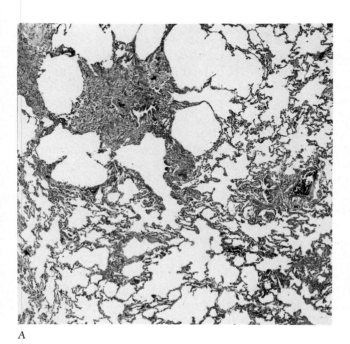

A

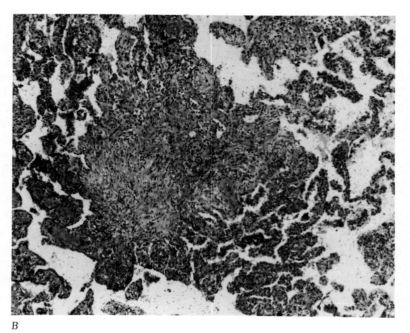

B

FIGURE 49-11 Histopathology in primary pulmonary histiocytosis X.   *A.* Low-power view showing stellate scar with retraction emphysema and cystic lesions; a narrowed, small airway is in the scar.   *B.* High-power view of an active area with a granuloma typical of histiocytosis X.

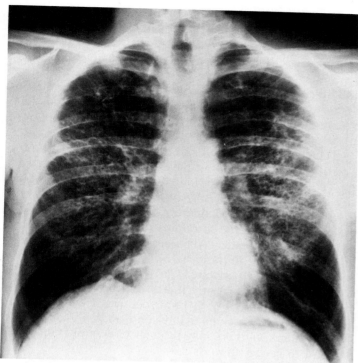

FIGURE 49-12 Primary pulmonary histiocytosis X in a 27-year-old male. Chest radiograph shows a reticular to reticulonodular midzonal infiltrate with sparing of the costophrenic angles. There is bilateral upper lobe fibrocytic disease, and volumes are maintained.

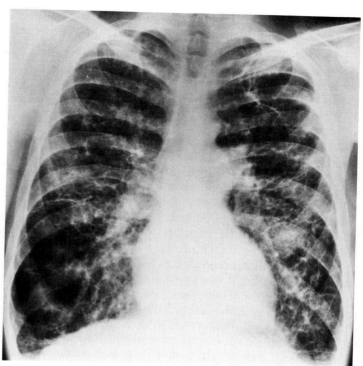

FIGURE 49-13 Chronic primary pulmonary histiocytosis X in a 37-year-old male. There is a diffuse "honeycomb" pattern with cystic lesions ranging from 1 to 3 cm. There are large upper and lower lobe bullae. Functional studies showed an elevated TLC with an increased RV/TLC. FEV_1/FVC was severely reduced, as was $D_{L_{CO}}$.

The diffusing capacity is decreased in nearly three quarters of patients, and nearly 80 percent have arterial hypoxemia, often that only becomes evident during exercise. In 10 to 15 percent of patients with acute disease, routine pulmonary function studies are entirely normal. Possibly because of bronchiolar lesions and the tendency to develop emphysema, obstructive airways disease is often a prominent feature of primary pulmonary histiocytosis X.

Chronic histiocytosis X is characterized by diffuse, either thin- or thick-walled cysts or cavities; bullae often occur at the lung bases (Fig. 49-13). Pulmonary function tests usually show that the VC is low, whereas TLC is either normal or increased, resulting in a markedly increased RV/TLC. In most patients with chronic histiocytosis X, the FEV_1/FVC is abnormal.

STRUCTURE-FUNCTION CORRELATES IN THE NATURAL HISTORY AND TREATED COURSE

Most patients with primary pulmonary histiocytosis X either stabilize or improve; 10 to 25 percent improve. Twenty to thirty percent of patients continue to deteriorate slowly, and ultimately, 10 to 20 percent die from the disease. Often deaths are 20 to 25 years after a slowly progressive disease. In general, young males have a more severe prognosis. In several series, the severity of the initial radiographic findings correlates with the subsequent pro-

gressive illness. However, severe disease is common. A markedly reduced $D_{L_{CO}}$ and an increased RV/TLC correlate with the development of cystic lesions, and patients with low values of $D_{L_{CO}}$ seldom improve and often deteriorate. Radiographic sparing of the costophrenic angles is stated to be a good prognostic sign. Corticosteroids have been extensively used in primary pulmonary histiocytosis X; they may speed the radiographic resolution but do not appear to alter the natural history of the disease.

OTHER INTERSTITIAL LUNG DISEASES

Inorganic Dust Diseases

Although this group of diseases constitutes the largest group of patients, few structural-functional studies exist. Further, it is difficult to make generalizations about radiographic-functional correlates because the clinical and pathologic forms of these diseases vary widely. Often mixed dusts are involved, and industrial bronchitis coexists with chronic airways disease due to cigarette smoking. However, in general, the radiographic appearances do correlate with overall pulmonary function even though variability is wide. Interestingly, the dust burden correlates poorly with the severity of functional impairment.

The accelerated and acute forms of silicosis (see Chapter 54) usually produce a pure restrictive ventilatory defect: D_{LCO} and lung compliance are decreased; arterial hypoxemia is present at rest and worsens with exercise. In individuals with asymptomatic simple silicosis, tests of ventilatory function are frequently normal. In individuals with simple silicosis who are symptomatic, the ventilatory patterns differ, sometimes being restrictive, other times obstructive, and sometimes mixed. In contrast, complicated silicosis is characterized by a restrictive pattern in which pulmonary compliance is low and arterial hypoxemia develops during exercise. In the terminal stage of silicosis, the restrictive ventilatory defect is usually severe, and arterial hypoxemia is pronounced.

Asbestos generally produces a restrictive ventilatory pattern with no evidence of obstructive airways disease on spirometry. A marked decrease in D_{LCO} precedes the changes in VC. Small airways disease is common, but not invariant, in early asbestosis. As the disease progresses, arterial hypoxemia ensues and the $P_{(A-a)O_2}$ widens, first during exercise and later while at rest. In general, the D_{LCO} correlates with overall severity of the disease, but neither the VC nor the D_{LCO} gives any indication of prognosis. Advanced asbestosis is characterized by marked restrictive ventilatory defects in which pulmonary compliance and lung volumes are low and arterial hypoxemia is present at rest.

Wegener's Granulomatosis

Wegener's granulomatosis can exhibit a variety of functional and structural pulmonary abnormalities. Although lung volumes and diffusing capacity are often low (in 30 to 40 percent), the most common functional abnormality is obstruction to airflow due to inflammatory disease of the large airways.

In patients with parenchymal disease, the lung volumes are often reduced. As a rule, lung volumes increase and airflow obstruction is relieved in response to treatment. But, in contrast, D_{LCO} often stabilizes or continues to decrease despite therapy.

CLINICAL AND FUNCTIONAL ASSESSMENT IN THE MANAGEMENT OF THE INTERSTITIAL DISEASES

With few exceptions, neither the symptoms nor their duration are of appreciable value in predicting the natural history or response to therapy of the interstitial diseases. Among the exceptions is exertional breathlessness that is slowly progressive over a long period of time; patients with this manifestation are not apt to show improvement when treated with corticosteroids. Also, in young individuals, the less the dyspnea, the more likely is a favorable response to corticosteroids; the same is true for those with acute disease (less than 1 month), particularly those with IPF. Symptoms are sometimes useful in assessing the response to therapy if they can be quantified, e.g., the number of stairs climbed or the distance walked. But because symptoms are notoriously unreliable in quantification and since most patients treated with corticosteroids undergo symptomatic improvement, more objective data, e.g., the chest radiograph or tests of pulmonary function, are needed to assess the response to therapy.

The chest radiograph can be useful in estimating the severity of disease and in predicting the response to therapy. The nodular or reticulonodular patterns that are usually seen early in the disease often signify an active alveolitis. In the absence of pleural disease, a ground glass pattern also generally correlates with active alveolitis, a stage of most interstitial diseases that is generally somewhat reversible. Similarly, several radiographic patterns correlate well with advanced, irreversible fibrosis, e.g., a coarsely reticular pattern intermingled with cystic lesions, retraction of hili, or honeycombing. However, even in the patient who seems to have end-stage fibrosis on the chest radiograph, there may be areas of alveolitis that will respond to corticosteroids.

In sarcoidosis, the chest radiograph is helpful in predicting the natural history of the disease: nearly 80 percent of those in radiographic stage I improve; 10 percent progress. In contrast, nearly 50 percent of patients in stage III sarcoidosis progress. Nevertheless, for the individual patient, these data are of limited help in prognosis. In general, the chest radiograph has great value for interstitial disease: it provides an objective basis for assessing the gross anatomy of the lungs and becomes a powerful tool when correlated with serial determinations of pulmonary function; although the chest radiograph can be useful in signaling changes in lung volumes or compliance, it cannot replace the functional assessment of interstitial disease.

At least in some of the interstitial diseases, e.g., IPF and sarcoidosis, a reasonably good correlation exists between the severity of certain functional abnormalities and the overall severity of the pulmonary disease. But, variability is so wide that values for an individual patient cannot be used to predict pulmonary pathology. Moreover, no pulmonary function tests can distinguish the severity of alveolitis, which may be responsive to treatment, from that of the fibrotic process, which is viewed as irreversible. The greatest value of pulmonary function studies in patients with interstitial disease is to track serial changes through sequential determinations. The vital capacity and the D_{LCO} appear to be the most sensitive parameters in sarcoidosis; measurements of gas exchange in conjunction with determinations of arterial blood-gas composition appear to be most sensitive in IPF. Rarely, if ever, can the results of these tests be translated to immediate clinical decisions; instead, they have to be correlated with the history, physical examination, and chest radiograph.

FUTURE

Two new tests, bronchoalveolar lavage (BAL) and gallium lung scanning, have emerged as possibly being useful in the staging and monitoring of the interstitial diseases. Bronchoalveolor lavage provides an easy and relatively noninvasive means for sampling repeatedly the cellular and soluble components of the lower respiratory tract. BAL seems to sample alveolar cells and, therefore, the severity of alveolitis. However, despite initial enthusiasm over the use of BAL in the clinical management of these diseases, its actual value remains to be established. Similarly, although there are data indicating that the intensity of gallium uptake by the interstitial diseases correlates with the severity of alveolitis, gallium lung scanning is still unproven in the management of these diseases. Like BAL, gallium lung scanning should be regarded as a research tool.

Radionuclide studies are on the horizon as an aid in the diagnosis and management of pulmonary vascular disease and cor pulmonale. Vasodilator therapy in pulmonary vascular disease is being intensively investigated, but its role in managing pulmonary hypertension in patients with interstitial lung disease has not been extensively explored.

BIBLIOGRAPHY

Allen DH, Williams GV, Woolcock AJ: Bird breeder's hypersensitivity pneumonitis: Progress studies of lung function after cessation of exposure to the provoking antigen. Am Rev Respir Dis 114:555–566, 1976.
  A clinical and physiological study of nine patients with bird breeder's organic dust disease followed up to 30 months after removal from the antigen. Functional outcomes are presented.

Braun SR, DoPico GA, Tsiatis A, Horvath E, Dickie HA, Rankin J: Farmer's lung disease: Long-term clinical and physiologic outcome. Am Rev Respir Dis 119:185–191, 1979.
  A study of the long-term effects of farmer's lung and the factors influencing outcome in 141 farmer's lung patients. Clinical, physiological, and radiographic data for a mean of nearly 15 years are presented.

Carrington CB, Gaensler EA, Coutu RE, Fitzgerald MX, Gupta RG: Natural history and treated course of usual and desquamative interstitial pneumonia. N Engl J Med 298:801–809, 1978.
  A prospective analysis of 93 patients classified as DIP or UIP. Data on clinical, physiological, and histologic correlates affecting the natural history and treated course of these diseases are presented.

Carrington CB, Gaensler EA, Mikus JP, Schachter AW, Burke GW, Goff AM: Structure and function in sarcoidosis. Ann NY Acad Sci 278:265–283, 1976.
  A structure-function correlative study of 59 patients with granulomatous lung disease; 47 had sarcoidosis. A comparison between grading of radiographs, lung histology, and pulmonary physiology was made.

Crystal RG, Fulmer JD, Roberts WC, Moss ML, Line BR, Reynolds HY: Idiopathic pulmonary fibrosis: Clinical, histologic, radiographic, physiologic, scintigraphic, cytologic, and biochemical aspects. Ann Intern Med 85:769–788, 1976.
  Clinical, radiographic, and physiological data are presented on 29 patients with IPF. Gallium lung scanning and bronchoalveolar lavage are introduced as monitors of the disease.

Crystal RG, Gadek JE, Ferrans VJ, Fulmer JD, Line BR, Hunninghake GW: Interstitial lung disease: Current concepts of pathogenesis, staging and therapy. Am J Med 70:542–568, 1981.
  A critical review of the interstitial disease. Lung lavage and gallium scanning are strongly presented.

Crystal RG, Roberts WC, Hunninghake GW, Gadek JE, Fulmer JD, Line BR: Pulmonary sarcoidosis: A disease characterized and perpetuated by activated lung T-lymphocytes. Ann Intern Med 94:73–94, 1981.
  A critical review of current concepts of the pathogenesis of sarcoidosis. Correlated radiographic structural data are presented.

DeTroyer A, Yernault JC: Inspiratory muscle force in normal subjects and patients with interstitial lung disease. Thorax 35:92–100, 1980.
  Inspiratory muscle mechanics are presented for 12 patients with diffuse interstitial lung disease.

DiMarco AF, Kelsen SG, Cherniack NS, Gothe B: Occlusion pressure and breathing pattern in patients with interstitial lung disease. Am Rev Respir Dis 127:425–430, 1983.
  A recent investigation of control of ventilation in diffuse interstitial lung disease.

Epler GR, McLoud TC, Gaensler EA, Mikus JP, Carrington CB: Normal chest roentgenograms in chronic diffuse infiltrative lung disease. N Engl J Med 298:934–939, 1978.
>   *A study of the prevalence of normal chest radiographs in patients with chronic interstitial lung disease. Reasons for biopsy and physiological data are presented.*

Fulmer JD, Roberts WC, Von Gal ER, Crystal RG: Small airways in idiopathic pulmonary fibrosis. J Clin Invest 60:595–610, 1977.
>   *An analysis of lung morphology and functional assessment of small airways in 19 IPF patients.*

Fulmer JD, Roberts WC, Von Gal ER, Crystal RG: Morphologic-physiologic correlates of the severity of fibrosis and degree of cellularity in idiopathic pulmonary fibrosis. J Clin Invest 63:665–676, 1979.
>   *A correlative study of 23 patients comparing severity of fibrosis or degree of cellularity with detailed physiological testing.*

Gibson GJ, Pride NB: Pulmonary mechanics in fibrosing alveolitis: The effects of lung shrinkage. Am Rev Respir Dis 116:637–647, 1977.
>   *A critical analysis of factors that determine lung mechanics in patients with advanced interstitial lung disease.*

Huang CT, Heurich AE, Rosen Y, Moon S, Lyons HA: Pulmonary sarcoidosis: Roentgenographic, functional and pathologic correlations. Respiration 37:337–345, 1979.
>   *A radiographic, physiological, pathologic correlative study of 81 patients with sarcoidosis. Open lung biopsy specimens were semiquantified as to fibrosis, cellularity, and granulomata and those data compared with radiographic and physiological data.*

Lourenco RV, Turino GM, Davidson LAG, Fishman AP: The regulation of ventilation in diffuse pulmonary fibrosis. Am J Med 38:199–216, 1965.
>   *A classic paper presenting an investigation of ventilation, work of breathing, and CO_2 response curves in 19 patients with diffuse interstitial disease.*

Marcy TW, Reynolds HY: Pulmonary histiocytosis X. Lung 163:129–150, 1985.
>   *A critical, up-to-date review of histiocytosis X. Pathogenesis and pathophysiology are excellent.*

Miller A, Teirstein AS, Jackler I, Chuang M, Siltzbach LE: Airway function in chronic pulmonary sarcoidosis with fibrosis. Am Rev Respir Dis 109:179–189, 1974.
>   *A study of 16 patients with chronic pulmonary sarcoidosis using maximal flow-volume curves. Twelve had major obstructive defects.*

Monkare S, Ikonen M, Haahtela T: Radiologic findings in farmer's lung: Prognosis and correlation to lung function. Chest 87:460–466, 1985.
>   *A critical analysis of radiographic patterns in acute and subacute farmer's lung. Radiographic findings were correlated with lung function and prognosis.*

Murphy, DMF, Fishman AP: Mushrooms and mushroom worker's lung, in Fishman AP (ed), Update: Pulmonary Diseases and Disorders. New York, McGraw-Hill, 1982, pp 230–242.
>   *A detailed review of one type of hypersensitivity pneumonitis that can progress to chronic interstitial fibrosis.*

Rosenberg DM, Weinberger SE, Fulmer JD, Flye MW, Fauci AS, Crystal RG: Functional correlates of lung involvement in Wegener's granulomatosis. Am J Med 69:387–394, 1980.
>   *A study of 22 patients with Wegener's granulomatosis to establish the usefulness of pulmonary function testing in the diagnosis and management of this disease.*

Tukiainen P, Taskinen E, Holsti P, Korhola O, Valle M: Prognosis of cryptogenic fibrosing alveolitis. Thorax 38:349–355, 1983.
>   *A retrospective analysis of 100 consecutive cases with IPF. Clinical, radiographic, physiological, histologic, and steroid response were correlated with prognosis.*

Turner-Warwick M, Burrows B, Johnson A: Cryptogenic fibrosing alveolitis: Clinical features and their influence on survival. Thorax 35:171–180, 1980.
>   *A retrospective analysis of 220 cases of IPF. The influence of corticosteroid therapy was assessed in terms of clinical, radiographic, and physiological response after 4 to 8 weeks of therapy.*

Widimsky J, Riedel M, Stanek V: Central haemodynamics during exercise in patients with restrictive pulmonary disease. Bull Eur Physiopathol Respir 13:369–379, 1977.
>   *Investigation of pulmonary hemodynamics at rest and exercise in patients with diffuse interstitial disease is presented and compared with similar data in pneumonectomy patients.*

Winterbauer RH, Hutchinson JF: Clinical significance of pulmonary function tests. Use of pulmonary function tests in the management of sarcoidosis. Chest 78:640–647, 1980.
>   *A critical analysis of the value of pulmonary function tests in the detection and management of sarcoidosis.*

Chapter *50*

Widespread Pulmonary Fibrosis

Margaret Turner-Warwick

Widespread fibrotic scarring occurs as a final stage of healing after many different types of injury to the lungs. In some patients, the injury evokes only a short-lived illness; in others, active disease smolders alongside the fibrosing process for many years. Progressive fibrosis sometimes occurs after the initiating injurious agent is no longer operative; at other times it continues as a process of progressive healing, the penalty for which is progressive deterioration in overall lung function. Whatever the sequence of events, the result is increasing breathlessness and often premature death.

In recent years our understanding of the factors stimulating fibroblast growth and collagen production has increased considerably. We also have some information on the enzymes which degrade collagen as well as their inhibitors. Nevertheless we still have very little knowledge about the ways in which the balance between collagen formation and dissolution is perturbed in various human pulmonary diseases. In particular, little is known about the factors promoting organization and fibrosis, on the one hand, and resolution, on the other, and much more has to be learned about the factors which allow progressive fibrosis in some cases but determine its arrest or stabilization without therapeutic intervention in others. In pulmonary medicine these events are often spread over many years, a fact that makes them hard to study in any meaningful way in animal models.

THE MAGNITUDE OF THE PROBLEM

In comparison with the prevalence in the community of nonfibrosing lung diseases, such as asthma, chronic obstruction of the airways, or lung cancer, fibrosing disorders are relatively uncommon. Interest in these disorders lies in the diversity of acute pathologies that cause them; their importance lies in early detection of the processes so that the fibrotic consequences may be prevented. In addition, study of chronic fibrotic lung diseases and their control provides insight into the fundamental issues of development and control of fibroblastic activity in tissue injury and repair.

ACUTE LESIONS RESULTING IN FIBROSIS

A wide range of acute injuries to the lung on occasion results in such widespread damage to the lung architecture that healing by fibrosis results. Some of the commoner agents are illustrated in Table 50-1.

It is also important to understand that a range of different initiating pathologic changes in the lung may progress to irreversible fibrosis if they persist for long periods. The reasons for their continuance are not always completely clear. In some, the initiating agent remains in the lungs (e.g., silica, asbestos). In others, persisting autonomous circuits that are no longer dependent on the primary agent (as, for example, in some cases of hypersensitivity pneumonitis) may be set up. In still others, the initial or persisting injury may interrupt the normal lung architecture and determine the progression to fibrosis. The variation in initiating pathologic processes in the lung and some of the recognized inducing agents are illustrated in Table 50-2.

It is important to understand that in many instances the causes of granuloma formation and chronic inflammatory exudates are unknown. In some instances, e.g., sarcoidosis, the clinical features are so well recognized that physicians often use the term as a "shorthand" and are tempted into the belief that it is therefore a "disease entity" with a single causal agent; this is unproved at the present time. In other instances of chronic inflammatory

TABLE 50-1
Some Acute Lesions of the Lung Resulting (on Occasion) in Widespread Pulmonary Fibrosis

Class of Injury	Type of Agent	Examples
Chemical	Oxygen	Prolonged use in high concentration
	NO_2, chlorine	Industrial accidents, silo fillers
Radiation		Therapeutic radiation
Medications	Hypersensitivity	Nitrofurantoin, gold
	Toxic	Bleomycin, busulfan, methotrexate
Inhaled gastric contents	Hydrochloric acid	Mendelsohn's syndrome
Infections	Viruses	Adenovirus pneumonia
	Bacteria	Septicemia, IV drug abuse, Legionnaires' disease
Organic dusts	Serum proteins	Pigeon breeder's lung
	Fungi	Acute farmer's lung
Exudates	Hemodynamic	Raised left atrial pressure
	"Immunologic"	Uremia
	"Toxic"?	Systemic lupus erythematosus

TABLE 50-2
The Range of Initiating Pathologies in the Lung Inducing Widespread Fibrosis

Pathology	Examples
Granuloma formation	Sarcoidosis
	Beryllium
	Extrinsic allergic alveolitis (organic materials)
Chronic exudates	Increase in left atrial pressure
	Damage to pulmonary capillaries by medical drugs, immunologic agents, infective agents
Fibrogenic agents	Silica, asbestos

exudates, some patients have associated immunologic as well as clinical characteristics, and these clusters of features are often identified under certain headings, e.g., systemic lupus erythematosus, rheumatoid disease, or systemic sclerosis. In none of these conditions is the causal agent(s) known.

In some instances, the lungs alone are affected, although some of the same immunologic features may occasionally be present; these are often termed *cryptogenic*, or *idiopathic*. However, strictly speaking, the systemic immunologic diseases, as well as sarcoid granulomatous disease, are also cryptogenic. "Lone" fibrosing alveolitis (FA) may describe better those instances in which apparently the lungs alone are affected. Whether the factors initiating and inducing persisting chronic inflammation in the lungs are similar or different in lone fibrosing alveolitis, compared with fibrosing alveolitis that is associated with connective tissue disorders (e.g., systemic lupus erythematosus, rheumatoid disease, and systemic sclerosis), is much debated but currently unknown. The histologic appearances are indistinguishable.

Just as a variety of more acute pathologies relating to known agents may progress to pulmonary fibrosis, several histologic variants of chronic inflammation are seen in the earlier stages of disorders that will progress to lone fibrosing alveolitis. These have been categorized according to the predominating inflammatory cell as a range of idiopathic chronic pneumonias. Thus *lymphocytic interstitial pneumonia (LIP)*, *plasma cell interstitial pneumonia (PIP)*, and *desquamative interstitial pneumonia (DIP)*

(now known to be macrophage accumulations) have all been described. These contrast with a mixed pattern of alveolar wall fibrosing inflammatory infiltrate that is associated with a variable intra-alveolar accumulate of macrophages termed *usual interstitial pneumonia (UIP)* (Fig. 50-1).

There is much debate as to whether these histologic variants represent "disease entities" or stages of the same condition. The argument is unresolved. There is some evidence in support of both views. Certainly DIP often has a more favorable outlook than UIP; some cases of LIP have immunologic abnormalities and may overlap with lymphomatous change; some cases of giant cell interstitial pneumonia (GIP) are now known to be associated with exposure to hard metal. There are now reports of cases of DIP which retain their identity for at least 7 to 8 years. On the other hand, some patients with typical DIP progress to UIP. Others have the typical changes of DIP and UIP in different areas of the same biopsy.

FACTORS INITIATING FIBROSIS RATHER THAN RESOLUTION

In most acute inflammatory processes of the lung, as in typical pneumococcal pneumonia, extensive intra-alveolar inflammation occurs together with inflammatory changes in the alveolar walls, but of a degree insufficient to cause necrosis and loss of lung architecture. These infections are quickly overcome within a week or two and usually resolve completely. But, when the initiating infective destruction is more severe, as in some staphylococcal pneumonias, necrosis and abscess formation occurs; this damage can heal only by fibrosis. Some of the more slowly resolving pneumonias heal by organization of the intra-alveolar exudate with fibroblastic proliferation and accretion of fibrous tissue laid on the walls of the alveolar space.

Under certain circumstances, damage to structures in the alveolar wall predominates: (1) when inhaled viable

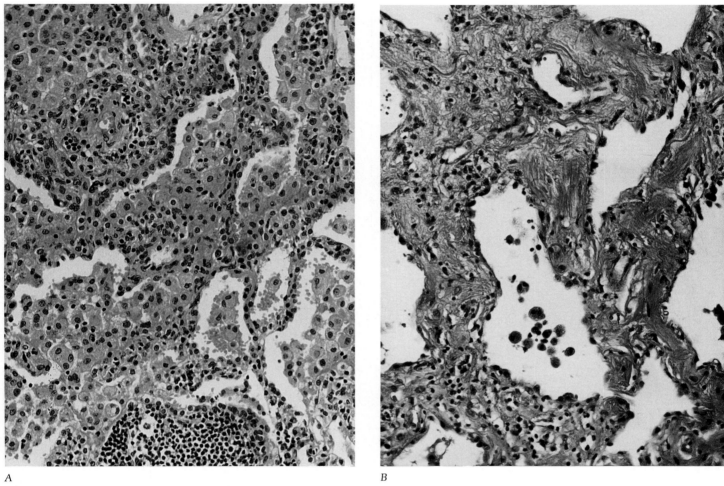

A

B

FIGURE 50-1 Histologic appearance of different types of chronic interstitial pneumonia of unknown cause. *A.* Desquamative interstitial pneumonia. The alveolar spaces are packed uniformly with large, mononuclear cells. The alveolar walls are thickened but without evidence of fibrosis; collections of lymphocytes are frequently seen. *B.* "Mural" fibrosing alveolitis (or usual interstitial pneumonia). The alveolar walls are grossly thickened by fibrosing with intermingled inflammatory cells, mainly lymphocytes and plasma cells.

organisms penetrate the alveolar epithelium and damage lung tissue; (2) when agents that retain their cytotoxicity after phagocytosis are taken up by macrophages and carried by them to the interstitial tissues rather than being cleared through the airways by the cilial escalator, e.g., inhaled dusts of many types, such as coal, silica, and asbestos; (3) when noxious agents or material reaches the lungs through the pulmonary circulation and becomes lodged in the pulmonary capillary bed, damaging the capillary epithelium and promoting an inflammatory exudate into the tissues.

THE EVOLUTION OF FIBROSIS

The evolution of fibrosis will, of course, depend on the type of acute pathology. In silicosis, whorls of collagen surround dust foci (Fig. 50-2) while the normal intervening lung is preserved. In sarcoidosis, fibrosis is often seen where conglomerate granulomata develop (Fig. 50-3). However, there are also many unexplained features. In lone cryptogenic fibrosing alveolitis (CFA) the earlier lesions can be followed by electron microscopy (Fig. 50-4*A, B, C*): initially there is an interstitial exudate; this progresses to an interstitial infiltrate of lymphocytes, plasma cells, fibroblasts, and histiocytes. Restoration of the pulmonary epithelium is reflected in the cuboidal type II pneumocytes spreading over the sites of damaged type I cells. Later, collagen fibers can be seen in both the thin and the thick parts of the alveolar wall, but the architecture is preserved. The pulmonary epithelium is often denuded, showing extensive areas of bare basement membrane; the alveolar architecture of the lung is destroyed, and large tracts of fibrosis with coexisting chronic mixed cell inflammation, often including lymphoid collection, are found. Residual airspaces may become lined with bronchiolar epithelium to form the histologic equivalent of the radiologic "honeycombed" lung.

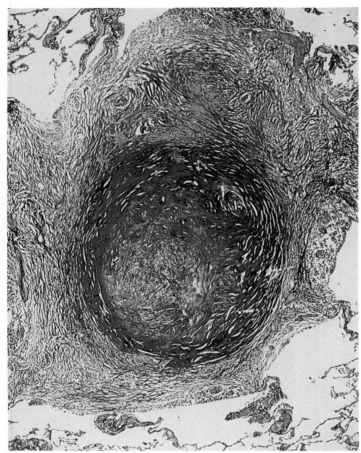

FIGURE 50-2 Histology of silicotic nodule of fibrosis in the lung. ×0.235.

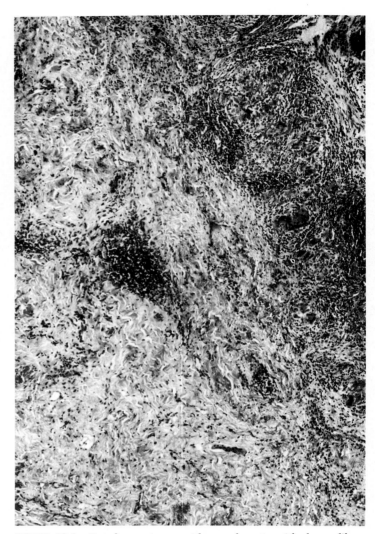

FIGURE 50-3 Conglomerate sarcoid granulomata with dense fibrosis.

THE PATHOGENESIS OF FIBROSIS

Cellular Interaction

The interrelationship between fibroblasts and macrophages has been studied for many years. Some years ago, Hepplestone and Styles showed that supernatants from macrophages cultured with silica stimulated an increased uptake of proline by fibroblasts. More recently, Lewis and Burrell showed that antilung antibody stimulates macrophages in the same way. Since then it has been shown that other agents, such as *Mycobacterium faeni*, stimulate macrophage activation and induce an accumulation of fibroblasts around them in unsensitized animals. Macrophage activation by many agents, including immune complexes, have the same effect.

In vitro studies of inflammatory cells obtained from normal and abnormal fibrosing lung conditions have increased our understanding, at a cellular level, of the events inducing fibrosis. "Activated" macrophages from patients with idiopathic pulmonary fibrosis (IPF) studied in vitro produce much greater amounts of fibronectin than do normal macrophages, and increased amounts of fibronectin can be found in lavage samples from these patients. The action of fibronectin is to regulate cell adhesion and spreading of a variety of cells including fibroblasts; it also acts as a chemotactic factor for these cells and works synergistically with other growth factors including fibroblast replication. Fibronectin appears to act as a competence factor that initiates the replication process, but other macrophage growth factors, acting as "progression factors," allow the replicative process to proceed.

Interestingly, fibronectin also seems to act as an opsonin for collagen. Therefore, it may facilitate the clearance of partially degraded collagen. Collagen is degraded by a variety of collagenases derived from both macrophages and neutrophils. These, in turn, are controlled by a range of collagenase inhibitors such as α_2 macroglobulins. Lymphocytes also appear to have a range of actions stimulating, attracting, and regulating fibroblast activity. The balanced control of collagen production against its

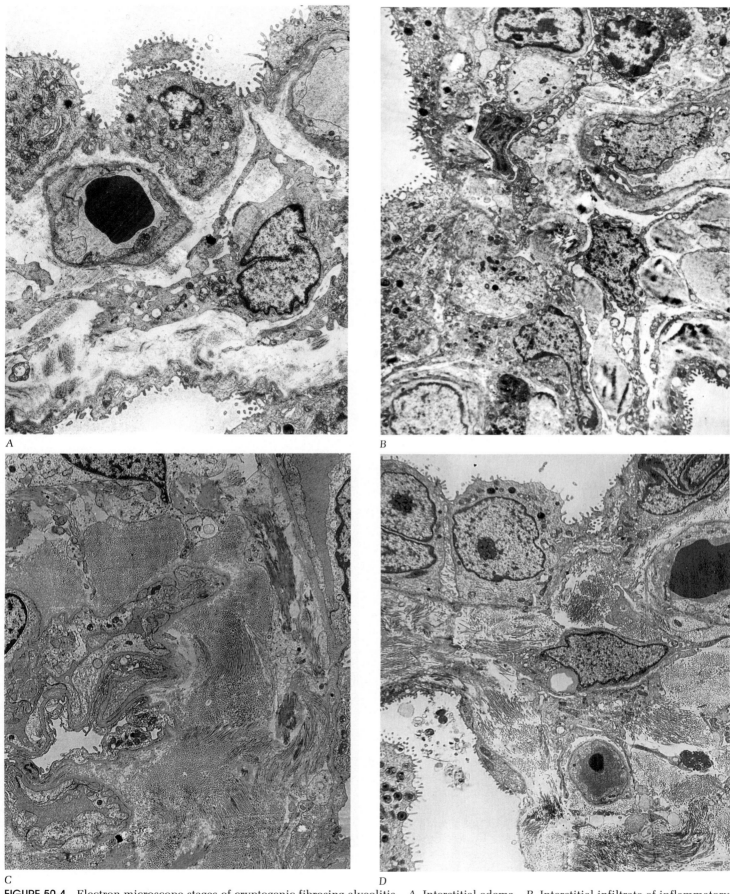

FIGURE 50-4 Electron microscope stages of cryptogenic fibrosing alveolitis. *A.* Interstitial edema. *B.* Interstitial infiltrate of inflammatory cells. *C.* Increasing infiltration by collagen and elastin. *D.* Disorganization of lung architecture with dense fibrosis. No areas of bare basement membrane denuded of pulmonary epithelium.

simultaneous dissolution forms a dynamic state continuously reshaping and restoring the tissue architecture.

Collagen turnover in normal and abnormal lung is a much more dynamic process than previously recognized. When the balanced controls in the normal lung have been completely dissected and understood, the likelihood of identifying the aberration responsible for progressive unexplained fibrosis of the lungs in disease will be much better than at present. Different types of collagen proliferate at different stages of lung inflammation and are related to the clinical reversibility of disease. When type II collagen predominates, patients with CFA tend to undergo radiographic and physiological improvement while taking corticosteroids. Improvement is less evident in patients in whom the increase is predominantly in type I collagen. Increased type III collagen in the lung is also reflected by increased amounts of procollagen type III in the circulation; improvement is associated with a decrease in levels.

Much remains to be learned about the fibroblast/collagen production/collagenase/collagenase inhibitor complex in relation to clinical aspects of fibrotic lung disease. Crystal (see Chapter 48) has recently drawn attention to important information about certain oncogenes and their function as cell growth factors or as receptors on cell membranes for growth factors. The techniques used in these oncologic studies are now being applied to fibrosing lung diseases.

Another fundamental deficiency in the understanding of fibrosing lung diseases is the role of angiogenesis in relation to fibrosis. Often, one of the more striking features of CFA is the intense proliferation of systemic blood vessels from the bronchial arteries (Fig. 50-5). Studies on the role of oncogenes in angiogenesis may also open the way to explaining the vascular proliferation in some progressive fibrosing pulmonary disorders, especially CFA.

INTRA-ALVEOLAR EVENTS

In addition to fibroblast-stimulating factors derived from macrophages, intra-alveolar fibrosis presumably also reflects the inefficiency of phagocytic cells in removing acute inflammatory exudates. Spencer has shown how some apparent fibrosis of the alveolar wall is, in fact, the result of an original deposit of a fibrous layer on the injured surfaces of the alveoli; this layer is subsequently incorporated into the alveolar wall by an overgrowth of type II pneumocytes, which proliferate to repair the damage. This pattern of healing leads to incorporation of collagen fibers into the thickness of the alveolar wall.

A recently described condition of *cryptogenic organizing pneumonia* is characterized by a loose fibroblastic proliferation into the alveolar spaces (as well as a similar process occasionally seen in terminal bronchioles). Special studies show a fine lattice of predominantly type III collagen. The condition appears to be very reversible, with rapid resolution while taking corticosteroids but with a tendency to relapse as the corticosteroids are withdrawn.

INTERSTITIAL EVENTS

Collagen is also deposited in sites where fibroblastic proliferation occurs between the basement membranes of the alveolar epithelium and the capillary epithelium, i.e., in the thick portions of the alveolar walls. The degree of collagen probably depends on the extent of the interstitial inflammatory exudate during the acute stages of disease. Even in those conditions where granulomas are the most striking feature, a more diffuse chronic inflammatory exudate is often also present, especially in hypersensitivity pneumonitis. Indeed, this component, although less florid, seems to be more important in determining later diffuse fibrosis.

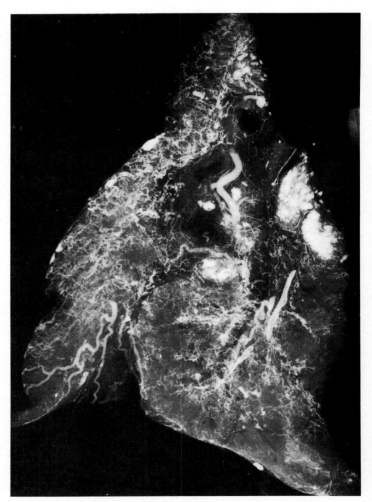

FIGURE 50-5 Exuberant bronchial arteries in widespread cryptogenic fibrosing alveolitis. Autopsy injection in bronchial arteries, 1 cm thick, sagittal section of right lower lobe.

Localization of Fibrosis

The site of deposition within the alveolar wall of immune complexes has also been studied experimentally by Brentjens et al. When complexes were inhaled, deposition occurred first on the alveolar basement membrane. When the complexes were injected intravenously and reached the lung through the circulation, they were deposited first on the basement membrane of the capillary epithelium. The site of subsequent fibrosis may therefore be influenced by the region of initial deposition.

INFLUENCE OF CYTOTOXICITY OF AGENTS ON FIBROSIS

Agents known to be associated with pulmonary fibrosis of varying patterns have differing cytotoxicity for macrophages. Silica, for instance, is more cytotoxic than asbestos. It is reasonable to suppose that these characteristics determine, to some extent, the pattern of fibrosis. Silica, for example, by killing cohorts of macrophages, with con-

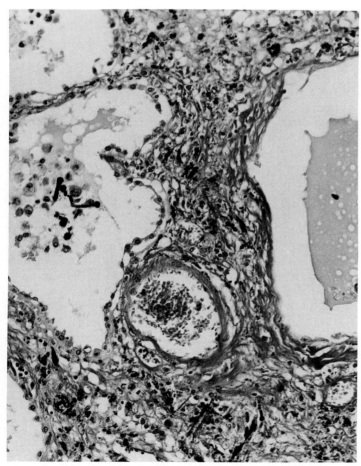

FIGURE 50-6 Asbestos. Histologic appearances showing diffuse thickening of alveolar walls by fibrosis and many asbestos bodies. Some alveoli show repair of pulmonary epithelium by type II pneumocytes *(left)*, others have lost epithelium and show a dense collagenous lining *(right)*.

sequent slowing of its own removal from the lung, persists locally and causes focal fibrosis (i.e., nodules). Fiber dimension is also likely to be important: if fibers cannot be ingested by macrophages, a more widespread in situ interstitial formation of collagen is to be expected, and this has been found (Fig. 50-6).

Immunologic Mechanisms

The role of antigens in the formation of fibrosis is not yet fully understood although circulating immune complexes have been demonstrated in idiopathic (cryptogenic) pulmonary fibrosis as well as in other fibrosing pulmonary disorders. The role of immune complexes in activated macrophages leading to the induction of fibrogenic factors has been mentioned above. Although many different animal models have been devised to investigate the role of antigen in the development of fibrosis, the conditions of exposure and the methods of sensitization are usually far removed from those pertinent to human disease. The granuloma of extrinsic allergic alveolitis may be explained possibly on the basis of immune complex deposition; however, evidence of such complexes is not normally found within granulomas in the human disease. Part of the granulomatous formation is likely to be a foreign body response to contaminants other than the specific antigen.

In some instances, tissue responses of delayed hypersensitivity, mediated by lymphocytes, also seem to contribute toward the pattern of granuloma formation. For instance, in some patients with acute pigeon breeder's lung, there is evidence of lymphocyte sensitization in terms of production of migration inhibition factor and lymphocyte transformation. The accumulation of macrophages under the influence of lymphokine is an attractively simple explanation for the histologic features of an acute granuloma, but the relation of this accumulation to the subsequent development of fibrosis has to be explained. Direct macrophage activation by *M. faeni* through the alternative pathway of complement activation may provide a nonimmunologic explanation for the development of fibrosis.

Efficient and complete removal of antigen by macrophages also depends upon adequate activation by T cells. When the function of these cells is impaired, as, perhaps, in sarcoidosis, or in certain immune-deficiency states, or in cigarette smokers, diminished macrophage function might allow persistence of the injurious agent and consequent fibrosis. This suggestion is an attractive one, and techniques are now available for it to be tested.

A number of immunologic responses seem to depend on the products of inflammation. For example, antifibrin antibody has been reported in patients with rheumatoid arthritis and may account for the continued activity of the lesions of rheumatoid arthritis. Antiglobulin (rheumatoid factors) developed against altered globulin may depend on the presence of immune complexes, and antibodies to nuclear components may be stimulated where there is considerable cell destruction, be this from host tissues or from inflammatory cells themselves. Anticollagen antibody- and lymphocyte-mediated immunologic reactions have also been demonstrated. Once developed, these antibodies could react with inflammatory products and account for persisting tissue reactions which, in turn, determine further fibrosis.

If, however, such autoallergic mechanisms were a major cause of persisting and progressive pulmonary disease, they would be detected quite consistently in advancing cases; but evidence of autoallergic mechanisms is uncommon. One possible reason for this discrepancy is that some individuals have a genetic predisposition to develop such autoantibody responses; the association between certain histocompatibility antigens in rheumatoid arthritis and systemic lupus erythematosus supports this theory. Thus, even though initial injury to the lung is caused by a large variety of agents or antigens, progressive fibrosis occurs only in those with a genetically derived pattern of responses which allows certain immunologic or inflammatory reactions to persist. There is a special opportunity to study genetically determined factors in the exceedingly rare cases of cryptogenic fibrosing alveolitis occurring in families; also, pulmonary fibrosis in ankylosing spondylitis has a very close association with B27 haplotype. Much work is now being done along these lines, and this should prove fruitful, not only in the field of respiratory medicine but also with respect to the wider problems of the causes of persisting chronic inflammation.

Multiple Factors

Just as genetic predisposition and immunologic factors may interrelate, multiple extrinsic agents may be necessary to promote progressive fibrosis. For example, inhaled bleomycin in animal models usually results in a short-lived, self-limiting, inflammation with transient and resolving fibrosis. Inhaled bleomycin, together with an inhaled high concentration of oxygen, results in a persisting and progressive fibrosis.

PROGRESSION OF FIBROSIS

The rate of development of fibrosis varies greatly, depending on the nature of the primary agent and also on the host. For instance, fibrosis in sarcoidosis affects fewer than 20 percent of those presenting with acute features, and within this group the rate of progression is very variable: some develop fibrotic shadows that persist unchanged for a decade or two; others progress to fibrotic contraction within as few as 5 or 6 years. In extrinsic aller-

gic alveolitis, progression from acute nodular shadowing to fatal fibrosis is also very variable but can be exceedingly rapid. In cryptogenic fibrosing alveolitis, some patients die within 12 months, while others live with grossly abnormal chest radiographs, but apparently arrested disease, for 30 years or more; the mean survival, however, is about 5 years. In the case of fibrogenic dusts, fibrosis usually develops more slowly, sometimes years after removal from exposure, presumably owing to the resident dust load in the lungs; the rate of development is extremely variable. Progression is related to many different factors: (1) persistence of the cytotoxic agent, (2) progressive healing, (3) foreign body reaction, (4) failure of clearance of normal environmental contaminants due to lung distortion, (5) development of antibodies to inflammatory products, and (6) genetic factors. All these factors have to be considered before assuming that persistence of the primary agent alone is responsible. Reconsideration of all these factors is important because their definition in individual patients may suggest new approaches to management.

THE DISTRIBUTION OF FIBROSIS

In spite of very extensive bilateral shadowing on the chest radiograph, fibrosis is virtually never universal. The pattern of distribution of fibrosis is frequently characteristic of a particular causal agent or condition.

The acute, noncaseating granulomas that occur in sarcoidosis or extrinsic allergic alveolitis are usually very widespread, affecting all regions of the lung, but in the chronic stages, fibrosis usually affects predominantly the upper lobes. In chronic sarcoidosis, a disease for which the etiology remains unknown, predominant fibrosis of the upper lobes is a clinical fact. Very little attention has been given to the anomalies of sarcoid fibrosis. These include not only the upper zone predominance, even though the preceding granulomas are much more widespread, but also the predominance of linear shadows and the very marked contraction of the upper lobes. It is probable that other explanations should be considered in addition to fibrosis of conglomerate sarcoid granulomates per se. For example, it is possible that some of the features are due to the obliterative effects of sarcoid lesions in the smaller airways. Bronchograms (Fig. 50-7) showing very marked distortion support this suggestion.

Organic dust diseases also cause greater structural damage to the upper lobes. The reasons for this preferential damage are speculative, but it is probable that the lesser ventilation and blood flow in the upper lobes, and possibly a slower lymphatic drainage, somehow contribute to delaying the clearance of particles that reach the interstitium.

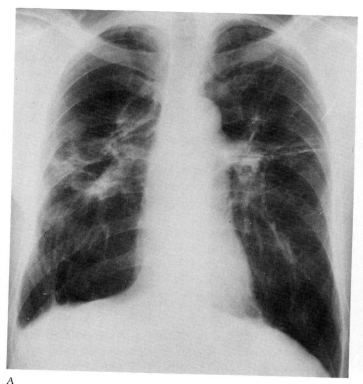

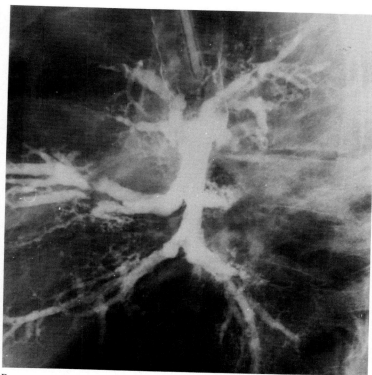

A

B

FIGURE 50-7 *A.* Chest radiograph of patient with fibrotic sarcoidosis. *B.* Bronchogram from the same patient showing multiple bronchial stenoses and airway distortion.

Some patterns seen in silicosis lend support to the suggestion that abnormal clearance mechanisms are involved. Silica characteristically results in whorled, nodular fibrosis. This exuberant fibrosis is generally attributed to the cytoxic effects of the dust on macrophages (Fig. 50-2). Silicotic nodules of the lungs predominate in the upper lobes (Fig. 50-8), but a predominantly basal distribution has been described among certain groups of Africans. This discrepancy has been ascribed to their working posture—bent double at the waist while hacking at the silicaceous rock—so that the lung bases are uppermost.

Upper zone fibrosis is also characteristic of *Mycobacterium tuberculosis* infections. A variety of explanations for the preferential growth of organisms in this position have been put forward, including relatively high P_{O_2} in the upper parts of the lungs and the slower clearance of particles. Among the other chronic disorders that preferentially damage the upper lobes is bronchopulmonary aspergillosis. In some instances, a sequence of radiographs taken early in the disease shows fleeting shadows (associated with a blood eosinophilia and a specific precipitating antibody) in random segments of the lung, sometimes the upper, and sometimes the lower, lobes. Later the pattern changes, and progressive fibrotic contraction of the upper lobe, associated with radiographic evidence of upper lobe bronchiectasis, ensues (Fig. 50-9).

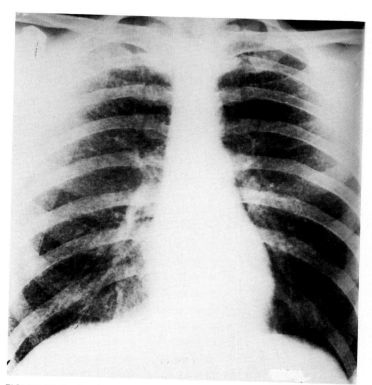

FIGURE 50-8 Predominant upper lobe distribution of nodular fibrosis in a patient with silicosis.

763

This localization is not associated with clinical evidence of secondary infection. Upper lobe fibrosis also occurs for quite unknown reasons in association with ankylosing spondylitis. One plausible, but unproved, hypothesis is that fixation of the posterior vertebrocostal joints prefer-

entially reduces upper lobe ventilation and normal clearance.

Preferential fibrosis of the lower lobes is equally characteristic of certain other disorders, such as asbestosis. An early report had suggested that the quantity of asbestos fibers is similar in the fibrotic lower and the nonfibrotic upper lobes. To account for localization of the lower lobes, an additional factor must be implicated. The quantitative distribution of asbestos fibers is now being reexamined using refined techniques of transmission electron microscopy combined with spectrophotometric analysis.

Basal fibrosis is also characteristic of cryptogenic fibrosing alveolitis (Fig. 50-10). In this condition, the more acute lesions also have a predominantly basal distribution. The most characteristic example of the latter is desquamative interstitial pneumonia. A basal distribution of fibrosis is also commonly seen in systemic sclerosis, rheumatoid arthritis, and subacute lupus erythematosus associated with fibrosing alveolitis. Although the causes of these conditions are unknown, their systemic distribution suggests that the pulmonary lesions are more likely to be dependent on circulating rather than inhaled agents. From these examples it is tempting to suggest that when injurious agents reach the lung through the pulmonary circulation, be these immune complexes, drugs, endotoxin, or other tissue-damaging material, areas of greatest perfusion will be predominantly affected; of course, under normal circumstances, these areas are the lung bases. A basal distribution of fibrosis is also found in chronic pulmonary congestion that has persisted for years because of a raised left atrial pressure; this distribution,

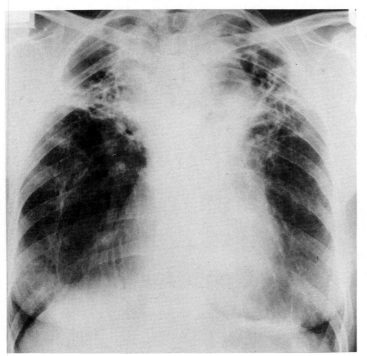

FIGURE 50-9 Contraction of the upper lobes following repeated episodes of "fleeting shadows" owing to *Aspergillus fumigatus* hypersensitivity (bronchopulmonary aspergillosis).

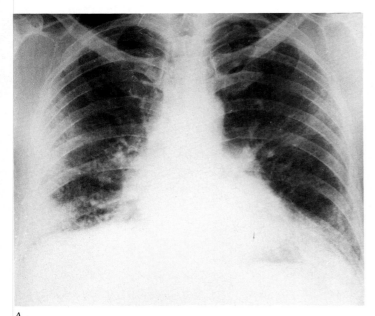
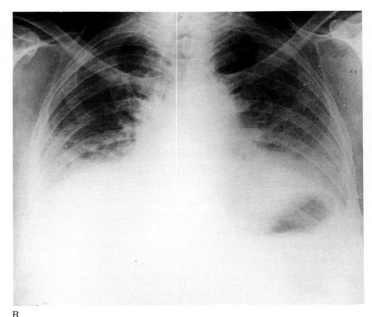

A   *B*

FIGURE 50-10 A patient with rapidly progressing cryptogenic fibrosing alveolitis in spite of corticosteroid therapy. A. July 1975: Predominant lower zone shadowing, normal mediastinal width. B. February 1976: Elevation of the diaphragms, extension of shadowing upwards, broadening of mediastinum.

too, presumably depends on changes in those regions of lung that have the greatest perfusion and are subjected to the greatest hydrostatic pressure.

In summary, fibrosing granulomas tend to be distributed preferentially in the upper lobes, whereas chronic capillary exudation from whatever cause, particularly when the upright position is maintained, in general predominantly affects the lower zones. The basal distribution

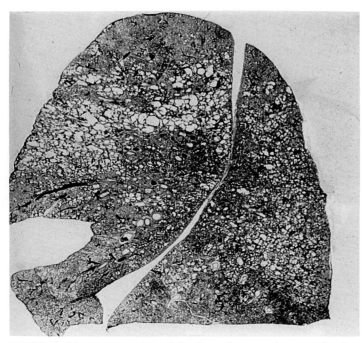

FIGURE 50-11 Macrosection of the lung showing the irregular distribution of fibrosis with honeycombing and the more normal central parts of the lung.

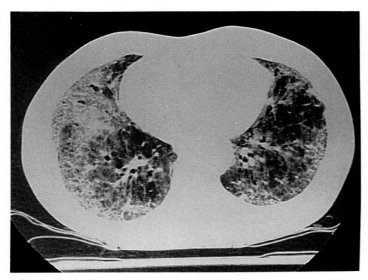

FIGURE 50-12 Computed tomography illustrating peripheral fibrosis of fibrosing alveolitis. The pattern does not shift when the patient's position is changed.

spreads upward as the severity and extent of capillary damage increases.

Other patterns of distribution are apparent on macrosections (Fig. 50-11) of the lungs or computed tomography (Fig. 50-12). In some individuals, the periphery of the lung is particularly affected, whereas the more central parts are relatively normal. This fact is important, because lung biopsies taken from the surface of the lung through the chest wall often show far more extensive fibrosis and disorganization than do transbronchial biopsies that come from more central areas.

THE RADIOLOGY OF FIBROSIS

The radiographic appearances of upper and lower lobe fibrosis reflect in a general way the distribution of features just described. The nodular shadows so characteristic of silicosis are distinctive (Fig. 50-8). Upper zone fibrosis is associated with elevation of the horizontal fissure; when fibrosis is bilateral, the trachea remains central. The hilar shadows are elevated, but the lower lobes tend to hyperinflate, so that the diaphragms remain in the normal position, albeit with a reduced range of movement (Fig. 50-9). By contrast, lower zone fibrosis leads to elevation of the diaphragms, and the distinction can be difficult between the patient who has failed to take a full inspiration and the one who is unable to do so (Fig. 50-10A). Extensive fibrosis often leads to a general broadening of the mediastinum simulating hilar or paratracheal gland enlargement (Fig. 50-10B). On occasion this has led to unnecessary, and potentially dangerous, mediastinoscopy. This procedure is hazardous because a large part of the shadows represent major vessels which are additionally enlarged in patients in whom parenchymal disease is associated with pulmonary hypertension. Often this error can be avoided by careful appraisal of the posteroanterior and lateral tomograms or CT scans.

Honeycombing on the chest radiograph correlates well with pathology on direct inspection of the lung. It is practical from the diagnostic viewpoint to distinguish *honeycombing*, which occurs irregularly within areas of marked fibrosis, from *honeycomb lung*, in which the cystic pattern is more uniformly distributed throughout the entire lung. Honeycomb lung occurs particularly in eosinophilic granuloma (Fig. 50-13), diffuse leiomyomatosis, tuberous sclerosis, and other very rare conditions such as pulmonary adenomatosis. In their early stages, all of these conditions may have a less extensive and less characteristic distribution than in the later stages.

Extensive fibrosis is sometimes associated with gross *destructive* emphysema in the nonfibrotic lobes, whereas in other instances the nonfibrotic lung remains relatively normal. The reasons for this difference have not been studied in detail. *Overdistention* (or *distension emphy-*

sema) of the lower lobes associated with upper lobe fibrosis leads to an increase in residual volume; the total lung capacity is relatively well maintained. If the lung architecture is preserved in the overdistended lower lobes, their performance is good, the balance between ventilation and perfusion is maintained, and the diffusing capacity for carbon monoxide is reasonably normal. On the other hand, extensive fibrosis, especially of the upper lobes, is sometimes associated with *destructive* emphysema of the lower lobes. This destructive emphysema is often seen in silicosis and sometimes in advanced fibrotic sarcoidosis. When this occurs, all the functional abnormalities associated with destructive emphysema can be found. In eosinophilic granuloma bullous cysts are often seen in the upper lobes in addition to the more commonly recognized honeycomb appearance. The radiographic picture (Fig. 50-13) is distinctive. The combination of destructive emphysema and fibrosis leads to very severe symptoms and functional impairment. By contrast, even extensive lower lobe fibrosis is much less frequently associated with extensive emphysema on the chest radiograph, although with the introduction of CT scanning this is now being found more frequently.

Computed tomography has transformed this radiographic visualization of lung fibrosis. Using this noninvasive technique, the distribution in the horizontal plane reveals the peripheral, central, or diffuse distribution of disease, and it distinguishes ventral from dorsal predominance. It also shows that many patients have a combination of fibrosis with intermingled emphysematous areas

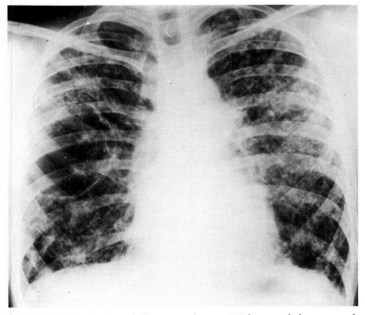

FIGURE 50-13 Eosinophilic granuloma. Widespread honeycomb lung with additional larger bullae.

quite unrecognized on posteroanterior (PA) lateral films. These observations improve our understanding of physiological measurements (Fig. 50-12). CT also reveals pulmonary abnormalities when the posteroanterior and lateral chest radiographs are entirely normal. It is essential to perform prone and supine radiographs to distinguish vascular pooling from true abnormalities.

SYMPTOMS AND PHYSICAL SIGNS OF FIBROSIS

The usual presenting symptom is breathlessness. Not uncommonly, it is associated with a dry, irritant, and persisting cough. The cause of the breathlessness is usually an increase in stiffness and presumably results from stimulation of receptors in the lungs (including the airways) rather than from a reduced arterial P_{O_2}.

The physical signs depend especially on distribution of fibrosis. Lower lobe fibrosis is usually associated with fine, end-inspiratory crepitations due probably to the opening of airways closed during expiration. Since airway closure occurs preferentially in the most dependent parts of the lung, crepitations disappear if the patient is examined in a position in which the lower lobes are uppermost. These fine, late crepitations should be distinguished from coarser ones occurring throughout inspiration and which sometimes continue into expiration; the coarser crepitations probably arise from bronchioles or small bronchi.

Finger clubbing occurs in about 60 percent of patients with cryptogenic fibrosing alveolitis and asbestosis but is much less common in other forms of widespread fibrosis. The explanation for finger clubbing in these disorders is unknown. In the lungs of patients with cryptogenic fibrosing alveolitis and finger clubbing, a correlation exists between the extent of proliferation on bronchial arteries into an exuberant fibrosis and the occurrence of clubbing (Fig. 50-5). Lower lobe fibrosis is more often associated with obvious finger clubbing than is fibrosis of the upper lobes. Moreover, clubbing sometimes precedes lung disease by many years, even though it is apt to strike in the late stages. Whether this early clubbing will prove to be an interesting marker for the genetics of fibrotic lung disease needs to be explored. This possibility is suggested because patients not infrequently remark that the fingers of other members of their family have a similar appearance to their own.

THE FUNCTIONAL CHANGES

The typical changes in pulmonary performance caused by widespread fibrosis are well recognized and are discussed in detail in Chapter 163.

MONITORING THE ACTIVITY OF THE DISEASE

Because the rate of progression of fibrosis is so variable, it must be separately assessed in each patient. This assessment is important in directing therapy for the following reasons. First, most treatments that are currently available have their own hazards; treatment should be reserved for those patients in whom it is certain that progression is occurring. Second and most important, if treatment is to be successful, it must be instituted at a stage when the tissue responses are still reversible. If treatment is withheld until fibrosis becomes established, it is bound to fail. Monitoring of the activity and progression in the early stages is imperative even though the patient has relatively few symptoms.

The mainstay of monitoring is on the basis of functional assessment. Usually serial simple tests suffice. These include determination of lung volumes, ventilation, and diffusing capacity of the lung for carbon monoxide. Should the patient's symptom of dyspnea be excessive for the degree of impairment in static lung function, serial exercise tests are often helpful, particularly the determination of the cost of exercise in terms of cardiac rate, O_2 uptake, and arterial P_{O_2}.

However, there remains a group of patients whose symptoms are at variance with objective exercise tests. In these patients, serial determinations of pulmonary compliance do not appear to be more sensitive, and serial assessment of pulmonary function is neither always concordant with clinical disability nor consistently sensitive enough to direct the adjustment of drug dosage.

Other measurements of activity of disease have received much attention in recent years. In some patients, the time-honored determination of erythrocyte sedimentation rate is helpful, but in others, it is often normal in spite of radiographic progression. Use of radioisotopes (gallium 67) has been suggested as a useful way to monitor activity in sarcoidosis, but it reflects particularly the activity of macrophage/histiocytes; therefore, it probably reflects the activity of granulomata rather than their tendency to progress to fibrosis. As noted above, only a minority of patients with sarcoidosis progress to fibrosis, and the activity of granulomata per se does not necessarily reflect the likelihood of identifying this minority subgroup. In one study, the extent of increase of gallium uptake before treatment did not predict whether corticosteroid treatment would induce complete clearing or leave residual fibrotic contractions. Likewise, concentrations of angiotensin-converting enzyme in serum appear to be raised equally in those patients in whom a normal chest radiograph can be restored by steroids and in those who have already developed some irreversible fibrosis. In CFA, a disorder in which the tendency to progressive fibrosis is far greater, gallium 67 scan counts are usually much less increased.

Bronchoalveolar lavage has received much attention as a method to monitor activity. Although in sarcoidosis increased lymphocyte counts are characteristic, those with evidence of fibrosis have greater numbers of neutrophils. Whether this feature is a contributory factor to fibrosis or develops as a consequence is unknown. In any event, an increased number of neutrophils in lavage samples is also characteristic of other forms of widespread fibrosis.

TREATMENT

At present, established pulmonary fibrosis is untreatable. However, prefibrotic acute tissue inflammation can often be suppressed by corticosteroids. As noted before, the exception to this general statement is the observed reversibility of increases in type III collagen in the lung. Thus, staging of fibrosis is important in establishing potential reversibility by treatment. Therapeutic agents have to be continued as long as the disease is active. In disorders in which activity can be assessed with some ease, such as sarcoidosis, alternate-day regimens have often, but not invariably, proved successful. In principle, such regimens should reduce the long-term side effects of corticosteroids; however, the value of alternate-day regimens is difficult to prove because they require very long follow-up of a large number of comparable cases.

Immunosuppressants such as cyclophosphamide have proved useful in arresting the progress of the disease in a few patients who responded only to unacceptably high doses of corticosteroids. A long-term, controlled trial of cyclophosphamide versus corticosteroids in cryptogenic fibrosing alveolitis has identified a number of patients who fail to respond to steroids but do respond to immunosuppressants. Penicillamine has also seemed to be of value in an occasional refractory patient: 4 of 18 cases showed objective improvement, having failed on corticosteroids alone; whether combination therapy will yield better results awaits formal study. Formal studies are difficult to plan because of the very different stages in the disease at which patients are first seen by their doctor, the variable rate of progression, and the relative rarity of these cases.

Improvement in therapy is likely to come from a better understanding of the sequence of events leading to progressive fibrosis and from the interruption of the circuits of tissue injury at an early stage when reversibility is still possible. A number of other agents that affect intracellular functions, such as aminoproprionitriles, and microtubule inhibitors, such as colchicine, have been proposed. But, as yet, they have no proved place in the management of pulmonary fibrosis.

CONCLUSIONS

Although widespread pulmonary fibrosis is relatively rare in the context of pulmonary disease in general, the problems that the disorder poses are far-reaching. The implications are great because a very wide range of agents induces fibrosis by a wide variety of pathogeneses. Understanding of these involves knowledge of the fundamental mechanisms of inflammation as well as of the mechanisms of tissue injury to immunologic triggers. Some of the potential interacting factors are illustrated in Fig. 50-14 and emphasize the potential central role of the alveolar macrophage. Whatever the pathogenesis, the rate of progression varies widely from patient to patient, and the proper assessment of when to treat, how to treat, in what drug dosage, and for how long requires much better methods for monitoring progression. As long as we are faced with cases of widespread irreversible fibrosis, we are facing our own failure. Only more intensive research can correct this deficiency.

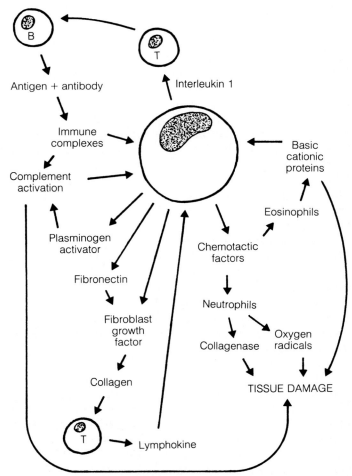

FIGURE 50-14 A summarization of some of the interrelating factors in the development of pulmonary fibrosis, emphasizing the probable central role of the alveolar macrophage.

BIBLIOGRAPHY

Agelli M, Wahl SM: Cytokines and fibrosis. Clin Exp Rheumatol 4:379–388, 1986.
A review of the characteristics of lymphocyte and monocyte cytokines which appear to be involved in regulating fibroblast recruitment, proliferation, and matrix synthesis.

Allison AC, Harrington JS, Birbeck M: Examination of the cytoxic effects of cilica on macrophages. J Exp Med 124:141–153, 1966.
A classic article demonstrating the cytotoxicity of silica on macrophages in vitro.

Bateman ED, Turner-Warwick M, Haslam PL, Adelmann-Gill BC: Cryptogenic fibrosing alveolitis: Prediction of fibrogenic activity from immunochemical studies of collagen types in the lung. Thorax 38:93–101, 1983.
The demonstration of type III and type I collagen in different proportions in different patients. Relatively greater amounts of type III collagen are associated with better response to corticosteroids.

Beattie J, Knox JF: Studies of mineral content and particle size distribution in the lungs of asbestos textile workers, in Davies CN (ed), Inhaled Particles and Vapors. London, Pergamon, 1961, pp 419–433.
Analysis of the distribution of asbestos in autopsy specimens from asbestos workers.

Bitterman BP, Rennard SI, Adelberg S, Crystal RG: Role of fibronectin as a growth factor for fibroblasts. J Cell Biol 97:1925–1932, 1983.
The demonstration that fibronectin is a growth factor for fibroblasts.

Bitterman BP, Rennard SI, Hunninghake GW: Human alveolar macrophage growth factor for fibroblasts. Regulation and partial characterization. J Clin Invest 70:806–822, 1982.
   The characterization of growth factor obtained from stimulated human alveolar macrophages in vitro.

Brentjens JR, O'Connell DW, Pawlowski IB, Hsu KC, Andres GA: Experimental immune complex disease of the lung. The pathogenesis of a laboratory model resembling certain interstitial lung disease. J Exp Med 140:105–125, 1974.
   The demonstration that immune complexes may induce certain patterns of interstitial lung disease.

Brown CH, Turner-Warwick M: The treatment of cryptogenic fibrosing alveolitis with immunosuppressant drugs. Q J Med 40:289–302, 1971.
   The demonstration that azathioprine and cyclophosphamide may be used as an alternative to steroids in the treatment of some patients with cryptogenic fibrosing alveolitis.

Burrell RG, Esber HJ, Hegadorn JE, Andrews CE: Specificity of lung-reactive antibodies in human serum. Am Rev Respir Dis 94:743–750, 1966.
   The demonstration that lung-reactive antibodies in human serum are not specific to lung tissue.

Caldwell JR, Pearce DE, Spencer C, Leder R, Waldman RH: Immunologic mechanisms in hypersensitivity pneumonitis. J Allergy Clin Immunol 52:225–230, 1973.
   The study of lymphocyte sensitization in hypersensitivity pneumonitis.

Carrington CB, Gaensler EA, Coutu RE, Fitzgerald MX, Gupta RG: Natural history and treated course of usual and desquamative interstitial pneumonia. N Engl J Med 298:801–809, 1978.
   A comprehensive article on the progression, fatality, and response to treatment of usual interstitial pneumonia (UIP) and desquamative interstitial pneumonia (DIP). This study indicates the better prognosis for patients with DIP.

Cegla UH, Kroidl RF, Meier-Sydow J, Thiel CL, Czarneck GV, Shreiber F: Therapy of the idiopathic fibrosis of the lung. Pneumologie 152:75–92, 1975.
   Uncontrolled study of corticosteroids, immunosuppressants, and penicillamine alone and in various combinations for idiopathic pulmonary fibrosis.

Clark JG, Greenberg J: Modulation of the effects of alveolar macrophages on lung fibroblast collagen production rate. Am Rev Respir Dis 135:52–56, 1987.
   A study of the factors that enable alveolar macrophages (AM) to function as effector cells that can either stimulate or inhibit lung fibroblast collagen production.

Corrin B, Dewar A, Rodriguez-Roison R, Turner-Warwick M: Fine structural changes in cryptogenic fibrosing alveolitis and asbestosis. J Pathol 147:107–119, 1985.
   A descriptive study of the histology of cryptogenic fibrosing alveolitis and asbestosis using electron microscopy.

Davies D: Ankylosing spondylitis and lung fibrosis. Q J Med 41:395–417, 1972.
   A clinical study on the association of ankylosing spondylitis and upper zone fibrosis, an association that remains unexplained.

Davison AG, Haslam PL, Corrin B, Coutts II, Dewar A, Riding WD, Studdy PR, Newman Taylor AJ: Interstitial lung disease and asthma in hard metal workers: Bronchoalveolar lavage, ultrastructural and analytical findings and results of bronchial provocation tests. Thorax 38:119–128, 1983.
   A description of the histology, electron microscope appearances, and lavage in hard metal workers, including the importance of giant cells.

Davison AG, Heard BE, McAllister WAC, Turner-Warwick M: Relapsing cryptogenic organizing pneumonitis. Q J Med 52:382–394, 1983.
   A descriptive study of unsolved organizing pneumonia of unknown cause, characterized by fibroblastic proliferation within alveolar spaces, responding dramatically to corticosteroids but relapsing on their withdrawal.

Dreisin RB, Schwartz MI, Theofilopoulos AN, Standford RE: Circulating immune complexes in the idiopathic interstitial pneumonias. N Engl J Med 298:353–357, 1978.
   A comparison of patients with idiopathic interstitial pneumonia with and without circulating immune complexes. The study demonstrates the better response of those with circulating complexes to corticosteroids.

Edwards JH: A quantitative study on the activation of the alternative pathways of complement by mouldy hay dust and thermophilic actinomycetes. Clin Allergy 6:19–25, 1976.
   A demonstration of alternative pathway activation by thermophilic molds responsible for farmer's lung.

Evered D, Whelan J (eds): Ciba Foundation Symposium New Series No. 114: Fibrosis. London, Pitman, 1985.
The report of the conference on fibrosis summarizing the many current aspects of the problems.

Fink JN, Moore VL, Barboriak JJ: Cell-mediated hypersensitivity in pigeon breeders. Int Arch Allergy Appl Immunol 49:831–836, 1975.
A study demonstrating the importance of cell-mediated hypersensitivity in pigeon breeder's lung.

Forgacs P: Lung sounds (origins of crepitations). Br J Dis Chest 63:1–12, 1969.
This study discusses the mechanism of production of various lung sounds, particularly crepitations.

Gadek JE, Kelman JA, Fells GA, Weinberger SE, Horwitz AL, Reynolds HY, Fulmer JD, Crystal RG: Collagenase in the lower respiratory tract of patients with idiopathic pulmonary fibrosis. N Engl J Med 301:737–747, 1979.
The demonstration of precollagenase in alveolar lavage material from patients with idiopathic pulmonary fibrosis.

Gandevia B, Mitchell CA: Small airways disease (bronchiolitis) following inhalation of proteolytic enzymes used in the detergent industry. Aust Ann Med 19:408, 1970.
An early study demonstrating the physiological evidence of small airways disease in workers from the detergent industry.

Hance AJ, Crystal RG: Idiopathic pulmonary fibrosis, in Flenley DC, Petty TL (eds), *Recent Advances in Respiratory Medicine, vol 3.* Edinburgh, Churchill Livingstone, 1983, pp 249–287.
An important comprehensive review of pathogenesis and treatment of idiopathic pulmonary fibrosis. A very comprehensive list of references.

Hansen PJ, Penny R: Pigeon breeders' disease. Study of the cell-mediated response to pigeon antigens by the lymphocyte culture technique. Int Arch Allergy Appl Immunol 47:498–507, 1974.
A study emphasizing the importance of cell-mediated responses in hypersensitivity pneumonitis distinguishing those with disease from those without.

Haslam PL, Thompson B, Mohammed I, Townsend PJ, Hodson M, Holborow EJ, Turner-Warwick M: Circulating immune complexes in patients with cryptogenic fibrosing alveolitis. Clin Exp Immunol 37:381–390, 1979.
A demonstration of circulating immune complexes in patients with fibrosing alveolitis, the correlates suggesting that their demonstration occurs in relatively early disease.

Hepplestone AG: The fibrogenic action of silica. Br Med Bull 25:282–287, 1969.
A study demonstrating the fibrogenic potential of macrophages stimulated by silica.

Hunter AM, Lamb D: Relapse of fibrosing alveolitis (desquamative interstitial pneumonia) after 12 years. Thorax 34:677–679, 1979.
A case report of desquamative interstitial pneumonia responding to treatment but relapsing after 12 years.

Kirk JME, Bateman ED, Haslam PL, Laurent GJ, Turner-Warwick M: Measurement of serum type III precollagen concentration in cryptogenic fibrosing alveolitis and its clinical relevance. Thorax 39:726–732, 1984.
The demonstration of type III procollagen in the serum of patients with fibrosing alveolitis with falling values correlating to the extent of improvement in lung function tests on treatment with steroids.

Kravis TC, Ahmed A, Brown TE, Fulmer JD, Crystal RG: Pathogenic mechanisms in pulmonary fibrosis collagen induced migration inhibition factor production and cytoxicity mediated by lymphocytes. J Clin Invest 58:1223–1232, 1976.
An in vitro study showing lymphocyte sensitization to collagen.

Laurent GJ, McAnulty RJ: Protein metabolism during bleomycin induced pulmonary fibrosis. Am Rev Respir Dis 128:82–88, 1983.
An experimental model of bleomycin lung fibrosis and the demonstration of rapid turnover of collagen.

Lewis DM, Burrell R: Induction of fibrogenesis by lung antibody-treated macrophages. Br J Ind Med 33:25–82, 1976.
A demonstration of induction of fibroblastic activity by macrophage activated by a lung antibody.

Liebow AA, Steer A, Billingsley JG: Desquamative interstitial pneumonia. Am J Med 39:369–404, 1965.
A classic article on the original description of desquamative interstitial pneumonia, its histology, and its clinical features.

Liebow AA: Definition and classification of interstitial pneumonias in human pathology, in Basset F, Georges R (eds), *Progress in Respiration Research, vol 8, Alveolar Interstitium of the Lung, Pathological and Physiological Aspects.* New York, Karger, 1975, pp 1–33.
A review of a number of interstitial pneumonias with predominance of different cell types including lymphocytes, macrophages, and plasma cells.

Lin YH, Haslam PL, Turner-Warwick M: Chronic pulmonary sarcoidosis. The relationship between lung lavage cell counts, the chest radiograph and standard lung function tests. Thorax 40:501–507, 1984.
The demonstration that as the chest radiograph in sarcoidosis shows more fibrosis, lavage neutrophils increase.

Line BR, Fulmer JD, Reynolds HY, Roberts WC, Jones AE, Harris EK, Crystal RG: Gallium 67 citrate scanning in the staging of idiopathic pulmonary fibrosis: Correlation with physiologic and morphologic features and bronchoalveolar lavage. Am Rev Respir Dis 118:355–365, 1978.
A comprehensive article on gallium scanning in evaluating the activity of disease in idiopathic pulmonary fibrosis.

Livingstone JL, Lewis JG, Reid L, Jefferson KE: Diffuse interstitial pulmonary fibrosis. Q J Med 33:71–103, 1964.
A descriptive article on the clinical, radiographic and histologic features of interstitial pulmonary fibrosis.

Martinet Y, Rom WN, Grotendorst GR, Martin GR, Crystal RG: Exaggerated spontaneous release of platelet-derived growth factor by alveolar macrophages from patients with idiopathic pulmonary fibrosis. N Engl J Med 317:202–209, 1987.
The accumulation of mesenchymal cells within the alveolar walls in patients with idiopathic pulmonary fibrosis may result partly from the exaggerated release of the potent mitogen platelet-derived growth factor by mononuclear phagocytes in the lower respiratory tract.

Moore VL, Fink JN, Barboriak JJ, Ruff LC, Schlueter DP: Immunologic events in pigeon breeders' disease. J Allergy Clin Immunol 53:319–328, 1974.
The cell-mediated responses in pigeon breeder's disease.

Phan SH: Fibrotic mechanisms in lung disease, in Ward P (ed), *Immunology of Inflammation.* New York, Elsevier, 1983, pp 121–162.
An overview of mechanisms of fibrosis in lung disease.

Quinones F, Crouch E: Biosynthesis of interstitial and basement membrane collagens in pulmonary fibrosis. Am Rev Respir Dis 134:1163–1171, 1986.
An investigation of the synthesis and matrix deposition of interstitial and basement membrane collagens in a rat model of bleomycin-induced pulmonary fibrosis.

Rennard SI, Crystal RG: Fibronectin in human bronchopulmonary lavage fluid: Elevation of patients with interstitial lung disease. J Clin Invest 69:113–122, 1982.
The demonstration of fibronectin in lavage fluid from patients with interstitial lung disease.

Reynolds HY: Lung inflammation: normal host defense or a complication of some diseases? Annu Rev Med 38:295–323, 1987.
A review of the normal interactions between alveolar macrophages, various opsonins, complement and chemotactic factors, and the responsiveness of polymorphonuclear leukocytes.

Reynolds HY, Fulmer JD, Kazmierowski JA, Roberts WC, Frank MM, Crystal RG: Analysis of cellular and protein content of broncho-alveolar lavage fluid from patients with idiopathic pulmonary fibrosis and chronic hypersensitivity pneumonitis. J Clin Invest 59:165–175, 1977.
One of the first descriptions of increases in neutrophils in lavage material from idiopathic pulmonary fibrosis.

Roschmann RA, Rothenberg RJ: Pulmonary fibrosis in rheumatoid arthritis: a review of clinical features and therapy. Semin Arthritis Rheum 16:174–185, 1987.
Approximately 30% to 40% of patients with rheumatoid arthritis demonstrate either radiographic or pulmonary function abnormalities indicative of interstitial fibrosis or restrictive lung disease.

Scadding JG: Fibrosing alveolitis. Br Med J 2:686, 1964.
A discussion of the genesis of the term fibrosing alveolitis and a justification for its use to designate a spectrum of fibrosing disease in the acinar parts of the lung.

Seal RME: Pathology of extrinsic allergic bronchiolo-alveolitis, in Basset F, Georges R (eds), *Progress in Respiratory Research, vol 8, Alveolar Interstitium of the Lung.* Basel/Paris, Karger, 1975, pp 66–73.
A description of the pathology of extrinsic allergic alveolitis emphasizing its involvement of small airways as well as acinar parts.

Spector WG, Heesom N: The production of granulomata by antigen-antibody complexes. J Pathol 98:31–39, 1969.
An analysis of the ratio of antibody-to-antigen–inducing granulomata, demonstrating that the latter tends to occur when antigen-antibody complexes are in equivalence.

Stack BHR, Choo Kang FJ, Heard BE: The prognosis of fibrosing alveolitis. Thorax 27:535–542, 1972.
A clinical study that considers the natural history of fibrosing alveolitis and its response to corticosteroids.

Tryka AF, Godleski JJ, Brain JD: Alterations in hamsters developing pulmonary fibrosis. Exp Lung Res 7:41–52, 1984.
An experimental model of lung fibrosis.

Turner-Warwick M: Systemic arterial patterns in the lung and clubbing of the fingers. Thorax 18:238–250, 1963.
A correlation of increase in bronchial artery size with finger clubbing, irrespective of the lung disease.

Turner-Warwick M: A perspective view of widespread pulmonary fibrosis. Br Med J 2:371–376, 1974.
An overview on clinical aspects of widespread pulmonary fibrosis posing some as yet unresolved questions on its distribution.

Turner-Warwick M: Future possibilities in therapeutic intervention, in Bouhuys A (ed), *Lung Cells in Disease.* Amsterdam, North Holland/Dekker, 1976, pp 329–340.
A review article speculating on various points at which aggressive fibrosis of the lung might be interrupted.

Turner-Warwick M, Burrows B, Johnson A: Cryptogenic fibrosing alveolitis: Clinical features and their influence on survival. Thorax 35:171–180, 1980.
A long term follow-up study of the natural history of fibrosing alveolitis, demonstrating a mean survival time of around 4 years.

Warrell DA, Harrison BDW, Fawcett IW, Mohammed Y, Mohammed WS, Pope HM, Watkins BJ: Silicosis among grindstone cutters in the north of Nigeria. Thorax 30:389–398, 1975.
Distribution of silicosis in the upper lobes of grindstone cutters in Nigeria.

Watters LC, King TE, Schwarz MI, Waldron JA, Stanford RE, Cherniack RM: A clinical, radiographic, and physiologic scoring system for the longitudinal assessment of patients with idiopathic pulmonary fibrosis. Am Rev Respir Dis 133:97–103, 1986.
A composite clinical-radiographic-physiologic scoring system is proposed for the estimation of the severity of underlying pathologic derangement in idiopathic pulmonary fibrosis and for the longitudinal quantitative assessment of clinical impairment in patients with IPF.

Watters LC, Schwarz MI, Cherniack RM, Waldron JA, Dunn TL, Stanford RE, King TE: Idiopathic pulmonary fibrosis. Pretreatment bronchoalveolar lavage cellular constituents and their relationships with lung histopathology and clinical response to therapy. Am Rev Respir Dis 135:696–704, 1987.
An evaluation of the relationship between the cellular constituents of bronchoalveolar lavage fluid and both the histopathologic abnormalities and the subsequent clinical response to corticosteroid therapy in 26 newly diagnosed, untreated patients with IPF. Pretreatment BALF lymphocytosis was associated with significant subsequent clinical improvement (p less than 0.002).

Chapter 51

Radiation Fibrosis

Theodore L. Phillips

Radiobiologic and Cellular Kinetic Principles

Histopathologic Changes in Human and Experimental Animal Lungs

Pathophysiology of Radiation Injury

Changes in Pulmonary Function

The Clinical Syndrome and Radiographic Findings

Time, Dose, Volume, and Other Modifying Factors

Treatment

Injurious effects of radiation treatment have been noted since the discovery of x-rays and have been a limiting factor in the application of radiation therapy to most clinical neoplasms. Indeed, the art and science of radiotherapy involves maximizing the cell-killing effect in tumor tissue while minimizing the volume and the extent of radiation damage to contiguous normal tissues.

Radiation therapy for neoplasms within the chest, on the chest wall, or in the breast began with the advent of kilovoltage equipment capable of penetrating and delivering significant doses to the structures deep within the thoracic cavity. The first reports of radiation injury to the lung appeared in the early 1920s when the syndrome of radiation pneumonitis was first described.

Radiation pneumonitis, more recently termed radiation pneumonopathy or radiation pleuropneumonitis, has occurred in the treatment of almost any tumor in which a significant dose of radiation reaches functioning pulmonary tissue. The syndrome is most apt to occur in patients with tumors in, or in the vicinity of, the lungs who remain alive for a long while after treatment and in whom irradiation has affected a portion of the lung. This category includes patients with carcinoma of the breast, in whom radiation portals often include the apex of at least one lung and a paramediastinal strip, as well as often a portion of the lung underlying the anterior chest wall. Segments of the apexes and the paramediastinal area are also often irradiated in patients with malignant lymphoma and, in particular, those with Hodgkin's disease. Patients with carcinoma of the esophagus and with mediastinal tumors, such as thymoma or germinoma, sometimes receive high doses to the adjacent lung. Occasionally, an injudicious treatment plan results in the delivery of a high dose to almost the entire lung. Patients with metastatic lesions to the lung are more likely to be exposed to irradiation of the whole lung for palliative or curative purposes than are patients with primary carcinoma of the lungs. They are also more likely to develop pneumonitis of the whole lung and to die from radiation pneumonitis.

Although the frequency of radiation pneumonitis has been categorized according to underlying disease entities, it is not reasonable to expect a specific incidence in any malignancy. The occurrence of radiation pneumonitis depends on the radiation dose delivered and on the volume of lung irradiated, as well as on the presence or absence of modifying influences. Although incidence rates in different reports of patients with carcinoma of the breast have ranged from a few percent to more than 70 percent, radiation pneumonitis is an avoidable complication of radiotherapy for carcinoma of the breast and symptomatic disease should occur in only a few percent of patients. In contrast, patients with malignant lymphomas and mediastinal primary disease, including carcinomas of the esophagus, require inclusion of a modest portion of the lung in the high-dose volume so that some degree of pneumonitis will occur in all patients. Even in this group, symptomatic pneumonitis is an avoidable complication. Patients who have bronchogenic carcinoma require that irradiation include portions of lung immediately surrounding the area involved by tumor. In these patients, pneumonitis is unavoidable and, in many instances, moderately symptomatic.

Fatal radiation pneumonitis is a complication either of injudicious, large-volume irradiation in the treatment of nonpulmonary disease, i.e., carcinoma of the esophagus, or of attempts at treating the whole lung, hemibody, or whole body for metastatic lesions. This entity should become rare now that information concerning the tolerance of the lung, and its modification by chemical agents, has made it possible to predict safe doses of irradiation.

Considerable variability exists in the appearance of changes on the chest radiograph, the occurrence of symptoms, and the incidence of death due to pneumonitis. In patients with Hodgkin's disease, radiologic evidence of pneumonitis occurs in as many as 65 percent of patients; in contrast, clinically evident pneumonitis occurs in only about 6 percent of patients, and the mortality rate is exceedingly low, i.e., 0.25 percent. The incidence of symptomatic pneumonitis is increased by retreatment or by whole lung irradiation, which can result in a 33 percent incidence and a 6 percent fatality rate.

The differential diagnosis of radiation pneumonitis is sometimes difficult. Accurate knowledge of the patient's prior treatment with radiotherapy can be of great help. It is particularly important to know the exact volume of lung that has been irradiated, to review the portal films, and to take into account the number of fractions as well as the overall time in which the radiation dose was delivered. Difficulty is likely to be encountered in the differential diagnosis when underlying changes due to the malignancy are present and when severe immunosuppression by whole body irradiation, or by systemic chemotherapy, has made the patient susceptible to secondary pulmonary infections with organisms such as *Pneumocystis carinii.* Other viral or bacterial pneumonias can also be confused with radiation pneumonitis, but, in general, they are associated with greater production of sputum that contains identifiable organisms. It is often necessary to obtain a sample by bronchoscopy or biopsy to determine if *P. carinii* or cytomegalovirus infection is present.

The etiology of pulmonary reactions in patients receiving bone marrow transplantation, the so-called white-lung syndrome, has been particularly difficult to ascertain. These patients receive a whole lung dose (usually 800 to 1000 cGy) that can cause radiation pneumonitis. In addition, they received a number of cytotoxic chemotherapeutic agents which intensify pneumonitis. Finally, they are often candidates for a graft-versus-host reaction that can add to the radiation damage. With the exception of this type of patient and the severely immunosuppressed patient, the differential diagnosis is usually made rather easily when the details of radiation are known.

RADIOBIOLOGIC AND CELLULAR KINETIC PRINCIPLES

Ionizing radiation causes tissue damage primarily by causing mitotic death in cells capable of proliferation. These dividing cells are either actively engaged in the cell cycle or are recruited into the cell cycle in response to radiation injury. Cells which are postmitotic, and cannot revert into cycle, usually do not show immediate radiation injury, but may die secondarily because of injury to other cells that are still engaged in proliferation. Radiation exposure also leads to intermitotic death in certain classes of lymphocytes.

Radiation injury occurs at doses which cause breaks in the DNA and in the chromosomes. Breaks may be single- or double-stranded; a very efficient mechanism exists for repair of single-stranded breaks. A lethal event is, in all likelihood, a double-stranded DNA break, which also is associated with a chromosome break that is either not repaired or else is repaired in an abnormal manner, leading to chromosomal aberrations. Damage to the chromatin leads to the loss of essential genetic information at the time of the next mitosis. It is highly likely that pieces of chromosome no longer attached to the centromere are lost to one daughter cell, or that material will be improp-

erly segregated. Although sufficient material coded by these segments of chromosome may be present in the cell for several cell divisions, ultimately cell division ceases and the cells become mitotically dead. Death does not necessarily occur at the first mitosis. Indeed, it may result after two, three, or more mitoses.

From this consideration of radiation injury and mitotic death, it is evident that cellular radiation injury, which results in histologic and, therefore, clinically evident radiation damage, will not be immediately apparent in cells which will undergo mitotic death. Although suppression of lymphocyte counts occurs within hours of radiation exposure, injury to other tissues is not evident until sufficient time for mitotic death ensues. In rapid renewal systems, such as the bone marrow or intestinal epithelium, the effects of injury are usually seen within a few days. This time extends to a few weeks in the reaction of skin and mucous membrane and is longer in most critical organs in which cell turnover is slower.

With the exception of lymphocytes, there do not appear to be any large cell populations within the lung which undergo immediate or intermitotic death. Most of the lung cells must undergo mitotic death. Therefore, the expression of injury in the lung is a function of the turnover rates of the cells that make up the lung, although initial edema, enzymatic changes, and flow alternatives can occur before cell death. Type I pneumocytes, which form the thin lining surface of the alveoli, appear to be fixed, postmitotic cells, although under some circumstances they may be capable of cell division. Their response to radiation injury can be explained by their replacement by the type II, or granular, pneumocytes. The type II cells are believed to be stem cells of the alveolar epithelium and are the principal source of pulmonary surfactant. Their turnover time has been determined to be 28 to 35 days in young mice. Although they normally divide at a rate needed to replace the cell population in the epithelium, they are capable of more rapid proliferation in response to injury, and they may be able to replace populations of both type II and type I cells.

The endothelial cells are slowly replaced through cell proliferation. In young mice, the doubling time of capillary endothelial cells in the lung has been estimated to be approximately 8 weeks. A reduction in this doubling time to approximately 4 weeks occurs after injury and in regenerating lung.

Alveolar macrophages have a short renewal time of approximately 1 week, but since they are capable of migrating into the lung from the pulmonary circulation, it is not clear whether this turnover time is due to actual proliferation time or time of ingress.

The cells of the bronchial epithelium appear to have a relatively short turnover time, between 1 and 3 weeks. These cells probably are capable of reducing this turnover time in response to injury.

Mitotic death leads to appreciable changes in pulmonary structure and function. Of primary importance are the changes in the alveolar walls. As indicated above, alveolar epithelial and endothelial cells appear to have turnover times ranging from 1 to 2 months. Thus, radiation injury that limits, or prevents, repopulation of the alveoli by these cells should be evidenced 2 to 4 months following radiotherapy because the cells go through one or more cell divisions in the normal renewal process. Accumulated injury speeds up the renewal process and leads to more rapid passage through mitosis and to mitotic death. The death of some critical cells increases the rate of proliferation of others; the result is a crescendo effect that produces a symptomatic pneumonitis.

The acute phase of radiation pneumonitis is associated with cellular depletion and mitotic death, as discussed above. The injury promotes the proliferation of cells within the irradiated area as well as the inward migration of cells that have multiple capabilities for enhancing healing and scar formation or for inducing regeneration of epithelium or capillary endothelium. Secondary bacterial or viral infections may stimulate another round of reparative attempts. Thus, the initial injury produced by radiation leads to delayed manifestations of cell death and of depletion of a critical cell population; secondary waves of repair and further injury subsequently give rise to chronic radiation fibrosis.

HISTOPATHOLOGIC CHANGES IN HUMAN AND EXPERIMENTAL ANIMAL LUNGS

The investigation of radiation pneumonitis in human beings has been hampered by the fact that most cases come to clinicopathologic investigation only in the last stages. Moreover, interpretation is often complicated by ancillary therapeutic measures, such as antibiotic and O_2 therapy, and by terminal infectious processes. Comparison of results from different institutions is also hampered by differences in time and dosage of radiation.

It has proved expedient to divide the histologic changes into three phases: the immediate phase, occurring 1 to 2 months following radiotherapy (Fig. 51-1); the intermediate phase, at 2 to 9 months; and the late phase, later than 9 months after irradiation. Although the histologic changes can be separated into these different time periods, in reality a continuum exists between the development of a lesion and its repair. Although a latent period occurs between the irradiation and the appearance of cellular injury, once this injury becomes manifest, the process of development and modification continues either until fibrosis occurs and stabilizes, or until the lesion resolves. The acute phase is characterized by vascular damage, congestion and edema, and cellular infiltration; in the subacute or intermediate phase, alveolar walls are infiltrated with cells and fibroblasts; the chronic phase is characterized by alveolar fibrosis and capillary sclerosis.

The consecutive stages of radiation injury to human lung during the first 6 months can be summarized in a morphologic timetable that consists of three phases: exudative, pneumonitic, and reparative. The exudative phase is usually seen during the first 30 days following radiotherapy. Endothelial and epithelial cell damage is associated with alveolar proteinosis and in some patients with hyaline membranes. In the pneumonitic phase, which occurs 1 to 3 months after radiotherapy, the type II cells are increased in number. These cells, as well as the pulmonary macrophages, fill the air sacs. This phase of injury resembles the alveolar damage that is associated with the usage of high levels of inspired O_2, as is often administered to patients dying of radiation pneumonitis. The reparative phase is characterized, except for special situations such as concurrent infections, by evidence of repair and reconstruction of the alveolar walls.

Experiments in animals have clarified the various phases of radiation pleuropneumonitis and its resolution, repair, or fixation. Examples of the histologic changes are shown in Figs. 51-2 and 51-3. In both figures, tissues were sampled from 3-month-old Sprague-Dawley rats that were raised and maintained in a specific pathogen-free colony, free of pulmonary infection. Four months after irradiation (Fig. 51-2B), the irradiated lung shows vascular congestion and occlusion, interstitial infiltration, and alveolar volume reduction. Six months following irradiation (Fig. 51-2C), the congestion and obliteration of capillaries is marked, and the reduction in alveolar volume is more marked. The number of type II pneumocytes is increased. At 12 months following irradiation (Fig. 51-2D), the volume of the alveoli is markedly reduced; many are completely obliterated, and their septa are markedly thickened by collagen and basement membrane material. The number of epithelial cells does not appear to be increased; some atypical type I and type II cells remain.

Electron micrographs show the process occurring in the subacute and chronic periods in greater detail (Fig. 51-3). Capillary injury with formation of blebs, as well as pericapillary edema, is seen 8 weeks after irradiation, i.e., when acute and subacute periods merge (Fig. 51-3B). Twenty weeks after irradiation (Fig. 51-3C), the changes are extensive and include the presence of atypical type II cells, damaged and regenerating capillaries, mast cell granular infiltrates, and collagen replacement. Fibroblasts and interstitial cells and their processes are also evident, as well as cellular debris, cellular processes, and lamellar bodies from type II pneumocytes. In other sections can be seen regenerating capillary epithelium, collagen, mast cell granules, and segments of interstitial fibroblasts (Fig. 51-3D). Twelve months following irradiation (Fig. 51-3F), some of the alveolar septa contain capillaries that are located within a thickened basement membrane containing

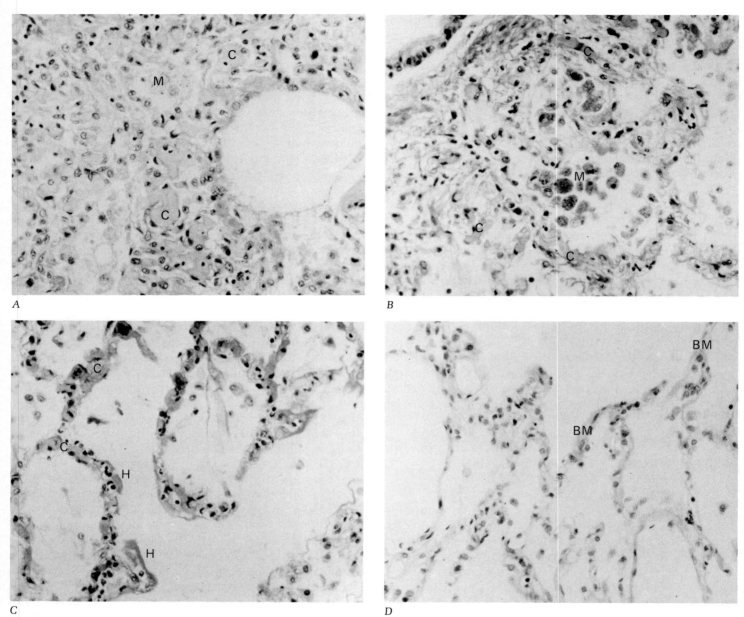

FIGURE 51-1 Histologic changes associated with acute radiation pneumonitis. *A.* Severe fatal pneumonitis in an autopsy specimen from a child who was treated for Wilms's tumor metastatic to the lung. Whole lung irradiation was used; severe dyspnea, cyanosis, and death followed the third course of actinomycin; patient was unresponsive to steroids. The specimen was obtained 4 months after administering 2150 cGy in 20 fractions. The alveoli are replaced by consolidation consisting of large alveolar macrophages (M) and a mononuclear cellular infiltrate. Many capillaries (C) are massively engorged and thrombosed. *B.* Autopsy specimen from a patient who died 2½ months after 2400 cGy in 18 fractions; actinomycin D was also administered. Large collections of large macrophages (M) in alveoli; atypical epithelial cells; septal thickening; engorged, thrombotic, and obstructed capillaries (C). Membranes line portions of alveoli, possibly secondary to autolysis. *C.* Another area of lung from patient in *B.* Thickening of alveolar walls is prominent. Basement, or hyaline, membranes (H) have been deposited in many alveolar septa. *D.* Surgical biopsy specimen from a patient 5 months after 3500 cGy in 37 fractions. The patient had experienced a bout of acute pneumonitis, which resolved completely on steroids, 6 weeks before. Some alveoli are normal in size and contain no cellular infiltrates. In others, septa show increase in thickening of basement membranes (BM) and in the number of cells in the interstitial space. ×74.

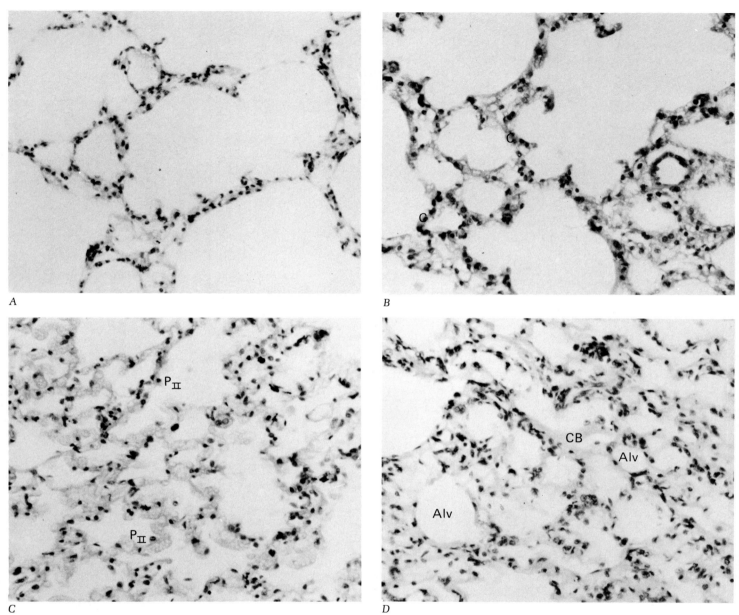

FIGURE 51-2 Histologic changes in rat lung (SPF Sprague-Dawley) irradiated at 3 months of age. *A.* Control unirradiated lung from a 5-month-old rat. *B.* Irradiated rat lung 4 months after 2000 cGy in one fraction to the left hemithorax. The capillaries (C) are engorged. Cellular infiltrates are prominent; lacking are inflammatory cells or macrophage collections. ×74. *C.* Rat lung 6 months after irradiation with 2000 cGy. Alveolar volume is decreased; capillaries are engorged and obstructed. The number of atypical type II pneumocytes (P_{II}) in the epithelium is increased. ×74. *D.* Rat lung 12 months after 2000 cGy. The reaction has now progressed to fibrosis. Many alveoli have been obliterated, and many of the residual alveoli (Alv) are small. The septa are markedly thickened by collagen and deposits of basement membrane material (CB). The number of epithelial cells is not increased, but some atypical type I and type II cells remain; interstitial infiltrates persist. ×74.

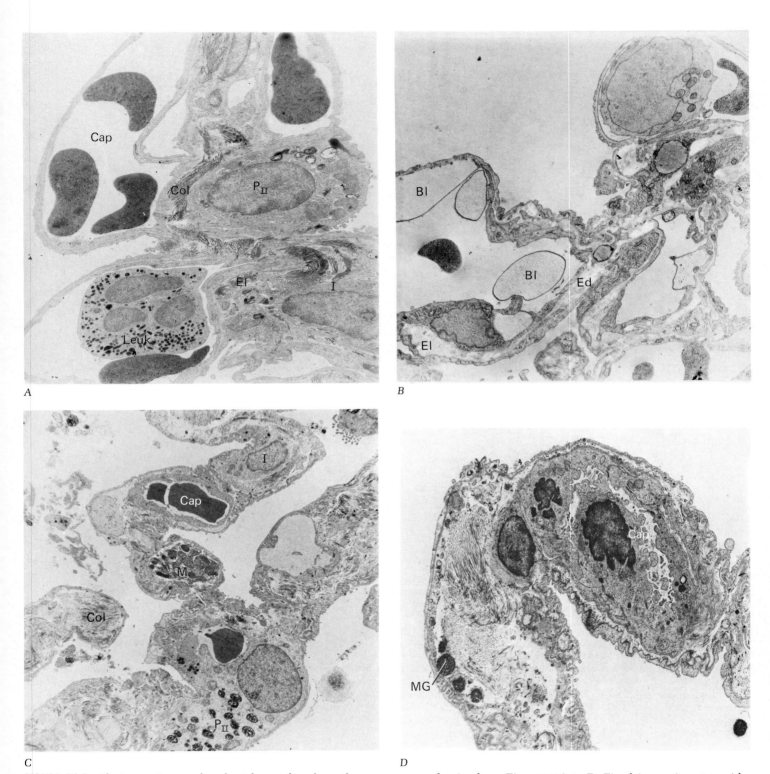

FIGURE 51-3 Electron micrographs of rat lung taken from the same group of animals as Figs. 51-2A to D. Fixed in osmium tetroxide, embedded in araldite. *A.* Control unirradiated lung. The capillary lumen (Cap) contains red cells and a polymorphonuclear leukocyte (Leuk). Collagen (Col), elastic fibers (El), an interstitial cell (I), and a type II pneumocyte (P_{II}) are also present. ×4950. *B.* Alveolar septum 8 weeks after 2000 cGy. The endothelium is abnormal and contains blebs (Bl). The pericapillary space is edematous (Ed). ×4950. *C.* Several alveolar septa 20 weeks after 2000 cGy. A new capillary (Cap), mast cell (M), type II pneumocyte within the septum (P_{II}), collagen (Col), and hyperplastic interstitial cell (I). ×2475. *D.* Alveolar septum partly replaced by collagen and mast cell granules (MG) and by an abnormal capillary (Cap), 6 months after irradiation. ×5050.

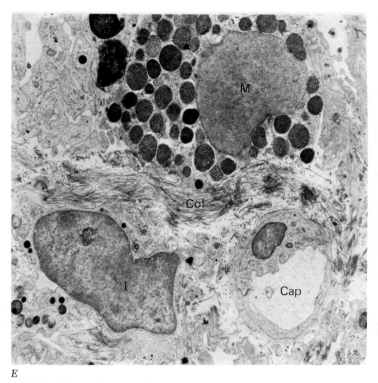

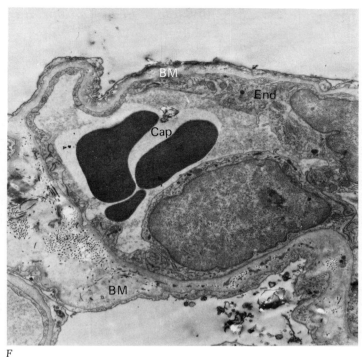

E

F

FIGURE 51-3 (continued) *E.* Portion of an alveolar septum showing regenerating capillary (Cap), mast cell (M), and interstitial cell (I) in close proximity to collagen production (Col), 6 months postirradiation. ×742. *F.* Alveolar septum 12 months after 2000 cGy. The capillary (Cap) is patent, but the endothelium (End) and the basement membranes (BM) are markedly thickened. ×4950.

collagen fibers, elastin, reticulin, and hypertrophied endothelium.

In summary, several cellular systems are involved in the accumulation and repair of radiation injury. The renewal rate of the type II pneumocytes and of the endothelium is relatively similar. Therefore, a delayed but concurrent appearance of injury is expected in both systems.

The response to injury in the first month after exposure is characterized by an increase in vascular permeability, with edema, and release of type II cell granules followed by scattered evidence of capillary blebbing and vacuolization. The number of type II pneumocytes decreases. The acute phase is followed by the subacute phase in which more advanced reaction and cell loss occur in the capillaries and type II cell injury is repaired. It is characterized by the infiltration of the alveolar spaces with mast cells, at least in the rat, and the accumulation of atypical type II pneumocytes, primarily along the alveolar lining; in the later phases of the subacute period, type II pneumocytes also accumulate in the interstitial spaces, in association with macrophages at higher doses. Collagen accumulates in the former vascular spaces. As this at-

tempt at repair proceeds toward the chronic period, the mast cells and fibroblastic infiltrates regress, and the alveolar septa are replaced by collagen and capillaries with thickened, hyalinized walls. The alveolar linings consist of both type II and type I pneumocytes. The end result is a marked reduction in capabilities of the affected alveoli to participate effectively in gas exchange.

PATHOPHYSIOLOGY OF RADIATION INJURY

Extensive work in the past 10 years using experimental animals including rats, mice, and rabbits has improved knowledge of the physiological and biochemical changes which precede and accompany the histologic and clinical patterns seen in radiation pneumonopathy. Alterations in the function of the type II pneumocytes, alveolar macrophages, endothelium, fibroblasts, and basement membrane have been quantitated and associated with radiation dose and time after exposure. The changes and the time of occurrence, as well as the dose required, are summarized in Table 51-1.

TABLE 51-1
Experimental Pathophysiology of Radiation Fibrosis

Cell Type	End Point	Change	Timing	Change	Timing	Dose, Gy
Type II	Surfactant in cells	Decreased	1–7 days	Increased	10–18 weeks	12–15
	Surfactant in alveoli	Increased	1–28 days	Normal	10–18 weeks	12–15
Alveolar macrophages	Number in alveoli	Decreased	1–3 weeks	Increased	2–6 months	10–30
	Phagocytic activity	Normal	All times			
	PLA	No data		Decreased	2–6 months	15–25
Endothelium	Permeability to proteins	Increased	1–24 hours	Increased	5–45 weeks	10–30
	Perfusion	Increased	1–15 days	Decreased 2.7% per Gy	30–150 days	10–30
	Angiotensin converting enzyme (ACE)	Unchanged	1–20 days	Decreased 4.2% per Gy	1–6 months	10–30
	Prostacyclin (PGI$_2$)	Decreased	1–15 days	Increased	1–6 months	10–25
	Plasminogen activator (PLA)	Unchanged	1–15 days	Decreased	1–6 months	10–30
Fibroblast	Collagen (HP)	Unchanged	1–15 days	Increased 2% per Gy	2–6 months	10–30
	Type I collagen (immunohistochemical)	No data		Dose-dependent increase	1 year	0–10
	Cell number	Unchanged	1–15 days	Increased	90–150 days	10–30
All (basal membranes)	Basal lamina GAG	Decreased	1 h–4 weeks	Normal to decreased	12 weeks	5–13
	Heparan sulfate GAG	Unchanged	1 h–1 week	Increased	4–12 weeks	5–13

NOTE: PLA = plasminogen activator; ACE = angiotensin converting enzyme; HP = hydroxyproline; GAG = glycosaminoglycans.

Type II pneumocytes play an important role in the early changes after irradiation. Release of surfactant with a decrease in the number of granules and an associated increase in alveolar surfactant occurs immediately at single doses above 12 Gy and increases up to 28 days. The levels in cells then increase and in the alveoli decrease back to normal by 18 weeks. In vitro experiments with cultured type II cells have shown that a large release of surfactant occurs at doses above 10 Gy without cell death. It is not clear that this release begins or potentiates the radiation injury to other cell types or is important in the final lesion, since the number of type II cells and the granule content is normal or elevated at the time of pneumonitis and fibrosis development.

Alveolar macrophages decrease in number for 1 to 3 weeks after irradiation, return to normal at 4 weeks, and then increase in number from 2 to 6 months related to doses between 10 and 30 Gy. Their phagocytic activity remains normal, even though the total number and thus total activity is reduced. Plasminogen activator activity (PLA) at 2 months after irradiation is reduced in macrophages at 25 Gy but not at 15 Gy. At 6 months it is reduced at both 15 and 25 Gy.

The endothelium is probably the most important site of injury by radiation histologically, and this is also true for physiological changes. Permeability to plasma proteins and fibrinogen is increased almost immediately after irradiation, and this leakiness persists up to 30 weeks after exposure to doses between 10 and 30 Gy. The accumulation of protein and fibrin in the alveoli probably contributes to the injury.

Perfusion measurements using labeled albumin microspheres show an initial increase up to 15 days and then a steady decrease with time to as low as 20 percent of control at 6 months with doses of 30 Gy. There is a clear dose-response relationship, the fractional perfusion decreasing 2.7 percent per gray.

Angiotensin converting enzyme (ACE), an index of endothelial function, decreases after 1 month, and the level is related to radiation dose with a decline of 4.2 percent per gray between 10 and 30 Gy. Prostacyclin (PGI$_2$) levels follow an opposite course. After an initial decrease to about 40 percent of normal, the prostacyclin level increases to as much as 10 times normal at 6 months, in inverse relation to perfusion. Thus the reduction which occurs in the number of endothelial cells is associated with decreased ACE and stimulation of PGI$_2$ release.

Plasminogen activator activity (PLA) associated with the endothelium is reduced beginning 1 month after irradiation and falls until 6 months. The level is related to dose over the range from 10 to 30 Gy at which it is <50 percent of normal.

Fibroblasts are a prominent component of the histologic picture and increase in number from 90 to 150 days.

The alveolar walls become hyalinized and the associated fibroblasts are normal, i.e., they do not have contractile or myofibroblast attributes. Associated collagen production as measured by hydroxyproline content of the lung increases from 2 to 6 months after exposure. The increase is about double at 6 months what it is at 2 months. The level is dose-related and increases at 2 percent per gray. Recently a quantitative scanning technique to measure type I collagen immunohistochemically has been developed. At 1 year after irradiation there is a dose-dependent increase in the amount at doses between 0 and 10 Gy.

Basal lamina glycosaminoglycans are also altered by irradiation. There is a decrease in the number of anionic sites 1 h to 4 weeks after exposure, with a return toward normal in 12 weeks. The heparan sulfate component is actually increased from 4 to 12 weeks after the irradiation.

It appears that the major physiological injury is to the endothelium and its function as well as to the basal laminae. Effects on type II cells are important but do not correlate with the time at which perfusion decreases. Surfactant may modify the level of injury or the time of its appearance, however.

CHANGES IN PULMONARY FUNCTION

Numerous evaluations of pulmonary function following irradiation have been conducted in human beings and in experimental animals. Bronchial function following radiotherapy has not been well studied. The turnover rate of the bronchial epithelium is rather short, and it is likely that bronchial irritation or denudation occurs following radiotherapy to the mediastinal region. This injury may lead to some asthmatic reactions, not only characterized by cough but also increased by sensitivity of the airway receptors and to airway spasm. Little is known concerning activity of the airways during the early period after radiotherapy has been initiated in humans.

The acute phase of radiation pneumonitis, i.e., from the time of radiotherapy until 2 months later, shows little change in pulmonary function until clinical symptoms appear. In patients receiving postoperative irradiation for carcinoma of the breast, Prato et al. (1977) performed repeated measurements of regional and total pulmonary blood flow and ventilation. Changes began about 25 days after the start of radiotherapy and reached a maximum about 150 days after the start of treatment. Of the static lung volumes, only the forced vital capacity and the expiratory reserve volume became abnormal after regional irradiation for carcinoma of the breast. All indexes of regional lung function assessed by radioisotopes 60 days or more after the start of treatment were abnormal. The indexes included ventilation per unit volume, blood flow to the ventilated alveoli, and blood flow per unit ventilated

lung volume. The greatest regional abnormality was in blood flow to ventilated alveoli. At 232 days after the beginning of irradiation, blood flow to ventilated alveoli and regional total lung function were still depressed. Blood flow in the irradiated area generally reached its nadir between 100 and 150 days after the start of radiation treatment. As discussed above, experimental studies in the rat have shown a similar time course.

As the volume of lung irradiated increases, the effects of irradiation become more generalized: decreases occur in vital capacity, inspiratory capacity, total lung capacity, residual volume, and the FEV_1.

In addition to changes in flow and in ventilation, changes occur in diffusing capacity. Gas exchange is impaired by 4 to 11 weeks after irradiation and remains depressed for 6 to 18 months. If the volume of lung that is irradiated is large enough, mild arterial hypoxemia ensues, and the alveolar-arterial difference in P_{O_2} widens. Both abnormalities tend to reverse within 6 to 18 months. As expected from diffuse pulmonary processes that stiffen the lungs, the arterial P_{CO_2} tends to fall.

The compliance of the lungs tends to decrease after irradiation, the larger doses resulting in marked reductions. The compliance of the chest wall is much less affected than the compliance of the lungs. The compliance begins to fall in humans at the time of acute pneumonitis and persists through the subacute and chronic fibrotic periods. These decreases in compliance and the increase in the work of breathing set the distinctive pattern of restrictive lung disease, i.e., rapid frequency, small tidal volumes, and net increases in minute ventilation. Workload stimulation accentuates the increases in minute ventilation.

Whether changes in the chest radiograph will precede changes in pulmonary function tests depends on the tests that are used and the extent of the irradiation injury. Diffuse injury to large areas of lung may be apparent by sensitive function test, e.g., closing volumes, before the chest radiograph becomes abnormal. The same is true of regional tests of blood flow using radioisotopes. On the other hand, local injury to the lung is not apt to cause serious derangement in conventional pulmonary function tests, e.g., diffusing capacity, unless severe. In time, diffuse injury evokes the pattern of restrictive lung disease: reduced lung volumes, low diffusing capacity, and hyperventilation, at rest and during exercise.

In summary, changes resulting from extensive acute and subacute radiation pneumonitis are reflected in tests of pulmonary ventilation, pulmonary blood flow, and alveolar-capillary gas exchange. For limited regional damage, which conventional tests are not designed to detect, radioisotopic determination of regional ventilation and blood flow is more sensitive. The results of these tests are useful in tracing the course of radiation pneumonitis and in predicting its outcome.

THE CLINICAL SYNDROME AND RADIOGRAPHIC FINDINGS

The clinical syndrome related to radiation injury of the lung depends on the amount of the lung that is irradiated and the doses delivered. In general, the irradiation of small volumes, the irradiation of volumes in the apical regions, and the use of fractionated doses below 2000 cGy will not result in symptomatic radiation pneumonitis. If the volume is somewhat larger, or if doses are in the range sufficient to cause acute pneumonitis, the first evidence may appear either radiographically or clinically or may be detected by a sensitive pulmonary function test of ventilation and perfusion.

Symptoms of radiation pneumonitis are absent during the first 1 to 2 months after radiotherapy is completed. Occasional patients develop signs of bronchial irritation during or immediately after radiotherapy, but usually a mild cough appears 6 weeks to 3 months following irradiation. This cough may be productive of a small amount of whitish to pinkish sputum. If larger volumes have been irradiated, cough is apt to be marked and to be associated with dyspnea, tachypnea, and a fever ranging from 30 to 40°C. Pneumonitis following whole lung irradiation usually evokes severe dyspnea, cyanosis, fever of about 40°C, and marked tachypnea.

If the irradiation has encompassed the whole lung or most of both lungs, these symptoms either progress to severe dyspnea and death or gradually subside. If the symptoms are reversible, they usually subside within a few days of supportive treatment and corticosteroids. Resolution is sometimes dramatic after corticosteroid treatment, so that an extremely ill patient becomes essentially asymptomatic within 24 h. Failure of the symptoms to subside during this interval carries the prospect of rapid progression to death.

Patients with normal baseline pulmonary function in whom the amount of irradiated lung is equivalent to less than one lung, and in whom the reaction to irradiation progresses, experience a gradual relief of symptoms as the acute exudative phase is succeeded by the subacute and chronic fibrotic phase. Cough, dyspnea, and tachypnea diminish.

Physical signs on chest examination are minimal, except in patients with severe reaction or whole lung pneumonitis who manifest evidence of consolidation. A pleural friction rub or evidence of small pleural effusion occasionally accompanies evidence of acute pneumonitis. The degree of respiratory discomfort is variable; after whole lung irradiation and radiation pneumonitis of both lungs, an adult respiratory distress syndrome may develop.

A mild leukocytosis and an increase in the erythrocyte sedimentation rate commonly accompany the abnormalities in pulmonary function tests. When the irradiated area is extensive, i.e., in cases where the volume irradiated has included one whole lung or is bilateral, arterial hypoxemia may occur.

Radiographic changes, as well as symptoms, of radiation pleuropneumonitis generally appear 1 to 3 months following treatment. The affected areas appear diffuse or hazy, and pulmonary markings are indistinct. The subsequent course, culminating in fibrosis and contraction, is shown in Fig. 51-4.

In Fig. 51-5 is shown the evolution of radiation pneumonitis in a patient treated postoperatively for carcinoma of the breast. Although the appearance is that of a generalized infiltration, in other patients the pattern is often nodular or alveolar, and an air bronchogram may be present.

The changes induced by irradiation are demarcated by a fairly sharp edge and are limited to the margins of the portal of irradiation. In some patients, pleural or pericardial effusion accompanies the pulmonary infiltrate. Adenopathy does not occur; nor should cavitation be seen unless necrosis occurs with a tumor in the irradiated portion of lung. These early changes of acute pneumonitis progress to a chronic and usually irreversible fibrosis. Shrinkage sometimes continues for more than 1 year following irradiation.

When the volume of lung included in the radiation portal is large and the dose is high, i.e., well above the threshold for development of radiation pneumonitis, the changes are severe but still restricted to the limits of the radiation volume. The patient depicted in Fig. 51-6 was treated for mediastinal germinoma with the very large portal shown in the portal film (Fig. 51-6A). Six months later (Fig. 51-6B) radiation fibrosis was evident in a configuration that corresponded to that of the radiation portal; functioning pulmonary volume was confined primarily to the left lung and to the right mid-lung region. Pleural effusion accompanied the pneumonitis on the right side. This patient was severely dyspneic, arterial hypoxemia was pronounced, and both the vital capacity and FEV_1 were low. This patient also demonstrated a severe reduction in perfusion (Fig. 51-6C).

Whole lung irradiation combined with a high dose to a small volume, such as the mediastinum and hilus, can cause generalized acute pneumonitis (Fig. 51-7). However, the area that is subjected to low-dose irradiation will clear completely, whereas the smaller area that receives a higher dose will undergo fibrosis.

Computed tomography (CT) scans of irradiated lung can show the extent of change more accurately than can plain chest films. In particular, they allow a three-dimensional view and estimate of the volume of lung involved. The changes consist of relatively dense consolidation confined to the field of radiation. The density is usually similar to tumor, and thus CT cannot separate fibrosis from tumor recurrence (Fig. 51-8).

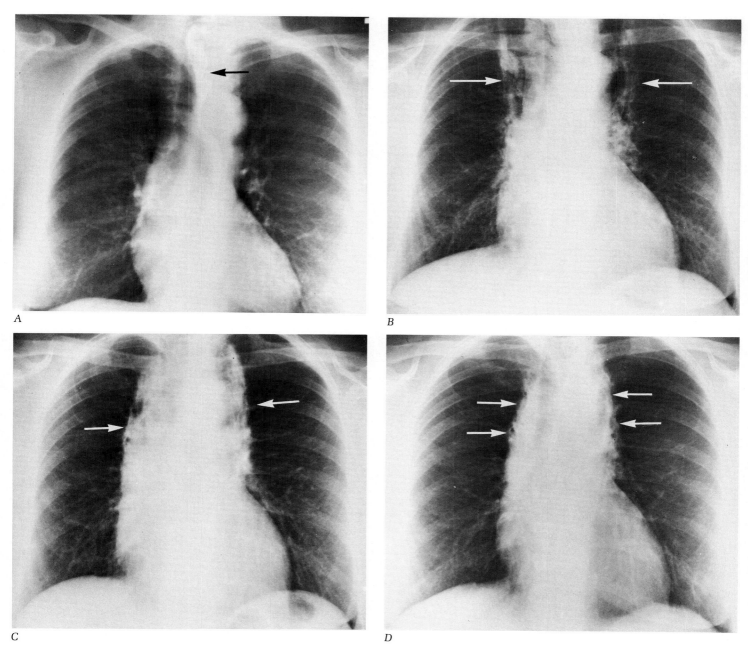

FIGURE 51-4 Development of asymptomatic pneumonitis and fibrosis in a 68-year-old female with carcinoma of the upper esophagus at the thoracic inlet. *A.* Chest and tumor (arrow) prior to radiotherapy. *B.* Onset of acute radiation pneumonitis changes in the paramediastinal areas (arrows) 3 months after 6000 cGy in 35 fractions. *C.* Radiation fibrosis (arrows) evident at 6 months after completion of treatment. *D.* Contracted permanent fibrosis (arrows) 2 years after radiotherapy.

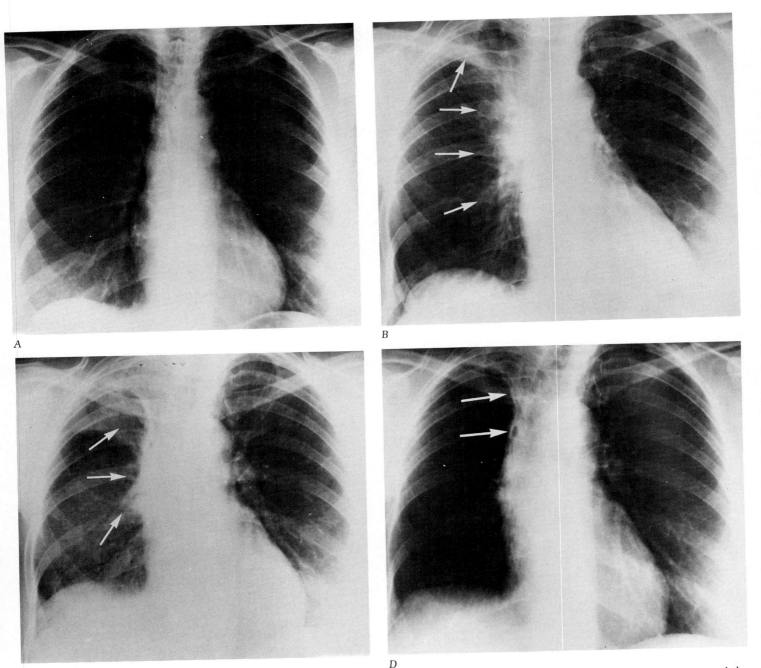

FIGURE 51-5 Woman with carcinoma of right breast given postoperative radiotherapy to the right chest wall, supraclavicular area, and the mediastinum; 3000 to 5000 cGy delivered to the lung in paramediastinal and apical areas. A. After mastectomy, but before radiotherapy. B. At the onset of cough and fever 4 months after completion of therapy. Soft infiltrates of acute radiation pneumonitis (arrows) are present. C. Three weeks later, as symptoms subsided. Early fibrosis on the right side (arrows). D. One year after radiotherapy showing residual fibrotic changes (arrows).

CT images have been used experimentally to quantitate radiation injury in animal models. An early increase in average density in Hounsfield units (HU) is associated with acute pneumonitis and a second increase with fibrosis and pleural effusion. The density is related to dose but does not occur at doses below those causing detectable functional changes and lethality.

Magnetic resonance imaging (MRI) has the potential to differentiate processes. In T1 weighted images the intensity ratio relative to muscle and to fat is lower than for tumor. It is also lower in T2 images, but the differential is less. Scans show a relatively low density infiltrate in the lung corresponding to the volume irradiated (Fig. 51-9).

Although patients receiving a dose of radiation that

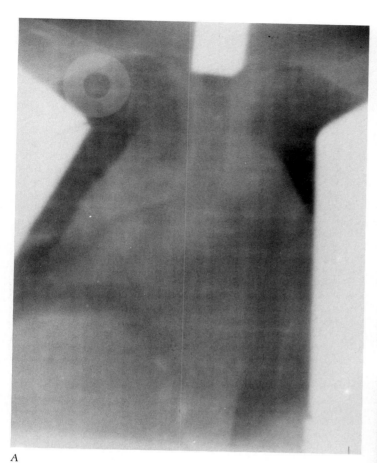

A

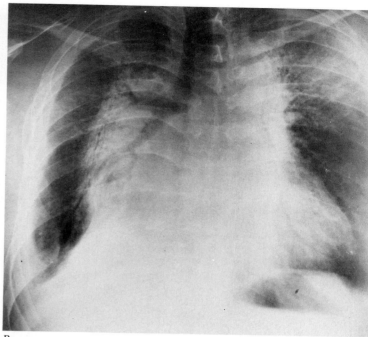

B

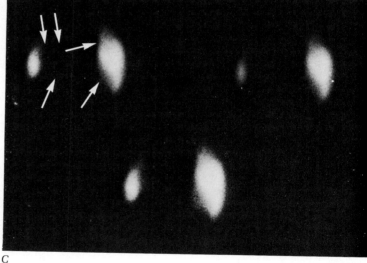

C

FIGURE 51-6 Patient treated for mediastinal germinoma in the thymic area with a large portal. *A.* Portal used to give 4000 cGy in 20 fractions. *B.* Radiation fibrosis evident with the shape of the portals 6 months after radiotherapy. Pleural effusion present. Probably persistent tumor at carina. *C.* Pulmonary scan performed with ^{99m}Tc-MAA showing decreased perfusion in most of the right lung and in the left apex, corresponding to the irradiation volume (arrows). Anterior view.

just suffices to cause radiation pneumonitis may show complete resolution of the pneumonitis, most patients show a gradual evolution of the process from the acute infiltration to a more sharply defined and dense permanent fibrosis. As fibrosis progresses, the appearance changes to that of linear streaks that radiate from the area of pneumonitis and of contraction toward either the hilus or the paramediastinal or apical regions (Fig. 51-10). After irradiation of lower lobe lesions, the diaphragm is often tented, and usually the pleura is thickened. Large losses in lung volume may cause a shift of the mediastinum toward the side of irradiation and deviation of the trachea. The fibrotic contracted upper lobe often causes hilar ele-

vation and other changes that resemble those of fibrotic pulmonary tuberculosis. The permanent changes of fibrosis take 6 to 24 months to evolve, but usually remain stable after 2 years. Cystic or bronchiectatic changes sometimes occur in large lobar, or whole lung, zones of fibrosis.

Complications of radiation pneumonitis and fibrosis include pleural effusion and occasionally spontaneous pneumothorax. Other complications usually are related to tumor response or tumor destruction, and include tracheoesophageal fistula in patients with carcinoma of the esophagus, bronchial obstruction in patients with carcinoma of the bronchus, and rib fractures in patients receiv-

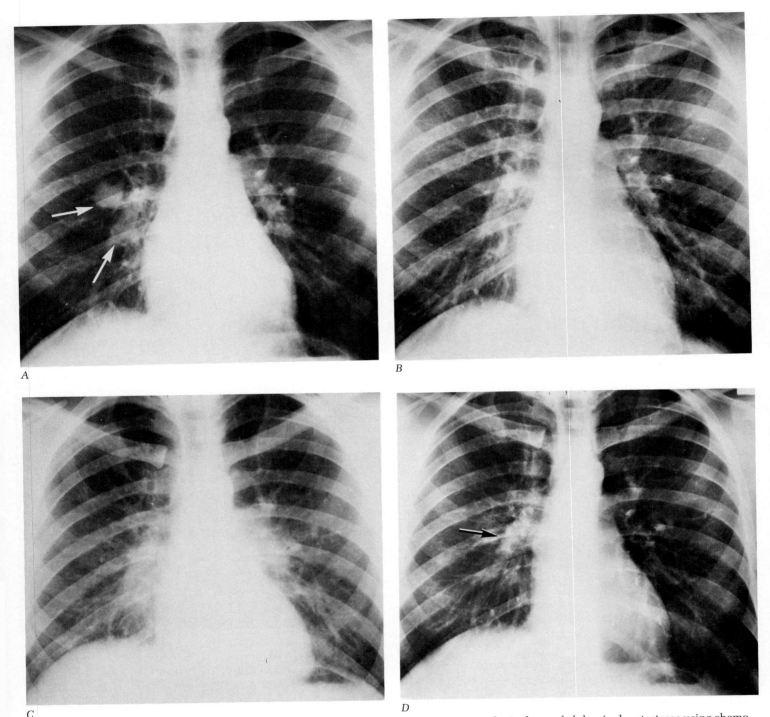

FIGURE 51-7 Patient treated for embryonal carcinoma of the testis with pulmonary, supraclavicular, and abdominal metastases using chemotherapy and radiotherapy. *A.* At onset of treatment with combination chemotherapy using cyclophosphamide, actinomycin D, vincristine, and mithramycin. Masses are present in the right hilus and middle lobe (arrows). *B.* Completion of radiotherapy 1500 cGy in 12 fractions to both entire lungs, and 4100 cGy to the mediastinum and right hilus in a total of 29 fractions. The masses have regressed. *C.* One month later, fever (40°C) and cough. Acute radiation pneumonitis involving both lung fields and right hilar area. *D.* Two weeks later on treatment with prednisone. Pneumonitis has cleared except in the right hilar area that received large doses of radiation (arrow).

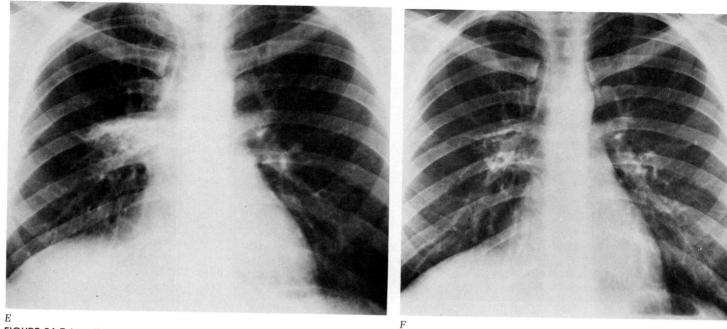

E   F

FIGURE 51-7 (continued) *E.* Six weeks later, the right hilar reaction is progressing toward fibrosis. *F.* One year later, residual, permanent asymptomatic fibrosis in the right hilar area, as well as elevation of the right diaphragm.

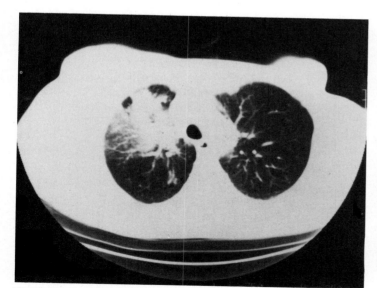

FIGURE 51-8 CT image with contrast of a patient after lung irradiation. The upper lobe on the right shows relatively dense consolidation limited to the field of irradiation.

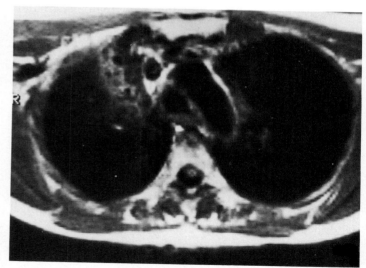

FIGURE 51-9 MRI of the same irradiated patient shown in the CT scan in Fig. 51-8. Gated scan, TE = 30 (TE = echo time). Areas of signal due to radiation pneumonitis are seen. The radiation fibrosis is relatively low in intensity compared to muscle.

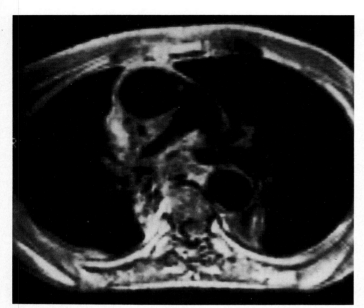

FIGURE 51-10 MRI image of patient in fibrotic phase after mediastinal irradiation. TR = 2000 (TR = repetition time), TE = 30. Contraction and distortion of the hilus are seen, and the radiation fibrosis is evident around the hilus. It is of moderate to low density.

ing high-dose chest wall irradiation. Rib fractures may also be secondary to the cough that accompanies radiation pneumonitis.

The major complications of radiation pneumonitis occur late in the disease and are secondary to persistent fibrosis of a large volume of lung. The patients are also vulnerable to unusual fungal infections and death. High-dose thoracic irradiation can also lead to acute and chronic pericarditis with secondary pericardial and pleural effusions. These secondary phenomena are distinct from the primary changes of radiation pneumonitis.

The possibility that pneumonitis may occur outside the radiation field has been extensively discussed. Nearly all instances which have prompted the discussions have proved to be attributable to secondary bacterial or fungal or viral infections or to scattering of the radiation dose. The explanation that mediastinal irradiation causes lymphatic obstruction that, in turn, produces bilateral changes beyond the limits of irradiation has been discounted; so has the possibility of an autoimmune response originating in unirradiated lung secondary to tissue destruction in the irradiated volume. In the author's experience, changes which were clinically, radiographically, and histologically consistent with radiation pneumonitis have not been observed in parts of the lung that do not lie within the radiation portal.

TIME, DOSE, VOLUME, AND OTHER MODIFYING FACTORS

In considering the clinical evidence of radiation pleuritis and pneumonitis—defined either by the presence of symptoms, the presence of functional changes, or the presence of radiographic findings—the volume that is irradiated, the radiation time, and the dose are critical elements. When small volumes of lung are irradiated, histologic and radiographic changes will occur, although the latter may be difficult to detect, unless MRI or CT studies are performed. If volumes large enough for radiographic detection are seen, at least regional changes in ventilation and perfusion will ensue. If larger volumes, equaling at least one-third to one-half the volume of one lung, are irradiated, then symptoms of cough, perhaps dyspnea, and occasionally fever, will accompany the functional and radiographic changes. Excessive whole lung irradiation can lead to severe pulmonary symptoms and/or death.

Radiation pneumonitis in small areas that are treated for nonpulmonary disease or for primary carcinomas of the lung is unavoidable because of the high dose required. When larger volumes are treated, tolerance must be predicted and injury avoided. Since there are insufficient data from patients to provide a quantitative prediction of radiation injury, a mouse model system has been devised. In this species, thoracic irradiation causes death from radiation pneumonitis between 100 and 160 days after treatment. The histologic picture and clinical syndrome is similar to that in humans. Using this technique, the following formula was derived:

$$\text{Total dose} = ED \times N^{0.38} \times t^{0.07}$$

where

$$ED = \text{equivalent single dose}$$
$$N = \text{number of fractions}$$
$$t = \text{time}$$

This equation has been used to equate the dose-time-fractionation number, for each patient who received irradiation to the whole lung at the University of California, San Francisco, for metastatic disease (with or without chemotherapy), to a single-dose equivalent in "rets." The validity of this formula has been substantiated by clinical observations on the incidence of radiation pneumonitis in patients treated with single exposures in a half-body palliative treatment technique. On the basis of this clinical evidence, this formula has been used (Table 51-2) to predict the risk of radiation pneumonitis after various total doses delivered in various numbers of fractions. In Table 51-2, the predicted risk of pneumonitis is presented as a function of the total dose and the number of fractions. The numbers in parentheses represent the risk at that dose and

TABLE 51-2
Percent Risk of Radiation Pneumonitis

Total Dose, cGy	Number of Fractions					
	5	10	15	20	25	30
1000	0 (0)	0 (0)	0 (0)	0 (0)	0 (0)	0 (0)
1250	0 (80)	0 (0)	0 (0)	0 (0)	0 (0)	0 (0)
1500	60 (100)	0 (15)	0 (0)	0 (0)	0 (0)	0 (0)
2000	100 (100)	20 (99)	0 (60)	0 (10)	0 (0)	0 (0)
2500	100 (100)	100 (100)	50 (100)	0 (95)	0 (70)	0 (15)
3000	100 (100)	100 (100)	100 (100)	85 (100)	10 (99)	1 (95)
3500	100 (100)	100 (100)	100 (100)	100 (100)	99 (100)	70 (100)
4000	100 (100)	100 (100)	100 (100)	100 (100)	100 (100)	100 (100)

NOTE: Numbers in parentheses refer to risk when actinomycin D is administered before, or during, irradiation. Based on the formula: Total dose = ED $\times$ N$^{0.38}$ $\times$ t$^{0.07}$ (see text).

number of fractions in the presence of a chemotherapeutic agent, such as actinomycin D, which potentiates effect on the lungs. Although cyclophosphamide, bleomycin, cisplatinum, and other drugs that are discussed below also potentiate, it must be borne in mind that the numbers were derived from patient information based on concomitant actinomycin D, but could reasonably be extrapolated to other drugs.

From this discussion it is clear that the time-dose relationships are extremely important in predicting radiation pneumonitis. Although total dose is important, even more important are the number of fractions into which this dose is divided and, to a smaller extent, the span of time over which the radiation is delivered. From the formula it can be seen that the exponent for number of fractions is much higher than for time. Therefore, the greater the number of daily fractions in which the radiation is delivered, the lower will be the damaging effect. Fractionation is different from dose rate, which refers to the output of the machine during radiotherapy. Dose rate certainly has an effect on lung tolerance: radiation delivered at 5 cGy/min is less damaging than at 30 cGy/min, which, in turn, is less damaging than 200 to 300 cGy/min. The lower dose rates are used in hemibody irradiation for palliation and in whole body irradiation for transplantation. In these circumstances, the tolerance of lung will be higher than stated in Table 51-2.

The tolerance dose of radiation will be modified by concomitant, prior, or subsequent chemotherapy. Actinomycin D potentiates the radiation effect, as does cisplatinum, whereas bleomycin, cyclophosphamide, vincristine, and doxorubicin hydrochloride (Adriamycin) add to radiation injury in the lung.

The extent to which underlying disease or superimposed infection during or after the time of irradiation influences the occurrence of radiation pneumonitis is unknown. Neither age nor underlying pulmonary disease has been shown to modify the radiation effects. Underlying impairment of pulmonary function will add to radiation damage and cause symptoms with smaller radiation volumes than in a patient with normal function. However, patients exposed to whole body irradiation and bone marrow transplantation for acute leukemias are more apt to develop radiation pneumonitis when the marrow is allogeneic from a well-matched donor, rather than syngeneic from an identical twin. This observation suggests that the presence of a graft-versus-host reaction augments the radiation effect to the lung.

TREATMENT

The best management of radiation pneumonitis is to avoid it whenever possible. Careful tailoring of the radiation fields so that high doses are delivered only to parts of the lung that are known, or suspected, of containing tumor will limit the areas of acute pneumonitis and late fibrosis. The use of higher energy beams or particle beams can further reduce the volume of lung that receives doses above the tolerance level (Table 51-2). Patients with poor pulmonary function (FEV$_1$ < 1.51) must be treated to more limited volumes. Even in situations that require irradiation of large volumes of lung—as with the use of a mantle field for treating Hodgkin's disease—doses above the tolerance level must be restricted to less than half of one lung if severe symptoms are to be avoided. If it is necessary to deliver whole lung irradiation, as for prophylactic treatment of patients with Hodgkin's disease in the hilus or of patients who have metastatic nodules of a radiosensitive tumor, then the absolute limits set out above must be followed in order to avoid severely symptomatic, or fatal, pneumonitis. Moreover, patients given single-dose whole body irradiation must have their total doses limited because of pulmonary tolerance. In essence, information is now available to define safe levels of whole lung irradiation and to correct these limits when chemotherapy has been given. Curative treatment to all but the most radiosensitive tumors requires doses above lung tolerance that will cause fibrosis. Volumes receiving their doses must be limited.

If acute pneumonitic symptoms do appear after irradiation of one entire lung, or both lungs, or large fractions of both lungs, three major methods of management are available: antibiotics, anticoagulants, and corticosteroids. In addition, the patient requires supportive care including, as necessary, medication for cough suppression and O_2 delivered by nasal catheter or mask. Intermittent positive pressure breathing has been tried, but neither its rationale nor its benefits are clearly established.

Although no controlled clinical trials in humans are available to prove the value of corticosteroids during irradiation or during the time of pneumonitis, corticosteroids given prophylactically generally fail to prevent pneumonitis. In mouse model systems they do increase the radiation dose for lethality by 20 percent and do delay death if given continuously. Death ensues when they are discontinued. A flare of pneumonitis is seen in humans who have received radiation doses above tolerance when corticosteroids are discontinued. Also, they are ineffective if given after fibrosis has become apparent clinically or radiographically. On the other hand, corticosteroids appear to be most effective when given at the start of the acute pneumonitis. Response rates have been reported to range from 20 to 100 percent. However, these data obscure the fact that response depends on the radiation dose. If the dose is far above the tolerance level, i.e., 5000 cGy delivered in 25 treatments compared to a tolerance level of 2500 cGy in the same number of treatments, then no amount of corticosteroids will reverse this reaction and it will progress inexorably toward fibrosis. Although the symptoms of fever and cough may be relieved somewhat, the underlying process will not be altered, and the irradiated lung will be destroyed. On the other hand, the patient who develops pneumonitis after whole lung irradiation at a dose close to tolerance can be expected to experience remarkable relief following corticosteroid treatment. A dose of 60 to 100 mg per day of prednisone often reduces the fever, decreases or eliminates cyanosis and dyspnea, and returns the chest radiograph to normal within a 24-h period. If response is not seen within the first 3 or 4 days, it is unlikely that further response will occur. Nonetheless, most experts recommend that treatment be contin-

ued over 3 to 4 weeks and that corticosteroids be tapered gradually. There is no evidence that corticosteroids can affect the subacute and chronic fibrotic phase.

Antibiotics have been tried both prophylactically and when pneumonitis develops. There is no evidence that this treatment modifies the process. Indeed, it occasionally allows the outgrowth of antibiotic-resistant organisms. Antibiotics should be reserved for patients showing positive cultures of specific organisms for which specific sensitivities can be established.

Because the basic lesion does involve occlusion and thrombosis of many small blood vessels, it was postulated that anticoagulant therapy might be of benefit. However, there is no experimental evidence to support this notion.

Experimental evidence exists that penicillamine can markedly reduce a number of changes in the lung of experimental animals induced by radiation. Treatment at nontoxic doses reduces PGI_2 production and increases ACE and PLA levels while it reduces collagen production. As yet this agent has not had large animal testing or human trials for this purpose, but it is of great interest.

On rare occasions, lobectomy or pneumonectomy is contemplated after whole lung irradiation with severe fibrosis. However, the feasibility of this undertaking will depend in large measure, on the total radiation dose that was delivered: doses above 5000 cGy will probably interfere too much with healing of the bronchial stump to allow pneumonectomy.

In summary, patients with radiation pneumonitis should simply be supported if the disease is asymptomatic even though it is radiographically manifest. A prediction of the degree of lasting deficit may be obtained by nuclear regional pulmonary ventilation and perfusion studies. Symptomatic patients in whom large areas are pneumonitic can often be made comfortable by cough suppressants and aspirin for fever. If the reaction involves a large volume of lung, symptomatic treatment is augmented by O_2 and high-dose corticosteroid therapy, e.g., prednisone 100 mg per day, tapered slowly over 3 weeks' time. Sputum cultures are obtained to rule out secondary infections, and the administration of O_2 is adjusted to keep arterial P_{O_2} within tolerable range without adding the additional insult of O_2 toxicity.

BIBLIOGRAPHY

Adamson IYR, Bowden DH, Wyatt JP: A pathway to pulmonary fibrosis: An ultrastructural study of mouse and rat following radiation to the whole body and hemithorax. Am J Pathol 58:481–498, 1970.
   The fundamentals of radiation changes at the ultrastructural level.

Bourgouin P, Cousineau G, Lemire P, Delvecchio P, Hebert G: Differentiation of radiation-induced fibrosis from recurrent pulmonary neoplasm by CT. J Can Assoc Radiol 38:23–26, 1987.
   CT permitted accurate differentiation between radiation fibrosis and recurrent tumor in all patients but two who had large pleural effusions.

Coggle, JE, Lambert BE, Moores SR: Radiation effects in the lung. Environ Health Perspect 70:261–291, 1986.

This article outlines the principles of radiobiology that can explain the time of onset, duration, and severity of the complex reactions of the lung to ionizing radiation.

Gross NJ: Pulmonary effects of radiation therapy. Ann Intern Med 86:81–92, 1977.

The cellular effects of irradiating the lungs are related to the histologic and clinical sequelae.

Gross NJ: Pulmonary effects of radiation therapy. Ann Intern Med 86:81–92, 1977.

A summary of the clinical findings and an excellent review of the problem.

Gross NJ: Experimental radiation pneumonitis. IV. Leakage of circulatory proteins onto the alveolar surface. J Lab Clin Med 95:19–31, 1980.

Evaluation of capillary and alveolar wall permeability using radiolabeled albumin.

Heiken JP, Ling D, Totty WG, Balfe DM, Emani B, Wasserman TH, Murphy WA, Glazer HS, Lee JK, Levitt RG: Radiation fibrosis: Differentiation from recurrent tumor by MR imaging. Radiology 156:721–726, 1985.

A comparison of the MRI parameters for tumor and radiation fibrosis with emphasis on the lung.

Jennings FL, Arden A: Development of radiation pneumonitis. Time and dose factors. Arch Pathol 74:351–360, 1960.

A classic experimental description of radiation pneumonopathy.

Jones PW, Al-Hillawi A, Wakefield JM, Johnson NM, Jelliffe AM: Differences in the effect of mediastinal radiotherapy on lung function and the ventilatory response to exercise. Clin Sci 67:389–396, 1984.

A prospective study of patients irradiated for Hodgkin's disease using classic pulmonary function tests.

Kaplan HS, Stewart JR: Complications of intensive megavoltage radiotherapy for Hodgkin's disease. Natl Cancer Inst Monogr 36:439–444, 1973.

An early important report on the complications of wide-field irradiation of the thorax.

Law MP: Vascular permeability and late radiation fibrosis in mouse lung. Radiat Res 103:60–76, 1985.

A study of vascular permeability and collagen content in irradiated mouse lung that establishes a relationship between protein in the alveoli and fibrosis.

Miller G, Siemann D, Scott P, Dawson D, Muldrew K, Trepanier P, McGann L: A semiquantitative probe for radiation-induced normal tissue damage at the molecular level. Radiat Res 105:76–83, 1986.

Immunochemical study using scanning of stained sections for type I collagen that shows great sensitivity.

Penney DP, Siemann DW, Rubin P, Shapiro DL, Finkelstein J, Cooper RA Jr: Morphologic changes reflecting early and late effects of irradiation of the distal lung of the mouse: A review. Scan Electron Microsc (Pt 1):413–425, 1982.

An excellent review of modern knowledge about the ultrastructural changes after irradiation of the lung is presented.

Phillips TL: An ultrastructural study of the development of radiation injury in the lung. Radiology 87:49–55, 1966.

The first detailed ultrastructural study of radiation changes in the lung presents data for rats exposed to 2000 cGy.

Phillips TL, Fu KK: Quantification of combined radiation therapy and chemotherapy effects on critical normal tissues. Cancer 37:1186–1200, 1976.

Summarizes data on the increase in radiation sensitivity seen in tissues when cytotoxic chemotherapy is given.

Prato FS, Kurdyak R, Saibil EA, Rider WD, Aspin N: Physiological and radiographic assessment during the development of pulmonary radiation fibrosis. Radiology 122:389–397, 1977.

An excellent study of patients undergoing therapeutic irradiation using radionuclide and standard function tests.

Rosenkrans WA Jr, Penney DP: Cell matrix interactions in induced lung injury. II. X-irradiation mediated changes in specific basal laminar glycosaminoglycans. Int J Radiat Oncol Biol Phys 11:1629–1637, 1985.

Demonstrates that basal laminar damage is an important component of radiation fibrosis.

Rubin P, Casarett GW: *Clinical Radiation Pathology.* Philadelphia, Saunders, 1968, pp 423–470.

This classic text reviews the entire clinical syndrome associated with radiation fibrosis.

Rubin P, Finkelstein JN, Siemann DW, Shapiro DL, Van Houtte P, Penney DP: Predictive biochemical assays for late radiation effects. Int J Radiat Oncol Biol Phys 12:469–476, 1986.
   A detailed review of this group's work on type II cells and alveolar surfactant is presented.

Travis EL, Harley RA, Fenn JO, Klubukowski CJ, Hargrove HB: Pathologic changes in the lung following single and multifraction irradiation. Int J Radiat Oncol Biol Phys 2:475–490, 1977.
   The histologic changes after radiation exposure of animals are described in great detail in this classic paper.

Tsao C, Ward WF: Plasminogen activator activity in lung and alveolar macrophages of rats exposed to graded single doses of gamma rays to the right hemithorax. Radiat Res 103:393–402, 1985.
   Reveals a linear dose-related decrease in plasminogen activator activity in lung tissue.

Tsao C, Ward W, Port C: Radiation injury in rat lung. I. Prostacyclin (PGI_2) production, arterial perfusion, and ultrastructure. Radiat Res 96:284–293, 1983.
   Pulmonary prostacyclin increases as perfusion of the irradiated lung decreases and fibrosis develops.

Van Dyk J, Hill RP: Post-irradiation lung density changes measured by computerized tomography. Int J Radiat Oncol Biol Phys 9:847–852, 1983.
   Lung density data from a patient and a series of irradiated mice are presented. Changes can be measured but occur only a short time before death.

Van Dyk J, Keane TJ, Kan S, Rider WD, Fryer C: Radiation pneumonitis following large single dose irradiation: A re-evaluation based on absolute dose to lung. Int J Radiat Oncol Biol Phys 7:461–467, 1981.
   Extensive dose-response function data on patients receiving a single radiation treatment.

Wara WM, Phillips TL, Margolis LW, Smith V: Radiation pneumonitis: A new approach to the derivation of time-dose factors. Cancer 32:547–552, 1973.
   A detailed analysis of the relationship of dose and number of exposures to the incidence of radiation injury.

Ward WF, Molteni A, Solliday NH, Jones GE: The relationship between endothelial dysfunction and collagen accumulation in irradiated rat lung. Int J Radiat Oncol Biol Phys 11:1985–1990, 1985.
   A good correlation between decreased perfusion and angiotensin converting enzyme activity is shown.

Ward WF, Molteni A, Tsao C, Solliday NH: Radiation injury in rat lung. Modification by D-penicillamine. Radiat Res 98:397–406, 1984.
   This drug appears to delay the onset of radiation-induced enzyme dysfunction.

Chapter 52

Pulmonary Disease Induced by Drugs

William J. Fulkerson, Jr. / Jon P. Gockerman

Patterns of Drug-Induced Lung Injury
  Pulmonary Vascular Disorders
  Adverse Airway Responses
  Pleural Disease
  Mediastinal Disease
  Neuromuscular Dysfunction
  Pulmonary Disease from Drug-Induced
    Systemic Lupus Erythematosus
  Hypersensitivity Syndrome
  Interstitial Pneumonitis

Clinical Problems of Commonly Used Drugs
  Methotrexate
  Bischlorethylnitrosourea (BCNU)
  Bleomycin
  Nitrofurantoin
  Amiodarone
  Combination and High-Dose Chemotherapy
  Radiation Therapy
  Pulmonary Oxygen Toxicity

Approach to the Patient

Drug-induced disease is a common problem in daily medical practice. Some adverse drug effects may be predictable pharmacologically. Overdosage, interactions with other drugs, or drug accumulation due to inadequate elimination or metabolism because of renal or hepatic disease may result in untoward or exaggerated effects. Frequently, however, drug-induced disease is difficult to explain based on the known biochemistry or pharmacology of a drug. Direct cytotoxicity of a drug or one of its metabolites may be responsible for organ injury, or a patient may experience an allergic or hypersensitivity reaction. Finally, idiosyncratic reactions may occur which can occasionally be attributed to genetically determined enzyme deficiencies. It is often difficult to define which of these general categories a drug-induced disease fits.

The lung has been increasingly recognized as a potential site of adverse drug reactions. The respiratory system is an excellent target for drug and chemical-induced injury because of its dual exposure to the circulation on the one hand and to the environment, through inspired air, on the other. The lungs are metabolically active and contain cellular systems capable of uptake, concentration, and metabolic alteration of pharmacologic agents and exogenously administered chemicals. Because of the high oxygen tension in the lung, this organ is also a potential site for damage if a drug is capable of oxygen radical production, either directly or as a by-product of metabolism. Drug-related reactions may vary with a patient's age or other co-morbid conditions.

As new and potentially toxic agents or combinations of drugs are released and recommended for clinical use for neoplastic disease, cardiac arrhythmias, rheumatic disease, and infections, the frequency and severity of drug-induced lung disease will likely increase.

PATTERNS OF DRUG-INDUCED LUNG INJURY

Pulmonary Vascular Disorders

Four types of disorders are included in this category: pulmonary edema, thromboembolic disease, pulmonary vasculitis, and pulmonary hemorrhage.

PULMONARY EDEMA

Pulmonary edema is a consequence of two basic pathogenetic mechanisms: increased permeability and hemodynamic (see Chapters 59 and 60). The pulmonary edema that results from increased permeability of the microvasculature of the lung is generally secondary to endothelial cell damage. Numerous drugs have been implicated in causing "permeability" (noncardiogenic) pulmonary edema (Table 52-1). For example, accidental or suicidal overdosage of aspirin has caused pulmonary edema in conjunction with normal cardiac function; as a rule, serum levels exceed 45 mg/dl. In animal models, salicylate toxicity has been shown to be accompanied by increased permeability of the pulmonary capillary bed. Acute, noncardiogenic pulmonary edema also occurs as a result of overdosage with narcotic agents (see Chapter 90).

Hemodynamic pulmonary edema is usually caused by left ventricular failure. Drugs that primarily affect myocardial function may acutely precipitate left ventricular failure, thereby giving rise to cardiogenic pulmonary edema (Table 52-2). For example, β-adrenergic antagonists sometimes cause heart failure by decreasing the ionotropy and chronotropy of the heart. Usually this occurs either in patients with preexisting heart disease or in individuals with other predisposing cause. α-Adrenergic agonists, such as metaraminol and phenylephrine, occasionally cause cardiogenic pulmonary edema, presumably by evoking an acute increase in left ventricular afterload. Verapamil also can depress myocardial contractility and precipitate pulmonary edema; diltiazem and nifedipine do this to a lesser degree.

TABLE 52-1
Pulmonary Edema, Noncardiogenic

Drug	Pharmacology	Comments	Therapy
Opiate derivatives or analogs (heroin, morphine, methadone, D-propoxyphene)	IV or po overdose; onset of symptoms within hours to minutes	Possibly related to histamine release, particulate material injury to capillary endothelium, or component of neurogenic pulmonary edema; frequent cause of death in addicts	O$_2$, mechanical ventilation with PEEP; physiological support
Acetylsalicylic acid	po (overdose); serum levels >45 mg/dl; onset within hours	Accidental or intentional overdose; experimental model has documented "leaky" pulmonary capillary membrane	Same as above
Chlordiazepoxide	IV overdose of tablets; onset within hours	Never reported with recommended dose or route of drug	Same as above
Ethchlorvynol	po; IV (overdose)	Overdosage only	Same as above
Colchicine	po (overdose); onset 24 h after overdose	Single case, massive overdose (150 mg)	Same as above
Protamine	IV; not clearly dose-dependent	Reports of noncardiac edema in 7 patients after coronary-artery bypass, 3 deaths	Same as above
Cytosine arabinoside	IV in patients with acute leukemia; not clearly dose-dependent but onset usually within 30 days of last dose	Autopsy and chart review indicating unexplained pulmonary edema in 33 patients who had received cytosine arabinoside; associated with gastrointestinal toxicity	Same as above
Tocolytic agents (isoxsuprine, terbutaline, ritodrine)	po, IV, probable dose- and duration-dependent	β agonists used in pre-term labor; rare event; several case reports document noncardiac etiology	Same as above
Amphotericin B (in association with leukocyte transfusion)	IV; not clearly dose-related	14 reactions in neutropenic patients concomitant with or shortly after leukocyte transfusions; possible amphotericin-induced lysis or transfused cells and secondary lung injury	Avoid combination by keeping administration separated by 12 h; physiological support
Miscellaneous Fluorescein, amitriptyline (overdose) hydrochlorothiazide, intravenous fat emulsion.		Rare but reasonably documented case reports; probable idiosyncratic reactions	Future avoidance; physiological support

NOTE: po = by mouth; IV = administered intravenously.

THROMBOEMBOLIC DISEASE

The use of oral contraceptives is a risk factor for venous thromboembolic disease (Table 52-3); this effect appears to be related most directly to the estrogenic potency of the particular drug. There also appears to be an additive risk in patients who take oral contraceptives and smoke cigarettes. A pulmonary embolic syndrome also occurs in main-line heroin abusers due to the particulate material used either to dilute the drug or to filter it before intravenous injection: talc, lactose, baking soda, starch, quinine, and maltose are commonly used as diluents; cotton fibers are often dislodged from the filtering material. The foreign material elicits a granulomatous foreign body reaction that obliterates the affected pulmonary microvessel. Another source of induced embolic phenomena is the injection of oil-based dye for lymphangiography; on rare occasions, this material has resulted in widespread occlusion

TABLE 52-2

Pulmonary Edema, Cardiogenic

Drug	Pharmacology	Comments	Therapy
Volume expanders (albumin, plasma protein fraction, hetastarch, dextran, isotonic or hypertonic saline)	IV, dose- and duration-dependent	Usually in setting of underlying cardiac or renal disease	Diuresis
β-Adrenergic antagonists (propranolol, nadolol, timolol, pindolol, metoprolol, atenolol)	po, IV, dose-dependent	Decreased inotropy and chronotropy in patients with preexisting heart disease	Avoidance, inotropes, diuresis
Calcium channel blocking agents (verapamil, diltiazem, nifedipine)	po, IV, sublingual dose- and duration-dependent	Decreased inotropy	Avoidance, inotropes, diuresis
α-Adrenergic agonists (metaraminol, phenylephrine, norepinephrine)	IV, dose- and duration-dependent	Increased afterload in patients with preexisting heart disease; high dose may induce a cardiomyopathy	Inotropes, diuresis

NOTE: IV = administered intravenously; po = by mouth.

TABLE 52-3

Pulmonary Thromboemboli, Vasculitis, Hypertension

Drug	Pharmacology	Comments	Therapy
Oral contraceptives (estrogen, progesterone)	po, IM, topical dose-dependent	Thromboemboli associated closely with estrogen concentration in contraceptives but also progesterone alone; isolated cases of nonthromboembolic pulmonary hypertension	Anticoagulation; discontinue drug
Oil-based lymphangiogram dye	Lymphatic administration; probably some dose dependency; increased risk with > 10 ml/limb	Oil microemboli in pulmonary arterioles; diffusion capacity falls in everyone, but symptoms in only 10%; usually those with preexisting lung disease	Oxygen; physiological support
Intravenous fat emulsion	IV	Fat microemboli and fat droplets in alveoli seen in preterm infants and neonates with respiratory distress	Discontinue drug if respiratory status deterioration is noted
Illicit drugs	IV of crushed tablets or with various particulate diluents	Talc, starch, soda, cotton, etc., may precipitate vascular obstruction, granulomatous vasculitis, and chronic interstitial fibrosis with capillary obliteration	Corticosteroids used occasionally in acute talcosis with questionable benefit
Adrenergic nasal sprays	Years of abuse	Autopsy reports showing interstitial fibrosis-pulmonary capillary obliteration	Discontinue drug
Protamine	IV; not clearly dose-dependent	Rare documentation of pulmonary hypertension, associated with development of thrombocytopenia	Physiological support

NOTE: po = by mouth; IM = administered intramuscularly; IV = administered intravenously.

of the pulmonary capillaries by lipid droplets within 24 to 48 h after injection. A similar reaction occasionally follows the use of fat emulsions administered intravenously in neonates.

PULMONARY VASCULITIS

Pulmonary vasculitis due to drug ingestion is uncommon. An anorexigenic agent (aminorex) which was sold over the counter for a while in Europe was associated with an intense pulmonary vasculitis that culminated in obliterative pulmonary vascular disease (see Chapter 64). On rare occasions, pulmonary vasculitis has also been attributed to other agents (Table 52-3). For example, obliterated pulmonary vessels have been found at autopsy in patients who have overused α-adrenergic nasal sprays; usually, the pulmonary vascular disease has been associated with interstitial fibrosis. The initiating mechanism for this reaction is enigmatic.

PULMONARY HEMORRHAGE

Pulmonary hemorrhage may complicate excessive systemic anticoagulation (Table 52-4), usually heparin overdosage for acute pulmonary embolism and infarction. Spontaneous pulmonary hemorrhage has also occurred in the course of overdosage with warfarin. Thrombolytic drugs can do the same. On occasion, hemothorax complicates the use of these drugs. Much less frequently, pulmonary hemorrhage occurs in the course of therapy with other pharmacologic agents. For example, in one patient, the initial manifestation of toxicity to nitrofurantoin was pulmonary hemorrhage. In a few instances, D-penicillamine therapy has been complicated by a combi-

nation of pulmonary hemorrhage and rapidly progressive glomerulonephritis that simulated Goodpasture's syndrome. In these instances, immunofluorescent stains applied to pulmonary or renal tissue consistently failed to show the characteristic linear staining for anti-GBM antibody (see Chapter 45), but in a few, interrupted immune complexes were found.

Adverse Airway Responses

Two major subsets of this category are bronchospasm and bronchiolitis.

BRONCHOSPASM

In patients with underlying hyperreactive airways, bronchospasm can be precipitated by numerous agents (Table 52-5). The most common offenders are β-adrenergic antagonists in patients with hypertension or ischemic heart disease: even antagonists that are relatively cardioselective can induce bronchospasm if given in sufficiently high dosage or when administered parenterally. Medications, such as methacholine, neostigmine, or succinylcholine, which have cholinergic properties, can also precipitate bronchospasm by upsetting the normal balance between cholinergic and adrenergic tone of the airways.

Severe bronchospasm is sometimes part of IgE-mediated anaphylaxis. Although the bronchospastic reaction is most often induced by penicillin and its congeners, it is a possible complication of any anaphylactic drug reaction.

Aspirin and other anti-inflammatory drugs that inhibit cyclooxygenase sometimes precipitate bronchospasm, particularly in patients with underlying asthma who have a history of atopy. Although the initiating

TABLE 52-4
Pulmonary Hemorrhage

Drug	Pharmacology	Comments	Therapy
Anticoagulants (heparin, warfarin, streptokinase, urokinase)	IV; SC; po	In setting of pulmonary emboli with infarction; pulmonary hemorrhage from warfarin usually associated with excessive anticoagulation	Reversal of anticoagulation
D-penicillamine	po; reported after 2–3 years of use	3 patients with Wilson's disease with concomitant glomerulonephritis, Goodpasture's syndrome, but no anti-GBM antibody; all 3 patients died	Discontinue drug; one patient given prednisone lived 6 months
Oil-based lymphangiogram dye, mineral oil (aspiration), nitrofurantoin		Single case reports where hemorrhage was prominent, probably as a manifestation of injury pattern described elsewhere in text	Discontinue drug; physiological support

NOTE: IV = administered intravenously; SC = administered subcutaneously; po = by mouth.

TABLE 52-5

Airways Disease

Drug	Pharmacology	Comments	Therapy
Acetylsalicylic acid	po; not clearly dose- or duration-dependent	Bronchospasm in 5–10% of asthmatic population; may be component of foods	Avoidance; bronchodilators for acute reactions; found in flavorings and many drug preparations
Nonsteroidal antiinflammatory drugs (indomethacin, ibuprofen, naproxen, fenoprofen, meclofenamate, phenylbutazone)	Same as above	Bronchospasm in aspirin-sensitive asthmatics	Same as above
Tartrazine (FDA yellow dye no. 5)	Same as above	Bronchospasm; common additive in foods and medications; 10% of aspirin-sensitive patients may react	Same as above
Sulfites	po, inhaled	Bronchospasm; preservative in foods and medications including some aerosol solutions for asthmatics	Same as above; avoid bronchodilator solutions and tablets containing sulfites
Chemotherapeutic agents (L-asparaginase, cisplatin)	IV, IM	Bronchospasm; more frequent when L-asparaginase is given IV rather than IM	Discontinue drug; corticosteroids; bronchodilators; in case of L-asparaginase an alternative bacterial source for the agent can be used
β-adrenergic antagonists (Nonselective: propranolol, nadolol, timolol, pindolol. Cardioselective: metoprolol, atenolol)	po; IV; ophth; dose- and route-dependent	Bronchospasm in patients with obstructive lung disease; cardioselective agents lose selectivity with higher dose	Avoidance; bronchodilators for acute reactions
Cholinergic agonists (carbachol, bethanecol, methacholine, pilocarpine)	po; SC; ophth; dose-dependent	Bronchospasm in susceptible patients; increase cholinergic tone in airways	Same as above
Neuromuscular blockers (d-tubocurarine, succinylcholine, atracurium)	IV; dose-dependent	Bronchospasm; possibly cause histamine release; succinylcholine may have muscarinic actions at high dose	Respiratory support; bronchodilators
Anticholinesterase drugs (edrophonium, neostigmine, pyridostigmine)	po, IM, IV; dose-dependent	Bronchospasm in susceptible patients by increasing cholinergic tone	Avoidance, bronchodilators, pralidoxime
Inhaled aerosols (metaproterenol and other β agonists, cromolyn, beclomethasone)	Inhaled; possibly dose- and duration dependent	Bronchospasm in asthmatics; probable irritant effect on airways; hypersensitivity possible with cromolyn; paradoxical β blockade with some β agonists	
Tween	po; no clear dose dependency	Bronchospasm in some asthmatics; emulsifier in foods and drugs	Avoidance
Prostaglandin $F_{2\infty}$	intrauterine	Bronchospasm in asthmatics; used for abortion induction	Avoidance, bronchodilators acutely
D-penicillamine	po; no definite dose dependence	Bronchiolitis obliterans in rare patients with rheumatoid arthritis	Discontinue drug; bronchodilators; corticosteroids
Anaphylaxis (any drug; most commonly penicillin)	Any route; not dose-dependent	IgE-mediated bronchospasm	Physiological support; bronchodilators; corticosteroids

NOTE: po = by mouth; IV = administered intravenously; IM = administered intramuscularly; SC = administered subcutaneously; ophth = ophthalmic administration.

TABLE 52-6
Pleural Inflammation and/or Effusion

Drug	Pharmacology	Comments	Therapy
Anticoagulants	Overdose	Hemothorax associated with traumatic rib fracture or rarely pulmonary embolus in setting of excessive anticoagulation	Reverse anticoagulant effect
Chemotherapeutic agents			
Bleomycin	Dose dependency at >450 mg	Associated with interstitial fibrosis	Discontinue drug; ? corticosteroids
Busulfan	Questionable dose dependency > 600 mg	Associated with interstitial fibrosis	Discontinue drug; ? corticosteroids
Methotrexate	po	Independent of hypersensitivity reaction	Discontinue drug
Mitomycin	IV; wks to mos.; not dose- or schedule-dependent	Seen in association with pulmonary fibrosis	Same as above
Procarbazine	po; seen with 2d or 3d drug exposure	Seen in association with hypersensitivity reaction	Same as above
Drug-induced SLE syndrome	See Table 52-10	Associated with other manifestation of lupus including hypersensitivity pulmonary infiltrates	Discontinue drug; corticosteroids
Ergot derivatives (methysergide, ergonovine)	po; mos on drug	Signaled by onset of dyspnea, pleurisy, and fever with pleural rub associated with interstitial fibrosis	Same as above
Ibuprofen	Months on drug	Single case; questionable association	Discontinue drug
Nitrofurantoin	po	Seen in association with hypersensitivity reaction	Same as above
Propranolol		Single case report of pleural thickening	Same as above
Radiation	Usually above 4000 cGy	Rare in relation to fibrosis; routinely seen with radiation of lung tissue	Same as above
Sodium morrhuate	IV into esophageal varices for sclerotherapy; no dose dependency	Mechanism not clear; associations not fully proven	Same as above

NOTE: po = by mouth; IV = administered intravenously.

TABLE 52-7
Mediastinal Alterations

Drug	Pharmacology	Comments	Therapy
Corticosteroids	Any route of administration; probable dose and time dependency	Referred to as lipomatosis due to increase in superior mediastinal fat	Discontinue drug
Diphenylhydantoin	po; no apparent dose dependency	As rare part of pseudo-lymphoma syndrome	Discontinue drug
Methotrexate	po; IV; intrathecal 20 mg/kg per week suggested dose dependency	Hilar adenopathy seen rarely in association with hypersensitivity reactions	Discontinue drug

NOTE: po = by mouth; IV = administered intravenously.

mechanism is unclear, the reaction is not IgE-mediated; one possible mechanism is overproduction of lipoxygenase products due to cyclooxygenase inhibition. Prostaglandin $F_{2\alpha}$, a lipoxygenase product used clinically for therapeutic abortions, sometimes precipitates bronchospasm.

Tartrazine (FDA yellow food dye no. 5) and sulfites used as preservative agents have evoked urticaria and asthma in certain individuals, most often in those who also are sensitive to aspirin; the mechanism responsible for these reactions is not IgE-mediated. A severe syndrome resembling anaphylaxis with bronchospasm has been described in some patients after the intravenous administration of radiocontrast dye; this reaction also does not appear to be immunologically mediated.

Inhaled medications, notably aerosols of cromolyn sodium, beclomethasone, and β-adrenergic agents, occasionally precipitate bronchospasm, presumably by an irritant effect on airways. Administration of high doses of β-adrenergic agents by aerosol occasionally evokes a paradoxical β-adrenergic blockade.

BRONCHIOLITIS

Bronchiolitis obliterans while taking penicillamine has occurred in several patients with rheumatoid arthritis. However, it has also occurred in other patients with rheumatoid arthritis who were not taking this agent. One explanation proffered to reconcile these observations is that penicillamine interferes with the healing of an inflammatory process in the distal bronchioles.

Pleural Disease

A variety of agents have been etiologically implicated in pleural pain, effusion, and thickening (Table 52-6). For example, pleural disease is the most common pulmonary manifestation of the drug-induced lupus syndrome (see Chapter 43): pleural pain occurs in nearly half of the patients with drug-induced lupus secondary to procainamide; pleural effusion occurs in approximately 10 percent

of these individuals. Effusions also occur as part of diffuse hypersensitivity responses to other agents.

Retroperitoneal fibrosis and pleural thickening and fibrosis occurred during treatment with practolol, a β-blocking agent that is no longer in clinical use. More recently, a single instance of pleural thickening associated with the use of propranolol has been described. Long-term use of methysergide, an ergot derivative, has been associated with retroperitoneal fibrosis, pleural effusion and fibrosis, and fibrotic thickening of cardiac valves; on rare occasions, ergonovine therapy has also been associated with pleural fibrosis.

Mediastinal Disease

Several medications can, on rare occasions, cause abnormalities in the mediastinum (Table 52-7). Pseudolymphomatous transformation of nodes occurs occasionally in the course of phenytoin therapy; mediastinal lymphadenopathy is an infrequent part of this syndrome and resolves quickly after the agent is discontinued. Methotrexate occasionally causes mediastinal lymphadenopathy as part of an acute pulmonary hypersensitivity reaction. Mediastinal lipomatosis frequently accompanies the prolonged use of pharmacologic doses of corticosteroids as part of a systemic cushingoid syndrome.

Neuromuscular Dysfunction

Within this category are two types of disorder: depression of the central nervous system (CNS) and neuromuscular blockade.

CNS DEPRESSION

Overdosage or idiosyncratic responses to sedatives, hypnotics, and narcotics causes central respiratory depression, alveolar hypoventilation, and subsequent respiratory acidosis (Table 52-8). Patients with underlying lung disease, especially those with preexisting hypercapnia, are often extremely sensitive to small doses of sedative or hypnotic agents.

TABLE 52-8
CNS Respiratory Center Dysfunction

Drug	Pharmacology	Comments	Therapy
Narcotics (cocaine, heroin, meperidine, methadone, morphine, pentazocine)	Seen with any route of administration and dose-dependent	Patients with elevated Pa_{CO_2} may be sensitive to small doses	Discontinue drug; respiratory support (naloxone)
Sedatives, tranquilizers (barbiturates, benzodiazepines)	Seen with any route of administration and dose-dependent	Mainly case reports often with overdose, more frequent with underlying respiratory disease	Respiratory support
Miscellaneous drugs (amitriptyline, gallamine, imipramine, ketamine, L-dopa, diphenoxylate HCl, promazine)	Seen with usual route of administration and probably dose-dependent	Mainly case reports in association with altered metabolic state impairing drug elimination	Same as above

NEUROMUSCULAR BLOCKADE

The administration of aminoglycoside antibiotics, penicillamine, or polymyxin B has been accompanied by weakness or paralysis of respiratory muscles, especially in patients with underlying neuromuscular disease and in patients who are hypocalcemic (Table 52-9). Other manifestations of neuromuscular blockade, such as weakness of extremities or ptosis, are often present. These agents seem to cause competitive inhibition of acetylcholine at the neuromuscular junction. Withholding the medications and correcting hypocalcemia usually restores muscle strength rapidly to baseline.

Pulmonary Disease from Drug-Induced Systemic Lupus Erythematosus

Many drugs have been implicated as the cause of the drug-induced lupus syndrome (Table 52-10). How they cause this syndrome is unknown. The clinical syndrome evoked by these agents satisfies the criteria for the diagnosis of lupus erythematosus: diffuse serositis, arthritis, and pulmonary manifestations are common; antinuclear antibodies are generally present even though antibodies to double-stranded DNA cannot be found. Pulmonary manifestations occur more often in the drug-induced syndrome than in spontaneous lupus erythematosus.

TABLE 52-9
Neuromuscular Dysfunction

Drug	Pharmacology	Comments	Therapy
Aminoglycosides (gentamicin, kanamycin, neomycin, tobramycin, streptomycin)	IM; IV; IP; effect seen in 10–30 min probable dose dependency	Seen mainly in setting of low serum Ca^{2+} and/or with preexisting muscular disease	Discontinue drug; IV calcium; neostigmine
Polymyxins	IM; IV; po; SC; topical within 1–26 h of administration	Seen in setting of underlying renal disease	Discontinue drug; not helped by calcium or neostigmine
Neuromuscular blockers (succinylcholine, trimethaphan camsylate, d-tubocurarine)	IV; dose dependency; onset within minutes to hours	Rare case report; usually associated with prolonged metabolism of drug in postanesthetic setting with unexpected prolonged or recurrent respiratory depression	Respiratory support

NOTE: IM = intramuscularly; IV = intravenously; IP = intraperitoneally; po = by mouth; SC = subcutaneously.

TABLE 52-10
Drug-Induced Systemic Lupus Erythematosus

Drug	Pharmacology	Comments	Therapy
Diphenylhydantoin	po; not dose or time-dependent		Discontinue drug; corticosteroids if clinical situation severe
Hydralazine	po; probably requires a dose of >100 mg/day for >1 month	Increased frequency in women, caucasians, and slow acetylators	Same as above
Isoniazid	po; not dose-dependent		Same as above
Procainamide	po; not dose-dependent, but increased frequency with duration of therapy >4 months	Slow acetylators at higher risk	Same as above
Other drugs (α-methyldopa, digitalis, ethosuximide, gold, griseofulvin, hydrochlorothiazide, mephenytoin, oral contraceptives, aminosalicylic acid, penicillin, phenylbutazone, primidone, propylthiouracil, reserpine, streptomycin, sulfonamides, tetracycline, trimethadione)		The above 4 drugs account for >80% of this drug-induced disease; the remaining drugs are case reports, and their causative relation to the disease is not completely confirmed	

NOTE: po = by mouth.

Approximately 50 percent of patients who take procainamide for over 2 months develop circulating antinuclear antibodies; fewer develop the clinical signs and symptoms typical of lupus. Pulmonary manifestations occur in approximately 50 percent of patients who develop the drug-induced syndrome; most have pleural pain, and 10 percent develop pleural effusions. About one-fourth of those who develop drug-induced lupus from procainamide also have radiographic evidence of a pneumonitis; discontinuing procainamide is usually followed within weeks by resolution of symptoms. Corticosteroids seem to promote resolution of the syndrome but are generally reserved for those with disabling symptoms. On rare occasions, symptoms persist for long periods of time following discontinuation of the procainamide.

The drug-induced lupus syndrome secondary to hydralazine usually occurs after chronic therapy using relatively high daily doses, i.e., for more than 3 months with an average daily dose of 300 to 400 mg per day. Although about 50 percent of those on chronic hydralazine therapy develop positive antinuclear antibodies, fewer than 5 percent develop the lupus syndrome. Pulmonary manifestations of the hydralazine-induced syndrome are not as common as with procainamide; i.e., only about 25 percent of patients with the hydralazine-induced syndrome develop pulmonary disease. As in the case of procainamide-induced lupus, pleural disease is more common than pneumonitis. A distinguishing feature of hydralazine-induced lupus is that the manifestations may persist for months or years after discontinuation of the drug. Corticosteroids are often used in the attempt to ameliorate the protracted course, but their value is unproven.

Hypersensitivity Syndrome

A number of medications can elicit a systemic hypersensitivity syndrome in which the lungs are also involved (Table 52-11). As a rule, the systemic allergic response consists of fever, urticaria, arthralgias, hypotension, and eosinophilia. The most common pulmonary manifestations of hypersensitivity are cough, shortness of breath, and chest pains; radiographically, there is evidence of pneumonitis, pleuritis, and pleural effusion. Antimicrobial medications, particularly the penicillins, sulfonamides, nitrofurantoin, and p-aminosalicylic acid, are common causes of this reaction; in some of these instances, the syndrome appears to be IgE-mediated.

Among the chemotherapeutic agents used for cancer, L-asparaginase causes a hypersensitivity syndrome that is mediated by IgE antibodies. Acute hypersensitivity reactions have also followed the use of *cis*-platinum. Bleomycin has also elicited acute severe reactions: an initial dose of bleomycin has occasionally been followed by hyperpyrexia, chills, diaphoresis, wheezing, and hypertension; in a few instances, death has ensued. Specific antibodies to bleomycin have not been implicated as the cause of this reaction, and it is possible that it represents a severe idiosyncratic reaction to the release of pyrogenic material.

Methotrexate-induced pulmonary disease may entail an allergic response since about half of these patients manifest eosinophilia in the peripheral blood; granulomas have been found in the occasional lung biopsies that have been performed. The pulmonary damage induced by methotrexate does not appear to be dose-related.

Bronchoalveolar lavage has been done in occasional patients in whom hypersensitivity reactions were probably drug-related. Lymphocytosis has been found. However, this finding is not specific for hypersensitivity reactions.

Interstitial Pneumonitis

Interstitial pneumonitis and/or fibrosis is the most common pattern of injury encountered with drug-induced pulmonary disease (Table 52-12). Although some interstitial inflammatory responses are part of drug-induced lupus syndromes and hypersensitivity reactions, more often, direct cytotoxic effects of a drug or its metabolic product on the endothelial, interstitial, or alveolar epithelial cells is the likely mechanism of injury. The cytotoxic reactions evoke an inflammatory response, commonly in the alveolus, that is characterized by the accumulation of macrophages, lymphocytes, and other inflammatory cells. Persistence of the inflammatory response leads to fibrin deposition within the alveolus and to interstitial inflammation and fibrosis.

These reactions can be acute, subacute, or chronic. In the *acute* form, the patients complain of shortness of breath and manifest a dry cough; commonly, they have a low grade fever. Chest radiographs show prominent interstitial markings, and airspaces are often opaque. Biopsies show the inflammatory infiltrates in the alveoli. The *subacute* form presents with similar, but more insidious, symptoms. Biopsies at this stage often show predominantly fibrin deposition and less intense inflammation. The chronic form of drug-induced interstitial lung disease is most common. Dyspnea on exertion has been gradual in onset. Frequently, there is a nonproductive cough. But, characteristically there is no fever. The chest radiograph shows diffuse interstitial reticulonodular infiltrates (Fig. 52-1). Mild arterial hypoxemia is common. Lung biopsy reveals alveolar inflammation in which chronic inflammatory cells predominate, proliferation of the epithelial type II pneumocytes, and intraluminal as well as interstitial fibrosis (Fig. 52-2). Three agents from this group warrant special mention: bleomycin, nitrofurantoin, and amiodarone.

Pulmonary interstitial disease secondary to bleomycin is one of the major adverse reactions associated with this drug and is dose-limiting. Electron microscopic and

TABLE 52-11

Hypersensitivity Pulmonary Infiltrate

Drug	Pharmacology	Comments	Therapy
Antibiotics			
Isoniazid	po	Rare event	Discontinue drug
Nitrofurantoin	po; hours to days after start of drug	Chest radiograph improved 48 h after stopping drug	Discontinue drug; corticosteroids
p-Aminosalicylic acid	po; 3–4 weeks after starting drug	Desensitization has been done	Discontinue drug
Penicillin	IM; weeks after starting drug	Old reports may be due to diluent used	Discontinue drug
Sulfonamides	po; topical, 5–7 days after starting drug		Discontinue drug
Tetracycline	po	Rare event	Discontinue drug
Cancer chemotherapy drugs			
Azathioprine	po; years on agent	Rare; and cases published very complicated	Discontinue drug
Methotrexate	po; IV; IT greater than 20/mg per week suggested dose dependency; onset days to weeks after start of drug	Primarily seen in children with acute lymphocytic leukemia; most patients improve	Discontinue drug
Procarbazine	po; seen with 2d or 3d drug exposure	Rapid improvement with drug withdrawal	Discontinue drug; corticosteroids
Miscellaneous drugs			
β-Adrenergic antagonist propranolol	po; months on drug	Rare case report	Discontinue drug
Carbamazepine	po; on drug for 1–3 months	Concomitant skin rash seen	Discontinue drug; ? corticosteroids
Chlorpropamide	po	Rare case report	Discontinue drug
Cromolyn	Aerosol; days to weeks on drug	Rare case reports in association with asthma	Discontinue drug
Diphenylhydantoin	po	Rare case reports	Discontinue drug
Gold salts	IM, weeks–months on drug; dose dependency 400–800 mg	Not totally clear if this is hypersensitivity reaction	Discontinue drug; ? corticosteroids
Hydrochlorothiazide	po	Rare case reports	Discontinue drug
Imipramine	po; days to wks on drug	Rare case reports	Discontinue drug
Nonsteroidal antiflammatory drugs (ibuprofen, naproxen, and sulindac)	po; wks on drug	Rapid improvement after stopping drug	Discontinue drug; ? corticosteroids

NOTE: po = by mouth; IM = intramuscularly; IV = intravenously; IT = intrathecally.

TABLE 52-12

Interstitial Pneumonitis/Fibrosis

Drug	Pharmacology	Comments	Therapy
Ganglion-blocking drugs (hexamethonium, mecamylamine, pentolinium)	po	Reported in setting of malignant hypertension and uremia; primarily of historic interest since rarely used	Discontinue drug
Cancer chemotherapy drugs			
Azathioprine	po; 1.5 to 24 months on drug	Rare case report; questionable association	Discontinue drug
Bleomycin	IM; SC; IV; clear dose relationship of 450 mg	Rare cases with first dose; increase risk with age, COPD,* radiation to lungs, use in combination chemotherapy protocols, and oxygen exposure	Discontinue drug; ? corticosteroid

TABLE 52-12 (*continued*)
Interstitial Pneumonitis/Fibrosis

Drug	Pharmacology	Comments	Therapy
Busulfan	po; ? dose dependency >600 mg	Rare in relation to use of agent	Discontinue drug
Chlorambucil	po; ? dose dependency at >2 g	Very rare in relation to use of agent	Discontinue drug
Cyclophosphamide	IV; po; ? dose dependency at 40–250 g; months to years on agent	Rare in relation to use of agent	Discontinue drug
Melphalan	po; years on drug	Limited improvement in few cases reported; rare in relation to use of agent	Discontinue drug
Mitomycin	IV, wks to months; not dose- or schedule-dependent	Possibly associated with concomitant use of vinblastine or vindesine, or oxygen exposure	Discontinue drug; corticosteroids
Nitrosoureas (BCNU, CCNU, MeCCNU,† Chlorozotocin)	IV (MeCCNU po) 1200–1500 mg/m² dose dependency with BCNU	Clear dose dependency with BCNU; preexisting lung disease is risk factor	Discontinue drug
Radiation	Dose dependency of 4000 cGy plus time dependency of 6–18 months	Limited to field of radiation; slow fibrosis taking months to finish	Respiratory support
Radioactive iodine	Years following treatment	Associated with extensive pulmonary metastases from thyroid cancer treated with ¹³¹I	Same as above
Miscellaneous drugs			
Adrenergic nasal sprays	Years of abuse	Rare	Discontinue drug
Amiodarone	po; ? dose dependency of >400 mg/day for months	Possibly causes pulmonary and systemic lipid storage disease and secondary inflammation	Discontinue drug; ? corticosteroids
Carbamazepine	po; months on drug	Rare case reports of this reaction in association with hypersensitivity reaction	Discontinue drug
Cromolyn	Aerosol	Rare case reports in association with hypersensitivity reactions in asthmatics	Discontinue drug
Diphenylhydantoin	po; months to years on drug	Very rare but well documented cases	Discontinue drug
D-penicillamine	po; 2–3 years on drug	Rare cases; some cases reported claiming hypersensitivity reaction	Discontinue drug; ? corticosteroids
Illicit drugs	IV	Due to agents used to "cut" drugs	? corticosteroids
Methysergide	po; months on drug	Rare in relation to retroperitoneal fibrosis; when occurs produces pleural fibrosis and effusions	? corticosteroids
Nitrofurantoin	po; dose dependency in range of 25–50 mg/day for 6 months–7 years	Not related to hypersensitivity reactions	Discontinue drug; ? corticosteroids
Oxygen	Concentration ≥60% and exposure time >48 h	May be worsened by concurrent or past drug use	Keep percent of O_2 as low as possible
Phenylbutazone	po	Rare	Discontinue drug

NOTE: po = by mouth; IM = intramuscularly; SC = subcutaneously; IV = intravenously.

*COPD = chronic obstructive pulmonary disease.

†MeCCNU = methyl CCNU.

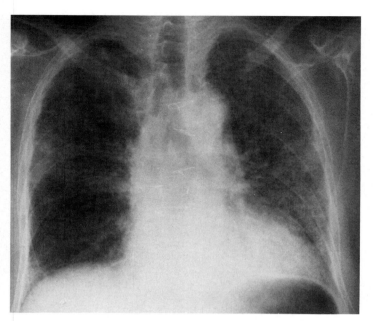

FIGURE 52-1 Chest radiograph showing diffuse increased interstitial markings and alveolar opacities in a patient who received a cumulative dose of 600 mg bleomycin for non-Hodgkin's lymphoma.

ultrastructural investigations in animals have shown that bleomycin causes necrosis of pulmonary endothelial cells and of type I pneumocytes followed by interstitial and alveolar edema, inflammation, and subsequent fibrosis. A cumulative bleomycin dose of over 450 mg, older age, underlying lung disease, exposure to hyperoxia, and concomitant or subsequent thoracic radiation therapy increase the risk of toxicity. Bleomycin is concentrated in the lung, but the actual mechanism of pulmonary injury is unclear. Whether oxygen radical production or specific direct immune reactions to lung tissues are the mechanism of action is uncertain.

Nitrofurantoin is the most common noncytotoxic drug that causes interstitial pneumonitis and fibrosis. The acute form of nitrofurantoin toxicity is the most common presentation. Because of the acute onset, the recurrence after rechallenge, and the rare association of a lupus erythematosus-like reaction, immunologic mechanisms have been suspected as the cause of the acute toxicity. However, attempts to implicate specific types of lymphocytes have proved inconsistent and inconclusive. In contrast, as in the case of bleomycin, the evidence favoring oxidant-mediated injury is more substantive.

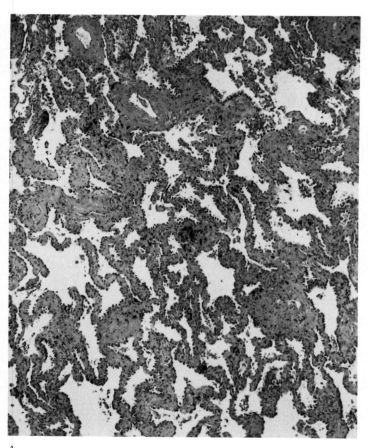

A

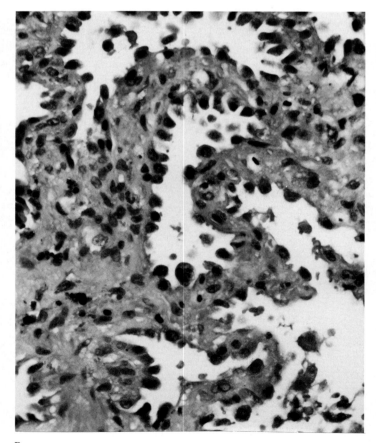

B

FIGURE 52-2 *A.* Low power magnification of left-lower lobe biopsy from patient in Fig. 52-1 demonstrating interstitial inflammation and thickening. ×57. *B.* Higher power view of same area showing type II pneumocyte proliferation and occasional atypical cells. ×357.

Amiodarone is another agent that causes interstitial pulmonary fibrosis, which is its most serious extracardiac side effect. The pulmonary toxicity appears to be dose-related; most patients manifesting this disturbance have taken a maintenance dose of over 400 mg per day. The onset of toxicity from the time of beginning amiodarone therapy is variable, anywhere from 1 month to 5 years.

The mechanism of amiodarone-induced pulmonary disease is unclear. Light-microscopic findings in these patients show accumulation of foamy macrophages within alveoli, thickening and fibrosis of the alveolar septum, and hyperplasia of type II pneumocytes. Electron micrographs of pulmonary tissue from patients with amiodarone pneumonitis have shown abnormal lamellar, or granular, inclusion bodies within distended lysosomes of macrophages, type II pneumocytes, endothelial cells, and interstitial cells. Similar lamellar inclusion bodies have also been seen in cells from extrapulmonary tissues. Amiodarone is an amphiphilic molecule, and other agents of this type have been shown to cause an increase in phospholipids in lung cells resulting in similar lysosomal inclusion bodies. Accumulation of phospholipids in cells may cause cellular injury followed by inflammation and fibrosis.

No evidence has been provided for immunoglobulin deposition in pulmonary tissue. Nor is there evidence of a drug-induced, lupus-type reaction. Although a hypersensitivity reaction to amiodarone has been suggested, it is difficult to reconcile with the prolonged course, i.e., 6 to 9 years, of amiodarone administration before clinical manifestations appeared.

CLINICAL PROBLEMS OF COMMONLY USED DRUGS

Methotrexate

Methotrexate is a folic acid antagonist which inhibits dihydrofolate reductase. It is used in the treatment of malignant and nonmalignant states. In recent years, it has become popular to use methotrexate in large dosages because toxicity can be prevented by leucovorin. It can be administered orally, intravenously, or intrathecally; no matter how administered, it seems capable of causing pulmonary complications.

Most pulmonary reactions caused by methotrexate are acute. They occur predominantly in children with acute lymphocytic leukemia. The pulmonary reaction is manifested by pneumonitis associated with fever, dry cough, dyspnea, hypoxemia, and bilateral pulmonary infiltrates. The syndrome often develops over 7 to 14 days. In some instances, a mild peripheral eosinophilia is present. Rarely have lung biopsies been done; these have shown inflammatory cells in the parenchyma, predominantly in the alveolar spaces and to a lesser extent in the interstitium. A few biopsies have shown granulomatous reactions with multinucleated giant cells. In many instances, regardless of whether the methotrexate is stopped, the patient improves in 10 to 14 days. In most of the patients, the acute lymphocytic leukemia is in remission when the pulmonary reaction is manifest. Rarely has this pulmonary reaction been seen in other malignant states, although it has been looked for carefully in trophoblastic tumors, osteogenic sarcomas, and cancers of the head and neck. An occasional instance of this pulmonary reaction has been found in benign situations, such as psoriasis; these have been associated with hepatic toxicity caused by methotrexate.

A dose of 20 mg per week has been proposed to be the threshold dose for causing the pulmonary reaction, but no additive effects of the drug have been seen with total doses of up to 6.5 g. The time interval to the onset of the pulmonary reaction can vary from days to years. Chest radiographs show alveolar infiltrates with occasional linear and reticulonodular areas. Rarely have pleural effusions and hilar lymphadenopathy been encountered. It has been estimated that about 10 percent of patients die from this reaction. The frequency of the pulmonary reaction is difficult to assess, but it appears to be less than 10 percent in children who are given methotrexate for acute lymphocytic leukemia and much less in other patients. Treatment of this disease remains confusing: some patients have improved when the drug was stopped, whereas others improved even though the drug was continued. The value of corticosteroids is unknown. At present, it seems reasonable to deal with the pulmonary reaction by stopping methotrexate and by giving corticosteroids if the clinical situation is severe. Except for acute lymphocytic leukemia there seems to be no other specific risk factor for the pulmonary reaction to methotrexate.

Bischlorethylnitrosourea (BCNU)

BCNU is an alkylating agent which is widely used in the treatment of lymphoma, myeloma, and brain tumors. It has been shown to cause pulmonary interstitial fibrosis which is dose-related: in brain tumor patients, the risk of developing an interstitial lung process with a cumulative dose of 1200 to 1500 mg/m^2 is 20 to 30 percent; the risk increases to 50 percent with cumulative doses that exceed 1500 mg/m^2. The clinical symptoms are similar to those seen in other interstitial processes including nonproductive cough, dyspnea, and tachypnea. Bibasilar crackles are present. Chest radiographs are abnormal in the majority of patients at the time that symptoms appear; they show linear and reticulonodular infiltrates. Pulmonary function studies are abnormal at the time of diagnosis; lung volumes and the diffusing capacity for carbon monoxide are low; it has been suggested that a decrease in the diffusing capacity for carbon monoxide is the earliest sign of toxicity. The possibility has been raised that preexisting pulmonary disease increases the risk of pulmonary toxicity. The additive risk of radiation therapy and combination chemotherapy is unclear. Age does not appear to influence toxicity.

Pathologic examination shows proteinaceous material and fibroblastic proliferation in alveoli. Type II pneumocytes undergo hyperplasia and metaplasia; the number of type I epithelial cells is increased. On rare occasion, eosinophilic infiltrates have been reported, but the process does not appear to be a hypersensitivity reaction.

The treatment for BCNU toxicity is to stop the drug. After stopping, between 60 and 80 percent of patients will stabilize or improve. Corticosteroids have been used but without clear evidence of benefit.

A number of other nitrosoureas are also in clinical use: chloroethylcyclohexylnitrosourea (CCNU), methylchloroethylcyclohexylnitrosourea (methyl CCNU), chlorozotocin, and streptozotocin. These agents are used in treating pulmonary and gastrointestinal cancers. All agents, except streptozotocin, have been reported to cause a similar pulmonary process as seen with BCNU. The clinical data with respect to the effect of dosage is unclear. In using a nitrosourea, the pulmonary status of the patient has to be carefully monitored. In the case of BCNU, the total dose should not exceed 1400 mg/m^2, and the diffusing capacity of carbon monoxide should be carefully monitored.

Bleomycin

Bleomycin is a microbial by-product that inhibits cell growth by causing single- and double-strand breaks in DNA. The agent is extremely useful in testicular cancer and lymphomas. Animal models show that bleomycin accumulates in the lungs and demonstrates a dose effect for pulmonary toxicity. The pulmonary toxicity does not depend clearly either on the schedule or route of administration, even though it has been suggested that pulmonary toxicity is slightly less when the drug is given intramuscularly than when it is given intravenously. At the outset, the process seems to be an inflammatory reaction that culminates in intra-alveolar and interstitial fibrosis that occurs at different times in different areas of the lung. Clinical use of bleomycin has caused death from pulmonary fibrosis. There are two clinical patterns showing similar clinical symptoms and pathology but differing in the dosage at which the events occur. Most common is the dose-dependent pattern; it is usually seen when the total dose of bleomycin given over any time period reaches the 450-mg range. The second pattern, the so-called acute pattern, occurs at lower doses; on rare occasions, it has occurred after a single initial dose. This acute pattern is generally seen in patients with additional risk factors, such as previous or concomitant radiotherapy to the chest, exposure to high oxygen concentrations, or old age.

The dose-dependent form of toxicity to bleomycin manifests itself initially by dry crackles; on rare occasions, rhonchi or a pleural friction rub is present. Often the chest radiograph at this time is entirely normal and the patient is asymptomatic. Over a time span of weeks to months, the patient then develops a dry cough, tachypnea, and dyspnea. At this juncture, the chest radiograph often shows diffuse lower lobe linear densities or nodular infiltrates; occasionally, an alveolar pattern is seen.

Although this chronic form is dose-related, the dosage levels at which toxicity is manifested depends on whether the patient has been previously radiated, or is given oxygen therapy, or is elderly. As a rule, about 15 percent of those who receive a cumulative dose of over 450 mg develop clinical pulmonary toxicity.

Attempts at the noninvasive diagnosis of bleomycin-induced lung injury using pulmonary function tests have yielded mixed results. Serial pulmonary function studies in humans receiving bleomycin have revealed decreasing lung volumes and abnormal diffusing capacities in all patients; however, no strict dose-response relationship has been found; nor is there a predictive value for subsequent toxicity. Further information is needed about the detection of pulmonary injury in a preclinical phase.

It is quite clear that radiotherapy given to the mediastinum or to the lung parenchyma predisposes to bleomycin toxicity. The acute reaction is most often seen in patients who have received extensive radiotherapy to their lungs; the added risk of serious pulmonary toxicity is about 20 percent in these patients. There is also a good correlation between bleomycin toxicity and the concomitant use of inspired mixtures that contain more than 39 percent oxygen. This correlation lends support to the concept that oxygen radical formation is a possible mechanism for the pulmonary injury.

Except for stopping the drug, the treatment of bleomycin toxicity is uncertain. Corticosteroids have been tried, but their effectiveness has not been proved. Most of the pulmonary toxicity caused by bleomycin depends on the extent of pulmonary disease that is present at the time of diagnosis: those patients in whom arterial P_{O_2} is low, and in whom radiographic changes are severe when the diagnosis of bleomycin toxicity is made, run a very high risk of dying. The likelihood that fibrosis will resolve is very slim, whereas the inflammatory response may resolve after the drug is discontinued. The earlier the pulmonary toxicity is detected and the agent stopped, the more likely is the response to be favorable. An important problem in dealing with bleomycin toxicity is to predict and detect early disease before the stage of irreversible fibrosis sets in.

Nitrofurantoin

Nitrofurantoin is a synthetic nitrofuran used for the treatment and prevention of urinary tract infections from susceptible organisms. The mechanism of its antimicrobial activity is unknown. This drug is available only in oral form. The incidence of adverse pulmonary effects from nitrofurantoin has been estimated to be approximately one in every 44,000 doses. Both acute and chronic reactions have been reported; the acute syndrome occurs approximately 10 times more often than the chronic. The two types of pulmonary disease present in different ways, probably because the pathogenetic mechanisms are also different. Pulmonary toxicity due to nitrofurantoin occurs in all age groups but most often in middle-aged to older women who take the drug for urinary tract infections.

The acute form of nitrofurantoin pulmonary toxicity is manifested by the sudden onset of fever, chills, cough, shortness of breath, wheezing, and occasionally chest pain, which may be pleuritic. The syndrome begins anywhere from hours to 8 to 10 days after starting the medication. Most patients give a past history of taking nitrofurantoin without difficulty; nitrofurantoin pulmonary toxicity is not dose-dependent. Crackles and wheezing are heard throughout the lungs. A peripheral eosinophilia is present in 20 to 30 percent of patients. The chest radiograph shows diffuse bilateral interstitial and occasional alveolar infiltrates. In one patient who died, autopsy showed the lungs to be heavy, congested, hemorrhagic, with a severe interstitial pneumonitis and fibrinous pulmonary edema. No immune complexes were seen in the lungs, even though the alveoli did contain a large number of plasma cells with surface markers for IgA.

If the syndrome is recognized and the drug is promptly discontinued, most patients improve rapidly. Corticosteroids are usually unnecessary. But an occasional patient has had persistent infiltrates even though the drug was discontinued; this type of patient has improved with corticosteroids.

Although the pathogenesis of the acute form is unclear, the acute onset, systemic symptoms, and rapid disappearance of the infiltrates after discontinuing the drug suggest an allergic or hypersensitivity phenomenon. Clinical patterns consistent with type I allergic reactions or type III reactions have been described. When incubated with pulmonary parenchymal cells for 12 h, nitrofurantoin caused injury to pulmonary cells that was exacerbated by hyperoxia and modified by antioxidant additives. Therefore, the possibility exists that production of superoxide radicals may contribute to acute injury caused by nitrofurantoin. However, the clinical patterns of response appear to be most typical of a hypersensitivity reaction.

Chronic pulmonary toxicity from nitrofurantoin is less common than the acute form. Only about 50 cases have been reported in the literature. Patients developed this disease after taking nitrofurantoin for from 6 months to 6 years, usually to suppress chronic or recurrent urinary tract infections. Clinically, the patient manifests insidious progression of dyspnea on exertion; a nonproduc-

tive cough is a common concomitant. Fever and systemic symptoms are unusual; so is chest pain. Crackles are present throughout the lungs. Peripheral eosinophilia is rare. Chest radiographs show diffuse interstitial infiltrates. Lung biopsy of patients with this type of reaction is nonspecific, revealing diffuse interstitial pneumonitis or fibrosis. The pattern is most typical of a cumulative cytotoxic drug effect; there is no evidence that a particular allergic diathesis causes the chronic reaction. Whether the formation of oxygen radicals plays a role in the chronic toxicity is speculative.

The chronic reaction to nitrofurantoin carries a poorer prognosis than the acute form. Eight to ten percent of patients who develop chronic nitrofurantoin toxicity die from their lung disease. However, most patients do show some resolution of infiltrates when the drug is discontinued. Corticosteroids have no proven role in therapy, although most patients who did not respond to simple discontinuation of the drug have received corticosteroids.

Amiodarone

Amiodarone is a new antiarrhythmic drug that is undergoing extensive clinical trial in the United States. A number of cardiac and extracardiac side effects have been described, and pulmonary toxicity appears to be the most serious extracardiac problem. The first report of pulmonary toxicity secondary to amiodarone was in 1980 despite 20 years of prior widespread use of the drug in Europe. Since that initial report, approximately 50 additional cases have been described. The incidence of amiodarone pulmonary toxicity in patients receiving the drug in the United States appears to be about 5 percent. Death occurs in about 25 percent of patients with amiodarone pulmonary toxicity. However, it must be recognized that these patients usually have had concomitant severe congestive heart failure. Toxicity appears to be dose- and duration-related: a dosage greater than 400 mg per day for months to years is necessary to develop toxicity. This may explain, in part, the lack of toxicity reports from European studies: the average daily dose in Europe ranges from 200 to 400 mg per day, whereas in the United States the average daily dose often exceeds 400 mg per day. In part, the larger doses in the United States are due to restriction of use to arrhythmias that are unresponsive to conventional therapy; as a rule, higher doses are needed to suppress these refractory arrhythmias.

The clinical findings of amiodarone pulmonary toxicity are nonspecific. The patients complain of dyspnea and nonproductive cough; fever or chills are rare. An occasional patient manifests muscle weakness or signs of a neuropathy. Thyroid dysfunction, hyperpigmentation, and asymptomatic corneal microdeposits have also been described. Peripheral eosinophilia and chest pain are uncommon. Chest radiographs show bilateral prominence of the interstitium that may progress to alveolar infiltrates (Fig. 52-3). Pleural effusions are uncommon. Pulmonary biopsies generally show nonspecific inflammation and pulmonary fibrosis (Fig. 52-4); in a few instances, as noted above, lipid accumulation in lung cells has been found. Similar inclusion bodies have been seen in dermal histiocytes, Schwann cells, muscle cells, fibroblasts, and corneal epithelial cells. Amiodarone may cause a generalized lipid storage disorder that may evoke a secondary inflammatory response. There is evidence in occasional patients that specific immune phenomena are involved in amiodarone toxicity. Although the question of a hypersensitiv-

ity syndrome has been raised, the evidence is inconclusive.

There are no clear predisposing factors other than dosage. Although the possibility has been raised that pre-existing pulmonary disease may predispose to amiodarone pulmonary toxicity, there is little support for this suggestion.

In most patients with amiodarone toxicity, stopping the drug early in its evolution leads to spontaneous resolution of the infiltrates. Although about one-half of the patients reported in the literature were given corticosteroids, there is no evidence that they were helpful.

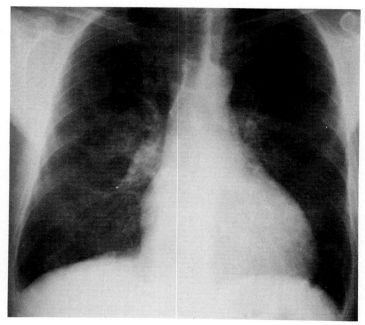

A

B

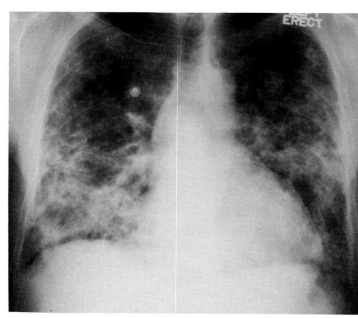

C

FIGURE 52-3   Chest radiographs of a 59-year-old male receiving amiodarone, 400 mg to 600 mg per day.   *A.* Baseline radiograph before therapy.   *B.* After 5 months of therapy. The patient was asymptomatic, but mild interstitial prominence is present. The drug was not discontinued.   *C.* Five months later. The patient was hypoxemic and dyspneic at rest, and the drug was stopped.

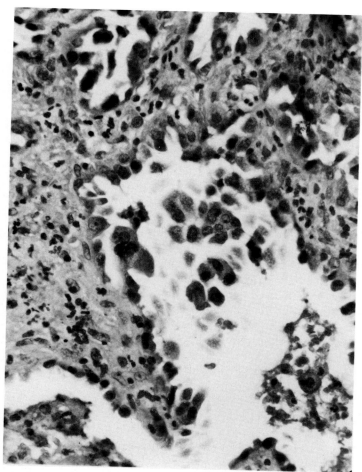

FIGURE 52-4 Lung biopsy from right lower lobe of patient in Fig. 52-3 showing interstitial inflammation and fibrosis. No lipid accumulation in lung cells was seen. ×275.

Once amiodarone toxicity is suspected, the major problem remains of dealing with the underlying cardiovascular problems. Since these patients have usually proved to be refractory to other antiarrhythmic drugs, some investigators have reintroduced amiodarone in lower doses and have achieved control of the arrhythmia without apparent pulmonary side effects. Others have reported occasional success after reintroducing a combination of amiodarone and corticosteroids. Not enough information is yet available to recommend either reintroduction of the drug in low dosage or the use of corticosteroids concomitantly in patients who have manifested pulmonary toxicity. Either of these trials should be undertaken with extreme caution and careful monitoring and only if alternative antiarrhythmic therapy is not feasible.

Patients who are taking amiodarone should be followed using serial chest radiographs to detect early asymptomatic interstitial changes. The value of serial pulmonary function tests is unsettled. However, in patients who are taking amiodarone, it seems reasonable to suppose that decrements in total lung capacity and diffusing capacity of more than 25 percent below baseline—without other apparent basis for change—may signal impending amiodarone toxicity.

Combination and High-Dose Chemotherapy

Current cancer chemotherapy relies either on combinations of drugs to attack the tumor cell at various metabolic points and/or on conventional chemotherapy in high doses to overcome the defense mechanisms of the tumor cell. To cope with the problem of bone marrow ablation that is entailed in high-dose chemotherapy, transplantation of autologous or allogenic bone marrow is done.

Combination chemotherapy programs that are used to treat non-Hodgkins's lymphoma often use bleomycin in conjunction with several other agents. In early studies using these combination programs, serious pulmonary toxicity was encountered when bleomycin doses were in the 150- to 200-mg range. Subsequently, lowering of the bleomycin dose in these protocols caused a marked drop in the frequency of the pulmonary toxicity. Similarly, mitomycin C elicits an increased frequency of pulmonary toxicity when used in conventional doses with vinca alkaloids. Therefore, care has to be taken in using combinations of drugs, even though dosages of individual drugs are less than those usually associated with toxicity.

In the case of allogenic bone marrow transplants, chemotherapeutic agents may play a role in causing interstitial pneumonitis. Most of these patients have been treated with combination chemotherapy before the transplant. They then receive high doses of agents, such as cyclophosphamide, followed by total body irradiation up to doses of 1400 cGy. The frequency of pulmonary complications is high in these patients, often exceeding 50 percent; in half of these, there is no known etiology. Therefore, it is assumed that the combinations of drugs plus radiation lead to the development of interstitial pneumonitis. Recently, cyclosporin A has been used instead of methotrexate to prevent graft-versus-host disease in patients following allogenic transplants. In these patients, there has been an unexpected drop in the incidence of interstitial pulmonary fibrosis. This change may reflect the avoidance of methotrexate. Other pulmonary reactions, such as noncardiogenic pulmonary edema, are not uncommon 7 to 14 days after transplantation. This may be due to endothelial cell injury from the high-dose chemotherapy and/or radiation with subsequent permeability changes resulting in pulmonary edema.

Radiation Therapy

Although therapeutic irradiation is not considered a "drug" in the usual sense, it is a frequently prescribed therapy for neoplastic disease in the chest; predictable side effects on the lung occur at doses exceeding 4000 cGy. This topic is considered elsewhere in this book (see Chapter 51).

Pulmonary Oxygen Toxicity

The lungs are the major target of oxygen toxicity (see Chapter 151). The mechanism of oxygen toxicity is felt to be generation of free-radical products during the process of oxidative metabolism in the lung. Antioxidant defenses exist, but in the setting of overwhelming oxygen exposure these defenses are exhausted. Free-radical products then attack cell membranes and destroy lipids and proteins.

APPROACH TO THE PATIENT

Patients with drug-induced lung disease present with a variety of symptoms and manifestations dependent on their underlying disease and the pattern of injury induced by the drug. Symptoms, physical findings, and radiographic manifestations are almost never specific for drug-induced disease although they will be supportive. Therefore, a high index of suspicion for possible drug toxicity is necessary. In most cases, if the diagnosis is not considered and the drug is continued, the patient's symptoms and pulmonary status will worsen. Laboratory tests are usually nonspecific. In some situations, such as drug-induced lupus, high titers of autoantibodies may strongly support the diagnosis. Chest radiographs are usually abnormal except in cases of neuromuscular dysfunction or airways disease. But, the patterns usually do not offer firm evidence for a particular diagnosis.

The differential diagnosis for patients with drug-induced lung disease obviously depends on the pulmonary manifestations. For patients who present with interstitial pneumonitis-fibrosis, among the other diagnostic possibilities are infection, tumor, fluid, hemorrhage, or other idiopathic interstitial diseases. Clinical events, dose dependency, and duration of therapy may bear upon the likelihood of these possibilities. In order to exclude diagnoses such as infection or tumor, pulmonary tissue for histologic examination may be needed. Although transbronchial biopsy via the fiberoptic bronchoscope may be helpful in diagnosing certain types of infection or lymphangitic tumor, this procedure usually does not settle the issue of interstitial inflammatory disease. Therefore, if the patient is a reasonable operative candidate, open lung biopsy is usually done in an attempt to establish the diagnosis. But, even the tissue obtained by open lung biopsy is apt to yield nonspecific histologic findings, so that the diagnosis remains one of exclusion.

Discontinuing the offending agent is obviously the primary treatment for any type of drug-related lung disease. Corticosteroids have been given to many patients with drug-induced disease, especially those who develop interstitial pneumonitis, but clear criteria for their use are not available. As a rule, corticosteroids are given to patients who have severe reactions that are believed to be due to drug-related inflammation.

Detection of drug-induced disease at a subclinical or asymptomatic phase is difficult. Patients receiving drugs that have some predictable percentage of toxicity require close surveillance entailing routine examination of the lungs and chest radiographs; serial determinations of lung volumes and diffusing capacities for carbon monoxide may prove to be helpful. Stopping the offending drug early in the course of injury affords the best prospects for full recovery of pulmonary function.

BIBLIOGRAPHY

Alarcon-Segovia D: Drug-induced lupus syndromes. Mayo Clin Proc 44:664–681, 1969.
A classic that summarizes clinical data on the drug-induced lupus syndromes.

Aronin PA, Mahaley MS, Rudnick SA, Dudka L, Donohue JF, Selker RG, Moore P: Prediction of BCNU pulmonary toxicity in patients with malignant gliomas: An assessment of risk factors. N Engl J Med 303:183–188, 1980.
A classic clinical study documenting the dose effect of BCNU in producing pulmonary fibrosis.

Brewis RAL: Respiratory disorders, in Davies DM (ed), *Textbook of Adverse Drug Reactions*. Oxford, Oxford University Press, 1981, pp 154–187.
An overview of the drug reactions involving the lung plus an excellent review of the general problem of drug reactions.

Brooks BJ Jr, Seifter EJ, Walsh TE, Lichter AS, Bunn PA, Zabell A, Johnston-Early A, Edison M, Makuch RW, Cohen MH et al: Pulmonary toxicity with combined modality therapy for limited stage small-cell lung cancer. J Clin Oncol 4:200–209, 1986.
In 80 patients with limited stage small-cell lung cancer treated in a randomized prospective trial, pulmonary toxicity was significantly more common with combined modality therapy than with chemotherapy alone (p = .017) and worse than expected with radiotherapy alone.

Camus PH, Jeannin L: The diseased lung and drugs. Arch Toxicol Suppl 7:66–87, 1984.
An attempt to explain the mechanism of interactions between drugs and pulmonary tissues.

Carson CW, Cannon GW, Egger MJ, Ward JR, Clegg DO: Pulmonary disease during the treatment of rheumatoid arthritis with low dose pulse methotrexate. Semin Arthritis Rheum 16:186–195, 1987.
Nine of 168 patients developed probable, or possible, methotrexate-induced pulmonary toxicity. All recovered completely with supportive care and/or corticosteroid therapy.

Comis RL, Kuppinger MS, Ginsberg SJ, Crooke ST, Gilbert R, Auchincloss JH, Prestayko AW: Role of single-breath carbon monoxide-diffusing in monitoring the pulmonary effects of bleomycin in germ cell tumor patients. Cancer Res 39:5076–5080, 1979.
Reports of serial pulmonary function testing in patients receiving bleomycin showing effects on lung volumes and diffusing capacity.

Cooper JAD, White DA, Matthay RA: Drug-induced pulmonary disease. Parts I–II. Am Rev Respir Dis 133:321–340, 488–505, 1986.
An excellent overview of drug reactions involving the lung.

Duprat G Jr, Chalaoui J, Sylvestre J, Robidoux A, Duranceau A: Pulmonary complications of multi-modality therapy for esophageal carcinoma. J Can Assoc Radiol 38:27–31, 1987.
A study of the incidence of pulmonary complications in 30 patients with cancer of the esophagus treated with multimodal therapy. Sequential measurements of $D_{L_{CO}}$ were more sensitive for detecting pulmonary damage than chest radiographs.

Ginsberg SJ, Comis RL: The pulmonary toxicity of antineoplastic agents. Sem Oncol 9:34–51, 1982.
A comprehensive review of the pulmonary toxicity of cancer chemotherapeutic agents.

Henningsen NC, Cederberg A, Hanson A, Johansson BW: Effect of long-term treatment with pro-caine amide. A prospective study with special regard to ANF and SLE in fast and slow acetylators. Acta Med Scand 198:475–482, 1975.
A classic regarding the SLE drug-induced syndrome due to procainamide.

Holmberg L, Boman G, Bottiger LE, Erickson B, Spross R, Wessling A: Adverse reactions to nitrofu-rantoin: Analysis of 921 reports. Am J Med 69:733–738, 1980.
Review of adverse reactions to nitrofurantoin over a 10-year period reported to the Swedish Adverse Drug Reaction Committee.

Kennedy JI, Myers JL, Plumb VJ, Fulmer JD: Amiodarone pulmonary toxicity. Clinical, radiologic, and pathologic correlations. Arch Intern Med 147:50–55, 1987.
In 15 patients with amiodarone pulmonary toxicity, an interstitial pneumonia with foamy alve-olar macrophages was the most common pathologic finding. However, neither foamy alveolar macrophages nor lamellated cytoplasmic inclusions reliably distinguish toxic from nontoxic patients.

Marchlinski FE, Gansler TS, Waxman HL, Josephson ME: Amiodarone pulmonary toxicity. Ann Intern Med 97:839–845, 1982.
Description of four patients with amiodarone pulmonary toxicity, with emphasis on microscopic findings of the pathologic reaction.

Martin WJ: Nitrofurantoin: Evidence for the oxidant injury of lung parenchymal cells. Am Rev Respir Dis 127:482–486, 1983.
Nitrofurantoin incubated with pulmonary parenchymal cells resulted in lung cell injury. The injury was exacerbated by hypoxia and decreased by antioxidants.

McCullough B, Collins JF, Johanson WG Jr, Grover FL: Bleomycin-induced diffuse interstitial pul-monary fibrosis in baboons. J Clin Invest 61:79–88, 1978.
An excellent animal study of drug-induced pulmonary fibrosis with bleomycin.

Myers JL, Kennedy JI, Plumb VJ: Amiodarone lung: pathologic findings in clinically toxic patients. Hum Pathol 18:349–354, 1987.
Lung biopsy and autopsy specimens of 12 patients with amiodarone pulmonary toxicity re-vealed that interstitial pneumonia was the most common manifestation of amiodarone lung. Foamy alveolar macrophages and cytoplasmic lamellar inclusions are characteristic, but nei-ther is specific.

Rakita L, Sobol SM, Mostow N, Vrobel T: Amiodarone pulmonary toxicity. Am Heart J 106:906–916, 1983.
Literature review of cases with data on findings with serial pulmonary function tests and experi-ence with rechallenge.

Slepian IK, Matthews KP, McLean JA: Aspirin-sensitive asthma. Chest 87:386–391, 1985.
Review of the clinical problem of aspirin-sensitive asthma and experimental evidence for pros-taglandin mediators.

Sostman HD, Matthay RA, Putman CE, Walker Smith GJ: Methotrexate-induced pneumonitis. Med-icine 55:371–388, 1976.
Analysis of seven original cases and literature of the clinical, radiographic, and pathologic features of methotrexate-induced lung disease.

Chapter 53

Primary Pulmonary Histiocytosis X

Edward C. Rosenow III

Primary pulmonary histiocytosis X is one of a group of closely related disorders now encompassed by the designation *histiocytosis X disease* (histiocytic reticulosis). Histiocytosis X disease is a benign disorder that includes Letterer-Siwe disease, Hand-Schüller-Christian disease, and eosinophilic granuloma, as well as primary pulmonary histiocytosis X. Not only do these entities have clinical features in common, but also one form not infrequently converts to another as it evolves. Histiocytosis X is neither hereditary nor familial in origin nor malignant nor related to the lipoid reticuloendothelioses. One shared pathologic feature is the presence, on histologic section, of eosinophilic granulomas that contain the histiocytosis X cell (see below).

In 1940 Lichtenstein and Jaffe first recognized the relationship between eosinophilic granuloma of bone, the histiocytic reticuloses of Letterer-Siwe disease, and Hand-Schüller-Christian disease. But it was not until 1951 that Lackey and Farinacci recognized that the entity encompassed a spectrum of disease: Letterer-Siwe disease almost invariably becomes evident before age 2 years, whereas Hand-Schüller-Christian disease is a disseminated histiocytic reticulosis in the older infant and young adult.

Primary pulmonary histiocytosis X is predominantly a disease of the third and fourth decades but has been reported in infants as well as individuals in their 70s. The incidence in males and females is about equal. Originally considered to be a rare disease, more than 1000 cases have now been reported. Primary pulmonary histiocytosis X is exceedingly uncommon in blacks and almost unheard of in Asians. Because of the presence of granulomas as well as eosinophils, it has been postulated that histiocytosis X is an autoimmune or hypersensitivity disease. Although neither hypothesis has been proved, the common findings of immune complexes and other immunologic abnormalities lend support to an immunologic basis for this disease. Along the same line, in Letterer-Siwe disease, the number of circulating suppressor T lymphocytes is decreased, and the ratio of helper T cells to suppressor T cells is abnormally high.

CLINICAL PRESENTATION

Approximately one-quarter of the patients with primary pulmonary histiocytosis X are asymptomatic, the disease being discovered on a routine chest radiograph. In the others, the presenting manifestations may be either pulmonary, systemic, or both. A nonproductive cough is the most common symptom; next in rank order are dyspnea and chest pain. Ten to twenty percent of patients, either initially or during the course of their disease, develop a pneumothorax; half of these develop recurrent or bilateral pneumothoraxes. Fever, wheezing, weight loss, and hemoptysis occur in a minority. Diabetes insipidus occurs in 15 percent, and eosinophilic granuloma of bone in 20 percent. There is no occupational or geographic predisposition to this disease. But the disease occurs predominantly in cigarette smokers; 97 percent of patients were smokers in one series and 80 percent in another.

The physical examination is usually unremarkable except for prolonged expiration in those with airways obstruction. Although clubbing of the digits does occur, its incidence is presumably low.

RADIOGRAPHY

The chest radiograph is abnormal in virtually all patients with proven histiocytosis X. The middle lung fields are consistently involved; involvement of the upper or lower lung fields is common but less consistent. The costophrenic angles are spared in more than three-quarters of the patients.

The patterns of the lesions seen on the chest radiograph vary considerably: from micronodular, nodular, or reticular on the one hand to cystic and honeycombing on the other (Figs. 53-1 to 53-5). Whether the disease uniformly begins in the micronodular (miliary) pattern and then progresses successively through the other stages, or if it sometimes begins with the cystic and honeycomb patterns, is unclear. Uncommonly the abnormalities are first manifested as nodules greater than 1 cm, as cavitating nodules, or in an alveolar pattern (Table 53-1).

TABLE 53-1
Abnormalities in the Chest Radiograph in Primary Pulmonary Histiocytosis X (50 Patients)*

	Incidence, Percent
Reticulation	94
Micronodules, <2 mm†	92
Cysts, <10 mm	50
Micronodules, 2 to 5 mm	40
Pneumothorax	14
Costophrenic angles	16
Pleural effusion	0
Hilar adenopathy	0
Alveolar infiltrates	0

*Based on Lacronique et al., 1982.

†In diameter.

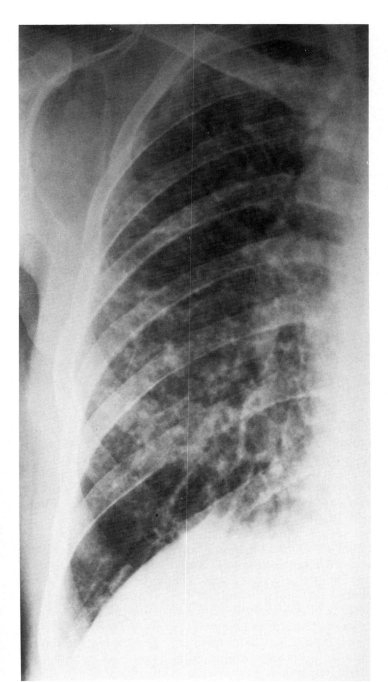

FIGURE 53-2 Primary pulmonary histiocytosis X in 28-year-old man. Micro- and macronodularity are associated with a lesser amount of reticular pattern. Small cysts are present at the apex.

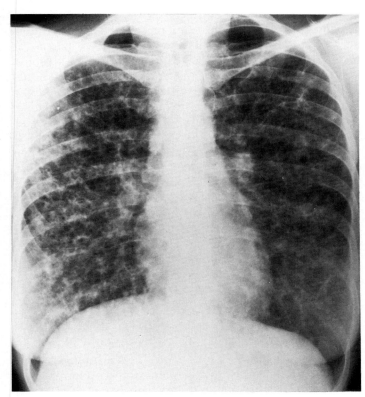

FIGURE 53-1 Primary pulmonary histiocytosis X. A diffuse reticular pattern with some micronodularity is present as well as bullae, both larger and smaller than 10 mm.

Radiographically, the lung volumes generally appear to be normal or increased according to the stage of the disease: hyperinflation is caused by large cysts that are believed to begin as bronchioles and then enlarge by air trapping and by bullae that are consequent to overdistension of lung in the vicinity of fibrotic and destroyed alveolar tissue; conversely, shrinkage of the lung volumes, as in advanced idiopathic interstitial fibrosis or sarcoidosis, is exceedingly uncommon. Hilar abnormalities occur in about one-quarter of the patients. Although sometimes these radiographic abnormalities can be identified as representing either lymphadenopathy or enlarged pulmonary arteries, in most instances the nature of the hilar abnormality is speculative.

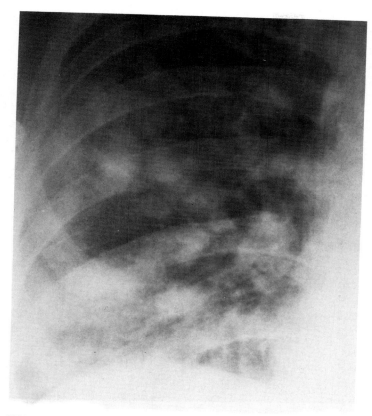

FIGURE 53-3 Primary pulmonary histiocytosis X in 36-year-old man. The pattern of the macronodules is predominantly alveolar.

From the radiographic picture, some prognostic guidelines can be established. The occurrence of large cysts and bullae and pneumothorax, as well as involvement of lungs in the costophrenic angles, dims the prognosis. However, the presence of large cysts and bullae does not preclude the possibility of stabilization or improvement. It is not uncommon for infiltrates to clear completely along with symptomatic improvement, either spontaneously or while the patient is taking corticosteroids. However, in many patients who improve symptomatically, the chest radiograph does not completely return to normal. Clear costophrenic angles at the outset seem to improve the prospect for complete resolution of the infiltrate.

PULMONARY FUNCTION

Although some abnormality in gas exchange is found in most patients with this disease, in about 15 percent of patients with primary pulmonary histiocytosis X, pulmonary function is normal. In some instances, a low diffusing capacity for carbon monoxide is the only detectable abnormality in pulmonary function, even though the chest radiograph is distinctly abnormal.

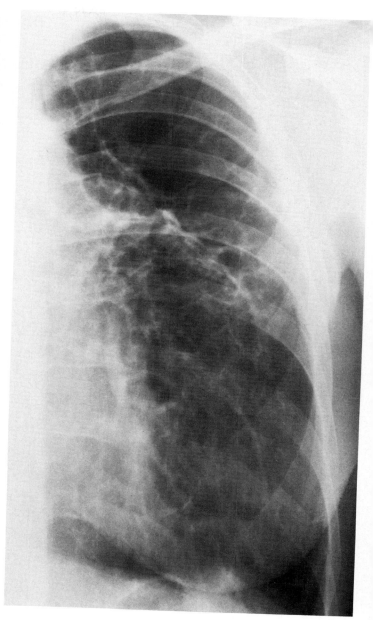

FIGURE 53-4 Primary pulmonary histiocytosis X in 62-year-old man. Late-stage bullous disease is evident.

Few comprehensive descriptions are available of pulmonary function in primary pulmonary histiocytosis X. However, obstructive lung disease is a characteristic feature of histiocytosis X, particularly in the later stages when bullae are present. In the early stages, obstructive airways disease is attributable to granulomatous involvement of the bronchioles. But, assignment of an etiology to the airways obstruction is often complicated by a history of cigarette smoking.

The degree to which abnormalities in gas exchange are reversible, either as a result of spontaneous resolution or as a result of corticosteroids, is unclear. In a study by

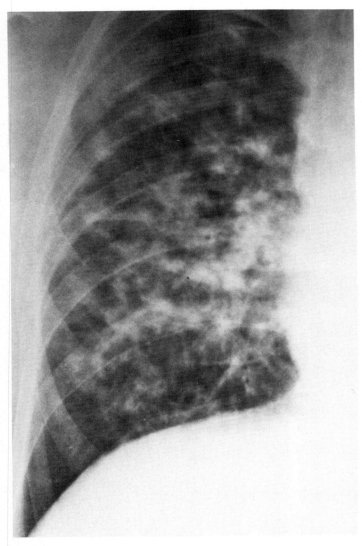

FIGURE 53-5 Primary pulmonary histiocytosis X in 46-year-old man. Both a reticular pattern and macronodularity are seen. The costophrenic angles are spared. Some small bullae are present.

Friedman et al. of 22 patients, and in our own experience (unpublished), little improvement occurs in the course of a 2-year period of follow-up.

PATHOLOGY

The lesions in the lungs may assume different forms: (1) discrete parenchymal infiltrates that range in size from miliary nodules to tumorous masses, (2) granulomatous polypoid lesions of the airways, (3) pleural plaques, and (4) "honeycomb lungs." The early parenchymal lesions are discrete and separated by normal lung. The usual lesion is 1 to 5 mm in diameter. About one-third of the nodules undergo necrosis and about one-half are associated

with honeycombing, primarily a consequence of destroyed alveolar walls and distortion produced by pulmonary fibrosis, and secondarily by air trapping distal to deformed bronchioles.

The histologic changes are unique to histiocytosis X (Figs. 53-6 and 53-7): for the diagnosis to be made, histiocytosis X cells must be seen. These histiocytes resemble Langerhans cells that are normally present in the skin but not in normal lung tissue; the possibility has been raised that the precursor of both of these cells is the mononuclear phagocytic system. In some instances, it is difficult to distinguish histiocytosis X cells from alveolar macrophages and fibroblasts. The cytoplasm of the histiocytosis X cell is pale and eosinophilic; the cell borders are indistinct and the nucleus is indented and elongated. The cell is not stained by p-aminosalicylic acid (PAS) and some-

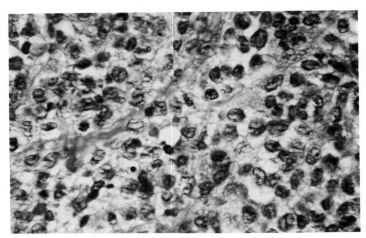

FIGURE 53-6 Lung tissue in primary pulmonary histiocytosis X. The histiocytosis X cells (Langerhans cell) are typical. A characteristic longitudinal groove is seen along the center of some cells. ×96.

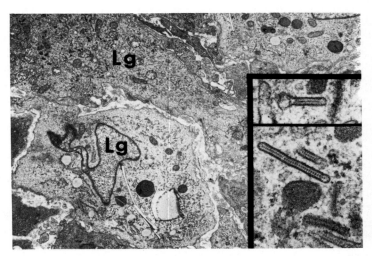

FIGURE 53-7 Electron micrograph of Langerhans cell (Lg) of the lung. Typical X bodies (Birbeck granules) are seen in the two inserts.

times shows mitotic activity. Within the histiocytosis X cell are "X bodies," or "Birbeck granules," that are 40 to 45 nm wide; their significance is unknown.

The histiocytosis X cell is rarely seen on histologic examination of the normal lung. But it does occur in the lungs of nearly one-fourth of patients with idiopathic pulmonary fibrosis and hypersensitivity pneumonitis. It is not found in sarcoidosis, inorganic pneumoconiosis, or pulmonary lymphangioleiomyomatosis. In contrast to the rarity of histiocytosis X cells in bronchoalveolar fluid from patients with other interstitial disorders, numerous histiocytosis X cells are recovered in the bronchoalveolar lavage fluid from most patients with primary pulmonary histiocytosis X.

Eosinophils are also found in about 80 percent of lung biopsies in primary pulmonary histiocytosis X. Eosinophilia is intense in about 15 percent and ranges from mild to moderate in the others. Other inflammatory cells, notably lymphocytes and polymorphonuclear leukocytes, contribute to the granulomatous response. Peripheral blood eosinophilia is exceedingly rare.

Commonly, the lesions of histiocytosis X include involvement of vessels and bronchioles, lymphoid proliferation to form follicles, and desquamation of cells into the alveolar spaces in the vicinity of the lesions. Next to each other are often found varying stages of activity, ranging from dividing histiocytosis X cells to fibrosis.

DIAGNOSIS

In the past, the diagnosis has been made by open lung biopsy in virtually all patients with primary pulmonary histiocytosis X. Some clinicians have felt comfortable in entertaining the diagnosis without histologic confirmation, as long as the characteristic radiologic pattern was present — including sparing of the costophrenic angles — particularly if a pneumothorax had occurred. Additional confirmation was supported by the finding of eosinophilic granulomas in the bone and diabetes insipidus.

At present, transbronchoscopic lung biopsy and bronchoalveolar lavage provide alternatives to open lung biopsy. The diagnostic yield from transbronchoscopic lung biopsy is indeterminate but is probably less than 50 percent. More apt to be diagnostic of pulmonary involvement in histiocytosis X is bronchoalveolar lavage (BAL), unless the disease is so inactive that the histiocytes are gone. For the diagnosis to be made by bronchoalveolar lavage, the characteristic histiocytosis X cell must be identified; this cell has not been seen in BAL fluid obtained from patients with any other entity. These cells account for 2 to 20 percent of the cells. Characteristically, the number and percentage of lymphocytes and/or polymorphonuclear leukocytes in the lavage fluid are also abnormally high. However, neither the quality nor quantity of cells pro-

vides a basis for prognosis. Nor has the gallium 67 scan proved to be either diagnostic or prognostic. The value of assessing the number of helper and suppressor T lymphocytes in the adult with primary pulmonary histiocytosis X has not yet been assessed.

COMPLICATIONS

Eosinophilic granuloma of the bone occurs in 4 to 15 percent of patients with primary pulmonary histiocytosis X. These values may be an underestimate since most patients do not undergo a bone survey unless there is bone pain. In 80 percent of adults with eosinophilic granulomas of bone, the lesions are solitary and involve the flat bones. The radiologic pattern in bone is not diagnostic of eosinophilic granuloma. Twenty percent of patients with eosinophilic granuloma of bone have pulmonary complications. Pulmonary involvement seems to occur early in the course of extrapulmonary disease or not at all.

Pneumothorax occurs in 10 to 20 percent of patients with primary pulmonary histiocytosis X; it favors young males who are less than 30 years of age. In most every instance, cysts and bullae are evident radiographically. Up to one-half of the pneumothoraxes are bilateral. It is very unusual for the pulmonary involvement of histiocytosis X to present as spontaneous pneumothorax if the chest radiograph is normal.

Diabetes insipidus occurs in 10 to 15 percent of patients with primary pulmonary histiocytosis X. The incidence is higher in those with Hand-Schüller-Christian disease. The possibility has been raised but remains unproven that the incidence of lymphoma is increased in patients with primary pulmonary histiocytosis X.

TREATMENT

Corticosteroids are the treatment of choice if there is evidence of progression of disease or potentially reversible symptoms such as dyspnea. However, it is difficult to assess the effects of therapy because of the propensity for spontaneous remission of the disease. Nearly two-thirds of patients with primary pulmonary histiocytosis X reverse, or stabilize either spontaneously or while taking corticosteroids. Most of the others remain symptomatic; in a few, the disease progresses to culminate in respiratory failure and cor pulmonale. Quitting smoking is mandatory.

In those who progress despite an adequate trial of corticosteroids, a trial of vinca alkaloids, such as vincristine or vinblastine, should be considered. These are the drugs of choice in treating disseminated disease. Symptomatic or progressively enlarging eosinophilic granuloma of the bone is treated either by excision, curettage, or radiation. Corticosteroids may also cause remission of lesions in bone.

PROGNOSIS

The prognosis of primary pulmonary histiocytosis X in the adult is very good. The overall mortality is estimated to be less than 5 percent—in contrast with estimates of 25 to 40 percent for disseminated histiocytosis X. Opportunistic infections are common in Letterer-Siwe disease but not in the other reticuloses.

BIBLIOGRAPHY

Basset F, Ferrans VJ, Soler P, Takemura T, Fukuda Y, Crystal RG: Intraluminal fibrosis in interstitial lung disorders. Am J Pathol 122:443–461, 1986.
 The histopathologic and ultrastructural features of intraluminal organizing and fibrotic changes were studied in open lung biopsies and autopsy specimens from 373 patients with interstitial lung disorders, including histiocytosis X (n-90).

Friedman PJ, Liebow AA, Sokoloff J: Eosinophilic granuloma of lung. Clinical aspects of primary pulmonary histiocytosis in the adult. Medicine 60:385–396, 1981.
 A review of 100 cases of eosinophilic granuloma diagnosed by open lung biopsy. The outcome was generally benign. The more severe manifestations, i.e., pneumothorax, fibrosis and honeycombing, and diabetes insipidus were found in young men. Smoking was far more common among these patients than in the general population.

Huhn D, König G, Weig J, Schneller W: Therapy in pulmonary histiocytosis X. Haematol Blood Transfus 27:231–237, 1981.
 Clinical findings and course of the disease are described in six patients with primary pulmonary histiocytosis X. Diagnosis was suspected because of a reticulonodular pattern on the chest radiograph or computed tomography of the lungs. Pulmonary function was impaired. In monitoring the course of the disease, repeated radiography and pulmonary function tests were of particular value.

Kawanami O, Basset F, Ferrans VJ, Soler P, Crystal RG: Pulmonary Langerhans' cells in patients with fibrotic lung disorders. Lab Invest 44:227–233, 1981.
 Langerhans cells were found in lung biopsies in one of nine control patients and in 20 of 160 patients with fibrotic lung disorders. Langerhans cells were not found in any of the 41 patients with sarcoidosis, the 35 patients with interstitial lung diseases associated with inhalation of inorganic dusts, the seven patients with pulmonary lymphangioleiomyomatosis, or the two patients with chronic eosinophilic pneumonia. In primary pulmonary histiocytosis X, histiocytosis X cells (HX cells) were seen in granulomas, in alveolar interstitium, between epithelial cells of the lower respiratory system, and in airspaces.

Komp DM: Long-term sequelae of histiocytosis X. Am J Pediatr Hematol/Oncol 3:165–168, 1981.
 Because of either continuously active disease or scarring of previously affected tissues, residual disabilities occur in more than half of children who survive histiocytosis X. Fatal outcomes from disabilities are seen particularly with primary pulmonary histiocytosis X, from either progressive fibrosis or complicating opportunistic infections.

Lacronique J, Roth C, Battesti J-P, Basset F, Chretien J: Chest radiological features of pulmonary histiocytosis X: A report based on 50 adult cases. Thorax 37:104–109, 1982.
 This study describes the chest radiographs of 50 adult patients with histologically verified histiocytosis X, proposes a radiologic classification, and examines the role of radiology in assessing the course and prognosis of the disease. Sparing of both costophrenic angles carries a good prognosis.

Lombard CM, Medeiros LJ, Colby TV: Pulmonary histiocytosis X and carcinoma. Arch Pathol Lab Med 111:339–341, 1987.
 Four patients who developed both pulmonary histiocytosis X and carcinoma of the lung are described. Bibliography refers to previous studies by same group on histologic and clinical features and course.

Prophet D: Primary pulmonary histiocytosis X. Clin Chest Med 3:643–653, 1982.
 After an overview of the clinical and pathologic features of the disease, the author reviews reports in the literature that used corticosteroids in therapy. Despite extensive use, the value of corticosteroids is unproven, but they are still tried empirically.

Chapter *54*

Occupational Pulmonary Diseases

Hans Weill / Robert N. Jones

The workplace has long been recognized as a source of potentially hazardous exposure. The lungs are the primary vital organs which are in direct contact with airborne contaminants, and it is not surprising that early recognition of occupational lung diseases was recorded centuries ago. Even the incomplete understanding of these hazards often led to the amelioration of the risks (rarely their elimination). However, an increasingly complex industrial society, with continuing introduction of new materials and processes, has added new risks which have become the legitimate concern of all members of society. Causal relations between environmental agents and respiratory diseases can often be suspected on the basis of anecdotal information (e.g., case reports). In most circumstances, however, the prevention of undesired health effects ultimately depends on the establishment of dose-response relationships, which provide quantitative estimates of risk for estimated conditions and levels of exposure. This leads to rational policy judgments regarding management of these risks. Decisions may then be made to avoid any exposure, when all estimated exposure-related risks are considered unacceptable. Or there may be very low risks that under certain conditions of exposure are considered reasonable and that compare favorably with many familiar and acceptable risks taken in our daily lives.

It is important as well to elucidate the mechanism and influence of host factors, which may provide information regarding the size and characteristics of any susceptible group of exposed workers. It may allow the avoidance of risk in a small, unduly sensitive group of workers. These data, providing information on the nature and quantitative aspects of risk, can be expected to provide the scientific basis for the determination that a material or process can be reasonably used within limits of practicality and economic feasibility or that substitution is required. This decision-making process must include those who are taking the risk, will invariably take into account the benefit to society of the material or process causing the risk, and will generally result in the taking of steps to reduce it.

The investigation of occupational lung disease must be multidisciplinary and requires expertise in pulmonary disease, epidemiology, statistics, physiology, immunology, cell biology, and environmental characterization. Sampling and measurement of airborne inhalants vary according to their type. Particulates are generally collected by personal gravimetric dust sampling to determine total and respirable fractions of dust to which the individual worker is exposed. It is sometimes possible to analyze for specific components of these dusts. Sampling periods are variable, but in general provide time-weighted average values. For asbestos, and for man-made mineral fibers (e.g., fibrous glass), individual fibers are counted under the microscope and expressed in terms of number per unit volume of air sampled. Vapors and gases can be sampled for average airborne concentrations with simple chemical devices or may be continuously monitored through the use of electronic physicochemical detectors, which provide data on instantaneous and peak levels of exposure.

Respiratory health is assessed in exposed individuals by clinical, radiographic, functional, and immunologic methods. An adequate occupational history must include a chronological account of all past jobs and exposure—not just information concerning current or last employment. It is of obvious importance to know that a welder with radiographic evidence of advanced silicosis has for many years worked in the holds of ships directly adjacent to sandblasting operations. Specific clinical patterns may lead to the identification of an exposure-related disease, as, for example, the symptoms of bronchoconstriction which have occurred in cotton textile workers after renewed dust exposure following an absence from work. Chest radiographs have become an important tool for the detection and quantitation of mineral dust exposure ef-

fects, and in population studies they have become particularly effective through the use of the International Labor Office (ILO) international classification.

Pulmonary function testing provides important information, both in the individual who is being monitored by serial studies, which reveal an unfavorable longitudinal course, and in investigations of populations, both cross-sectional and prospective, where lung function becomes an important response variable which can be correlated with other biologic indicators as well as estimates of exposure. Studies to date have generally shown that simpler lung function measurements (primarily, well-standardized spirometric testing) have provided information at least as useful as more complex tests (e.g., pulmonary diffusing capacity or airways resistance). This is fortunate, since the latter may be difficult to apply in the occupational health monitoring of exposed workers or in large epidemiologic surveys. Even when looking for the early effects of mineral dust exposure (e.g., asbestos), there is good evidence that such reactions can be detected by measurements of ordinary ventilatory function. This appears to be a logical consequence of the initial peribronchiolar tissue reactions of particulate materials which have been deposited in the respiratory bronchioles. The proper timing of lung function measurements in relation to exposures can enhance the sensitivity of the tests. The demonstration that a postshift ventilatory function decline in cotton-dust-exposed workers occurs early in the work week has been strikingly helpful in the detection of this adverse effect. Pulmonary function testing following an inhalation challenge, which has clearly demonstrated a late (4- to 6-h) drop in ventilatory function, often without a detectable immediate bronchoconstrictor response, has been helpful in the understanding of clinical patterns in many forms of occupational asthma.

Since a number of occupational diseases of the airways and pulmonary parenchyma are based on immunologic mechanisms, measurements to detect abnormal humoral antibodies and cellular immunity are finding wide application in the investigation of individuals and groups exposed to potentially allergenic inhalants. These procedures will range from simple skin-prick testing, through assays for specific IgE (radioallergosorbent test, or RAST), to newer in vitro tests of cell-mediated immunity.

Data collected in the studies of populations are used by the epidemiologist and statistician to assess the presence, determinants, and magnitude of the risk to respiratory health caused by specific occupational exposures. Confounding factors, such as age, cigarette smoking, and atopy, can be dealt with by multiple regression analyses. The time-response relationship will vary from the immediate reaction following the inhalation of an irritant gas to a delay of many years before the appearance of an environmentally induced malignant effect or fibrosis due to mineral dust.

The principal causes of occupational pulmonary disorders fall into three major categories: (1) mineral (inorganic) dusts, causing diffuse fibrosis or deposition with only limited cellular reaction, and including metal dusts and fumes which may cause a wide spectrum of lung disorders, ranging from acute pneumonia to diffuse granuloma and fibrosis; (2) organic dusts, which may cause hypersensitivity pneumonia or asthma; and (3) gases and chemical vapors, which may cause acute and chronic airways and alveolar inflammatory injury, through an irritant mechanism, or occupational asthma in susceptible workers. In addition, particulate or gaseous materials may be carcinogenic.

COAL WORKER'S PNEUMOCONIOSIS

Coal worker's pneumoconiosis (CWP) is the result of deposition of coal dust in the lungs. Its simple form is usually asymptomatic, although the dust can produce chronic bronchitis. In a small percentage of cases, progressive massive fibrosis (PMF) may develop. The risk of subsequently developing PMF is related to the severity (category) of simple CWP. After termination of exposure, simple disease does not advance, but complicated massive disease may progress after exposure ceases, with potential for respiratory failure and a fatal outcome. The disease is intensified by inhalation of free silica; silica increases the risk of and enhances progression to PMF. The complicated disease is often associated with evidence of autoimmune serologic reactions.

The development of chronic pulmonary disease in coal miners has been recognized for centuries. In the late nineteenth century, the dust disease of miners was simply classified as *pneumoconiosis*. The opinion was strongly held that free silica was the cause until later developments in the United Kingdom, notably Wales, clarified the roles of free silica and coal dust in the etiology of the disease. In the early twentieth century, it was thought that CWP was no longer a problem because of the effectiveness of preventive measures, but by 1935 a great increase in CWP was reported in the United Kingdom. The change was related to the introduction of machinery which increased coal production but raised the concentration of coal dust within the mines. Cases of silicosis were reported in coal miners, but it was recognized that others engaged in operations which did not involve exposure to crystalline free silica were developing pneumoconiosis. The appearance of pneumoconiosis in coal trimmers, specialized longshoremen who carried coal, established this point and led to the specific diagnosis *coal worker's pneumoconiosis*.

Pathology

The disease follows exposure to high concentrations of coal dust and is more likely to occur in miners who cut coal of high rank, notably anthracite, in which the volatile component is as low as 5%. The earliest pulmonary dust foci are located adjacent to the walls of the respiratory bronchioles. The dust macules produce little fibrosis, but damage the adjacent fine airways, predisposing to focal or centrilobar emphysema, which may be difficult to distinguish (Fig. 54-1). While there continues to be controversy about whether destructive forms of emphysema are the result of simple CWP, there is increasing evidence that coal dust exposure does increase the risk of centrilobular emphysema.

The disease is observed in two stages: the simple coal macule, in which there is little fibrous reaction, and the complicated type, in which large masses containing carbon and scar are present (Fig. 54-2). The macular lesions may enlarge and coalesce to form broad sleeves along the respiratory bronchioles. The simple lesions are usually complicated by focal emphysema, which may be the result of excessive inspiratory traction upon or weakening of the wall of the respiratory bronchiole. If exposure continues, the disease may progress. Simple lesions will usually stabilize on termination of exposure and have been said to partially regress (not considered likely), but complicated massive lesions remain active and are associated with lobar contraction and distortion of bronchial and pulmonary structure. In PMF, gross bronchial and vascular occlusions are noted. Bland excavation of the masses has occurred. A small percentage of such cases is still associated with infections by tubercle bacilli and atypical mycobacteria.

PATHOGENESIS

The tissue changes of CWP largely represent the cellular response to the dose of inhaled dust. The relationship can be distorted by two principal factors: autoimmunity and the presence of other fibrogenic dusts. In coal-induced, as in other pneumoconioses, the dangerous element is respirable dust with particles substantially less than 10 μm in diameter. A great excess of particles 1 to 3 μm in diameter results in heavy alveolar deposition and accumulation in the zones adjacent to the walls of the respiratory bronchioles. Coal dust is almost completely composed of carbon and rarely contains more than 10 percent (usually less than 5 percent) free silica. Silicotic lesions are uncommon, except in those who work at the borders of the coal seams and use high-energy machines which penetrate neighboring veins of rock. This is more likely to occur in anthracite workers (Fig. 54-3). Excessive silica dust exposure can affect transportation workers whose power-driven cars travel at rapid rates over rails that have been

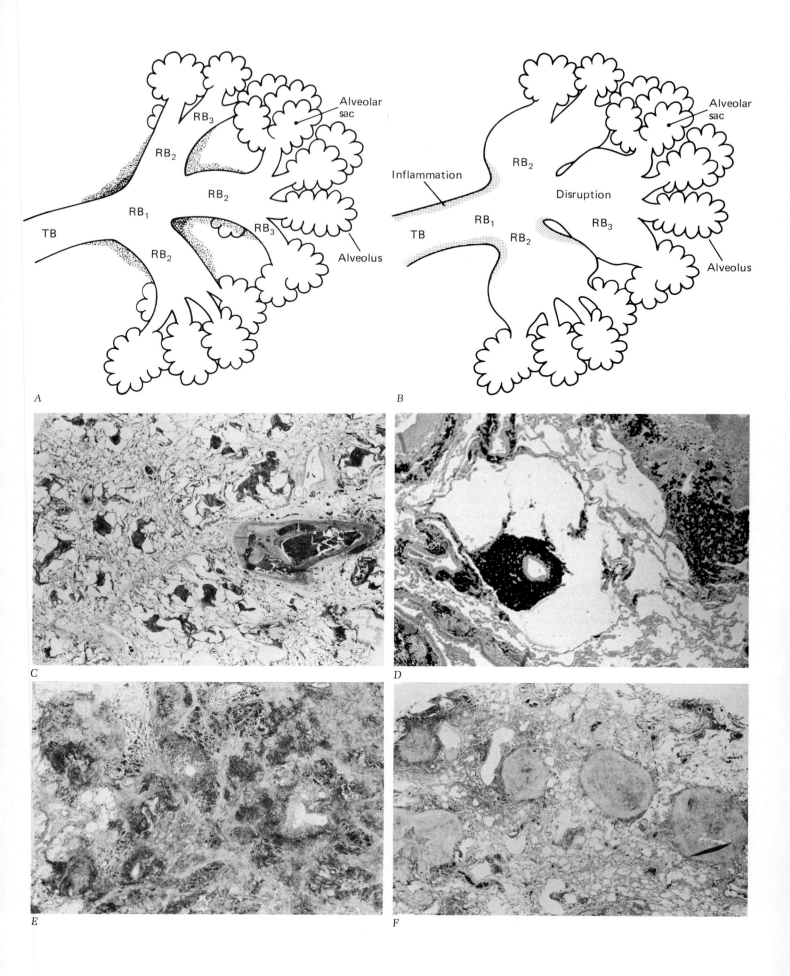

A

B

C

D

E

F

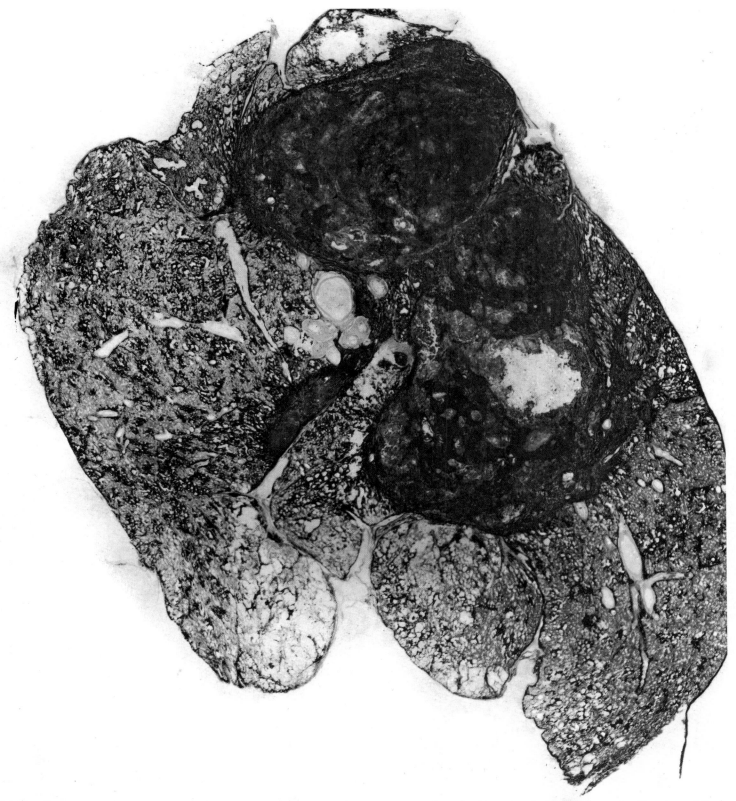

FIGURE 54-2 Massive pneumoconiosis in a 59-year-old coal miner of 30 years. Pulmonary hypertension, cor pulmonale. *(Courtesy of Professor J. Gough.)*

◀ **FIGURE 54-1** Microscopic changes in coal miner's pneumoconiosis. *A.* Schematic representation of coal macule (shaded area around respiratory bronchioles) (RB). *B.* Contrast with A. In centrilobular emphysema, local inflammation causes disruption of terminal bronchioles. *C.* Coal macules and focal emphysema. Geographic view (×2.5). *D.* Coal macule (×350). *E.* Section of lesion of progressive massive fibrosis. Geographic view (×2.5). *F.* Caplan's nodules in a coal miner's pneumoconiosis (×2.5). *(C to F, courtesy of Professor A. G. Heppleston.)*

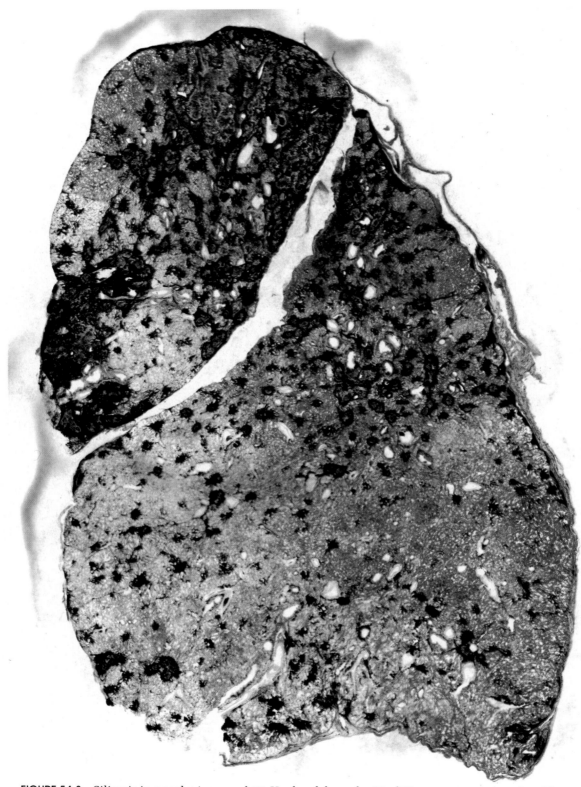

FIGURE 54-3 Silicosis in a coal miner, aged 56. Hard rock borer for 17 of 39 years as a mine worker. The silicosis is classic for the rock worker and distinct from the coal nodules and emphysematous changes of the miner who works on the coal face. *(Courtesy of Professor J. Gough.)*

covered with sand to prevent electrical explosions of gases.

The controversy about the role of silica in CWP has abated in the face of quantitative information from dust sampling, demonstrating dose-response relationships in low silica-containing coal dust exposures, and the demonstration of distinctive tissue reactions which differ from those of silicosis. Tuberculosis is uncommon and does not account for the changes of CWP. Other chronic infections are rare. Immunologic disorders and the development of autoimmune antibodies are often present, but specific collagen-vascular disorders other than rheumatoid arthritis are uncommon. It appears that the increased dust burden accounts for the higher incidence of CWP in this century and is responsible for the frequency of autoimmune serologic reactions.

In a minority of cases, typical silicosis may occur. Bronchitis is more common in coal miners than in the general population and cannot be explained on the basis of excessive cigarette smoking alone. The "industrial" bronchitis may represent a nonspecific response of the bronchial mucous membrane to prolonged heavy exposure to any irritating dust or chemical.

CLINICAL

Simple CWP is not likely to be responsible for significant respiratory symptoms in the absence of other complicating dust-related effects, such as industrial bronchitis. Long-term workers (a survivor group) are usually in good functional condition; their symptoms may be limited to irritative cough, wheezing, and sputum production. Respiratory symptoms may be more severe in those individuals who have retired from coal work, who make up a population which has been replaced because of PMF, more severe chronic obstructive disease, or other diseases. Dyspnea on effort is usually associated with complicated pneumoconiosis or smoking-related advanced chronic obstructive pulmonary disease (COPD). In such individuals, bronchitic symptoms are more severe, and melanoptysis may occur from excavated lesions. Complicated disease may be progressive and predisposes to recurrent infections and pulmonary hypertension and cor pulmonale. A small percentage of the patients with CWP develop symptomatic cavitary tuberculosis.

RADIOGRAPHY

The importance of standardized reading and interpretation of chest radiographs was recognized before World War II. Following the war, a system evolved under the aegis of the International Labor Office, supplemented by the International Union Against Cancer (UICC), for classifying chest radiographic changes in the pneumoconioses. The current version is the ILO 1980 Classification, which includes both written descriptions and illustrative radiographs. The reader determines if the chest radiograph shows opacities consistent with pneumoconiosis, notes their sizes and shapes, and then considers the extent of involvement of the lungs. In simple CWP (Fig. 54-4), the individual lesions are read as small opacities, rounded, or irregular, or both, and classified by size. Rounded opaci-

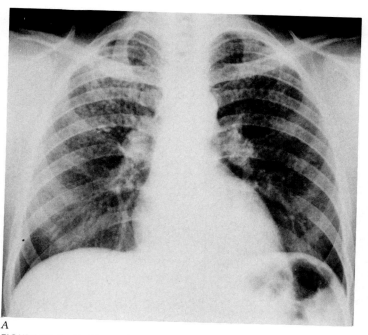

A

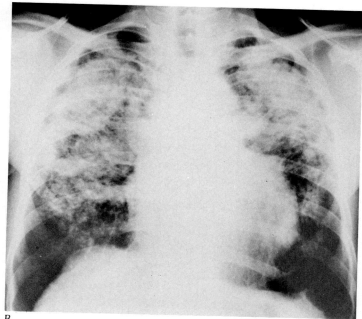

B

FIGURE 54-4 Radiographic changes in a coal miner's pneumoconiosis. *A.* Simple stage showing diffuse nodular lesions. *B.* Complicated stage, with progressive massive fibrosis and bullous emphysema. *(Courtesy of Dr. J. F. Wiot.)*

ties less than 1.5 mm are designated "p"; "q" opacities range from 1.5 to 3 mm; and "r" range from 3 to 10 mm. The finest irregular or linear lesions are "s"; with increasing coarseness, the lesions are classed as "t" and "u". The profusion (concentration) of these lesions within the lungs is read as an average in categories 0, 1, 2, or 3 (Fig. 54-5). The classification is expanded, however, since the reader gives an initial reading and then a final impression of the profusion of the lesions. For example, on a film ultimately considered to have category 1 profusion of small opacities, 1/2 ("one-slant-two") indicates that profusion category 2 was seriously considered. With 1/0, profusion category 0 was considered. A reading of 1/1 indicates no serious consideration of either adjacent category. The four major categories of the original system have thus been divided each into three subcategories, to form 12 divisions of the continuum from an appearance of exceptional normalcy, 0/ − , to one of exceptionally high profusion of small opacities, 3/ + . The characteristic opacities observed in simple CWP are rounded in type. It has been

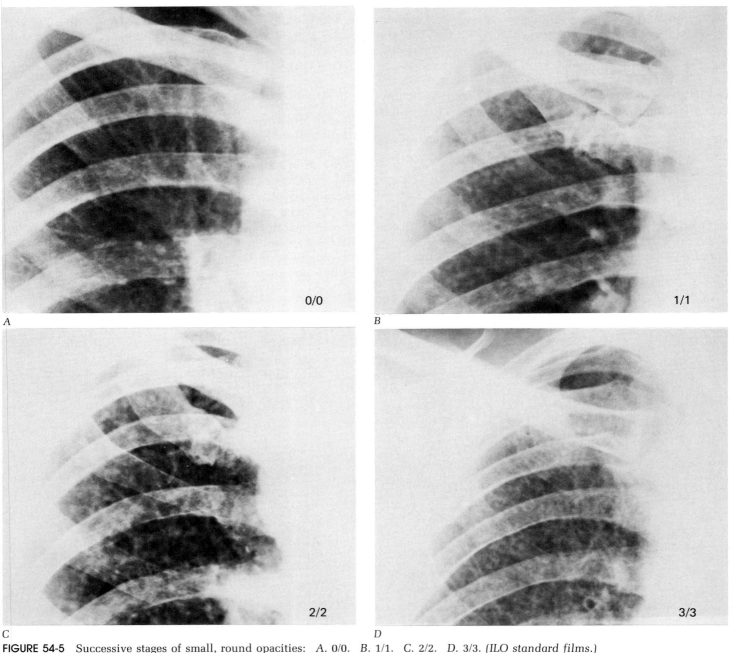

FIGURE 54-5 Successive stages of small, round opacities: *A.* 0/0. *B.* 1/1. *C.* 2/2. *D.* 3/3. *(ILO standard films.)*

suggested, but not resolved, however, that irregular small opacities may also be seen in simple CWP, that this appearance is the result of diffuse fibrosis and/or emphysema, and that their presence has unfavorable physiological implications.

Massive lesions are classified on the basis of their size. Lesions greater than 1 cm, with aggregate diameter less than 5 cm, are in category A; lesions of aggregate diameter greater than 5 cm, but covering less than the area of the upper third of the right lung, are B; and C opacities have an aggregate area equal to or exceeding the upper third of the right lung. The classification also grades pleural abnormalities and has symbols for loss of cardiac silhouette and diaphragm. Symbols are supplied for other findings, and room is provided on the standard form for comments about the individual film. The ILO classification has proved invaluable for monitoring exposed miners (allowing for intervention before progressive changes occur), for assessing the efficacy of dust control, and for studying epidemiology.

This method of standardized reading of chest radiographs has been validated in studies relating radiographic changes to pulmonary function, pathology, and the dust content of the lungs. Large studies of miners have found that the actual dust content correlates well with the extent and progression of simple CWP, as judged on the radiograph.

PULMONARY FUNCTION

Most studies have found no consistent abnormalities of ventilatory function that are attributable to simple CWP. Other measures of lung function have shown modest abnormalities, including, at times: increase in residual volume, reduction in pulmonary diffusing capacity in the presence of p opacities, increase in A-a oxygen gradient, an increased V_D/V_T ratio, and frequency dependence of compliance. The industrial bronchitis is said to involve the central airways and may result in some reduction in maximum expiratory flow indicators (e.g., FEV_1), although the effect of dust on these measures is found to be far less than that of smoking. In those who develop complication or progressive massive fibrosis, evidence of restrictive and obstructive disease may become striking, the relative proportions depending on the respective contributions of fibrosis, airway distortion, and chronic bronchitis and pulmonary emphysema. Gas-exchange disturbances may lead to respiratory failure and cor pulmonale.

Diagnosis

The diagnosis of CWP depends on the history of exposure and the changes noted on the chest radiograph. The appearance of simple nodular disease or massive changes in an exposed coal worker is sufficient to establish the presence of pneumoconiosis. The nature of the pneumoconiosis depends on the type of exposure. The question of silicosis or mixed pneumoconiosis can usually be determined from knowledge of the source of the dust and the course of the disease. As with other pneumoconioses, lung biopsy is not usually required for diagnosis. Sputum examination can demonstrate coal pigment, but this alone does not establish the diagnosis of CWP.

Treatment

In common with the other mineral dust diseases, effective management depends on prevention, usually through dust control, since there is no specific treatment for the coal deposits and the massive change within the lungs. Symptomatic bronchitis with bronchospasm can be relieved with antitussive and bronchodilator drugs. Complicating infections can be treated with general antibiotics, or in the case of tuberculosis, with specific antituberculosis drugs. In those individuals who have autoimmune disorders, notably rheumatoid arthritis, some aspects of the disease can be suppressed with anti-inflammatory drugs.

As suggested, the prevention of CWP requires effective ventilation of the mines. If the dust concentration is reduced, the deposition of respirable dust within the lungs will be reduced, and the risk of developing pneumoconiosis during an ordinary working lifetime will become small. Those who are engaged in especially dusty work, or who are periodically exposed to significant concentrations of free silica, should be provided with well-fitting respirators that can be comfortably used for the exposure periods. Early simple radiographic findings may not require termination of all exposure, depending on such factors as age and economic considerations, but enlargement of nodules on serial films should exclude the worker from all dusty trades.

Prognosis

Mortality studies have shown that reduced survival in relation to coal dust exposure is attributable to excess deaths from PMF, COPD and, perhaps, gastrointestinal neoplasms. Simple CWP does not appear to lead to increased mortality, except in those who, in past years, contracted their disease early in life (now unlikely, as a result of relatively low current exposures). The prognosis is therefore good for patients with simple disease, but the complicated disease, although uncommon, is progressive and produces disorders of respiratory function. Tuberculosis usually responds well to treatment in complicated CWP, but the massive disease has often progressed to cardiorespiratory insufficiency.

GRAPHITE

Graphite is mined as crystalline or amorphous carbon mixed with impurities, including free silica. Both mining and processing are dusty jobs and can lead to pneumoconiosis strongly resembling CWP. It has been noted that the simple form of graphite pneumoconiosis may include extensive zones of alveoli filled with carbon-laden macrophages. Associated diffuse interstitial fibrosis and massive fibrosis have been reported in graphite workers. In some cases suspected of being graphite pneumoconiosis, the fibrotic progressive changes have been related to rather high concentrations of inhaled free silica. Another related substance producing the same type of pneumoconiosis is carbon black, which is used as a filter and coloring agent in phonograph records and as a coloring agent in older printing processes. Graphite has similar uses in printing and foundry work and as a coloring agent and lubricant. It is used in the rubber industry and in carbon electrodes. It is an important constituent in metal mixtures and alloys and is well known in its use in pencils. Accumulations of graphite within the lungs may predispose to infection with atypical mycobacteria.

SILICON

The compounds of silicon are heavily concentrated within the rocks and soil of the earth's surface. The most common is silicon dioxide, known as free silica when uncombined with other chemical species. Of the varieties of free silica—crystalline, cryptocrystalline, and amorphous—the crystalline is most commonly associated with human pulmonary disease. In crystals of free silica, there is regular orientation of the atoms of silicon and oxygen. The orientation is random in the amorphous substance. The most common form of crystalline silica is quartz, found in granite, sandstone, and sand. Cristobalite and tridymite are other kinds of crystalline free silica which appear after exposure of amorphous silica to high temperatures. Flint and chalcedony are examples of cryptocrystalline silica; opal and diatomaceous earth are varieties of amorphous silica.

The physical properties of quartz as rock and sand are responsible for its widespread use in industry. Its hardness and resistance to thermal and chemical change are useful in structural and abrasive applications. It can be converted to glass by superheating. Fine rock crystal is used in electronics because it is extremely sensitive to pressure (piezoelectric effect). The relation of silica dust exposure, in mining, grinding, pottery manufacture, construction, and abrasive production, to excessive pulmonary disease was well recognized from the middle of the nineteenth century when the term *pneumoconiosis* was coined to designate diseases in which dust was retained within the lungs, with or without fibrous reaction.

Amorphous Silica

Natural amorphous silica, such as diatomite, also known as kieselguhr, is mildly fibrogenic after a long period of exposure. By heating, however, it can be converted into very toxic species of crystalline silica. The crude substance is extracted by open mining methods and later may be heated (*calcined*) at temperatures ranging from 800 to 1100°C to eliminate organic residues. The final products are fine and coarse powders that are widely used in filtration of organic and inorganic liquids and as insulating substances. Above 800°C, amorphous silica (less than 2% quartz) is converted to crystalline cristobalite in high concentration (20 to 60%). Toxic dust exposure is severe for mill hands and baggers; in one series, 25 percent of workers with more than 5 years of exposure had silicosis. The severe, accelerated disease encountered is related to the length of exposure to high concentrations of cristobalite. The clinical, physiological, and pathologic features of the disease will be described with those of other forms of accelerated silicosis. Dust suppression and the enclosure of dust-generating processes can prevent this type of silicosis. The current threshold limit value (TLV) for untreated diatomite is 20 million particles per cubic foot (MPPCF). For the calcined substance, it should be one-half that calculated for quartz.

SILICOSIS

Silicosis is the pulmonary fibrosis produced by respirable dust containing crystalline free silica. In most occupations carrying this risk, decades of exposure produce disseminated, discrete, small hyalinized nodules throughout the lungs. Silicosis in the stage of isolated small foci of fibrosis is termed *simple silicosis*. In some persons, the focal lesions coalesce to form masses of scar tissue, which can efface the architecture of large areas, contracting and distorting the lungs. That process is called *progressive massive fibrosis* and is a feature of other pneumoconioses. Silicosis in which the process of coalescence has begun is called *complicated silicosis*, a term which nowadays is devoid of its older implication of superinfection with tuberculosis. For clinical reasons it is also useful to identify several kinds of silicosis distinguished mainly by differences in the intensity of the causative exposures, with resultant differences in behavior of the disease. *Ordinary silicosis* is contracted after decades of moderate exposure in such jobs as hard rock mining or granite quarrying. Most of its sufferers are old men with simple silicosis. *Accelerated silicosis* is contracted after years of exposure to the higher concentrations produced by sandblasting or silica flour production, with suboptimal respiratory protection. Its sufferers are younger and face a higher risk of complicated silicosis. *Acute silicosis* has been seen after months to a few years of unprotected exposure to high concentrations: this variety of silicosis is rapidly progressive and usually fatal, but is now fortunately rare.

History

Silicosis was not distinguished from other forms of pneumoconiosis, nor they from chronic lung diseases in general, until the advances in pathology and bacteriology of the second half of the last century. It was named by Visconti in 1870. The incidence of the disease and its complications increased early in this century when the use of pneumatic mining drills and other machines and tools powered by high-energy sources raised the concentration of respirable dust particles in the workplace. Dust suppression measures, such as wet methods of mining and stonecutting, were then applied and shown to be efficacious in reducing disease incidence and severity. For a long time, it has been known that disabling or fatal silicosis occurs in response to grossly unhygienic working conditions, and so it is eminently preventable. Unfortunately, this knowledge has never been universal, nor has it been particularly durable. Succeeding generations of physicians and industrial hygienists have had to "rediscover" silicosis; and each new circumstance of occupational exposure seems to go unscrutinized until the health costs become obvious.

Occupational Exposure

Silicosis is the result of the cellular reactions which follow the inhalation, peripheral deposition, and retention of free silica particles. Peripheral deposition is maximal when particles are 0.5 to 3 μm in diameter. Respirable dust containing free silica is produced in many activities: mining and quarrying; extraction and processing of ores, rocks, and other quartz-containing substances; cutting and dressing stone; manufacture of pottery, porcelain, ceramic, and glass; preparation of ground silica and its compounding and use in mixtures such as paints and abrasive powders; removal of foundry molds and boiler scale; production, installation, and cleaning of refractory bricks; calcination of siliceous material prior to use in filtering; and manufacture of cement-based pipe and building and roofing materials. This list includes the major sources of silica exposure, but it is not exhaustive. Most sources involve mixed exposure to silica and other toxic or inert dusts. Dust exposure is intensified with increased activity, particularly when inadequate or faulty protective devices are used in enclosed spaces.

Dust samples can be collected using area samplers through which air is drawn at a rate of 1 ft^3/min (approximately 28 L/min). Respirable silica concentrations are estimated from the particle size distribution and percent silica known to obtain in the area. For respiratory health surveys, individual exposure levels may be measured with personal gravimetric samplers equipped with size-selective cyclones and attached to the workers' clothing in the breathing zone. The commonly used sampler operates at an airflow rate of 1.7 L/min and collects particles smaller than 10 μm in diameter on a millipore filter. The dust samples are weighed on a fine electrobalance and analyzed for percent crystalline free silica by x-ray diffraction.

Pathogenesis

The particles that reach the alveoli are cleared by phagocytosis and carried by secretions and ciliary motion up the airways. These defenses are overcome when deposition of particles within the airspaces is excessive. The toxic effect of crystalline free silica following phagocytosis has been visualized by transmission electron microscopy. The precise mechanism of toxicity remains unexplained, but the particles destroy the intracellular organelles; the phagosomes rupture, leading to enzymatic autolysis. The cellular products and residues stimulate migration of other macrophages and cells of fibroblastic potential. If the alveolar load is not overwhelming, plaques composed of inflammatory and necrotic cells form near the orifices of the respiratory bronchioles. Interstitial localization of particles is related to injury of lining cells and is followed by passage of some silica through the lymphatics to the lymph nodes, where typical nodules develop. The rare finding of particles or nodules in distant viscera is evidence of limited bloodstream dissemination of the mineral. The silicosis patient's liability to active infection by mycobacteria and fungi is probably the direct result of toxic injury to macrophages. Macrophages that survive silica dusting in vitro show reduced abilities to kill or suppress microbes. Tuberculosis or other infection is now rarely responsible for instances of progression from simple to complicated silicosis. The risk of progression in groups is roughly correlated with cumulative dose of silica, but the cause of progression in the individual patient is usually unknown.

Pathology

The alteration of bronchopulmonary structure in silicosis is related to the rates of mobilization and destruction of macrophages and of the conversion of connective tissue cells into fibroblasts. In uncomplicated, slowly progressive disease, the silicotic nodules produce little change in the intervening, uninvolved tissue. The nodules undergo fibrosis with hyaline degeneration and slowly enlarge (Fig. 54-6). Calcification of nodules is relatively uncommon. In simple disease, the lesions are usually not visible on chest radiographs until 20 years after the initial exposure.

Heavier exposure to respirable free silica produces an accelerated response. In sandblaster's silicosis, the lesions

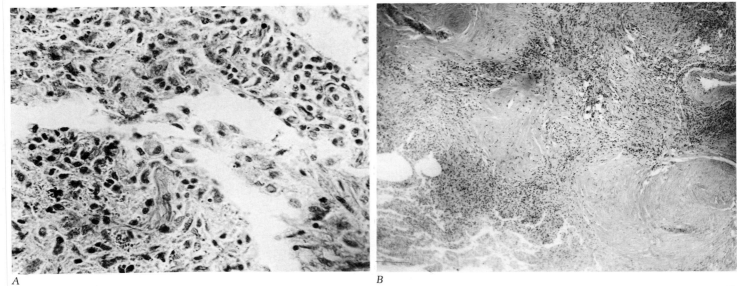

FIGURE 54-6 Classic simple silicosis. *A.* The alveolar walls are thickened by organization of luminal contents and accretion into the wall (H&E, ×390). *B.* The laminated silicotic nodules obliterate the parenchyma and are contiguous with the advancing margin of interstitial pneumonitis in the lower left of picture (H&E, ×47).

frequently appear as early as 4 to 8 years after first exposure. The nodules are cellular, and zones of diffuse fibrosis are common. Massive fibrosis of complicated silicosis is common and appears early. Very heavy exposure to respirable free silica produces early diffuse tissue reactions. Enclosed and poorly protected workers have developed visible disease in 6 to 9 months. Florid, so-called acute silicosis develops, in which the airspaces are filled with dead and dying macrophages. A diffuse interstitial reaction takes place in which few nodules are seen. In extreme cases, the intra-alveolar debris strongly resembles the lipoproteinaceous material of pulmonary alveolar proteinosis and has similar histochemical properties.

Complicated silicosis is characterized by masses composed of fibrous and acellular material usually situated within the upper lobes in chronic disease. Enlargement of the masses is associated with lobar contraction, and distortion and obstruction of bronchial branches. Compensatory emphysema occurs; the development of large bullae at the bases is common. There is apparent reduction of nodulation in association with these changes. Enlargement of lymph nodes is common in accelerated and advanced silicosis. Eggshell calcification of lymph nodes may be found in either simple or complicated silicosis and seems more related to duration than severity of disease. Patchy pleural thickening over the upper lobes is often noted in advanced silicosis. Bleb and bulla formation are responsible for occurrences of pneumothorax complicating advanced silicosis. In advanced, complicated disease with severe distortion of the vascular bed leading to pulmonary hypertension, cor pulmonale will develop.

Clinical Features

In ordinary silicosis, related symptoms occur late (if at all) and are long preceded by abnormalities of the chest radiograph. Cough and expectoration are common in patients with simple silicosis; most such patients also have a lengthy history of cigarette smoking. Since long exposures to a variety of fibrogenic and nonfibrogenic dusts have been shown to cause industrial bronchitis and since the development of silicosis proves that the individual has sustained excessive dust exposures, chronic bronchitis in a silicotic should be considered at least partly attributable to the occupational exposure.

Complicated disease can ultimately reduce the mass of functioning tissue and distort airways and blood vessels. It is often associated with chronic productive cough and effort dyspnea. The patient may become increasingly susceptible to lower respiratory infection by ordinary bronchial pathogens. Loss of weight and generalized weakness are common in advanced complicated silicosis.

Symptoms appear earlier in accelerated disease, which often develops within 10 years of onset of exposure. Complication occurs earlier and more often. In acute disease, the packing of airspaces with macrophages and the interstitial reaction lead to early and progressive dyspnea on exertion and generalized weakness and wasting. Cellular necrosis is rarely associated with fever in the absence of infection.

The physical findings vary with the state of the disease. Simple nodulation produces no signs, but rales are heard with diffuse involvement of airspaces and interstitial infiltration. Rhonchi are produced by bronchial distortion and secretions. Clubbing is not a sign of silicosis; cyanosis is seen only in advanced disease. Ventilatory failure and cor pulmonale are end stages of complicated or acute silicosis.

INFECTIOUS COMPLICATIONS

Bouts of lower respiratory infection by pyogenic bacteria are frequent in complicated silicosis. Acute or recurrent bronchitis in the silicosis patient should be treated the same way as exacerbations of ordinary chronic bronchitis. The silicosis patient should receive the one-time immunization against pneumococci and annual immunizations against influenza virus. In the past, tuberculosis was thought to be the main cause of progressive massive fibrosis. This association has become less frequent, but the old relationship of massive disease and mycobacteria was found in a recent study of silicotic sandblasters. Mycobacterial disease was found in 25 percent of these workers, but about 50 percent of the casual organisms were nontuberculous, mostly *Mycobacterium kansasii*. In the same group of patients, there was an excess of other granulomatous infections. Of 100 patients, two had nocardiosis, two had cryptococcosis, and one had sporotrichosis.

IMMUNOLOGY

The fairly rapid development of multiple well-circumscribed peripheral nodules (0.5 to 5.0 cm in diameter) which resemble metastatic tumors was first described in coal miners with rheumatoid arthritis. In miners with serum positive for rheumatoid factor, the pulmonary lesions may precede joint involvement. Smaller, apparently simple silicotic nodules may rapidly enlarge with activity of rheumatoid arthritis and then partially clear in response to adrenal corticosteroids. Histologic examination shows that lesions contain thin layers of dust in addition to the necrotic collagen and active inflammatory zone of rheumatoid nodules. Cavities may be formed by expectoration of necrotic material. The nodules may stabilize or calcify. Later experience has shown that serologic tests for autoimmunity (antinuclear antibody) are frequently positive (over 40 percent) in the accelerated silicosis of sandblasters. In this group of patients, about 10 percent have clinical autoimmune connective tissue diseases, including rheumatoid arthritis, localized and general scleroderma, and systemic lupus erythematosus. Studies of cellular immunity are under way using alveolar macrophages and lymphocytes obtained from bronchial washings through the flexible bronchoscope.

CHEST RADIOGRAPHY

The patterns of reaction seen on the chest radiograph correspond with the pathology previously described (Fig. 54-7). The radiographic images of silicotic nodules are

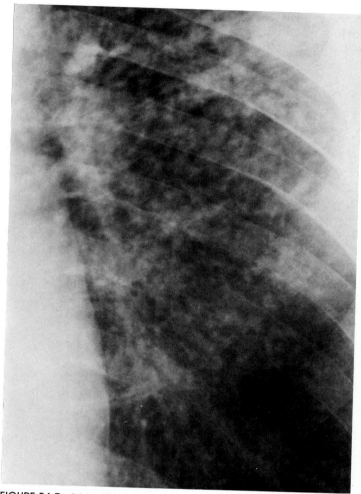

FIGURE 54-7 Magnified radiograph showing corresponding appearances of silicosis in a sandblaster.

rounded small opacities, less than 10 mm and usually 1.5 to 3 mm in diameter. In early simple silicosis, these opacities may be seen only in the upper lung zones. Within a zone, however, the spacing appears relatively uniform, not grouped like the typical distribution of infectious granulomas. This fact, and the uniformity of opacity size in the individual case, are quite useful in differentiating silicosis from infectious granulomas and hematogenous carcinomatosis. The experienced physician can sometimes suspect silicosis (even without exposure history) from the radiographic abnormalities in a case of proven tuberculosis, based on finding uniform size and distribution of small opacities in zones remote from the obvious loci of infection. Miliary tuberculosis, of course, also produces uniform nodulation, but it differs dramatically from silicosis in its clinical features. Healed lesions of "miliary histoplasmosis" (an inhalational disease, not a hematogenous one) may be numerous and widespread, but the opacities are less uniform in distribution and size and are more likely to be densely calcified. Calcified lymph nodes in silicosis usually show the eggshell pattern of enhanced peripheral calcification, even if there is coexisting granulomatous infection. In infection without silicosis, nodes calcify in a stippled or uniformly dense pattern.

Pneumoconiotic large opacities (diameter greater than 10 mm) are the defining lesions of complicated silicosis (Fig. 54-8), and bilateral symmetry and upper-zone predominance are their typical radiographic features. There is also a strong tendency to remain rounded and to remain separated from the pleural surfaces (by a 1- or 2-cm zone of subpleural blebs, the thin walls of which may sometimes be seen). Any unilateral large opacity, especially one that abuts the pleural surface, suggests cancer or infection, even in the patient with severe simple silicosis. Cavitation in an otherwise typical large opacity suggests infection, although it may prove to be caused by ischemic necrosis.

The now rare acute silicosis (Fig. 54-9) presents a radiographic appearance of bilateral consolidations, often with linear small opacities in less-involved areas. Lymph node enlargement is relatively common.

The ILO 1980 Classification (see preceding section), a descendant of systems devised for grading coal worker's pneumoconiosis, is also used to define and quantify the radiographic abnormalities of silicosis. This is an absolute necessity in population research, and it is helpful in describing and reporting clinical cases. In simple silicosis, the size of the nodules, the lung zones involved, and the intensity of involvement (profusion) are recorded. The profusion on a 12-point scale is determined by reference to a set of standard radiographs. Large opacities are categorized by combined size. Allowance is made for notation of other abnormalities of the heart, lungs, pleural spaces, and chest cage.

LUNG FUNCTION

Pulmonary function is well preserved in simple silicosis. Reduced airflow rates can usually be explained by other factors such as heavy cigarette smoking and postinflammatory changes in the airways, but bronchitis from prolonged, heavy dust exposure should be considered. An exception is simple silicosis manifest radiographically by very profuse fine nodules (less than 1.5 mm in diameter): this appearance is usually the result of rapidly developing disease, and is often associated with reduction of vital capacity, total lung capacity, pulmonary diffusing capacity, and oxygen uptake, but with little effect upon airflow. In complicated silicosis, obstruction to airways and structural distortion can lead to reduced airflow. Hyperinflation is found in many cases: restriction is prominent only in far-advanced disease.

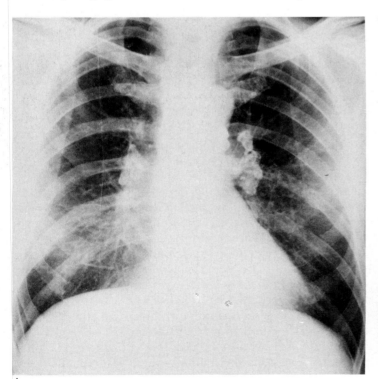

A

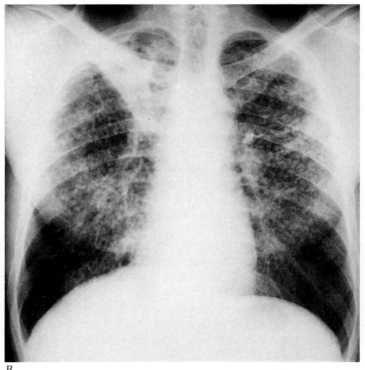

B

FIGURE 54-8 Silicosis. *A.* Silicosis, with minimal nodulation, after 20 years of sandblasting. Tuberculin reaction negative. Film shows eggshell calcification of hilar lymph nodes. *B.* Silicomycobacteriosis (*M. kansasii*). Extensive bilateral nodular disease with focal coalescence is present in the upper lobes. The right upper lobe contains a cavity.

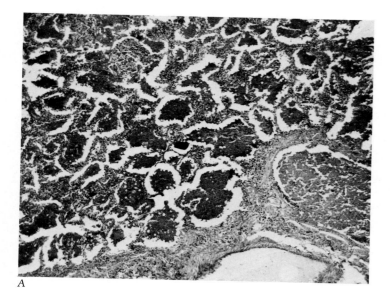

Ventilation-perfusion (V/Q) imbalance is the usual cause of arterial hypoxemia at rest and exercise in chronic disease; until late in the course, V/Q abnormalities are responsible for observed reductions in pulmonary diffusing capacity. In end-stage disease, arterial hypoxemia, CO_2 retention, and pulmonary hypertension with cor pulmonale frequently coexist.

Diagnosis

Silicosis is usually diagnosed by "ordinary medical means," that is, without resort to biopsy. The diagnosis can be made by meeting three criteria:

1. There is an exposure history that connotes a substantial risk of present silicosis.
2. The radiograph bears abnormalities consistent with silicosis.
3. There is no sound reason for believing that some other condition is responsible for the radiographic abnormalities.

Lung biopsy is required to prove the diagnosis when there is serious uncertainty about meeting one or more of the above criteria. Open biopsy is usually needed, unless bronchoscopic biopsy confirms a diagnosis such as infection or neoplasm. The deficiencies of bronchoscopic biopsy to establish silicosis are the small size of the specimen (precluding tissue mineralogy) and the possibility that it is unrepresentative of the whole lung. The latter objection would seem unimportant if the specimen were reported as showing fibrosis and crystals, but the mechanics of transbronchial peripheral lung biopsy require that the forceps' jaws straddle the carina between daughter bronchi, and the tissue is thus from a proximal part of the lung, an area to which dust is preferentially cleared and sequestered. Indeed, the pathologic diagnosis *anthracosilicosis* is frequently reported in biopsy specimens from the lungs of smokers or city dwellers who have had no occupational dust exposure. Anthracosilicosis simply means "soot in the lung," not silicosis.

The pathognomonic lesion of silicosis is the mature silicotic nodule, described above. Tissue diagnosis may also be made when less-well-defined and -well-organized lesions are seen, provided there are substantial amounts of silica associated with the pathology—again pointing to the need for generous amounts of representative tissue.

Treatment

There is no specific treatment for silicosis. Current experimental drugs, e.g., polyvinyl pyridine-N-oxide (PVPNO), are designed to prevent destruction of macrophages, but they are not ready for use in patients. Some complications of silicosis respond to treatment. Ordinary tuberculosis

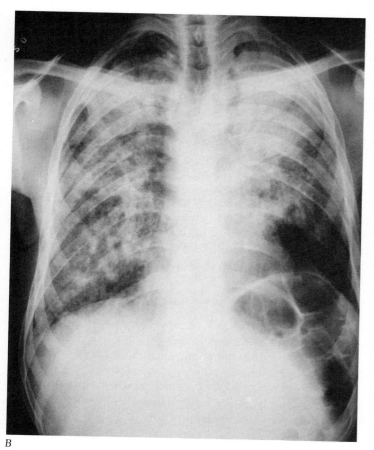

FIGURE 54-9 Silicosis. *A.* Florid acute silicosis. Alveolar proteinosis is simulated by this form of silicosis. The diffuse alveolar filling is striking. The bronchiole in the lower right contains a coagulum (H&E, ×47). *B.* Corresponding chest radiograph of acute silicosis showing advanced consolidation of parenchyma. Air bronchograms are present in the upper lobes.

can be successfully treated with isoniazid (INH) and rifampin, although the higher chance of relapse argues for two or more years of therapy rather than the shorter courses in general use. The atypical mycobacteria other than *M. avium-intracellulare* (Battey bacillus) also respond to specific chemotherapy. Continued worsening of PMF during treatment does not necessarily indicate failure of antimicrobial therapy, but withdrawal of therapy in the face of radiographic worsening requires courage and demands meticulous follow-up for clinical and laboratory evidence of bacteriologic relapse. The high risk of developing PMF as a consequence of tuberculosis warrants an aggressive approach to prophylaxis. The patient with simple silicosis and a positive tuberculin test should be given INH. The patient with complicated silicosis, positive tuberculin test, and negative sputum cultures is a candidate for INH and rifampin. The optimal duration of prophylaxis has not been established, but treatment for periods longer than a year seems indicated, since macrophage defenses are permanently impaired.

The corticosteroids have produced partial clearing on chest radiographs and have improved pulmonary function in some individuals with coexisting connective tissue diseases. They have also temporarily slowed the advance of acute silicosis with diffuse consolidation of airspaces and interstitial cellular reaction.

Pneumothorax is treated in the ordinary way, but the silicotic lung is sometimes difficult to reexpand when fibrosis is severe. Cor pulmonale occurs in end-stage silicosis when no treatment affords much relief of dyspnea.

Prognosis

Silicosis can, and not infrequently does, worsen despite cessation of dust exposure. It is ordinarily quite slowly progressive, however, and the elderly patient with mild simple silicosis has a good chance of escaping significant functional impairment from the disease. Even complicated silicosis, despite the frightening appellation *progressive massive fibrosis*, may enter a long and relatively stable period.

The risk of worsening, however, is positively correlated with radiographic severity of disease at the start of the observation period. In a study of determinants of radiographic progression in sandblaster's silicosis, the risk was greater for those with larger cumulative silica exposures, for younger patients (who must have received higher average exposures to have developed disease at an earlier age), and for blacks of any age (who may have received larger exposures in the past). Smoking, or the presence of serum antinuclear antibody or rheumatoid factor activity, had no detectable effect. The prognosis in acute silicosis is negative. Death usually occurs within 1 to 2 years of diagnosis.

Connective tissue diseases tend to be incompletely expressed when they complicate silicosis, and so seem to have better prognosis than when they occur de novo. In particular, the development of even extensive scleroderma is not often a prelude to severe visceral involvement. Similarly, the silicosis patients' rheumatoid arthritis, although inflammatory, seems to seldom produce conspicuous deformities or severe debility.

SILICATES OTHER THAN ASBESTOS

Silicates are composed of silica bound chemically with other inorganic compounds, usually the oxides of aluminum, calcium, iron, potassium, magnesium, or sodium. Abundant in rock, clay, and soil, the silicates form most of the surface of the earth. Tetrahedral silica units (SiO_4) recur regularly throughout the minerals. The silicates are most commonly encountered as asbestos, mica, talc, clays, and slate. The principal risk of pneumoconiosis arises from free silica or asbestos which may be present in the dust produced during extraction, processing, and use of these substances.

The discussions below assume inhalant exposure. Because talc and other silicates are often used as fillers in tablets and capsules, intravenous drug abuse can produce hematogenous lung exposure. This can result in a diffuse vasculocentric granulomatous interstitial disease, with large amounts of inorganic foreign material in the lesions.

Talc

Talc is a hydrous magnesium silicate which is rarely found in the pure state. It is commonly extracted from mines in which the rock is rich in quartz or fibrous silicates. Finer grades of talc are used as cosmetic powders. The crude varieties of the mineral are in common use as fillers. The lubricating power of talc is also employed to separate surfaces in the rubber industry and the manufacture of roofing materials.

Talc pneumoconiosis occurs (Fig. 54-10) in talc miners and rubber workers. It has also been reported after heavy and frequent personal application to the human body. The reactions usually develop slowly. Nodular and diffuse fibroses have been regarded as responses to contaminating quartz or asbestos (tremolite), but the tissue content of free silica is usually low (0.1%). Foreign-body granulomas have been produced by pure talc. Coalescence of pulmonary nodules occurs and may be further complicated by cavitation. Pleural plaques are common in tremolite talc workers (Fig. 54-11). Symptomatic respiratory difficulties and a restrictive ventilatory functional disorder with impaired gas exchange are associated with diffuse fibrosis. Irritative bronchial symptoms and effort

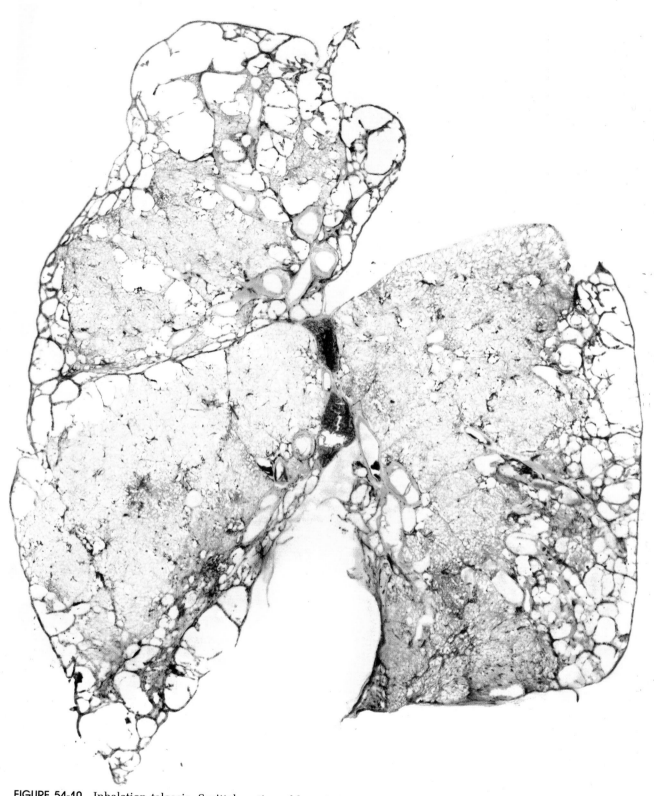

FIGURE 54-10 Inhalation talcosis. Sagittal section of lung in a 60-year-old rubber worker with 20 years of exposure. Diffuse fibrosis and bullous emphysema. Multifocal papillary adenoma, bilateral. *(Courtesy of Dr. S. Moolten.)*

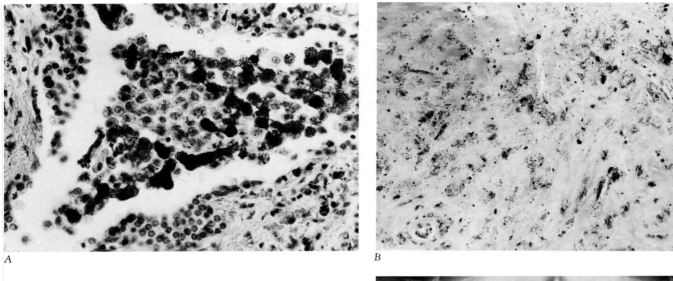

A

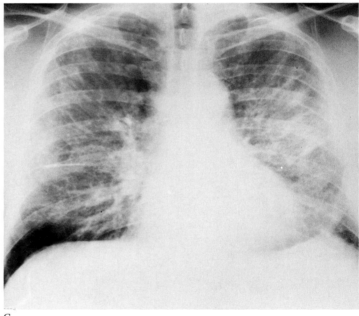

B

C

FIGURE 54-11 Inhalation talcosis. *A.* Tremolite fibers within alveoli and macrophage response (×290). *B.* Mineral deposits and diffuse fibrosis (×117). *C.* Advanced pulmonary fibrosis with pleural plaques after tremolite. *(A and B, courtesy of Dr. P. Daroca, Jr.)*

dyspnea are consequences of progressive massive disease. Clubbed fingers occur late with diffuse disease. Increased incidence of neoplasms has been reported in talc miners. The diagnosis of talcosis is usually established on the basis of the exposure history and the radiograph, and lung biopsy is rarely required. If fresh lung tissue is obtained, a portion should be reserved for mineralogic and electron-microscope studies.

Kaolin and Other Clays

The clays are mixtures of hydrated aluminum silicates which contain many impurities, including quartz. Fine-textured clay is used in ceramic and brick manufacture and for building. Kaolin (china clay), which has medical and cosmetic as well as industrial uses, is obtained by

open-pit and underground mining. After drying, bagging and loading are carried out in a dusty atmosphere in which particle diameters range from 0.5 to 2.0 μm. Pneumoconiosis is rare unless very high concentrations of dust are inhaled for many years, or quartz admixture is excessive. Some clays are rich in montmorillonite. Fuller's earth is composed mainly of the calcium compound and contains little quartz. There is little evidence that dust per se evokes strong tissue reactions. Progressive massive disease strongly suggests exposure to free silica. Bentonite contains over 85% sodium montmorillonite, but the admixture of free silica from sandstone and shale may be greater than 15% with an excess of cristobalite. Dust exposure during milling and drying of bentonite is now listed as one of the causes of silicosis.

Sillimanite

This fibrous mineral is composed of aluminum silicates and is used in brick and porcelain manufacture. Positive chest radiographic changes without disability have been reported only once in workers with prolonged exposure.

Mica

The varieties of mica are made up of hydrated groups of aluminum, potassium, and magnesium silicates. The substance shows a characteristic slate structure, which fractures into thin layers. It is used mainly for electrical insulation. Heavy exposure during underground extraction from granite rock has produced silicosis. The powdered mica itself irritates the bronchi and may produce pneumoconiosis resembling that of coal workers.

Slate

This term refers to clays and sedimentary rocks that split easily into layers. Slate contains mica and quartz. Miners, quarriers, and handlers of slate are at risk of developing silicosis. The severity of the disease is related to the free silica content which ranges from 7 to 35%.

Cement

Portland cement, which is a mainstay of the construction industry, is composed of limestone, clay, and gypsum, a hydrated calcium sulfate. The free silica content is low, and the hydrated particles are large. Although cement dust does not cause pneumoconiosis, obstructive airways disease is reported as excessive in workers who produce the material. No such risk has been detected in users of cement.

ASBESTOS-RELATED HEALTH EFFECTS

The use of asbestos increased from the time that this mineral was discovered a century ago to its peak consumption in the late 1970s. Its commercial use was followed closely by the recognition of several important adverse effects on the health of exposed workers. Asbestos-associated diseases are now more in the public awareness than any other group of occupational disorders. The recent reduction in use of this mineral is in large part related to these exposure-related diseases.

The term *asbestos* generally applies to the group of naturally occurring fibrous silicates with crystalline structure whose commercial value depends on high tensile strength, flexibility, acid resistance, and ability to withstand high temperatures. The primary commercial types have included chrysotile (magnesium silicate), crocidolite (sodium and iron silicate), amosite and, of more regional importance (mined and used in Finland), anthophyllite,

which is similar in composition to amosite. Serpentine mineral is mined predominantly in the Province of Quebec, Canada, and in the Soviet Union, and produces chrysotile asbestos. The amphiboles are mined primarily in South Africa, with the production of crocidolite and amosite. The use of asbestos (more than 90 percent of production is chrysotile), while decreasing in the industrialized world, is for economic reasons increasing in slowly developing countries.

Sources of Exposure

Although most of the health effects associated with asbestos exposure have been recognized in occupationally exposed individuals, risk of secondary exposures, either in the neighborhood of uncontrolled asbestos emissions or through domestic transmission of asbestos fiber by individuals occupationally exposed, has also been demonstrated.

Occupational exposures can be categorized into three major groups: mining and milling, manufacturing, and product use. Exposures to asbestos during its mining and milling have been most prevalent in Canada, the Soviet Union, and Africa. However, asbestos has also been mined to a lesser extent in the United States, Australia, Italy, Cyprus, Finland, and other countries. The most important worldwide use of asbestos today is in the manufacture of asbestos cement products for construction. Such products include flat and corrugated siding, shingles, and pressure or sewerage pipe. While chrysotile is the predominant fiber type in the manufacture of these products, crocidolite continues to be used in many parts of the world (including the United States), particularly in pipe and bulkhead manufacture. A second major use of asbestos continues to be in the manufacture of friction materials, although substitution has been possible for some brake linings. The asbestos textile industry has decreased in importance in recent years, but asbestos textiles continue to be produced for such purposes as fireproof curtains and fire-resistant clothing.

Asbestos insulation is no longer manufactured, with synthetic fibers and other substitutes replacing asbestos for insulating materials. Hazardous exposures have occurred in those occupations utilizing these asbestos products, particularly in insulators, installing new insulation, and continuing in the construction trades during demolition of buildings. Exposures have also resulted in disease in marine engineers (insulation around boilers and pipes in ships' engine rooms) and shipyard workers who were exposed in new ship construction and repair operations. While asbestos-associated disease was recognized on both sides of the Atlantic in the early years of the century, as the result of manufacturing exposures (primarily textiles), many of the important health effects associated with asbestos exposure became widely known in the United

States as the result of epidemiologic studies of insulators in the 1960s. It is important to recognize that currently some of the heaviest potential exposures to dust containing asbestos fiber result from the demolition of buildings containing old asbestos insulation and other materials and in the refitting of ships similarly constructed with the liberal use of asbestos. Special protective safeguards must be taken in these operations.

Pathogenesis

The two important potential effects on health related to exposure to asbestos dust are fibrosis and tumor. To initiate the cellular responses which lead to disease, fiber must come into contact with and be retained at the target organ site. It has become apparent that deposition and retention of fiber depend to a great extent on fiber size and shape, particularly on aerodynamic diameter. A unique characteristic of asbestos is its capability of continually dividing along the long axis of the fiber. This results in particles, which may have diameters of far less than 1 μm

and yet lengths of over 100 μm, still having the potential of inhalation, alveolar deposition, and retention. It has been suggested that amphibole asbestos, which characteristically has straight thin fibers, has greater potential for deposition deep within the lung, while chrysotile, being more "curly," is more likely to be intercepted at points of airway branching, although chrysotile may also be deposited and retained deep within the lung substance. Some fibers when deposited in the tissue become coated with a ferrous proteinaceous material, and these are then called asbestos bodies or, more nonspecifically, ferruginous bodies.

Only a portion of asbestos fibers can be detected by light microscopy; the greater number are of a size that make them detectable only by electron microscopy. Asbestos fibers less than 3 μm in diameter can be considered "respirable." As with nonfibrous particles, many asbestos fibers are cleared by way of the mucociliary escalator. Fibers deposited deep within the lung may be partially or completely (depending upon their size) engulfed by alve-

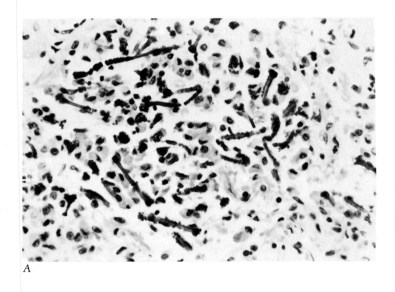

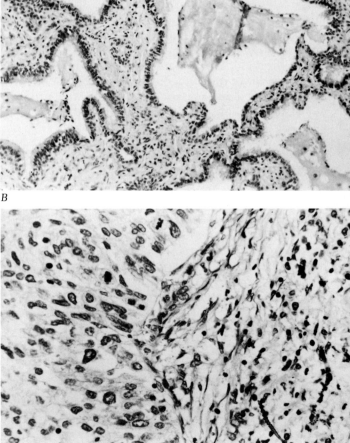

FIGURE 54-12   Microscopic changes in asbestosis.   A. Early macrophage response. Numerous asbestos bodies (×290).   B. Interstitial fibrosis and honeycomb lung (×117).   C. Asbestosis and bronchogenic carcinoma. Asbestos body is present (×290). *(Courtesy of Dr. P. Daroca, Jr.)*

olar macrophages (Fig. 54-11). Some fibers may then be cleared through the lymphatics, and some penetrate to the visceral and parietal pleural surfaces. It is of considerable interest that the effect of asbestos on the macrophage differs from that of silica, and the former is, in fact, less toxic. Through a mechanism not entirely understood, fibroblasts are stimulated, and fibrosis may occur in the lungs and pleura. All commercially important types of asbestos undoubtedly can exert the range of fibrotic and tumorigenic health effects. However, there appear to be quantitative differences in their potential to result in these diseases. These differences may very well be based on their differing physical configuration (e.g., fiber diameter, straight versus curled shape) with consequent differing dose of respirable particles and retention in the tissue. In addition, although commonly thought of as indestructible, chrysotile asbestos particularly may be degraded in the tissue, and magnesium may be leached out. This could be the explanation for the less common finding of chrysotile fibers in ferruginous bodies; most of these bodies can be shown to have an amphibole fiber as their core.

The mechanism by which asbestos exerts its tumorigenic effect is unknown, but in the case of bronchogenic carcinoma, it is strikingly enhanced by the synergistic action of cigarette smoking.

Fibrotic Effects

In the early 1900s, it was recognized that individuals occupationally exposed to asbestos dust were at risk of de-

veloping diffuse pulmonary fibrosis, termed *asbestosis* (Fig. 54-12). Pathologically, the early changes include cellular infiltrations of the alveolar walls, very often predominantly in proximity to the respiratory bronchioles. Bronchiolar walls may be thickened and narrowed. Macrophages are present, and peribronchiolar fibrosis appears. Ultimately, the fibrosis becomes diffuse and involves the interstitium. Ferruginous bodies should be identifiable within the histologic reaction. There is progressive destruction of the normal alveolar architecture and contraction of the lungs.

Clinically, the most prominent symptom is exertional dyspnea frequently associated with severe nonproductive cough. Mucoid sputum is present when there is the commonly associated chronic bronchitis. Auscultation of lungs reveals inspiratory crackles (rales), and as the disease progresses, there is obvious reduction in lung inflation. Clubbing of the fingers has been said to be common in patients with asbestosis, and while not unusual in the authors' experience, it is by no means invariably present. Progressive disease may ultimately result in respiratory failure with cardiac complications.

The chest radiograph plays a major role in the assessment of the presence and extent of diffuse pulmonary effects of asbestos dust exposure. Characteristically, linear or irregular small opacities are first observed in the lower lung zones and, while they remain most prominent in these areas, will be detected throughout both lungs (Fig. 54-13). There is generally gradual reduction in lung vol-

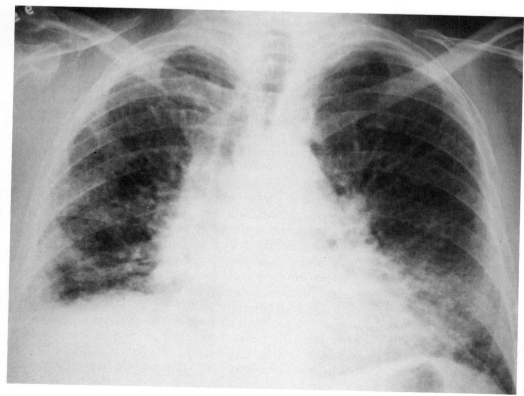

FIGURE 54-13 Diffuse linear or irregular small opacities within both lungs, most prominent in the lower lung zones. Lung volumes are small as indicated by the high diaphragms.

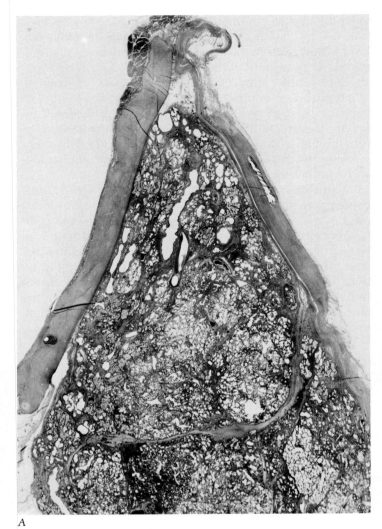

A

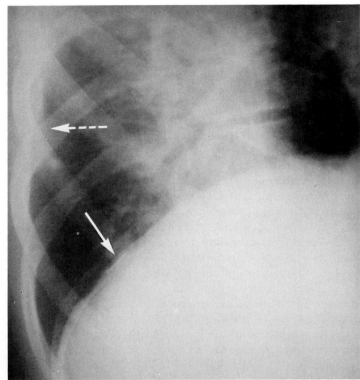

B

FIGURE 54-14 Hyaline plaque on pleural surface. *A.* Advanced asbestosis with overlying pleural plaque. *B.* Radiograph showing hyaline plaque on pleural surface (dashed arrow). Calcified plaque on diaphragm (solid arrow). *(A, courtesy of Dr. M. Kuschner)*

umes with high diaphragms. The radiographic appearance is not distinguishable from that encountered in the other pulmonary fibrotic conditions. As with the other pneumoconioses, the international classification has been found to be useful in the studies of exposed populations and, as an epidemiologic tool, permits the quantitation of dust effects on the pulmonary parenchyma and pleural surfaces.

While a number of conditions produce pulmonary fibrosis in association with diffuse or focal pleural thickening, this combination should alert the physician to the possibility of asbestos-related disease. Pleural changes in association with asbestos exposure may be present in the absence of the above-described lung changes. Focal hyaline pleural plaques are often recognized along the lateral chest walls or on the diaphragms (Fig. 54-14). These plaques must be carefully distinguished from normal soft-tissue, or "companion," shadows which are symmetrically visible along the chest walls. Hyaline plaques may calcify and provide an important clue to past asbestos

exposure. In addition to these focal pleural changes, a diffuse pleural reaction, unilateral or bilateral, has been recognized among the benign pleural complications of asbestos exposure. There may be an exudative pleural effusion which can be recurrent; this effect appears to be quite rare. It is obviously of considerable importance to rule out the possibility that such an effusion is associated with a mesothelioma or pleural metastases from primary pulmonary or intra-abdominal carcinomas.

The classic pulmonary physiological pattern which has been associated with asbestosis includes reduction in lung volumes, impaired gas exchange with hypoxemia made worse by exercise, a low pulmonary diffusing capacity, reduced compliance, and the absence of airflow obstruction. It is important to recognize that these physiological impairments are present in well-established disease, generally easily recognized on physical examination and by radiograph. The early effects of asbestos dust inhalation may also affect lung volumes but, in addition, may result in limitation of expiratory flows, presumably as the result of the peribronchiolar reaction in the earliest stages of this disorder. It is for this reason that ordinary spirometric measurements are adequately sensitive for the detection of early physiological changes resulting from asbestos dust exposure. Pleural plaques and most instances of diffuse pleural thickening do not affect pulmonary function, and they are therefore not expected to produce symptoms of respiratory impairment. The less common instance of prominent generalized pleural thickening may reduce lung volume on the basis of *fibrothorax*. The latter may, at times, be the result of an unrecognized asbestos-related benign exudative pleural effusion.

Asbestosis, as it is currently enountered, is now recognized to be very slowly progressive. Radiographic evidence of progression may require comparison of films taken several years apart (4 to 6 years would not be uncommon). Since progression is related to exposure dose and level of disease (profusion of small opacities on chest film), the lower exposures in recent decades, and lesser extent of disease when now diagnosed explain the slow progression described.

The diagnosis of asbestosis depends on the weighing of exposure history, clinical and physiological findings, and the radiographic pattern. Lung histopathology is most often not available, and lung biopsy is rarely justifiable for the purpose of making this diagnosis. If tissue is, however, available (e.g., surgery for other purposes), the pathologic diagnosis depends on the presence of diffuse fibrosis *and* ferruginous bodies; neither alone is sufficient. In practice, the diagnosis of asbestosis most heavily depends on an appropriate exposure history and radiographic evidence of lung fibrosis. The presence of pleural plaques or diffuse thickening without parenchymal abnormalities does not justify the diagnosis (they indicate *exposure*, not asbestosis). The term *pleural asbestosis* is invalid and should not be used.

The question of whether asbestos exposure can cause chronic obstructive pulmonary disease continues to be raised. As indicated previously, physiological and pathologic evidence indicates that there is bronchiolar involvement as a result of asbestos exposure. There is no evidence, however, to support the view that clinically significant airways obstruction results from this exposure. When present in an asbestos-exposed individual, it is most likely the consequence of another factor, usually smoking.

Neoplastic Effects

The increased risk for the development of bronchogenic carcinoma in workers exposed to asbestos dust was suggested in 1935 and established with the report of a British epidemiologic study in 1955. In the 1960s, it was suggested that this excess risk was essentially limited to those asbestos workers who were also cigarette smokers. More

recently, it has become accepted that, while substantially lower, the risk of lung cancer in nonsmokers is also elevated. Most (but not all) epidemiologic studies have demonstrated an excess risk of lung cancer in occupationally exposed individuals, but estimation of the extent of this risk has varied from one study to another, usually related to different parts of the asbestos industry. Perhaps the most difficult question has been whether the excess lung cancer risk is limited to those individuals who also have diffuse scarring of the lungs (asbestosis) or whether exposed individuals without evidence of pulmonary or pleural disease also carry such an increased risk. Many investigators still believe that the carcinoma risk is associated with asbestosis but, because of nonspecificity of the malignant tumor and the frequent presence of other causal factors (cigarette smoking), the question cannot be definitely answered for the individual case. Limited evidence does suggest that in an asbestos-exposed population, the absence of indicators of asbestosis (on radiograph, pulmonary function) will probably be associated with no detectable increase in lung cancer risk.

The synergistic role of cigarette smoking in association with asbestos exposure in the production of excess lung tumors is not in dispute. While there is some suggestion that adenocarcinomas occur in greater frequency among asbestos-exposed individuals, cell-type specificity for asbestos-related tumors has not been demonstrated. In general, the development of lung cancer among previously exposed individuals presents a clinical picture similar to that seen in the general population, with the exception that there is frequently diffuse pulmonary fibrosis, limiting even further the potential successful management of this disease (Fig. 54-15). The results of treatment are poor. There is inconsistent evidence of an association between occupational exposure to asbestos and gastrointestinal and laryngeal tumors, the latter more likely representing a true causal association. Any risk of developing these malignant effects is far lower than for lung cancer.

Malignant mesothelioma of pleural and peritoneal surfaces is a rare, bulky tumor which varies histologically and is frequently difficult to diagnose even with biopsy specimens available (Fig. 54-16). The association between this tumor and past (often distant) asbestos exposure was initially suggested by case reports in the 1940s and the 1950s, and it was established in 1960 by a report of mesotheliomas appearing in individuals occupationally and residentially exposed to the dust of South African crocidolite mines. Asbestos remains the only known occupational cause of this tumor. The tumor is invariably fatal and extends locally, but it may also produce distant metastases. Mesothelioma is usually not associated with well-established diffuse pulmonary fibrosis, although microscopic evidence of focal fibrosis is not uncommon. There may, however, frequently be evidence of asbestos exposure with fibers and ferruginous bodies demonstrable

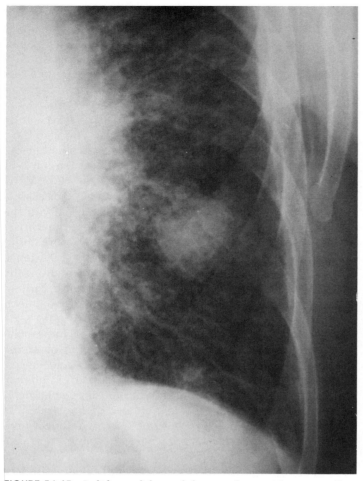

FIGURE 54-15 Left lower lobe nodular neoplasm with surrounding pulmonary fibrosis (asbestosis).

the larger-diameter crocidolite fibers and chrysotile are less hazardous because they are less likely to be peripherally deposited and retained. Lower risk associated with chrysotile may also be related to its tissue solubility. For whatever reason, the occurrence of mesothelioma in individuals who have had long exposure to the dust of Quebec chrysotile mines is infrequent. That there are cases at all has been suggested by some to be related to the tremolite contamination (an amphibole mineral) of the chrysotile mines. As regards mesothelioma risk in relation to fiber type, an enlarging body of epidemiologic evidence from all major types of asbestos exposure (mining, manufacturing, and product use) confirms the greater hazard of crocidolite.

The clinical picture of patients with mesothelioma is nonspecific. Presenting complaints frequently include chest pain, shortness of breath, fatigue, and weight loss. The radiograph often reveals a large pleural effusion and occasionally will demonstrate lobulated densities on the pleural surface. The effusion is commonly bloody. Pathologically, cell types include epithelial or tubulopapillary, mesenchymal, or sarcomatous, polygonal, and mixed. Histologically, it may be difficult to differentiate these tumors from secondary deposits of primary carcinomas (particularly adenocarcinoma) elsewhere. Pleural fluid cytology and needle biopsy of the pleura are not useful in establishing the diagnosis. Surgical biopsy specimens may suggest the diagnosis of mesothelioma, but at times they will not be definitive. Confirmation may await the postmortem examination which excludes a primary tumor of the lungs, gastrointestinal tract, or elsewhere. Surgical excision, radiotherapy, and chemotherapy have generally been unsuccessful. A fatal outcome can usually be expected within 1 or 2 years of the diagnosis.

Epidemiologic Studies and Dose-Response Relationships

Epidemiologic investigations of exposed workers have depended on either clinical, radiographic, and physiological evaluation of individuals for evidence of pulmonary and pleural dust effects or on mortality studies directed primarily at the malignant effects of exposure. Where past exposure dose has been estimated, these studies have usually demonstrated that the asbestos-associated health effects are dose-related. Through retrospective estimation of cumulative asbestos dust exposure, dose-response curves have been constructed for asbestosis in mining and milling, as well as for manufacturing exposures. These relationships hold for both radiographic and physiological evidence of abnormality. In population studies, radiographs and pulmonary function tests appear to be equally sensitive in detecting early dust effects, but in individuals either one or the other may become abnormal first. There is some evidence that a threshold level of exposure exists

in the lung after systematic search. In retrospective studies, varying proportions of cases have had no previous identifiable occupational, household, or residential exposure to asbestos. While there remains some difference of opinion concerning the importance of fiber types, most investigators agree that crocidolite exposure is more likely to result in these tumors than is chrysotile exposure. There has been no significant smoking association.

Among the major problems in understanding mesothelioma and its relationship to asbestos exposure is whether some of the neighborhood exposures which have been incriminated were not only brief but also low-level. Certainly the household exposures are likely to have been moderate or high in dose, on an intermittent but recurring basis. Most often, the asbestos exposure reported occurred between 20 and 40 years prior to the clinical onset of the disease. It is of interest that the thinner crocidolite asbestos fibers mined in Northwest Cape, South Africa, have been far more likely to produce mesotheliomas in exposed individuals than the thicker crocidolite fibers from the Transvaal. This observation has led to the suggestion that

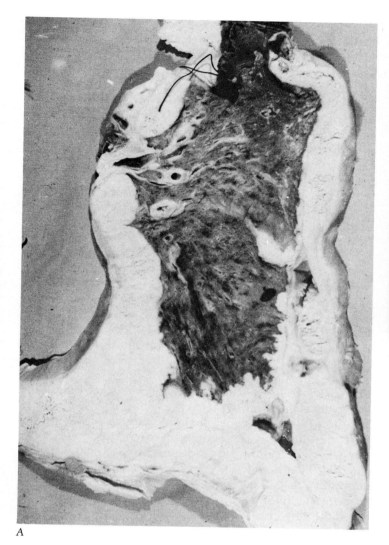

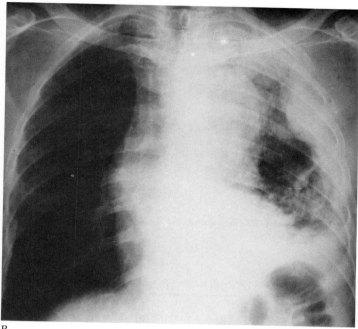

FIGURE 54-16 Pleural mesothelioma. *A.* Lung encased by meso-thelioma with invasion of parenchyma by malignant tumor. *B.* Mesothelioma encasing left lung, including its medial aspect. *(A, courtesy of Dr. J. Kuschner.)*

below which the effects of asbestos are not detectable, but lifetime follow-up is needed to confirm this suggestion. As indicated previously, mortality studies have shown different magnitudes of risk for the development of bron-chogenic carcinoma in differing exposed populations. With exposure dose taken into account, to the extent pos-sible, it appears that lung cancer risk is greatest in asbes-tos textile manufacturing, intermediate in asbestos ce-ment product manufacturing, and lowest in mining and milling and friction materials production (Fig. 54-17). The mix of fiber types used in these parts of the industry does not explain the demonstrated risk gradient. Where dose has been estimated, however, these studies generally indi-cate that the risk of lung cancer is dose-related, at times with an apparent threshold for a *detectable* increase in lung cancer risk.

The concept of a threshold level for carcinogenic ex-posures is highly controversial and for practical purposes can be discussed only within the framework of detection during the lifetime of exposed workers, using available epidemiologic methods. While scientific evidence does not permit the conclusion that there is a theoretical threshold for carcinogenesis, there is also no evidence that proves that there is none. It is therefore reasonable that prudent scientists and those responsible for public health have adopted a linear, no-threshold model upon which to base public policy regarding occupational and environ-mental carcinogenesis. While limited data indicate that the risk for developing mesothelioma among exposed in-dividuals is also dose-related, it is likely that the nature of the dose-response relationship is different. Lower expo-sures than are associated with demonstrable excess of lung cancer may be causally related to this tumor. Clarifi-cation of these relationships will remain elusive in view of the uncertainties of estimating exposure and the rela-tive infrequency of mesothelioma (approximately 1500 cases in the United States per year, in contrast to 130,000 cases of lung cancer annually).

The obvious importance of detecting dose-response relationships and possible threshold levels of exposure is

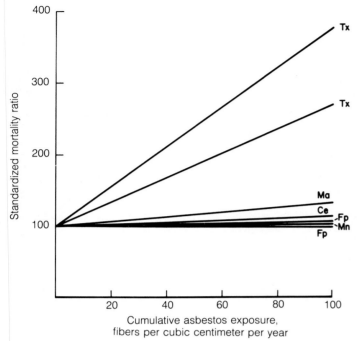

FIGURE 54-17 Estimated lung cancer dose-response relationships from seven epidemiologic studies. Tx = textiles; Ma = manufacturing; Ce = asbestos cement; Mn = mining, Fp = friction products.

to reduce the risk of these exposure-related diseases. These relationships will never apply uniformly to all individuals because of differences in host responsiveness, perhaps genetically or immunologically determined. Ultimately, the determination of an adverse dust effect in an individual for medical or compensation purposes must be based on competent medical judgment.

Prevention: Monitoring of Exposed Workers

Since in general the asbestos-related diseases described above are not effectively treatable, the basis for management must be prevention. Prevention of these disorders requires careful monitoring of both airborne asbestos dust levels to which the worker is exposed and respiratory health. The current method for measurement of airborne asbestos in the workplace in the United States and United Kingdom is the membrane filter fiber count. The current standard in both countries for permissible asbestos dust exposure is two fibers per milliliter as a time-weighted average over an 8-h work shift. In the United Kingdom, there is a separate standard for crocidolite exposure of 0.2 fibers per milliliter, or one-tenth the chrysotile standard. There continues to be understandable anxiety that the current standard is not fully protective, and efforts are under way to effect further lowering of this occupational standard.

Dust levels are best controlled by engineering methods, which provide negative pressure in areas where dust is generated, and enclosure of dusty operations. Wetting processes, whenever possible, are also helpful. Least satisfactory is the wearing of personal protective devices (masks), which are generally not tolerated by workers on a regular long-term basis, but may be useful for jobs associated with only intermittent brief exposures. In demolition and ship-refitting work where very high exposures to asbestos dust are likely, elaborate protection must be provided, which usually will include an air-supplied respirator effectively sealing the worker off from the immediate work environment.

As has already been indicated, both the chest radiograph and simple ventilatory function tests are very helpful in following exposed workers for the purpose of detecting an adverse response affecting their respiratory health. In general, chest radiographs and pulmonary function measurements should be performed regularly, but at less-frequent intervals than previously considered necessary. Two- to three-year intervals are probably adequate. The radiographs should be of good quality, taken with a high kilovoltage technique, and interpreted by experienced readers, perhaps in a central location. Comparisons should be made with previous films in order to assess progression and increase the sensitivity of detecting early changes. Spirometry must be performed according to the accepted standards, by an experienced operator who is familiar with techniques for obtaining maximum effort and who demands reproducibility of the expiratory flow curves. The operator must be familiar with calibration of the instrument, and this procedure should be performed routinely. Just as with the classification for radiograph reading, standards have now been accepted which outline the minimum requirements for apparatus and technique of spirometry (ATS).

MAN-MADE MINERAL FIBERS (MMMF)

The increasing use of fibrous glass and other synthetic fibers has resulted, at least in part, from the desirability of reducing asbestos use in insulation and other products. Recent attention to energy conservation has also enhanced the wide use of these fibers. Understandably, a watchful eye has been focused on the possibility that adverse health effects, not unlike those associated with asbestos exposure, might result from these occupational exposures. In fact, until recently, animal and human data have been extremely encouraging, since it has appeared that no such effects result from exposure to man-made mineral fibers.

There are plausible reasons why these fibers could be expected to be free of the consequences of exposure to the naturally occurring fibrous minerals. They do not have the capability of continually dividing along their long axis, producing very thin diameter fibers (a capability of asbestos), which would increase the likelihood of respirability and alveolar deposition. Also, they have generally been shown to be far less durable in lung tissue than asbestos. However, the largely negative early studies of exposed workers must be interpreted in light of the limited follow-up time and limited commercial reliance on thin diameter glass fibers. Other synthetic fibers, such as ceramic fibers, which are more durable in the lung, until very recently have not been evaluated by animal studies, and there are still no human data available.

Animal studies reported in the last few years indicate that under certain conditions (not necessarily simulating human exposure situations), fibrotic and neoplastic effects may be produced. Occupational exposure to thin glass fibers has been associated with the presence of low-level diffuse, small, irregular opacities on chest radiographs of smoking workers. An excess of lung cancer mortality has been found in workers producing mineral wool and fibrous glass. Whether fiber exposure is responsible for the results of these studies is not yet clear owing to confounding exposures and the absence of a fiber exposure-response relationship in the mortality studies. These studies do not prove that MMMF exposure in the workplace constitutes a definite risk of malignant or nonmalignant respiratory disease. Elucidation of this important potential risk will result from further research, which is under way.

METALS

Metallurgy is an ancient industry based on the useful properties of metals. These substances can usually be recognized by their strength, weight, toughness, malleability, and ductility. Their ability to conduct heat and electricity is universally employed in modern living. Metallic ores are mixed by a process that exposes workers to mixed dusts, including that of the matrix. Smelting of the ore exposes the operator to respirable dust particles, including fumes with elements less than 1 μm in diameter. Such exposure in enclosed spaces can lead to acute pulmonary disease or, after longer periods, to progressive lung fibrosis, inert dust deposits, or granulomatous disease. Respiratory diseases associated with metal exposures are now quite rare. They are included here because these exposures do still occur, so their potential effects must be recognized and their cause(s) considered in the appropriate clinical circumstances.

Metal Fume Fever

Metal fumes (zinc, copper, magnesium) and, less commonly, metal dusts (copper) can produce an acute self-limited disease. The illness is most frequently encountered during welding, working at brass foundries, and the smelting of zinc. Several hours after exposure cough, dry throat, and tightness of the chest appear, with chills, fever, and leukocytosis. These symptoms are followed by sweating, weakness, nausea, and then recovery within 24 h. The fever may be the result of metal particles acting on leukocytes to produce pyrogens. Affected workers often described themselves as "galvanized," referring to the zinc coating of iron which melts to emit fumes during welding. Heating surfaces painted with products containing zinc compounds can produce the same symptoms. Tolerance to metal fumes has been described, but is lost in part with absence from work. The benign course of the disease distinguishes it from acute intoxication with cadmium fumes and the pulmonary edema and bronchopneumonia which follow acute and heavy exposure to fumes and dusts of mercury and other metals.

Cadmium

Cadmium, an anticorrosive malleable metal extensively used in electroplating and the production of alloys, is extracted from zinc ores. While processing this ore or other substances containing cadmium, workers are exposed to respirable dust and fumes. The hazard is increased if the exposure occurs (welding, soldering) in enclosed spaces.

There is little warning before severe or fatal symptoms appear. The acute disease is uncommon, but has mortality of 15 percent; it is a severe chemical pneumonia which is preceded by pulmonary edema. Survivors recover completely, but in fatal cases, metaplasia of the lining of the alveolar spaces and renal cortical necrosis have been demonstrated. In acute animal experiments, destructive emphysema has been produced with heavy cadmium exposures.

It has been claimed that chronic pulmonary disease has followed repeated short exposures to low concentrations of fumes and dusts of cadmium compounds over a period of years. The suggestion that emphysema encountered in cadmium workers is a consequence of such exposure lacks firm scientific support. Prolonged exposure has been associated with proteinuria and renal tubular acidosis, and the Fanconi syndrome has been reported; diffuse interstitial fibrosis of the kidneys with atrophy of tubules and glomeruli has been demonstrated. Related renal changes, anemia, osteoporosis, and renal calculi have been noted.

The symptoms of chronic disease are weakness, weight loss, breathlessness, and anosmia. Chronic renal insufficiency may occur, but death in renal failure is unusual. Pulmonary hypertension is uncommon. The diagnosis depends on the history of exposure and the course of the disease.

The treatment of the acute disorder is symptomatic. Corticosteroid therapy is beneficial when given early. Removal from exposure to cadmium is required in chronic cases. Prevention of the disease depends on reducing exposure to cadmium by control of ventilation and prevention of contamination of food and water. Workers who have been exposed to cadmium should be examined annually.

Beryllium

Interest in beryllium increased with the discovery that chronic pulmonary disease was caused by its compounds, notably the oxide, in the production of fluorescent lamps (Fig. 54-18). The abandonment of this type of manufacture has reduced the incidence of the chronic illness. The risk of acute beryllium pulmonary disease is now low, but since the metal is toxic in small quantities, it must be handled with great care in enclosed spaces.

Pulmonary disease associated with beryllium mining is uncommon and is related to exposure to the other materials such as free silica rather than beryl ore. Beryllium is the fourth lightest element and has important physical properties. It is strong, hard, and resistant to heat and corrosion. It yields neutrons upon bombardment by alpha particles. It is translucent to x-rays. Its oxide has high thermal conductivity. With few exceptions, beryllium compounds vaporize at low temperatures. The phosphorescence of beryllium oxide when acted upon by external radiation was responsible for its use in illumination. Today, the greatest use of the substance is in the production of metal alloys. It is an important agent in nuclear

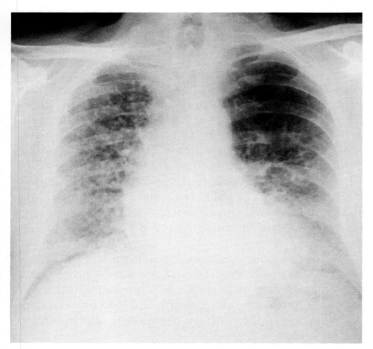

FIGURE 54-18 Chronic berylliosis in a janitor who fragmented burned-out fluorescent lamps for many years. *(Courtesy of Dr. P. Epstein.)*

energy research, and it also is used in the production of electronic and x-ray tubes. It is employed in vehicles and instruments used in space exploration.

In the production of metal alloys, a master alloy of copper and beryllium containing 2% beryllium is made. In several cases of acute beryllium pneumonitis, the alloys contained 1% of the light metal, and the respirable atmospheric concentrations ran from 3.55 to 21.2 $\mu g/m^3$. In another acute case, the respirable exposure was 45 μg in 20 min. Cases of chronic disease followed dry surface grinding with dust concentrations of 89 to 194 $\mu g/m^3$.

Beryllium enters the body by inhalation. In combination with protein it is widely distributed through the bloodstream lodging in liver, spleen, and bone, from which it is slowly excreted. Through broken skin, the metal crystals produce granulomatous ulcers.

The acute form of beryllium disease remains uncommon and is usually the result of an accidental exposure. It may be limited to irritative changes in the upper airways, but bronchiolitis, pneumonia, and pulmonary edema with mortality of 10 to 15 percent can occur. Perforation of the nasal septum has been reported. The illness may be extended for as long as a year; a fatal outcome has occurred in a small proportion of cases. Apparent recovery from the acute disease has been followed by the development of chronic disease without additional exposure. Chronic disease can be complicated by acute flare-ups.

The chronic disease is more likely to occur without a preceding acute phase and has appeared usually within 5 years but as long as 20 or more years after termination of exposure to beryllium. The disease has occurred in individuals who handled the contaminated clothes of workers exposed to smoke fumes from a neighboring plant. Chronic pulmonary disease is progressive with periodic intervals of remission. Complete cure of the illness is unknown, but radiographic changes can be present without symptoms. The disease usually produces a granulomatous pneumonitis which progresses to pulmonary fibrosis. The principal symptom is dyspnea on exertion. In the end stages, pulmonary hypertension is followed by cor pulmonale in association with pulmonary insufficiency. Beryllium with cellular reactions is also found in lymph nodes, liver, spleen, and kidney. Calculi can form in the lung and parotid glands but are most common in kidneys; cases of renal failure have been reported. Marked weight loss can occur in both acute and chronic forms of the disease.

In the chronic disease, increased serum globulin, elevated uric acid levels, and hypercalcemia have been reported. Immunologic changes have been attributed to beryllium, including delayed skin sensitivity (patch test) to solutions of beryllium compounds. This test, however, is no longer employed because of the risk of sensitizing subjects and exacerbating underlying chronic disease. Inhibition of macrophage migration by sensitized lymphocytes has been demonstrated; it is likely that cell-mediated hypersensitivity is the underlying mechanism for chronic beryllium disease.

The pathology of beryllium disease has been extensively studied. Patients dying in the acute phase of the disease show edematous changes and inflammatory infiltration of the pulmonary parenchyma. In the subacute disease, granuloma formation has been identified. In chronic disease, tissue has been obtained by biopsy and autopsy. In addition to the lungs, lymph nodes can be obtained by mediastinoscopy and may show granuloma or fibrosis indistinguishable from the tissue reactions of sarcoidosis. The tissue should be examined for beryllium; the finding of elevated levels supports the diagnosis. A negative beryllium assay does not, however, preclude this diagnosis. The presence of beryllium in urine indicates beryllium exposure, but the material is excreted over long periods of time after inhalation and does not indicate the presence of disease. In progressive disease, a late pathologic reaction is *honeycomb lung*, often associated with cor pulmonale. The chronic disease can involve the myocardium, muscles, skin, and bones.

The diagnosis of the disease depends on the history of the exposure and characteristic reactions. If there is doubt about the exposure, biopsy of a lymph node and/or lung should provide the needed information. There is no specific treatment for this disorder, but the granulomatous form can respond to treatment with adrenal corticosteroids and remissions may be induced.

The important requirement for the elimination of beryllium disease is the prevention of exposure of the worker to the metal. The use of industrial beryllium increased more than 15-fold from 1950 to 1969. Since this versatile and useful material is employed in many industrial operations, the possibility of beryllium disease should be considered in dealing with acute chemical pneumonia and chronic diffuse pulmonary illness which gives rise to granulomatous or fibrotic patterns. Whether beryllium is a human lung carcinogen is controversial; evidence on this point is conflicting.

Hard Metal (Tungsten and Cobalt)

Special tools required for cutting hard materials are often made of tungsten carbide and cobalt. The fine powder produced in preparing these instruments has been associated with the development of acute and chronic pulmonary disorders.

The chronic disease remains rare; it is a diffuse intramural and intra-alveolar pulmonary fibrosis in which particles probably of tungsten carbide can be demonstrated. Although most authorities consider cobalt the likely cause, there is no correlation between tissue concentra-

tions and the severity of the disease. The acute illness resembles asthma, disappears following termination of exposure, and recurs at work. Bronchodilators relieve the acute attacks, but the permanent effects of recurrent acute episodes are unknown. Both atopic and nonatopic persons are affected. There is also an acute pneumonic disorder, which usually occurs after a year or two of exposure. Termination of exposure may lead to complete resolution or to arrest of the process. Histologic studies have demonstrated the presence of desquamative fibrosing alveolitis.

The chronic disease is usually demonstrated in workers with more than 10 years of exposure in the industry. Its rare occurrence raises the question of the specificity of the fibrosis, but there are common characteristics such as length of exposure, age of the worker, and presence of respirable metallic particles. The variety of respiratory disorders associated with this type of work justifies the introduction of effective dust control.

Aluminum

Exposure of workers to aluminum dust in the form of stamped flakes of the metal has been reported as a cause of pulmonary fibrosis in Germany and England. The disease was explained by the reaction of the metal with water, with release of aluminum hydroxide and hydrogen. The lack of similar cases in the United States and Canada has led to experimental studies of the effects of aluminum metallic powders on the lungs of small animals. The work showed that the size and collagen content of lesions were directly related to the dose and the artifact of intratracheal injection. Transient alveolar proteinosis was frequently noted. The mechanism for fatal pulmonary fibrosis following exposure to pyroaluminum powder has not yet been discovered. Indeed, it is still uncertain whether aluminum per se causes pulmonary fibrosis. No evidence of fibrosis has been found in persons who work in aluminum reduction plants.

The processing of aluminum oxide from bauxite for use as an abrasive was associated by Shaver with accelerated nonnodular interstitial fibrosis. Shaver's disease is frequently complicated by pneumothorax and is often fatal. Apparently, only furnace workers have developed the disease. Bauxite at temperatures of 2000°C produces fumes containing 60% alumina (Al_2O_3) and 25% silica, with 12% iron and magnesium oxides. This evidence supports the view that Shaver's disease is a variety of accelerated silicosis.

Iron and Iron Oxide

Heavy exposure to iron and iron oxide dust and fumes occurs during arc welding and hematite mining. A positive chest radiograph is rare with less than 10 years of work, and usually occurs after heavy dust exposure in mines or enclosed spaces. The disease is usually asymptomatic unless complicated by bronchitis. The typical chest radiograph shows dense nodules (atomic number 26) up to 2 mm in diameter that are widely distributed throughout the lungs. Kerley B lines may be visible, but massive coalescence of nodules is not an anticipated consequence of this exposure. Microscopic examination shows iron particles and active macrophages usually in perivascular foci, but collagenous fibrous reaction is absent unless the inspired dust has also contained respirable free silica as in mining and foundry work.

Pulmonary function is usually normal. Obstructive ventilatory disorders are usually explained by exposure to tobacco smoke, but the possibility of industrial bronchitis should be considered.

The diagnosis is based on the history of prolonged exposure to iron or iron oxide fumes and the radiographic appearance. The appearance of massive lesions on the chest film of a miner should suggest coexisting silicosis. The incidence of bronchogenic carcinoma is not increased in these workers.

Other Inert Dusts

A group of metals of high atomic number (AN) with high-density particles produce spectacular changes on the chest radiograph, but no collagenous fibrosis or clinical symptoms. The inhaled particles of the inert dusts are usually surrounded by foci of macrophages. The group includes zirconium (AN 40), tin (AN 50), antimony (AN 51), and barium (AN 56). Although these substances are extracted by mining, the dust in this operation is mixed, and the principal risk is from neighboring quartz. Industrial processing creates high concentrations of dust and fumes. The density of the deposits favors early visualization, and positive chest radiographs with nodules up to 3 mm in diameter have been seen after 3 years of continuous exposure. Kerley B lines are often present. Pulmonary function is not impaired as the result of exposure to these dusts. The diagnosis depends on the history of specific exposure and the pattern of disease on the chest radiographs.

Free admixture of other substances may account for the development of symptoms in workers with "inert" dusts. The separation of antimony from arsenic in the ore is difficult, and the latter may be responsible for irritation of skin and upper respiratory and intestinal tracts. Although antimony has produced severe irritation of the upper airways, deposits of its dust within the small airspaces do not produce fibrosis. Some of the inert dusts are widely used for toilet and household purposes. The possibility of reactions in the airways and airspaces to prolonged dust exposure has been investigated for zirconium and its compounds, but no adverse effect upon the human lung has been reported.

IRRITANT GASES

Irritant gases (and irritant mists and vapors) produce their major effects on the mucosae of the upper and lower respiratory tracts. Serious injuries by these agents usually extend to the alveoli and result in pulmonary edema. The pathologic and clinical pictures, and the indicated treatments, are sufficiently similar to permit single discussions of these features for all the listed irritants.

The scope of this chapter limits consideration to the common industrial inorganic irritants, the organic irritants, and phosgene. Many organic chemicals have irritant toxicity, especially aldehydes, acids, and acid anhydrides. Isocyanates are also irritants, although their sensitizing properties have received more study. Smoke inhalation is in part an irritant injury by aldehydes and nitrogen oxides from natural fuels and by other volatile or gaseous compounds from synthetics.

Ammonia

Ammonia (NH_3) is a colorless gas with a specific gravity 0.6 times that of air. It is extremely soluble in water, and large volumes of the material can be stored and transported as "ammonia water." Ammonia is also stored and transported under pressure as liquid ammonia. The material is widely used industrially, e.g., in the synthesis of fertilizers, plastics, and explosives, and is also used as a commercial refrigerant. Some home cleaning solutions contain ammonia, the chief hazard in this use being burns of the skin or eyes from splashing.

Ammonia is so intensely irritating to the eyes, nose, and throat that is impossible to voluntarily inhale concentrations dangerous to the lower respiratory tract. Serious lung injuries are therefore limited to large spills, drenchings, or accidents in which the victim is unable to escape the gas, sometimes because of blinding.

Sulfur Dioxide

Sulfur dioxide (SO_2) is a colorless gas with a specific gravity 2.23 times that of air. It is almost as soluble and irritating as ammonia, and serious lower respiratory injuries are comparably rare. SO_2 is used in the production of sulfates and sulfites, as a fumigant and food and beverage preservative, and as a commercial refrigerant. It is stored and shipped under pressure as a liquid.

Hydrogen Chloride

Hydrogen chloride (HCl) in the anhydrous state is a colorless gas with specific gravity 1.27 times that of air. In air the gas rapidly becomes hydrated, forming dense white fumes consisting of small droplets. This is *hydrochloric acid mist*, the form in which the gas interacts with the respiratory tract. Hydrochloric acid (as the aqueous solution) is used extensively in industry, but opportunities for exposure to high concentrations of the gas or mist are limited. The agent is included here because it is liberated in large quantities from burning polyvinyl chloride (PVC), a plastic widely used in home and office furnishings, and in pipes and electrical insulation. Exposure under fire conditions is likely to be complex and include smoke particulates, carbon monoxide, and nitrogen dioxide. Products of heated or burned plastics may continue to evolve after control of flames and dissipation of smoke and so may constitute a particular hazard to fire fighters who remove respiratory protection devices during clean-up operations.

Chlorine

Chlorine (Cl₂) is a greenish-yellow gas with a specific gravity 2.5 times that of air. It is widely used in the chemical and plastics industries in enormous quantities. It is shipped under pressure as the liquid, by truck, train, and boat. Large spills have occurred in urban and rural areas, and there is a continuing danger of mass casualties from such accidents.

Chlorine is dangerous in much lower concentrations than either hydrogen chloride or hydrochloric acid mist. Despite its intermediate solubility, it produces strong and immediate eye and upper respiratory irritation. In still air chlorine can diffuse away from a spill, the concentration gradient providing some warning of impending heavy exposure. In light wind, the gas may form a "rolling cloud," the leading edge of which contains a potentially lethal concentration of chlorine. In this form the gas was used with its greatest effect in World War I. Higher winds disperse the cloud, and rain hastens the decline in gas concentration.

Phosgene

Phosgene (COCl₂) is colorless and has a specific gravity 1.4 times that of air. In contrast to the preceding irritants, it is poorly perceptible, its faint odor resembling that of mown hay. This deceptive quality, and a toxicity comparable to that of chlorine, led to its use as a war gas. Phosgene is an important intermediate in synthetic reactions, and is used in the production of plastics. It is also generated when chlorinated hydrocarbons are heated and is a minor decomposition product of heated PVC. The gas may be produced in dangerous concentrations when carbon tetrachloride fire extinguishers are used in enclosed spaces. Welders are at risk of phosgene exposure when heating surfaces that are damp with chlorinated degreasing agents (e.g., trichlorethylene).

Nitrogen Dioxide

Nitrogen dioxide exists in two forms at body temperature, NO₂ and N₂O₄. The composition of the mixture, called *nitrous fumes*, is determined by temperature. Nitrogen dioxides are heavier than air, are detectable by a reddish brown color and pungent odor, but are only moderately irritating to the eyes and upper respiratory tract. They are produced by the action of nitric acid on organic materials, evolve from heated nitric acid, and are produced by combustion of a variety of substances containing the nitrous radical (including celluloid, guncotton, and dynamite). Both acetylene and electric arc welding can produce the nitrogen dioxides, but dangerous concentrations are reached only in enclosed and unventilated areas. Nitrogen dioxides are also produced when grasses and hay are stored, and lethal injuries have occurred when farm workers entered incompletely ventilated silos. *Silo-filler's disease* is the term applied to the injury received in these circumstances. Gassing may also occur when nitric acid is spilled on a wood floor or when an acid spill is cleaned up by absorption with sawdust.

Clinical and Pathologic Features

The locus of respiratory tract injury depends on solubility and on the strength and speed of irritation produced. Ammonia produces immediate and intense burning sensations in the eyes and upper airway; phosgene is poorly perceptible. Anyone exposed to dangerous concentrations of ammonia, sulfur dioxide, hydrogen chloride, or chlorine, and not immediately overcome or trapped, is impelled rapidly to get away from the chemical. The poorly soluble nitrogen dioxides and phosgene can penetrate to the alveoli while producing minimal irritation of eyes, nose, and throat. The latter agents may thus be tolerated in concentrations that (often hours after exposure) produce fatal pulmonary edema.

Several of the irritants are quite reactive chemically, and in high concentrations are directly corrosive to flesh. This has led some to the erroneous conclusion that the respiratory mucosal injury is a simple chemical "burn." That this is not so can be inferred from:

1. The low concentrations at which these gases injure living mucosal tissues, compared to the high concentrations required to produce any detectable alteration in dead flesh
2. The common histologic appearance of the reaction, regardless of which of several chemically dissimilar agents causes the injury
3. The latent period between exposure and illness found in some injuries caused by the less soluble irritants
4. The rapid recovery in most instances of sublethal injury
5. The fact that experimental burns of the lower respiratory tract are rapidly and uniformly fatal

The pathologic change produced by the irritants is an inflammatory reaction dominated by capillary damage and edema. In the airways, there is reddening, swelling of mucous membranes, and increased mucous secretion. If edema is severe, the mucosa is dissected from supporting tissues and sloughed, leaving denuded areas. Respiratory secretions are mucoid and bloody, later becoming purulent if bacterial infection supervenes. Pulmonary edema produced by these agents is fibrinous or hemorrhagic.

Respiratory insufficiency is the immediate cause of death in fatal exposures to irritant gases. If damage to the deeper airways is widespread, the secretions and edema can produce marked inhomogeneity of ventilation. The resulting abnormality, mismatching ventilation and perfusion, produces hypoxemia in all cases and hypercapnia in severe cases. Pulmonary edema is usually also present (Fig. 54-19) when the deeper airways are extensively damaged, but the alveolar injury is likewise nonuniform. Chest radiographs may show diffuse bilateral consolidation, widespread patchy infiltrates resembling severe

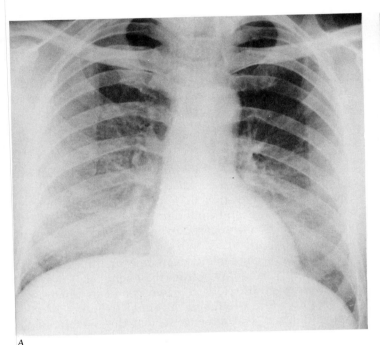

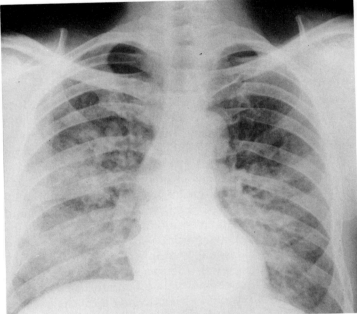

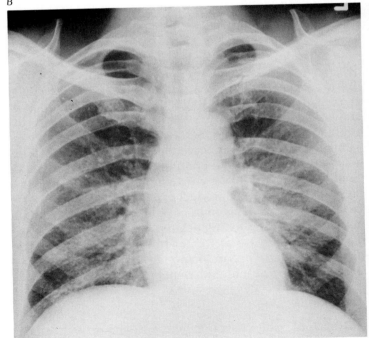

FIGURE 54-19 Accidental exposure of 55-year-old mechanic to spill of liquid Cl_2, followed immediately by coughing and dyspnea. *A.* Day of exposure. Bilateral alveolar infiltrates, most marked on right. *B.* Two days later. Progression of alveolar infiltrates. *C.* Seven days later. Incomplete resolution of infiltrates associated with persistent shortness of breath.

bronchopneumonias, or areas of consolidation separated by areas of apparent overinflation. Lung volumes, estimated from radiographic appearance, are often reduced in the early stages of acute injury.

In the presence of severe respiratory failure, lung function is rarely measured in the hours following injury. The hypoxemia produced by maldistribution of ventilation is correctable by administration of O_2, except when very severe. With increasing degrees of airway and alveolar obstruction and interstitial edema, pulmonary compliance must fall. Hypercapnia can develop when underventilated and nonventilated lung units cannot be balanced by overventilated units, and the increasing work of ventilation imposed by falling compliance hastens this development. Hypoxemia may be protracted and severe, however, with normal or subnormal arterial CO_2 tensions. Although dyspnea usually parallels pulmonary injury, gassed subjects occasionally show central cyanosis in the absence of overt respiratory distress.

The clinical course following acute exposure is similar in these agents, with important exceptions for phosgene and nitrogen dioxide. The latter agents may have a long latent period, occasionally lasting 12 h or more, between exposure and injury. Symptoms, and radiographic and functional abnormalities, may recur up to 6 weeks after apparent recovery from nitrogen dioxide injury (see below).

Whichever agent is responsible, the gassed patient often complains of burning of eyes, nose, and throat, coughing, chest tightness, and shortness of breath. Upper airway or laryngeal symptoms predominate in ammonia injuries, and chest symptoms in phosgene or nitrogen dioxide injuries. Nausea, vomiting, and headache are frequent after acute exposure to any irritant. Physical findings may include tachypnea, tachycardia, fever, sweating, cyanosis, inflammation of conjunctivae and visible parts of the respiratory tract, hoarseness or aphonia, and rhonchi, rales, or wheezes. Fever may occur shortly after severe gassing and does not always signify infection. Cardiac irregularities can occur in the absence of hypoxemia in some cases, and sudden death sometimes occurs in the treated patient. Hypotension in the case of nitrogen dioxide injury can be caused or aggravated by the systemic absorption of nitrates and nitrites, and the absorption of nitrites can also produce methemoglobinemia (important exceptions to the usual lack of systemic toxicity of common irritants). Acid-base disturbances are caused by respiratory failure or its effects on circulation and tissue respiration, rather than the chemical properties of the irritant or its metabolites.

Treatment

Treatment of the acute injury is similar for all irritants. The injured person is removed from contact with the gas and should be kept as quiet as circumstances permit. In case of drenching with liquid agents, these should be washed off with water. Oxygen should be provided as soon as possible.

Persons showing signs of laryngeal or lower respiratory injury should then be placed under close medical observation, preferably in a hospital. The possibilities of worsening in early hours, dissociation of dyspnea and hypoxemia, and unanticipated arrhythmias, make hospitalization the prudent course.

Following interruption of exposure, the first priority is relief of hypoxemia. Ventilation must be established and maintained. Oxygen toxicity is not seen after short-term administration by mask, and this should be applied early in first-aid efforts. In the ventilated patient, however, parsimony of O_2 administration is desirable: arterial O_2 tensions below 60 mmHg should be corrected to that level, but not much higher when more than 40% inspired O_2 is required. Otherwise, elevated arterial tension is obtained at the cost of unacceptably high inspired O_2 concentrations, and so may reduce the chance of survival in severe lung injury. The physician should also be aware of special situations in which higher arterial O_2 tension may be temporarily desirable, such as methemoglobinemia in nitrogen dioxide poisoning or carboxyhemoglobinemia in complex exposures from fires.

Severely ill patients may need mechanical ventilation. The preferred method is by cuffed tube and a volume ventilator. Arterial hypoxemia that is inadequately or marginally corrected by mask O_2 delivery is the commonest indication for intubation and mechanical ventilation. In the presence of this indication, there is no justification for waiting to see if hypercapnia is going to develop. Tidal volumes of about 12 ml/kg should be given; by recruiting units marginally ventilated at lower tidal volumes, arterial blood oxygenation is often improved without increasing the inspired O_2 concentration. Pressure-cycled ventilators can be used successfully, but they require constant attention because of the low lung compliance and the often copious, bloody secretions that characterize this injury. Oral endotracheal tubes with large diameters are preferred, to facilitate suctioning; a long, narrow nasotracheal tube is a poor choice for initial management. In view of the often rapid recovery from even severe bronchial and lung injury, tracheostomy can usually be avoided, but it may be needed when secretions are overwhelming in volume and tenacity. Laryngeal edema, which may be encountered in ammonia or sulfur dioxide gassing, can also force tracheostomy.

Another indication for ventilation is the demonstration of worsening oxygenation over a period of observation; elective intubation and mechanical ventilation should be done whenever it is clear that these will soon be needed. Ventilatory support is also required when there is visible tiring of the severely dyspneic patient, just as when an asthmatic tires dangerously during a severe attack. Rising arterial CO_2 levels (except where relief of overventilation is due clearly to improvement in pulmonary edema) also warrant mechanical ventilation.

Positive end-expiratory pressure (PEEP) and continuous positive airway pressure (CPAP) are adjuncts to ventilator treatment of hypoxemia. Both work by increasing lung volume beyond the effects of a given tidal volume and may be expected to work best in those patients with small lung volumes and reduced compliances. Both methods offer a potential improvement in oxygenation that becomes important only when potentially toxic levels of inspired oxygen are being required. The patient with satisfactory arterial O_2 tension on 40 or 50 percent inspired O_2 does not need PEEP or CPAP. PEEP and CPAP often produce falls in cardiac output, arterial pressure, and urine flow, and they should not be used except in circumstances where these risks are outweighed by the hazards of O_2 toxicity.

Hypotension and shock may be produced by the effects of gassing per se, usually in the setting of severe lung injury (adult respiratory distress syndrome), by nitrate and nitrite absorption in nitrogen dioxide injury, or by associated injuries. All patients, but especially those who cannot speak (unconscious, aphonic, or intubated), should be carefully examined for occult trauma. Sudden deterioration of vital signs in a ventilator-dependent patient calls for a rapid check to exclude machine malfunction, tube displacement, and pneumothorax. In severe gassings with pulmonary edema, one should not automatically apply the dictum that the first step in treatment of hypotension is volume expansion. The initial correction of hypoxemia should be followed by clinical assessment of extracellular fluid volume. If this is manifestly low, then volume expanders may be cautiously given. If volume is not manifestly low, expansion should be avoided. If the heart rate is acceptable, vasopressor drugs should be tried in the hypotensive patient who is neither hypoxemic nor obviously hypovolemic.

Methemoglobinemia is managed with methylene blue: 50 mg may be given intravenously over 5 to 10 min, and may be repeated as needed for methemoglobin concentrations above 20 to 30%. Carboxyhemoglobinemia calls for high arterial O_2 tensions (to aid clearance). The potential occurrence of these conditions makes it desirable to be able to measure the methemoglobin and carboxyhemoglobin levels, or to know the actual oxyhemoglobin saturation. It should be remembered that the "saturation" reported by some laboratories is a value derived from O_2 tension and pH measurements, not a measured value. The same saturation would be reported even if hemoglobin were absent or entirely saturated with carbon monoxide.

There is no rationale for inhalation of buffers or neutralizing solutions after irritant gas injury. Recovery is ordinarily rapid without corticosteroids; although there is no compelling evidence to support their value in the acute phase, there is apparently no risk in their use for a brief period, and so they are often given in cases of serious injury. Bronchodilators may be tried when wheezing or other evidence of obstruction is prominent; the risk of arrhythmias is minimized when hypoxemia and acid-base disturbances are corrected first. A parenteral drug, such as aminophylline by continuous or intermittent infusion, is preferable in severe injury.

Antibiotics should be given to patients with lower respiratory injuries. Reviews of war gas injuries, and of civilian gas injuries before the antibiotic era, document the important roles of secondary infection and suppuration in delayed fatality or permanent impairment. Such outcomes are now rare. Penicillin has been used with success, and erythromycin, tetracycline, and cephalosporins can be used if the patient is allergic to penicillin. Aminoglycosides, carbenicillin, or drugs intended for anaerobic infections should be reserved for specific indications warranting their use. The Gram stain of sputum or tracheal secretions is usually necessary to interpret cultures of the same materials, especially after several days of penicillin. Whichever antibiotic is used, 2 or 3 weeks of treatment is desirable. The cardinal rule is to remain alert for signs of unsatisfactory response, usually a return of fever and increasing sputum purulence.

Rapid improvement is the ordinary course, even in severe injury. Ventilated patients will begin to show falling gradients between alveolar and arterial O_2 tensions, increasing compliance (as shown by decreasing pressures required to deliver the tidal volume), reduced volume of secretions, and improvement in radiographic appearance. Weaning from the ventilator is almost never a problem, especially when prolonged hypocapnia has been avoided by use of a dead-space extension tube when needed. The patient is ready for weaning when arterial O_2 tension is close to 100 mmHg on inspired O_2 of 40% or less, when vital capacity is greater than or equal to 20 ml/kg, and when the volume of secretions is not prohibitive. These criteria are only rough guides, and management should be changed in appropriate ways if longitudinal observation of the patient suggests delayed or unusually rapid recovery or if there are nonrespiratory complications (e.g., bleeding). Radiographic resolution and decreasing symptoms permit discharge of the hospitalized patient.

In the special case of nitrogen dioxide gassing, some patients have a sudden recrudescence of respiratory symptoms 2 to 6 weeks after apparent recovery. Miliary infiltrates may be seen on the previously clear chest radiograph, and the recurrent respiratory failure can be severe or even fatal. This phase of the illness apparently corresponds to the development of bronchiolitis obliterans. (Experimental evidence suggests a risk of this disorder after gassings with other insoluble irritants, such as ozone or phosgene, and a few cases have been reported after ammonia injury.) Patients subject to this risk must receive clear instruction, given at the time of treatment of the initial injury, to report recurrent symptoms (cough, chest tightness, dyspnea) without delay. The condition may be completely reversed by a short course of oral corticosteroids in relatively high dosage.

Prognosis

Complete recovery is the expected outcome in acute irritant gas injury, but cases of persistent respiratory disease and impairment have been reported for each of the listed agents. It is probable that extensive and severe injury can sometimes lead to irreversible respiratory tract disease. Ammonia, sulfur dioxide, and nitrogen dioxide have been particularly implicated as likely to produce permanent damage after intense exposure and severe injury of the lungs.

BRONCHIOLITIS OBLITERANS

This topic is considered elsewhere in this book (Chapter 77) with particular reference to infections in childhood. However, the causes of bronchiolitis obliterans are many (Table 54-1) and include chemical injuries. The affected parts of the lungs are the terminal bronchioles and some of the respiratory bronchioles to which they give rise. Respiratory insufficiency is a long-term consequence of widespread, patchy necrosis and denuding of bronchiolar epithelium that is repaired by tufts of fibroblastic granulation tissue. These polypoid masses cause partial occlusion of the terminal airways and air trapping, and result in honeycombing of the lungs (Fig. 54-20). The commonest functional impairments are fixed airways obstruction, increase or reduction of lung volume, and maldistribution of inspired air, the last being responsible for any observed reduction in gas transfer.

TABLE 54-1
Some Causes of Bronchiolitis Obliterans

Inhalation of irritant gases, especially oxides of nitrogen
Viral pneumonia and bronchiolitis
Connective tissue diseases
Adverse reaction to certain drugs (e.g., penicillamine)
Uremia
Organization of hyaline membranes or after O_2 toxicity in the neonate
Chronic graft-versus-host reaction
Intrauterine pneumonia
Idiopathic

OCCUPATIONAL BRONCHITIS

Chronic bronchitis, whether or not it is associated with airflow limitation, is multifactorial in its etiology. While cigarette smoking is its single most important cause, allergy, socioeconomic factors (which may include general environmental factors such as indoor air pollution), and childhood respiratory infections are highly probable additional contributors to risk. The role of occupational exposures in causation of chronic bronchitis, particularly when associated with airways obstruction, has been controversial. This is so because the evidence to support a causal association has generally not been strong, the effect detected is often substantially less in magnitude than smoking, and compensation issues are difficult to deal with in the face of a nonspecific disease and the presence of multiple causal factors.

The emerging (but incomplete) data base on occupational bronchitis deals primarily with mineral and organic dust exposures; little is known yet about the risks which may result from long-term continuous or episodic exposures to low or moderate concentrations of irritant chemical vapors or gases in the workplace. The current state of the evidence that causally links specific dusts with chronic airways effects is taken up in the relevant sections of this chapter. There seems little doubt that both chronic bronchitis (excess mucous secretion) and chronic airflow limitation can be caused by long-term exposure to coal and grain dust. Probably, bronchitis has been the result of past exposures to cotton dust in the textile industry, but whether disabling airways obstruction is also a consequence of this exposure is not yet clear. Longitudinal studies of working populations, more sensitive than cross-sectional investigations, will, in coming years, undoubtedly add greatly to our knowledge regarding the contribution of workplace exposures to chronic airways disease in the population.

OCCUPATIONAL ASTHMA

Definitions

Asthma is a disease characterized by recurrent attacks of diffuse airway obstruction, caused by bronchial muscle spasm, edema, and mucous hypersecretion, accompanied by attacks or exacerbations of respiratory symptoms. Although the diagnosis does not always require demonstration of an immunologic mechanism, it is inappropriate in those cases in which obstruction only follows such other causes as pulmonary edema, respiratory infections, or chemical (toxic) bronchitis.

In occupational asthma, the attacks are caused by workplace exposures to one or more allergens or other inducers of asthma. In effect, all cases of occupational

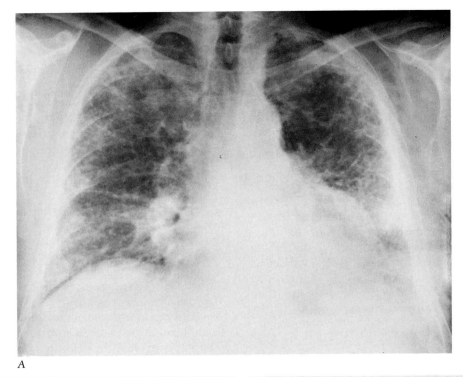

A

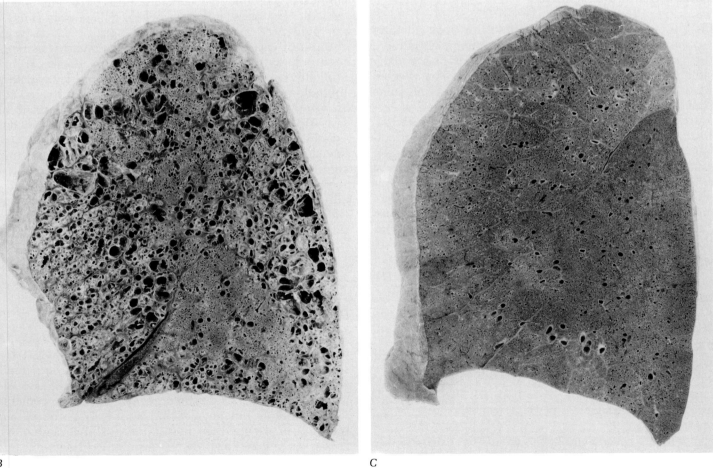

B   C

FIGURE 54-20 Bronchiolitis obliterans in a 63-year-old man who had been exposed to a wide variety of unidentified fumes in his jobs, which included welding. *A.* Chest radiograph. Diffuse pulmonary fibrosis and honeycombing, most marked in the peripheral portions of the lungs. *B.* Sagittal section of lung from same patient showing markedly dilated airspaces. Microscopic sections revealed bronchiolitis obliterans and chronic interstitial pulmonary fibrosis. *C.* Normal lung from a 43-year-old man who died suddenly. The difference between *B* and *C* in the alveolar portions of the lungs is striking. *(Courtesy of Dr. R. Ochs.)*

asthma are "extrinsic" in the sense of having an identifiable external cause.

The diagnosis of occupational asthma has two necessary elements:

1. A showing that the patient has asthma, as defined above
2. A showing that the attacks are related to workplace exposures

The Diagnosis of Asthma

The documentation of marked variation in bronchial function requires repeated observations over a substantial period. Variable obstruction may be documented by serial lung function testing or serial chest examination. It is not enough to show that, on a given day, a patient has reversible airways obstruction. Many patients with chronic obstructive lung disease show modest improvement in lung function tests after bronchodilator use, but over long periods of observation a fairly constant degree of obstruction is found. Acute bronchitis, of infectious or chemical cause, usually improves spontaneously and rapidly, and the convalescent patient frequently has bronchodilator responsiveness and nonspecific bronchial hyperresponsiveness (NSBH). The patient with asthma shows marked variation in bronchial function, either apparently spontaneous or provoked by allergen exposure.

Wheezing and shortness of breath are the classic symptoms of asthma, but the kind and severity of symptoms vary from patient to patient. Prominent complaints of cough, chest tightness, mucoid sputum, exertional shortness of breath (only), and even easy fatigability, are sometimes elicited from patients who deny attacks of wheezing with breathlessness. These are considered equivalents of the usual asthma symptoms when they accompany declines and abate with improvements in airways function.

Histamine and methacholine testing for NSBH have become common, although the drug and delivery method of choice, and even the best criterion of positive response, have yet to be determined. In the absence of NSBH, ambiguous symptoms are probably not caused by allergic respiratory disease. This is not exactly the same as saying that a negative test for NSBH rules out asthma; specific antigen challenge has been positive when NSBH is absent, but this is quite rare, and most such patients are asymptomatic at the time of testing. Pharmacologic testing for NSBH is preferred. Alternative methods (cold air, saline, distilled water, exercise), as usually applied, are dichotomizing, and are thus less sensitive to large and potentially important differences between persons, or in the same person at different times.

Testing for specific IgE antibody using skin tests or radioallergosorbent (RAST) systems can demonstrate sensitization. This does not by itself prove a diagnosis of asthma, for many persons with specific IgE antibodies do not have allergic disease. Moreover, some patients with undoubted asthma have uniformly negative skin and RAST reactivity.

In summary, the diagnosis of asthma ordinarily depends on observing, over a long period, provoked or unprovoked attacks that admit of no better explanation. Simple spirometry and chest physical examination are primary objective tests for airways obstruction, and serial application is required. Other laboratory tests, however helpful in etiologic diagnosis, are ancillary.

The Diagnosis of Occupational Asthma

Given that the patient has asthma, the essential element in the further diagnosis of occupational asthma is the demonstration of a significant and reproducible decline in airways function that is temporally related to ordinary levels of occupational exposure. Contrary to a frequently expressed notion, this does not require precise identification of the offending agent. In order of increasing specificity, the inciting circumstance might be identified as the workplace, a specific work area, a particular task, exposure to a group of substances, or exposure to a single substance. The greater the specificity, the easier to identify a single causative agent. But it is the clarity and consistency of the temporal relationship that supports the diagnosis.

Obviously, the diagnosis will not be made unless someone suspects that there is a connection between the respiratory ailment and the patient's work. In some cases this suspicion comes from the physician's knowledge of a particular sensitizing agent associated with the job or workplace. More often, it arises because the patient recognizes some temporal relationship between workplace exposures and symptoms. This recognition may occur only after the physician has asked the appropriate questions.

A symptom pattern of work relatedness may be obvious or obscure. It is more likely to be obvious when the onset of asthma occurs shortly after starting a new job or task or when symptoms recur minutes after each exposure to the causative agent, rather than hours later. It is difficult to perceive the connection when symptoms occur mainly at night, especially if they recur on successive nights after the latest workday, giving no weekend respite. For this reason one should inquire whether symptoms abate over longer periods off work: vacations, labor disputes, layoffs, maintenance shutdowns.

Occasionally, a history of work relatedness will prove misleading. A worker with ordinary asthma may improve on vacations because of absence from geographically restricted pollens or the family pets. A worker with marked NSBH may have bronchial symptoms from workplace exposures to cold air or potent airborne irritants.

Suspecting occupational asthma, the physician should look for objective evidence of a relationship between workplace exposures and recurrences of airways obstruction. Recordings made by the worker using a disposable peak flowmeter, both during and away from work, can be examined for relationships to workplace exposures. The primary modes of objective documentation are the chest examination and spirometry, the latter being preferable because of its greater sensitivity. Invalid testing, however, is worse than having no spirometry at all: the instrument used should provide a graphic record, to permit assessment of test quality.

The observations may be made before and after the work shift, looking for substantial declines (e.g., >15 percent of preshift FEV_1); or on Friday morning and Monday morning, looking for weekend recovery; or on the first and last mornings of longer absences from work, again looking for recovery. Equivocal results call for repeated testing, not a search for more-sensitive lung function tests or less-stringent criteria. Notice that this approach does not require precise identification of a causative agent, nor the knowledge or cooperation of the employer. When there is strong suspicion of a particular causative agent, and active cooperation of the employer, the focus and timing of observations can be refined.

The foregoing assumes regular, or at least frequent, exposures. Great difficulties are presented when exposures are irregular and infrequent, especially when some are so slight as to be subclinical in their effects. Such cases are likely to elude suspicion (and diagnosis) altogether.

Challenge Testing

Inhalation challenge with the suspected material is an accepted method of etiologic diagnosis (Fig. 54-21). It is most useful when a single agent is the likely cause and when that agent is highly irritating as well as allergenic, e.g., formaldehyde, phthalic anhydride, or isocyanates. Sophisticated testing involves the production, measurement, and maintenance of subirritant concentrations, so that an observed bronchial reaction may be imputed to enhanced susceptibility, usually allergy. Gases, vapors, or liquids that can be dispersed in a fine solvent aerosol are most suitable for this approach. Insoluble solids and colloids are difficult to disperse, control, and measure.

Some useful studies have been done by trying to imitate certain working conditions in laboratory exposures. This may be the only way to make observations when there is no access to either the workplace or a challenge chamber, or when the substance is too complex to screen for allergy to all its components. Unless, however, the concentrations can be measured or otherwise controlled, there is a risk that inappropriate exposure levels will give misleading results.

In some cases, such as occupational asthma in a grain elevator worker, it is usually not important to prove which of the dozens of grains or their contaminants is the offending agent, even supposing there is only one (an unlikely supposition).

The candidate for challenge testing must have relatively good lung function, both for safety and to avoid

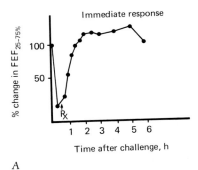

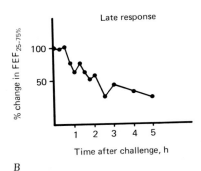

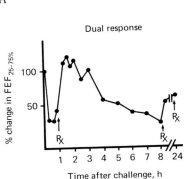

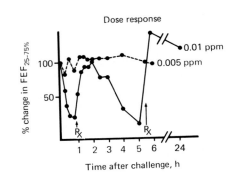

FIGURE 54-21   Patterns of change in ventilatory function following 15-min inhalation challenge with toluene diisocyanate (TDI).   *A.* Immediate response.   *B.* Late response.   *C.* Dual response.   *D.* Dose response.

false-positive results. Persons with moderate or severe obstruction can develop large declines in expiratory flow rates from slight decreases in the caliber of their already narrowed airways. The candidate must also be able to tolerate withdrawal from bronchodilators, atropine, antihistamines, cromolyn, and steroids, for a period of up to several days, depending on the agent.

As with testing for NSBH, there is as yet no consensus on the best lung function test for detecting an adverse response, nor on what percentage decline is minimal evidence of a positive test. The FEV_1 has advantages of easy performance and wide acceptance, and a persistent decline of 20 percent from baseline is persuasive evidence of an adverse effect.

Causative Agents

A discussion of causative agents has been deferred until now to reinforce an important point: a sound diagnosis of occupational asthma can be made without identifying the agent. As set forth above, the orderly sequence is to show that the patient's illness is asthma and then to show that attacks are temporally related to workplace exposures. At that point, the diagnosis of occupational asthma is made, with or without suspicions as to the agent.

Knowledge of common occupational allergens is helpful, however, in several respects. Attempts to show work relatedness of attacks may be focused on one or a few substances, allowing certainty that exposure(s) did in fact occur in the period of observation. For agents with good skin test and RAST antigens, these tests may be helpful. Most importantly, knowledge that a patient or group of workers is exposed to a potent sensitizer should allow detection of disease and interruption of exposure at an earlier stage, reducing the risk of more severe or chronic manifestations.

A list of all substances ever said to have caused occupational asthma would be long, somewhat misleading because of erroneous reports, and useless in cases of yet undiscovered causes. The incomplete listing that follows contains selections made because of asthma induction potency or large numbers exposed; the listing is also intended to suggest the diversity of potential occupational settings for respiratory sensitization.

1. *Simple synthetic organic chemicals.* Formaldehyde, isocyanates, aliphatic polyamines (e.g., epoxy hardeners), acid anhydrides (phthalic, trimellitic), and p-phenylene diamine and p-aminophenol (fur dyes).
2. *Inorganic salts.* Salts of platinum group metals, nickel, chrome, cobalt.
3. *Drugs and pharmaceuticals.* Especially antibiotics; methyldopa, psyllium, enzymes, hormone extracts.
4. *Biologic substances.* Grains and flours; shellfish and sea squirts; mammalian danders, urine, and dejecta;

feathers and bird droppings; unroasted coffee; castor beans; vegetable gums; certain woods; colophony (pine resin); mushrooms; detergent (bacterial) enzymes; and insects, worms, weevils, and mites.

Some of these materials are also known to cause hypersensitivity pneumonia. A few cause rare lung disorders, e.g., pulmonary hemorrhages from trimellitic anhydride, hard metal disease from cobalt. As a general rule, materials known to cause one kind of respiratory hypersensitivity should be suspected of being able to cause others.

Platinum salts are potent sensitizers in the epidemiologic sense of "potency," producing reactivity in more than half the exposed workers in some studies. Castor bean is also highly potent: it requires only trace amounts to sensitize. Many grains are of low potency in both respects. Toluene diisocyanate (TDI) produces asthma in about 5 percent of regularly exposed workers. Formaldehyde, considering its exceptionally wide and intensive use, must be a very weak sensitizer.

IgE antibodies have been demonstrated for most of the listed agents. TDI is an exception. Recent studies suggest that TDI alters native proteins or glycoproteins, which thereby acquire antigenicity. This phenomenon could explain the failure to produce good skin test or RAST antigens by simple coupling of isocyanate moieties to albumin, and it points to a profitable line for more general investigations of mechanisms of sensitization.

Mechanisms and Dose Response

The mechanisms of occupational asthma are varied and frequently unknown. Although the immunologic basis for several of the forms is established, frequently clinical and pulmonary function information is extrapolated to suggest, but by no means prove, that occupational asthma is caused by an immunologic mechanism. A late response to an inhalation challenge does not confirm an immunologic basis for bronchoconstriction, nor is this mechanism excluded. Irritant effects are undoubtedly important in a number of conditions that resemble asthma, although defining a threshold level for an irritant is difficult and may vary because of host factors. There are individuals who have hyperreactive airways and respond to low levels of an irritant inhalant on the basis of a nonimmunologic mechanism. In addition to allergic and irritant effects of an inhalant, the probability that dusts (and perhaps gases or vapors) cause bronchoconstriction by way of direct pharmacologic mediator-releasing mechanisms must also be considered. An atopic individual may be more likely to respond with bronchoconstriction to inhalants that produce asthma on the basis of nonimmunologic mechanisms because such an individual has hyperreactive airways. The increasing use of methacholine inhalation challenge will undoubtedly provide further information in regard to identifying and standardizing criteria for potential reactors. While cigarette smoking enhances the risk for the development of chronic fixed airways obstruction, it appears to have little influence on the acute constrictor response in occupational asthma.

A careful accumulation of biologic and environmental data frequently leads to the establishment of dose-response relationships in occupationally induced respiratory disease, including asthma. This was demonstrated when significant reductions of proteolytic enzyme dust levels in detergent plants resulted in reversal of an adverse longitudinal effect on lung function. Levels of exposure also correlated with enzyme skin test reactivity, with resulting reduction in sensitization rates when effective dust control had been accomplished in this industry. There is evidence for exposure-related abnormalities of lung function in both coffee workers and TDI producers, and the evidence persists after excluding the asthmatic members of the study populations—suggesting a subclinical effect of asthmagenic inhalants.

In addition to the relationship between atmospheric levels of inhalants and the long-term overall effect on airways function, a dose-response relationship can also be shown with those materials known to produce an acute constrictor response, such as TDI vapor. The level of TDI exposure has been related to the degree of acute ventilatory response during a working shift. In spite of the frequently stated opinion that sensitized workers cannot tolerate even minute levels of TDI in their working environment, inhalation challenge tests have shown a threshold level of exposure, below which no bronchial reaction can be detected.

Treatment and Prevention

Standard methods for the treatment of asthma are effective and include such newer modalities as cromolyn and inhaled, poorly absorbed corticosteroids. Pretreatment with cromolyn has been shown to block both the immediate and late bronchoconstrictor response in the laboratory and might be tried in those individuals for whom continuing exposure cannot be avoided. However, the ultimate preventive measure in occupational asthma is the removal of the affected worker from the job environment. While this step is often necessary in order to prevent the periodic recurrences of asthma, increasingly effective control of environmental inhalants by modern industrial hygiene techniques is making it possible for many workers to remain in the improved occupational environment. Engineering dust and vapor suppression is the most effective way of lowering the average concentration of the atmospheric inhalant. The most difficult exposure to control is the short intermittent peak that generally results from equipment or operational malfunction. These "spills" or other short exposures are often responsible for the symptoms of occupational asthma. While respiratory protection is useful in some instances, it is difficult to apply prior to the time such an unpredictable exposure occurs. Changes in product formulation may play a role in reducing exposure to the injurious inhalant. This was demonstrated by the detergent-enzyme-induced asthma where the enzyme portion of the product was made less dusty by an encapsulation procedure. If, in spite of vigorous attempts, exposures cannot be controlled to the point where individual symptoms or excess decline of ventilatory function are prevented, then the worker must be removed from all further exposure. In certain industrial situations this is not easily accomplished, as in many chemical plants, where exposure to most airborne chemicals can be demonstrated in all portions of the installation.

Prognosis

Reliable information on the risk of chronic ill health from occupational sensitization is meager. The best epidemiologic studies have examined the outcome of western red cedar asthma in British Columbian workers. Those who remained in sawmill jobs remained symptomatic, with more NSBH and poorer lung function than those who changed jobs. Of those who left the sawmills but were still available for examination, about half still had manifestations of asthma, and many of these were not atopic.

The authors' clinical experience with occupational asthma of other causes suggests a generally favorable prognosis, and this seems to be the view of many writers. It is probable, however, that bad outcomes can occur in any kind of occupational asthma, although some agents may be worse than others. On a percentage basis, this is apt to be rare because of the presumably large numbers of persons who quit noxious environments after relatively short exposures, because of symptoms but before a diagnosis can be made.

BYSSINOSIS

For more than a century, it has been known that dust exposure in cotton textile mills can lead to a respiratory disorder termed *byssinosis*. This disease was first described in the Lancashire mills in Britain, but received little attention until the 1950s, first in the United Kingdom and subsequently in the United States, and in other textile-producing countries around the world. Exposures to flax and hemp were recognized to produce similar respiratory symptoms.

Clinical Features

Characteristically, affected cotton textile workers experience chest tightness, breathlessness, or cough after an absence from work, such as the weekend. There is initially improvement on subsequent working days. Symptoms which first occur on Mondays (or other day which is the beginning of the work week) later are present on additional days of the week. A questionnaire was developed by Richard Schilling to grade the severity of byssinosis, utilizing this natural history of the process. The symptoms are the result of airways obstruction. The physiological indicator of an acute respiratory response to cotton dust is worsening of a measure of airways obstruction (most commonly the FEV_1) over the working shift. It has been suggested that ultimately dust-related fixed airways obstruction occurs, although chronic airflow limitation has not been adequately correlated with the acute byssinotic response (by which this occupational disorder has been identified), nor has it been related to estimates of cotton exposure. Cigarette smoking, present in most exposed individuals with chronic airways obstruction, has been an important confounder.

The risk of byssinosis (the acute response) has been shown to be related to exposure dose and early processing jobs (opening, picking, carding) by several studies. In addition, there have been differences in byssinosis risks among mills (after controlling for differing exposure levels), which may be explained by such factors as grade of cotton processed, extent and type of contaminating microorganisms (gram-negative endotoxin producers), or work practices. Even after all the currently known controlling variables have been taken into account, a "mill effect" may remain as an annoying reminder of our ignorance of the etiologic agents for these respiratory effects. Despite this ignorance, however, a substantial reduction in dust levels in textile mills has resulted in the expected decline in byssinosis prevalence in this industry.

Epidemiologic and Pathologic Studies

In addition to exposure dose, weaker influences, and residual mill effect, smoking has been found to be a risk factor in byssinosis. Atopy, while not generally considered an important predisposing host factor, may play a role in some instances of variable airflow limitation in textile workers; a number of exposed workers develop positive skin reactions and RAST tests to cotton dust extract. Studies have shown that cotton dust exposure in textile mills is associated with chronic bronchitis, but not emphysema. The evidence that cotton dust exposure results in or contributes substantially to chronic airways obstruction is inconclusive. Such an association is, however, not implausible and is currently under investigation by longitudinal study of a large textile worker cohort. Several recent mortality studies have failed to demonstrate significant increases in cause-specific mortality in workers who had been employed in the cotton textile industry.

Prevention

Worker surveillance supplements dust control in the prevention of byssinosis. The current cotton dust standard mandates a permissible exposure limit (in yarn production) of 0.2 μg of elutriated dust per cubic meter of air, a level that promises to greatly reduce the risk of byssinosis. All workers have periodic pulmonary function measurements before and after the working shift of the first day back following their days off, and standardized questions are administered which serve to identify the complex of symptoms which indicate byssinosis. These data are used to make a decision on removal from further exposure. Smoking should be particularly discouraged in cotton dust-exposed workers.

OCCUPATIONAL PULMONARY CANCER

It has been estimated that while less than 5 percent of all cancers in humans are due to occupational exposures, a substantial proportion of these can be expected to occur in the lungs. Smoking is by far the most important lung carcinogen in our society. Smoking and occupational carcinogens interact to increase the risk of lung cancer, and the tumor itself bears no marker to indicate its cause. When a worker with substantial risks from both occupation and smoking develops lung cancer, it is impossible to determine which factor caused the cancer, or whether both did so in concert.

Animal studies can predict that a substance is a lung carcinogen, and epidemiologic evidence can estimate the level of excess risk under varying conditions of exposure to known human carcinogens. The usual induction time, or latency period, is 20 or more years after first exposure, explaining why there is often delay in recognizing causes of lung cancer.

Asbestos, the best known and most important occupational cause of respiratory cancers, has been discussed elsewhere in this chapter. Ionizing radiation exposure in uranium miners has produced substantial excess risk of lung cancer in the past. The risk is related to exposure dose and is greatly enhanced by cigarette smoking. Inorganic arsenic exposure, encountered in copper, zinc, and lead smelting, increases lung cancer risk. Other metal exposures with demonstrated risk of lung malignant disease include chromates and nickel. The chloroethers, notably bis-chloromethyl and probably chloromethyl ether, used in organic solvents in the chemical industry are causes of pulmonary neoplasms, apparently small cell carcinomas.

The carcinogenic properties of coal tar have been amply demonstrated by the epidemiologic studies of coke oven workers in the steel industry who have a dose-related risk of excess lung cancer mortality. Workers engaged in the curing of tires in the rubber industry have also been shown to have been at increased risk of lung cancer. In these and coke oven workers, the specific carcinogen(s) has not been identified; polycyclic aromatic hydrocarbons are reasonable suspects. As indicated previously, whether beryllium is a lung carcinogen is uncertain; the evidence indicates that coal dust and silica are not.

BIBLIOGRAPHY

Becklake MR: Asbestos-related diseases of the lung and pleura. Current clinical issues (editorial). Am Rev Respir Dis 126:187–194, 1982.
  A review, with 100 references.

Becklake MR, Irwig L, Kielkowski D, Webster I, de Beer M, Landau S: The predictors of emphysema in South African gold miners. Am Rev Respir Dis 135:1234–1241, 1987.
  Study of South African gold miners showing exposure response relationship between mining service and airflow limitation measured by lung function tests.

Davies R, Blainey AD: Occupational asthma: Classification and clinical aspects. Sem Respir Med 5:229–239, 1984.
  A recent review, with 125 references. (Ignore tabulation of ammonia et seq. and listing of meat wrappers under polyurethane exposure.)

Doll R, Peto R: *The Causes of Cancer. Quantitative Estimates of Avoidable Risks of Cancer in the United States Today.* New York, Oxford University Press, 1981.
  A review of preventable cancers, occupational and otherwise; commissioned by the U.S. Congress' Office of Technology Assessment.

Hughes JM, Weill H: Asbestos exposure—quantitative assessment of risk. Am Rev Respir Dis 133:5–13, 1986.
  Quantitative approaches to asbestos-related cancers.

International Labour Office: Guidelines for the Use of ILO International Classification of Radiographs of Pneumoconioses. Occupational Safety and Health Series, No. 22 (Rev). Geneva, International Labour Office, 1980.
  Explanation of the classification, sold with the set of standard radiographs, both of which are needed to use the system.

McDonald JC (ed): *Recent Advances in Occupational Health.* New York, Churchill Livingstone, 1981.
  Agent-specific reviews, and chapters on methods of study.

Parkes WR: *Occupational Lung Disorders,* 2d ed. London, Butterworths, 1982.
  An encyclopedic work, strongest in the mineral dust diseases.

Seaton A: Coal and the lung (editorial). Thorax 38:241–243, 1983.
  Current problems in the understanding of coal worker's pneumoconiosis.

Weill H (ed): International Conference on Byssinosis. Chest 79(suppl):1S–136S, 1981.
  Reports, reviews, and controversies.

Weill H, Turner-Warwick M (eds): *Occupational Lung Diseases. Research Approaches and Methods.* New York, Dekker, 1981.
  Research methodology, an understanding of which is often needed to fully assess contributions to the medical and scientific literature on occupational lung diseases.

World Health Organization: Biological effects of man-made mineral fibres. Proceedings of a WHO/IARC Conference, Copenhagen, April 20–22, 1982. Geneva, World Health Organization, 1984.
  A two-volume work by international contributors, reporting all recent research in this area.

Ziskind M, Jones RN, Weill H: Silicosis: state of the art. Am Rev Respir Dis 113:643–665, 1976.
  Review article, with 127 references.

Chapter 55

The Lungs in Some Inborn Errors of Metabolism

Masazumi Adachi / Bruno W. Volk

The so-called storage diseases are genetic disorders in which deposits of abnormal biochemical compounds occur in various organs as a result of specific enzyme deficiencies. These diseases are rare, and most are transmitted as an autosomal recessive trait.

Although many viscera and the central nervous system have been extensively studied in these disorders, comparatively little attention has been paid to the lungs, except to note that the "stored" material is sometimes deposited in the interalveolar septa or alveoli, that these pathologic changes occasionally lead to pulmonary hypertension and severe pulmonary arteriosclerosis, and that, in some instances, characteristic alterations in the lungs can be demonstrated on radiographic examination.

NIEMANN-PICK DISEASE

Niemann-Pick disease is characterized by excessive accumulation of sphingomyelin in the cells of reticuloendothelial and parenchymal tissues of the viscera and/or the brain. Six types have been described according to the age of onset, clinical course, and pathologic and biochemical features. All but one type (type F) are autosomal recessive disorders. Type F may be inherited in a sex-linked mode. Reticular or reticulonodular abnormalities occur in the lungs of most patients afflicted with this disease.

Clinical Features

Type A, the most common type, is an acute disorder that affects infants and involves viscera and the nervous system. Almost one-half of affected infants are of Jewish extraction. The onset is insidious, and the children manifest difficulties in feeding and fail to thrive during the early months. The infants show progressive psychomotor deterioration and hepatosplenomegaly. The chest radiograph (Fig. 55-1) shows diffuse reticular infiltration. The infants generally die within the second year of life.

Type B is a chronic infantile form without neurologic involvement. It is less common than types A and C. These

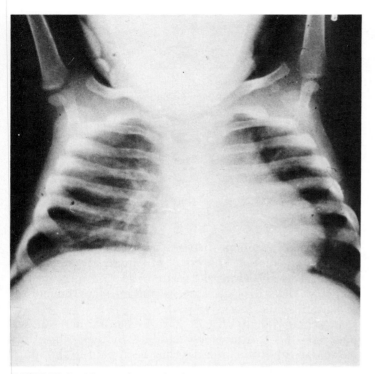

FIGURE 55-1 Chest radiograph of a patient with Niemann-Pick disease (type A) showing bilateral diffuse reticular infiltration.

infants often have hepatosplenomegaly and lymphadenopathy which may develop as early as those with type A. However, most patients are in good health until late infancy. The children often develop recurrent pulmonary infection and die during the juvenile stage.

Type C is the second most common type of this disorder. It involves viscera and the central nervous system. The initial symptoms usually occur after the first or second year and occasionally after the sixth year. Psychomotor deterioration is progressive. Hepatosplenomegaly is less striking than in the previous two types. The patients usually die within the fifth and fifteenth years of life; they occasionally survive to adolescence.

Type D is a variant of type C that occurs in descendants of persons from Nova Scotia. However, in contrast to type C, the children in this group develop jaundice early in life which disappears as the disease progresses.

Only a few cases of the adult form (type E) have been reported. These patients have no clinical symptoms even though abnormal lipid accumulations occur in various organs, including the lungs. Type F is characterized by childhood onset of splenomegaly, lack of neurologic involvement, and diminished activity of heat labile sphingomyelinase.

Pathologic Features

The lungs, particularly in type A, are frequently increased in weight and their cut surfaces show yellow mottling.

The liver is markedly enlarged and reaches two to three times the expected weight for the age. Cut surfaces are diffusely yellow, although the original architecture is usually preserved. The weight of the spleen is often five to six times normal, and sections show a yellow color with peculiar salmon-pink spots representing malpighian bodies. The lymph nodes are also enlarged. The brains of the patients in types A, C, and D are uniformly reduced in size. On section, the cortex is atrophic, and the gray matter is deep, but the white matter is relatively preserved.

Histology

Although some patients have no respiratory disturbances, foamy cells are usually contained in the pulmonary septa and alveoli in most cases (Fig. 55-2). These cells measure 15 to 90 μm in diameter and contain a single nucleus; the cytoplasm contains numerous fine vacuoles (Fig. 55-3). Similar foamy cells are observed in various organs and the nervous system. Although the foamy cells are characteristic of this disease, they are not diagnostic without histochemical proof of sphingomyelin. Because the cytoplasmic vacuoles seen in routine sections represent a partly soluble material that has been dissolved during the histologic preparations, frozen sections are often required for analysis.

Ultrastructure

The foamy cells are filled with round to oval cytoplasmic bodies that range from 0.5 to 5 μm in diameter; these bodies are membrane-bound and contain loosely arranged membranous structures (Fig. 55-4). Histochemical preparations for lysosomal enzymes reveal reaction granules in the cytoplasmic inclusion bodies, indicating that they are the residua of a cellular effort to eliminate the accumulated lipid material.

Biochemical Features

An increase in the sphingomyelin content of the viscera and/or brain from 2 to more than 30 times normal is the basis for the diagnosis of this disorder. This accumulation is most marked in types A and B. The cholesterol content of the viscera is also usually increased.

A deficiency of sphingomyelinase is the primary defect in types A and B, while a partial deficiency of the enzyme is detected in type C by isoelectric focusing technique. Acidic phospholipase C deficiency is found in types A, B, and C of Niemann-Pick disease in cultured fibroblasts. Using somatic cell hybridization studies, a different gene mutation in Niemann-Pick variants is observed by restoration of sphingomyelinase activity by fusion of type C skin fibroblasts to type A or B, but not other fusion combinations. Total sphingomyelinase activity in types D and E appears to be normal, and no specific deficiency has been shown.

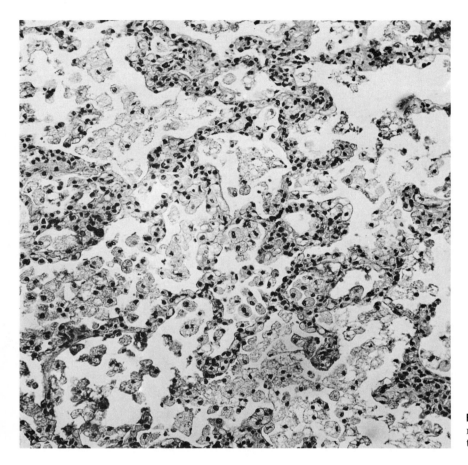

FIGURE 55-2   Sections from lung of a patient with Niemann-Pick disease (type A) exhibiting foamy cells in the alveoli. H&E, ×200.

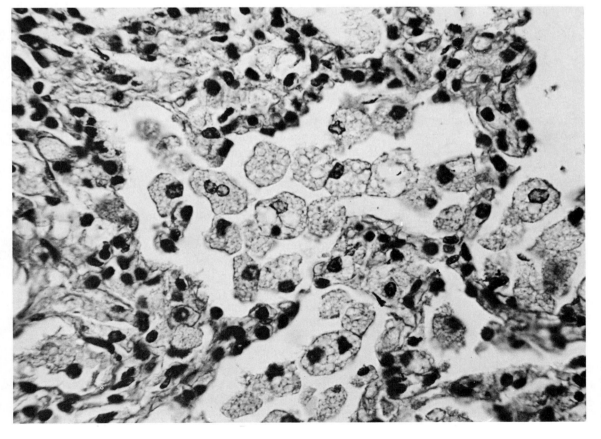

FIGURE 55-3 Under higher magnification, the foamy cells contain one or two nuclei and numerous fine vacuoles. H&E, ×640.

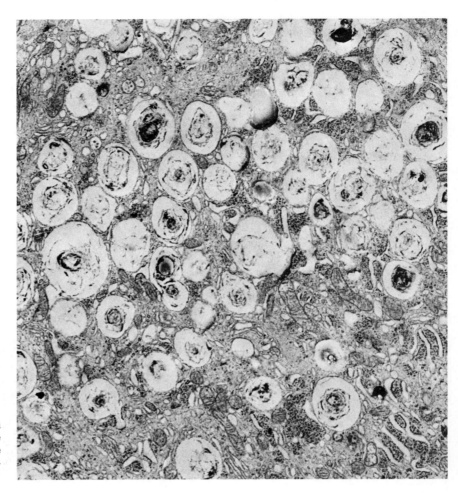

FIGURE 55-4 Electron micrograph of a portion of a foamy cell from a patient with Niemann-Pick disease containing cytoplasmic inclusion bodies which are membrane-bound and contain loosely arranged membranous structures. ×7200.

Diagnosis

Once suspicion of the disease is aroused, biochemical assays should be made for sphingomyelin and sphingomyelinase in fresh blood samples and frozen tissue. An ultramicrochemical assay for sphingomyelinase has permitted the examination of single cells with either fluorogenic or radioactive substrates. Thin layer chromatography in chloroform-methanol-water extract of formalin fixed tissue for phospholipid can also be performed. The peripheral smear, bone marrow aspiration, and biopsy of a lymph node or liver should be examined for foamy cells by special histochemical preparations. Radiologic examination of the chest sometimes reveals the characteristic infiltrates (Fig. 55-1).

GAUCHER'S DISEASE

Gaucher's disease is a hereditary disorder which is transmitted as an autosomal recessive trait. It is characterized by the accumulation of glucosyl ceramide in various organs associated with a deficiency of β-glucosidase.

Clinical Features

Three types of this disorder are usually recognized: type 1, the adult form, is most common and usually occurs in Ashkenazi Jews; it is a chronic disorder that may start comparatively soon after birth and usually lasts into childhood. It differs from the other types in its lack of neurologic manifestations. Type 2 is the acute form; it occurs in infants and is characterized by progressive neurologic deterioration. The incidence in Jewish families is less than in type 1. Type 3 is the subacute variety; it occurs in juveniles and presents a more protracted course of neurologic involvement than does type 2.

Some patients with the adult form (type 1) die early in life from thrombocytopenia, severe anemia, and pulmonary infections. Hepatosplenomegaly and Gaucher cells in the bone marrow are regular features. The concentration of acid phosphatase in serum is markedly increased. Pulmonary hypertension and severe pulmonary arteriosclerosis occur in a few patients. The reticular pattern of pulmonary infiltration that is characteristic of Niemann-Pick disease is rare. Repeated episodes of bone pain are common, and fractures after minor trauma sometimes lead to permanent deformity. Osteolytic changes are frequently seen by radiologic examination.

In type 2, the children develop normally until 3 to 6 months of age. Thereafter, splenohepatomegaly and lymphadenopathy become prominent, and Gaucher cells are found in the bone marrow. High levels of acid phosphatase in serum sometimes occur as early as 3 months of age. Progressive psychomotor deterioration then sets in, and the patients die within 2 years.

Type 3 presents a more protracted course of neurologic changes. Patients with type 3 also show splenomegaly and often a slowly progressive hepatomegaly. The children often display pulmonary infiltration on radiologic examination. However, the typical reticular pattern is rarely seen. Osteolytic lesions are frequent. About one-half of the patients with this type have been reported from four interrelated families from the province of Norrbotten in northern Sweden. The mode of inheritance is also consistent with an autosomal recessive trait.

E Rosette forming peripheral lymphocytes are defective in Gaucher's disease, which is caused by serum factors, one of which is ferritin found elevated in the patients. It might play a role in the high incidence of cancer in Gaucher patients. The Gaucher gene has been identified on a small segment at the end of the long arm (1q42-1qter) of human chromosome 1. Despite the fact that the three types show major phenotypic differences, the genes of these types express at least two functional domains. Namely, one domain would alter the enzyme such that neurologic disease resulted. Another domain would result in nonneurologic disease. The immunoblotting method used in differentiating one clinical type from another is still controversial.

Pathologic Features

The spleen, liver, and lymph nodes are markedly enlarged. Gaucher cells are the histologic hallmark of this disease (Fig. 55-5). They are round or polygonal in shape and measure 20 to 80 μm in diameter. The cytoplasm shows many fibrils of varying sizes or gives an appearance of striation. The cells are primarily derived from the reticuloendothelial system. An unusual cardiac and renal involvement with pulmonary hypertension in a 25-year-old black woman who had Gaucher's disease since 1 year of age has been reported.

Although the typical pulmonary infiltrate is seen on chest radiograph, it has rarely been reported. Severe involvement of lung in adult Gaucher also has been reported in three patients who had a long-standing history since infancy followed by juvenile onset of dyspnea. Their lungs are heavy, and the cut surfaces disclose diffuse interstitial infiltrate. Gaucher cells are found in the alveolar septa perivascularly, or they fill up alveoli and thus obliterate air exchange. Glomoid lesions in pulmonary arteri-

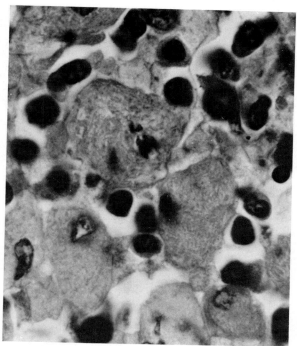

FIGURE 55-5 Gaucher cells from an infant with Gaucher's disease. They contain numerous fibrils and appear striated. H&E, ×1090.

oles with dilatation of postglomoid vessels form angiomatoids typical of grade A3 hypertensive pulmonary vascular disease (Fig. 55-6), and numerous marrow emboli of various ages containing Gaucher cells are also reported.

Malignant tumors associated with Gaucher's disease have been found in 35 out of 275 patients. The associated malignancies are myeloma, Hodgkin's disease, acute myelogenous leukemia, lymphatic leukemia, and carcinoma of the lung, breast, kidney, liver, colon, pancreas, skin, mouth, larynx, prostate, and brain.

Histochemically, the Gaucher cells show characteristic reactions staining pink to red with the modified periodic acid-Schiff stain for cerebroside.

Ultrastructure

The Gaucher cells contain cytoplasmic inclusion bodies which are pleomorphic structures surrounded by a single limiting membrane. These inclusions, called Gaucher bodies, contain tubular structures measuring 120 to 250 Å in diameter (Fig. 55-7), each of which consists of 10 to 12 fibrils in a characteristic arrangement. The inclusion bodies are derived from the cisternae of the endoplasmic reticulum. Acid phosphatase preparations disclose reaction granules within the Gaucher bodies, which indicate a lysosomal character of the inclusion material. Experimentally, Gaucher bodies have been produced in mice by administration of conduritol-β-epoxide which is an inhibitor of nonmammalian β-glucosidase.

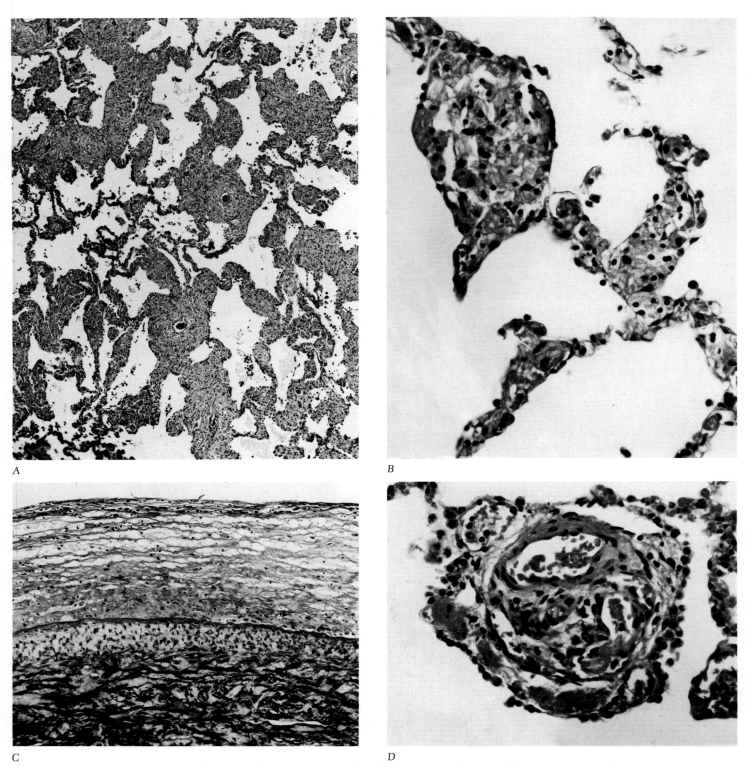

FIGURE 55-6 *A* and *C*. Low- and high-power photomicrographs of pulmonary parenchymal infiltration by Gaucher cells. The vascular bed appears to be absent in much of the tissue and what remains shows distension of capillaries with blood. *B*. Atherosclerotic lesion from the main pulmonary artery. *D*. Glomoid lesion in a pulmonary arteriole with dilatation of postglomoid vessels forming an angiomatoid, typical of grade A3 hypertensive pulmonary vascular disease. *(Courtesy of Dr. GM Hutchins, Am J Med 65:356, 1978.)*

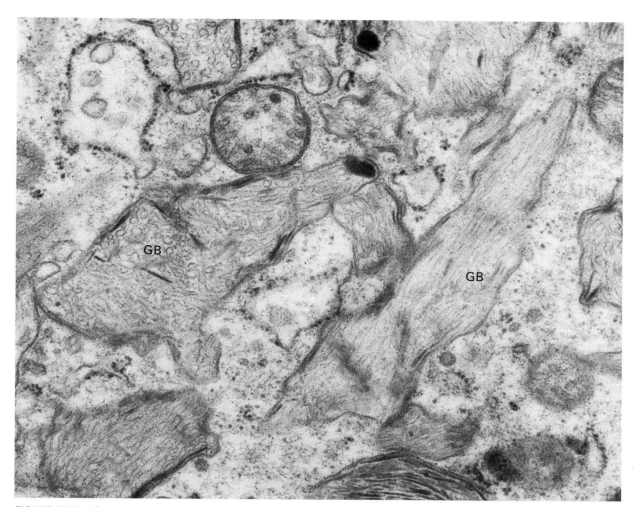

FIGURE 55-7   Electron micrograph of a portion of a Gaucher cell showing pleomorphic Gaucher bodies (GB) which contain tubular structures. ×43,000.

Biochemical Features

The organs of patients with the three types of Gaucher's disease almost always have a marked increase in the concentration of glucose-1-ceramide, occasionally exceeding 100 times normal. The enzyme defect in Gaucher's disease is a deficiency of β-glucosidase which catalyzes the cleavage of glucose from glycosyl ceramide.

Bone marrow transplantation in severe Gaucher's disease was successful in restoring β-glucosidase in mononuclear white blood cells and plasma with complete engraftment of the enzymatically normal donor cells; yet Gaucher cells persisted in bone marrow. This 8-year-old patient with type 3 Gaucher's disease died of sepsis 13 months after bone marrow transplantation.

Diagnosis

In all suspected cases, there should be a careful radiologic survey of the lungs and bones, identification of Gaucher cells in smears from the bone marrow, and assays of β-glucosidase in leukocytes, or cultured fibroblasts. Should liver biopsy or splenectomy be undertaken, enough fresh frozen tissue (1.0 g) should be preserved for determination of glycosyl ceramide and activity of β-glucosidase. Portions of these tissues should also be studied histologically and electron microscopically.

G_{M1} GANGLIOSIDOSIS

Clinical Features

Three types are recognized: type 1 is an infantile form with generalized gangliosidosis, accompanied by bone involvement and psychomotor retardation manifested shortly after birth. Early in the disease, the lungs are unremarkable; later, bronchopneumonia is common, and the patients usually die of bronchopneumonia before the age of 2 years. Radiologically, abnormalities similar to Hurler's disease are observed after 6 months. Foamy cells are demonstrable in smears of bone marrow. Type 2 is a juvenile form with later onset, milder bone abnormalities, and progressive motor and mental deterioration. The average life span varies from 3 to 10 years. Visceral histiocytosis is less common, but neuronal lipidosis occurs more often than in type 1. Type 3 is an adult form with juvenile onset of progressive cerebellar dysarthria and slow but progressive motor and intellectual impairment. Thus far, no patients have expired.

Pathologic Features

The liver, spleen, and kidneys are usually increased in size and weight. The lungs generally appear normal.

The most striking histologic finding is the presence of foamy histiocytes in many visceral organs. In the lungs, these cells are observed in the alveoli and septa. The ma-

terial in the cytoplasmic vacuoles consists of complex proteolipid compounds.

Ultrastructure

The foamy cells in the lungs and other organs contain membrane-bound inclusions which consist of a moderately electron-dense material mixed with fine granules (Fig. 55-8).

Ultrastructural studies of rectal mucosal biopsy proved to be useful in that the storage material was found in the plasma cells in G_{M1} gangliosidosis as well as other neuronal storage diseases.

Biochemical Features

Deficiency in G_{M1} ganglioside β-galactosidase causes G_{M1} ganglioside to accumulate in the different organs. The de-

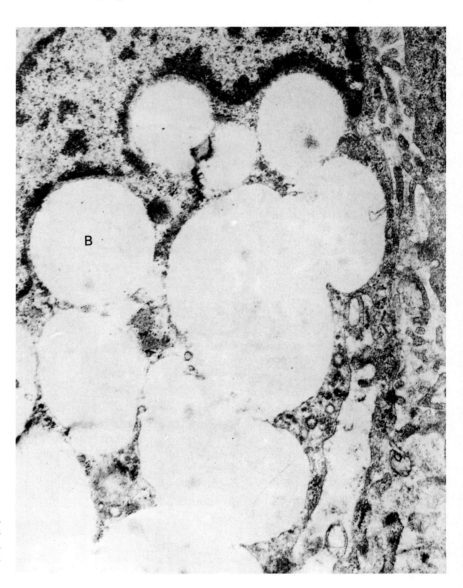

FIGURE 55-8 Electron micrograph of a portion of a foamy cell from a patient with G_{M1} gangliosidosis showing cytoplasmic membrane-bound inclusion bodies (B) which contain electron-lucent material mixed with fine granules. ×15,000.

ficiency of β-galactosidase apparently also interferes with the degrading process of mucopolysaccharides.

Diagnosis

The disease can be confirmed by analysis of β-galactosidase activity in leukocytes, urine, and skin. In heterozygotes, intermediate levels of the enzyme can be demonstrated.

SULFATIDE LIPIDOSIS (METACHROMATIC LEUKODYSTROPHY)

Six categories of sulfatide lipidosis have been identified according to the age of onset of clinical manifestations. The clinical manifestations reflect striking changes in the white matter of the brain.

Pathologic Features

Grossly, the visceral organs are unremarkable. Microscopic changes, characterized by metachromatic inclusion bodies in the cytoplasm, are widespread and affect the lung. The metachromatic granules are with histiocytes in the interalveolar septa, but not in the alveolar spaces or in the vascular walls in the septa. Ultrastructural examination indicates that the cytoplasmic inclusion bodies are composed primarily of lamellar structures and irregular whorls.

Biochemical Features

Patients afflicted with this disease show a marked increase in the concentration of cerebroside sulfatides in the brain and viscera secondary to reduced activity of arylsulfatase A and to a lesser degree in the activity of arylsulfatase B; arylsulfatase C is affected only in the sixth form, which begins with respiratory difficulty in early infancy and is characterized by progressive psychomotor deterioration.

Diagnosis

The most important diagnostic procedure is the determination of arylsulfatase A activity in the leukocytes, or cultured skin fibroblasts. Analysis for sulfatase A in the urine is rapid and simpler but less reliable.

KRABBE'S DISEASE (GLOBOID CELL LEUKODYSTROPHY)

Clinical Features

Three clinical forms of Krabbe's disease have been observed according to the age of onset. In most patients, the disease occurs in early infancy exhibiting the first clinical symptoms at 3 to 6 months of age. The disease is characterized by progressive psychomotor deterioration that generally culminates in death within 2 years. A late infancy form is rare and shows mental deterioration, pyramidal signs, and visual impairment manifested at the age of 2 to 6 years. The duration of this type is about 1 to 5 years. In the adult form, the main clinical manifestation consists of visual impairment which starts between the ages of 10 and 35 years. They exhibit slowly progressive motor deterioration, lasting between 2 and 10 years. The disease appears to be inherited in an autosomal recessive pattern.

Pathologic Features

Gross pathologic changes are generally confined to the brain. The white matter of all lobes is extensively affected, whereas the cortices and deep gray matter are relatively preserved.

Although the visceral organs appear normal, giant cells, similar to globoid cells in the nervous system, also occur in the lungs, lymph nodes, spleen, and bone marrow. The globoid cells, which are derived from histiocytes, are characterized by large, round cell bodies containing several peripherally placed nuclei (Fig. 55-9) which measure from 20 to 50 μm in diameter and are filled with cytoplasmic fine granules. Animal models

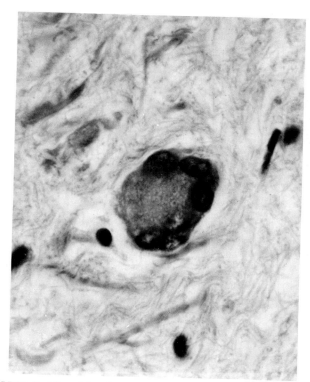

FIGURE 55-9 The globoid cell from a child with Krabbe's disease is characterized by large, round cell bodies containing several peripherally placed nuclei and many cytoplasmic fine granules. H&E, ×1100.

with Krabbe's disease such as sheep, dog, and twitcher mouse have been observed.

Biochemical Features

Deficient activity of galactocerebroside β-galactosidase, leading to a marked increase in the galactosyl ceramide concentration in the white matter of the brain, appears to be the primary enzyme defect in this disorder.

Diagnosis

In infants suspected of having Krabbe's disease, serum, leukocytes, or cultured fibroblasts should be studied for activity of galactocerebroside β-galactosidase.

FABRY'S DISEASE (GLYCOSPHINGOLIPID LIPIDOSIS)

Fabry's disease is the only sphingolipidosis that is transmitted by the gene on the X chromosome which controls the deficient hydrolytic enzyme, α-galactosyl hydrolase. The clinical picture results from the progressive accumulation of galactosyl-galactosyl-glucosyl ceramide in most visceral organs as well as in the brain.

Clinical Features

The initial manifestations appear in childhood and adolescence and are usually of two kinds: severe pain and telangiectases. The pain is often in the form of a lightning or burning sensation in the fingers and toes that extends to the palms and soles, respectively. Attacks of abdominal or flank pain simulate those of appendicitis or renal colic. The telangiectases are symmetric, involve the superficial layers of the skin, do not bleach on pressure, and are progressive. The oral mucosa, conjunctivae, hips, back, thighs, buttocks, penis, and scrotum are most commonly involved; the area between the umbilicus and the knees is less often, but severely, affected. Some patients develop pulmonary disorders which range from obstructive disease of the airways to diffuse interstitial disease. Pulmonary function tests in older patients may reveal significant airflow obstruction, reduced diffusing capacity, and a reduction in the $V_{max,25\%}$ values. Pulmonary complications are a frequent cause of death. These clinical manifestations are usually observed in humans. However, the clinical features are also noted in isolated cases of heterozygous women.

Pathologic Features

The lungs are increased in weight, and the cut surfaces are often congested and edematous. Multiple vacuoles are present in the alveolar epithelium, in the smooth muscles of the bronchi, within endothelial cells of the capillaries and arterioles, and in the smooth muscles of the arterioles.

Ultrastructural examination shows that both the capillary endothelium and the alveolar type II cells contain laminated inclusions with a periodicity of 50 to 60 Å. This pattern contrasts with the variable periodicity of the lamellar bodies that the type II cells contain in the normal lung.

Cytoplasmic inclusion bodies in the ciliated epithelial cells and goblet cells stain darkly in toluidine blue. Ultrastructurally, these inclusion bodies are limited by a single membrane and contain electron-dense lamellae arranged in either parallel or concentric fashion. Alveolar macrophages are devoid of these inclusions.

Biochemical Features and Diagnosis

The primary enzyme defect is the absence of an α-galactosyl hydrolase. Affected males can be identified by demonstrating an increase in trihexosyl ceramide and by assaying hydrolase activity in serum, leukocytes, tears, and cultured skin fibroblasts.

MUCOPOLYSACCHARIDOSES

The term mucopolysaccharidosis (MPS) refers to a group of genetic diseases manifested by abnormal tissue deposition of acid mucopolysaccharide (glycosaminoglycans). Seven major forms of the disease have been recognized: Hurler's syndrome (MPS I), Sheie's syndrome (MPS IS, formerly V), Hunter's syndrome (MPS II), Sanfilippo's syndrome (MPS III), Morquio's syndrome (MPS IV), Maroteaux-Lamy syndrome (MPS VI), and Sly syndrome (MPS VII).

The most severely affected patients (except for those with type IS) commonly have respiratory involvement, particularly obstructive disease of the airways. All forms, but type II, in which the mode of inheritance follows an X-linked recessive pattern, are autosomal recessive traits.

Pathologic Features

The affected organs vary with the type, but despite extensive involvement of other viscera, the lungs are rarely affected grossly.

In type I, histologic alterations are seen in almost all organs, including the lungs. The characteristic feature is the presence of an abnormal deposited material in cells that are variously called clear cells, gargoyle cells, Hurler's cells, or balloon cells. They are large, oval, or polygonal, measure 20 μm in diameter, and contain pale central nuclei. Frozen sections exhibit metachromatic material in toluidine blue stain and give positive reactions in Alcian blue preparations. The histologic changes in types II and III are similar to those of type I. The histologic findings in the other types are less well documented.

On ultrastructural examination, the gargoyle cells characteristically contain round or oval inclusion bodies which are membrane-bound and display an electron-lucent or low electron-dense material, occasionally mixed with fine granules or lamellae.

Biochemistry

Types I and IS show a deficiency of α-L-iduronidase and increased urinary excretion of dermatan sulfate and heparan sulfate. The deficiency in type II involves iduronate sulfatase. Dermatan sulfate and heparan sulfate are also excreted in urine in type II. Although about 80 percent of the extracted mucopolysaccharide is dermatan sulfate in type I, in type II that portion is about 55 percent. In type III, there are four enzymatic steps involved to excrete and accumulate heparan sulfate only: they are heparan N-sulfatase in type IIIA, N-acetyl-α-D glucosaminidase in type IIIB, acetyl CoA:α-glucosaminide-N-acetyltransferase in type IIIC, and N-acetyl-α-D-glucosaminide-6-sulfatase in type IIID. The enzymatic defect of type IV is galactosamine-6-sulfate sulfatase in IVA and β-galactosidase in IVB and shows increased levels of keratan sulfate in urine. Type VI reveals a deficiency of arylsulfatase B and increased urinary excretion of dermatan sulfate, while in type VII defective degradation of dermatan sulfate and heparan sulfate is due to a deficiency of β-glucuronidase.

Diagnosis

The excretion of mucopolysaccharides in the urine is markedly increased. Although metachromatic material can be demonstrated in polymorphonuclear leukocytes and lymphocytes, the diagnosis can be established only by measuring urine mucopolysaccharides with precise identification of the substances excreted. The defect of enzyme of each type should be studied in leukocytes, serum, or fibroblasts.

GLYCOGEN STORAGE DISEASE

Among the major groups of glycogen storage disorder (GSD), Pompe's disease (GSD, type II) frequently shows cardiorespiratory disturbances. Hypotonia, which often develops by 2 months of age, is the cardinal feature of this disorder. The heart is markedly enlarged, and heart failure is common. Most patients die within the first year of life. However, a few survive up to 15 years. The disease is transmitted as an autosomal recessive trait.

Pathologic Features

The heart is markedly enlarged and increased in weight. About one-fifth of the patients show thickening of the endocardium similar to that seen in endocardial fibroelastosis. The liver is also enlarged. The lungs and brain are grossly unremarkable.

There is a massive accumulation of glycogen granules

in the cytoplasm of the parenchymal cells of most organs, including the lungs. Alveolar foamy macrophages are filled with glycogenlike material (Fig. 55-10). It is also present in smaller amounts in cartilage cells, mucus, and bronchial epithelial cells. Ultrastructurally, the cytoplasmic inclusion bodies are membrane-bound and contain electron-dense glycogen granules.

Biochemistry

Patients with Pompe's disease show massive accumulation of tissue glycogen due to a deficiency in an acid maltase (α-1,4-glucosidase).

Diagnosis

The diagnosis can be established by the presence of increased tissue glycogen concentration and deficiency of α-1,4-glucosidase. The urine, muscle biopsies, and cultured fibroblasts are also useful in diagnosis.

DISORDERS OF AMINO ACID METABOLISM

Amongst the various types of amino acid metabolic disorders, only maple syrup urine disease (leucinosis, branched-chain ketonuria) is occasionally associated with bouts of respiratory embarrassment for which there is no infectious process. In affected infants, respiratory distress develops within the first week of life. The infants often become apneic and require respiratory assistance. Severe psychomotor deterioration and episodes of seizures occur during the course of the disease, and the children usually die from intercurrent infections within the first year. However, some patients, with the help of a synthetic diet, survive up to 13 years of age. The clinical features are consistent with an autosomal recessive inheritance.

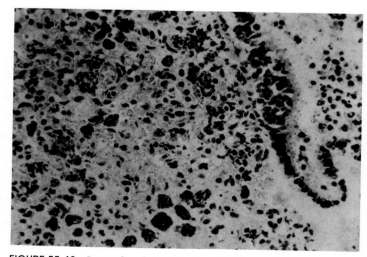

FIGURE 55-10 Intra-alveolar and interstitial macrophage laden with glycogen granules (black granules). Best's glycogen stain. (*Courtesy of Dr. H. Spencer, 1985.*)

Despite severe clinical symptoms in early life, at autopsy only the brain shows specific changes; grossly, it exhibits microcephaly and microgyria; histologically, it shows a deficiency in myelin sheaths, presumably a result of reduced synthesis of proteolipids.

Biochemical Features

An excessive amount of three amino acids (leucine, isoleucine, and valine) and branched-chain keto acids in the plasma suggests a failure in the oxidative decarboxylation of the derivatives of these amino acids.

Diagnosis

The maple syrup odor of the urine can be detected within the first weeks of life. Although the odor is clinically the most distinctive sign of this disease, the diagnosis should be verified by studies of the amino acids and keto acids in blood and urine.

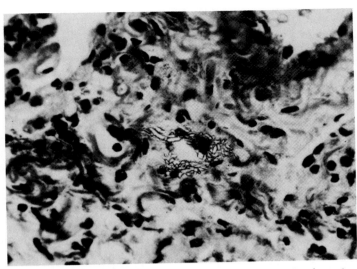

FIGURE 55-11 Cystinosis of the lung showing crystals of cystine containing reticuloendothelial cells surrounding pulmonary vessels. (*Courtesy of Dr. H. Spencer, 1985.*)

CYSTINE STORAGE DISEASE (LIGNAC-FANCONI DISEASE)

This disorder reveals widespread pathologic changes in many organs. The mode of inheritance is considered to be a simple Mendelian recessive character.

Clinical Features

The children afflicted with this disease frequently show severe rickets, dwarfism with marked photophobia, or amino aciduria, and they die from infection or renal diseases.

Pathologic Features

The disease affects the bones, kidneys, lymph nodes, spleen, liver, and lungs. The deposits provoke no cellular reactions nor do they alter pulmonary functions. The deposits may be mistaken for calcium with von Kóssa's stain if they contain traces of cystine. The cystine is water soluble and is best fixed in absolute alcohol. In tissue sections,

the crystals are birefringent and form clumps of radiating needlelike crystals when treated with concentrated sulfuric acid and phosphotungstic acid. The crystals in the lungs are distributed mainly within the peribronchial and periarterial reticuloendothelial cells in alveolar septa (Fig. 55-11).

CONCLUSIONS

Enzyme replacement therapy for these storage diseases is not available at present. However, the birth of children afflicted with inborn errors of metabolic disorders can be predicted by prenatal diagnosis through amniocentesis and analysis of enzyme activity of cultured amniotic cells. Advice recommending genetic counseling, therefore, seems to be one of the important functions of the physician in those instances where parents are homozygotes and may produce a baby afflicted with one of these disorders.

BIBLIOGRAPHY

Adachi M, Volk BW: Methodology: Histochemistry, in Volk BW, Schneck L (eds), *The Gangliosidoses.* New York, Plenum, 1975, pp 249–264.
  Histochemical procedures and the characteristics of the various lipids and other chemical compounds that constitute the cytoplasmic inclusions of the different storage diseases.

Bach G, Eisenberg F Jr, Cantz M, Neufeld EF: The defect in the Hunter syndrome: Deficiency of sulfoiduronate sulfatase. Proc Natl Acad Sci USA 70:2134–2138, 1973.
  Sulfoiduronate sulfatase deficiency is implicated in the pathogenesis of Hunter's syndrome.

Besley GTN, Hoogeboom AJM, Hoogeveen AM, Kleijer WJ, Galjaard H: Somatic cell hybridization studies showing different gene mutations in Niemann-Pick variants. Hum Genet 54:409–412, 1980.
  Somatic cell hybridization discloses a different gene mutation in type C Niemann-Pick disease.

Beutler E, Kuhl W, Sorge J: Glucocerebrosidase "processing" and gene expression in various forms of Gaucher disease. Am J Hum Genet 37:1062–1070, 1985.

Immunoblotting is used to differentiate among the clinical types of Gaucher's disease.

Brady RO, Barranger JA: Glucosylceramide lipidosis: Gaucher's disease, in Stanbury JB, Wyngaarden JB, Fredrickson DS, Goldstein JL, Brown MS (eds), *The Metabolic Basis of Inherited Disease,* 5th ed. New York, McGraw-Hill, 1983, pp 842–856.

A critical review of Gaucher's disease which includes patients from four interrelated families with type 3.

Brady RO, Kanfer JN, Mock MB, Fredrickson DS: The metabolism of sphingomyelin. II. Evidence of an enzyme deficiency in Niemann-Pick disease. Proc Natl Acad Sci USA 55:366–369, 1966.

Sphingomyelinase deficiency is implicated in the pathogenesis of type A Niemann-Pick disease.

Brady RO, Kanfer JN, Shapiro D: Metabolism of glucocerebroside. II. Evidence of an enzyme deficiency in Gaucher's disease. Biochem Biophys Res Commun 18:211–225, 1965.

Deficiency of β-glucosidase is reported to catalyze the cleavage of glucose from glycosylceramide in Gaucher's disease.

Cagle PT, Ferry GD, Beaudet AL, Hawkins EP: Pulmonary hypertension in an 18-year-old girl with cholesterol ester storage disease (CESD) [clinical conference]. Am J Med Genet 24:711–722, 1986.

As in Gaucher's disease, cholesterol ester storage disease can elicit pulmonary hypertension.

Choplin RH, Theros EG: Pulmonary involvement in diseases of other systems. Radiol Clin North Am 22:673–685, 1984.

The radiographic pattern is helpful in developing an appropriate differential diagnosis for the predominantly extrapulmonary diseases.

Dancis J, Hutzler J, Levitz M: The diagnosis of maple syrup urine disease (branched-chain ketoaciduria) by the in vitro study of the peripheral leukocyte. Pediatrics 32:234–238, 1963.

Branched-chain ketoacids were found in in vitro studies of the peripheral leukocytes from patients with maple syrup urine disease.

Desnick RJ: Gaucher disease: A century of delineation and understanding. Prog Clin Biol Res 95:1–30, 1982.

A depiction of the growth of ideas about this disease and a delineation of the genetic aspects that await clarification.

Desnick RJ, Sweely CC: Fabry's disease: α-Galactosidase A deficiency, in Stanbury JB, Wyngaarden JB, Fredrickson DS, Goldstein JL, Brown MS (eds), *The Metabolic Basis of Inherited Disease,* 5th ed. New York, McGraw-Hill, 1983, pp 906–944.

A comprehensive review of Fabry's disease and of relevant diagnostic procedures.

Devine EA, Smith M, Arredondo-Vega FX, Shafit-Zagardo B, Desnick RJ: Chromosomal localization of the gene for Gaucher disease. Prog Clin Biol Res 95:511–534, 1982.

The structural gene for human GBA has been identified on chromosome 1 using somatic cell hybridization techniques for gene mapping. The results of this study localize the gene for GBA to the narrow region, 1q42 leads to 1qter.

Gal AE, Brady RO, Barranger JA, Pentchev PG: The diagnosis of type A and B Niemann-Pick disease and detection of carriers using leukocytes and a chromogenic analogue of sphingomyelin. Clin Chim Acta 104:129–132, 1980.

In type B Niemann-Pick disease the level of sphingomyelinase activity is slightly higher than that of type A.

Huijing F, van Creveld S, Losekoot G: Diagnosis of generalized glycogen storage disease (Pompe's disease). J Pediatr 63:984–987, 1963.

Investigations on the deficiency of acid maltase (α-1,4-glucosidase) in generalized glycogen storage disease (Pompe's disease).

Kreese H, Paschke E, Von Figura K, Gilberg W, Fuchs W: Sanfilippo disease type D: Deficiency of N-acetylglucosamine-6-sulfatase required for heparan sulfate degradation. Proc Natl Acad Sci 77:6822–6826, 1980.

Using skin fibroblasts from two patients who had symptoms of the Sanfilippo syndrome (mucopolysaccharidosis III) the authors found that it is the sulfatase activity directed toward heparan sulfate (and not keratan sulfate) that is deficient in these patients.

Lee RE: The pathology of Gaucher disease. Prog Clin Biol Res 95:177–217, 1982.

From an experience with 275 patients, the authors describe the various types of systemic and pulmonary involvement in this disease. They call attention to the high incidence of malignant tumors in patients with type I disease.

Levade T, Salvayre R, Douste-Blazy L: Sphingomyelinases and Niemann-Pick disease. J Clin Chem Clin Biochem 24:205–220, 1986.
In the first part of this review, the properties of normal mammalian sphingomyelinase are reviewed. In the second part, the classification of Niemann-Pick disease, the characteristic features of each type, and the biologic tools used for the diagnosis are reported.

Matsumoto T, Matsumori H, Taki T, Takagi T, Fukuda Y: Infantile G_{M1} gangliosidosis with marked manifestation of lungs. Acta Pathol Jpn 29:269–276, 1979.
In a 14-month-old boy with G_{M1} gangliosidosis who died of respiratory insufficiency, there was a marked accumulation of foam cells in the alveolar spaces as well as widespread visceral involvement by similar cells.

O'Brien JS: The Gangliosidoses, in Stanbury JB, Wyngaarden JB, Fredrickson DS, Goldstein JL, Brown MS (eds), *The Metabolic Basis of Inherited Disease*, 5th ed. New York, McGraw-Hill, 1983, pp 945–969.
A comprehensive review of gangliosidoses.

Paakko P, Ryhanen L, Rantala H, Autio-Harmainen H: Pulmonary emphysema in a nonsmoking patient with Salla disease. Am Rev Respir Dis 135:979–982, 1987.
Severe centrilobular emphysema affecting primarily the lower lobes is reported in a Finnish patient with Salla disease, a recessively inherited disorder of sialic acid metabolism that leads to intralysosomal accumulation of free sialic acid in cells of various tissues.

Rappeport JM, Ginns EI: Bone marrow transplantation in severe Gaucher's disease. N Engl J Med 311:84–88, 1984.
Allogeneic bone-marrow transplantation of normal cells was done in an 8-year-old patient with type 3 Gaucher's disease in an attempt to alter his progressive deterioration. There was no clinical improvement.

Rodriguez FH, Hoffmann EO, Ordinario AT, Baliga M: Fabry's disease in heterozygous women. Arch Pathol Lab Med 109:89–91, 1985.
The authors correlate the clinical, pathologic, enzymatic, and ultastructural findings in a 42-year-old woman with the heterozygous form of Fabry's disease.

Rosenberg DM, Ferrans VJ, Fulmer JD, Line BR, Barranger JA, Brady RO, Crystal RG: Chronic airflow obstruction in Fabry's disease. Am J Med 68:898–905, 1980.
Seven patients with Fabry's disease were found to have significant obstruction to airflow. Their airway epithelial cells, obtained by bronchoscopy, demonstrated that these cells contained inclusion bodies consistent with deposits of ceramide trihexoside.

Schneider EL, Epstein CJ, Kaback MJ, Brandes D: Severe pulmonary involvement in adult Gaucher's disease. Am J Med 63:475–480, 1977.
Instances of severe pulmonary involvement in adult Gaucher's disease.

Smith RRL, Hutchins GM, Sack GH, Ridolfi RL: Unusual cardiac, renal and pulmonary involvement in Gaucher's disease: Interstitial glucocerebroside accumulation, pulmonary hypertension and fatal bone marrow embolization. Am J Med 65:352–360, 1978.
In a 25-year-old woman with Gaucher's disease, the pulmonary findings included pulmonary arterial hypertension, accentuated basilar deposition of glucocerebroside in the interstitium of alveolar septum, and fatal bone marrow embolization.

Spencer H: *Pathology of the Lung.* New York, Pergamon, 1985, pp 753–754.
Pulmonary pathology in glycogen storage and Lignac-Fanconi diseases.

Suzuki K, Suzuki K: The twitcher mouse. A model of human globoid cell leukodystrophy (Krabbe's disease). Am J Pathol 111:394–397, 1983.
Description of an animal model for Krabbe's disease.

Volk BW, Schneck L: *The Gangliosidoses.* New York, Plenum, 1975.
Excellent review of gangliosidoses.

Wise D, Wallace HJ, Jellinek EH: Angiokeratoma corporis diffusum: A clinical study of eight affected families. Q J Med 31:177–206, 1962.
Cases with Fabry's disease develop pulmonary airway obstruction to diffuse interstitial disease and pulmonary complications.

Yamano T, Shimada M, Okada S, Yutaka T, Kato T, Yabuuchi H: Ultrastructural study of biopsy specimens of rectal mucosa. Arch Pathol Lab Med 106:673–677, 1982.
Importance of electron microscopy of rectal mucosa proved useful in making the diagnosis in a variety of neuronal diseases.

NOTES

Appendixes

Respiratory Questionnaire

Name _____ Social security no. _____ Date _____

Plant _____ Sex ___ Date of birth _____ Age _____

Questionnaire administered by _____

I. Occupational history: Please list entire work history starting with present job and going back to first job. (Use extra sheet if necessary.)

Industry (or company) and location	From	To	Specific job

	Yes	No	Number of years
A. Have you ever worked in a dusty job?			
1. In a mine?			
2. In a quarry?			
3. In a foundry?			
4. In a pottery?			
5. In a cotton, flax, or hemp mill?			
6. With asbestos?			
7. In a brick plant?			
8. As a sandblaster?			
9. In the manufacture of glass, ceramics, or abrasives?			
10. In other dusty jobs?			
Specify _____			
B. Have you ever worked with chemicals?			
1. Solvents?			
Specify _____			
2. Acids?			
Specify _____			
3. Lead?			
4. Plastics?			
Specify _____			
5. TDI?			

	Yes	No

II. Previous illnesses
  A. Have you ever had any of the following problems?
    1. Asthma?
    2. Emphysema?
    3. Chronic bronchitis?
    4. Pneumonia?
    5. Tuberculosis?
    6. Pleurisy?
    7. Heart trouble of any type?
III. Symptoms
  A. Cough
    1. Do you usually cough first thing in the morning?
    2. Do you usually cough at other times during the day or night?

Skip 3 to 6 if answer to 1 and 2 is "no." Answer if "yes."

    3. Do you cough on most days for as much as 3 months of the year?
    4. For how many years have you had this cough?
      Less than 2 years _____
      2 to 5 years _____
      5 years or more _____
    5. Do you cough more on any particular day of the week?
      If yes, which day? _____
    6. Do you cough during any particular season of the year?
      If yes, which season? _____

  B. Sputum
    1. Do you usually bring up phlegm, sputum, or mucus from your chest first thing in the morning?
    2. Do you usually bring up phlegm, sputum, or mucus from your chest at other times of the day or night?

Skip 3 and 4 if answer to 1 and 2 is "no." Answer if "yes."

    3. Do you bring up phlegm, sputum, or mucus from your chest on most days for as much as 3 months of the year?
    4. For how many years have you raised phlegm, sputum, or mucus from your chest
      Less than 2 years _____
      2 to 5 years _____
      5 years or more _____

  C. Wheezing
    1. Does your breathing ever sound wheezy?
    2. Have you ever had attacks of shortness of breath with wheezing?
    3. Have you ever had a feeling of tightness in your chest?

Skip 4 to 6 if answer to 1, 2, or 3 is "no." Answer if "yes."

    4. At what age did wheezing first occur? _____
    5. How frequently does wheezing occur?
      Daily _____
      Nightly _____
      A few times per week _____
      A few times per month _____
      A few times per year _____
    6. Is it worse on any particular day of the week?
      What day? _____

D. Breathlessness
  1. Do you get short of breath when walking on level ground?
  2. Do you get short of breath while walking up stairs?
  3. How many flights of stairs can you climb up without stopping?
     1 to 2? _____
     2 to 3? _____
     More than 3? _____
E. Hemoptysis
  1. Have you ever coughed up blood from your chest? If yes, when was the last time this happened? _____

IV. Smoking
  A. Smoking (currently)
    1. Do you now smoke regularly (cigarettes, pipe, cigars)?

Skip 2 to 6 if answer to 1 is "no." Answer if "yes."

    2. How old were you when you started smoking?
       _____
    3. For how many years have you smoked regularly?
       _____
    4. How many cigarettes do you now smoke each day?
       _____
    5. How much pipe tobacco do you now smoke each week?
       _____
    6. How many cigars do you now smoke each day?
       _____

  B. Smoking (formerly)
    1. Have you ever smoked regularly?

Skip 2 to 7 if answer to 1 is "no." Answer if "yes."

    2. How old were you when you started smoking regularly?
       _____
    3. For how many years did you smoke regularly?
       _____
    4. How long ago did you last quit smoking?
       Months _____
       Years _____
    5. How many cigarettes did you usually smoke per day?
       _____
    6. How much pipe tobacco did you usually smoke per week?
       _____
    7. How many cigars did you usually smoke per day?
       _____

V. Additional comments

Appendix *B*

Normal Values

TYPICAL VALUES FOR A 20-YEAR-OLD, SEATED MAN*

Ventilation (BTPS)

Tidal volume, L	0.50
Frequency, breaths/min	12
Minute volume, L/min	6.00
Respiratory dead space, ml	150
Alveolar ventilation, L/min	4.20

Lung Volumes (BTPS)

Inspiratory capacity (IC), L	3.00
Expiratory reserve volume (ERV), L	1.50
Vital capacity (VC), L	4.50
Residual volume (RV), L	1.50
Functional residual capacity (FRC), L	3.00
Total lung capacity (TLC), L	6.00
Residual volume/total lung capacity $\times$ 100 (RV/TLC%)	25

Mechanics of Breathing

Maximum voluntary ventilation (MVV), L/min	170
Forced expiratory volume in 1 s ($FEV_1/FVC\%$)	83
Forced expiratory volume in 3 s ($FEV_3/FVC\%$)	97
Forced expiratory flow during middle half of FVC ($FEF_{25-75\%}$), L/s	4.7
Forced inspiratory flow during middle half of FIVC ($FIF_{25-75\%}$), L/s	5.0
Static compliance of the lungs (Cst,L), L/cmH_2O	0.2
Compliance of lungs and thoracic cage, L/cmH_2O	0.1
Airway resistance at FRC (Raw), $cmH_2O/L/s$	1.5
Pulmonary resistance at FRC, $cmH_2O/L/s$	2.0
Airway conductance at FRC (Gaw), $L/s/cmH_2O$	0.66
Specific conductance (Gaw/V_L)	0.22
Work of quiet breathing, $(kg \cdot m)/min$	0.5
Maximum work of breathing, $(kg \cdot m)/breath$	10
Maximum inspiratory pressure, mmHg	75
Maximum expiratory pressure, mmHg	120

Distribution of Inspired Gas

Single-breath N_2 test (ΔN_2 from 750 to 1250 ml in expired gas), % N_2	<1.5
Alveolar N_2 after 7 min of breathing O_2, % N_2	<2.5
Closing volume (CV), ml	400
CV/VC $\times$ 100%	9
Closing capacity (CC), ml	1900
CC/TLC $\times$ 100%	32
Slope of phase III in single-breath N_2 test, % N_2/L	<2

*Height = 165 cm; weight = 64 kg; body surface area = 1.7 m².

Pulmonary Blood Flow

Cardiac output, L/min	5.40
Virtual venous admixture/cardiac output $\times$ 100%	<7
Anatomic venous admixture/cardiac output $\times$ 100%	<3

Gas Exchange

O_2 consumption at rest (STPD), ml/min	240
CO_2 output at rest (STPD), ml/min	192
Respiratory exchange ratio (R), CO_2 output/O_2 uptake	0.8

Alveolar Gas

$P_{A_{O_2}}$, mmHg	105
$P_{A_{CO_2}}$, mmHg	40

Arterial Blood

Pa_{O_2}, mmHg	95
Sa_{O_2}, %	98
pH	7.41
Pa_{CO_2}, mmHg	40
Pa_{O_2} while breathing 100% O_2, mmHg	640
$P(A-a)_{O_2}$, mmHg	10

Alveolar Ventilation-Perfusion

Alveolar ventilation, L/min	4.20
Pulmonary capillary blood flow, L/min	5.40
Alveolar ventilation/blood flow ($\dot{V}_A/\dot{Q}$)	0.8
Physiological dead space/tidal volume $\times$ 100 (V_D/V_T, %)	<30
Alveolar-arterial P_{O_2}, mmHg	10

Diffusion

Diffusing capacity at rest for CO, single-breath ($DL_{CO_{sb}}$), ml CO/min/mmHg	32

Control of Ventilation

Ventilatory response to hypercapnia, L/min/mmHg	>0.5
Ventilatory response to hypoxia, L/min per ΔS_{O_2} (%)	>0.2
Arterial blood P_{O_2} during moderate exercise, mmHg	95

Pulmonary Hemodynamics

Pulmonary blood flow (cardiac output), L/min	5.40
Pulmonary artery pressure, mmHg	25/8
Pulmonary capillary blood volume, ml	100
Pulmonary "capillary" blood pressure (wedge), mmHg	<10

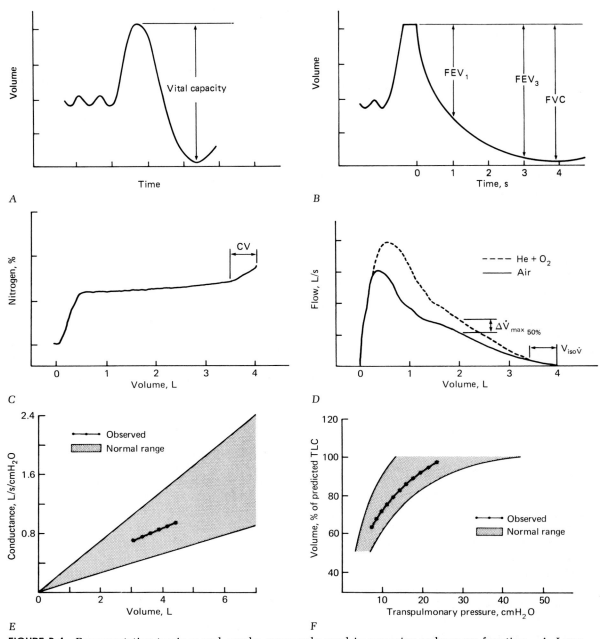

FIGURE B-1 Representative tracings and graphs commonly used in assessing pulmonary function. *A.* Lung volumes (vital capacity). *B.* Mechanics of breathing (forced expiratory volumes). *C.* Distribution (closing volumes). *D.* Flow-volume curves for breathing air and a helium-oxygen mixture. *E.* Mechanics of breathing (airway conductance). *F.* Mechanics of breathing (compliance of lungs).

Prophylaxis for Influenza and Pneumococcal Pneumonia

Influenza Vaccine
   The Viruses
   Individuals at Risk
   Options for Preventing Influenza

Pneumococcal Vaccine

Vaccines are now available to prevent influenza and pneumococcal pneumonia in individuals who might have difficulty in coping with them under conventional medical management or are particularly vulnerable to respiratory infection.

INFLUENZA VACCINE

In May 1986, the Immunization Practices Advisory Committee (ACIP) of the Centers for Disease Control (CDC) issued its annual advisory concerning Recommendations for the Use of the Influenza Vaccine During the Year 1986–1987. The following draws heavily on the CDC report. Even though the nature of the vaccine is destined to change somewhat almost from year to year, the general guiding principles for the use of this vaccine will probably remain unchanged. The CDC report for each year should be consulted for changes and details.

Influenza is a major threat to life among certain high-risk patients. It is responsible for about 10,000 patients in a nonepidemic year and for more than 30,000 after a severe epidemic. Killed influenza vaccine can prevent the illness if the viruses represented in the vaccine correspond closely in antigenic structure to the anticipated wild-type strain: the vaccine has proved to be completely effective in about two-thirds of recipients and has attenuated the disease in others whom it failed to protect completely.

The Viruses

Influenza A viruses are classified into subtypes based on two antigens: hemagglutinin (H) and neuraminidase (N). Three subtypes of hemagglutinin (H1, H2, H3) and two

subtypes of neuraminidase (N1, N2) are recognized among influenza A viruses that have caused widespread human disease. Immunity to these antigens, especially hemagglutinin, reduces the likelihood of infection and the severity of disease if infection does occur. However, there may be sufficient antigenic variation (antigenic drift) within the same subtype over time, so that infection or vaccination with one strain may not induce immunity to distantly related strains of the same subtype. Although influenza B viruses have shown much more antigenic stability than influenza A viruses, antigenic variation does occur. For these reasons, major epidemics of respiratory disease caused by new variants of influenza continue to occur, and the antigenic characteristics of current strains provide the basis for selecting virus strains included in each year's vaccine.

Individuals at Risk

"High-risk" persons may become deathly ill during a bout of influenza because of either associated health problems or age. Not only are they apt to require hospitalization for their illness but mortality rates are apt to be inordinate. The high mortality is due not only to the pneumonia but also to the final strain that the disease imposes on the underlying chronic pulmonary or cardiopulmonary disease. Influenza is a serious epidemiologic problem for the increasing number of elderly and for certain groups of younger individuals who are particularly susceptible to the disease, e.g., neonates who have survived respiratory intensive care, patients with cystic fibrosis, and individuals who have undergone organ transplantation.

Options for Preventing Influenza

Two measures are available to prevent influenza: (1) immunoprophylaxis using vaccines; and (2) chemoprophylaxis (as well as chemotherapy) using the antiviral drug amantadine hydrochloride (Symmetrel).

VACCINATION

The best protection for the high-risk individuals is vaccination, *each year*, before the start of the influenza season. High-risk individuals include those for whom influenza would have dire consequences and those who have an inordinate potential for infection. Vaccination is also used for individuals with a strong interest in avoiding influenza, in reducing the severity of disease if it should befall them, or minimizing chances of transmitting infection to high-risk individuals in their environments.

Inactivated Vaccine

Influenza vaccines are made from highly purified egg-grown viruses that have been rendered noninfectious ("inactivated"). Influenza vaccine contains three virus strains (two type A and one type B) that represent influenza viruses currently circulating in the world and believed likely to occur in the United States in the winter ahead. The potency of the vaccine is adjusted with two goals in mind: (1) to evoke minimal systemic and febrile reactions; and (2) to elicit hemagglutinin-inhibition antibody titers that probably would protect them against infection by strains like those in the vaccine or by related variants. Although the elderly, the very young, and patients with certain chronic diseases may develop lower postvaccination antibody titers than young adults—and thus be more susceptible to upper respiratory tract infection—influenza vaccine can still be effective in preventing lower respiratory tract involvement or other complications of influenza.

Recommendations for Use of Inactivated Vaccine

Influenza vaccine is recommended for individuals at high risk who are 6 months of age or older, for the medical personnel who care for them, for primary providers of care in the home setting, for children receiving long-term aspirin therapy, and for other persons who wish to decrease their chances of acquiring influenza illness. Vaccine composition for 1987–1988 and doses are given in Table C-1. Guidelines for the use of vaccine are given below for different segments of the population. Any vaccine left over from the previous year should not be used: although the current influenza vaccine often contains one or more antigens used in previous years, immunity declines during the year following vaccination. Therefore, a history of vaccination in any previous year with a vaccine containing one or more antigens included in the current vaccine does not preclude the need for revaccination for the 1987–1988 influenza season to provide optimal protection.

TABLE C-1

*Influenza Vaccine Dosage by Age of Patient— United States, 1987–1988 Influenza Season**

Age Group	Product†	Dosage‡, ml	No. Doses	Route§
6–35 months	Split virus only	0.25	2¶	IM
3–12 years	Split virus only	0.5	2¶	IM
Older than 12 years	Whole or split virus	0.5	1	IM

*Vaccine contains 15 μg each of influenza A/Taiwan/1/86 (hemagluttinin 1, neuraminidase 1); influenza A/Leningrad/360/86 (hemagluttinin 3, neuraminidase 2); and influenza B/Ann Arbor/1/86 hemagluttin antigens in each 0.5 ml. Manufacturers include Connaught Laboratories (Swiftwater, Pennsylvania) (Fluzone, whole or split; distributed by E. R. Squibb, Princeton, New Jersey), Parke-Davis (Fluogen; Morris Plains, New Jersey), and Wyeth Laboratories (Influenza Virus Vaccine, Trivalent, split; Philadelphia, Pennsylvania). Manufacturer's phone numbers for further information are Connaught, (800) 822-2463; Parke-Davis, (800) 223-0432; and Wyeth, (800) 321-2304.

†Because of the lower potential for causing febrile reactions, only split (subvirion) vaccine should be used in children. When used according to the recommended dosage, split and whole virus vaccines produce similar immunogenicity and side effects in adults.

‡Because children are accessible when pediatric vaccines are administered, it may be desirable to administer influenza vaccine to high-risk children simultaneously with routine pediatric vaccine or pneumococcal polysaccharide vaccine, but in a different site. Although studies have not been done, no diminution of immunogenicity or enhancement of adverse reactions should be expected.

§The recommended site of vaccination is the deltoid muscle for adults and older children. The preferred site for infants and young children is the anterolateral aspect of the thigh.

¶Two doses are recommended for maximum protection with at least 4 weeks between doses. However, if the individual received at least one dose of influenza vaccine between the 1978 to 1979 and 1986 to 1987 influenza seasons, one dose is sufficient.

NOTE: IM = intramuscular.

SOURCE: Prevention and Control of Influenza. Recommendations of the Immunization Practices Advisory Committee. Centers for Disease Control. Ann Intern Med 107:521–525, 1987.

TABLE C-2

Influenza Vaccination: High-Priority Target Groups for Special Vaccination Programs

Greatest medical risk of influenza-related complications

Adults and children with chronic disorders of the cardiovascular or pulmonary systems that are severe enough to have required medical follow-up or hospitalization during the preceding year.

Residents of nursing homes and other chronic-care facilities (i.e., institutions housing patients of any age with chronic medical conditions).

Moderate medical risk of influenza-related complications

Otherwise healthy individuals 6 years of age or older.

Adults and children with chronic metabolic diseases (including diabetes mellitus), renal dysfunction, anemia, immunosuppression, or asthma severe enough to require regular medical follow-up or hospitalization during the preceding year.

Children receiving long-term aspirin therapy, who may be at risk of developing Reye's syndrome following influenza infection.

Potentially capable of nosocomial transmission of influenza to high-risk persons

Physicians, nurses, and other personnel who have extensive contact with high-risk patients (e.g., primary-care and certain specialty clinicians, staff of intensive-care units, particularly neonatal intensive-care units).

Providers of care to high-risk persons in the home setting, e.g., family members, visiting nurses, volunteer workers.

Other groups

Any person who wishes to reduce the likelihood of acquiring influenza infection.

A pregnant woman with a medical condition that increases her risk of complications from influenza should be vaccinated as long as she has no egg allergy. Waiting until after the first trimester is a reasonable precaution to minimize the theoretical possibility of teratogenicity. However, it may be undesirable to delay vaccination of a pregnant woman with a high-risk condition who will be in the first trimester of pregnancy when the "influenza season" usually begins.

The preferred route of vaccination is intramuscular. The recommended site of vaccination is the deltoid muscle for adults and older children and the anterolateral aspect of the thigh for infants and young children.

High-Priority Target Groups

The highest priority for vaccination is directed toward the two high-risk groups in Table C-2.

Persons Who Should Not Be Vaccinated

Inactivated influenza vaccine should not be given to persons who have an anaphylactic sensitivity to eggs. Persons with acute febrile illnesses usually should not be vaccinated until their temporary symptoms have abated.

Timing of Influenza Vaccination Activities

For high-risk persons who are readily accessible, such as those in chronic-care facilities or work sites, vaccination is optimally undertaken in November. Earlier vaccination, i.e., in September and October, is warranted if (1) regional experience indicates earlier-than-normal epidemic activity, (2) hospitalized high-risk patients are discharged between September and the time that influenza activity begins to decline in their community, or (3) persons have been recommended for vaccination but will not be seen again until after November.

Children who have not been previously vaccinated require two doses of vaccine with at least 1 month between doses. Programs for childhood influenza vaccination should be scheduled so the second dose can be given before December. Vaccine can be given to both children and adults up to and even after influenza virus activity is documented in a region, although temporary chemoprophylaxis using amantadine may be indicated when influenza outbreaks are occurring.

Side Effects and Adverse Reactions

Because vaccines contain only noninfectious viruses, they cannot cause influenza. The most frequent side effect of vaccination, which occurs in fewer than one-third of vaccines, is soreness around the vaccination site for up to 1 to 2 days. Systemic reactions have been of two types:

1. Fever, malaise, myalgia, and other systemic symptoms of toxicity that, although infrequent, most often affect persons such as young children who have had no exposure to the influenza virus antigens contained in the vaccine. These reactions begin 6 to 12 h after vaccination and can persist for 1 to 2 days.

2. Immediate, presumably allergic, responses, such as flare and wheal or various respiratory tract symptoms of hypersensitivity, which may occur extremely rarely after influenza vaccination. These symptoms probably result from sensitivity to some vaccine component—most likely residual egg protein. Although current influenza vaccines contain only a small quantity of egg protein, the vaccine is presumed capable of inducing hypersensitivity reactions in individuals with anaphylactic hypersensitivity to eggs, and such persons should not be given influenza vaccine. This includes individuals who, after eating eggs, develop swelling of the lips or tongue or experience acute respiratory distress or collapse, or persons who have a documented IgE-mediated hypersensitivity reaction to eggs, including those who, from occupational exposure to egg protein, have developed evidence of occupational asthma or other allergic response. Unlike the 1976 swine influenza vaccine, subsequent vaccines, which have been prepared from other virus strains, have not been associated with an increased frequency of Guillain-Barré syndrome.

Simultaneous Administration of Other or Childhood Vaccines

There is considerable overlap in the target groups for influenza and pneumococcal vaccination. Pneumococcal and influenza vaccines can be given at the same time at different sites without increased side effects, but it should be emphasized that, whereas influenza vaccine is given annually, pneumococcal vaccine should be given only once.

AMANTADINE HYDROCHLORIDE (SYMMETREL)

Specific therapy for influenza A by treatment with amantadine is indicated for individuals who seek medical attention promptly after the abrupt onset of troublesome symptoms of an acute respiratory infection during an influenza A epidemic. For high-risk individuals for whom influenza vaccine has not been used or has not prevented infection, early treatment with amantadine should help to reduce the severity and duration of illness.

Amantadine is the only drug currently approved in the United States for the specific prophylaxis and therapy of influenza virus infections. This drug appears to interfere with the uncoating step in the virus replication cycle and also reduces virus shedding. Amantadine is 76 to 90 percent effective in preventing illnesses caused by circulating strains of type A influenza viruses, but it is not effective against type B influenza. When administered within 24 to 48 h after onset of illness, amantadine reduces the duration of fever and other systemic symptoms, allowing for a more rapid return to routine daily activities and improvement in peripheral airway function. Although it may not prevent infection, persons who take the drug may still develop immune responses that will protect them when exposed to antigenically related viruses.

Although amantadine chemoprophylaxis is effective against influenza A, under most circumstances, it should not be used in lieu of vaccination for two reasons: (1) it confers no protection against influenza B; and (2) patient compliance could be a problem for continuous administration throughout epidemic periods, which generally last 6 to 12 weeks.

Recommendations for Amantadine Prophylaxis

Amantadine prophylaxis is particularly recommended to control outbreaks presumably due to influenza A. The drug should be given as early as possible after recognition of an outbreak in an effort to reduce the spread of the infection. When the decision is made to give amantadine for outbreak control, it is desirable to administer the drug to all residents of the affected institution. Amantadine prophylaxis should also be offered to unvaccinated staff who provide care to high-risk residents of chronic-care institutions or hospitals experiencing a presumed influenza A outbreak.

Amantadine prophylaxis is also recommended in the following situations:

1. As an adjunct to late immunization of high-risk individuals. It is not too late to immunize even when influenza A is known to be in the community. However, since the development of an antibody response following vaccination takes about 2 weeks, amantadine should be used in the interim. The drug does not interfere with antibody response to the vaccine.

2. To reduce spread of virus and maintain care for high-risk persons in the home setting. Persons who play a major role in providing care for high-risk persons in the home setting (e.g., family members, visiting nurses, volunteer workers) should also receive amantadine for prophylaxis when influenza A virus outbreaks occur in their communities, if such persons have not been appropriately immunized.

3. For immunodeficient persons. To supplement protection afforded by vaccination, chemoprophylaxis is also indicated for high-risk patients who may be expected to have a poor antibody response to influenza vaccine, e.g., those with severe immunodeficiency.

4. For persons for whom influenza vaccine is contraindicated. Chemoprophylaxis throughout the influenza season is appropriate for those few high-risk individuals for whom influenza vaccine is contraindicated because of anaphylactic hypersensitivity to egg protein or prior severe reactions associated with influenza vaccination.

5. For prophylactic use in other situations (e.g., unimmunized members of the general population who wish to avoid influenza A illness). This decision should be made on an individual basis.

Recommendations for Amantadine Therapy

Amantadine should be considered for therapeutic use, particularly for persons in the high-risk groups who develop an illness compatible with influenza during known or suspected influenza A activity in the community. The drug should be given within 24 to 48 h of onset of illness and should be continued until 48 h after resolution of signs and symptoms.

Precautions in Using Amantadine

Special precautions should be taken when amantadine is administered to persons with impaired renal function or those with an active seizure disorder (see "Dosage" below). The safety and efficacy of amantadine for children under 1 year of age have not been fully established.

Dosage

The usual adult dosage of amantadine is 200 mg per day; splitting the dose into 100 mg twice daily may reduce the incidence of side effects (Table C-3). Amantadine is not

TABLE C-3

Amantadine Hydrochloride* Dosage, by Age of Patient and Level of Renal Function

Age Group	Dosage†
No recognized renal disease	
1–9 years‡	4.4–8.8 mg/kg/day once daily or divided twice daily. Total dosage should not exceed 150 mg/day.
10–64 years§	200 mg once daily or divided twice daily.
≥65 years	100 mg once daily.¶

Creatinine clearance, ml/min 1.73 m²	Dosage
Recognized renal disease	
≥80	100 mg twice daily
60–79	200 mg/100 mg on alternate days
40–59	100 mg once daily
30–39	200 mg twice weekly
20–29	100 mg thrice weekly
10–19	200 mg/100 mg alternating every 7 days

* Amantadine hydrochloride (Symmetrel®) is manufactured and distributed by E.I. DuPont de Nemours and Company [Medical Department phone number (800) 441-9861, or in Delaware (302) 992-3273].

†For prophylaxis, amantadine must be taken each day for the duration of influenza A activity in the community (generally 6 to 12 weeks). For therapy, amantadine should be started as soon as possible after onset of symptoms and should be continued for 24 to 48 h after the disappearance of symptoms (generally 5 to 7 days).

‡Use in children under 1 year has not been evaluated adequately.

§Reduction of dosage to 100 mg per day is also recommended for persons with an active seizure disorder, because such persons may be at risk of experiencing an increase in the frequency of their seizures when given amantadine at 200 mg per day.

¶The reduced dosage of 100 mg per day for persons 65 years of age or older without recognized renal disease is recommended to minimize the risk of toxicity, because renal function normally declines with age, and because side effects have been reported more frequently in the elderly when a daily dose of 200 mg has been used.

metabolized and is excreted unchanged in the urine. Because renal function normally decreases with age, and because side effects have been reported more frequently among older persons, a reduced dosage of 100 mg per day is generally advisable for persons aged 65 years or older to minimize the risk of toxicity. Persons 10 to 64 years old with an active seizure disorder may also be at risk of increased frequency of seizures when given amantadine at 200 mg per day rather than 100 mg per day.

Side Effects and Adverse Reactions

Five to ten percent of otherwise healthy adults taking amantadine report side effects such as insomnia, lightheadedness, irritability, and difficulty concentrating. These and other side effects may be more pronounced among patients with underlying diseases, particularly those common among the elderly; provisions for careful monitoring are needed for these individuals so that adverse effects may be recognized promptly and the drug reduced in dosage or discontinued, if needed. Since amantadine is not metabolized, toxic levels can occur in individuals in whom renal function is sufficiently impaired.

PNEUMOCOCCAL VACCINE

The original vaccine against disease caused by *Streptococcus pneumoniae* (pneumococcus) was licensed in 1977 and contained 14 serotypes. It was succeeded in 1983 by a 23-valent polysaccharide vaccine. The increase in efficacy afforded by the 23-valent vaccine is modest. Although virtually all epidemiologic studies to date are based on the 14-valent vaccine, the results are considered to be applicable to the 23-valent vaccine. There is still no consensus about the efficacy of the pneumococcal vaccine. Nonetheless, evidence is mounting in favor of vaccinating high-risk patients. The following material and recommendations draw heavily on the Report of the Immunization Practices Advisory Committee of the Centers for Disease Control.

The estimated number of cases of pneumococcal pneumonia per year ranges from 150 to 750 per 1000, and the case-fatality rate is about 5 percent. *S. pneumoniae* is the most common cause of pneumonia, meningitis, and otitis media in the western world. Bacteremia, which occurs in about 20 to 25 percent of all patients, is associated with a high mortality. Before antibiotics became available, mortality from bacteremia was about 75 percent, approaching 100 percent in the elderly. Since the advent of antibiotics, mortality has decreased, and leveled off, at about 25 to 30 percent (reports vary from 13 to 52 percent). The two principal factors that predispose to pneumococcal pneumonia are underlying disease and old age. However, pneumococcal pneumonia occurs in all age groups: in adults, its incidence increases gradually among those over 40 years old, with a twofold increase in incidence among those over 60 years old.

Patients with certain chronic conditions are clearly at increased risk of developing pneumococcal infection, as well as experiencing more severe pneumococcal illness. These conditions include: sickle cell anemia, Hodgkin's disease, multiple myeloma, cirrhosis, alcoholism, nephrotic syndrome, renal failure, chronic pulmonary disease, splenic dysfunction, and history of splenectomy or organ transplant. Other patients may be at greater risk of developing pneumococcal infection or having more severe illness because of diabetes mellitus, congestive heart failure, or conditions associated with immunosuppression. Patients with cerebrospinal fluid (CSF) leakage complicating skull fractures or neurosurgical procedures can have recurrent pneumococcal meningitis.

The importance of preventing pneumococcal bacteremia is underscored by the increasing frequency of penicillin resistance and by failure of sophisticated management in the intensive-care setting to improve survival. However, the extent to which the vaccine will be effective in this regard remains to be settled.

Pneumococcal Polysaccharide Vaccines

The new pneumococcal vaccine is composed of purified, capsular polysaccharide antigens of 23 types of *S. pneumoniae* (Danish types 1, 2, 3, 4, 5, 6B, 7F, 8, 9N, 9V, 10A, 11A, 12F, 14, 15B, 17F, 18C, 19A, 19F, 20, 22F, 23F, and 33F). Each polysaccharide is extracted separately and combined into the final product. Each dose of the new vaccine contains 25 μg of each polysaccharide antigen.

The 23 bacterial types represented in the current vaccine are responsible for 87 percent of bacteremic pneumococcal disease in the United States reported to the CDC in 1983, compared with 71 percent for the previous 14-valent formulation. Studies of the cross reactivity of human antibodies against related types suggest that cross protection may occur among some of these types (e.g., 6A and 6B).

Although the new polysaccharide vaccine contains only 25 μg of each antigen, compared with 50 μg of antigen in the old 14-valent vaccine, a study of 53 adults reveals comparable levels of immunogenicity of the two vaccines. Most healthy adults show a twofold or greater rise in type-specific antibody, as measured by radioimmunoassay, within 2 to 3 weeks after vaccination. In contrast, the vaccine is generally less antigenic for children under 2 years old than are other vaccinees. However, because the precise protective titers of antibody for any of these serotypes have not been established, measuring antibody levels in vaccinated persons is not indicated.

Effectiveness of Pneumococcal Polysaccharide Vaccines

In the 1970s, two randomized controlled trials were conducted in populations with a high incidence of disease in

South Africa and New Guinea using newly formulated pneumococcal vaccine. Both studies demonstrated significant reductions in the occurrence of pneumonia in these young, healthy populations.

However, other subsequent randomized controlled trials of pneumococcal vaccine in older-aged U.S. adults showed less satisfactory results. One was of outpatients over 45 years old; the second, of inpatients of a chronic-care psychiatric facility. In neither study was there any difference in the occurrence of respiratory morbidity and mortality between those vaccinated and those given a placebo. Nor did a Veterans' Administration Cooperative Study using high-risk ambulatory patients support the use of vaccine.

A major difficulty in comparing the results of epidemiologic studies is the different populations used, the different criteria for identification of pneumococcal infections, and the varied statistical treatment of the data. Methodologies are also far from uniform. For example, one recent approach assessed the efficacy of pneumococcal vaccine by comparing the distribution of serotypes of pneumococci isolated from the blood of vaccinated and unvaccinated persons, i.e., *S. pneumoniae* isolates from the blood of persons who receive the 14-valent vaccine were compared with blood isolates from unvaccinated persons. Among individuals more than 60 years old without either underlying illness or chronic pulmonary disease, chronic heart disease, or diabetes mellitus, the estimated efficacy of the vaccine ranged between 60 and 80 percent; the efficacy was lower among individuals with cirrhosis or renal failure.

Few studies of the efficacy of pneumococcal vaccine have been conducted in children. However, in one small, nonrandomized study of children and young adults 2 to 25 years old who had sickle cell anemia or who had undergone splenectomy, the occurrence of bacteremic pneumococcal disease was significantly reduced by immunization with an 8-valent vaccine.

The duration of protection induced by vaccination is unknown. Although antibody titers remain high 5 years after immunization, how long the high titers will persist after vaccination is not known.

Recommendations for Use of Inactivated Vaccine
Mounting evidence favors the more extensive use of pneumococcal vaccine.

Adults
Vaccination is particularly recommended for the following:

1. Adults with chronic illnesses, especially cardiovascular disease and chronic pulmonary disease, who are seriously compromised by respiratory infections.

2. Adults with chronic illnesses specifically associated with an increased risk for pneumococcal disease or its complications. These include splenic dysfunction or anatomic asplenia, Hodgkin's disease, multiple myeloma, cirrhosis, alcoholism, renal failure, CSF leaks, and conditions associated with immunosuppression.

3. Older adults, especially those aged 65 and over, who are otherwise healthy.

Children
Vaccination is particularly recommended for the following:

1. Children aged 2 years and older with chronic illnesses specifically associated with increased risk for pneumococcal disease or its complications. These include anatomic or functional asplenia, such as sickle cell disease or splenectomy, nephrotic syndrome, CSF leaks, and conditions associated with immunosuppression.

2. Recurrent upper respiratory diseases, including otitis media and sinusitis, are not considered indications for the use of vaccine in children.

General Considerations
When elective splenectomy is being considered, pneumococcal vaccine should be given, if possible, at least 2 weeks before the operation. Similarly, when immunosuppressive therapy is being planned, as in patients who are candidates for organ transplants, the interval between vaccination and initiation of immunosuppressive therapy should be as long as possible.

Although vaccine failures have been reported in some of these groups, especially those who are immunocompromised, vaccination is still recommended for such persons because they are at high risk of developing severe disease.

Adverse Reactions
About half of those given pneumococcal vaccine develop mild side effects, such as erythema and pain at the injection site. In less than 1 percent of those given pneumococcal vaccine, fever, myalgias, and severe local reactions have been reported. Severe adverse effects, such as anaphylactoid reactions, have rarely been reported—about 5 per million doses administered.

Revaccination
It should be emphasized that pneumococcal vaccine should be given only once to adults. Arthus' reactions and systemic reactions have been common among adults given second doses and are thought to result from localized antigen-antibody reactions involving antibody induced by previous vaccination. Therefore, second or "booster" doses are not recommended, at least at this time. Data on revaccination of children are not yet sufficient to provide a basis for comment.

Persons who have received the 14-valent pneumococcal vaccine should not be revaccinated with the 23-valent vaccine, as the modest increase in coverage does not warrant the possible increased risk of adverse reactions. However, when there is doubt or no information on whether a person has ever received pneumococcal vaccine, the vaccine should not be given.

Precautions

The safety of pneumococcal vaccine for pregnant women has not been evaluated. It should not be given to otherwise healthy pregnant women. Women at high risk of pneumococcal disease ideally should be vaccinated before pregnancy.

BIBLIOGRAPHY

American Lung Association: Update: Pneumococcal polysaccharide vaccine usage—United States. ATS News, Spring, 1985.

A strong endorsement, by the Subcommittee on Prevention of Pneumonia and Influenza of the American Thoracic Society, of the Immunization Practices Advisory Committee, United States Public Health Service. The new 23-valent vaccine should be given to individuals either at high risk of developing pneumococcal pneumonia or who would be in serious jeopardy if pneumococcal pneumonia supervened on an underlying chronic disorder, including chronic pulmonary disease.

Bolan G, Broome CV, Fracklam RR, Plikaytis BD, Fraser DW, Schlech WF III: Pneumococcal vaccine efficacy in selected populations in the United States. Ann Intern Med 104:1–6, 1986.

In an analysis of 1634 bacteremic infections, the pneumococcal vaccine proved to be efficacious, to some degree, in all the immunocompetent groups. This study supports the use of pneumococcal vaccine.

Health and Public Policy Committee, American College of Physicians: Pneumococcal vaccine. Ann Intern Med 104:118–120, 1986.

Endorses the use of pneumococcal vaccine.

LaForce FM, Eickhoff TC: Pneumococcal vaccine: The evidence mounts. Ann Intern Med 104:110–112, 1986.

In favor of vaccinating high-risk patients.

Prevention and control of influenza. Recommendations of the Immunization Practices Advisory Committee. Centers for Disease Control. Ann Intern Med 107:521–525, 1987.

An update of information on the vaccine and antiviral agent available for prevention and control of influenza. It extends the 1985 report in several different ways: (1) updating of the influenza strains in the vaccine for 1986–1987; (2) immunization and amantadine prophylaxis for household members who provide home care for high-risk persons; (3) optimal time for conducting routine vaccination programs; (4) concurrent administration of influenza vaccine and childhood vaccines; (5) immunization of children receiving long-term aspirin therapy; and (6) other sources of information about influenza and control measures. It also includes a selected but comprehensive bibliography.

Simberkoff MS, Cross AP, Al-Ibrahim M, Baltch AL, Geiseler PJ, Nadler J, Richmond AS, Smith RP, Schiffman G, Shepard DS et al: Efficacy of pneumococcal vaccine in high-risk patients: Results of a Veterans' Administration Cooperative Study. N Engl J Med 315:1318–1327, 1986.

A report of a cooperative study to test the effectiveness of pneumococcal vaccine in preventing vaccine-serotype Streptococcus pneumoniae infections in high-risk ambulatory patients (not hospitalized bacteremic patients). The study was unable to prove efficacy of pneumococcal vaccine in this high-risk population. The authors suggest that chronically ill patients, who are most susceptible to infection, may have an impaired immune response to the pneumococcal vaccine. (See also Letters to the Editor, N Engl J Med 316:1272–1273, 1987.)

Update: Pneumococcal polysaccharide vaccine usage—United States. MMWR 33:273–281, 1984.

Recommends pneumococcal vaccine for adults with chronic illnesses "who sustain increased morbidity with respiratory infections" and for those "with chronic illnesses specifically associated with an increased risk for pneumococcal disease or its complications."

Appendix *D*

Terms and Symbols in Respiratory Physiology

GENERAL SYMBOLS

P
: Partial pressure in blood or gas.

$$P_{O_2} = \text{partial pressure of } O_2$$

$\overline{X}$
: A bar over the symbol indicates a mean value.

$$\overline{P} = \text{mean pressure, as distinct from instantaneous pressure}$$

$\dot{X}$
: A time derivative (rate) is indicated by a dot above the symbol.

$$\dot{V}_{O_2} = O_2 \text{ consumption per unit time}$$
$$\dot{V}_{CO_2} = CO_2 \text{ production per unit time}$$

% X
: Percent sign preceding a symbol indicates percentage of the predicted normal value.

X/Y %
: Percent sign following a symbol indicates a ratio function with the ratio expressed as a percentage. Both components of the ratio must be designated.

$$FEV_2/FVC \% = 100 \times FEV_1/FVC$$

X_A, X_a
: A small capital letter or a lowercase letter on the same line following a primary symbol is a qualifier to further define the primary symbol. When small capital letters are not available on typewriters or to printers, subscript capital letters may be used.

$$X_A = X_A$$

$P_{ECO_2}, \dot{V}_{Dan}$
: Additional qualifiers of the primary symbol may be identified as shown.

GAS PHASE SYMBOLS

Primary Symbols

V
: Volume of gas.

$\dot{V}$
: Flow of gas.

F
: Fractional concentration of a gas.

Common Qualifying Symbols

I
: Inspired.

$$V_I = \text{inspired volume}$$

E
: Expired.

$$V_E = \text{expired volume}$$

A
: Alveolar.

$$V_A = \text{alveolar volume}$$
$$\dot{V}_A = \text{alveolar ventilation per unit time}$$

T
: Tidal.

$$V_T = \text{tidal volume}$$

D   Dead space.

$\qquad$ V_D = volume of dead space

$\qquad$ $\dot{V}_D$ = dead space ventilation per unit time

B   Barometric.

$\qquad$ P_B = barometric pressure

L   Lung.

STPD   Standard conditions: temperature 0°C, pressure 760 mmHg, and dry (0 mmHg water vapor).

BTPS   Body conditions: body temperature and ambient pressure, saturated with water vapor at these conditions.

ATPD   Ambient temperature and pressure, dry.

ATPS   Ambient temperature and pressure, saturated with water vapor at these conditions.

an   Anatomic.

p   Physiological.

f   Respiratory frequency, per minute.

max   Maximum.

t   Time.

BLOOD PHASE SYMBOLS

Primary Symbols

Q   Volume of blood.

$\dot{Q}$ Blood flow.

$\qquad$ $\dot{Q}$ = cardiac output, L/min

C   Concentration in the blood phase.

$\qquad$ C_{N_2} = concentration of N_2 in blood, ml of N_2 per 100 ml of blood

S   Saturation in the blood phase.

$\qquad$ S_{O_2} = saturation of hemoglobin with O_2, percent

Qualifying Symbols

b   Blood, in general.

$\qquad$ Cb_{O_2} = concentration of O_2 in blood, ml of O_2 per 100 ml of blood

a   Arterial.

$\qquad$ Ca_{O_2} = concentration of O_2 in arterial blood, ml of O_2 per 100 ml of blood

c   Capillary.

$\qquad$ Cc_{O_2} = concentration of O_2 in capillary blood, ml of O_2 per 100 ml of blood

c′   Pulmonary end-capillary.

$\qquad$ Pc'_{CO_2} = partial pressure of CO_2 in end-capillary blood, mmHg

v   Venous.

$\qquad$ Cv_{O_2} = concentration of O_2 in venous blood, ml of O_2 per 100 ml of blood

$\bar{v}$ Mixed venous.

$$C\bar{v}_{O_2} = \text{concentration of } O_2 \text{ in mixed venous blood, ml of } O_2 \text{ per 100 ml of blood}$$

VENTILATION AND LUNG MECHANICS TESTS AND SYMBOLS

Static Lung volumes[1]

PRIMARY COMPARTMENTS (SEE FIG. 163-1)

RV	Residual volume. Volume of air remaining in the lungs after maximum expiration.
CV	Closing volume. Volume of air remaining in the lungs at onset of airways closure (see Fig. 163-30). Often expressed as a fraction of VC, that is, CV/VC %.
ERV	Expiratory reserve volume. Maximum volume of air expired from the resting end-expiratory level.
V_T	Tidal volume. Volume of air inspired or expired with each breath during quiet breathing. When tidal volume is used in gas-exchange formulations, this symbol is used. When indicating a subdivision of lung volumes, the symbol TV may be used.
IRV	Inspiratory reserve volume. Maximum volume of air inspired from the resting end-inspiratory level.
V_L	Volume of the lung, including the conducting airways.

Lung Capacities[2]

IC	Inspiratory capacity. The sum of IRV and TV.
IVC	Inspiratory vital capacity. Maximum volume of air inspired from the point of maximum expiration.
VC	Vital capacity. Maximum volume of air expired from the point of maximum inspiration.
FRC	Functional residual capacity. Sum of RV and ERV. FRC is the volume of air remaining in the lungs at the resting end-expiratory position.
TLC	Total lung capacity. Volume of air in the lungs after maximum inspiration. Also, the sum of all volume compartments of the lungs.
RV/TLC %	Residual volume to total lung capacity ratio, expressed as a percentage.
CC	Closing capacity. Closing volume plus residual volume, often expressed as a ratio of TLC, that is, CC/TLC %.

Forced Respiratory Maneuvers during Spirometry[3]

FVC	Forced vital capacity. The maximum volume of air forcibly expired from the maximum inspiratory position.
FIVC	Forced inspiratory vital capacity. Maximum volume of air forcibly inspired starting from a maximum expiration.
FEV_t	Timed forced expiratory volume. Volume of air expired in a specified time in the course of the forced vital capacity maneuver.

$$FEV_1 = \text{volume of air expired during the first second of the FVC}$$

FEV_t/FVC %	Ratio of time forced expiratory volume to forced vital capacity, expressed as a percentage.
FEF_x	Forced expiratory flow, related to some portion of the FVC curve. Modifiers refer to the amount of the FVC that has been expired at the time of measurement.
$FEF_{200-1200}$	Forced expiratory flow between 200 and 1200 ml of the FVC (formerly called the maximum expiratory flow rate).
$FEF_{25-75\%}$	Forced expiratory flow during middle half of the FVC (formerly called the maximum midexpiratory flow rate).
PEF	Peak expiratory flow. Highest value for expiratory flow.
$\dot{V}max_{x\%}$	Maximum flow when x percent of the FVC has been expired.

$$\dot{V}max_{75\%} = \text{flow (instantaneous) when 75 percent of the FVC has been expired}$$

[1] Expressed at BTPS unless otherwise specified. Asterisks indicate values obtainable by spirometry.

[2] Combinations of volumes for practical purposes.

[3] All values at BTPS unless otherwise specified.

$\dot{V}max_{x\%TLC}$ Maximum flow when x percent of the TLC remains.

$$\dot{V}max_{75\%TLC} = \text{flow (instantaneous) when the lungs contain 75 percent of the TLC}$$

FET_x Forced expiratory time required to expire a specified FVC.

$$FET_{95\%} = \text{time required to expire the first 95 percent of the FVC}$$
$$FET_{25-75\%} = \text{time required to expire the } FET_{25-75\%}$$

FIF_x Forced inspiratory flow. As in the case of the FEF, appropriate modifiers designate the volume at which flow is being measured. Unless otherwise specified, the volume qualifiers indicate the volume inspired from RV at the point of measurement.

$$FIF_{25-75\%} = \text{forced inspiratory flow during the middle half of the FIVC}$$

$I\dot{V}max_{x\%}$ Maximum inspiratory flow (instantaneous) when x percent of the FIVC has been inspired.

$I\dot{V}max_{x\%TLC}$ Maximum inspiratory flow (instantaneous) when the lungs contain x percent of the TLC.

MVV   Maximum voluntary ventilation. Volume of air breathed during maximum breathing efforts during a specified time period. Formerly called maximum breathing capacity. If breathing frequency is set by the examiner, it is indicated by the qualifier.

$$MVV_{60} = \text{MVV at a breathing frequency of 60 per minute}$$

Measurements Related to Ventilation

$\dot{V}_E$ Expired volume per minute (BTPS).

$\dot{V}_I$ Inspired volume per minute (BTPS).

$\dot{V}_{CO_2}$ Carbon dioxide production per minute (STPD).

$\dot{V}_{O_2}$ Oxygen consumption per minute (STPD).

R   Respiratory exchange ratio, the ratio of CO_2 output to O_2 intake in the lungs.

$\dot{V}_A$ Alveolar ventilation per minute (BTPS).

$\dot{V}_D$ Ventilation per minute of the physiological dead space (BTPS) defined by the equation

$$\dot{V}_D = \dot{V}_E \frac{Pa_{CO_2} - PE_{CO_2}}{Pa_{CO_2} - PI_{CO_2}}$$

V_D Volume of the physiological dead space, calculated as $\dot{V}_D/f$.

$\dot{V}_{Dan}$ Ventilation per minute of the anatomic dead space, that portion of the conducting airway in which no significant gas exchange occurs (BTPS).

V_{Dan} Volume of the anatomic dead space (BTPS).

$\dot{V}_{DA}$ Ventilation of the alveolar dead space (BTPS), defined by the equation

$$\dot{V}_{DA} = \dot{V}_D - \dot{V}_{Dan}$$

V_{DA} The alveolar dead space volume, defined as

$$V_{DA} = \dot{V}_{DA}/f$$

Mechanics of Breathing[1]

PRESSURE TERMS

Paw   Pressure at any point along the airways.

Pao   Pressure at the airway opening.

Ppl   Pleural pressure.

P_A Alveolar pressure.

Pbs   Pressure at the body surface.

Pes   Esophageal pressure; used to estimate Ppl.

P_A − Ppl   Transpulmonary pressure.

---

[1] All pressures expressed relative to ambient pressure unless otherwise specified.

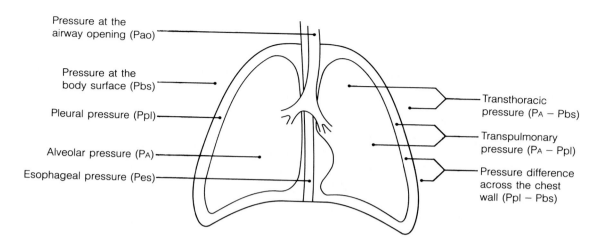

Pressure at the airway opening (Pao)

Pressure at the body surface (Pbs)

Pleural pressure (Ppl)

Alveolar pressure (PA)

Esophageal pressure (Pes)

Transthoracic pressure (PA − Pbs)

Transpulmonary pressure (PA − Ppl)

Pressure difference across the chest wall (Ppl − Pbs)

Ppl − Pbs	Transthoracic pressure, pressure difference across the chest wall.
Paw − Ppl	Transbronchial pressure, estimated as difference between airway and pleural pressures.

FLOW-PRESSURE RELATIONSHIPS[1]

R	General symbol for frictional resistance, defined as the ratio of pressure difference to flow.
Raw	Airway resistance, calculated from pressure difference between airway opening (Pao) and alveoli (PA) divided by the airflow, $cmH_2O/L/s$.
RL	Total pulmonary resistance, measured by relating flow-dependent transpulmonary pressure to airflow at the mouth.
Rti	Tissue resistance (viscous resistance of lung tissue), calculated as difference between RL and Raw.
Rus	Resistance of the airways on the upstream (alveolar) side of the point in the airways where intraluminal pressure equals Ppl, i.e., equal pressure point. Measured during a forced expiration.
Rds	Resistance of the airways on the downstream (mouth) side of the point in the airways where intraluminal pressure equals Ppl, i.e., equal pressure point. Measured during a forced expiration.
Gaw	Airway conductance, reciprocal of Raw.
Gaw/VL	Specific conductance, airway conductance, expressed per liter of lung volume at which Gaw is measured.
$\dot{W}$	Rate of work or power. Expressed either in kpm/min or J/s (watt).

VOLUME-PRESSURE RELATIONSHIPS

C	General symbol for compliance of the lungs, chest wall, or total respiratory system. Volume change per unit change in applied pressure. For the lungs, the applied pressure is the pressure difference across the lungs, or transpulmonary pressure, Pao − Ppl; for the chest wall, the applied pressure is the transthoracic pressure, Ppl − Pbs; for the entire respiratory system the applied pressure is Pao − Pbs.
Cdyn	Dynamic compliance. Value for compliance determined at time of zero gas flow at the mouth during uninterrupted breathing. The respiratory frequency appears as a qualifier.

$$Cdyn_{40} = \text{dynamic compliance at a respiratory frequency of 40 per minute}$$

Cst	Static compliance, value for compliance determined on the basis of measurements made during a period of zero airflow.
C/VL	Specific compliance. Compliance divided by the lung volume at which it is determined, usually FRC.
E	Reciprocal of compliance (elastance).
Pst	Static pulmonary pressure at a specified lung volume.

$$Pst_{TLC} = \text{static recoil pressure of the lung measured at TLC (maximum recoil pressure)}$$

W	Mechanical work of breathing.

[1]Unless otherwise specified, all resistance measurements assumed to be made at lung FRC.

DIFFUSING CAPACITY TESTS AND SYMBOLS

D_{L_X}, D_X — Diffusing capacity of the lung expressed as volume (STPD) of gas (x) uptake per minute per unit alveolar-capillary pressure difference for the gas used. A modifier can be used to designate the technique:

$$D_{L_{CO_{sb}}} = \text{single-breath CO diffusing capacity}$$
$$D_{L_{CO_{ss}}} = \text{steady-state CO diffusing capacity}$$

D_M — Diffusing capacity of the alveolar-capillary membrane (STPD).

θ — Reaction rate coefficient for red blood cells. Determined as the volume of gas (STPD) which will combine per minute with 1 unit volume of blood per unit of gas tension. If the specific gas is not stated, θ is assumed to refer to CO and is a function of existing O_2 tension.

V_C — Capillary blood volume. This should be Qc for consistency with other symbols, but Vc is entrenched in the literature. In the equation which follows for $1/D_L$, Vc represents the effective pulmonary capillary blood volume, i.e., capillary blood volume in intimate association with alveolar gas.

$1/D_L$ — Total resistance to diffusion, including resistance to diffusion of test gas across the alveolar-capillary membrane, through plasma in the capillary, and across the red blood cell membrane ($1/D_M$), the resistance to diffusion with the red cell arising from the chemical reaction of the test gas and hemoglobin ($1/\theta V_C$), according to the formulation

$$\frac{1}{D_L} = \frac{1}{D_M} + \frac{1}{\theta V_C}$$

D_L/V_A — Diffusion per unit of alveolar volume. D_L is expressed STPD, and V_A is expressed in liters, BTPS.

BLOOD GAS SYMBOLS

Symbols for these values are readily composed by combining general symbols. Some examples include the following.

Pa_{CO_2} — Arterial CO_2 tension, torr (mmHg)

Sa_{O_2} — Arterial O_2 saturation, percent

Cc'_{O_2} — Oxygen content of pulmonary end-capillary blood, ml of O_2 per 100 ml of blood

$PA_{O_2} - Pa_{O_2}$, $P(A\text{-}a)_{O_2}$ — Alveolar-arterial difference in the partial pressure of O_2 mmHg

$Ca_{O_2} - C\bar{v}_{O_2}$ — Arteriovenous O_2 content difference, ml of O_2 per 100 ml of blood

PULMONARY SHUNT SYMBOLS

$\dot{Q}s$ — Flow of blood via shunts. Usually determined as percent of cardiac output ($\dot{Q}$) while breathing 100% O_2, according to the equation

$$\frac{\dot{Q}s}{\dot{Q}} = \frac{Cc' - Ca}{Cc' - C\bar{v}}$$

where

$$\frac{\dot{Q}s}{\dot{Q}} = \text{``anatomic'' venous admixture}$$

and

Cc'_{O_2} = O_2 content of end-capillary blood
Ca_{O_2} = O_2 content of arterial blood
$C\bar{v}_{O_2}$ = O_2 content of mixed venous blood, usually assumed to be 4.5 to 5.0 ml/100 ml of blood

NOTES

Index

Abdomen: motion of, 2273
Abdominal muscles and expiration, 2269–2270, 2272
Abdominal surgery
  and pleural effusions, 2147–2148
  pulmonary function effects of, 2415
ABPA (see Aspergillosis, allergic bronchopulmonary)
Abscess
  hepatic: from *E. hystolitica*, 1668–1670
  lung (see Lung abscess)
  mediastinal, 2075
  peritonsillar, 1453
  subphrenic
    and pleural effusions, 2148
    and spontaneous pneumothorax, 2175
  tuboovarian, 1618
Absidia: infection with (see Mucormycosis)
Acanthamoeba: aspiration pneumonitis from, 1670
Acanthosis nigricans, 367, 384
  and neoplasms, 384
Acceleration in lungs, 177
  convective, 177
  local, 177
Acclimatization to altitude, 140–141, 251–252, 255
Acebutolol: small vessel vasculitis induced by, 1146
Acetaminophen sodium salicylate: asthma and, 1303
Acetazolamide
  for alveolar hypoventilation, 1343
  and bicarbonate excretion, 1191
  in chronic hypercapnia, 287, 1197
  in cor pulmonale therapy, 1015
  effects of, 166–167
  and sleep apnea, 1356
Acetone, 207
Acetylcholine
  in airway smooth muscle regulation, 123
  as neurotransmitter, 134
  and sleep, 147
  as vasodilator, 985
Acetylcysteine
  in acute respiratory failure treatment, 2294
  for cystic fibrosis, 1284, 1285
Acetylene, 207
Acetylsalicylic acid (see Aspirin)
Acid anhydrides: asthma induced by, 857
Acid-base balance, 1189–1194
  kidneys in, 1190–1192
  monitoring in mechanical ventilation, 2363
Acid-base disturbances (see Metabolic acid-base disturbances; Respiratory: acid-base disturbances)
Acid-base map, 1192

Acid-fast stains for Mycobacteria, 1812–1813
Acidosis (see Metabolic acidosis; Respiratory acidosis)
Acidphosphatase in alveolar macrophages, 705
Acinar adenocarcinoma, 1915, 1921, 1924, 1935
  (See also Adenocarcinoma)
Acinar capillary sheet: blood flow through, 44
Acinar pathway: length of, 54–55
Acinetobacter spp.
  antibiotics for, 1403
  nosocomial infection with, 1436, 1747
  stains of, 1399
A. antritatus: nosocomial pneumonia from, 1491
A. lwoffi: nosocomial pneumonia from, 1491
Acini
  anatomy of, 17, 1250
  development of, 62, 64
  function in parenchyma, 33
  number of, 29
  plasma cells in, 27
Acinic cell tumors, 2017
Acne: drug-induced, 374
Acquired immunodeficiency syndrome (AIDS)
  antiviral research, 1687–1689
  and ARDS, 1697
  AZT for, 1666, 1688–1689
  bacterial infections in, 1696
  bronchoalveolar lavage in, 433, 1405, 1690, 1752
  bronchoscopy in, 453, 1405, 1467, 1690, 1700
  candidal infection in, 1684, 1686, 1692, 1696
  case definition for surveillance purposes, 1684–1685
  CDC classification of HIV infection, 1686
  coccidioidomycosis in, 1696, 1786, 1787
  cryptococcosis in, 1421, 1453, 1460, 1696, 1769–1771
  Cryptosporidium infection in, 1676–1679, 1684, 1686, 1696
  cytomegalovirus infection in, 1395, 1397, 1421, 1460, 1661, 1666, 1672, 1684, 1685, 1687, 1690, 1691, 1695, 1701, 1749, 1755
    coexistent with *P. carinii*, 1460, 1661, 1666, 1672, 1755
  dementia in, 1684, 1685, 1686
  diagnostic approach to pulmonary disease, 1690–1692
  differential diagnosis: radiography, 1691, 1692
  among drug abusers, 1456, 1467, 1686–1687, 1690, 1695, 1698

Acquired immunodeficiency syndrome (AIDS) (*Cont.*)
  endoscopist risk, 462
  and eosinophilic pneumonia, 686
  epidemiology of, 1685–1687
    in Africa, 1687, 1695, 1697–1698
    in New York City, 1686–1687
  etiology of, 1687–1689
    (See also Human immunodeficiency virus)
  fungal infections in, 1421, 1453, 1460, 1684–1686, 1691, 1695–1696, 1761, 1769–1771, 1780
  gallium lung scanning in, 1691, 2553, 2554
  among hemophiliacs, 1686, 1687
  among heterosexuals, 1686–1687
  histoplasmosis in, 1684, 1685, 1686, 1691, 1696, 1780
  among homosexuals, 1683, 1686–1687, 1698
  immunologic defect in, 1689–1690
  incidence of, 1683, 1685
  infection control precautions, 1699–1701
  Kaposi's sarcoma in, 1467, 1658, 1683, 1684, 1685, 1686, 1690, 1691, 1692, 1697–1700, 2025, 2026, 2028
    epidemic, 1698
    pulmonary, 1698–1699
    (See also Kaposi's sarcoma)
  Legionella infection in, 1395, 1421, 1696, 1697
  leishmaniasis, 1679
  lymphomas, primary malignant lung, 2050, 2052
  mycobacterial infection and disease in, 1395, 1421, 1467, 1684, 1686, 1691, 1695, 1701, 1753, 1800, 1812, 1817, 1838–1839, 1858, 1859, 1863, 1864, 1867
  nocardial infections in, 1696, 1753
  nonHodgkin's lymphoma and, 1684, 1685, 1686, 1691
  open lung biopsy in, 1691–1692
  pleural involvement in, 1697
  pneumonia in, 1393, 1394–1395, 1397, 1460, 1538, 1745–1747, 1749, 1752–1753, 1755, 1758
    bacterial, 1696
    diagnostic approach, 1690–1692
    diagnostic studies, 1400, 1401, 1402, 1690–1692
    fungal, 1695–1696
    lymphocytic interstitial, 1684, 1685, 1686, 1691, 1692, 1697
    P. carinii, 1394–1395, 1397, 1421, 1460, 1657–1666, 1683, 1684, 1685, 1686, 1690, 1691, 1692–1695, 1697, 1700, 1701, 1752, 1755
    treatment for, 1664–1666, 1693–1695